MEDICAL MICROBIOLOGY

MEDICAL MICROBIOLOGY

A Guide to The Laboratory Diagnosis and Control of Infection

Edited by

ROBERT CRUICKSHANK

C.B.E., M.D., F.R.C.P., F.R.C.P.E., D.P.H., F.R.S.E.

Emeritus Professor of Bacteriology, University of Edinburgh.
Formerly Adviser in Bacteriology, Scottish Home and Health Dept., and
S.E. Regional Hospital Board (Scotland), and
Senior Consultant in Bacteriology, Royal Infirmary, Edinburgh.

Assistant Editors

J. P. DUGUID

M.D., B.Sc., F.C.Path.

Professor of Bacteriology, University of Dundee

R. H. A. SWAIN

M.A., M.D., F.R.C.P.E., F.C.Path., F.R.S.E.

Reader in Virology, University of Edinburgh.
Visiting Consultant in Virology
The Royal Infirmary and the City Hospital, Edinburgh.

ELEVENTH EDITION

REVISED REPRINT

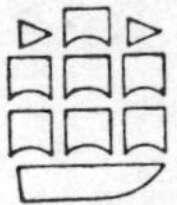

CHURCHILL LIVINGSTONE

EDINBURGH AND LONDON

1972

First Edition	1925
Second Edition	1928
Third Edition	1931
Fourth Edition	1934
Fifth Edition	1938
Sixth Edition	1942
Seventh Edition	1945
Reprinted	1946
Eighth Edition	1948
Reprinted	1949
Reprinted	1950
Ninth Edition	1953
Reprinted	1956
Reprinted	1959
Tenth Edition	1960
Reprinted	1962
Eleventh Edition	1965
Revised Reprint	1968
Reprinted	1969
Reprinted	1970
Reprinted	1972
E.L.B.S. Edition first published .	1965
Reprinted	1968, 1969, 1970

ISBN 0 443 00135 9

Printed in Great Britain

PREFACE

It has been agreed that this eleventh edition of what was formerly *A Handbook of Practical Bacteriology* by Mackie and McCartney should now be called *Medical Microbiology* and should cater as much for the needs of medical students and doctors as for bacteriologists and laboratory technicians. Consequently, there has been a rearrangement of the subject-matter into five parts, of which Part I deals with the microbial cell and the general principles of infection and immunity; Parts II and III are concerned with the aetiology, laboratory diagnosis and epidemiology of bacterial infections and of viral and some fungous and protozoal infections; Part IV, on applied microbiology, is aimed particularly at the senior medical student, the house officer and the general practitioner; and Part V is the "methods" section of special interest to microbiologists and technical staff.

Our objective was a comprehensive textbook to cater for the needs of all those concerned with the laboratory diagnosis and control of infection in man. We were particularly conscious of the usefulness, for countries where communicable disease is still the major contributor to sickness and death, of an all-purpose textbook on medical microbiology which could be a vade mecum for teachers and students alike in the many new Medical Schools in these countries. We were therefore gratified to know that this new edition will be included in the English Language Book Society for developing countries.

The whole text has been thoroughly revised and rearranged and a number of new illustrations have been added. There has been further subdivision of chapters dealing with bacterial and viral infections, and new chapters have been added on the classification and identification of bacteria, laboratory diagnosis of common infective syndromes, biochemical tests in bacterial identification and biological standardisation and measurement. We were fortunate in having in the department for a year Dr. Nancy Hayward, of Melbourne, who undertook a drastic revision of the chapter on culture media. We have also had most valuable comments, corrections and constructive suggestions from many laboratory colleagues both at home and abroad. Although too numerous to mention individually, we gladly extend our thanks to them collectively.

For this edition, Professor J. P. Duguid and Dr. R. H. A. Swain have acted as Assistant Editors and have taken a large share of the burden of subediting and proof reading. Dr. R. R. Gillies, who has been responsible for the preparation of the index, and all the contributors, whose responsibilities for new, or the revision of existing, chapters are indicated in the List of Contributors, have in our numerous round-table discussions helped in welding this textbook into what I hope will be a worthy successor to the earlier editions.

In preparing the revised reprint of the eleventh edition of this book we have been guided by letters from our many friends who drew attention to errors of detail and typography. For this help we are most grateful and we have used it to good advantage to secure a fuller measure of consistency in the use of scientific terms and bibliographical references. We have also been able to introduce modern concepts of brucellosis into Chapter 23 and to incorporate the new standards required for the examination of milk into Chapter 55.

To Mr. W. G. Henderson and to Mr. A. D. Lewis are due our grateful acknowledgements for their advice in the preparation of this text. We also wish to add our warmest thanks to Mrs. Mona Wilson for her acute perception and the ruthless exclusion of errors that had managed to escape the eyes of our many readers in the past.

Edinburgh, 1968 R. Cruickshank.

LIST OF CONTRIBUTORS

and the topics for which they have had main or shared responsibility in preparation or revision

COGHLAN, Joyce D., B.Sc., Ph.D.
Brucella; leptospira; bacteriology of water, food and air.

COLLEE, J. G., M.D., M.C.Path.
Pasteurella; clostridia; use of culture media; tests employed in bacterial identification; biological standardisation and measurement.

CRUICKSHANK, R., *C.B.E.*, M.D., F.R.C.P., F.R.C.P.E., D.P.H., F.R.S.E.
Acquired immunity and prophylactic immunisation; neisseria, corynebacterium; mycobacterium; haemophilus; bordetella; cholera vibrio; spirillum.

DUGUID, J. P., M.D., B.Sc., F.C.Path.[1]
Bacterial morphology and classification; bacterial genetics; mechanisms of infection; pathogenic fungi; staining methods; sterilisation.

GILLIES, R. R., M.D., D.P.H., M.C.Path.
Streptococcus; pneumococcus; salmonella; shigella; escherichia; other enterobacteriaceae; proteus; pseudomonas; loefflerella; bacteroides; donovania; actinomyces; nocardia.

GOULD, J. C., B.Sc., M.D., F.R.C.P.E., M.C.Path., F.R.S.E.[2]
Staphylococcus; phage-typing; protozoa; laboratory diagnosis of common infective syndromes; antimicrobial agents.

HAYWARD, Nancy J., B.Sc., Ph.D.[3]
Culture media.

SLEIGH, J. D., M.B., Ch.B., M.C.Path.[4]
Anthrax; laboratory diagnosis of common infective syndromes; sterilisation.

SWAIN, R. H. A., M.A., M.D., F.R.C.P.E., F.C.Path., F.R.S.E.
Viruses and their cultivation; all chapters on specific viruses and virus infections; psittacosis and lymphogranuloma; rickettsia; bartonella; mycoplasma (PPLO); treponema; borrelia; microscopy; immunological and serological methods; care and use of laboratory animals.

WEIR, D. M., M.D.
Infection and immunity; immunological and serological methods.

WILKINSON, J. F., M.A., Ph.D.[5]
Bacterial physiology; bacteriophage; tests employed in bacterial identification; physical and chemical methods.

[1] Department of Bacteriology, University of Dundee.
[2] Central Microbiological Laboratories, Edinburgh.
[3] Department of Microbiology, Monash University, Prahran, Victoria, Australia.
[4] Pathology Department. Dunbartonshire Area Laboratory, Vale of Leven Hospital, Alexandria, Dunbartonshire.
[5] Sub-department of General Microbiology, Department of Agriculture, University of Edinburgh.

[illegible] CONTRIBUTORS [illegible]

and the chapters for which they have been mainly responsible
[illegible]

[illegible], Ph.D.
Brucella; leptospira; bacteriology of water, food and air.

[illegible], M.D., M.C.Path.
Pasteurella; clostridium; use of culture media; tests employed in bacterial identification; biological standardisation; antibacterial treatment.

CRUICKSHANK, R., C.B.E., M.D., F.R.C.P., F.R.C.P.E., D.P.H., F.R.S.E.
Acquired immunity and prophylactic immunisation; neisseria; corynebacterium; mycobacterium; haemophilus; bordetella; cholera vibrio; spirillum.

DUGUID, J. P., M.D., B.Sc., F.C.Path.
Bacteria: morphology and classification; bacterial genetics; mechanisms of infection; pathogenic fungi; staining methods; sterilisation.

GILLIES, R. R., M.D., D.P.H., M.C.Path.
Streptococcus; pneumococcus; enterobacteria: shigella; escherichia; salmonella; klebsiella; proteus; pseudomonas; bacteroides; [illegible]

[illegible], B.Sc., M.D., F.R.C.P.E., M.C.Path., F.R.A.C.P.
Staphylococcus; plague; typhus; protozoa; laboratory diagnosis of common infective syndromes; antimicrobial agents.

[illegible], B.Sc., Ph.D.
Culture media.

SLEIGH, J. D., M.B., Ch.B., M.C.Path.
Anthrax; laboratory diagnosis of common infective syndromes; sterilisation.

SWAIN, R. H. A., M.A., M.D., F.R.C.P.E., F.C.Path., F.R.S.E.
Viruses and their cultivation; all chapters on specific viruses and virus infections; rickettsiae and lymphogranuloma; rickettsiae; bartonella; mycoplasma (PPLO); treponema; borrelia; microscopy; immunological and serological methods; care and use of laboratory animals.

[illegible], M.D.
Detection and primary [illegible] immunological and serological methods.

WILKINSON, J. F., M.A., Ph.D.
Bacterial physiology; bacteriophages; tests employed in bacterial identification; physical and chemical methods.

[illegible] Department of Bacteriology, University of Dundee.
[illegible] Central Microbiological Laboratories, Edinburgh.
[illegible] Department of Microbiology, Monash University [illegible] Microbiology Department and [illegible] Laboratory, [illegible] Alexandria, Dunbartonshire.
[illegible] Department of General Microbiology, Department of Agriculture, University of Edinburgh.

CONTENTS

Part I

MICROBIAL BIOLOGY; INFECTION AND IMMUNITY

Part II

PATHOGENIC AND COMMENSAL BACTERIA

Part III

VIRUSES AND OTHER MICROORGANISMS

Part IV

APPLIED MICROBIOLOGY

PART V

TECHNICAL METHODS

PART I

MICROBIAL BIOLOGY: INFECTION AND IMMUNITY

CHAPTER 1

MICROBIOLOGY AND MEDICINE

MICROBIOLOGY is one of the younger biological sciences. Although its paternity is rather nebulous, the first productive seed was implanted by a French chemist, Louis Pasteur, who a century ago was persuaded to turn his inquisitive mind from a study of tartrate crystals to the troubles that were affecting the wine industry in France. Pasteur, brooding over the age-old phenomenon of fermentation, which has given us both bread and wine, was not prepared to accept the pontifical pronouncements of the leading chemists of the day that this was a chemical reaction. Having satisfied himself that the souring of milk was due to the formation of lactic acid by multiplying bacteria, he proceeded to turn sugar into alcohol with only ammonia and some organic salts as a source of nutriment for the growing yeast cells. He concluded his paper in 1857 with these words: "Alcoholic fermentation is an act correlated with the life and with the organization of these (yeast) globules, and not with their death or their putrefaction".

In his early work in microbiology Pasteur also made the fundamental observation that certain bacteria (which he called *anaerobic*) would grow only in the absence of oxygen, a momentous discovery at a time when oxygen was still regarded as the essential elixir for all living creatures. A few years later, his monograph on "The Study of Wines" and his demonstration of the value of differential heating—or *pasteurisation* as we now call it—revolutionised the whole wine and beer industry of Europe and established the importance of microbiology in industry.

Joseph Lister, an English surgeon working in Scotland, saw in Pasteur's work on fermentation a possible explanation of the tragic fate that befell so many of his patients who after injury or amputation were dying like flies of hospital gangrene and "blood poisoning ". By placing an antiseptic dressing over the open wound, he prevented bacteria in the environment from getting access to the susceptible tissues and so satisfied himself that putrefaction or sepsis was caused, like fermentation, by these invisible but living microbes which Leeuwenhoek, two centuries earlier, had called his "little animals". A little later, the surgeon Ogston, in Aberdeen, showed that grape-like clusters of cocci, which he named staphylococci, were the common cause of abscesses.

In an era dominated by the physical sciences it required great courage and pertinacity as well as ingenuity and technical skill for these pioneers in microbiology to persuade their fellows of the validity of the new gospel. However, they had strong support from one of the outstanding physicists of the day, John Tyndall, who interested himself in the new biological science and gave us intermittent sterilisation (or *tyndallisation*); he was, incidentally, one of the first observers to note the antibacterial properties of the mould penicillium. About this time Robert Koch, a country doctor in Germany, became painfully aware of the havoc which a disease called "splenic fever" was causing among the sheep and cattle of the farming community. By most ingenious methods devised in a home-made laboratory, Koch was able to prove that a large square-ended rod was constantly present in the blood of animals dying of splenic fever, that this microbe could be grown and purified from contaminants on nutrient jelly, and when injected into laboratory animals could reproduce an infection identical with that which killed the cow and the sheep. This was the first wholly satisfying evidence that a specific germ, the anthrax bacillus, was the cause of a specific disease. And so, by 1880, the new science of microbiology was firmly founded and its importance in the economy of men, animals and industry was beginning to be appreciated.

Mention may be made here of two early offshoots of this science—immunology and virology—in which Pasteur was involved. He was the first to extend Jenner's protective *vaccination*, a word coined by Pasteur in honour of Jenner's work with cowpox, by the use of living attenuated cultures of pathogenic microbes against important infections like anthrax, swine erysipelas and chicken cholera, and today the *attenuated vaccine* is being used with outstanding success in such diverse diseases as tuberculosis, yellow fever, poliomyelitis, dog distemper and contagious abortion of cattle.

Pasteur's contribution to virology was equally fertile. From his boyhood days in the Jura hills, he had known of the horrible deaths that might follow the bite of a wolf or a mad dog, and in due course he turned his attention to the aetiology of rabies. After some false trails, his assistant Roux eventually injected some of the infective material into the brain of a dog, which fourteen days later developed rabies. Thus the use of selective living tissue for the growth of viruses—which today is practised on an enormous scale—was born in Pasteur's laboratory and this experimental work with rabies led on to the anti-rabies vaccine which was his last great effort in the field of immunology. Later, the demonstration of bacterial toxins by both French and German workers was the precursor of antitoxin therapy by von Behring, leading on to Ehrlich's concept of "magic bullets" and so to our modern chemotherapy.

This brief historical sketch illustrates the importance of microbiology as an applied science, particularly in fermentation processes and in infectious diseases. The term *microbiology* (as originally used by Pasteur) is preferred to *bacteriology* since it includes in the present context viruses, fungi and protozoa in addition to bacteria. Only a small proportion of the myriads of microorganisms that abound in nature are disease-producing or *pathogenic* for man; most of the microorganisms present on the skin and mucous membranes are non-pathogenic and are often referred to as *commensals* (table companions), or if they live on food residues, as in the intestine, they may be called *saprophytes*. The term saprophyte is, however, commonly used in a wider sense to denote free-living bacteria in soil, water and decaying matter. In contrast, a *parasite* may be defined as a microorganism or some larger species (*e.g.* worms) that lives in or on, and obtains its nourishment from, a living host, and is potentially pathogenic. Some of the commensal bacteria which constitute the resident flora of the skin and mucous membranes may also be potentially pathogenic in the sense that they may initiate infection under certain circumstances, as when coliform bacilli from the gut set up infection in the urinary tract or when mouth streptococci become attached to diseased heart valves and cause endocarditis.

Medical microbiology is concerned with the aetiology, *pathogenesis* (mode of infection), laboratory diagnosis and treatment of infection in the individual and with the *epidemiology* (study of mass disease) and control of infection in the community. It therefore has close links with several other disciplines into which the training of the doctor has been divided to form the medical curriculum, *e.g.* pathology, clinical medicine and surgery, pharmacology and therapeutics, and preventive medicine.

The changes that occur in the host's tissues as the result of infection are often recognised by the pathologist as specific or pathognomonic of a particular pathogenic microorganism, *e.g.* the circumscribed boil of the staphylococcus, the spreading cellulitis of the streptococcus, the red liver-like appearance (hepatisation) of the lung in pneumococcal pneumonia, the tubercles and the subsequent necrotic changes (called caseation) of tuberculosis, the aortic disease and granulomata (gummata) of syphilis, and the typical intestinal ulcerations of typhoid fever and the dysenteries. But the prudent pathologist will usually seek to confirm his diagnosis of the cause of these macroscopic changes by taking smears and cultures from the lesions to demonstrate the microscopic germ. The pathology of infection provides a fascinating but relatively unexplored field of study since it includes the affinity of pathogens for particular tissues and the initiation of infection as well as the characteristic tissue reactions.

Microbiology has a close link with curative medicine in regard to the precise diagnosis and the rational treatment of microbial diseases. Certain infections are not ordinarily transmissible from one person to another, *e.g.* the urinary tract infections or subacute bacterial endocarditis, and for these the term *endogenous* (or *autogenous*) infection may be used although an autogenous infection, for example, a boil resulting from infection with a staphylococcus on the victim's skin or nose may be *infectious* in the sense of being transmissible to another person. Most of the common fevers—measles, whooping-cough, chicken pox, etc.—are *infectious* or *communicable* diseases. However, certain infections that are transmissible from animal hosts to man, called the *zoonoses*, are not ordinarily communicable from man to man, *e.g.* bubonic plague, brucellosis, rabies.

The doctor engaged in the care of sick patients, be he general practitioner, surgeon or other medical specialist, will often be able to identify the pathogenic microorganism from the special clinical features of an infection and will accordingly prescribe the appropriate treatment. Sometimes the patient presents with a fever but no characteristic signs or symptoms that will allow the doctor to make a precise diagnosis; this pyrexia of unknown—or uncertain—origin (P.U.O.) will require laboratory help to elucidate the cause of the fever. Even when the doctor identifies the infection from the patient's signs or symptoms—sore throat, acute diarrhoea, pneumonia, meningitis—he will still need laboratory help since many of these syndromes are caused by different kinds of microorganisms, *e.g.* acute diarrhoea may be due to a wide range of pathogenic bacteria, viruses and protozoa. Moreover, some of these pathogenic bacteria which are ordinarily sensitive to certain anti-microbial drugs, may acquire drug-resistance. Therefore with modern selective *chemotherapy* the effective treatment of the patient with a clinical infection requires the early isolation and identification of the infecting microorganism. In other words, the doctor has to identify and treat specific infections rather than clinical syndromes. When an infection is not amenable to chemotherapy as is the case with the toxic infections and most virus infections, *antisera* containing neutralising antibodies against the pathogenic agent (either specially prepared in animals like the horse or derived from human blood *i.e.* gamma globulin) may be used either to treat the patient as in diphtheria or to give temporary protection to a person exposed to the risk of infection as in measles.

Microbiology is closely concerned with the *epidemiology* and control of infection in any community where the transmission and disease-producing capacity of the infecting microorganisms is facilitated by environmental or host factors: *e.g.* overcrowding, contaminated food, drink or air, malnutrition, tissue damage. The term epidemiology has in the past been applied particularly to the study of the factors contributing to the endemic or epidemic prevalence of an infectious or communicable disease; but, as the name implies, it is concerned with the study of any community disease or disability and in recent years we have seen the application of epidemiological methods to many non-infective conditions. As a medical science it is particularly concerned with aetiological factors and it has had remarkable successes in their elucidation among both infectious and non-infectious diseases. Thus, the evidence that cholera and typhoid fever were due to living agents spread by water was produced from epidemiological data collected respectively by John Snow, a London anaesthetist and William Budd, a West Country doctor, 20 years or more before the aetiological agents were identified, pellagra was shown by Goldberger to be a deficiency disease long before vitamins were defined while in our own time, heavy cigarette smoking has been proved to be causally related to lung cancer although the carcinogenic agent has not yet been identified.

In the study of the sources and modes of spread of infectious diseases, microbiology has demonstrated the importance of *carriers*; that is, individuals who, while not showing any clinical symptoms of infection, carry and disperse a pathogenic microorganism and so contribute to the dissemination of infection in a community. Again, tests for the presence of antibodies to specific pathogens or their toxins have shown that latent or inapparent infections may play a large part in raising the resistance of a community to epidemic outbursts of disease. With a good knowledge of the epidemiology of a specific communicable disease, the Health Officer concerned with preventive medicine knows what measures for its control are most likely to be effective and here again, in the field of prophylactic immunisation, the microbiologist has been a most valuable partner.

Most of the major pestilences—typhus and typhoid fever, plague, cholera, smallpox and yellow fever—that used to decimate armies and beleaguered cities or spread like wild-fire round the world are now being controlled by good environmental sanitation, by the destruction of insect vectors such as louse, flea and mosquito, or by prophylactic vaccination. However, some of these great plagues, together with other global infections like malaria, tuberculosis and leprosy, the diarrhoeal diseases and the pneumonias, still take a heavy toll of life and health in most of the developing countries. Pandemics of influenza still occur and respiratory infections are still the major cause of sickness in most countries.

A community infection of a special kind still occurs among patients congregated in hospitals. Although the consequences of hospital cross-infection are much less serious than they were in Lister's day, we are reminded of the aphorisms of two great hospital reformers of the nineteenth century—Florence Nightingale's pungent comment that "the first requirement of any hospital (is) that it do the sick no harm" and Sir James Y. Simpson's conclusions after a most remarkable epidemiological survey of deaths from infection following amputations that "in treatment of the sick, there is ever danger in their aggregation and safety only in their segregation; and our hospitals should be constructed so as to avoid . . . the former and secure . . . the latter condition". We are still far from achieving these worthy objectives. It is pertinent in these days when teaching hospitals are becoming the repositories of ageing patients with degenerative diseases to remind medical students and doctors that acute and chronic infections are still responsible for more than a third of all the illnesses requiring medical care and that in the most susceptible group of children under 5 years of age, infections account for over 80 per cent. of the total sickness.

Microbiology developed originally as an applied science of particular importance in medicine, agriculture and industry. But it soon became obvious that the bacterial cell and its products had many attractions for the general biologist, the chemist, the physicist, the geneticist, the pharmacologist and other specialists as well as the bacteriologist, immunologist and pathologist. In its free living form, the bacterial cell with its simple food requirements, rapid growth and remarkable hardiness, and its great range of enzymes and diffusible products has become very acceptable for detailed study and, in the past few decades, bacterial physiology (sometimes called microbial chemistry) has made many contributions to advances in our knowledge of cellular and molecular biology. Together with bacteriophage (its own particular parasite) the bacterial cell has been specially useful in advancing the science of genetics while the biochemist interested in enzymology finds it a most valuable granary. Although many of the developments in general microbiology are not immediately relevant to medicine, it is essential that the medical student should have some understanding of the anatomy and physiology of the bacterial cell and this aspect of microbiology is discussed in the chapters that follow.

FURTHER READING

BROCK, T. D. (1961). *Milestones in Microbiology*. Trans. Englewood Cliff, N.J. London: Prentice Hall.

BULLOCH, W. (1960). *The History of Bacteriology*. London: Oxford University Press.

BURNET, F. M. (1962). *Natural History of Infectious Disease*. 3rd ed. Cambridge: University Press.

DUBOS, R. (1950). *Louis Pasteur, Free Lance of Science*. Boston: Little Brown.

GODLEE, R. J. (1917). *Lord Lister*. London: Macmillan.

KRUIF, DE P. (1958). *Microbe Hunters*. London: Hutchinson.

MAUROIS, A. (1959). *The Life of Sir Alexander Fleming, Discoverer of Penicillin*. London: Cape.

SMITH, T. (1934). *Parasitism and Disease*. Princeton: University Press.

WINSLOW, C. E. A. (1943). *The Conquest of Epidemic Disease; a Chapter in the History of Ideas*. Princeton: University Press.

ZINSSER, H. (1937). *Rats, Lice and History*. London: Routledge.

CHAPTER 2

MORPHOLOGY OF BACTERIA

Microorganisms may be defined as living creatures that are microscopical in size and relatively simple, often unicellular in structure. The diameter of the smallest body that can be resolved and seen clearly with the naked eye is about 100 μ (1 μ, or micron = 0·001 millimetres). All but a few of the microorganisms are smaller than this and a microscope is therefore necessary for their observation. The light microscope under optimal conditions can resolve bodies down to 0·2 μ in diameter, and this includes all microbes except the viruses, most of which are even smaller. The electron microscope has a limit of resolution better than 0·0005 μ (*i.e.* 0·5 mμ or millimicron = 5 Angström Units), and can resolve even the smallest viruses (0·01 μ diam.). It should be noted, however, that when bacteria or fungi are allowed to grow undisturbed on a solid or semi-solid substrate, their numerous progeny accumulate locally to form masses, or *colonies*, which are readily visible to the naked eye.

Living material, or protoplasm, is organised in units known as *cells*. Each cell consists of a body of protoplasm, the *protoplast*, enclosed by a thin semipermeable membrane, the *plasma membrane* or *cytoplasmic membrane*, and also, in most cases, by an outer, relatively rigid *cell wall*. The protoplast is differentiated into a major part, the *cytoplasm*, and an inner body, the *nucleus*, which contains the hereditary determinants of character, the *genes*, borne on thread-like *chromosomes*.

The bodies of higher plants and animals are multicellular, with interdependence and specialisation of function among the cells, the different kinds of cells being segregated in separate tissues. Many microorganisms, on the other hand, are unicellular, existing as single self-sufficient cells, unattached to their fellows. Other microorganisms grow as aggregates of cells joined together by their cell walls in clusters, chains, rods, filaments (hyphae) or mycelia (*i.e.* meshworks of branching filaments), and some grow as a *plasmodium*, *i.e.* a multinucleate mass of cytoplasm. Generally, these morphologically multicellular microbes are physiologically unicellular, each cell being self-sufficient and, if isolated artificially, being able to nourish itself, grow and reproduce the species. Some specialisation of cell function, approaching that of true multicellular organisms, is encountered in colonies of moulds and higher bacteria; thus, certain cells, which form an aerial mycelium, are specialised for the formation and dissemination of spores, and are dependent for their nutrition on the activities of other cells comprising a vegetative mycelium.

The majority of microorganisms may be classified in the following large biological groups: (1) Algae, (2) Protozoa, (3) Slime moulds, (4) Fungi proper, or *Eumycetes*, including the moulds and the yeasts, (5) Bacteria, or *Schizomycetes* ("fission fungi"), (6) *Rickettsiales*, (7) *Mycoplasmatales*, and (8) Viruses, or *Virales*. The algae (except the blue-green algae), the protozoa, slime moulds and fungi include the larger and more highly developed microorganisms; their cells have the same general type of structure and organisation, described as *eucaryotic*, that is found in the cells of higher plants and animals. The bacteria and the closely related blue-green algae, the organisms of the mycoplasma and rickettsia groups and the so-called "viruses" of the psittacosis-lymphogranuloma-trachoma group include the smaller microorganisms having a simpler form of cellular organisation described as *procaryotic* (Stanier & van Niel, 1962). The viruses are the smallest of the microorganisms; the infectious virus particles, or *virions*, have a relatively simple structure that is not comparable with that of a cell, and their mode of reproduction is fundamentally different from that of cellular organisms.

Since the algae and slime moulds contain no species of medical or veterinary importance, they will not be dealt with in this book. The main differential characters of the other groups are as follows:

Protozoa.—These are non-photosynthetic unicellular organisms (a few are colonial) with protoplasm clearly differentiated into nucleus and cytoplasm. They are relatively large microorganisms, with transverse diameters mainly in the range 2–100 μ. Their surface membranes vary in complexity and rigidity from a thin, flexible membrane in amoebae, which allows major changes in cell shape and the protrusion of pseudopodia in the movements of locomotion and ingestion, to a relatively stiff pellicle in ciliate protozoa, which preserves a characteristic shape to the cell. Most free-living, and some parasitic species have the mode of nutrition typical of animals, that called *holozoic*: they capture, ingest and digest internally solid masses or particles of food material. Many protozoa, for instance, feed on bacteria. Protozoa, therefore, are generally regarded as the lowest forms of animal life, though certain flagellate protozoa are very closely related in their morphology and mode of development to photosynthetic flagellate algae in the plant kingdom. Some free-living protozoa are *saprophytic*, absorbing soluble nutrient substances derived from dead plant or animal material, or from the excretions of plants and animals. Many protozoa are *parasitic* and live in and derive their nourishment from the body of an animal host; some of these parasites ingest masses of solid material whilst others absorb soluble nutrients through their cell surface. Malaria parasites, for instance, both absorb soluble nutrients from the host and ingest masses of host-cell cytoplasm. Protozoa reproduce asexually by binary fission or multiple fission (schizogony), and some also by a sexual mechanism. Some species exhibit a definite life cycle with both sexual and asexual phases, and some form round, thick-walled resting cells, or "cysts", which are important for the persistence and spread of the organism through the environment, where conditions may be unfavourable to survival of the vegetative forms.

Fungi.—These are non-photosynthetic microorganisms possessing relatively rigid cell walls. They are saprophytic or parasitic, and take in soluble nutrient substances by diffusion through their cell surfaces. When solid food materials are utilised, these are first broken

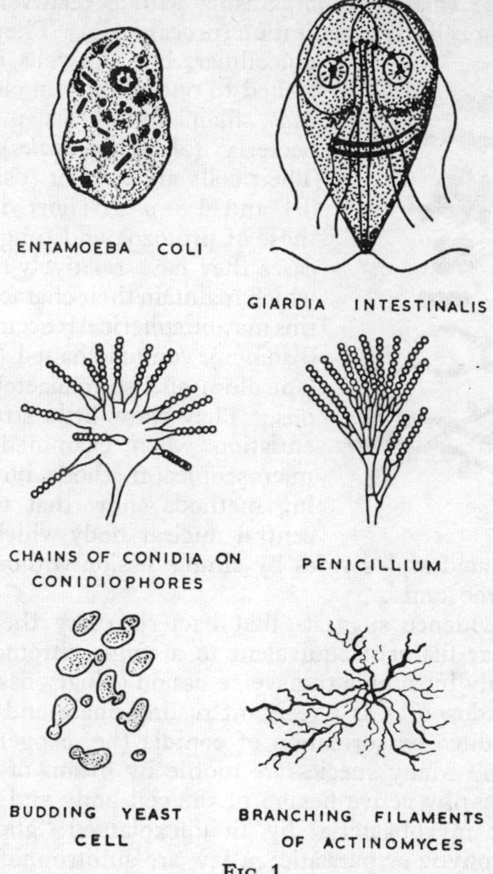

FIG. 1

down to soluble products by enzymes secreted extracellularly by the fungus. Except for the flagellate spores and gametes of the primitive aquatic species, fungi are non-motile. *Moulds* grow as branching filaments (hyphae), usually between 2 and 10 μ in width, which interlace to form a meshwork (mycelium). The hyphae are *coenocytic* (*i.e.* have a continuous multinucleate protoplasm), being non-septate or else septate with a central pore in each cross-wall. Moulds reproduce by the formation of various kinds of sexual and asexual spores that develop from the vegetative (feeding) mycelium or from an aerial mycelium that effects their airborne dissemination. *Yeasts* are ovoid or spherical cells that reproduce asexually by budding and also, in many cases, sexually with the formation of sexual spores. They do not form a mycelium, although the intermediate *yeast-like fungi* may form a pseudomycelium consisting of chains of elongated cells. The higher fungi of the class *Basidiomycetes* (mushrooms), which produce large fruiting structures for aerial dissemination of spores, play no part in infection of man or animals, though some species, e.g. *Amanita phalloides*, are poisonous when eaten.

Bacteria are small microorganisms with a relatively simple and primitive form of cellular organisation (procaryotic). They are generally unicellular, but the cells may grow attached to one another in clusters, chains, rods, filaments or, as in the "higher bacteria" (*Actinomycetales*), a mycelium. Their cells are smaller (usually between 0·4 and 1·5 μ in short diameter) than those of protozoa and fungi, and in most cases they have relatively rigid cell walls which maintain their characteristic shape; this may be spherical (coccus), rod-shaped (bacillus), comma-shaped (vibrio), spiral (spirillum and spirochaete), or filamentous. They show little structural differentiation when examined by ordinary microscopical methods, but special staining methods show that they possess a central nuclear body which contains deoxyribonucleic acid and divides by simple fission without evidence of mitosis or chromosomes.

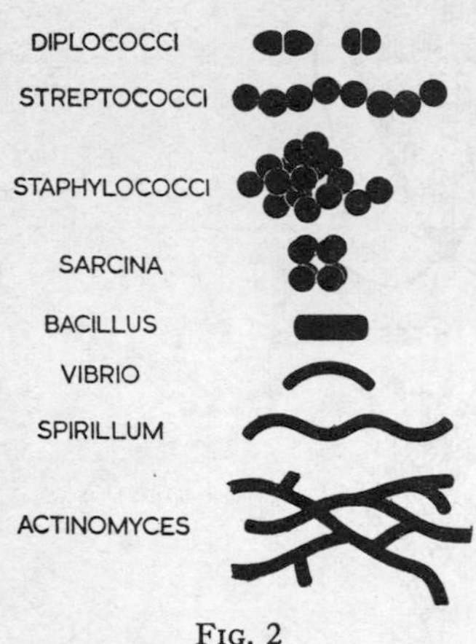

FIG. 2

Genetical evidence suggests that bacteria carry their genes on a linear or circular filament equivalent to a single chromosome. They reproduce mainly by simple transverse fission (binary fission). Certain species form endospores as a resistant resting phase and some (actinomycetes) reproduce by formation of conidia (i.e. exogenously formed asexual spores). Many species are motile by means of flagella, some (the spirochaetes) by active flexion of the cell body and some (*e.g.* the non-pathogenic myxobacteria) by an unexplained "gliding" process. Most are saprophytic or parasitic; a few are autotrophic and a few are photosynthetic (*vide infra*). (The photosynthetic bacteria, or "green" and "purple" bacteria, carry out a special kind of photosynthesis which differs from that of the blue-green algae and the higher algae and plants in that it does not involve the production of oxygen.) Autotrophic and photosynthetic bacteria are inhabitants of soil and water, and are harmless to man and animals.

Bacteria are *parasitic* when they live on or in, and gain their nourishment, including organic nutrient compounds, from the body of a living animal or plant host. Non-parasitic and free-living bacteria include: (1) those that are *saprophytic*, *i.e.* absorb soluble organic nutrients derived from the *dead* bodies and excretions of plants and animals, (2) those that are *autotrophic*, *i.e.* nourish themselves on inorganic substances, deriving their carbon from CO_2 and their energy by oxidation of an inorganic nitrogen, sulphur or iron compound, and (3) those that are *photosynthetic*, *i.e.* obtain their carbon from CO_2 and their energy from sunlight. Parasitic and saprophytic bacteria are described as *heterotrophic* because, in contrast with the autotrophs and photosynthetic bacteria, they obtain their carbon and energy from the dissimilation of organic compounds.

Bacteria (together with the blue-green algae, *Rickettsiales* and *Mycoplasmatales*) are distinguished from the higher microorganisms, plants and animals by the simpler organisation of their cells. These are described as being *procaryotic*, in contrast with the cells of the higher organisms, which are termed *eucaryotic*. The main distinguishing features of the procaryotic cell are as follows. (1) Its nucleus appears as a simple, homogeneous body not possessing a nuclear membrane separating it from the cytoplasm, nor a nucleolus, nor a spindle, nor a number of separate non-identical chromosomes. (2) It lacks the internal membranes isolating the respiratory and photosynthetic enzyme systems in specific organelles, comparable with the membrane-bounded mitochondria and chloroplasts of eucaryotic cells. Thus, the respiratory enzymes in bacteria are located mainly in the peripheral cytoplasmic membrane and their effective functioning is dependent upon the integrity of the cell protoplast as a whole. (3) Its rigid cell wall contains as its main strengthening element a specific mucopeptide substance not found in eucaryotic organisms. This mucopeptide is the "target" of the antibacterial actions of penicillin and lysozyme.

Rickettsiales are simple unicellular organisms that are rod-shaped, spherical or pleomorphic. They are generally similar to, though smaller than bacteria, but they are still resolvable by the light microscope (*i.e.* over 0·2 μ in diam.) and most species are not filterable through bacteria-stopping filters. The majority are strict parasites that can grow only in the living tissues of a suitable animal host, usually intracellularly. A few exceptional species (e.g. *Bartonella bacilliformis*, which is also exceptional in being flagellate and motile) can grow in cell-free nutrient media containing body fluids. The organisms of psittacosis and trachoma, previously classed as viruses, are now included in this order.

Mycoplasmatales (pleuropneumonia-like organisms, or PPLO) are procaryotic cellular organisms that differ from bacteria in their smaller size, their lack of a rigid cell wall, and their consequent extreme pleomorphism and great sensitivity to the osmotic tension in the environment. Cell size is variable and the viable elements range from 0·15 to over 1 μ in diameter, the smallest being capable of passing through bacteria-stopping filters. Mycoplasmas can be cultivated on artificial cell-free nutrient media enriched with serum and they are the smallest and simplest organisms capable of autonomous growth. Most are parasites of man or animals, but one known species is a saprophyte present in soil and sewage.

Viruses are the smallest and simplest of all the microorganisms and different species range in size from 0·01 to 0·3 μ in diameter. Most are "ultramicroscopic" (*i.e.* are smaller than can be resolved by the light microscope, under 0·2 μ in diam.) and are filterable through bacteria-stopping filters. All species are strictly parasitic and are capable of growing only within the living cells of an appropriate animal, plant or bacterial host; none can grow on an inanimate nutrient medium. A few bacteria and the rickettsiae resemble viruses in their inability to grow elsewhere than in living cells, but the viruses are distinguished from these organisms by having an entirely different method of growth and reproduction.

Viruses lack biosynthetic and energy-yielding enzymes for the manufacture of their molecular components, and possess only one kind of nucleic acid, either ribonucleic acid (RNA) or deoxyribonucleic acid (DNA), instead of both as do cellular organisms. The infectious virus particle, "elementary body", or *virion*, introduces its nucleic acid into the host cell and the viral nucleic acid organises the synthetic systems of the host cell to manufacture viral molecular components (principally nucleic acid and protein) which are ultimately assembled to form a new generation of complete infectious virus particles.

The viruses that infect and parasitise bacteria are named *bacteriophages* or *phages*. "Virulent" phages undergo free development inside the host bacterium, which after a short interval undergoes *lysis* (disruption) and liberates the resultant crop of infectious phage particles. "Temperate" phages become reduced within the host bacterium to a latent form, or *prophage* (believed to be the phage DNA incorporated in the bacterial chromosome), which is reproduced *pari passu* with the bacterium through many generations. Occasionally the prophage becomes vegetative and a crop of infectious phage particles is produced, with consequent lysis of the bacterium. A bacterium carrying latent prophage is termed *lysogenic*.

The bacteria and viruses play the most important part in the causation of human infective disease. Protozoal infections are more prevalent in tropical and subtropical countries, whilst the common fungal infections are mainly superficial (*e.g.* skin infections) and often of minor severity.

The remainder of this chapter and Chapter 3 will be devoted to the general biology of the bacteria. That of the other groups of microorganisms will be dealt with in Chapters 5 and 31–41.

MORPHOLOGICAL STUDY OF BACTERIA

Microscopical examination is usually the first step taken for the identification of an unknown bacterium. The bacterium may be allocated to one or other of the major groups when its *morphology* and *staining reactions* have been observed. The morphological features of importance are the size, shape and grouping of the cells, and their possession of any distinctive structures such as endospores, flagella (or motility), capsules and intracellular granules. Staining reactions are observed after treatment by special procedures such as the Gram and Ziehl-Neelsen stains, the different kinds of bacteria being shown in separate colours due to their different permeability to certain decolourising agents. A preparation stained by one of these methods usually suffices for observation of the general morphology of the bacterium, but some morphological features can be demonstrated only by the application of further special stains. (For a full discussion of the principles of different staining procedures, see Lamanna and Mallette, 1959.)

The optical, or light microscope (employing visible light) is generally sufficient for making the observations of shape, staining reaction and special morphology that are required for the identification of a bacterium. The electron microscope, which has contributed much new information about the fine structure of the bacterial cell, is rarely required for diagnostic work. It may be valuable, however, in enabling demonstration of certain structures of taxonomic importance, *e.g.* fimbriae, which cannot be demonstrated with the light microscope.

Unstained Preparations of Living Organisms.—The morphology of bacteria can be studied in the first place by examining them microscopically in the unstained condition, suspended in a thin film of fluid between a glass slide and coverslip (*i.e.* in an "unstained wet film"). In this way their general shape can be seen and their motility determined. Certain very slender bacteria, however, such as the spirochaetes, are so feebly refractile that they cannot be seen by the ordinary microscopic methods, and *dark-ground illumination* or *phase-contrast microscopy* is necessary for their demonstration.

For the study of the development of individual organisms and the growth of bacteria in colonies, the "agar-block" method of Ørskov, and the microscope-incubator may be used. These methods enable living bacteria to be observed at intervals during their actual growth on a suitable substrate, and present a more natural picture than other procedures involving manipulations that may sometimes create artificial appearances.

Stained Preparations.—The microscopical examination of fixed and stained preparations is usually an essential routine procedure. The bacteria are more readily discovered and studied when immobilised by fixation and darkly stained in contrast with the bright background. *Simple staining* is effected by the application of a watery solution of a single basic dye, *e.g.* methylene blue, methyl violet or basic fuchsin, or sometimes along with a mordant, *e.g.* dilute carbol fuchsin. The coloured, positively charged cation of the basic dye combines firmly with negatively charged groups in the bacterial protoplasm, especially with those of the abundant nucleic acids. The stain is retained through a subsequent washing with water for the removal of excess dye from the slide. Acidic dyes, having coloured anions, do not stain bacteria strongly except at very acid pH values, and thus can be used for "negative staining" (see below). Cells or structures that stain with basic dyes at normal pH values are described as *basophilic* and those that stain with acidic dyes as *acidophilic*.

Prior to staining, the film or smear of bacteria must be fixed on the slide. *Fixation* is usually effected by heat; the slide is first thoroughly dried in air and then heated gently in a flame. Vegetative bacteria are thereby killed, rendered permeable to the stain, stuck to the surface of the slide and preserved from undergoing autolytic changes. Chemical fixatives are used for sections of infected tissue and films of infected blood, since they cause less damage to the tissue cells; they include formalin, mercuric chloride, methyl alcohol and osmic acid.

It should be noted that the bacterial cell wall is not stained by ordinary methods and the coloured body seen corresponds to the cell protoplasm only. This is usually much shrunken as a result of drying. Chains of stained bacteria thus show the coloured bodies separated by gaps that are the sites of unstained, connecting cell walls.

Beaded and *Bipolar Staining*.—Certain bacteria do not colour evenly with simple stains. Thus, the diphtheria bacillus shows a "beaded" appearance, with alternating dark and light bars. The plague bacillus shows "bipolar staining", the ends being more deeply coloured than the centre. The uneven staining may be due to the manner in which the protoplasm shrinks when the cell is dried and fixed.

"*Negative*" or *Background Staining* is of value as a rapid method for the simple morphological study of bacteria. The bacteria are mixed with a substance such as India ink, or nigrosin, which, after spreading as a film, yields a dark background in which the bacteria stand out as bright, unstained objects.

Silver Impregnation methods are utilised for the staining of spirochaetes, especially for demonstrating these organisms in tissues. The slender cells are thickened by a dark deposit of silver on their surface.

Impression Preparations are used for cytological studies when it is desired to avoid the distortion of cell structure and colonial arrangement inevitable in the normal procedure of preparing a smear, drying it and fixing it by heat. Bacteria, newly spread on the surface of an agar medium, or grown on agar to form small colonies, are fixed ***in situ*** without drying, to a slide or coverslip. This is done by allowing a chemical fixative to diffuse through the agar from below. The fixed bacteria adhere to the glass when the agar is removed and can then be stained.

Staining Reactions.—The staining reactions of bacteria are of the greatest importance in their differentiation and identification. *Gram's staining reaction* has the widest application, dividing all bacteria into two categories, named "Gram-positive" and "Gram-negative", according to whether or not the organisms resist decolourisation with acetone, alcohol or aniline oil after staining with a para-rosaniline (triphenylmethane) dye, *e.g.* methyl violet, and subsequent treatment with iodine. The Gram-positive bacteria resist decolourisation and remain stained a dark purple colour. The Gram-negative bacteria are decolourised, and then counterstained light pink by the subsequent application of basic fuchsin, safranine, neutral red or dilute carbol fuchsin. In routine diagnostic work a Gram-stained smear is often the only preparation examined microscopically, since it shows clearly the general morphology of the bacteria as well as revealing their Gram-reaction. It should be noted that species which are characteristically Gram-positive, may appear Gram-negative under certain conditions of growth; thus, some show an increasing proportion of partly or wholly Gram-negative cells in ageing cultures on nutrient agar. On the other hand, characteristically Gram-negative species do not produce cells that stain Gram-positively in correctly treated smears.

Gram-reactivity appears to reflect a fundamental aspect of cell structure and is correlated with many other biological properties. Thus, the different species of a single genus generally show the same reaction. Gram-positive bacteria are more susceptible than Gram-negative bacteria to the antibacterial actions of penicillin, acids, iodine, basic dyes, detergents and lysozyme, and less susceptible to alkalies, azide, tellurite, proteolytic enzymes, lysis by antibody and complement, and plasmolysis in solutes of high osmotic pressure.

The mechanism of the Gram stain is not fully understood. Gram-positive organisms are able to retain basic dyes at a higher hydrogen-ion concentration than the Gram-negative species, showing an isoelectric point of pH 2–3 as compared with pH 4–5. The more acidic character of their protoplasm, which is enhanced by treatment with iodine, may partly explain their stronger retention of basic dye. It has also been suggested that the difference in Gram reaction depends upon a difference in the permeability of the cell wall or the cytoplasmic membrane. After staining with methyl violet and treatment with iodine, a dye-iodine complex, or "lake", is formed within the cell, which is insoluble in water but moderately soluble and dissociable in the acetone or alcohol used as the decolouriser. Under the action of the decolouriser, the dye and iodine diffuse freely out of the Gram-negative cell, but not from the Gram-positive cell, presumably because the latter's surface is less permeable to the decolouriser or its iodine solute. It has recently been suggested by Salton (1963), that dehydration by the decolouriser and the action of the iodine play an important part in selectively decreasing the porosity of the cell wall of Gram-positive organisms. Whatever the complete mechanism of the reaction may be, Gram-positivity appears to depend upon the integrity of the cellular structure and the presence in the cell of a specific magnesium ribonucleate-protein complex (and perhaps also of other specific compounds). Thus, Gram-positive bacteria become Gram-negative if they are ruptured mechanically, or if their magnesium ribonucleate is removed by autolysis or by treatment with bile salt or the enzyme ribonuclease. From cytological studies it seems that Gram-positive staining colours the whole cell, including the cell wall, but chemical analysis of isolated cell walls has not shown them to contain magnesium ribonucleate.

The *acid-fast staining reaction*, as revealed by the Ziehl-Neelsen method is of value in distinguishing a few bacterial species, *e.g.* the tubercle bacillus, from all others. These "acid-fast" bacteria are relatively impermeable and resistant to simple stains, but when stained with a strong reagent (basic fuchsin in aqueous 5 per cent. phenol, applied with heat), subsequently resist decolourisation by strong acids, *e.g.* 20 per cent. sulphuric acid. Any decolourised non-acid-fast organisms are counterstained in a contrasting colour with methylene blue or malachite green.

The acid-fast bacteria have an exceptionally rich and varied content of lipids, fatty acids and higher alcohols, and their acid-fastness has been attributed to this. When the lipids, including those firmly bound in the protoplasm, are removed by treatment with suitable solvents, the cells are no longer acid-fast. One of the lipids peculiar to acid-fast bacteria exhibits the property of acid-fastness in the free state; this is a wax *mycolic acid*, a high molecular weight hydroxy acid containing carboxyl groups. The mere presence of such a substance in the cell is not by itself sufficient to explain acid-fastness, since the character is lost when the cell is ruptured by mechanical means or autolysis. Acid-fastness therefore depends on the structural integrity of the cell, its content of lipids and, possibly, a special anatomical disposition of the lipids.

THE ANATOMY OF THE BACTERIAL CELL

The essential structures of the bacterial cell are shown in Figure 3. The *protoplast*, *i.e.* the whole body of living material (protoplasm), is bounded peripherally by a very thin, elastic and semipermeable membrane called the *plasma membrane*, or *cytoplasmic membrane*. Outside, and closely covering this, lies the rigid, supporting *cell wall*, which is porous and relatively permeable. Cell division occurs by the development, from the periphery inwards, of a transverse cytoplasmic membrane and a transverse cell wall, or *cross wall*.

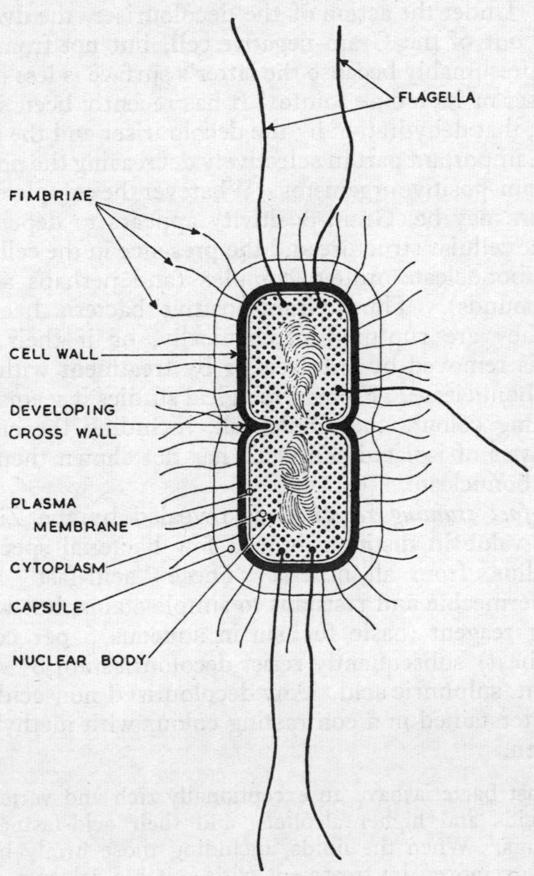

FIG. 3
The structure of the bacterial cell.

The *cytoplasm*, or main part of the protoplasm, consists of a watery sap packed with large numbers of small granules called *ribosomes*, which are visible only with the electron microscope. The "nucleus", more properly called the *nuclear body* or *chromatin body*, is centrally placed; it appears homogeneous with the light microscope and, usually, as a skein of parallel fibres in ultrathin sections under the electron microscope. In rapidly growing cells, nuclear replication and division proceed a little in advance of cell division, so that two, four or even more nuclei are seen within a single 'cell' as demarcated by transverse cell walls.

In addition to these essential structures, other intracellular and extracellular structures may be present in particular species of bacteria, in some cases only under particular conditions of growth. In the cytoplasm, for instance, there may be present *inclusion granules* consisting of volutin, lipid, glycogen or starch, or membranous bodies called *mesosomes*. Outside the cell wall, there may be a protective gelatinous covering layer called a *capsule* or, when it is too thin to be resolved with the light microscope ($<0{\cdot}2\ \mu$), a *microcapsule*. Soluble large-molecular material may be dispersed by the bacterium into the environment as *loose slime*. Some bacteria bear, protruding outwards from the cell wall, one or both of two kinds of filamentous appendages, *flagella*, which are organs of locomotion, and *fimbriae*, which appear to be organs of adhesion. Because they are exposed to contact and interaction with the cells and humoral substances of the body of the host, it is the surface structures of bacteria, the cell wall, capsule or microcapsule, flagella and fimbriae, that are most likely to have a special role in the processes of infection.

The methods of demonstration, the composition and the functional roles of the various bacterial cell structures are reviewed briefly below. Further details may be obtained from the books edited by Spooner and Stocker (1956) and Gunsalus and Stanier (1960).

Cytoplasm of Bacteria.—The cytoplasm of the bacterial cell is a viscous watery solution, or soft gel, containing a variety of organic and inorganic solutes, and numerous small granules called *ribosomes*. The ribosomes are 10–30 mμ in diameter and number tens of thousands per cell. They correspond to the microsomes of animal and plant cells, consist mainly of protein and ribonucleic acid (RNA) and are the sites of manufacture of the enzymes and other proteins of the bacterium, the specificity of these proteins being determined by *messenger RNA* transmitted to the ribosomes from the nucleus. The cytoplasm of bacteria differs from that of the higher eucaryotic organisms in not containing an endoplasmic reticulum of membranes bearing microsomes, in not containing mitochondria and in not showing signs of internal mobility, *e.g.* cytoplasmic streaming, the formation, migration and disappearance of vacuoles, and amoeboid movement.

Nuclear Bodies.—In unstained bacteria, and in bacteria stained by the usual methods, the protoplast shows no differentiation into nucleus and cytoplasm. However, by a special method it is possible to demonstrate the presence of bodies that correspond to nuclei, although differing morphologically from the organised nuclei of the eucaryotic cells of animals and plants. After suitable fixation, the bacteria are treated with hydrochloric acid to reduce the staining affinity of the cytoplasm by removing its content of ribonucleic acid; on subsequent staining the nuclear bodies become deeply coloured and the cytoplasm only slightly coloured. The nuclear bodies are usually oval or elongated and lie transversely in the cell. They react positively to the Feulgen test for deoxyribonucleic acid (DNA), the essential constituent of the nuclei of the higher organisms. Unlike the intracellular storage granules described below, they are constantly present in all cells and under all conditions of culture. The nuclear bodies appear to increase by growth and simple fission, and not by mitosis; they show no evidence of possessing an outer nuclear membrane separating them from the cytoplasm, a nucleolus or separate chromosomes. Genetic evidence obtained from studies of conjugation in one species, *Escherichia coli*, suggests that all the genes of a bacterium are carried in a single linkage group, or chromosome. The appearance of the nuclear body in ultrathin sections examined with the electron microscope is compatible with the bacterial chromosome occurring as a very long thin fibre folded backwards and forwards on itself in the form of a skein. Only a single nuclear body is present in some cells, whilst in others, as a result of nuclear division preceding cell division, two, four or even more nuclear bodies may be present.

Inclusion Granules.—In many species of bacteria, round granules are observed in the cytoplasm. These are not permanent or essential structures, and may be absent under certain conditions of growth. They appear to be aggregates of substances concerned in cell metabolism, *e.g.* an excess metabolite stored as a nutrient reserve. Generally, they are present in largest amount when the bacteria have access to an abundance of energy-yielding nutrients, and diminish or disappear under conditions of energy-source starvation (Wilkinson & Duguid, 1960). They consist of volutin, lipid, glycogen, starch, or sulphur. Volutin and lipid granules, 0·1–1·0 μ in diameter, are seen in many parasitic and saprophytic bacteria, and their demonstration may assist in the identification of certain organisms; thus, the diphtheria bacillus may be distinguished from related bacilli found in the throat by its content of volutin granules.

Volutin granules (syn. *metachromatic* or *Babes-Ernst* granules) have an intense affinity for basic dyes. With toluidine blue or methylene blue, they stain *metachromatically* a red-violet colour, contrasting with the blue staining of the bacterial protoplasm. By special methods, *e.g.* Neisser's and Albert's, employing also iodine and/or a counterstain, the granules can be demonstrated with even greater colour contrast; their staining, unlike that of the protoplasm generally, is not bleached by the iodine or displaced by the counterstain. The metachromatic staining of volutin granules is thought to be due to their content of polymerised inorganic polyphosphate. This is an energy-rich compound which may act as a reserve of energy and phosphate for cell metabolism. Volutin granules are slightly acid-fast, resisting decolourisation by 1 per cent. sulphuric acid; they are more refractile than the protoplasm and are sometimes distinguishable in unstained wet films. By electron microscopy they appear as very opaque, clearly demarcated bodies.

Lipid granules are recognised by their affinity for fat-soluble dyes such as Sudan black. Thus, by Burdon's method they are coloured black in contrast to the remaining protoplasm, which is counterstained pink with basic fuchsin. The granules are spherical, of varying size and highly refractile, being easily seen in unstained preparations. They are slightly acid-fast and may be stained by the modified Ziehl-Neelsen method used for spores. They resist staining by basic dyes and appear as unstained spaces in bacteria treated with simple stains or by Gram's method. Lipid granules resemble endospores (see below) in their acid-fast staining and their resistance to simple stains, but are distinguished by their staining with Sudan black, their smaller size and their frequent occurrence in numbers of more than one per cell. In the bacteria so far subjected to chemical analysis, the granules appear to consist mainly of polymerised β-hydroxybutyric acid (or poly-β-hydroxybutyrate). The manner in which the lipid content of bacteria varies with the conditions of culture suggests that this substance may act as a carbon and energy storage product.

Polysaccharide granules that stain with iodine like either glycogen (red-brown) or starch (blue) can be seen in the cytoplasm of certain bacteria. Many other species, e.g. *Escherichia coli*, do not form granules visible with the light microscope but, when grown with abundant carbon- and energy-yielding nutrients, show a diffuse staining of their cytoplasm with the periodic acid-Schiff stain for polysaccharides. In *Esch. coli* this cytoplasmic polysaccharide is glycogen and it is present as minute granules visible as clear areas under the electron microscope.

Mesosomes are intracytoplasmic bodies of unknown function that have been seen with the electron microscope in some ultrathin sections of bacteria. They consist of a convoluted membrane. In some cases the membrane is seen to be derived by invagination from the plasma membrane.

Plasma Membrane (Cytoplasmic Membrane).—The bacterial protoplast is limited externally by a thin, elastic *plasma membrane*, which is 5–10 mμ thick, consists mainly of lipo-protein and is visible in some ultrathin sections examined electron-microscopically. It constitutes an osmotic barrier impermeable to many small molecular solutes and is responsible for maintaining the differences in solute content between the cytoplasm and the external environment. It permits the passive diffusion inwards and outwards of water and certain other small molecular substances, especially lipid-soluble ones, and it also effects actively the selective transport of specific nutrient solutes into the cell and that of waste products out of it. In addition to the enzymes, or *permeases*, responsible for the active uptake of nutrients, it contains also many other kinds of enzymes, notably respiratory enzymes and pigments (cytochrome system), certain enzymes of the tricarboxylic acid cycle and, probably, polymerising enzymes that manufacture the substances of the cell wall and extracellular structures. The plasma membrane has little mechanical strength and is supported by the enclosing cell wall to which it normally adheres very closely.

Cell Wall.—The cell wall is the covering layer that encases the protoplast and lies immediately external to the plasma membrane. It is 10–25 mμ thick, strong and relatively rigid, though with some elasticity, and openly porous, being freely permeable to solute molecules smaller than 10,000 in molecular weight and 1 mμ in diameter. It is responsible for supporting the weak plasma membrane against the high internal osmotic pressure of the protoplasm (usually between 5 and 25 atmospheres) and for maintaining the characteristic shape of the bacterium, *e.g.* coccal, bacillary, filamentous or spiral. From a mechanical point of view the cell wall may be likened to the outer cover, and the plasma membrane to the inner tube of the pneumatic tyre of a motor car.

The integrity of the cell wall is essential to the viability of the bacterium. If the wall is weakened or ruptured, the protoplasm swells from osmotic imbibition of water, bursts the weak plasma membrane and escapes. The bacterium thus becomes disintegrated and dies. The process of lethal disintegration and dissolution is termed *lysis*. When the rupture occurs locally in some part of the cell wall and a bubble of protoplasm is extruded there, the process is called *plasmoptysis*.

When intact bacteria, particularly Gram-negative bacteria, are placed in a solution of very high solute concentration and osmotic pressure, water may be withdrawn osmotically from the protoplast to the extent that this shrinks, detaching and retracting the plasma membrane from the cell wall. This process is called *plasmolysis*. A similar process takes place when bacteria are dried, as in preparing a dry film on a microscope slide. Plasmolysis may be reversible or it may be lethal.

The cell wall plays an important part in *cell division*. A transverse partition of cell wall material grows inwards, like a closing iris diaphragm, from the lateral wall at the equator of the cell and forms a complete *cross wall* separating two daughter cells. Splitting of the cross wall occurs immediately or at some time after its formation and results in liberation of the daughter cells. In cases where bacteria grow firmly attached together in clusters (*e.g.* staphylococci), pairs (*e.g.* pneumococci), chains (*e.g.* streptococci) or rods and filaments (e.g. *Bacillus anthracis*), the attachment depends on the cell walls remaining in continuity, *i.e.* without splitting of cross walls, for the duration of several generations after cell division.

The cell wall is not seen in conventionally stained smears examined with the light microscope; it generally remains unstained and lies, invisible, outside the stained shrunken bacterial protoplast. It can be demonstrated by special staining methods but most readily and clearly by electron microscopy; it is seen both in ultrathin sections and, as an empty fold surrounding the shrunken protoplast, in whole-cell preparations shadowcast with heavy metal.

The chemical composition of the cell wall (Salton, 1960; Strominger, 1962) differs considerably between different bacterial species, but in all species the main strengthening component (the "basal structure") is a *mucopeptide* (glycopeptide) substance. The mucopeptide is composed of acetylglucosamine and acetylmuramic acid molecules linked alternately in a chain, the acetylmuramic acid molecules each carrying a short peptide side-chain containing D- and L-alanine, D-glutamic acid and either L-lysine or diaminopimelic acid. The wall also contains some other components (collectively called the "special structure") whose nature and amount vary with the species and whose role is unknown. In Gram-positive bacteria the special structure is generally simple and minor in amount; *e.g.* in *Staphylococcus aureus* it consists of teichoic acid (ribitol phosphate polymer) and glycine, and makes up only about 20 per cent. of the weight of the wall. In Gram-negative bacteria it is complex and large in amount, *e.g.* in *Escherichia coli* it comprises lipid, polysaccharide, protein and lipopolysaccharide (endotoxin) and makes up over 80 per cent. of the wall weight.

The presence of a muramic acid-containing mucopeptide has recently been demonstrated in rickettsiae and "viruses" of the psittacosis group, and this is taken to indicate that these organisms are phylogenetically related to the bacteria rather than to true viruses, in which muramic acid has not been found.

The cell wall, and in particular its basal mucopeptide component, is the target of the action of a variety of antibiotics and other antibacterial agents. Penicillin, bacitracin, novobiocin, oxamycin (D-cycloserine) and gentian violet are known to interfere with particular stages in the manufacture of the mucopeptide, and bacteria growing in their presence form defective cell walls (and cross walls) and, as a result, undergo lysis and die. The body defence substance, *lysozyme*, which lyses bacteria of many species, dissolves the mucopeptide by cleaving the acetylglucosamine from the acetylmuramic acid molecules. Bacteriophages possess a lysozyme-like enzyme that effects their initial penetration into the bacterium and, after they have reproduced, causes lysis of the bacterium.

It should be noted, moreover, that bacteria themselves possess enzymes, called *autolysins*, able to hydrolyse their own cell-wall substances. Under some unfavourable physiological conditions the autolysins may act to bring about massive lysis, but normally their action is kept in check and is probably confined to the minor removal of wall substance necessary for remodelling of the cell wall in the course of growth.

Weakening, removal or defective formation of the cell wall is involved in the production of the abnormal forms called *spheroplasts*, *free protoplasts*, *pleomorphic involution forms* and *L-forms* (see below).

Capsules, Microcapsules and Loose Slime.—Many bacteria are surrounded by a discrete covering layer of a relatively firm gelatinous material that lies outside and immediately in contact with the cell wall. When this layer, in the wet state, is wide enough (0·2 μ, or more) to be resolved with the light microscope, it is called a *capsule*. When it is narrower, and detectable only by indirect, serological means, or by electron microscopy, it may be termed a *microcapsule* (Wilkinson, 1958). The capsular gel consists largely of water and has only a small content (*e.g.* 2 per cent.) of solids. In most species, the solid material is a complex polysaccharide, though in some species its main constituent is polypeptide or protein.

Loose slime, or *free slime*, is an amorphous, viscid colloidal material that is secreted extracellularly by some non-capsulate bacteria and also, outside their capsules, by many capsulate bacteria. In capsulate bacteria the slime is generally similar in chemical composition and antigenic character to the capsular substance. When slime-forming bacteria are grown on a solid culture medium, the slime remains around the bacteria as a matrix in which they are embedded and its presence confers on the growths a watery and sticky, "mucoid" character. The slime is freely soluble in water and, when the bacteria are grown or suspended in a liquid medium, it passes away from them and disperses through the medium.

Demonstration.—Capsules and slime have little affinity for basic dyes and are usually invisible in films stained by ordinary methods, *e.g.* Gram's and Leishman's. Capsules are most likely to be visualised by these stains, as either clear or coloured haloes, when the bacteria are contained in blood, pus or serous fluid. Special methods are available for the "positive" or "negative" staining of capsules, some being applied to dry, and some to wet films. Since capsules consist largely of water, they shrink very greatly on drying. For this reason, dry-film methods of demonstrating capsules are unreliable; the capsules may shrink so much that they become invisible or, on the other hand, shrinkage artefacts may give the appearance of capsules on non-capsulate bacteria. The most reliable method of demonstration is by "negative" staining in wet films with India ink; the carbon particles of the ink make a dark background in the film, but cannot penetrate the capsule, which thus appears as a clear halo around the bacterium. When bacteria that have been grown on solid medium are being examined for capsules, it is important that they should first be washed or suspended for a sufficient time in water to ensure the removal of any loose slime. Loose slime can be observed when films are made directly from the solid medium.

Because of their low solid content and tendency to shrink greatly on drying, capsules and microcapsules are not easily demonstrated with the electron microscope. A large capsule is commonly seen only as an indefinite narrow zone of slight opacity that blurs the otherwise clear-cut edge of the cell wall. Microcapsules may not be seen at all and for this reason the presence of microcapsules has generally to be deduced from serological evidence that the cell-wall antigen (*e.g.* the O, or somatic antigen in enterobacteriaceae) is masked by a covering layer (*e.g.* of K, or "capsular" antigen).

In attempting to demonstrate capsules it should be remembered that their development is often dependent on the existence of favourable environmental conditions. Thus, their size may vary with the amount of carbohydrate in the culture medium available for nutrition of the bacteria. In the later stages of growth in artificial culture (*e.g.* 12–24 hr.) they may become reduced in size due to carbon and energy starvation or they may disappear due to the accumulation in the medium of capsule-degrading enzymes (*e.g.* hyaluronidase in the case of *Streptococcus pyogenes*).

Function.—Little definite is known about the functions of capsules and microcapsules, but it is probable that their principal action is in protecting the cell wall against attack by various kinds of antibacterial agents, *e.g.* bacteriophages, colicines, lysozyme and other lytic enzymes, that otherwise would more readily damage or destroy it. In the case of certain capsulate pathogenic organisms (*e.g.* pneumococcus, pyogenic streptococci, anthrax bacillus and plague bacillus) good evidence has been obtained to show that the capsule protects the bacteria against ingestion by the phagocytes of the host. The capsule is thus an important agent determining virulence and non-capsulate mutants of these bacteria are found to be non-virulent. In some organisms the capsule contains more than one functional component. Thus, *Streptococcus pyogenes*, which under favourable conditions of growth forms an anti-phagocytic capsule composed of hyaluronic acid, usually possesses also a second surface substance, M protein, which inhibits either the ingestion or the intracellular digestion of the cocci by the phagocytes; the M protein occurs in association with the hyaluronic acid capsule or, when the latter is absent, by itself in the form of a microcapsule. In *Bacillus anthracis* the capsule (polymer of D-glutamic acid) protects the bacteria not only against phagocytosis but also, to some extent, against the action of a bactericidal basic polypeptide present in animal tissues.

The capsular substance is usually antigenic (see below) and the capsular antigens play a very important part in determining the immunological specificity of bacteria.

Flagella and Motility.—Motile strains of bacteria possess filamentous appendages known as *flagella*, which effect screw-like propulsive movements and act as organs of locomotion. The flagellum is a long, thin filament, twisted spirally in an open, regular wave-form. It is about 0·02 μ thick and is usually several times the length of the bacterial cell. It originates in the bacterial protoplasm and is extruded through the cell wall. According to the species, there may be one or several (*e.g.* 1–20) flagella per cell, and in elongated bacteria the arrangement of the flagella may be *peritrichous*, or *lateral*, when they originate from the sides of the cell, or *polar*, when they originate from one or both ends. Where several occur on a cell, they may function coiled together as a single "tail". Flagella consist largely or entirely of a protein, *flagellin*, belonging to the same chemical group as myosin, the contractile protein of muscle. They can be demonstrated easily and clearly with the electron microscope, particularly in metal-shadowed preparations or preparations "negatively" stained with phosphotungstic acid (PTA), usually appearing as simple fibrils without internal differentiation. In some PTA preparations the flagellum appears as a hollow tube formed of helically twisted fibrils, and the flagella of some bacteria, *e.g.* vibrios, have an outer sheath; but bacterial flagella do not have the complex structure of the flagella and cilia of plants and animals, which in all cases consist of two central and nine peripheral fibrils contained in a tube-like sheath. They are invisible in ordinary preparations by the light microscope, but may be shown by the use of special staining methods that involve mordanting and deposition of stain, and in special circumstances by dark-ground illumination. Because of the difficulties of these methods, the presence of flagella is commonly inferred from the observation of motility.

Motility may be observed either microscopically or by noting the occurrence of spreading growth in semi-solid agar medium. On microscopic observation of wet films, motile bacteria are seen swimming in different directions across the field, with a darting, wriggling or tumbling movement. True motility must be distinguished from a drifting of the bacteria in a single direction due to a current in the liquid, and also from Brownian movement, which is a rapid oscillation of each bacterium within a very limited area due to bombardment by the water molecules.

Among the spirochaetes, motility appears to be a function of the cell body, since flagella do not occur. The most characteristic movement is a fast spiral rotation on the long axis with slow progression in the axial line; movements of flexion and lashing movements may be observed. Some spirochaetes possess an axial filament and others a band of fibrils wound around their surface from pole to pole. It has been suggested that these structures may contribute to motility, either through being themselves contractile or by acting as stiffeners for recoil against the contractile protoplast.

Function.—It is not known with certainty what advantage a bacterium derives from its capability of active locomotion. Motility may be beneficial in increasing the rate of uptake of nutrient solutes by continuously changing the environmental fluid in contact with the bacterial cell surface. Random movement and dispersion through the environment may be beneficial in ensuring that at least some cells of a strain reach every locality suitable for colonisation. There is, moreover, good evidence that the movement of many bacteria is *directed* by tactic responses of the organism towards localities favourable to growth and away from unfavourable regions. Thus, bacteria tend to migrate towards regions where there is a higher concentration of nutrient solutes and away from regions containing higher concentrations of disinfectant substances. Motile aerobic bacteria show positive aerotaxis and migrate towards regions where there is a higher concentration of dissolved oxygen; anaerobes migrate away from such regions.

It may be supposed that the power of active locomotion will assist pathogenic bacteria in penetrating through viscid mucous secretions and epithelial barriers, and in spreading throughout the body fluids and tissues, but it must be noted that many non-motile pathogens (*e.g.* brucellae and streptococci) are not any less invasive than motile ones.

Fimbriae.—Certain Gram-negative bacilli, including saprophytic, intestinal commensal and pathogenic species in the family *Enterobacteriaceae*, possess filamentous appendages of a different kind from the flagella. These are called *fimbriae*, and they occur in some non-motile, as well as in some motile strains. They are far more numerous than flagella (*e.g.* 100–500 being borne peritrichously by each cell) and are much shorter and only about half as thick (*e.g.* varying from 0·1 to 1·5 μ in length and having a uniform width between 4 and 8 mμ). They do not have the smoothly curved spiral form of flagella and are mostly more or less straight. They cannot be seen with the light microscope but are clearly seen with the electron microscope in metal-shadowed preparations and preparations negatively stained with phosphotungstic acid.

Most potentially (*i.e.* genetically) fimbriate strains of bacteria readily undergo a reversible variation between a fimbriate phase and a non-fimbriate phase and this variation is affected by the conditions of growth. The fimbriate phase becomes predominant, and the majority of bacilli in the culture fimbriate, as a result of prolonged culture or serial (48 hourly) subculture, in static liquid medium incubated aerobically. The non-fimbriate phase predominates and cultures consist entirely or almost entirely of non-fimbriate bacilli when growth is carried serially on a solid culture medium.

Function.—There is evidence that fimbriae may function as organs of adhesion. The possession of fimbriae confers on bacilli the power of adhering firmly to solid surfaces of various kinds, including those of the cells of animals, plants and fungi. Comparable non-fimbriate bacilli do not adhere when they collide with such surfaces. The adhesive property may be of value to the bacteria in holding them in nutritionally favourable micro-environments. Moreover, bacteria growing in stagnant liquid medium under air are assisted by the possession of fimbriae to grow attached together in the form of a *pellicle* that floats on the surface of the medium where the growth is greatly enhanced by the free supply of atmospheric oxygen.

Haemagglutination.—The majority of fimbriate bacteria bear fimbriae of a type that enables them to adhere to, among other kinds of tissue cells, the red blood cells of many animal species (*e.g.* to guinea-pig, fowl, horse and pig red cells very strongly, to human cells moderately strongly, to sheep cells weakly and to ox cells scarcely at all). If a drop of a concentrated suspension of fimbriate bacilli is mixed for a few minutes with a drop of a suspension of red cells, preferably guinea-pig red cells, the adhering bacilli bind the red cells together in clumps visible to the naked eye. A simple haemagglutination test can thus be used to determine whether a culture contains fimbriate bacilli.

There exist different kinds of fimbriae having different adhesive properties. The commonest kind (*e.g.* in escherichia, salmonella and shigella organisms) is about 8 mμ in width, and it may be recognised by the observation that its adhesive and haemagglutinating actions are completely and specifically inhibited by the addition of a small amount (0·1–0·5 per cent.) of D-mannose to the test mixture (*i.e.* its activities are mannose-sensitive). In addition to, or instead of such fimbriae, some klebsiella and serratia organisms possess "thin" fimbriae, about 5 mμ in width; these do not agglutinate red cells unless the cells are first heated or tanned, and their adhesive properties are unaffected by mannose. Proteus organisms possess a third kind of fimbriae, which have mannose-resistant haemagglutinating activity against untreated red cells of certain species. A few salmonella organisms (e.g. *S. gallinarum* and *S. pullorum*) possess a fourth kind of fimbrae, apparently devoid of all haemagglutinating and adhesive properties. It should be noted also that some bacteria, *e.g.* a minority of strains of *Esch. coli*, possess haemagglutinating factors (mannose-resistant) that are not associated with fimbriae.

For further information see Duguid and Gillies (1957) and Duguid, Anderson and Campbell (1966).

Bacterial Reproduction.—Among the "lower" or true bacteria, multiplication takes place by *simple binary fission*. The cell grows in size, usually elongating to twice its original length, and the protoplasm becomes divided into two approximately equal parts by the ingrowth of a transverse septum from the plasma membrane and cell wall. In some species, the cell wall septum, or cross wall, splits in two and the daughter cells separate almost immediately. In others, the cell walls of the daughter cells remain continuous for some time after cell division and the organisms grow adhering in pairs, clusters, chains or filaments. If cross wall splitting is thus delayed in an organism in which the cross walls of successive cell divisions are all formed in parallel planes, the cells will be grouped in pairs, chains, rods or filaments. If it is delayed in an organism which forms successive cross walls in different planes, *e.g.* ones at right angles to each other, the cells will be grouped in pairs and either cubical or irregular clusters. Under favourable conditions, growth and division are repeated with great rapidity, *e.g.* every half-hour, so that one individual may reproduce thousands of millions of new organisms in less than a day. *E.g.* a bacterium dividing in two every 20 min. multiplies about 1,000,000,000-fold in 10 hr. Among the spirochaetes, transverse fission occurs as in other bacteria.

In the "higher" or mycelial bacteria, growth takes place by extension of the vegetative filaments, and multiplication by transverse division of these into shorter forms, or by the liberation of numerous conidia (*vide supra*) which later germinate and give rise to fresh mycelia.

Some observers have described more complex processes of reproduction among bacteria and postulated life cycles comprising different morphological phases. In many cases, however, the forms presumed to be "intermediate phases" have in fact been degenerate involution cells, and the evidence at present available does not warrant acceptance of such views. Sexual reproduction does not occur commonly in bacteria, but genetical evidence has been obtained that, in a few varieties, the conjugation of two individual cells and genetic recombination may rarely occur.

Bacterial Spores.—Some species, particularly those of the genera *Bacillus* and *Clostridium*, develop a highly resistant resting-phase, or *endospore*, whereby the organism can survive in a dormant state through a long period of starvation or other adverse environmental condition. The process does not involve multiplication: in *sporulation*, each vegetative cell forms only one spore, and in subsequent *germination* each spore gives rise to a single vegetative cell.

Sporulation.—Although it has been suggested that spores are formed spontaneously, as an intermediate stage in a bacterial life cycle, it seems more likely that sporulation occurs as a response to starvation. It does not take place as long as conditions continue to favour maximal vegetative growth, but occurs when growth is being arrested, as in the later stages of artificial culture. In certain species, sporulation can be induced by depletion of the supply of one of the nutrients necessary for vegetative growth, *e.g.* the carbon and energy source, the nitrogen source, sulphate, phosphate or iron salt: at the same time, the process requires a continued supply of other minerals (K, Mg, Mn and Ca salts) and favourable conditions of moisture, temperature, pH, oxygen tension, etc. The spore is formed inside the parent vegetative cell (hence the name "endospore"). It develops from a portion of protoplasm near one end of the cell (the "forespore"), incorporates part of the nuclear material of the cell and acquires a thick covering layer, the "cortex", and a thin, but tough, outer "spore coat" consisting of several layers. The appearance of the mature spore varies according to the species, being spherical, ovoid or elongated, occupying a terminal, subterminal or central position, and being narrower than the cell, or broader and bulging it. Finally, the remainder of the parent cell disintegrates and the spore is freed.

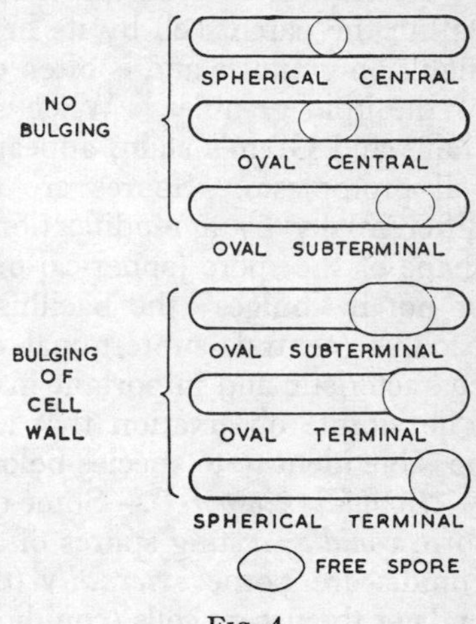

FIG. 4
The shape and situation of spores in the bacterial cell.

Viability.—Spores are much more resistant than the vegetative forms to injurious chemical and physical influences, including exposure to disinfectants, drying and heating. Thus, their killing requires application of moist heat at 100°–120° C. for a period (*e.g.* 10 min.) although heating at 60° C. would suffice to kill the vegetative cells. Spores may remain viable for many years, either when in the dry state or in moist conditions unfavourable to growth, as in absence of nutrients sufficient to maintain the minimal metabolism of the vegetative form. The high resistance of spores has been attributed to several factors in which they differ from vegetative cells: the impermeability of their cortex and outer coat, their high content of calcium and dipicolinic acid, their low content of water (maybe 5–20 per cent.), and their very low metabolic and enzymatic activity.

Germination of the spore occurs when the external conditions become favourable to growth by access to moisture and nutrients, in particular to trigger nutrients such as L-alanine, inosine or glucose in certain *Bacillus* species. Spores that have survived exposure to severe adverse influences such as heat are found to be much more exacting than normal spores in their requirements for germination. For this reason, specially enriched culture media are used when testing the sterility of materials, such as surgical catgut, which have been exposed to disinfecting procedures. In the process of germination, the spore swells, its cortex disintegrates, its coat is broken open and a single vegetative cell emerges.

Demonstration.—In unstained preparations the spore is recognised within the parent cell by its higher refractility. It is larger than lipid inclusion granules and is often ovoid, in contrast to the spherical shape of the lipid granules. When mature it resists colouration by simple stains and Gram's stain, appearing as a clear space within the stained cell protoplasm. Spores are slightly acid-fast and may be stained differentially by a modification of the Ziehl-Neelsen method. The shape of the spore (spherical or ovoid), its size, as judged by whether or not it "bulges" the bacillus containing it, and its position in the bacillus (central, subterminal or terminal) are features that may be characteristic and important in the identification of a bacterial species. The simple observation that a bacterium is a *spore-former* limits its possible identity to species belonging to a very few genera.

Conidia (*exospores*).—Some of the mycelial bacteria (*Actinomycetales*) form *conidia*, resting spores of a kind different from endospores. The conidia are borne *externally* (extracellularly) by abstriction from the ends of the parent cells (conidiophores) and are disseminated by the air or other means to fresh habitats. They are not specially resistant to heat and disinfectants.

Pleomorphism and Involution.—In the course of growth, bacteria of a single strain may show considerable variation in size and shape, forming a proportion of cells that differ grossly from the normal, *e.g.* swollen, spherical and pear-shaped forms, elongated filaments and filaments with localised swellings. This pleomorphism occurs most readily in certain species (e.g. *Streptobacillus moniliformis*, *Pasteurella pestis*), in ageing cultures on artificial medium and, especially, in the presence of antagonistic substances such as penicillin, glycine, lithium, chloride, sodium chloride in high concentrations, and organic acids at low pH. The abnormal cells are generally regarded as degeneration or *involution* forms; some are non-viable, whilst others may grow and revert to the normal form when transferred to a suitable environment. In many cases the abnormal shape seems to be the result of defective cell-wall synthesis; the growing protoplasm expands the weakened wall to produce a grotesquely swollen cell comparable to a spheroplast (see below), which later usually bursts and lyses.

Spheroplasts and Free Protoplasts.—If bacteria have their cell walls removed or weakened while they are held in a medium of high enough solute content (*e.g.* 0·2–1·0 M sucrose with 0·01 M Mg^{++}) to prevent them imbibing water by osmosis, they may escape being lysed and, instead, may become converted into viable spherical bodies. If all the cell-wall material has been removed from them, the spheres are *free protoplasts*. If they remain enclosed by an intact, but weakened residual cell wall, they are called *spheroplasts*. Protoplasts, for example, are readily liberated from the Gram-positive bacillus, *Bacillus mega-*

terium, by dissolution of the cell walls with egg-white lysozyme. Spheroplasts are readily produced from Gram-negative bacilli such as *Escherichia coli* by growing the organism in the presence of a substance, *e.g.* penicillin, bacitracin, oxymycin or glycine, that specifically inhibits synthesis of the mucopeptide component of the cell wall. A similar result may be obtained by culturing certain bacteria on medium lacking a nutrient, *e.g.* diaminopimelic acid, lysine or hexosamine derivative, that they require specifically for cell-wall synthesis.

Protoplasts and spheroplasts are osmotically sensitive; they vary in size with the osmotic pressure of the suspending medium and if the medium is much diluted, *e.g.* until isotonic with body fluids, they swell up, burst and perish by lysis. If maintained in an osmotically protective nutrient medium, they remain viable and continue to metabolise, synthesise and grow. Protoplasts enlarge but do not multiply. Spheroplasts, when kept on an osmotically protective agar medium containing a cell wall inhibitor such as penicillin, may multiply by fission or budding and reproduce through many serial subcultures. The spheroplasts of Gram-negative bacilli, because they retain a residual wall structure, are not as osmotically sensitive as free protoplasts and are often capable of growing on an ordinary agar culture medium. Protoplasts have not been found capable of re-forming their cell walls and reverting to normal bacterial morphology, but spheroplasts commonly revert *en masse* when transferred to culture medium lacking the cell wall inhibitor. Spheroplast cultures have sometimes been called "unstable L-forms" on account of their resemblance in colonial and cellular morphology to the stable L-forms of bacteria (see below).

L-forms of bacteria.—These are abnormal growth forms derived by variation, usually in the laboratory, from bacteria of normal morphology, *e.g.* cocci, bacilli or vibrios. They differ from the parent bacteria in lacking a rigid cell wall and, in consequence, regular size and shape, but they are nevertheless viable and capable of growing and multiplying through an indefinite series of cultures on a suitable artificial nutrient medium. They are soft protoplasmic bodies, generally spherical or disc-like, but also extremely variable in shape, and they range in size from minute bodies about 0·1 μ in diameter to large ones of 10–20 μ. The smallest *viable* forms are about 0·3 μ in diameter and can occasionally pass through bacteria-stopping filters. Some L-forms may be entirely devoid of a cell wall, and others, like spheroplasts, possess an intact cell wall that is weakened by absence of a strengthening component (mucopeptide).

Colonies of L-form organisms on agar media are small and have a characteristic 'fried egg' appearance; they have a dark, thick centre, where many of the organisms embed themselves and grow within the agar, and a lighter peripheral zone with a lace-like texture consisting of organisms lying on the surface of the agar together with oily excretory droplets (probably containing cholesterol). In liquid media, growth is usually in the form of clumps. Because of their fragility, microscopical examination of L-forms is best done while they are *in situ* on the agar medium, a coverslip being applied to a block of agar bearing the growth. If desired, the organisms can be stained after fixation by a fixative that is allowed to diffuse through the agar.

Origin.—Some bacteria, e.g. *Streptobacillus moniliformis* and *Bacteroides* spp. give rise spontaneously to L-forms even when grown in an optimal culture medium. In many other species, L-form growth may be induced by culture in the presence of an inhibitor of cell wall synthesis, such as penicillin, or by deprivation of a nutrient essential for cell wall synthesis, *e.g.* diaminopimelic acid, or by destruction of the cell wall with antibody and complement.

Maintenance.—Though L-forms of some species may be grown on ordinary culture media, even in liquid medium, generally a special medium must be used: *e.g.* a soft agar medium containing meat infusion and 20 per cent. horse serum. Agar apparently gives mechanical support to L-bodies embedding themselves and multiplying by lobulation within it. Some L-forms require a medium with a large content of sucrose or sodium chloride for osmotic protection, as described for the maintenance of spheroplasts.

Reversion to the bacterial form.—True, or stable L-forms, even if their origin was induced by exposure to penicillin or other cell-wall inhibitor, continue to reproduce as L-forms through repeated subcultures in the absence of cell-wall inhibitor, and do not give rise to revertants of normal bacterial morphology. Unstable L-forms, *e.g.* growths of penicillin-induced spheroplasts, generally revert *en masse* to the normal bacterial form within a few hours of culture in the absence of the inducing agent. Transitional L-forms give rise occasionally to small numbers of bacterial revertants.

Role.—Although they have many resemblances to the pathogenic mycoplasma organisms, L-forms should probably be regarded as laboratory artefacts, degenerate growths that do not occur or survive to any important extent in natural habitats. They are non-pathogenic to laboratory animals.

REFERENCES

Duguid, J. P. & Gillies, R. R. (1957). Fimbriae and adhesive properties in dysentery bacilli. *J. Path. Bact.*, **74**, 397.

Duguid, J. P., Anderson, E. S. & Campbell, I. (1966). Fimbrial and adhesive properties in salmonellae. *J. Path. Bact.*, **92**, 107.

Gunsalus, I. C. & Stanier, R. Y. (1960). *The Bacteria*, Vol. I, (Structure). New York: Academic Press.

Lamanna, C. & Mallette, M. F. (1959). *Basic Bacteriology*, 2nd ed., p. 116. Baltimore: Williams & Wilkins.

Salton, M. R. J. (1960). Surface layers of the bacterial cell. In *The Bacteria*, Vol. I, ed. I. C. Gunsalus & R. Y. Stanier, p. 97. New York: Academic Press.

Salton, M. R. J. (1963). The relationship between the nature of the cell wall and the Gram stain. *J. gen. Microbiol.*, **30**, 223.

Spooner, E. T. C. & Stocker, B. A. D. (1956). Bacterial anatomy, *Symposium Soc. gen. Microbiol.*, p. 6, Cambridge.

Stanier, R. Y. & van Niel, C. B. (1962). The concept of a bacterium. *Arch. Mikrobiol.*, **42**, 17.

Strominger, J. L. (1962). Biosynthesis of bacterial cell walls. In *The Bacteria*, Vol. III, ed. I. C. Gunsalus & R. Y. Stanier, p. 413. New York: Academic Press.

Wilkinson, J. F. (1958). The extracellular polysaccharides of bacteria. *Bact. Rev.*, **22**, 46.

Wilkinson, J. F. & Duguid, J. P. (1960). The influence of cultural conditions on bacterial cytology. *Int. Rev. Cytol.*, **9**, 1.

CHAPTER 3

THE GROWTH AND NUTRITION OF BACTERIA

BACTERIA, when inoculated into a suitable medium and incubated under appropriate conditions, grow at a very rapid rate. In this sense, the term "grow" refers to the fact that there is an increase in the number of cells present, in other words, there has been multiplication of cells rather than an increase in size of each bacterium. This is the result of the normal method of division of a "true" bacterium which is by binary fission. It is important to realise how rapid growth may be under favourable circumstances when a cell may double every 20 min. If this rate were maintained for 24 hr., the progeny of a single cell would be about 1×10^{21} cells and would have a mass of approximately four thousand tons. The conditions used for culture never permit such a rate of multiplication for more than a short time, generally because of an insufficiency of food or nutrients.

When a culture of an organism is inoculated into a fresh growth medium, the inoculum used will usually contain a comparatively small number of cells which may multiply by a factor of a million-fold or more during growth. If the number of cells present at different times after inoculation is measured, it is possible to draw a growth curve in which it is usual to plot the logarithm of the number of bacteria against time. Two types of growth curve can be drawn according to the nature of the measurement of cell numbers used. A *total count* will measure the number of cells present irrespective of whether they are living or not. On the other hand, a viable count measures only those cells capable of growing and hence of producing a colony on a suitable solid growth medium. Typical growth curves are shown in Fig. 5. Four main phases of growth can be recognised.

1. **The Lag Phase.**—In this period there is no appreciable multiplication of cells although they may increase considerably in size and show marked metabolic activity. The length of this phase varies according to the condition and number of cells in the inoculum and it can be looked upon as representing the time taken for the organism to adapt itself to growth in the fresh medium. The cells in an inoculum may be so depleted of enzymes, metabolic intermediates, and other factors, that some time is required for these materials to build up to their optimal levels. Alternatively, if the new medium is different in composition to that in which the inoculum was growing previously, entirely new enzymes may require to be synthesised by the process of induction or by the selection of mutants.

2. **The Log or Exponential Phase.**—In this period, the cells divide at a constant rate and, as a result of growth by binary fission, there is a linear relationship between the logarithm of the number of cells and time. Cells in the log phase must have a very high rate of metabolism and, as a result of their adaptation to the maximum rate of synthesis and growth possible, they may be considerably more sensitive

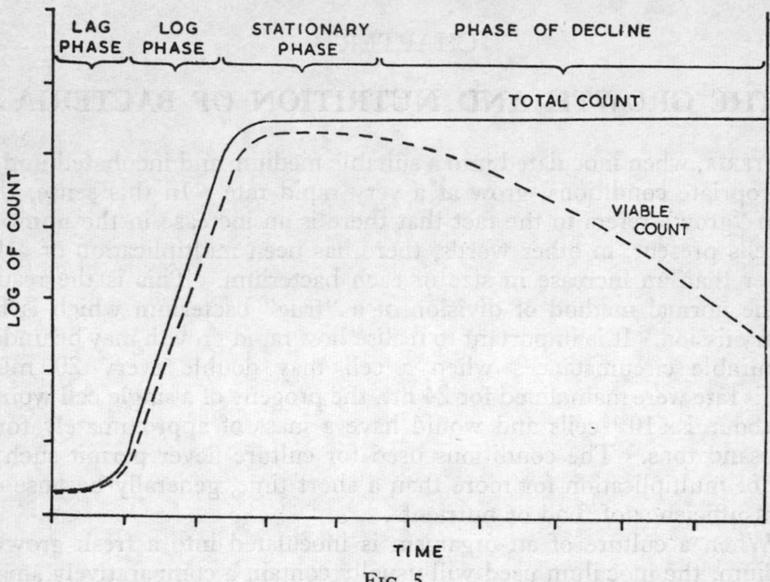

Fig. 5

Continuous line = Total number of bacteria alive and dead.
Interrupted line = Total number of tiring bacteria.

to the effect of antimicrobial agents. The actual rate of growth will be determined by the generation time (the time between divisions) of the bacterium under the particular environmental conditions used. The nature of some of the environmental factors affecting the rate of growth will be considered later.

3. **The Stationary Phase.**—After several hours, there is a decrease in the rate of growth until the number of cells eventually stays constant and the culture passes into the stationary phase. This cessation of growth is most commonly caused by the exhaustion of an essential nutrient in the medium, although another factor may be the accumulation of toxic waste products, *e.g.* acids produced by the fermentation of sugars.

4. **The Death or Decline Phase.**—After a variable period of time in the stationary phase, the cells in a culture begin to die—that is they become incapable of growth when transferred to a fresh medium. This can be seen in Fig. 5 as an increasing divergence between the total count of living and dead cells and the viable count of living cells only. The causes of this death or loss of viability are various, the main determinant being the factor causing the cessation of growth in the stationary phase. If this cause is the accumulation of toxic products, there may be a very small stationary phase followed by rapid death. In some cases, there may be a rapid fall in the total count as well as the viable count. The reason for this is that some microorganisms are very prone to digest themselves so that they eventually lyse liberating their cytoplasmic contents into the environment; this process is known as autolysis. Another common occurrence in this phase of growth is the

appearance of bizarre cell shapes together with a change of staining characteristics. For example, cells in the stationary phase and decline phase often change from Gram-positive to Gram-negative.

Growth of the type discussed above, in which an inoculum is placed in a culture vessel, is known as *batch culture* and is the usual method of growing bacteria in the laboratory. However, it is possible to use an "open" system in which there is a continuous supply of fresh nutrients into the culture vessel and a continuous removal of grown bacteria by means of a constant level device. This method of culture—called *continuous culture*—has been used recently for research and industrial purposes and it may correspond more truly with the situation occurring in some diseases of man and animals.

In order to identify and study a bacterial species, it is necessary to grow the organism under laboratory conditions and it is therefore essential to know its growth requirements. Two conditions must be fulfilled: (i) Suitable nutrients must be supplied: (ii) The physical conditions must be as near optimum as possible for the organism under consideration.

Bacteria differ widely in the nutritional requirements and the physical conditions needed for growth, and it is therefore of great importance to understand these factors.

BACTERIAL NUTRITION

The growth of bacteria is dependent on an adequate supply of suitable food materials, the specific nutrient requirements varying in the different species according to their natural environmental adaptations. Some species are able to grow under a wide range of conditions, but others, especially the more strictly parasitic (*e.g.* gonococcus) are very exacting and restricted in their requirements. Whilst it is hardly possible to reproduce exactly the natural environmental conditions of pathogenic bacteria, suitable artificial culture media have been devised for the great majority.

The chemical composition of all bacteria is essentially similar, the principal components being as follows:—

1. High molecular weight organic compounds, usually polymers, such as proteins, nucleic acids, polysaccharides and lipids. These make up at least 80 per cent. of the dry weight of bacteria.

2. Low molecular weight organic compounds such as coenzymes, prosthetic groups and intermediary metabolites. These make up about 10 per cent. of the dry weight of bacteria.

3. Inorganic compounds such as water and mineral salts.

The study of comparative biochemistry has shown how similar living organisms are in their component chemical units as well as in the mechanisms by which these components are formed—the process of metabolism. This concept is generally referred to as "The Unity of Biochemistry". Thus the nucleotide and amino acid components of nucleic acids and proteins are the same in bacteria as in mammals or higher plants, and their synthetic pathways are usually very similar. It is evident that nutrients must be provided in the medium for the synthesis of the components outlined above, and that they must therefore provide both the structural units required as well as energy for the formation and polymerisation of these structural units, for the maintenance of membrane equilibria, for motility and for other energy-requiring processes in the cell. In view of the similarity of the chemical components of all microorganisms, the different nutrient requirements that are found must reflect different synthetic abilities. The transformation of simple nutrients into the complex constituents of bacteria involves the formation in stages of various intermediate substances of increasing chemical complexity, each stage in the synthesis being catalysed by an appropriate enzyme. Any interference with an intermediate metabolite or with its associated enzyme will inhibit growth by preventing the metabolite from being used for further synthesis.

It is by such interferences that many antiseptics, chemotherapeutic drugs and antibiotics bring about the inhibition of growth or killing of the organism. For example, the sulphonamide series of drugs act by preventing the conversion of the growth factor *p*-aminobenzoic acid into a coenzyme form related to folic acid which is required for essential synthetic reactions within the cell, and in the absence of this coenzyme the cell dies. It soon became evident that *p*-aminobenzoic acid and the sulphonamide nucleus have a very similar chemical structure and compete for the same site on the enzyme responsible for the further metabolism of *p*-aminobenzoic acid—a process known as *competitive inhibition.* It has been possible to produce many antimicrobial drugs by preparing chemical analogues of other essential growth factors although unfortunately few of these have had much practical value in the treatment of infections. However, it is probable that many antimicrobial drugs act in this way and much research is being done to identify the sites of this action. It is known that penicillin inhibits the final transpeptidation in the synthesis of the mucopeptide of the bacterial cell wall, but the nature of the inhibition is uncertain.

If we consider the basic elements making up the chemical components of a living organism, it is evident that the main elements required for growth are carbon, hydrogen, oxygen and nitrogen, with sulphur and phosphorus being required in somewhat smaller amounts and other elements such as sodium, potassium, magnesium, iron and manganese in considerably smaller amounts. Since hydrogen and oxygen can be supplied in the water essential for any growth, it is evident that carbon and nitrogen are the main bulk elements required.

The Carbon Source for Growth.—Some non-parasitic bacteria are able, like the plants, to utilise carbon dioxide as the main source of carbon and are called autotrophs (or lithotrophs). Energy is obtained in these organisms by the oxidation of inorganic compounds (chemosynthetic autotrophs) or from sunlight (photosynthetic autotrophs). The majority of bacteria, however, including all the parasitic species, require organic nutrients such as carbohydrates, amino acids, peptides or lipids to serve as the sources of carbon and energy. These organisms are called heterotrophs (or organotrophs), and they obtain their energy by the breakdown of the organic carbon source or sources. They differ widely in the range of organic compounds that can be used. Thus some bacteria are remarkably versatile as evidenced by the fact that some species of the genus *Pseudomonas* can utilise any one of over a hundred organic compounds (sugars, acids, alcohols, etc.) as the sole source of carbon and energy. On the other hand, many bacteria are much more specific in their requirement.

The Nitrogen Source of Growth.—Bacteria differ widely in the nature of their requirement for nitrogen, reflecting differences in their ability to synthesise the main nitrogenous structural units—amino acids and nucleotides. Thus some are able to grow on an ammonium salt as the sole source of nitrogen, while others require a variety of amino acids and nucleotides preformed in the medium.

The Requirement for Growth Factors.—As mentioned previously, essential metabolites such as coenzymes and prosthetic groups are required by all bacteria. They must be synthesised by the cell or be provided, at least in a simplified form, in the growth medium. If required as nutrients, these substances are called "growth factors" or "bacterial vitamins" and they are usually only needed in very small amounts, their function being catalytic rather than structural. They are diverse substances with regard to their chemical nature and in many cases they are identical with the vitamins required for mammalian nutrition (*e.g.* thiamine, riboflavine, nicotinic acid, pyridoxine, *p*-aminobenzoic acid, folic acid, biotin, cobamide, etc.).

Under appropriate conditions in synthetic media, the amount of bacterial growth is linearly proportional to the concentration of a growth factor, essential amino acid or nucleotide whose supply is deficient in relation to other nutrients. This is the principle of microbiological assay, wherein the amount of a growth factor, amino acid, or nucleotide is measured according to the amount of the growth that it supports, *e.g.* assay of cobamide (vitamin B_{12}) using *Lactobacillus leichmanii.* The method has the advantage of specificity and high sensitivity. In the case of vitamins it is possible to determine as little as 0·001 μg. per ml., and in some cases (*e.g.* biotin, cobamide) considerably less.

Inorganic Salts for Growth.—Bacteria require a supply of inorganic salts for growth, particularly phosphate and sulphate among the anions and sodium, potassium, magnesium, iron, manganese and calcium among the cations.

Nutritional Evolution

It has been shown that bacteria differ widely in their requirements for amino acids, nucleotides and growth factors and therefore in their synthetic capacities. Some, especially among the non-parasitic species, have comprehensive synthetic abilities and are therefore *non-exacting* nutritionally; they are able to synthesise all their structural units from the carbon and energy source and inorganic salts. For example, *Escherichia coli* can grow on a "simple synthetic medium" which contains only glucose (carbon and energy source), ammonium sulphate (nitrogen and sulphur source), phosphate buffer, potassium chloride, magnesium chloride and traces of other inorganic salts; alternatively, an amino acid such as alanine might serve as the combined source of carbon, energy and nitrogen. Other bacteria, in the course of evolution towards a strictly parasitic mode of life, have increasingly obtained their amino acids, nucleotides and growth factors from the tissues of their host, and have lost the power of synthesising these compounds. Many species are thus nutritionally exacting (e.g. *Streptococcus pyogenes*) and can grow in a synthetic medium only if it contains a wide range of different amino acids, nucleotides and growth factors. This process of nutritional evolution to increasing dependence upon nutrients in the environment can be paralleled in the laboratory by the selection of mutants. An enzyme catalysing a step in the synthesis of an amino acid, nucleotide or growth factor, may be lost as a result of gene mutation (p. 94) and the variant strain thus becomes nutritionally exacting in respect of the substance which the parent strain can synthesise for itself.

THE PHYSICAL CONDITIONS REQUIRED FOR GROWTH

As stated previously, bacterial growth can be extremely rapid. If a cell can double its size and divide within 30 minutes, it must therefore be capable of synthesising its own weight of cell material within this period. In order to do this, it must have a very rapid rate of metabolism together with a correspondingly rapid uptake of nutrients and disposal of waste products. It can do this only on account of its small size, which gives it a very large surface for absorption and excretion in relation to its volume. But the very rapid growth that can occur in the log phase is possible only under certain restricted environmental conditions: it is most important to understand these thoroughly.

The Influence of Oxygen and Redox Potential

The majority of bacteria are described as *facultative anaerobes* because they are able to grow either aerobically, *i.e.* in the presence of air and free oxygen, or anaerobically, in its absence. Certain other species will grow only in the presence of air or free oxygen, and are described as *strict* or *obligate aerobes*. Still others will grow only in the absence of free oxygen and are usually killed in its presence; these are known as *strict anaerobes*. In the latter case, the ultimate determining factor is the state of oxidation of the environment, this being best described in terms of the oxidation-reduction, or "redox" potential. A sufficiently low redox potential for the growth of strict anaerobes is usually provided by placing the culture medium in an atmosphere of hydrogen, with the complete exclusion of free oxygen (*e.g.* in a McIntosh and Fildes anaerobic jar). It has been suggested that in the presence of oxygen a strict anaerobe is liable to produce toxic peroxides which it cannot destroy owing to lack of catalase, an enzyme present in most aerobes and facultative anaerobes. Finally, there is a group of organisms which grow best in the presence of a trace only of free oxygen and often prefer an increased concentration of carbon dioxide; these are called *microaerophilic.*

The natural environment of a bacterium is determined by its oxygen and redox potential requirements. Thus, a strict aerobe like the tubercle bacillus will grow best in a well-aerated environment such as the animal lung, and a strict anaerobe like *Clostridium welchii* requires an anaerobic environment such as in the contents of the intestine or in dead tissue in a lacerated wound.

As stated previously, heterotrophic bacteria obtain their energy by the breakdown of the carbon and energy source. The aerobic or anaerobic nature is related to the aerobic or anaerobic nature of this metabolism. Thus aerobes obtain most of their energy by a series of coupled oxido-reductions in which the ultimate electron-acceptor is atmospheric oxygen; in this *aerobic respiration,* the carbon and energy source may be completely oxidised to carbon dioxide and water. Energy is obtained by the production of energy-rich phosphate bonds and their transfer to adenosine diphosphate (ADP) to form adenosine triphosphate (ATP) during the passage of electrons through the electron-transport system. This process is known as oxidative phosphorylation. The electron-transport systems of microorganisms are often very similar to those occurring in higher organisms and involve pyridine nucleotide coenzymes, flavoproteins, cytochromes and cytochrome oxidase.

Anaerobes, on the other hand, oxidise compounds at the expense of some electron acceptor other than oxygen. In some instances, an inorganic compound capable of reduction such as nitrate or sulphate acts as the electron acceptor; this process is known as *anaerobic respiration* and energy is again produced mainly during the passage of electrons from the substrate to the inorganic electron acceptor. However, anaerobic growth probably occurs more commonly by the carbon and energy source acting both as the electron donor and the electron acceptor in a series of oxido-reductions. This process is known as *fermentation* and it leads to the formation of a variety of waste products such as ethanol in yeasts and organic acids and alcohols in bacteria, *e.g.* lactic acid in the lactobacilli and streptococci, and a mixture of lactic, acetic, formic and succinic acids in the enterobacteria. Carbon dioxide and, in some cases hydrogen, is commonly produced and therefore fermentation is usually accompanied by the production of both acid and gas. The nature of the fermentation product is also of significance in the classification of bacteria. During the process of fermentation, energy-rich phosphate bonds are produced by the introduction of inorganic phosphate into intermediates on the fermentation pathway, a process known as substrate-level phosphorylation. The energy-rich phosphate groups so produced are transferred on to ADP to form ATP under the influence of the appropriate enzyme. It should be noted that the amount of energy produced from a given amount of carbon and energy source under anaerobic conditions is considerably less than that produced under aerobic conditions and therefore growth of a facultative anaerobe is usually much more abundant aerobically.

The Influence of Carbon Dioxide

It is now recognised that all bacteria require the presence of a small amount of carbon dioxide for growth, an amount normally provided by the atmosphere or by oxidation and fermentation reactions within the cell itself. Some bacteria, however, require a much higher concentration of carbon dioxide (5–10 per cent.), which must be provided in the environment of the culture medium (e.g. *Brucella abortus*, when first isolated from the body).

The Influence of Temperature

(*a*) *On Growth.*—For each species there is a definite temperature range within which growth takes place. The limits are the "maximum" and "minimum" temperatures, and an intermediate "optimum" temperature can usually be recognised at which growth is most rapid. In the laboratory, bacteria are grown at this optimum temperature in a thermostatically controlled *incubator*. The optimum temperature of a bacterium is approximately that of its natural habitat, *e.g.* about 37° C. in the case of organisms that are parasitic on man and warm-blooded animals. These, and many saprophytes of soil and water, which grow best at between 25° and 40° C., are termed *mesophilic*. Some mesophiles have a wide growth temperature range (*e.g.* 5°–43° C. for *Pseudomonas pyocyanea*), whilst others are more restricted (*e.g.* 30°–39° C. for *Neisseria gonorrhoeae*). None of them grows appreciably at temperatures below 5° C., (as in a domestic refrigerator at 3°–5° C.), and few at more than 45° C.

A group of soil and water bacteria, the *psychrophiles*, grow best at temperatures below 20° C., usually quite well at 0° C. and in some cases, slowly, down to about −7° C. on unfrozen media. Their importance lies in their ability to cause spoilage of refrigerated and frozen food, though none is pathogenic. Another group of non-parasitic bacteria, the *thermophiles*, grow best at high temperatures between 55° and 80° C., and have minimum growth temperatures ranging from 20° to 40° C. (facultative thermophiles), or even above 40° C. (strict thermophiles). These organisms are important as a cause of spoilage in under-processed canned foods, since many form spores of exceptionally high heat-resistance.

(*b*) *On Viability.*—Heat is an important agent in the artificial destruction of microorganisms, the effect depending under moist conditions on the coagulation and denaturation of cell proteins, and under dry conditions, on oxidation and charring. Among the bacteria that are parasites of mammalian animals, non-sporing forms in the presence of water generally cannot withstand temperatures above 45° C. for any length of time. The time of exposure to heat that is necessary for killing is shorter the higher the temperature, and various other factors influence the exact amount of heating required. Thus, bacteria are more susceptible to "moist heat", *e.g.* in hot water or saturated steam, than to "dry heat", *e.g.* in a hot-air oven. They are rendered more susceptible by the presence of acid, alkali or any chemical disinfectant, and less suceptible by the presence of organic substances such as proteins, sugars and fats, and also by their own occurrence in large numbers. The *thermal death point* of a particular organism may be defined as the lowest temperature that kills it under standard conditions, within a given time, *e.g.* ten minutes. Under moist conditions, it lies between 50° and 65° C. for most non-sporing mesophilic bacteria, and between 100° and 120° for the spores of most sporing species (*e.g.* about 105° C. for *Cl. tetani* and 115° C. for *Cl. botulinum*). The extreme limit of resistance to moist heat is shown by the spores of a non-pathogenic, strictly thermophilic bacillus, *B. stearothermophilus*, whose killing requires exposure to 121° C. for 10–35 minutes. With dry heat, the 10-minute thermal death points of the different sporing bacteria are mostly between 140° and 180° C.

At low temperatures some species die rapidly, but the majority survive well. Cultures of the latter may be preserved for long periods at between 3° and 5° C. in a domestic-type refrigerator, or in the frozen state as between −20° and −70° C. in a "deep freeze" cabinet. The process of freezing kills a proportion of the bacterial cells present, and this is least if freezing is effected rapidly (*e.g.* by use of solid carbon dioxide).

The Influence of Moisture and of Desiccation

Four-fifths by weight of the bacterial cell consists of water and, as in the case of other organisms, moisture is absolutely necessary for growth. Drying in air is injurious to many microbes, and the different species vary widely in their ability to survive when dried under natural conditions, as in infected exudate smeared on clothing or furniture, and converted to dust. Thus, the gonococcus, *Treponema pallidum* and the common cold virus appear to die almost at once, while the tubercle bacillus, *Staph. aureus* and the smallpox virus may survive for several months. Bacterial endospores survive drying especially well; for instance, those of *Bacillus anthracis*, when dried on threads, have survived for over sixty years.

Even delicate, non-sporing organisms may survive drying for a period of years if they are desiccated rapidly and completely, preferably while frozen, and thereafter maintained in a high vacuum (0·01 mm. Hg., or less) in a sealed glass ampoule which is stored at room temperature in the dark. This is the basis of the *lyophilisation* or "freeze-drying" process of preserving bacterial cultures in the laboratory.

The Influence of Hydrogen-ion Concentration

This is an essential factor in bacterial metabolism and growth. The majority of commensal and pathogenic bacteria grow best at a neutral or very slightly alkaline reaction (pH 7·2 to 7·6). Some bacteria, however, flourish in the presence of a considerable degree of acidity and are termed *acidophilic*, e.g. *Lactobacillus*. Others are very sensitive to acid, but tolerant of alkali, e.g. *Vibrio cholerae*. Strong acid or alkali solutions, *e.g.* 5 per cent. hydrochloric acid or sodium hydroxide, are rapidly lethal to most bacteria, the mycobacteria (*e.g.* tubercle bacillus) being exceptional in resisting them.

The Influence of Light and other Radiations

Darkness is a favourable condition for growth and viability. Ultraviolet rays are rapidly bactericidal, *e.g.* direct sunlight or radiation from a mercury vapour lamp. Even diffuse daylight, as it enters a room through window glass, significantly shortens the survival of micro-organisms and may be of hygienic importance. Bacteria are also killed by Cathode and Röntgen rays, and by radium emanations.

The Influence of Osmotic Pressure

As a result of the presence of a semi-permeable cytoplasmic membrane, bacteria resemble other cells in being subject to osmotic phenomena. Relatively, however, they are very tolerant of changes in the osmotic pressure of their environment and can grow in media with widely varying contents of salt, sugar and other such solutes. This is partly a reflection of the thickness and mechanical strength of their cell walls. For most species the upper limit of sodium chloride concentration permitting growth lies between 5 and 15 per cent., though *halophilic* (or osmophilic) species occur which can grow at higher concentrations up to saturation. The latter are saprophytes whose importance lies in their ability to cause spoilage of food preserved with salt or sugar. Sudden exposure of bacteria to solutions of high concentration (*e.g.* 2–25 per cent. sodium chloride) may cause *plasmolysis*, i.e. temporary shrinkage of the protoplast and its retraction from the cell wall due to the osmotic withdrawal of water; this occurs much more readily in Gram-negative than in Gram-positive bacteria. Sudden transfer from a concentrated to a weak solution, or to distilled water, may cause *plasmoptysis*, i.e. swelling and bursting of the cell through excessive osmotic imbibition of water.

The Influence of Mechanical and Sonic Stresses

Although their cell walls have considerable strength and some elasticity, it is possible to rupture and kill bacteria by exposure to mechanical stresses. A bacterial suspension may be largely disintegrated by subjection to very vigorous shaking with fine glass beads, or to supersonic or ultrasonic vibration (9000–200,000, and over 200,000 cycles per second, respectively). These measures are used in isolating the large molecular components of the cell.

CHAPTER 4

CLASSIFICATION AND IDENTIFICATION OF BACTERIA

MORPHOLOGICAL CLASSIFICATION

The main groups of bacteria are distinguished by microscopical observation of their morphology and staining reactions, initially in a Gram-stained preparation. They can be classified simply as follows:

I. **Lower Bacteria.**—Simple, generally unicellular structures, never in the form of a mycelium or sheathed filaments.

1. Cocci—spherical or nearly spherical cells.
2. Bacilli—relatively straight rod-shaped (cylindrical) cells.
3. Vibrios—curved rod-shaped cells ("comma-shaped").
4. Spirilla—spirally twisted, non-flexuous rods.
5. Spirochaetes—thin, spirally twisted, flexuous filaments.

II. **Higher Bacteria.**—Filamentous organisms, some being sheathed and some growing with branching to form a mycelium. May have certain cells specialised for reproduction; *e.g.*

Actinomycetes—simple branching filaments forming a mycelium; may form conidia; non-motile.

Cocci

The main groups of cocci are distinguished according to their predominant mode of cell grouping and their reaction to the Gram stain. The following groups correspond with biological genera:

(1) *Diplococcus.*—Cells mainly adherent in pairs and slightly elongated in axis of pair; Gram-positive (e.g. *D. pneumoniae*).

(2) *Streptococcus.*—Cells mainly adherent in chains, due to successive cell divisions occurring in the same axis; Gram-positive (e.g. *Strept. pyogenes*).

(3) *Staphylococcus.*—Cells mainly adherent in irregular clusters, due to successive divisions occurring irregularly in different planes; Gram-positive (e.g. *Staph. aureus*).

The genus *Micrococcus*, comprising only non-pathogenic species, is similar to *Staphylococcus*, though some of its species differ in size, in being motile or in being only weakly Gram-positive.

(4) *Gaffkya.*—Cells mainly adherent in plates of four (tetrads), or multiples thereof, due to division occurring successively in two planes at right angles; Gram-positive (e.g. *Gaff. tetragena*).

(5) *Sarcina.*—Cells mainly adherent in cubical packets of eight, or multiples thereof, due to division occurring successively in three planes at right angles; Gram-positive (e.g. *Sarc. lutea*).

(6) *Neisseria.*—Cells mainly adherent in pairs and slightly elongated at right angles to axis of pair; Gram-negative (e.g. *N. meningitidis*).

(7) *Veillonella.*—Generally very small cocci arranged mainly in clusters and pairs; Gram-negative (e.g. *Veill. parvula*).

The different cocci are relatively uniform in size, about 1 μ being the average diameter. Some species are capsulate and a very few are motile. It should be noted that a pure growth will usually show, in addition to the predominant cell grouping (*e.g.* clusters or long chains), a number of single cocci, pairs and very short chains.

Bacilli

The primary subdivision of the rod-shaped bacteria is made according to their staining reactions by the Gram and Ziehl-Neelsen methods, and whether or not endospores are formed. Some of the groups thus distinguished include several biological genera, and these can be recognised only by study of their physiological characters in artificial cultures.

(1) The *Acid-fast Bacilli.*—In giving an acid-fast staining reaction by the Ziehl-Neelsen method, members of the genus *Mycobacterium*, including the tubercle bacillus, are distinguished from all other bacilli.

(2) The *Gram-positive Spore-forming Bacilli.*—Apart from some rare saprophytic varieties, the only bacteria to form endospores are those of the genera *Bacillus* (aerobic) and *Clostridium* (anaerobic). They are primarily Gram-positive, but very liable to become Gram-negative in ageing cultures. The size, shape and position of the spore may assist recognition of the species; *e.g.* the tetanus bacillus is characterised by its bulging, spherical, terminal spore ("drum-stick" form).

(3) The *Gram-positive Non-sporing Bacilli.*—These include several genera. *Corynebacterium* is distinguished by a tendency to slight curving and club-shaped or ovoid swelling of the bacilli, and their arrangement in parallel and angular clusters due to the snapping mode of cell division. *Erysipelothrix* and *Lactobacillus* are distinguished by a tendency to grow in chains and filaments, and *Listeria* by the occurrence of motility and flagellation.

(4) The *Gram-negative Bacilli.*—These include numerous genera belonging to the families *Pseudomonadaceae*, *Achromobacteraceae*, *Enterobacteriaceae*, *Brucellaceae* and *Bacteroidaceae*. *Pseudomonas* is distinguished by its polar flagellation, whereas motile members of the other families are peritrichously flagellate.

Vibrios and Spirilla

Vibrios are recognised as short, non-flexuous curved rods (e.g. *V. cholerae*) and spirilla as non-flexuous spiral filaments (e.g. *Sp. minus*). They are Gram-negative and mostly motile, having polar flagella and showing very active, "darting" motility.

Spirochaetes

The spirochaetes are slender, flexuous spiral filaments, and their staining reaction, when demonstrable, is Gram-negative. They are distinguished from the spirilla in being capable of active flexion of the cell body and in being motile without possession of flagella. The different varieties are recognised by their size, shape, wave form and refractility, observed in the natural state in unstained wet films by dark-ground microscopy (See Fig. 6). The pathogenic species are classified in three genera:

(1) *Borrelia.*—Larger and more refractile than the other pathogenic spirochaetes, and more readily stained by ordinary methods; coils large and open, with a wave-length of 2–3 μ; a leash of 8–12 fibrils, each about 0·02 μ thick, is seen twisted round the whole length of the protoplast, by electron microscopy (e.g. *Borr. recurrentis*).

(2) *Treponema.*—Thinner filaments in coils of shorter wave-length (*e.g.* 1·0–1·5 μ), typically presenting a regular "corkscrew" form; feebly refractile and difficult to stain except by silver impregnation methods; by electron microscopy, a leash of 3–4 fibrils is seen wound round the protoplast within the cell wall (e.g. *Tr. pallidum*).

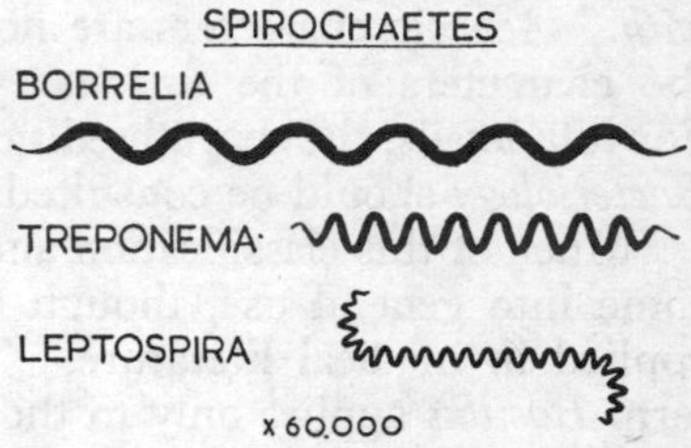

Fig. 6

(3) *Leptospira.*—The coils are so fine and close (wave-length about 0·5 μ) that they are barely discernible by dark-ground microscopy, though clearly seen winding round a single axial filament by electron microscopy. One or both extremities of the spirochaete are "hooked" or recurved, so that it may take the shape of a walking-stick, an S or a C (e.g. *L. icterohaemorrhagiae*).

Actinomycetes

These mycelial bacteria, or *Actinomycetales*, include three main genera:

(1) *Actinomyces.*—Gram-positive, non-acid-fast, tending to fragment into short coccal and bacillary forms, and not forming conidia; anaerobic (e.g. *Actinomyces israelii*).

(2) *Nocardia.*—Similar to *Actinomyces*, but aerobic and mostly acid-fast (e.g. *Noc. farcinica*)

(3) *Streptomyces.*—Vegetative mycelium not fragmenting into short forms; conidia formed in chains from aerial hyphae (e.g. *Streptomyces griseus*).

BIOLOGICAL CLASSIFICATION

Whilst observations of morphology and staining reactions are sufficient to distinguish the main groups of bacteria, the biological classification of bacteria is based on a consideration of all kinds of observable characters, including physiological, immunological and ecological ones.

At present no standard classification is universally accepted and applied. The older systems based mainly on morphological characters are quite inadequate for detailed classification. Thus, the term *Bacillus* was used in the past as a generic name for all rod-shaped bacteria, e.g. *Bacillus anthracis*, *B. tuberculosis* and *B. coli*, but the bacillary organisms clearly require subdivision into many separate genera in view of their heterogeneity. A system of classification and nomenclature of the bacteria was introduced some years ago by the Society of American Bacteriologists following the accepted rules of biological classification, and has since been elaborated by American systematists. A brief outline of this system is given, *but only those orders, families and genera which are of special importance in medical and veterinary bacteriology are dealt with.* Generic characters are not detailed, but these are indicated by the characters of the various type-species quoted in later chapters. For full details, the seventh edition of Bergey's *Manual of Determinative Bacteriology* should be consulted.

Much of this classification and many of the names given below have come into general use, though older designations are sometimes still applied in medical literature. Thus, in the new system the generic term *Bacillus* applies only to those rod-shaped bacteria that are spore-forming and aerobic, but its older use for a diversity of rod-shaped organisms is still current. It is, of course, quite correct to use the term "bacillus" as the common or vernacular name for any rod-shaped bacterium, and the common names such as "anthrax bacillus", "tubercle bacillus" and "colon bacillus" in place of the international scientific names (viz. *Bacillus anthracis*, *Mycobacterium tuberculosis* and *Escherichia coli*). In this book the new names of the American system are in general given priority, but the older conventional designations are indicated and also certain biological names used commonly by British writers. Abbreviations of generic names, e.g. "*B*"., "*Myco.*", etc., used throughout the text of the book are those adopted in the following summary.

ORDERS OF BACTERIA (CLASS SCHIZOMYCETES)

PSEUDOMONADALES.—Cells rigid, in form of straight, curved or spiral rods; rarely coccoid. Usually occur singly, though rarely in pairs or chains. Usually motile, possessing polar flagella. Gram-negative.

EUBACTERIALES.—Cells rigid, and spherical or straight rod-shaped in form. Occur singly, or in pairs, clusters, chains or filaments. Motile with peritrichous flagella or non-motile. Endospores formed in one family (*Bacillaceae*). Gram-positive or Gram-negative. Not acid-fast.

ACTINOMYCETALES.—Cells rigid, and rod-shaped or filamentous, with a tendency to branching; may grow as a mycelium which may develop aerial conidia, oidiospores or sporangiospores, and so give mould-like colonies. Mostly non-motile. Usually Gram-positive and some species acid-fast.

SPIROCHAETALES.—Cells flexuous, slender and spiral-shaped. Motile by flexion of the cell body. Do not possess flagella. Gram-negative.

MYCOPLASMATALES (Pleuropneumonia-like organisms).—Cells soft, fragile and highly pleomorphic. Reproduce by fission of filaments and large bodies into coccoid elementary bodies that are filterable. Non-motile. Gram-negative. Grow on agar media and so differ from the filterable viruses.

PSEUDOMONADALES

FAMILIES

Pseudomonadaceae.—Cells are straight rods, occasionally coccoid. May form a water-soluble pigment (*e.g.* green or brown) or a water-insoluble pigment (*e.g.* yellow or red).

Spirillaceae.—Cells are rigid, curved or spiral rods.

Further families in this order include most of the photosynthetic and autotrophic species of bacteria.

Genera

Pseudomonadaceae

Pseudomonas.—e.g. *Ps. aeruginosa* (*Ps. pyocyanea*).

Spirillaceae

Vibrio.—e.g. *V. comma* (*V. cholerae*).
Spirillum.—e.g. *Sp. minus.*

EUBACTERIALES

FAMILIES

Achromobacteraceae.—Cells rod-shaped and Gram-negative. Non-pigmented or forming yellow, orange or brown pigments. Grow well on ordinary peptone media. Few species can ferment sugars to give acid; glucose is usually attacked oxidatively if at all.

Enterobacteriaceae.—Cells rod-shaped and Gram-negative. Grow well on ordinary peptone media. Actively ferment glucose, and in many cases lactose and other sugars, producing acid, or acid and visible gas (CO_2 and H_2).

Brucellaceae.—Cells small, coccoid to rod-shaped, and Gram-negative. Obligate animal parasites. Many fail to grow on ordinary peptone media, requiring addition of body fluids. Many lack power to ferment sugars.

Bacteroidaceae.—Cells rod-shaped or filamentous, and Gram-negative. Most are strict anaerobes and many require enriched culture media for growth. Parasites of mammals, especially of the alimentary canal.

Micrococcaceae.—Cells spherical and Gram-positive; occur singly and in pairs, tetrads, cubical packets and irregular clusters. Many form a non-water-soluble yellow, orange or red pigment. Mostly non-motile. (*Sarcina ureae* alone forms endospores.)

Neisseriaceae.—Cells spherical to elliptical, and Gram-negative; occur mainly in pairs, with long axes parallel, or in clusters. Non-motile. Parasites of mammals.

Lactobacillaceae.—Cells are cocci or rods occurring singly, in pairs and in chains. Gram-positive. Mostly non-motile. Facultatively or strictly anaerobic. Actively ferment sugars with lactic acid as main product.

Corynebacteriaceae.—Cells rod-shaped or club-shaped; Gram-positive. Mostly non-motile.

Bacillaceae.—Cells rod-shaped and usually Gram-positive. Form endospores. Many are motile.

Genera

Achromobacteraceae

Alcaligenes.—e.g. *Alc. faecalis.*

Enterobacteriaceae

Escherichia.—e.g. *Esch. coli.*
Aerobacter.—e.g. *Aero. aerogenes, Aero. cloacae.*
Klebsiella.—e.g. *Kl. pneumoniae.*
Paracolobactrum.—e.g. *Par. coliforme.*
Serratia.—e.g. *Serr. marcescens* (*B. prodigiosus*).
Proteus.—e.g. *Pr. vulgaris.*
Salmonella.—e.g. *S. typhosa* (*S. typhi*) and *S. enteritidis.*
Shigella.—e.g. *Sh. dysenteriae.*

(*Note.*—In this book the above classification of the Enterobacteriaceae has been modified so that the genera conform more closely with the groups proposed by the Enterobacteriaceae Subcommittee of the International Committee on Bacterial Nomenclature and Taxonomy. The genera *Aerobacter* and *Paracolobactrum* are omitted and the following genera included:

Citrobacter.—e.g. *Cit. freundii.*
Cloaca.—e.g. *Cloaca cloacae.*
Hafnia.—e.g. *Hafnia alvei.*

Thus, *Aerobacter aerogenes* is included in the genus *Klebsiella* as *Kl. aerogenes* and *Aerobacter cloacae* in the genus *Cloaca.* The *Paracolobactrum* organisms are regarded as lactose non-fermenting variants in the genera *Escherichia, Citrobacter, Klebsiella, Cloaca* and *Hafnia.*)

Brucellaceae

Pasteurella.—e.g. *P. pestis.*
Bordetella.—e.g. *Bord. pertussis.*
Brucella.—e.g. *Br. melitensis.*

Haemophilus.—e.g. *H. influenzae.*
Actinobacillus.—e.g. *Actinobacillus lignieresi.*
Moraxella.—e.g. *Morax. lacunata.*

Bacteroidaceae

Bacteroides.—e.g. *Bacteroides fragilis.*
Fusobacterium.—e.g. *F. fusiforme.*
Sphaerophorus (or *Necrobacterium*).—e.g. *Sph. necrophorus.*
Streptobacillus.—e.g. *Streptobacillus moniliformis.*

Micrococcaceae

Micrococcus.—e.g. *Micro. ureae.*
Staphylococcus.—e.g. *Staph. aureus.*
Gaffkya.—e.g. *Gaff. tetragena.*
Sarcina—e.g. *Sarc. lutea.*

Neisseriaceae

Neisseria.—e.g. *N. meningitidis, N. gonorrhoeae.*
Veillonella.—e.g. *Veill. parvula.*

Lactobacillaceae

Diplococcus.—e.g. *D. pneumoniae.*
Streptococcus.—e.g. *Strept. pyogenes.*
Peptostreptococcus.—e.g. *Peptostrept. putridus.*
Lactobacillus.—e.g. *Lacto. acidophilus.*

Corynebacteriaceae

Corynebacterium.—e.g. *C. diphtheriae.*
Listeria.—e.g. *List. monocytogenes.*
Erysipelothrix.—e.g. *Ery. insidiosa.*

Bacillaceae

Bacillus.—e.g. *B. anthracis.*
Clostridium.—e.g. *Cl. tetani.*

ACTINOMYCETALES

FAMILIES

Mycobacteriaceae.—Cells rod-shaped, but rarely filamentous or branching. Do not form conidia or other kinds of spores.

Actinomycetaceae.—Cells filamentous and branching. Grow as a mycelium which may fragment into short rod or coccoid forms, and reproduce by budding or by spores formed through fragmentation of the mycelium and in some cases from aerial hyphae.

Streptomycetaceae.—Cells filamentous and branching. Grow as a mycelium which does not fragment. Conidia are borne on sporophores, in many cases aerial.

GENERA

Mycobacteriaceae

Mycobacterium.—e.g. *Myco. tuberculosis.*

Actinomycetaceae

Actinomyces.—e.g. *Actinomyces israelii.*
Nocardia.—e.g. *Noc. madurae.*

Streptomycetaceae

Streptomyces.—e.g. *Streptomyces griseus.*

SPIROCHAETALES

GENERA OF THE FAMILY TREPONEMATACEAE (THE SMALL SPIROCHAETES)

Borrelia.—*Borr. recurrentis.*
Treponema.—e.g. *Tr. pallidum.*
Leptospira.—e.g. *L. icterohaemorrhagiae.*

MYCOPLASMATALES

GENERA

Mycoplasma.—e.g. *M. mycoides.*

CLASS MICROTATOBIOTES

This class contains the smallest of living organisms, all obligate parasites and capable of growth only in the living tissues of an appropriate host, usually intracellularly. It includes two orders:

RICKETTSIALES.—Individual organisms are over 0·2 μ in diameter, resolvable by the light microscope and not filterable through bacteria-stopping filters, except for a few species with filterable phases. Gram-negative. Only a few species can grow on cell-free nutrient media.

VIRALES.—Individual organisms are mostly less than 0·2 μ in diameter, ultramicroscopic and filterable. All are obligate intracellular parasites, and none grows on inanimate or cell-free nutrient media.

There is no generally accepted classification of the viruses into genera and species (but see p. 83 et seq).

RICKETTSIALES

GENERA

Rickettsia.—e.g. *R. prowazekii.*
Coxiella.—e.g. *Cox. burnetii.*
Ehrlichia.—e.g. *Ehrl. ovina.*

Cowdria.—e.g. *Cowdria ruminantium.*

Bedsonia.—e.g. the viruses of psittacosis, lymphogranuloma, trachoma and inclusion conjunctivitis.

Bartonella.—e.g. *Bart. bacilliformis.*

Haemobartonella.—e.g. *Haemobartonella muris.*

Anaplasma.—e.g. *An. marginale.*

SYSTEM OF IDENTIFICATION OF BACTERIA

1. **The Morphology and Staining Reactions of Individual Organisms** generally serve as a preliminary criterion, particularly for placing an unknown species in its appropriate biological group. A Gram-stained smear is first examined and this suffices to show the Gram reaction, size, shape and grouping of the bacteria, whether they possess endospores, and the shape, size and intracellular position of such spores. An unstained wet film is examined with the dark-ground microscope for observation of the exact morphology of delicate spirochaetes, and an unstained wet film, or "hanging drop" preparation is examined with the ordinary microscope for observation of motility. When it is possible that the organism is a mycobacterium or a nocardia, a preparation is stained by the Ziehl-Neelsen method to demonstrate the acid-fast staining reaction.

In medical bacteriology the microscopic characters of certain organisms in pathological specimens may be sufficient for diagnostic identification, *e.g.* tubercle bacilli in sputum, or *Treponema pallidum* in exudate from a chancre. Morphology among the bacteria usually fails, however, to differentiate allied organisms, *e.g.* the meningococcus, gonococcus and *Neisseria catarrhalis*, and further tests must be applied, as below.

2. **Cultural Characters,** including the growth requirements and the appearance of cultures to the naked eye, are further criteria assisting identification, but may also be insufficient to differentiate species; *e.g.* different species of *Salmonella* produce indistinguishable colonies. A *culture* is a growth of bacteria prepared in the laboratory on an artificial nutrient medium, or *culture medium.* Attempts are made to grow (to "cultivate" or "culture") the bacterium on media of different compositions, *e.g.* a glucose-ammonia-inorganic salts mixture, or meat infusion or meat infusion plus blood, incubated under a variety of conditions, *e.g.* at different temperatures, at different pH values, in the presence of atmospheric oxygen (i.e. aerobically) or in its absence (*i.e.* anaerobically). The range of the conditions supporting growth is characteristic of particular organisms. The ability or inability of the organism to grow on medium containing a selective inhibitor (*e.g.* bile salt, optochin, bacitracin, low pH, high pH, tellurite) may also be of diagnostic significance.

The appearances of growths in liquid culture media, *e.g.* nutrient broth, are generally not distinctive, usually there is a uniform turbidity in the liquid and a little deposit at the bottom. Much more value attaches to observations of the appearance of the discrete masses of

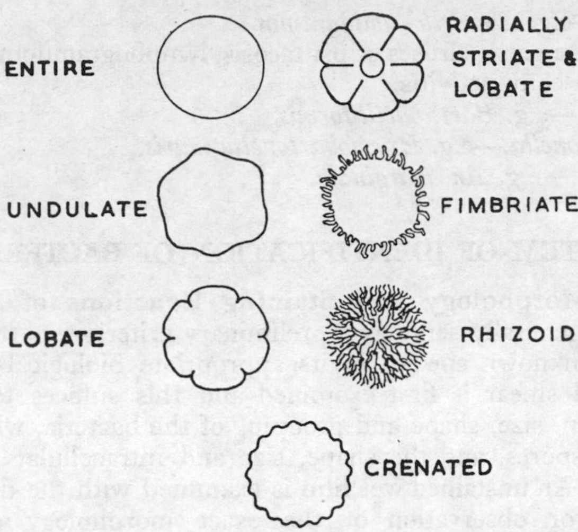

Fig. 7

growth, or *colonies*, that can be grown from isolated bacteria on the surface of solid culture medium such as nutrient agar. Attention is paid to the size of the colonies (diameter in mm.), their outline (whether circular and entire, or indented, or wavy, or rhizoid), their elevation (low convex, high convex, flat, plateau-like, umbonate, or nodular), their translucency (clear and transparent, or translucent, or opaque), whether they are colourless, white or otherwise pigmented, and whether they produce any change in the medium (*e.g.* haemolysis in a blood-containing agar medium).

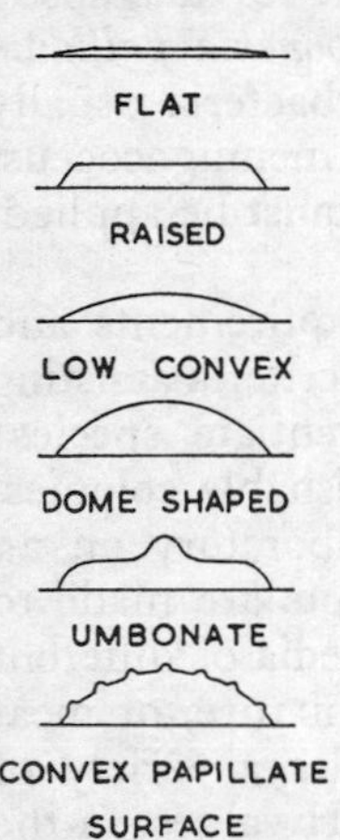

Fig. 8
The elevation of bacterial colonies.

3. **Biochemical Reactions,** *e.g.* the fermentation of various carbohydrates. Species that cannot be distinguished by morphology and cultural characters may exhibit distinct differences in their biochemical reactions, *e.g.* typhoid and paratyphoid bacilli. Different species or types may, however, resemble one another in fermentative properties, *e.g.* certain serotypes of the *Salmonella* group.

The most commonly used biochemical tests involve the observation of whether or not a growth of the bacterium in liquid nutrient medium will ferment particular "sugars" (*e.g.* glucose, lactose, mannitol) with the production of acid, detected by change of colour of an indicator dye present in the medium, or of acid plus gas; gas production is detected by the collection of a bubble in a small inverted tube (Durham tube) immersed in the medium. Other tests involve observation of the ability of a bacterium to produce particular end-products, *e.g.* indole, H_2S, and nitrite, when grown in suitable culture media, and of whether it possesses certain enzymic activities, *e.g.* oxidase, catalase, urease, gelatinase, collagenase, lecithinase, or lipase.

4. **Antigenic Characters.**—In bacteriology, species and types can often be identified by specific "antibody reactions" observed in *serological tests.* These reactions depend on the fact that the serum of an animal immunised against a microorganism contains specific antibodies (for the homologous species or type) which react in a characteristic manner with the particular microorganism. Such antisera, for example, may agglutinate or clump the homologous organism in test-tube experiment, and this effect can be observed with the naked eye. An unknown bacterium may thus be identified by demonstrating its reaction with one out of a number of standard known antisera.

It should be noted here that the serum of a person suffering from a bacterial infection may also exhibit specific antibody reactions. The nature of the infection may thus be diagnosed by demonstrating that the patient's serum agglutinates one out of a number of known laboratory cultures, *e.g.* the Widal reaction in enteric fever (see Chapter 18).

5. **Typing of Bacteria: Bacteriophage Sensitivity.**—A single bacterial species with a particular set of pathogenic activities may nevertheless include strains belonging to a variety of different *types* that are distinguishable in minor characters. Recognition of the type of a strain isolated from a patient may be of value in epidemiological studies relating to the source and spread of the infection in the community. In some pathogenic species, the "typing" of strains may be done by special biochemical or serological tests. Another important method of typing is by testing the susceptibility of the culture to lysis by each of a set of type-specific, lytic bacteriophages.

6. **Animal Pathogenicity.**—In the case of pathogenic organisms, *e.g.* the tubercle bacillus, that are virulent to, and produce characteristic lesions in laboratory animals, the inoculation test provides a reliable method of identification.

In many cases animal pathogenicity tests are controlled by the use of specific neutralising antisera and the pathogenic organisms are thereby identified with a high degree of specificity. Thus, the final identification of a diphtheria bacillus may be made by injecting culture material intradermally into two guinea-pigs, one of which has been protected by prior injection of specific antiserum to diphtheria toxin (a soluble poisonous protein secreted by the bacilli). The development of an inflammatory and necrotic skin reaction in the unprotected, but not in the protected animal identifies the culture as an organism producing diphtheria toxin. The tetanus bacillus is identified similarly by a test in mice that proves its production of the specific tetanus toxin. Strains of *Clostridium welchii* may be "typed" by demonstration of the set of specific toxins they produce; in this case the culture fluid is mixed with specific antiserum before injection.

7. **Antibiotic Sensitivity.**—The organism is tested for its ability to grow on artificial nutrient media containing different antibiotic and chemotherapeutic agents in different concentrations. In the *disk diffusion test*, the culture to be examined is inoculated confluently over the

surface of an agar plate and 6–10 paper disks or tablets containing different antibiotics are placed on different areas of the plate. Antibiotic diffuses outwards from each disk into the surrounding agar and produces a diminishing gradient of concentration. On incubation the bacteria grow on areas of the plate except those around the drugs to which they are sensitive, and the width of each growth-free "zone of inhibition" is a measure of their degree of sensitivity to the drug.

In a few cases, reactions are sufficiently uniform among the strains of a species, and distinctive from those of related species, to be valuable in the identification of the species (*e.g.* bacitracin sensitivity in *Streptococcus pyogenes*, and optochin sensitivity in the pneumococcus). Commonly, however, there are marked differences in antibiotic sensitivity between different strains of a species. Information about the sensitivity patterns of strains ("antibiograms") isolated from patients is required as a guide to the choice of drug for therapy and may also be used as an epidemiological marker in tracing hospital cross-infections.

IDENTIFICATION IN MATERIAL CONTAINING A MIXTURE OF BACTERIA: ISOLATION IN PURE CULTURE

Most of the identifying tests in the categories described above are valid only if made with a pure preparation or pure culture of a single kind of bacterium (*i.e.* a population of cells consisting exclusively of the progeny of a single ancestral cell). Specimens of material collected for diagnostic purposes from the bodies of patients include many (*e.g.* of faeces, sputum and throat secretion) that contain a wide variety of resident commensal bacteria as well as any pathogenic or potentially pathogenic species. Specimens of other materials, *e.g.* blood, pus, cerebrospinal fluid and urine, that are free from a resident commensal flora, are likely to be infected with only a single pathogenic species; but these specimens are liable sometimes to contain other bacteria as a result of secondary infection from the body surfaces or contamination in the course of collection.

Useful information may be obtained from certain examinations made on mixed infective material. Thus, microscopical examination reveals the morphology and staining reactions of the different organisms and also allows an assessment to be made of the relative numbers of each kind present (such an assessment is more reliable than one made from examination of a culture of the material because the conditions of culture may selectively favour the growth of some species and inhibit that of others). When material containing a mixture of bacteria is cultured by "plating", *i.e.* by inoculating it very thinly on the surface of a plate (Petri dish) of solid culture medium such as nutrient agar, the different bacteria are seen to grow as separate *colonies*, each of which is usually a *pure culture* descended from a single inoculated cell. Useful information relating to the identity of the different bacteria and their relative numbers in the specimen may be obtained by noting the appearances of the colonies. When a selective culture medium is used the occurrence of growth is suggestive of the identity of the bacteria growing, but it must be remembered that other kinds of bacteria incapable of growth on this medium may also be present in the specimen. Anaerobic bacteria will not grow or be recognised in cultures incubated aerobically, in the ordinary way.

Most other identifying tests can be performed only after the unknown bacterium has been isolated in pure culture. Isolation is generally done by Koch's procedure, following the preparation of plate cultures bearing well separated colonies (see Chapter 48). A single colony, suspected from its appearance of being that of a significant or pathogenic organism, is "picked" with an inoculating wire-loop and subcultured by itself in a tube or plate of fresh, sterile culture medium. (It is a useful practice in certain circumstances to examine microscopically a stained smear of the residue of the colony that has been "picked".) If there is any doubt about the purity of a supposedly pure culture, it should be plated out again on fresh medium, the colonies in the subculture should be examined to confirm their uniform appearance and one of these colonies should be picked and subcultured to give, through a second purification, a final 'pure culture'.

The morphological and cultural characters of the organism should, where necessary, be confirmed in examinations of the pure culture and the pure culture is then used in tests for examination of its biochemical reactions, antigenic characters, bacteriophage type, pathogenicity for laboratory animals, and antibiotic sensitivity reactions.

In some types of investigative work it is desirable to store pure cultures of strains for later reference. This is best done by the *freeze-drying* procedure; the organisms are held dried and *in vacuo* in a sealed ampoule and remain alive, though not metabolising or growing, for very long periods. Otherwise, the organism should be subcultured on a suitable *maintenance medium* and stored under conditions, *e.g.* in the dark at room temperature or in a refrigerator at 4° C., conducive to their maximal survival.

In addition to preliminary microscopical and cultural examinations, there are some special identifying tests that may be made directly on pathological specimens containing mixtures of bacteria. Use of the fluorescent antibody staining method makes it possible on microscopical examination to recognise and identify individual bacteria according to their antigenic character, thus with a high specificity comparable to that of conventional serological tests. Material containing commensal bacteria as well as a suspected pathogen, may be injected into a laboratory animal where only the pathogen may be capable of producing a fatal infection. Antibiotic sensitivity tests by the disk diffusion method are sometimes usefully performed on the primary diagnostic culture plate that grows the whole mixture of organisms present in the specimen; if this *primary sensitivity test* is made, results are sooner available for reporting to clinicians.

REFERENCE

Breed, R. S., Murray, E. G. D. & Smith, N. R. (1957). *Bergey's Manual of Determinative Bacteriology*, 7th ed. Baltimore: Williams & Wilkins.

CHAPTER 5

VIRUSES

GENERAL CONSIDERATIONS

AMONG the common contagious illnesses of man and animals there are many for which no bacterial cause has been found. These diseases have been known clinically throughout the centuries; smallpox has been recognised as a deadly infection since pre-Christian times and Hippocrates was perfectly familiar with the swollen neck in mumps. At the beginning of the present century it was realised that an agent present in the tissues or blood of such cases could transmit the infection in the absence of bacteria. Pasteur in 1884, when he failed to detect bacteria in infective material from rabid dogs, said that he was tempted to believe that the cause of the disease was "a micro-organism infinitesimally small".

In 1892 Pasteur's theory was confirmed, though in a different disease, by Iwanowsky, who showed that the mosaic disease of tobacco plants was caused by a minute agent which was so small that it was ultramicroscopic and would pass through the pores of a filter that would not permit the passage of any known bacterium. In 1898 the vesicle fluid from cases of foot and mouth disease in cattle was shown by Loeffler and Frosch to contain an infectious agent that was similarly filterable. In 1901 it was proved that yellow fever in man was caused by a filterable virus carried by mosquitoes. From these discoveries it soon became apparent that there were a number of virus agents which could pass through bacteria-stopping filters and still retain their powers to cause disease in animals and human volunteers. Viruses were therefore originally recognised as ultramicroscopic and filter passing.

During the years that followed, many similar minute filter-passing organisms were found to be widely distributed throughout the animal and plant kingdoms, causing mild as well as severe diseases and often being carried latently in their hosts without giving rise to any obvious signs of harm. In man it was shown that viruses cause not only such serious illnesses as smallpox, poliomyelitis, encephalitis, infectious hepatitis and pneumonia but that they are also responsible for many familiar minor infections including the common cold, influenza, mumps, measles and chickenpox, and a whole host of other conditions. Amongst the many important virus diseases of animals are foot and mouth disease and rinderpest in cattle, distemper and rabies in dogs, and fowl pest in poultry.

Not only do viruses clearly cause many infectious illnesses, but it has been realised gradually that they also play a part, perhaps with the aid of other factors, in the production of certain types of tumours. Rous in 1911 discovered that certain sarcomata in fowls could be transmitted with cell free filtrates of the tumours and since that time an impressive list of tumours has been compiled in which viruses undoubtedly play a causative role. These viruses are known as *oncogenic viruses* and they include the agents that cause warts in man, fibromas, papillomas and related tumours in rabbits and domestic and wild animals, mammary carcinomata, leukaemias, and parotid tumours (polyoma virus) in mice, and leucosis in poultry (Andrewes, 1964a).

Many insects suffer from virus diseases, *e.g.* epizootics of jaundice in silk worms and sac brood in bees have been the cause of much economic loss. Insects are however perhaps more notorious as the *vectors* of viruses that attack man, animals and plants. Some viruses can multiply within their bodies without harming them and often the virus is carried through the whole of the life cycle of the insect. Thus lice, ticks, flies and mosquitoes transmit viruses within human and animal communities and can carry infection from plant to plant. Again, nematode worms that are parasitic in pigs spread the swine influenza virus, and other nematodes that infest plants play an important part in the transmission of infection to vines and cereals. (At least one virus that affects the roots of tomato plants, also attacks and kills the larvae of its vector the Southern Root Knot Nematode.)

When plants are affected by viruses, one of the characteristic effects is a mottling or "mosaic" of the leaves that may be followed by withering and death of the plant. There are more than three hundred viruses recognised as pathogenic for plants and many, for example the tobacco mosaic virus, the tomato bushy stunt virus and the virus of "X" disease of potatoes, are of great economic importance. One plant virus, the tulip mosaic virus, however, is virtually harmless and is responsible for the beautiful coloured mottlings and pencillings on the petals of tulip flowers. It has been known for many years and the Dutch and Turkish artists of the sixteenth and seventeenth centuries took great pleasure in depicting these variegated tulips.

That bacteria too are subject to infection by viruses was realised when Twort in 1915 and d'Herelle in 1917 independently observed the phenomenon of the transmissible lysis of bacteria. This was demonstrated in the following way: a few drops of liquid faeces from a case of bacterial dysentery were added to a tube of broth which was incubated overnight; filtration of this culture through a porcelain candle yielded a bacteria-free filtrate which, when added in very small quantities to a young culture of *Shigella shigae*, produced clearing and lysis of the bacteria after incubation for several hours. d'Herelle was able to show that this lysed culture possessed a similar lytic property towards a fresh culture and he was able to carry the effect through more than fifty successive transfers; he thought the effect was caused by "an invisible microbe that is antagonistic to the dysentery bacillus" and suggested that this was a minute parasite of bacteria propagating and multiplying at the expense of the bacterial cells. He called the microbe "bacteriophage", a name now frequently abbreviated to *phage*, and his view that it was a virus has been confirmed beyond all doubt. Bacteriophages can also be recognised by their ability to produce a clearing of an area when spotted on to a confluent growth of the host bacterium on an agar plate. The clear area is known as a *plaque*; it is often produced by a single phage particle and is therefore analogous to a bacterial colony. Bacteriophages have the great advantage that they can be easily propagated and counted and moreover their hosts, the bacterial cells, lend themselves readily to study at biochemical and genetic levels. It is for these reasons that our knowledge of the mechanisms of phage infection and reproduction is far more advanced than our knowledge of the corresponding mechanisms in animal viruses. There is therefore a tendency to regard phages as model viruses and to adapt the methods used successfully in their study to the more complex relationships between the animal virus and its host cell (Hayes, 1963).

The new biological science of *Virology* comprises the study of both the infecting microorganism and its host. The four main divisions of the subject comprise (1) the viruses of man and animals, (2) the bacteriophages, (3) the viruses of insects and worms, and (4) the viruses of plants. In these pages where attention is focused on the medical and veterinary infections we shall deal only with the first two of these divisions of virology.

Approximate Sizes of Viruses and Reference Objects

	Diameter or width × length in mμ
*Staphylococcus	1000
*Rickettsia prowazekii	475
Bedsonia organisms	330-490
Pox viruses	300–250
Mumps and Newcastle viruses	80–340
*Pleuropneumonia organisms	150
Rabies virus	150
Measles virus	140
Herpes simplex viruses	120
Influenza groups of viruses	100
Adenovirus groups	100
T2 bacteriophage of *E. coli*	95 × 65
Rous sarcoma virus	65
Lymphocytic choriomeningitis virus	50
Tobacco mosaic virus	300 × 15
Rabbit papilloma virus	45
Arthropod-borne viruses	40
Poliovirus and enteroviruses	28
Foot and mouth disease virus	25
*Haemoglobin molecule	15 × 3
*Albumin molecule	10 × 2·5

Microorganisms above the line are visible with the optical microscope.

* For reference.

FUNDAMENTAL CHARACTERS OF VIRUSES

Viruses differ fundamentally from bacteria in that: they are small in size and consequently are able to pass through filters that retain bacteria; they can grow only in living cells; they resist the action of antibiotics and some agents that destroy bacteria; and they have reproductive processes that are quite different from the simple binary fission of bacteria. A virus particle contains only one kind of nucleic acid and is covered by a protein coat.

Small Size and Filterability

The unit used for the measurement of virus size is the millimicron (mμ), *i.e.* a one-thousandth part of a micron (μ) or 0·000001 mm. The Angström unit (Å), which is one-tenth of millimicron (0·0000001 mm.), is often used as a measure for very small structures such as virus capsomeres, and macromolecules. In the preceding list the sizes of various representative viruses are given together with those of reference objects.

Individual virus particles are known as *virions* (the old term, which is still used, was *elementary bodies*). They may vary in diameter from 300 to 25 mμ; the largest are about half the size of the smallest bacterium and the smallest are about the size of large protein molecules. Virions over 200 mμ in diameter are within the resolving power of the light microscope and can be demonstrated in stained films or sections taken from the lesions of virus diseases such as smallpox.

Measurement.—The most frequently used method for estimating virus size is by direct observation under the electron microscope. Viruses that are far beyond the limits of the resolution of the light microscope can be seen and photographed in this instrument, which is capable of resolving objects as small as 3Å (0·3 mμ) in diameter (see Chapter 44). The usual method of making the measurements is to include in a suspension of purified virus some latex particles of known size (*e.g.* 250 mμ); in electron micrographs the known and the unknown particles can be measured with accuracy and the size of the virus is determined with precision. One advantage of electron-microscopical examination of viruses is that the shape as well as the size can be determined. In this way it has been found that the vaccinia virus particles are brick-shaped, that influenza viruses have a filamentous as well as a spherical form, and that most bacteriophages have a sperm-like morphology, with a polyhedral head and a tail. The crystalline nature of plant viruses and the crystal-like lattice arrangement of the component subunits of some human viruses such as those of the adenovirus group are clearly seen in electron micrographs. In ultra-thin sections of infected cells it is possible under the electron microscope to follow the morphological changes *in situ* in the host cell as the virus multiplies.

Originally viruses were measured by their capacity to pass through filters. Many types of filter have been used for this purpose, but the best are made from collodion and these have replaced the older diatomaceous earth filters of Berkefeld and the Chamberland porcelain candles. Filtration methods, however, have no high degree of precision in virus measurement and have for the most part been replaced by newer techniques. Nevertheless, filtration does have a special use in measuring a very small virus when it is contained in a material contaminated with so much host cell protein that other methods cannot be used.

A third method by which virus size can be determined is by estimating the rate at which the particles fall in a suspending fluid; large particles being heavier fall faster than small ones. This relationship between particle size and rate of sedimentation follows Stokes' law and holds good even when forces many times greater than that of gravity are applied to a virus preparation in a fast-moving centrifuge. From values for the density and viscosity of the medium, the distance from the axis of rotation and the speed in r.p.m., the diameter of the virus particle can be calculated (p. 863).

The Structure of Viruses

Intrinsically a virus particle is composed of an inner core of either DNA or RNA (but not both) surrounded by a shell of protein which is referred to as a capsid. All the plant viruses contain RNA and the vast majority of bacteriophages so far described contain DNA, but in the case of the animal viruses about one-half contain RNA and have been called *riboviruses* while the other half contain DNA and have been named *deoxyviruses* (Cooper, 1961). The influenza, enteric and arthropod-borne groups are riboviruses and the pox, herpes and adenoviruses are deoxyviruses.

The protein shell appears to act as a protective covering for the underlying nucleic acid. When it is removed, as for example by cold phenol extraction, the exposed nucleic acid remains infective for a time and can by itself initiate virus growth if it is introduced into a susceptible host cell. Although naked viral nucleic acid is only stable for short periods of time and is considerably less infective than the complete virion, it contains the genetic material that is responsible for the transmission of heritable characters and the production of new virus. The proportion of nucleic acid to protein in the virus particle varies greatly with different viruses; the DNA content of the T2 phage is about 40 per cent. of its dried weight and that of the vaccinia virus about 6 per cent. The RNA content of the polioviruses is 20–30 per cent. and that of the influenza virus only about 1 per cent.

The chemical composition of the larger animal viruses is rather more complex. The influenza viruses, for example, in addition to their proteins and RNA contain 4–6 per cent. polysaccharide with galactose, mannose and fucose as monomer components, 11 per cent. phospholipids, which include cephalin, sphingomyelin and lecithin, and 6 per cent. cholesterol. It is probably at the end of the growth cycle that the components of these viruses are assembled at the periphery of the host cell from whose wall the virion obtains the lipid constituents for its own covering membrane. These lipid-containing surface structures often make the virions readily disintegrated by organic solvents such as ether and for this reason they have been referred to as *lipoviruses* (Cooper, 1961). Ether-sensitive viruses include the influenza, herpes and arthropod-borne groups whilst the enteric, adeno, papilloma and polyoma viruses, which have no peripheral lipid components, are ether-resistant. As might be expected, the ether sensitivity of viruses seems to go hand in hand with sensitivity to bile salts and other surface active agents. These two properties are so sharply defined that they are valuable in the differentiation and classification of the various animal virus groups.

The pox group of viruses are even more complex and one member, the vaccinia virus, contains 6 per cent. lipids in addition to its protein and DNA, as well as certain enzymes such as phosphatase, catalase and lipase which are present as part of the virion together with coenzymes such as biotin, riboflavine and adenine-flavine dinucleotide. Vaccinia virus particles have, however, no normal metabolic activity when freed from their host cells. A number of pox viruses including the vaccinia virus are very resistant to ether whilst some are sensitive and others react in an intermediate way; the different behaviour of members of the group may depend on whether the lipid constituents are situated on the surface or lie deep in the virion protected by a resistant outer membrane.

The protein shell (capsid) of the virus particle (virion) is built of a number of subunits or *capsomeres* which are, according to the virus species, spherical, wedge-shaped, or in the form of hollow prisms (Fig. 9). The nucleic acid of the core is in the form of one or more helical strands. The disposition of capsomeres in the shell confers a variety of patterns so that a virus may have cubic, helical, or a combined and complex symmetry (Wildy & Horne, 1963). In the case of some of the larger viruses this assembly is surrounded by one or more membranes though no such covering is found in the smallest viruses.

Viruses with cubic symmetry have a hexagonal outline due to the fact that their capsomeres are arranged in a geometrical configuration that is a regular solid with 20 equilateral triangular faces, *i.e.* an *icosahedron.* This figure is described as having 5.3.2 rotational symmetry and imposes a definite number of capsomeres on each side of its triangular faces (Caspar & Klug, 1962). The total number of capsomeres of a virion may be calculated from the formula $10(n-1)^2+2$ where n is the number of capsomeres between and including those on any five-fold rotational axis. From this it has been found that the number of capsomeres of various groups of viruses falls into the series 12, 42, 92, 162 or 252. Viruses known to have icosahedral symmetry have the following number of capsomeres; ϕx174 bacteriophage 12, poliovirus 42(?) warts and polyoma viruses 42, reovirus 92, herpes group of viruses 162, the group of adenoviruses 252.

Of the viruses having a helical symmetry, that of tobacco mosaic disease has been most fully investigated. This virus is in the form of a hollow rigid rod 300×17 mμ and is composed of a helical core of RNA to which about 2000 wedge-shaped capsomeres are attached so that there are $16\frac{1}{3}$ on each turn of the spiral. Helical symmetry is also found in some of the animal viruses, notably in the influenza and measles groups. In these the capsid is composed of one or more helical strands of RNA covered by many capsomeres. The long thread of the capsid is hollow, but unlike that of the tobacco mosaic virus is flexible and it is wound upon itself to give a spherical mass which has a whorled appearance under the electron microscope. This capsid is enclosed by a membrane through which protrude a large number of regularly arranged projections in which resides the enzyme that confers the characteristic haemagglutination property of these viruses.

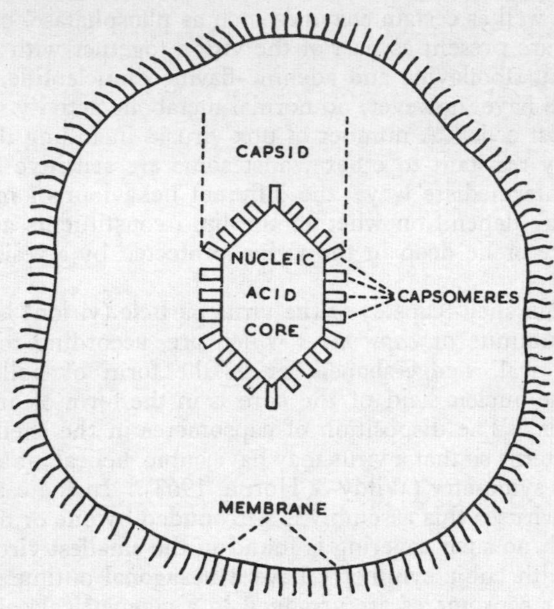

FIG. 9

Modified from a diagram by R. W. Horne (1963).
Scientific American, 208.50

A yet more complex symmetry is that of some of the larger viruses, notably those of the pox group. The particle of the vaccinia virus is surrounded by one or more membranes that envelop a peripheral protein layer within which is situated a dumbell-like structure into the hollows of which fit dense central bodies. Negatively stained particles are seen to contain hollow tubular structures 7–9 mμ in diameter but it is in doubt whether they are truly multiple or merely parts of a single thread. In the case of the contagious pustular dermatitis (orf) virus the thread seems to be arranged in a figure-of-eight pattern and may be continuous, but in some pox viruses the appearance is that of multiple angular strands. It cannot yet be said whether these strands are capsids or capsomeres.

The structure of bacteriophages, notably the so-called "T-even" phages of *E. coli* is more complex and sophisticated than that of any virus so far considered (Horne & Wildy, 1962; Champe, 1963). The basic design is sperm-shaped with a polyhedral head and a cylindrical tail. Although phages from different sources may vary morphologically,

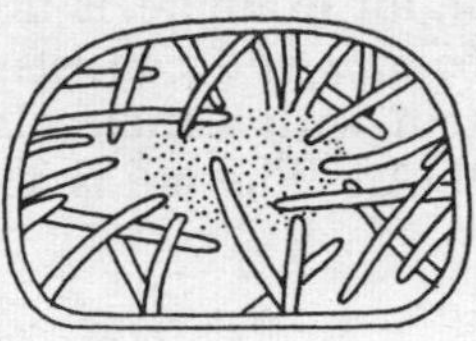

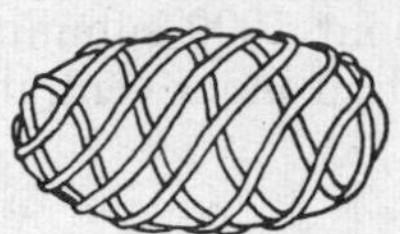

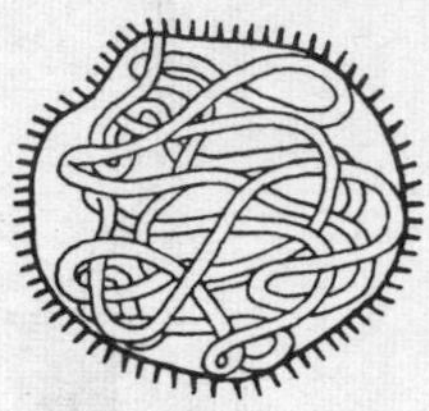

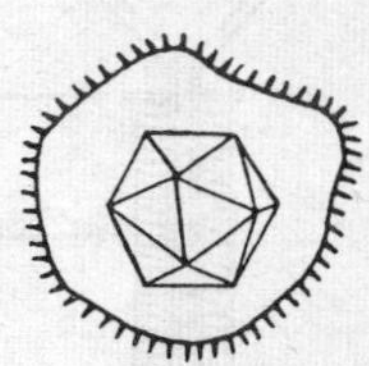

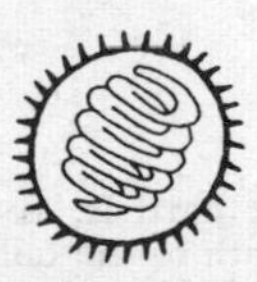

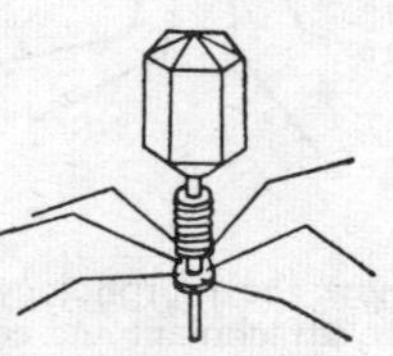

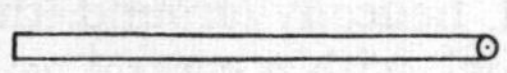

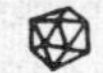

FIG. 10

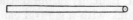

Modified from a diagram by R. W. Horne (1963). *Scientific American*, 208.49

particularly in the length and thickness of the tail, by far the majority (with the exception of the ϕx174 of *E. coli* and *Shigella*) have these two basic components.

The head of the T2 phage of *E. coli*, for example, is in the form of a bipyramidal hexagonal prism 100×65 mμ and consists of an outer shell of about 1000 subunits of a protein with a molecular weight of 80,000 and an inner central mass of DNA. The tail is about 100 mμ

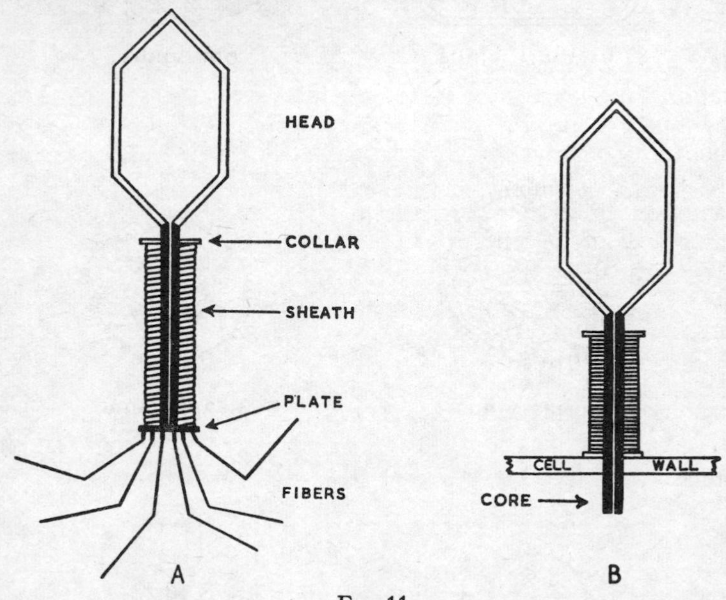

FIG. 11

To show the morphology of a T-even phage particle, A before, and B after, attachment and contraction of the sheath of the tail. (Modified from a diagram by Champe 1963.)

long and 25 mμ wide and is composed of a contractile sheath surrounding a central hollow core. The sheath is constructed from some 140–200 subunits of a second protein with a molecular weight of 54,000; the subunits are arranged helically around the cylindrical protein core which is about 7 mμ thick with a central canal 2·5 mμ in diameter. At the distal extremity of the tail is a hexagonal plate to which six fibres are attached. These tail fibres are 130 mμ long and 2 mμ wide and are composed of subunits of a protein that has a molecular weight of not less than 100,000. In the intact phage the tail fibres are folded around the tip of the tail, but when the initial contact with the bacterium is made they are freed to combine with specific receptor areas on the bacterial surface (see Figs. 11A and 13). This stage is followed by the contraction of the sheath of the tail to less than half of its original length and the extrusion of the central core through the bacterial wall to enable the transference of the DNA to the host cell (see Figs. 11B and 13).

Reaction to Physical and Chemical Agents

Outside the body, and at room temperature, many viruses are extremely labile and may survive for only a few hours. Such is the case with the viruses of influenza, mumps and measles, and in these diseases great care must be taken to ensure that the specimens under investigation are frozen with a minimum delay. Other viruses, such as the smallpox and poliomyelitis viruses, are much hardier and may survive under ordinary atmospheric conditions for many days, weeks or even months.

Heat.—The viruses causing disease in man and animals are in general readily inactivated by moderate heat (56°–60° C. for 30 min.) though there are some notable exceptions—homologous serum jaundice and poliomyelitis viruses. Like bacteria, viruses are resistant to extremes of cold, and, in fact, freezing at $-35°$ C. or $-70°$ C. is a satisfactory method for their preservation and is much used in the laboratory. The majority of viruses are also well preserved by drying from the frozen state, using the method of freeze-drying. By this means, virus vaccines are preserved in an active form for long periods before use to immunise against such diseases as smallpox and yellow fever.

pH Variation.—Viruses remain viable as a rule within the range of pH 5 to 9, but are destroyed by extreme acidity or alkalinity. Certain of their properties, however, like haemagglutination (*vide infra*) may be profoundly disturbed by variations of a few tenths of a pH unit.

Glycerol.—In a 50 per cent. solution of glycerol, ordinary non-sporing bacteria are killed comparatively quickly, but many viruses remain alive in this fluid for several months or even years. The preservation of the vaccinia virus used prophylactically against smallpox is accomplished by means of glycerol. Other viruses that can be kept for long periods in glycerol at 4° C., or lower temperatures, are those of poliomyelitis, rabies and herpes simplex. On the other hand, some viruses, *e.g.* the rinderpest virus and the psittacosis group of agents survive for less time in glycerol than certain bacteria.

Bactericidal Agents.—The most efficient disinfectants for use against viruses are oxidising agents such as hydrogen peroxide, potassium permanganate and hypochlorites, and organic iodine derivatives. Formaldehyde may also be used but is slower in its action. Phenol and certain cresol disinfectants such as lysol are active against only a few viruses and are not to be recommended for material contaminated by the poliomyelitis or smallpox viruses.

Antibiotics and Chemotherapeutic Substances such as sulphonamides, penicillin, streptomycin and the tetracyclines have no effect on true viruses. The fact that the agents of the psittacosis-lymphogranuloma group are susceptible to these drugs has been an important consideration in their being classified as rickettsiales instead of as viruses. Originally, viruses were "purified", *i.e* separated from bacteria in contaminated fluids such as sputum or faeces, by filtration through a bacteria-stopping filter, but now it has been found easier to use antibiotics; these (*e.g.* penicillin and streptomycin) are added to the material to kill the bacteria and they leave the viruses unharmed.

There are, however, a number of substances that are able to inhibit virus reproduction. A recent trial has shown that N-methylisatin β-thiosemicarbazone has a valuable prophylactic effect in protecting house contacts of cases of smallpox. The use of 5-iodo-2 deoxyuridine, which inhibits the synthesis of viral DNA, has recently been used therapeutically in human infections with the herpes simplex and vaccinia virus, but its clinical effects seem to be rather uncertain.

THE REPRODUCTION OF VIRUSES

The mechanism of virus reproduction has been most closely analysed in the phage-bacterium system because it is much easier to control experimental conditions for this system than for virus infections of higher organisms. Indeed the phage-infection model has been used for many fundamental studies on the mechanism and regulation of specific nucleic acid and protein synthesis in living organisms (Hayes, 1963). If infection of a bacterium by a phage causes the lysis of the host cell, the phage is said to be *virulent*. The cycle of the vegetative reproduction of virulent phages can be divided into various stages (see Fig. 12).

1. *Phage Adsorption and Replication* (Fig. 13)

Stage A.—The first event is the random collision of the phage particle with the bacterium.

Stage B.—Adsorption of the phage now occurs between complementary surfaces on the tail and the superficial layers of the bacteria by a process that is so highly selective that the surface components of the bacterial cell exhibit more specificity in this respect than they do in serological reactions. With some phages, adsorption requires also the presence of specific co-factors, particularly inorganic ions and amino acids.

Stage C.—Following adsorption a lysozyme-like enzyme, which is a component of the phage tail, is activated and this dissolves a localised portion of the bacterial cell wall. (If sufficient phages are adsorbed on to a single cell, leakage through the holes may be great enough to produce immediate lysis—so-called "lysis from without".) The sheath of the tail of the phage then contracts and the DNA inside the head is extruded down its central canal and passes through the bacterial cell wall and cytoplasmic membrane to reach the cytoplasm of the host cell. As has already been explained, the contractile sheath of the tail consists of 140–200 protein subunits, each of which seems to be associated with a molecule of a nucleoside triphosphate and a bound calcium ion. The process of contraction is associated with the action of an enzyme which hydrolyses the nucleoside triphosphate with the concomitant release of inorganic phosphate and a calcium ion. The energy produced in this reaction is used for the contraction of the sheath, presumably by an alteration in the protein of the sheath similar to that which occurs in the muscle protein of higher animals. The protein components of the phage can be considered as a disposable micro-syringe whose purpose is to protect the phage nucleic acid and to inject it into a new host cell.

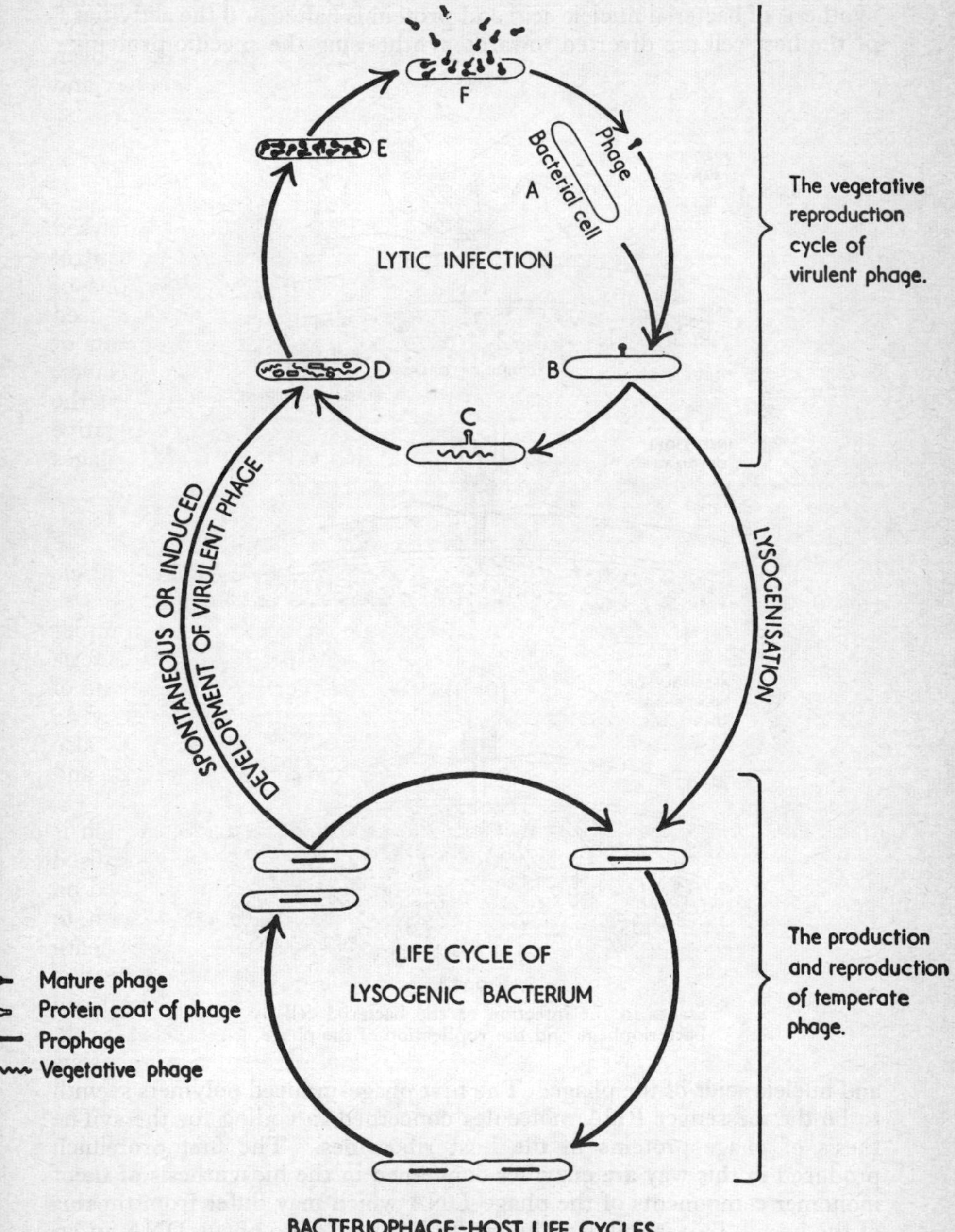

FIG. 12.

2. *Phage Multiplication*

Stage D.—After attachment to the bacterium there is a period—the "*eclipse phase*"—amounting to about half the total division cycle, when no phage can be detected within the host cell. During this phase the synthesis of bacterial nucleic acid and protein is halted and the activities of the host cell are diverted towards synthesising the specific proteins

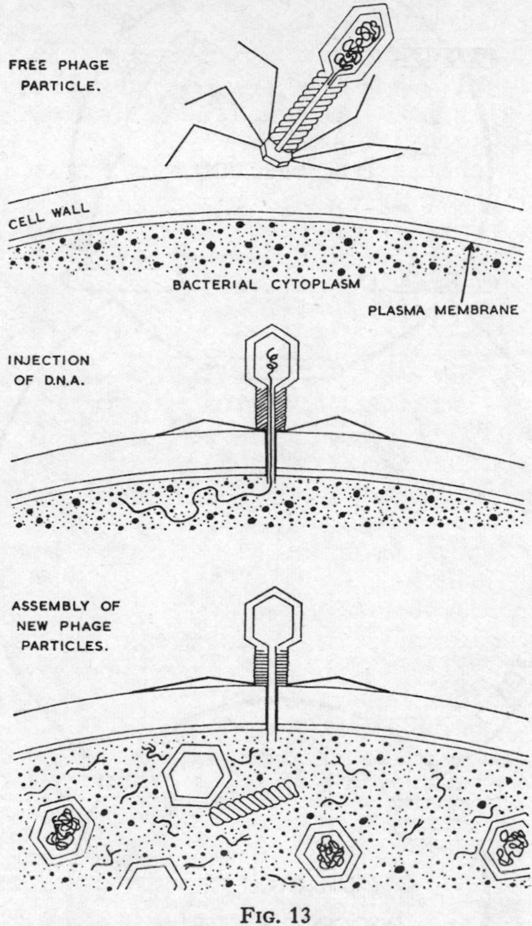

Fig. 13

Stages in the infection of the bacterial cell by bacteriophage and the replication of the phage.

and nucleic acids of the phage. The first phage-induced polymers seem to be the messenger RNA molecules concerned in coding for the synthesis of phage proteins in the host ribosomes. The first proteins produced in this way are enzymes concerned in the biosynthesis of the monomer components of the phage DNA which may differ from those of the host. This is followed by multiplication of the phage DNA and production of the structural proteins of the mature bacteriophage. The view that the various components of the phage are formed separately and that they are assembled towards the end of the reproductive cycle is confirmed by electron micrographs of infected bacteria and by biochemical and immunological evidence.

Stage E.—Phage components are assembled to form the mature particles which accumulate within the cell.

3. *Bacterial Lysis* (*lysis from within*)

When the number of mature phages within the cell reaches a critical level the bacterium lyses liberating the virus particles which may then attack further cells. The mechanism producing the lysis of the bacterium seems to be that of an accumulation of a soluble lysozyme induced in the later stages of phage growth.

Each cycle of phage reproduction may occupy 20–60 min. and in this time a single phage may produce 200 or more progeny. The precise number of new particles liberated from a single infected bacterium is known as the "burst size" and is characteristic for each phage strain.

Phage Specificity and Phage-Typing

Generally speaking phages are exceedingly specific for the host bacteria in which they can multiply. Indeed, their specificity in this respect often allows a finer differentiation between types of a species of bacterium that can be obtained by any other methods. This phenomenon is therefore often used to subdivide single bacterial species into "phage-types" according to the number and nature of the phages capable of causing their lysis, and has provided much valuable information on the spread of strains of staphylococci, salmonellae, etc. in epidemiological studies of infection in the community. The phage-typing of the staphylococcus is discussed in greater detail in Chapter 9.

The usual mechanism of the host specificity seems to lie in the process of attachment between the superficial layers of the bacterium and the tail fibres of the phage. Usually it is found that the virus will adsorb only to susceptible bacteria. It is assumed that the specific nature of this attachment is due to complementary structures in the tail of the phage (probably in the tail fibres) and in a component of the bacterial cell wall. The nature of the cell wall receptors for the *T phages* of *E. coli* has been analysed; in some cases the lipopolysaccharide of the O somatic antigen is responsible whilst in others the lipoprotein layer of the cell wall may provide the areas of attachment. However, in some phages, the host specificity does not lie solely in the adsorption process. Thus the *Vi* phages used for the typing of typhoid bacilli adsorb to all strains of *Salmonella typhi* irrespective of their type. However, a *Vi* phage will *multiply* only in a typhoid bacillus of the homologous specific type, so that if applied at a low concentration at which "lysis from without" cannot occur, it forms plaques of lysis (from within) only with this type. The reason for the specificity in such systems is unknown, but probably it must lie in some phase after the entry of the phage DNA into the host.

Lysogeny and Temperate Phages.—Infection of a bacterium with phage may result in no perceptible damage to the host cell, and in this case the phage is said to be *temperate* (Fig. 12). The initial stages of adsorption of the phage and injection of the DNA are the same as for virulent phage. However, in some of the infected bacterial cells, no breakdown of the means of bacterial growth and reproduction occurs; instead the bacterium apparently divides normally. Such cells are carrying no detectable phage, but all the progeny of the infected bacterium carry the potentiality of producing further phages and lysing at some later generation. Each cell must contain a component forming part of its genetic constitution which reproduces synchronously with the bacterium and which is capable of forming mature phage. This component is known as *prophage*, the process is known as lysogenisation, and the host bacterium is said to be *lysogenic*.

Although a temperate phage suspension will lyse a large proportion of the susceptible bacteria and so will form plaques, some of the bacterial cells will be lysogenised and thus become resistant, growing as colonies within the plaque. These resistant colonies can be shown to carry prophage since they have the capacity to develop spontaneously vegetative temperate phages. This process can be induced to the vegetative phase much more efficiently by various non-specific environmental factors such as ultraviolet light. Thus the prophage-vegetative system has the characteristics of an episome (see p. 94). Lysogenic bacteria are immune to infection by phage of the type already carried as prophage. There is thus an analogy between lysogenicity and the "latent infection" shown by animal viruses.

Phages are important agents in *transduction* in bacteria, for bacterial genetic material can be carried accidentally from host cells of one genotype to host cells of another genotype by a temperate phage. In other cases (lysogenic conversion) the prophage itself confers the new properties. For instance, non-toxigenic strains of *Corynebacterium diphtheriae* become toxigenic when lysogenised by certain phages, and similarly salmonellae may acquire new somatic antigens. Bacteriophages can thus be regarded as important factors in bacterial ecology.

The Multiplication of Animal Viruses

A purified suspension of virus particles washed free from contaminating host material is biologically inert and has none of the metabolic activities that characterise living cells. When such a suspension is injected into a susceptible host, however, the virus invades the cells and multiplies within them. The first stage of infection is adsorption of the virus particle on to the surface of the host cell. The influenza virus for instance possesses the enzyme neuraminidase which combines with mucopolysaccharide on the cell surface and thus enables the particle to attach itself. No exact knowledge is yet available of the means by which this virus invades but it is probable that the particle disintegrates on the cell surface and that only its ribonucleic acid passes through the cell wall. (What happens at this stage to the other components of the virus, such as the haemagglutinin and lipid, is unknown.)

The cell membrane of an animal cell is very much less rigid and is considerably more active than that of the bacterial cell so that virus penetration may not need the succession of events in the syringe mechanism employed by bacteriophages. Although neuraminidase facilitates attachment of the virion, penetration frequently occurs without its aid and it must be assumed that the host cell itself plays an active part in drawing in, or ingesting, the virus nucleic acid. One hypothesis is that when there is close contact between the virus and cell surfaces there is fusion of the opposing two lipoprotein membranes and the establishment of a homogeneous mass which is then engulfed by a process similar to that of pinocytosis by which non-phagocytic cells are able to ingest fluid droplets. Once within the cell the influenza virus RNA begins to initiate development of new viral material at a site in or close to the nucleus and after an *eclipse period* the cell is induced to produce a substance with the properties of the viral core. Simultaneously there occurs in the cytoplasm a different synthetic process that produces haemagglutinating particles containing protein but no nucleic acid. These two virus components migrate from the sites of their formation to the periphery of the cell where they are assembled to form new virus particles, probably with the active participation of processes initiated in the host cell membrane. The new virions are released in small numbers by a slow continuous leaking process and as they leave the host cell they acquire from the cell membrane an outer lipid covering layer which binds their components together. Viruses assembled at or on the host cell membrane are, by virtue of the lipid content of their covering membrane, easily disrupted by ether (Franklin, 1962). The virus of herpes simplex appears to have a somewhat similar method of replication although in the early phases of its growth cycle, synthesis of viral DNA and of protein occurs within the nucleus and continues until the capsid is assembled and covered by a single membrane. The particles seem to acquire a second membrane from the nuclear membrane as they enter the cytoplasm whence they are released without apparent damage to the host cell.

There is, as yet, little information available on the means by which other animal viruses attach themselves to and penetrate their host cells but there is evidence that the poliovirus disintegrates at the cell surface to release its RNA. In the case of the vaccinia virus, however, the particles are found within the host cell walls with their outer membranes intact within an hour of first contact.

Some animal viruses have the same profound effect on their host cells that a virulent phage has on a susceptible bacterium, and the reproductive cycle ends with gross damage and total destruction as the cell bursts to liberate large numbers of new particles. The pox viruses produce this effect in the skin and the damage may be so profound that severe clinical manifestations of the disease become apparent.

Other animal viruses multiply rapidly but damage the tissues mildly so that the affected cells may survive for quite long periods and the illness may be less severe. In some circumstances, *e.g.* in herpes infections in the skin of the face, a state of equilibrium may be reached similar to that established between a temperate phage and lysogenic bacterium. Such latent infections continue for long periods and it is only under the action of external stimuli, such as exposure to ultraviolet light or metabolic disturbance, that the herpes virus or the prophage are activated once more to damage their host cells and give rise to obvious effects.

Virus Tropisms.—Many animal viruses have a marked affinity for special organs and it has been customary to group them together according to their particular tissue predilections. Thus viruses were classified as dermotropic, neurotropic, pneumotropic, enterotropic and viscerotropic, but these tropisms are seldom absolute and vary as the virus is grown in the laboratory. For example the strains of the poliomyelitis virus used in Sabin's oral vaccine have changed so completely that they have lost their neurotropism and no longer damage nerve cells although they retain their enterotropism and multiply freely in the cells of the intestinal tract. Frequently a lesser variation in tissue tropism occurs in the laboratory and this indeed happens whenever a newly isolated virus is adapted to grow in any unfamiliar cell system. Tissue tropisms are *not* closely related to the other properties of a virus and thus constitute only one of a number of minor criteria used in virus taxonomy.

Little is known of the factors that determine the susceptibility or resistance of any particular tissue to an individual virus, but the surface configuration and chemical structures of the cell membrane are important factors just as they are in the bacterium phage system. In the case of the poliovirus Holland and Hayer (1962) have shown that a specific receptor (probably an insoluble lipo-protein complex) is present in the membrane of susceptible nerve cells and that it is absent from organs and tissues not normally attacked.

Inclusion Bodies.—During the course of multiplication, many viruses are associated with the appearance of large distinctive structures known as inclusion bodies. They may be situated either in the cytoplasm, or in the nucleus or, as in the case of measles, in both. The inclusion bodies are often acidophilic and usually appear as pink masses in smears or sections stained with Giemsa's stain or with Mann's eosin methyl-blue stain; basophilic inclusions are characteristic of the psittacosis-lymphogranuloma group. In size they vary from 1 to 30 μ in diameter. In certain infections the inclusion body is intimately concerned with the reproductive cycle and can be seen to contain large numbers of virus particles when it is examined electron-microscopically. During the early stages of the formation of an inclusion the elementary bodies are held within it in a jelly-like matrix.

Intracytoplasmic inclusion bodies are often so characteristic in their appearance that their presence in tissues is of diagnostic significance. One large inclusion, the Negri body, is up to 20 μ in diameter and acidophilic; its presence in the nerve cells of the hippocampus of the dog's brain justifies the presumptive diagnosis of rabies. Rather smaller multiple inclusions are found in the cells of hosts infected with the vaccinia virus and are known as Guarnieri bodies. Very large inclusions known as Bollinger bodies are characteristic of fowl-pox and those of molluscum contagiosum are so large ($20 \times 30\ \mu$) that they are easily visible in sections of the skin seen under the low power microscope.

Intranuclear inclusions are acidophilic and may be of two types; Cowdry Type A is granular in appearance and of variable size, and is found in herpes simplex, zoster, varicella and yellow fever; Type B, which is more circumscribed and sometimes multiple, is found in poliomyelitis, adenovirus infections and Rift Valley fever.

The fundamental characters described can be used to place the great majority of animal viruses into eight main groups. These are (1) the *poxviruses*, so-called from the skin lesions they produce, (2) the *myxoviruses* named from their affinity for mucus, (3) the *herpesviruses* named from the creeping lesions of shingles, (4) the *adenoviruses* which were first found inhabiting adenoid lymphatic tissue, (5) the *reoviruses* associated with respiratory enteric infections, (6) the *arboviruses* which are arthropod-borne, (7) the enteroviruses together with the rhinoviruses are now to be called "*picornaviruses*" (pico implies a very small virus and RNA, of course, indicates the nucleic acid content). (8) the papilloma (PA), polyoma (PO), vacuolating agent (VA), *papovaviruses*. A more complete classification of the viruses of vertebrate hosts is given (Andrewes, 1963) on p. 83 *et seq.*

A Summary of the Fundamental Characters of the Eight Main Groups of Animal Viruses (after Andrewes, 1962)

Virus Group	Nucleic Acid	Size in mμ	Number of Capsomeres	Membrane covering capsid	Maturation at cell surface	Ether Sensitivity
1. Poxviruses	DNA	300 × 250	?	+	0	+ or 0
2. Myxoviruses	RNA	100 – 300	?	+	+	+
3. Herpesviruses	DNA	120	162	+	0	+
4. Adenoviruses	DNA	60 – 85	252	None	0	0
5. Reoviruses	RNA	75	92	None	0	0
6. Arboviruses	RNA	40	?	?	+	+
7. Picornaviruses	RNA	20 – 30	42?	None	0	0
8. Papovaviruses	DNA	25 – 45	42	?	0	0

Pathogenesis.—The point at which a virus enters the host's body and the course of its subsequent growth is determined partly by the nature of the virus itself and partly by the resistance or susceptibility of the cells concerned. When the virus multiplies it may spread only from cell to cell producing a small focal lesion, as for example a wart or a single molluscum contagiosum body. Viruses deposited on mucous membranes of the respiratory tract, however, may multiply and spread over much larger areas producing, in the nose, a common cold or in the trachea and bronchi an attack of influenza. The mode by which the virus spreads over the mucosae is probably by a combination of the cilia-motivated flow of infected mucus and the migration of virus-laden leucocytes.

In other infections the virus may spread from its site of primary multiplication to the local lymph nodes. This often happens in primary cutaneous vaccination against smallpox when the axillary lymph glands enlarge. In severe infections with such viruses as those of smallpox or poliomyelitis, the process continues even further and virus is liberated into the lymph channels and carried thence into the blood stream to give rise to viraemia and the generalisation of infection throughout the whole body. These events mark the conclusion of the "incubation period" of the disease and during the next few days prodromal signs, particularly fever and malaise, occur as the "target organs" are being invaded by the virus. When massive areas of the target organs have been destroyed by the virus the severe clinical form of the illness becomes obvious, *e.g.* the skin rash of smallpox and the paralysis in poliomyelitis. The damage that viruses do to tissues usually takes the form of degenerative changes in foci of virus-infected cells; these foci are surrounded by an outpouring of inflammatory cells that are predominantly monocytic. The nature of the degenerative changes depends on the type of the cell involved and on whether the virus multiplies in the nucleus or the cytoplasm; the anterior horn cells in the spinal cord in paralytic poliomyelitis show granulation of the cytoplasm and severe nuclear damage, whereas the epithelial cells in the epidermis in smallpox show ballooning of the cytoplasm and later break down to form vesicles. Some viruses do not destroy the host cells but stimulate them to proliferation and to form tumours; in man, the warts virus produces a small, innocent, localised papilloma whilst in mice polyoma viruses give rise to multiple highly malignant neoplasms.

Infectivity.—Viruses, as a group, are highly pathogenic in minute doses. Serum from a case of infectious hepatitis injected in a dose of less than 0·1 ml. has been known to transmit the disease. A millionth part of 1·0 ml. of a 10 per cent. brain suspension from an infected monkey is sufficient to infect another animal with yellow fever.

Epidemics are particularly characteristic of many virus diseases. Influenza assumes major epidemic proportions at irregular intervals of three to five years and at roughly forty-year intervals sweeps over the whole world, as is witnessed in the pandemic of 1918-19 and the Asian influenza of 1957. Smallpox is notorious for the ease and rapidity with which it spreads and for the severity of the epidemics it causes. Amongst animals, foot and mouth disease and fowl pest have an amazing power to spread not only from one host to the next but from one geographical location to another.

The transmission of virus infections may occur in many ways. Direct transmission by contact between persons is responsible for the spread of the inclusion conjunctivitis virus which inhabits the human genital tract and spreads from one consort to another during sexual intercourse; later it reaches the eyes of a baby as it passes through the birth canal. Similarly the virus of molluscum contagiosum spreads by direct contact of skin to skin. Spread by means of the ingestion of infected food or drink is the main method by which polioviruses and other enteroviruses reach new victims after leaving the body of the previous host in the faeces. Droplets of infected mucus sneezed out by patients suffering from common colds or influenza possibly convey the infection through the air and may be inhaled by the next person in the chain of infection. Dust contaminated with the organism of Q fever may be breathed in and give its recipient an attack of pneumonia. (It should be noted, however, that there is very little good evidence available to indicate the relative importance of droplets, dust, contact and other *possible* mechanisms in the spread of the respiratory tract viruses.) A dog may bite a victim and introduce directly into the tissues the rabies virus which is present in its saliva. Mosquitoes, ticks and other arthropod vectors carry viruses for long periods in their bodies and when they bite man they are able to infect him by the injection of the virus in their saliva.

Virus Haemagglutination

Some viruses, notably those of the influenza group, cause the agglutination of the red blood cells of man, fowls, guinea-pigs and other animals. Virus particles attach themselves to the surface of these cells by means of enzymatic groups which react with a mucopolysaccharide substrate in exactly the same way as they adhere to the surface of the epithelial cells of the bronchioles.

When red blood cells are added to a virus suspension each cell becomes speckled with many adherent virions; often one particle is attached to one or more cells forming a bridge between them and fastening them together. In this way the cells are agglutinated into masses which fall rapidly in the suspending fluid to settle on the bottom of the tube in an irregular ragged pattern. Once the cells have been agglutinated, and when the substrate in the *receptor areas* has been exhausted, dissociation occurs and the virus is liberated. Red blood cells treated in this way are permanently damaged and can no longer be agglutinated by the virus, which is unaltered by the process and retains its power to agglutinate fresh cells.

Haemagglutination is probably a model of the first stage of the natural infection of cells, because the mucopolysaccharide substrate which enables the virus to attach itself to the red cell envelope, is also found on the surface of the epithelial cells of the respiratory tract. In this way the influenza virus can be intimately applied to the surface of its host cell and has only to traverse the cell wall to initiate infection. The mucopolysaccharide substrate is also present in mucus from the intestine, ovarian cysts, milk, urine and serum; it is often referred to as a "non-specific inhibitor" of virus action. A similar enzyme is also found in some bacteria, notably the cholera vibrio and *Cl. welchii*; it is usually called the "receptor destroying enzyme" (RDE). The property of haemagglutination resides in the virus particle itself; in the case of the influenza virus it is formed early in the reproductive cycle and can be demonstrated in immature, or "incomplete" virus, which is not yet infective.

The haemagglutination reaction is important in laboratory work because it provides a simple and rapid method by which virus can be detected in egg and tissue culture fluids. Furthermore infected cells in tissue cultures adsorb red blood cells to their surfaces (haemadsorption) and are thus shown to be harbouring virus. Haemagglutination is also the basis of a method of virus purification. Virus in crude infected fluids is adsorbed on red cells which are then sedimented; after removal of the supernatant the virus is eluted into a small volume of clean fluid and the erythrocytes are removed by slow centrifugation.

Haemagglutination is found in other groups of viruses. Poxviruses give the reaction, but their haemagglutinin is distinct from the intact infective virus. The haemagglutinin of the vaccinia virus is destroyed by lecithinase (*e.g.* α toxin of *Cl. welchii*) and is a lipoprotein; it is a much smaller particle than the virus itself and can be separated from it by centrifugation or adsorption with red blood cells.

The arthropod-borne viruses which cause such infections as dengue, yellow fever, Japanese B and other types of encephalitis also possess haemagglutinins, as also does the mouse pneumonia virus (PVM). These haemagglutinins appear to have a reversible state of equilibrium with erythrocytes; they are inhibited by lipids and are very sensitive to slight variations of pH. The members of the group of adenoviruses agglutinate the red blood cells of monkeys, mice, and rats. Certain types of ECHO viruses agglutinate human group O erythrocytes and in the process the red cell receptors are exhausted.

Haemagglutination reactions of many of these types are used in antibody estimations. Viruses when mixed with antibodies lose their power to agglutinate red blood cells; the extent to which a serum is able to inhibit haemagglutination is a measure of its antibody content. *Haemagglutination inhibition* tests are highly specific and are particularly valuable in serological work with the variants of the influenza viruses.

Interference

When animals are inoculated with certain viruses they may become resistant for a while to the effects of a second and more virulent virus. The injection of Rift Valley Fever virus into monkeys, in which it causes only a mild illness, protects them against the challenge of a lethal dose of the yellow fever virus and similarly the benign lymphocytic choriomeningitis virus excludes the effects of infection with the poliomyelitis virus. The viruses in these examples of interference are unrelated and are distinct immunologically.

There are, however, many other instances of interference where the two viruses are more closely related and in these the phenomenon can be clearly demonstrated in experiments with chick embryo and tissue cultures. Thus previous infection with influenza A virus precludes subsequent invasion by another influenza A virus, or the mumps or Newcastle viruses. There is some evidence to suggest that interference may occur under natural conditions in man, for if patients convalescent from infection with dengue type I virus are challenged with the immunologically distinct dengue II virus they can be shown to have some resistance.

Interference has frequently been observed to occur between viruses and their own mutants; the dermotropic vaccinia virus suppresses the growth of its neurotropic variant, and non-encephalitogenic strains of the herpes simplex virus protect the rabbit against virulent encephalitogenic strains.

The interfering action of living viruses may be due to a variety of causes. Enzymatically active virus may destroy or occupy all the receptor areas on the host cell and thus prevent access by the second virus; or the interfering virus may compete successfully for the control of enzyme systems and nucleic acid synthesis within the cell, leaving no metabolic processes available for the second virus. It is also possible that the mechanism of escape of the interfering virus from the cell is blocked and that this prevents invasion by the challenging virus. In short, if the cell is occupied by an interfering virus a second virus may be unable to enter.

It must be remembered, however, that there are some occasions when two viruses can invade and multiply in the same cell simultaneously without interference occurring. When one virus is situated in the nucleus and the other in the cytoplasm both can reproduce unhindered, *e.g.* herpes simplex and vaccinia, measles and poliomyelitis.

Killed virus as well as living virus possesses the power to interfere. Heat at 56° C. and exposure to ultra-violet light destroy the infectivity of a virus without affecting its capacity for interference.

Interferon.—The mechanisms of viral interference became more clearly understandable when Isaacs and Lindemann (1957) showed that virus-containing cells release a soluble substance which has the power to reproduce the effects of an interfering virus. This substance they named "*interferon*" and their first observations showed that influenza virus inactivated by heat or ultra-violet light was able to stimulate the cells of growing fragments of chick chorio-allantoic membrane to release interferon in considerable amounts. It was soon discovered, however, that many different animal viruses possessed this property and that interferon production also occurs when cells are infected with living viruses. Deoxyviruses such as the poxviruses as well as riboviruses such as the myxoviruses, and the arbo- and enteroviruses can all stimulate interferon production. No matter which virus initiates the reaction, the interferon produced is always essentially the same substance. It must be emphasised that interferon is a host cell product.

Interferon differs from the original virus in many ways. It is much smaller, it is not neutralised by specific viral antisera, and it cannot be adsorbed on to erythrocytes. The interferon particle is composed of protein with a molecular weight of 20,000—34,000 and a trace of carbohydrate; it is non-dialysable and contains *no* nucleic acid (Lampson *et al.*, 1963). Interferon is destroyed by proteolytic enzymes but is insensitive to non-proteolytic enzymes such as amylase, lipase and deoxyribonuclease. Although it is a protein, it is not antigenic, even when injected together with adjuvants. It is stable over the pH range 2—11 and its ability to withstand pH 2 is useful in distinguishing it from inactivated viruses. Purified interferon is adsorbed strongly to glass, paper, starch, and agar but not to polypropylene vessels. It can be eluted from glass by the use of bovine albumin or Tween 80. The production of interferon in cell cultures is inhibited by cortisone, a finding that may offer an explanation of the way this drug is able to enhance the severity of so many virus infections. There is some evidence to suggest that interferon production may be a general response to the introduction of foreign nucleic acids into the host cell.

When a cell has been invaded by a virus the interferon produced diffuses to neighbouring cells and confers on them a temporary resistance which limits the spread of infection and probably plays a part in the recovery from disease. Cells that have been treated with interferon can still take in the virus particle which, however, is unable to multiply. The action of interferon is entirely on the host cell and it is without any direct effect on the virus. The exact mode of its action is not yet understood but it is likely that it inhibits some oxidative process that supplies the vital energy for the synthesis of viral DNA or RNA, possibly by uncoupling phosphorylation from oxidation. Oxygen tension plays a critical role in the production of interferon. If oxygen in the atmosphere is replaced by nitrogen little or no interferon is produced. Conversely if a high oxygen tension pertains, as when mice are infected with influenza virus and held in an atmosphere of 50 per cent. oxygen, they fail to produce interferon in their lung tissues and suffer an increased mortality and die earlier than control animals kept in the ordinary atmosphere.

Cancer cells and the cells of very young chick embryos are insensitive to the anti-viral actions of interferon and this may be related to the fact that both these two types of cells are able to carry out the glycolysis of glucose under anaerobic conditions and that they do not require oxidative phosphorylation for their energy requirements. It is probable that the interferon mechanism is developed by the cells only after the first third of embryonic life and if this is true it would offer an explanation of the great susceptibility of early embryonic tissues to virus infections. This could also explain why mothers infected with the rubella virus during the first three months of pregnancy are very liable to have babies with congenital abnormalities, whereas others infected later in pregnancy only rarely have abnormal children. The ability of a virus to stimulate interferon production is closely and inversely related to its virulence and to the optimum temperature for its growth. Avirulent strains of the poliomyelitis and measles viruses are known to cause considerable interferon production, but wild and virulent strains of these viruses stimulate little or no interferon reaction by the host cell. Viruses with high optimal temperatures for growth, *e.g.* Newcastle disease virus at 42° C. and fowl plague virus at 39° C., are less sensitive to interferon than those that grow at lower temperatures, *e.g.* some arboviruses at 35° C. and common cold viruses at 32° C. It is generally true that virulent viruses with high optimal growth temperatures are weak inducers of interferon production in the host cell (Isaacs, 1962).

Since interferon is non-toxic, non-antigenic and active against many different viruses it may have an important role to play in medicine. If interferon is injected locally it will prevent infection of the human skin with the vaccinia virus, but its value as a therapeutic agent in established virus disease has yet to be determined.

The Cultivation of Animal Viruses

To cultivate viruses it is always necessary to provide living host cells; no inanimate culture medium can meet the growth requirements of a virus and there is no evidence that reproduction ever takes place outside a living cell. Host cells are usually provided in one of three forms:

(1) The experimental animal.
(2) Chick embryos.
(3) Tissue cultures.

Animal Inoculation was at one time the only method available, but has now been largely replaced by newer methods. In general, animal inoculation techniques depend for their success on the demonstration of a recognisable disease or death after a defined time interval. The presence of inclusion bodies of characteristic morphology in the animal's tissues provides additional evidence of virus infection. The poliomyelitis virus, for example, after intraspinal or intracerebral inoculation causes typical paralytic disease in the monkey, while the variola or smallpox virus causes the formation of lesions in the scarified skin or cornea of the rabbit (Paul's Test) accompanied by the appearance of multiple eosinophilic intracytoplasmic inclusions in the epithelial cells. Since these methods are slow and full of technical difficulties, they are employed only when no other means is available. When animals are suspected of rabies, brain tissue is taken at autopsy and is inoculated intracerebrally in mice and rabbits; if virus is present the animals develop encephalitis and die seven to ten days later. Coxsackie viruses are identified by their unique property of causing severe myositis and paralysis in suckling mice. In yellow fever, antibodies in the serum are detected and titrated by their power to protect mice against a lethal dose of the virus.

Chick Embryos provide more satisfactory hosts for they are clean and bacteriologically sterile; they also have the advantage that they lack any protective specific immune mechanism to counteract virus infection. Vaccinia and the other pox viruses together with the herpes simplex virus all produce lesions on the chorio-allantoic membrane which are highly characteristic and easily recognisable with the naked eye. Influenza viruses multiply in the cells of the embryo's lungs and in the cells lining the allantoic cavity and they are recognised by their haemagglutination and haemadsorption properties. The bedsoniae and rickettsiae grow well in the yolk sac and usually kill the embryos within well defined time limits.

Tissue Cultures of human or simian cells are the most frequently used and are relatively simple to prepare in the large quantities that are required by modern diagnostic virological methods. Suspensions of cells dispersed from tissue fragments or from bulk cultures of cell lines such as HeLa, are obtained by tryptic digestion The cells adhere to the walls of the test-tubes and grow out to form a sheet, or *monolayer*, which is easily observed *in situ* under the low power objective of the microscope.

The details of the techniques of egg cultivation and tissue culture are given in Chapter 57.

THE ASSAY OF ANIMAL VIRUSES

The presence of a virus in infected tissues or exudates is demonstrated by the methods of cultivation already described and by the observation of changes in whatever host system is employed. But it is often essential in medical diagnostic work, in fundamental studies of the growth of viruses, and in observing activity of antibodies and antiviral agents, to have some means of estimating accurately the numbers of virus particles.

There are many methods for counting, the most direct is that of spraying a fine aerosol of the virus-containing fluid on to electron microscope grids. The droplets of the aerosol are of known volume as estimated by physical measurements or the inclusion of known numbers of reference latex particles in the virus suspension; the virus particles contained are deposited in a circumscribed area so that they can be counted on the electron-micrograph. Of course, preparations of this sort give only a total count which includes both living and dead virus particles; if a viable count is needed an estimate must be made of the infectivity of the particles.

The numbers of infective virus particles can be counted by inoculating a series of gradually diminishing doses of the viruses into groups of susceptible animals, eggs, or tissue cultures.

The Cytopathic Effect (CPE) of the virus on the host cell is much used for the determination of the infectivity titre of a virus suspension. Viruses as they grow in tissue cultures produce different effects varying from rapid and complete necrosis of the host cells in 48 hours to a slow rounding off and minor types of degeneration appearing many days after infection. The CPE is easily observed with the low-power objective of the light microscope and is given by nearly all the major groups of animal viruses. Sometimes the effects are characteristic for the virus concerned, as for example the giant cells and syncytia formed when tissue cultures are infected with the herpes or measles viruses. The infectivity titre of a virus culture can be determined by the inoculation of a series of diminishing amounts of it into a sufficient number of tissue cultures and the definition of the minimal dose needed to produce a CPE.

A point is reached where a given dose of the virus produces a recognisable effect in one-half of the inoculated hosts. When, as usually happens, none of the inocula used gives exactly a 50 per cent. incidence of infection, the size of the inoculum that would have done so may be calculated by the formulae mentioned in Chapter 52. The 50 per cent. incidence of infection represents the end point of a virus titration; the inoculum giving this result in animals is known as the LD50 (50 per cent. lethal dose), the EID50 (for infectivity in eggs), or the TCD50 (for tissue culture effects).

The plaque counting technique offers another convenient method of estimating the number of living virus particles. If a suitable dilution of a virus is added to a confluent sheet of susceptible cells growing in a Petri dish visible plaques appear wherever the virus attacks and lyses the cells. When a virus particle enters a single cell, it multiplies and destroys the cell, and then spreads to contiguous cells; the process is then repeated until a visible area of clearing (*a plaque*) results. With small virus inocula each plaque represents a single infective virus particle and by counting the plaques that result from a given volume of a virus dilution an estimate can be made of the total number of plaque forming units (*i.e.* infective virus particles) present. The proportion of the total number of particles as estimated under the electron microscope to the number of plaque forming units (*i.e.* viable virus particles) gives an estimate of the "*plating efficiency*" of the virus preparation. Under optimal conditions bacteriophages have a very high plating efficiency (1·0) and each particle may be infective, but with animal viruses (*e.g.* vaccinia) the infectivity may be much lower because some of the viruses may be inactive or some of the host cells insusceptible. With plant viruses the plating efficiency is usually poor and a hundred or more particles are needed to establish infection. Plaque counting methods have a general application in experiments with bacteriophages and with animal viruses growing in tissue culture monolayers. A very similar method is used for those animal viruses that produce lesions on the chorio-allantoic membrane of the chick embryo and is known as the *pock counting technique.*

These assay methods rely on the infectivity of virus particles to reveal their presence but there are other properties that can be used for this purpose.

Haemagglutination is one such property that is frequently used in estimations of the number of virus particles present in the fluids of egg cultures of the myxoviruses. The haemagglutinin titre of a virus fluid gives an index of the number of virus particles present, but the figure obtained is often higher than that obtained in infectivity experiments. This apparent discrepancy is due partly to the fact that immature or "incomplete" virus particles acquire the property of haemagglutination before they become fully infective and partly to the fact that virus particles exposed to heat or other physical agents retain their power to agglutinate red blood cells long after losing their ability to reproduce. Myxo- and arboviruses as they grow induce a change in their host cells so that red blood cells attach themselves to the cell walls. This phenomenon is known as *haemadsorption* and is of special value in the assay of para-influenza viruses.

Antigenic components that can be detected by serological methods, such as complement fixation, precipitation, or haemagglutination inhibition are also often used in virus assay and provide the means whereby the potency of an antigen can be gauged before use in diagnostic antibody tests. By mixing gradually diminishing amounts of the virus with a fixed quantity of a suitable antiserum the amount of virus can be determined by the manner and degree with which the two reagents combine together. In tests of this type the antigen concerned is usually the protein of the viral capsid.

Metabolic Effects.—The multiplication of many viruses (notably the polioviruses) damages the host cells so profoundly that their normal metabolic processes cease. In tissue cultures this effect becomes obvious because the damaged cells can no longer liberate acid and the phenol red indicator of the culture medium fails to change colour in the same way as it does in control uninfected cultures. This colour change is used to titrate the activity of enteroviruses in tissue cultures and also to estimate the power of antibodies to check virus growth.

VIRUS MUTATION

Although some animal viruses such as those of mumps and measles are remarkably stable over many years, others, like the influenza virus A, show a striking lability with a marked tendency to variation and mutation of some of their characters. In a growing population of the latter viruses mutation occurs constantly and there is a continuously active process of selective proliferation and survival which determines the character of the dominant virus. There is much laboratory evidence to prove that new virus forms emerge as a result of this process. Mutant viruses can differ from the parent strains in many ways; they may have an increased rate of reproduction, altered haemagglutinating characters, increased or diminished pathogenicity or modified antigenic structure. It is its high mutability and the plasticity of its antigenic structure that enables the influenza virus A to assume a new form at irregular intervals and to initiate frequent epidemics.

In contrast, other mutants remain antigenically stable but lose the pathogenicity of the parent strain; such mutants are referred to as being "attenuated". Thus the vaccinia virus has retained antigens of the variola virus but has lost its power to produce smallpox, and the 17D strain still contains the antigens of the yellow fever virus although it lacks its virulence. Both these mutants are of great importance because they can be used safely as highly efficient immunising agents.

The isolation of mutants of this type from other viruses is a matter of importance because vaccines containing live virus impart a fuller measure of durable immunity than do those containing killed virus. The selection of an attenuated mutant is usually accomplished by passing large doses of the original virus in a series of rapid transfers in an unfamiliar host, so that any fast-growing mutant will have optimal conditions for survival. When a mutant reproduces more rapidly than the parent strain it can be separated in a pure clone from a single virus particle. This can be done by making "limiting infective dilutions" and transferring to a new host, or by plating on a monolayer of cells in tissue culture, using the plaque technique.

By these methods, attenuated mutants have been obtained from the three poliomyelitis viruses and have been used in the living state as vaccines for oral administration. Using egg cultivation methods, attenuated strains of the rabies virus (Flury strain), the canine distemper virus, and the rinderpest virus have been obtained and have provided efficient vaccines for veterinary use.

Recombination.—If a host cell is confronted by two animal viruses simultaneously, there are three possible outcomes: (*a*) both viruses may enter and multiply without either influencing the other; (*b*) entry of one virus may inhibit the multiplication of the second (interference); (*c*) the presence of the first virus may influence the reproductive processes of the second and *vice versa*, so that the progeny develop characters derived from both the parent viruses. In the third eventuality a genetic transfer of material between the two growing closely related viruses has occurred and is referred to as a process of *recombination.* It has been shown for example that the neuropathogenicity of a variant of influenza virus A (NWS) can be transferred under these circumstances to another influenza virus (MEL) that lacks this quality. Recombination has been most intensively studied in the group of influenza viruses, but has been induced between vaccinia and rabbit pox, and in strains of the psittacosis virus. It is not known how frequently hybrids of this type occur under natural conditions but the mechanism may offer an explanation for the evolution of new viruses. For further reading on the subject of virus genetics the reader is referred to a review of the work of Burnet (1959) and to Fenner & Sambrook (1964).

ANTIVIRAL IMMUNITY

Resistance to infection with viruses depends on the same defence mechanisms that operate against bacteria. Viral infection is consistently followed by the development of specific antibodies that can be measured by the usual immunological methods, such as complement fixation, neutralisation and precipitation. Natural immunity, together with species-specific resistance, is as familiar in virus diseases as it is in bacterial infections. The rôle of antibodies in overcoming viral infections lies principally in their power to combine with the invading microorganism and to prevent it gaining access to the host's cells. In this way they are less efficient than antitoxins, which combine rapidly and avidly with bacterial toxins, but far more effective than the humoral antibodies in such infections as tuberculosis or typhoid fever. In the rare condition of hypogammaglobulinaemia, children do not develop antibodies after receiving inoculations of antigens nor after recovery from measles, mumps, chickenpox, or Jennerian vaccination. And yet these conditions are no more severe than in ordinary children and after recovery the children are clinically resistant to re-infection or re-vaccination. Viral immunity must rest on other factors besides humoral antibodies, and it seems probable that cellular resistance together with interference and interferon production by other viruses may be of importance. The rôle of phagocytic cells and the value to the host of non-specific factors such as complement is still undetermined.

The outstanding feature of all virus infections is the intracellular situation of the growing virus; here it is protected by the cell membrane which is an impervious barrier to circulating antibodies. It is this circumstance which renders ineffective the therapeutic use of antiserum once a virus infection is established; in paralytic poliomyelitis, for example, antibodies given in the form of convalescent serum or as gamma-globulin do not benefit the patient, because they cannot reach the virus as it grows within the horn cells of the spinal cord. The real value in medicine of antibodies lies in their capacity to neutralise the virus *before* it reaches the host cells. Thus the early prophylactic use of human gamma globulin is highly effective in preventing the establishment of clinical infection in persons recently exposed to measles or infective hepatitis.

Some virus infections are followed by a prolonged immunity that may persist for life, while in others it may last for only a few months. A prolonged immunity is characteristic of measles, mumps, smallpox, yellow fever and second attacks of these diseases are extremely rare. It is significant that in all these diseases there is a phase of viraemia and often a long incubation period. Probably the long incubation period allows time for a secondary antibody response to become effective before the stage at which symptoms of the infection would become apparent. After multiplication in a primary focus of infection for about ten days, the virus overflows into the bloodstream; it is then carried to fresh host cells at a distance where it may multiply to produce a rash and provide a powerful secondary stimulus to antibody production. Viruses that give long-lasting immunity are almost invariably antigenically stable and it is rare for them under natural circumstances to vary or mutate.

One explanation of the reasons for the long persistence of a solid immunity may be that the virus remains alive in a modified form within affected cells to act continually as a stimulus to antibody formation. It must, however, be stated that whenever such events have been proved to occur, as in herpes simplex infection around the lips in man, or in benign lymphocytic choriomeningitis infections in mice, there is, instead of a solid immunity, a marked tendency to relapse with recrudescence of clinical lesions.

Limited immunity of short duration occurs most frequently in conditions where there is no evidence of a viraemic phase and where the infecting virus has a marked tendency to antigenic variation. Influenza, the common cold, and many other viral infections of the upper respiratory tract are followed by immunity of very short duration and second attacks of these illnesses occur very frequently. They are infections of surface mucous membranes and the viruses reach the host cells directly by the inhalation of infected particles without being exposed to antibodies or virucidal mechanisms in the bloodstream. Immunity to influenza and the common cold is further limited by the existence of multiple immunological types of the viruses. An attack of influenza is, of course, followed by the development of specific antibodies, but these are of limited effectiveness in protecting the individual, partly because the next virus may be of a novel antigenic type and partly because there is little opportunity for contact between virus and antibody. It is possible that the small measure of immunity that does follow an attack of influenza is mediated by antibodies present in the nasal secretions.

Although humoral antibodies arising after a viral disease are accepted as a very important factor in increasing the individuals' resistance and in preventing a virus from reaching the host cells it must be remembered that other protective mechanisms also operate. One of these is the mechanism of hypersensitivity in which the host cells themselves are rendered resistant to invasion by the infecting virus. The importance of allergy in resistance to viral infections is not yet well understood but for further information the reader should consult Beveridge (1963).

CLASSIFICATION OF THE VIRUSES OF VERTEBRATE HOSTS

The extent of our knowledge is not yet sufficient to warrant the use of the Linnaean binomial nomenclature used for bacteria. It is, however, possible to group the viruses of vertebrate hosts according to some of their outstanding properties and to distinguish the individual members of the groups. There has been international agreement that the following criteria should be used in the classification (Andrewes, 1963).

1. Morphology, size, and methods of reproduction.
2. Chemical composition and physical properties.
3. Immunological properties.
4. Susceptibility to physical and chemical agents.
5. Natural methods of transmission.
6. Host, tissue and cell tropisms.
7. Pathology and inclusion body formation.
8. Symptomatology (deliberately placed last as of minor importance).

Using these criteria, over 350 animal viruses have been placed in eight main groups most of which are divided into sub-sections of closely related species. In some cases the name of the group is followed by the suffix "virus" and a descriptive adjective is added. Such Latinised names are only applied to a few viruses and as yet they are but little used.

Group I.—Pox viruses (about 20 types)

(*a*) Variola-like viruses:
Poxvirus variolae (smallpox virus)
Poxvirus officinalis (vaccinia virus)
Poxvirus bovis (cow-pox virus)
Poxvirus muris (ectromelia virus)
Poxvirus cuniculi (rabbit-pox virus)
Poxvirus simiae (monkey-pox virus)

(*b*) Pox viruses affecting ungulates:
Contagious pustular dermatitis (orf) virus
Papular stomatis (bovine) virus
Horse pox virus — Swine pox virus
Goat pox virus — Camel pox virus
Sheep pox virus

(*c*) Avian pox viruses:
Poxvirus avium (fowl-pox virus)
Pigeon-pox virus
Canary-pox virus

(*d*) Myxoma-like viruses:
Rabbit myxoma virus — Rabbit fibroma virus

(*e*) Miscellaneous:
Molluscum contagiosum virus
Para-vaccinia virus (? milkers nodes)

GROUP 2.—Myxoviruses (about 20 types)

(*a*) True influenza viruses:
Myxovirus influenzae A
Myxovirus influenzae B
Myxovirus influenzae C
Myxovirus pestis galli (fowl plague)
Influenza virus A porci (swine influenza)
Influenza virus A equi (horse influenza)
Influenza virus A anatis (duck influenza)

(*b*) Paramyxoviruses (multiform viruses):
Myxovirus parotitidis (mumps virus)
Myxovirus multiforme (Newcastle virus)
Myxovirus para-influenzae 1 (sendai virus)
Myxovirus para-influenzae 2 (croup associated virus)
Myxovirus para-influenzae 3 (haemadsorption virus)
Myxovirus para-influenzae 4
Simian myxovirus (SV5).

(*c*) Measles virus
Canine distemper virus
Rinderpest virus

(*d*) Avian tumour viruses:
The viruses of fowl lymphomatosis, myeloblastosis, erythroblastosis, sarcomata and osteopetrosis

GROUP 3.—Herpesviruses (about 35 types)

(*a*) *Herpesvirus hominum* (herpes simplex virus)
Herpesvirus varicellae (varicella and zoster)
Herpesvirus suis (pseudo-rabies virus)
Herpesvirus simiae (virus B)
Herpesvirus cuniculi (virus III)

(*b*) Cytomegaloviruses:
  Inclusion or salivary virus of man
  Inclusion virus of guinea-pigs

(*c*) Avian viruses:
  Infectious laryngotracheitis (ILT)

(*d*) Miscellaneous:
  Lumpy skin disease virus
  Infectious bovine rhinotracheitis virus

GROUP 4.—Adenoviruses (about 145 types)

Human adenoviruses (at least 31 serotypes)
Simian adenoviruses (at least 11 serotypes)
Canine hepatitis virus
Fowl strain (GAL)
Mouse strain

GROUP 5.—Reoviruses

Human respiratory and enteric disease viruses (three serotypes)

GROUP 6.—Arboviruses (about 150 types)

(*a*) Group A:
  Equine encephalomyelitis viruses (Eastern, Western and Venezuelan)
  Semliki Forest virus
  Chikungunya virus
  Sindbis virus
  and eight other named viruses

(*b*) Group B:
  Yellow fever virus
  Dengue (several serotypes) viruses
  St. Louis encephalitis virus
  Japanese B encephalitis virus
  Murray Valley fever virus
  Louping ill virus
  Russian tick-borne encephalitis virus
  Kyasanur Forest Disease virus
  and at least 17 other named viruses

(*c*) Group C:
  Marituba virus and five others all from the Amazon

(*d*) Bunyamwera group and seven other viruses

(*e*) Culicoides-borne viruses:
  African horse sickness viruses (seven or more serotypes)
  Blue tongue viruses (11 serotypes)

(*f*) Small groups. 25 viruses fall into 9 groups and 13 others show no close relationship to any other arboviruses (*e.g.* the two serotypes of the sandfly fever virus)

GROUP 7.—Picorna viruses (*pico* indicates very small and RNA the type of nucleic acid). About 100 types.

These viruses include the large group formerly known as enteroviruses

(*a*) *Poliovirus hominis*: 3 serotypes
(*b*) *Poliovirus muris* (mouse encephalomyelitis virus Theiler)
(*c*) Coxsackie A viruses: 24 serotypes
(*d*) Coxsackie B viruses: 6 serotypes
(*e*) ECHO viruses: 30 serotypes
(*f*) Enteroviruses of
cattle (ECBO): at least 3 serotypes
swine (ECSO): at least 5 serotypes
cats (ECCO)
birds (ECAO): several serotypes
(*g*) JH, 2060 (ECHO 28) cold viruses
(*h*) Rhinoviruses
(*i*) Teschen disease virus
(*j*) Foot and mouth disease virus: 5 serotypes
(*k*) Encephalomyocarditis viruses
EMC, COL SK, MENGO and other strains
(*l*) Encephalomyelitis viruses of mice
FA and GD VII strains

GROUP 8.—Papova viruses

This group contains the papilloma and polyoma viruses and vacuolating agent of monkeys (Hence PA – PO – VA)

Papilloma (warts) in man
Rabbit papilloma virus
Papilloma viruses of cattle, goats, horses, dogs and other animals
Vacuolating agent of monkeys (SV 40)

Unclassified Viruses.—There exist a considerable number of viruses that as yet cannot be placed in the main groups. In particular the rabies virus seems to stand alone and the virus of benign lymphocytic choriomeningitis is difficult to place although it may be close to the viruses of hepatitis and pneumonia of mice. There is insufficient information available to place the viruses of human infectious hepatitis and homologous serum jaundice in any group although it may transpire that they belong to the picornaviruses. Similarly the respiratory syncytial and rubella viruses have not been studied sufficiently to decide in which groups they should be classified.

For further information on animal viruses and their relationships to one another the reader should consult Andrewes (1964b).

REFERENCES

ANDREWES, C. H. (1962). Classification of viruses of vertebrates. *Advanc. Virus Res.* **9**, 271.

ANDREWES, C. H. (1963). Recommendations on virus nomenclature. *Virology*, **21**, 516.

ANDREWES, C. H. (1964a). Tumour-viruses and virus tumours. *Brit. med. J.*, i, 653.

ANDREWES, C. H. (1964b). *Viruses of Vertebrates*. London: Baillière, Tindall & Cox.

BEVERIDGE, W. I. B. (1963). Acquired Immunity: Viral Infections. Chapter 6 in *Modern Trends in Immunology*. London: Butterworth.

BURNET, F. M. (1959). *Genetic interactions between animal viruses. The Viruses*, vol. 3, p. 275. New York: Academic Press.

CASPAR, D. L. D. & KLUG, A. (1962). Physical principles in the construction of regular viruses. *Cold Spring Harbour Symposium on Basic Mechanisms in Animal Virus Biology*, **27**, 1. New York: Long Island Biological Association.

CHAMPE, S. P. (1963). Bacteriophage reproduction. *Ann. Rev. Microbiol.*, **17**, 87.

COOPER, P. D. (1961). A chemical basis for the classification of animal viruses. *Nature (Lond.)*, **190**, 302.

FENNER, F. & SAMBROOK, J. F. (1964). The genetics of animal viruses. *Ann. Rev. Microbiol.*, **18**, 47.

FRANKLIN, R. W. (1962). The significance of lipids in animal viruses. *Progr. med. Virol.*, **4**, 1.

HAYES, W. (1963). *The bacteriophage model. Chap. 2. Mechanisms of Virus Infection.* Ed. Wilson Smith. London: Academic Press.

HOLLAND, J. J. & HAYER, B. H. (1962). Early stages of enterovirus infection. *Cold Spring Harbour Symposium on Basic Mechanisms in Animal Virus Biology*, **27**, 101. New York: Long Island Biological Association.

HORNE, R. W. & WILDY, P. (1962). Recent studies on the structure of viruses by electron-microscopy using negative staining techniques. *Brit. med. Bull.*, **18**, 199.

ISAACS, A. (1962). Production and action of interferon. *Cold Spring Harbour Symposium on Basic Mechanisms in Animal Virus Biology*, **27**, 343. New York: Long Island Biological Association.

ISAACS, A. & LINDEMANN, J. (1957). Virus interference. *Proc. Roy. Soc.*, **147**, 258.

LAMPSON, G. P., TYTELL, A. A., NEMES, M. M. & HILLEMAN, M. R. (1963). Purification and characterisation of chick embryo interferon. *Proc. Soc. exp. Biol. (N.Y.)*, **112**, 468.

WILDY, P. & HORNE, R. W. (1963). Structure of animal virus particles. *Progr. med. Virol.*, **5**, 1.

CHAPTER 6

BACTERIAL GENETICS AND VARIATION

LIKE other organisms, bacteria in general breed true and maintain their characters constant from generation to generation, yet at the same time show variations of particular characters in a small proportion of their progeny. Because of the great rapidity of bacterial reproduction, such variations are frequently encountered in the laboratory, even during relatively short periods of cultivation.

The characters that a bacterium exhibits at a given time (*i.e.* its phenotype) are determined both by its genetic constitution (genotype) and by environmental conditions which influence the contemporary expression of the genetic potentialities. The observed characters of a pure growth are thus liable to two kinds of variation: (1) *heritable variation* due to change in genetic constitution, *e.g.* by mutation, transduction, lysogenic conversion, transfer of an episome, or genetic recombination through cell conjugation, and (2) *non-heritable variation* due to change in the environmental conditions, *i.e.* environmentally impressed modifications and enzymic inductions and repressions.

Bacteria reproduce by asexual binary fission, normally maintaining their genetic constitution unaltered through successive generations. The hereditary cell components that determine the inherited characters, are called "genes"; they are thought to correspond to specific segments of a deoxyribonucleic acid (DNA) molecule in the bacterial nucleus. The bacterial cell contains a large number of different genes, probably over 1000. Each gene is capable of ensuring its own replication and also of directing the formation of a particular substance or enzyme which is responsible for some of the inherited characters. Duplication of the genes must precede cell division, and there must be a mechanism for ensuring that each daughter cell receives a complete and identical set. In the higher organisms, the genes are borne in fixed linear order along the thread-like chromosomes in the nucleus, and during mitotic cell division the latter are split longitudinally and segregated in two equal sets. Bacteria must have a comparable mechanism and this probably comprises a single linear or ring-like chromosome located in their DNA-containing nuclear bodies.

Mutation.—Replication of the cell's set of genes is usually an exact process. However, in a small proportion of cell divisions a mutation may occur, a gene accidentally being lost or altered. The mutant cell and its progeny then continue to reproduce with the new genetic constitution; correspondingly, they exhibit a sudden change of character which is heritable and, apart from the possibility of an occasional reverse mutation, permanent. Bacteria are thought to be "haploid", *i.e.* possessing only a single set of genes; the effect of a mutated gene is thus not masked by that of an unmutated partner, as may occur in the higher, diploid organisms.

Spontaneous Mutations of unknown cause seem to be responsible for most of the heritable variations observed in bacteria. Any gene is liable to undergo spontaneous mutation. The mutation rate of a given kind of gene in a given organism is fairly constant, but different genes show different rates, mostly between once per 10^4 and once per 10^{10} cells per generation. One large bacterial colony of about 10^9 cells, the product of a similar number of cell divisions, is thus liable to contain thousands of mutant cells of different kinds, including many cells changed in the more readily mutating genes and a few changed in the less readily mutating.

The mutations that have been studied most thoroughly are ones in which the microorganism loses or gains the ability to synthesise an essential metabolite, *e.g.* a particular amino acid, and thus also the ability to grow in the absence of a supply of that substance as a nutrient component of the culture medium. Many organisms, e.g. *Esch. coli*, can grow on a simple defined culture medium that contains glucose as the sole source of carbon and energy, ammonium chloride as the sole source of nitrogen, and certain inorganic salts. They have this ability because they are genetically endowed with the power of forming all the different enzymes that are needed to enable them synthesise from these simple nutrients each of the large variety of organic compounds required for the construction and functioning of their cells. Such organisms are termed *prototrophic*. Occasionally, prototrophic organisms undergo mutation to *auxotrophic* forms; these can grow on the simple medium only if this is supplemented with a particular nutrient compound, *e.g.* a particular amino acid or vitamin. The specific nutritional requirement reflects the fact that the organism has lost the power of forming either the enzyme immediately responsible for synthesis of the required compound or else an enzyme responsible for synthesis of a precursor of the compound. Studies of mutations of this kind, *e.g.* those of Beadle and Tatum (Beadle 1945) with the fungus *Neurospora crassa*, have indicated that the formation of each specific enzyme is determined by the action of a different specific gene; this is the "one-enzyme, one-gene" hypothesis. A mutation destroying or restoring the activity of a particular gene exerts its specific effect on the phenotypic properties of the organism through the consequential loss or gain to the organism of the power of producing the corresponding enzyme.

Other commonly observed mutations include: (1) variation in fermentative ability, involving loss or gain of the power to ferment a given substrate (*e.g.* as occurs in the "late" fermentation of lactose by *Esch. coli mutabilis* and *Sh. sonnei* after 2–8 days' incubation in a lactose-containing medium); (2) drug resistance variation, *i.e.* the acquisition of increased resistance to the antibacterial action of sulphonamide, penicillin, streptomycin or other drug; (3) loss of the capacity to form capsules, usually with associated loss of virulence, antigenic type specificity and mucoid colony character (*e.g.* in *Diplococcus pneumoniae*); (4) loss of the capacity to form the O somatic antigen, with associated loss of virulence, type specificity and smooth colony texture (*e.g.* as in the smooth-to-rough, or S-R, variation in salmonellae); (5) loss of the capacity to form flagella with associated loss of motility (*e.g.* in salmonellae); (6) exaltation or attenuation of virulence (*e.g.* as in the origin of attenuated living vaccines); (7) loss of sensitivity to a particular bacteriophage or colicine; and (8) acquisition of resistance to toxic waste products accumulating in artificial cultures (*e.g.* the variation of *Br. abortus* to R-type cells having an increased resistance to the inhibitory metabolite, D-alanine, which accumulates in cultures with DL-asparagine as nitrogen source). Many character changes result in an associated change of colonial morphology, as in size, pigmentation and texture. Mutants arising in a growing colony may therefore form visibly distinctive sectors or papillae in the colony.

Phase Variation.—Some heritable variations are readily reversible and occur with relatively high frequency in either direction (*e.g.* once per 1000 cell divisions). The variation of certain Gram-negative bacilli between a fimbriate and a non-fimbriate phase, and the phase variation of flagellar antigens in *Salmonella* are of this kind. It has been suggested that their mechanism differs from that of true gene mutation.

Induced Mutations and Mutagenic Agents.—The rate of almost any mutation may be increased greatly, *e.g.* 10–100,000 fold, by exposure of the resting or dividing cells to X-rays, ultraviolet radiation, nitrogen mustard, peroxides, acriflavine, nitrous oxide, ethyl methane sulphonate, manganous chloride and certain other substances. The induced mutations are undirected, the nature of the new character not being determined by the nature of the mutagenic agent.

Environmental Selection of Mutants.—The rate of most mutations is so low that the small proportion of mutant cells originating in a culture usually remains undetected and does not alter the gross characters of the culture. Indeed, most kinds of mutation are harmful or lethal, and these cells die out. Only those mutants are detected whose altered genetic constitution fits them better than the parent strain for growth and survival under the concurrent cultural conditions. Such mutants increase in number relative to the parent-type cells until they predominate in the culture and so make the new character manifest. In nature, mutation and environmental selection have probably been the main means effecting the evolution and differentiation of bacterial varieties specially adapted to life in the different habitats.

Many conditions may be selective for a mutant. (1) A given culture medium favours those mutants that can utilise its constituents more rapidly or completely than the parent-type cells. When they originate in a growing colony, such mutants may form distinctive "secondary colonies", or "papillae", due to their greater growth (*e.g.* the lactose-fermenting mutants of *Esch. coli mutabilis* and *Sh. sonnei* on a lactose medium). A mutant that has gained the ability to synthesise for itself an essential growth factor is selected absolutely by cultivation in a synthetic medium that lacks that factor and so cannot support growth of the parent-type cells. (2) A lethal or growth-inhibiting condition is highly selective for mutants having increased resistance to that condition, *e.g.* the presence of an antibiotic, bacteriophage or toxic waste product of metabolism. Thus, cultivation on nutrient agar containing streptomycin will give a growth of streptomycin-resistant mutants without growth of the sensitive parent-type cells. (3) Repeated passage of a pathogenic bacterium through animals of a given species is selective for mutants that have an increased ability to survive and multiply in this species, and thus are exalted in virulence. Repeated passage in another species is selective of mutants that are better fitted for survival and growth in this second species, and thus are often attenuated in virulence for the former host species.

(4) When a bacterium is cultivated in the laboratory, the nutritional and other conditions of growth are likely to be very different from those of the natural habitat to which it is specifically adapted. For this reason, in a culture, mutations can commonly occur that give rise to mutant organisms better suited for growth under the conditions of the artificial culture than the parent, "wild-type" organism. On continued subcultivation such mutants are liable to outgrow and replace the parent form. For example, pathogenic bacteria manufacture substances such as capsules, aggressins and toxins, that enable them to survive and overcome the action of the body's defence mechanisms, *e.g.* phagocytosis. In artificial culture media they are not exposed to these defence mechanisms, so that mutants lacking the ability to form the aggressive substance are not at a disadvantage and indeed may benefit from being relieved of the nutritional burden of synthesising the substance. Thus, non-capsulate mutants of pathogens such as the pneumococcus and the anthrax bacillus commonly replace the parent capsulate form during repeated subcultivation in the laboratory. (It should be noted that in addition to being capable of undergoing this mutation to a heritably non-capsulate form, the anthrax bacillus is also capable of undergoing an environmentally induced non-heritable change to a form without capsules; it does this when grown on medium devoid of serum or added bicarbonate, and the bacilli form capsules again when returned to a serum medium.)

Avoidance of mutations in laboratory work.—When a bacterial strain is being maintained in the laboratory for reference or other purposes for which its properties must be kept unchanged, attention should be paid to avoiding the emergence and outgrowth of mutants. (1) This is best done by *freeze-drying* a pure culture obtained as soon as possible after the first isolation of the strain. The organism is preserved in a dormant state *in vacuo* and thus kept in its original genetic form for as long a time as required. (2) If moist cultures are to be kept, they should be grown on a *maintenance medium*, *e.g.* Dorset's egg for enterobacteria and cooked meat broth for sporing anaerobic bacilli. This ensures prolonged survival at room or refrigerator temperature, *e.g.* for several years, and so obviates the need for repeated subculture. (3) When repeated subculture cannot be avoided, it should not be done by mass subinoculation, which may allow progressive multiplication of mutants in the successive cultures, but by plating out on each occasion and inoculating the subculture from a single typical colony. The rationale of this procedure is the assumption that in the course of any one subculture the outgrowth of mutants will not be sufficiently advanced to make it likely for a colony of a mutant to be picked.

Since environmental selection is normally essential for the detection of mutants, it is sometimes suggested that the pertinent environmental influence is required to induce the variation or direct its character. However, it can be shown that these mutations are undirected and occur spontaneously in the absence of the environmental condition that is subsequently selective; *e.g.* streptomycin-resistant mutants originate as readily in the absence of streptomycin as in its presence, although they only emerge as dominant in the latter case.

Other Mechanisms of Heritable Variation.—Less common mechanisms are transformation by free DNA, transduction by bacteriophage, lysogenic conversion, episome transfer, and recombination by cell conjugation. In these cases, a *directed* change is produced in the genotype of a susceptible strain through receipt of genetic material derived from a donor strain possessing the character to be acquired. So far, each of the mechanisms has been demonstrated in only a few kinds of bacteria and the extent to which each is important in the production of variations in natural environments is unknown.

Transformation by free DNA.—Free soluble deoxyribonucleic acid derived from a suitable donor strain has been found capable of transforming the nature of the capsular antigen, the degree of drug-sensitivity and other characters in strains of *D. pneumoniae*, *H. influenzae*, *B. subtilis* and other species. The DNA acts as a gene, or collection of genes, and enters the recipient bacterium, becoming by recombination incorporated in its nucleus and thereafter reproducing in step with cell multiplication. In the type transformation of the pneumococcus, cells of one antigenic type, *e.g.* type 2, are changed into another antigenic type, *e.g.* type 3 or 6. Capsulate, or "S"-form cells of type 2 are first allowed to undergo spontaneous mutation to a non-capsulate "R"-form that lacks type specificity and does not revert spontaneously to the S-form. A small proportion of the R cells are then transformed to S cells of a chosen type (*e.g.* type 3 or 6) by mixture with the transforming substance derived from donor S cells of that type. The latter is supplied as heat-killed S cells, cell-free extracts of the S culture, or purified DNA obtained from the S cells. The few cells transformed to encapsulation are detected either by selective culture of the DNA/R-cell mixture in broth with anti-R antibody or by inoculation of the mixture subcutaneously into mice, where the R cells are destroyed by phagocytosis while the S cells multiply and produce septicaemia.

Phage-mediated Transduction.—This is a heritable change effected through the agency of a temperate bacteriophage. The transducing gene, or group of genes, is derived from a donor bacterial culture that either is lysogenic (*i.e.* carrying phage) or else has been infected with phage; it leaves the donor bacterium in a liberated phage particle that has accidentally incorporated it, and enters the recipient bacterium when this is infected by the phage. The recipient cell may by recombination exchange the transduced gene for its own corresponding gene, eliminating the latter. Single antigenic, nutritional, fermentative or drug-resistance properties may thus be transduced between different *salmonellae* (e.g. *S. typhi* may acquire the flagellar antigen of

S. typhimurium), *Shigella*, *Escherichia coli*, *Staphylococcus aureus* and other organisms. Usually only a very small proportion (*e.g.* 1 in 10^5) of the phage-treated cells acquire any particular character by transduction and only a very small proportion (*e.g.* 1 in 10^6) of the phage particles derived from the donor bacteria carry a transducing gene and are able to transmit the character.

The type of transduction just described, and the commonest type, is called *generalised*, or *non-specific* transduction, because any of a wide variety of characters may be transmitted by a particular phage. A different kind of transduction, termed *limited* or *specific transduction* is produced by the lambda (λ) phage of *Escherichia coli* strain K12. The λ phage is incapable of transducing any genetic character of the donor bacterium other than that of the power of fermenting galactose. When in its prophage state the λ phage is attached to the bacterial chromosome adjacent to the genetic loci controlling galactose fermentation, and when the lysogenic donor bacteria are induced, as by ultraviolet irradiation, to form and liberate infectious phage particles, a small proportion (*c.* 1 in 10^6) of these particles incorporate a fragment of bacterial chromosome containing the galactose loci in exchange for part (*c.* a quarter) of the phage genetic material.

Lysogenic Conversion.—A temperate bacteriophage may confer certain properties on its bacterial host by virtue of the presence and activity of its own (*i.e.* phage) genetic material. When a susceptible bacterial culture is infected with the phage, the new properties are acquired by every bacterial cell that becomes lysogenised, *i.e.* contracts stable heritable phage infection. They are retained by the bacterium and all its progeny for as long as these remain lysogenic, *i.e.* parasitised by the phage in the prophage state. The prophage reproduces in association with the bacterial chromosome and acts as if it were a group of bacterial genes. If the prophage is lost from the bacterium (*e.g.* by mutation) and the lysogenic state is thus ended, the acquired properties are also lost.

When a bacterium becomes lysogenised it normally acquires two new heritable properties: (1) an immunity to lytic infection by the corresponding infectious phage, and (2) the potentiality of giving rise to infectious phage when it is *induced* artificially or spontaneously. In addition to these properties, special properties are conferred by certain kinds of phages. Thus a non-virulent strain of the diphtheria bacillus may acquire toxigenicity, *i.e.* the power of producing the toxin responsible for virulence, by infection and lysogenisation with the β phage derived from a virulent strain. Again, some salmonella organisms are converted by lysogeny with certain phages to produce a different kind of surface antigen: *e.g.* salmonellae having the O antigens 3, 10 produce instead the O antigens 3, 15 when they are lysogenised with phage ε15, and the O antigen 34 when further lysogenised with phage ε34; similarly, salmonellae with O antigens 2, 12, or 4, 5, 12, or 9, 12 produce additionally the O antigen 1 when lysogenised with phage ι.

Recombination by Cell Conjugation.—A form of gene recombination resembling in some respects that of sexual reproduction has been found to occur rarely in certain strains of some bacterial species, e.g. *Esch. coli.* It requires contact and conjugation between living parent cells of suitable mating types, at least one of which must possess a fertility factor, *e.g.* the F factor (see below). The recombination cannot be induced in one parent by cell-free extracts of the other. Apparently, the donor cell (either F+ or Hfr, see below) and the recipient cell (commonly F−) become attached to one another, and part of the chromosome of the former is transferred into the latter. Chromosomal cross-over may then occur in the diploid or partly diploid zygote and a process of segregation finally yields a haploid daughter cell with a genetic constitution derived partly from each parent. Recombination by cell conjugation has also been observed between *Esch. coli* organisms as donors and salmonella and shigella organisms as recipients.

Transfer of Episomes.—An episome is a genetic element that determines the possession of a dispensable property in bacteria and that is additional to, and can be reproduced and transmitted independently of the genetic material of the bacterial chromosome. A bacterium may lose the episome irreversibly by mutation and may acquire it only by conjugation or transduction from another bacterium that already harbours it. The episome may occur in one or other of, and alternate between, two states: (1) an *autonomous* state, in which it is located in the cytoplasm of the bacterium and replicates independently of the chromosome, and (2) an *integrated* state, in which it is located on the chromosome and is reproduced only *pari passu* with the chromosome. Examples of episomes are the fertility factor, F, of *Esch. coli*, colicinogenic factors and, probably, resistance transfer factors.

The *fertility factor*, *F*, confers on *Esch. coli* organisms the property of "maleness", or donor ability in conjugation (see above). Cells designated F+ carry the F factor in the autonomous form. They have the power of conjugating readily and frequently with F− cells, *i.e.* cells lacking the F factor, and can within a short time convert a majority of them to the F+ state by "infecting" them with the F factor. F+ donor cultures, although giving a high frequency of conjugation with F− cultures, give rise to only a very small proportion of genetic recombinants, *e.g.* 1 in 10^6.

Cells designated Hfr ("high frequency of recombination") carry the F factor in the integrated form, *i.e.* attached to the chromosome. They not only conjugate with F− cells at high frequency, but also produce genetic recombinants at high frequency, *e.g.* 1 in 100 cells. They differ from F+ cells in being unable to transmit the F factor by infection into F− conjugant cells. F+ cells occasionally mutate to the Hfr form and Hfr cells to the F+ form.

Colicinogenic factors are the genetic elements that confer on enterobacteria the power of producing the protein antibiotic substances called colicines. Like the F factor, some colicinogenic factors spread readily by "infection" in the course of cell conjugation, *i.e.* from colicinogenic (col+) bacteria to non-colicinogenic (col−) bacteria. In salmonellae, cell conjugation is promoted by the presence of certain colicinogenic factors in one of two organisms in a mixture, and this may lead to chromosome transfer and genetic recombination.

Resistance transfer factors.—The power of resisting the antibacterial action of antibiotic drugs has in a few cases been shown to be transmissible by infection through cell contact between different strains of *Shigella flexneri*, *Salmonella typhimurium* and *Esch. coli.* The genes, or resistance factors, that confer resistance to the different drugs, are carried together on an element called the resistance transfer factor; this behaves like an episome and is passed from resistant to sensitive cells within a very short time (*e.g.* within a few minutes) of cell contact.

Non-Heritable Variation.—The influence of environmental conditions may directly modify morphologic, metabolic and other properties without involving a change of genetic constitution. Such modifications of phenotype are temporary and non-heritable. All the exposed cells of identical genotype and responsive physiological state are affected simultaneously. They maintain their altered character as long as they are exposed to the inducing condition, but on withdrawal of this influence rapidly revert to their original state, *e.g.* within a few hours or within 1–10 generations of growth. Examples of such *environmentally impressed modifications* include: (1) the suppression of flagellation and motility in *Salmonella* during cultivation on agar containing 0·1 per cent. phenol; (2) the development of pleomorphic involution cells during growth in unfavourable conditions, *e.g.* in *P. pestis* cultures on medium containing 3 per cent. of sodium chloride; (3) the increased formation of capsular polysaccharide during growth on media with a relative excess of utilisable carbohydrate (*e.g.* in *Klebsiella*); and (4) the failure of capsule formation in *B. anthracis* when cultures are grown in the absence of serum or bicarbonate.

Enzymic inductions are a special form of non-heritable variation, and a common and important mechanism enabling bacteria to exploit fully the different nutrients that they successively encounter. Many enzymes, termed "inducible" or "adaptive", are formed in significant amount only when growth takes place in the presence of their specific substrate, which thus acts as their inducer. The enzymic activity is not exhibited by a washed suspension of non-growing bacteria taken from a medium lacking this substrate. When such unadapted cells are grown in the presence of the substrate, they produce the enzyme after a brief interval, *e.g.* beginning its production in less than 1 min. Examples of inducible enzymes include those fermenting various carbohydrates in *Esch. coli* and other species; the enzymes, or *permeases*, responsible for the uptake of specific nutrients, including carbohydrates, from the environment; and penicillinase in *B. cereus.* Evidence obtained in the study of the inducible β-galactosidase of *Esch. coli* suggests that the enzyme's substrate and inducer (*e.g.* lactose) exerts its effect by interfering with a normally present repressor substance that otherwise acts on the genetic material of the bacterium, preventing synthesis of the enzyme.

Enzyme repression.—The amount of the formation of enzymes engaged in the synthesis of intermediate metabolites, such as amino acids, is regulated by the mechanism of *repression.* When a sufficiency of the metabolite accumulates within the cell, whether as a result of its synthesis intracellularly or of its uptake as a nutrient from the environment, the metabolite represses the further manufacture of the enzymes specifically responsible for its synthesis. The mechanisms of induction and repression ensure that the bacterium does not waste energy and nutrients in producing unnecessary enzymes.

Drug Resistance Variation

Variations conferring on bacteria an increased resistance to the action of chemotherapeutic and antibiotic drugs are of great importance in medicine because they may lead to failure in the drug therapy of infections. Failure of therapy may, however, be due to a variety of causes, *e.g.* (1) incorrect identification of the causative pathogen, (2) failure of the antibiotic to penetrate in adequate amounts into the lesion, (3) protection of a drug-sensitive pathogen, *e.g.* a penicillin-sensitive *Strept. pyogenes*, as a result of simultaneous infection with a drug-destroying bacterium, *e.g.* a penicillinase-producing *Staph. aureus*, and (4) secondary infection from an exogenous or endogenous source with a different, drug-resistant organism, *e.g. Staph. aureus* or *Ps. pyocyanea* from the hospital environment, or commensal *Candida albicans* from the intestine. Most commonly, however, failure is due to (5) the emergence, during treatment, of a drug-resistant variant of the originally sensitive, infecting organism, or (6) primary infection with a drug-resistant variety of a species of organism that is generally susceptible to the drug used.

Occurrence of Drug Resistance Variation in Bacteria in Patients under Treatment.—Drug-resistance variation, generally by spontaneous genetic mutation, may take place in a drug-sensitive bacterium while it is growing in the body of the patient before or during treatment with the drug. This occurs commonly, for example, in tubercle bacilli during therapy with streptomycin, isoniazid or para-aminosalicylic acid and in almost any kind of bacterium during therapy with streptomycin, and it sometimes occurs in *Staph. aureus* during therapy with erythromycin or novobiocin. After a favourable initial response to the drug, associated with destruction of the sensitive parent-type organisms, the infection relapses due to the proliferation of the drug-resistant mutant cells. The number of viable organisms in the lesion and exudate (*e.g.* sputum or urine) thus shows a "fall and rise" fluctuation. Evidence from a variety of genetical experiments suggests strongly that the majority of such instances of drug-resistance variation are due to *spontaneous gene mutation.* As a rule, a mutation confers resistance to a single drug only, and a bacterium that becomes resistant to one drug remains sensitive to other unrelated drugs. Only a very small number of resistant mutant cells are originally produced, *e.g.* 1 per 10^5–10^9 parent-type cells, but these mutants multiply selectively in the presence of the drug and soon outnumber and replace the parent-type cells which are being destroyed by the drug.

In some kinds of infection the emergence of drug-resistant mutants may be prevented by *double-drug therapy*, *i.e.* treatment with two different drugs given simultaneously. Thus, the treatment of pulmonary tuberculosis with streptomycin and isoniazid in combination has been almost uniformly successful in cases of the disease in which the infecting bacilli were initially fully sensitive to both drugs. The apparent reason for the success of double-drug therapy is that resistance to each drug requires mutation in a different gene and the chances of these two mutations occurring simultaneously in the same bacterial cell are infinitesimally small. (In general, the probability of a double mutation is equal to the product of the individual mutation rates of the two genes.) In tubercle bacilli, mutants resistant to streptomycin arise at the rate of about 1 per 10^6 parent-type cells and mutants to isoniazid at about the same rate. Such mutant cells, with resistance to a single drug, are therefore likely to be already present before the start of therapy in all patients with clinical tuberculosis, except those, *e.g.* children with early primary infection or patients with tuberculous meningitis, in whom the total population of tubercle bacilli is very small. The single-resistance mutants are likely all to be killed if the patient is given the two drugs simultaneously, the streptomycin-resistant cells being killed by the isoniazid and the isoniazid-resistant cells by the streptomycin. Cells resistant to both streptomycin and isoniazid could be expected to arise only by the simultaneous occurrence of the two different mutations, and thus at the rate of only about 1 per 10^{12} parent-type cells. Since the total bacterial population of the lesions of a patient is probably usually less than 10^{12} it is very unlikely for even a single such "double mutant" to appear.

In cases where a drug-sensitive pathogen is present in a part of the body, such as the throat or intestine, in which drug-resistant commensal bacteria may be present, there is the possibility that it could acquire a drug-resistance character by the transfer of genes from one of the latter organisms. Transfer might take place by transformation, transduction or recombination, or by infection with a resistance transfer factor. Evidence has been obtained that, in certain cases, pathogenic *Sh. flexneri* and *S. typhimurium* organisms have, while in the intestine of carriers, acquired multiple drug resistance by infection with a *resistance transfer factor* derived from commensal *Esch. coli* organisms.

In the past, claims have been made that drug-resistance variation commonly arises as a *physiological adaptation* in bacteria, the adaptation being induced by contact with the drug in all the bacterial cells exposed to it. There is, however, no good evidence that adaptation is responsible for any instance of resistance variation observed to take place under clinical conditions. In special experiments *Bacillus cereus* has been shown to acquire resistance to penicillin *in vitro* by adaptively increasing its production of the penicillin-destroying enzyme, penicillinase. A brief contact with a small concentration of penicillin was found to stimulate one strain of *B. cereus* to increase its production of penicillinase about 300-fold and so to become capable of growth in the presence of a 100-fold higher concentration of penicillin than it was originally

(Pollock, 1957). Since induction is achieved within a very short time, *e.g.* several minutes, after first exposure to the drug, bacteria that can acquire resistance in this way will normally not be distinguished from ones that are inherently and originally resistant.

Infection of Patients with Strains already Drug-Resistant.—The patient may be infected originally, or become infected secondarily during the course of drug therapy, with a strain of a pathogenic bacterium that is already drug-resistant before being acquired from its exogenous source. Such an organism may be a variant that has recently mutated to resistance in another patient receiving the drug, *e.g.* as in cross-infection with streptomycin-resistant coliform and tubercle bacilli, or it may be a variety of organism that is inherently resistant and has existed in this form since before the time that the drug was first discovered and used, *e.g.* penicillinase-producing strains of *Staph. aureus.*

(Penicillin-sensitive strains of *Staph. aureus* undergo mutations *in vitro* that confer on them an increased tolerance of penicillin. These penicillin-resistant mutants do not form penicillinase. They appear to be non-virulent and mutants of this kind do not emerge *in vivo* or cause clinical infections. The "penicillin-resistant" strains of *Staph. aureus* that are found in clinical infections are all strains that produce penicillinase and so destroy penicillin. Apart from the effect of their penicillinase, they have no special power of resisting or tolerating the action of penicillin and, indeed, they are sensitive to, and destroyed by the "penicillinase-resistant" penicillins such as methicillin and cloxacillin. Penicillin-sensitive staphylococci have never been found to give rise to mutants of this penicillinase-producing type and the penicillinase-producers are therefore considered to be an originally distinct variety of the staphylococcus.)

Primary and secondary infection with already resistant variant strains and varieties of pathogenic organisms are especially likely to occur in patients in hospital, *e.g.* in mothers and babies in maternity hospitals. The presence together in a hospital of many patients who have lesions capable of harbouring pathogenic organisms and who are subjected to treatment with antibiotic drugs, provides conditions that selectively favour the proliferation and dissemination of virulent "hospital strains" of bacteria with multiple resistance to the antibiotics in common use. These multi-resistant organisms are distributed in large numbers into the hospital environment and new patients are thus exposed to heavy infection with them. A further source of "hospital staphylococci" is provided by the medical, nursing and domestic staff; the skin and nostrils of these persons are subject to frequent contamination with traces of spilt antibiotic, some in the form of airborne dust, or aerosol, so that they become selectively favourable to the carriage of drug-resistant strains of *Staph. aureus* (Gould, 1958).

For general reading on the subject of microbial genetics, the books of Hayes (1962, 1964), Hayes and Clowes (1960) and Jacob and Wollman (1962) are recommended. A good discussion on some problems of drug resistance in the treatment of patients in hospital is given by Lowbury (1962).

REFERENCES

BEADLE, G. W. (1945). Biochemical genetics. *Chem. Rev.*, 37, 15.

GOULD, J. C. (1958). Environmental penicillin and penicillin-resistant *Staphylococcus aureus*. *Lancet*, i, 489.

HAYES, W. & CLOWES, R. C. (1960). Microbial genetics, *Tenth Symp. Soc. gen. Microbiol.* Cambridge: Cambridge University Press.

HAYES, W. (1962). Genetics of microorganisms. *Brit. med. Bull.*, 2, 1-84.

HAYES, W. (1964). *The Genetics of Bacteria and their Viruses.* Oxford : Blackwell.

JACOB, F. & WOLLMAN, E. L. (1962). *Sexuality and Genetics of Bacteria.* New York and London: Academic Press.

LOWBURY, E. J. L. (1962). Drug resistance and the response to therapy. *Scientific Basis of Medicine Annual Reviews*, p. 57. London: The Athlone Press of the University of London. Distributed by Constable & Co. Ltd.

POLLOCK, M. R. (1957). Penicillin-induced resistance to penicillin in cultures of *Bacillus cereus*. *Ciba Foundation Symposium on Drug Resistance in Micro-organisms*, ed. by G. E. W. Wolstenholme & Cecilia M. O'Connor, p. 78. London: Churchill.

CHAPTER 7

INFECTION AND RESISTANCE TO INFECTION

INFECTION is the invasion of the tissues of the body by microorganisms. The animal body is continually exposed to contact with numerous microorganisms of many different species, including commensals which grow on its skin and mucous membranes, and saprophytes which grow in the soil and elsewhere. The blood and tissue fluids contain nutrients sufficient to sustain profuse growth of many of these species. However, the normal (non-immunised) body possesses a series of defence mechanisms that enable it generally to resist microbial invasion of its tissues and give it a ***natural immunity*** or ***innate resistance*** towards most microorganisms. This resistance is a genetic endowment of an entire species with respect to a particular agent. The immunity is sometimes absolute, so that all individuals are entirely resistant and in other instances relative and varying in degree between one individual and another. The native defence mechanisms are of tremendous importance to the daily welfare of the body. These mechanisms are non-specific in that each is operative against a variety of microbe species. They include mechanical barriers to the entry and spread of microbes, the antibiotic action of the normal commensal flora, microbicidal substances present in the body fluids and secretions, microbicidal substances liberated from tissue cells damaged by the infective process, and phagocytosis by microphages (polymorphonuclear leucocytes) and macrophages (*e.g.* fixed reticulo-endothelial cells and wandering monocytes). The defences do not need to be of an aggressive nature, that is, the host may simply fail to supply, for example, a sufficiently high oxygen tension in a particular organ or an essential nutrient for a bacterium or an enzyme system required by a particular virus.

Pathogenic microbes are specially adapted and endowed with mechanisms for overcoming the normal body defences in one or more animal species, and can thus invade the germ-free tissues and fluids. Some pathogens invade only the surface epithelium, skin or mucous membrane, but many invade more deeply, spreading through the tissues and/or disseminating by the lymphatic and blood streams. In some cases a pathogenic microbe can infect an entirely healthy individual, whilst in other cases infection occurs only if the body defence mechanisms are deranged by some locally or systemically debilitating condition, *e.g.* wounding, intoxication, chilling, fatigue, malnutrition, administration of cortisone, adrenalin, etc., and various predisposing diseases and functional disorders. Certain organisms that are saprophytic or commensal organisms of the gut, e.g. *Cl. welchii* or *Esch. coli*, can damage healthy tissues when outside the gut. When an organism succeeds in overcoming the normal body defences, the infection usually progresses until specific immunity mechanisms become operative, for example that involving the formation of humoral antibodies specific for the invading microbe or its poisonous products.

NORMAL NON-SPECIFIC DEFENCE MECHANISMS

Mechanical Barriers.—The skin and mucous membranes are important mechanical barriers to the entry of microbes into the tissues. The skin is the more resistant barrier because its outer horny layer hinders access of the microbes and their toxins to the living epithelial cells. Microbes are removed mechanically from the mucous membranes of the respiratory, alimentary and urinary tracts; they are trapped in the sticky mucous secretion covering the membrane and this is regularly removed by ciliary action or by peristalsis and evacuation. Infection often follows a disorder of this function, as in the obstructed urinary tract or in a bronchus blocked by excessive mucus. Within the body, the spread of microbes may be limited by dense cellular or fibrous tissues, or by the gelatinous intercellular cement substance (hyaluronic acid) or by a meshwork of fibrin deposited in the infected tissues as part of their inflammatory reaction.

Antagonism of Indigenous Flora.—The antibiotic activity of the normal commensal flora of the mucous membranes may be important in denying access of potentially pathogenic organisms. Thus, the salivary streptococci produce substances (*e.g.* hydrogen peroxide) that are lethal to the diphtheria bacillus and the meningococcus. During the childbearing period, the commensal *Lactobacillus acidophilus* (Döderlein's bacillus) ferments glycogen derived from the vaginal epithelium and produces a highly acid vaginal secretion which is inhibitory to many kinds of bacteria, including streptococci and staphylococci. When the normal commensal flora of the intestine, particularly the lactobacilli, is eliminated by oral administration of a broad-spectrum antibiotic drug, a serious infection may follow due to a drug-resistant *Staph. aureus* or *Candida albicans* previously excluded by the commensals.

Bactericidal Substances.—It has been known for a long time that body fluids, especially the blood, can suppress putrefaction. The responsible factors are even now often only vaguely characterised (see Skarnes & Watson, 1957). Microbicidal substances are normally present in the body secretions, tissue fluids and blood serum. *Long-chain fatty acids, e.g.* oleic acid, which are present in the slightly acid (pH 5–6) secretion of the skin, are lethal to many bacteria within an hour or two of their contact with the skin, e.g. *Strept. pyogenes* and *C. diphtheriae*; bacteria normally resident on the skin, e.g. *Staph. aureus* and *Staph. albus*, are better adapted to withstand the action of these acids. *Lactenin* is a protein present in milk (*e.g.* human, cow) which is selectively bactericidal for *Strept. pyogenes* and may thus protect against puerperal mastitis and neonatal throat infection. The *hydrochloric acid* and low pH (*e.g.* 1–2) of the gastric juice is lethal to a majority of ingested microbes and serves as an important protection for the intestinal canal.

Lysozyme.—This mucolytic enzyme, first recognised by Fleming in 1922, occurs in various animals in the tissue and body fluids except the cerebrospinal fluid, aqueous humour, sweat and urine. Human tears contain a large amount, and egg white is a rich commercial source of the enzyme. This enzyme is a basic protein that splits sugars from the mucopeptide component of the bacterial cell wall so that the cell contents leak out (Salton, 1957). Lysozyme acts most strongly on certain saprophytic Gram-positive bacteria, e.g. *Micrococcus lysodeikticus* and *B. megaterium*, though in certain conditions it may affect pathogens such as staphylococci and anthrax bacilli, and it accelerates the lysis of Gram-negative pathogenic bacteria under the action of antibody and complement. The mucous secretions probably contain several other microbicidal substances besides lysozyme.

Basic Polypeptides.—A variety of basic proteins, derived from tissue and blood cells damaged in the course of infection and inflammation, which can act upon the cell wall and cause bacillary disintegration, have been described in the tissues and fluids of animals. This group includes polyamine derivatives of tissues called spermine and spermidine (Hirsch & Dubos, 1952) which kill tubercle bacilli and *Staph. aureus*, and protamine and histone acting as antibacterial agents in inflammatory exudates. The basic proteins are probably the active constituent of the antibacterial substances derived from leucocytes and thus leukin and endolysin described by Metchnikoff probably owe their antibacterial activity to basic proteins. It may be noted that a group of highly effective antibiotics, including tyrothricin, gramicidin, bacitracin and the polymyxins are all polypeptides.

Properdin.—The anti-bacterial factors discussed above are in general active against Gram-positive bacteria and do not require for their activity a heat labile protein complex of serum called complement (p. 124). Pillemer and his co-workers in 1954 described a germicidal high molecular weight protein constituent of normal serum (0·02 per cent. of the total serum proteins) that was active against Gram-negative bacteria. This substance, called properdin, is thought not to be an antibody although it requires complement and Mg^{++} ions for its activity. Properdin also participates in the destruction of protozoa, abnormal red cells and certain viruses. These diverse activities of the properdin system and its presence in normal serum suggest that it is one of the factors responsible for natural resistance (Pillemer, 1956). There is however some doubt as to the identity of this substance as a single entity and some workers suggest that properdin represents a group of antibodies that are heat-labile, high-molecular-weight gamma globulins.

Anti-viral Substances.—The nasal secretions and serum of normal persons have the ability to neutralise certain viruses, including those of influenza A and B, vaccinia, mumps and Newcastle disease. These activities may be due to the diversion of the viruses from the susceptible cells (haemagglutination inhibition see p. 74) and also to the effect on the virus of properdin and, in some instances, acid and alkaline phosphatase enzymes (perhaps because some viral constituent essential for infectivity is active only in the phosphorylated form). The effect of interferon, an inhibitory agent released by virus infected cells, is described on p. 75.

The metabolism of the leucocytes and other cells in inflamed tissue can ultimately cause a local accumulation of lactic acid and carbon dioxide, and a depletion of oxygen, conditions that are unfavourable for the growth of bacteria such as the tubercle bacillus and *Staph. aureus*.

Phagocytosis.—The phagocytes are "eating cells" which are specialised for the pursuit, capture, ingestion and intracellular destruction of invading microbes (phagocytosis). Metchnikoff in 1905 first realised the importance of these cells in resistance to infective agents. They include the polymorphonuclear leucocytes and large mononuclear leucocytes of the blood (70 per cent. of the total WBC, 3500–7000 cells per c. mm. in man) and the fixed macrophages of the reticulo-endothelial system (*e.g.* sinusoidal cells of spleen, liver, bone marrow and lymph nodes, adventitial cells of blood vessels and histiocytes of connective tissue). Polymorph leucocytes and monocytes migrate from the blood vessels in inflamed tissues, apparently guided by diffusible factors from the irritant or the damaged tissue cells, and accumulate to attack the bacteria causing a local infection. The fixed macrophages of the reticulo-endothelial system are mainly responsible for eliminating bacteria from the blood and lymph. Most microorganisms attract polymorphonuclear leucocytes, as do the products of tissue injury. Phagocytes can most readily entrap bacteria when they are supported on a cellular or fibrous surface (*surface phagocytosis*); the deposition of a fibrin meshwork in inflamed tissue assists phagocytosis by providing supporting surfaces. When the phagocytes are freely suspended in fluid, *e.g.* oedema fluid, the opsonic activity of antibody and complement is generally required to make phagocytosis possible. It should be noted that the effect of opsonins (p. 125) seems to be in part related to the neutralisation of the strong electro-negative charge on the surface of many microorganisms. Thus any protein deposited on an organism will assist phagocytosis, antibody protein functioning particularly efficiently because of its specific affinity for the organism.

Susceptible bacteria die and disintegrate within an hour or two after their ingestion, partly due to the secretion of acid (pH 3–5) in the vacuole surrounding them and probably also due to the action of lysozyme and other digestive enzymes. Cohn and Hirsch (1960 *a* & *b*) showed that cytoplasmic granules of polymorphs contained many enzymes (acid and alkaline phosphatases, ribonuclease and β-glucuronidase) as well as a major part of the antibacterial protein, *phagocytin*, present in the polymorphs. The granules of polymorphs spontaneously lyse following phagocytosis of bacteria, and phagocytin, and other enzymes are probably liberated into the vacuoles around the ingested bacteria. Phagocytin has an antibacterial effect on a wide range of organisms, both Gram-positive and Gram-negative.

The strong bactericidal action of monocytes (macrophages) is still unexplained, since monocytes do not possess significant amounts of phagocytin or lysozyme.

Many pathogenic bacteria are able to survive and multiply inside the phagocyte, thus causing its death and lysis, and eventually escape from it (*e.g.* tubercle bacillus, brucellae and salmonellae). For general reference to phagocytosis see Rowley (1962) and for resistance mechanisms in general see Symposium on Mechanisms of Non-specific Resistance to Infection (1960).

ACQUIRED NON-SPECIFIC DEFENCE MECHANISMS

The injection of endotoxin (p. 107) derived from Gram-negative bacteria is known to stimulate resistance of the host to infection with a wide range of *antigenically unrelated* microorganisms. A similar effect is also found after the injection of various mycobacteria and brucellae.

Numerous studies have shown that there is markedly increased phagocytic activity of the reticulo-endothelial system following such treatment although direct evidence of intensified intracellular microbicidal activity is lacking. It seems possible that this effect may involve both the synergistic effect of multiple humoral factors and cellular changes associated with parasitisation of the reticulo-endothelial system.

THE INVASIVE MECHANISMS OF PATHOGENIC BACTERIA

Bacteria that infect the animal body must have means of overcoming their host's defence mechanisms, of protecting themselves against the bactericidal substances in the body fluids and of avoiding ingestion or intracellular destruction by phagocytes. Such protection is generally afforded by the special nature of their outermost covering, *i.e.* capsule, microcapsule or somatic antigens. If this covering is lost by gene mutation or enzymatic digestion, or becomes coated with antibody and complement, the bacterium is rendered non-virulent. Thus, virulent pneumococci isolated from infected animals possess polysaccharide capsules that render them relatively resistant to capture and ingestion by phagocytes; non-capsulate mutant strains derived by artificial culture in the laboratory are susceptible to phagocytosis and are non-virulent. Some pathogens, e.g. *Strept. pyogenes* and *Staph. aureus*, secrete *leucocidins*, i.e. phagocyte-destroying toxins, and some, e.g. *S. typhi*, produce substances that inhibit the migration of leucocytes. The factors that enable certain pathogens such as the tubercle bacillus to survive and grow within phagocytes have not yet been defined.

Whilst some pathogens normally enter the body through a wound, others may require mechanisms for breaching the epithelial barriers and for assisting spread through the tissues. Thus, some species produce toxins that destroy the epithelial cells (e.g. *C. diphtheriae*), some produce a "spreading factor" such as hyaluronidase which dissolves the hyaluronic-acid cement substance of tissues (e.g. *Strept.*

pyogenes), and some produce a fibrinolysin which induces solution of the fibrin clots deposited as barriers to the spread of infection (e.g. *Strept. pyogenes*). Many pathogenic bacteria, especially when growing in the tissues, liberate diffusible substances (termed "aggressins") which, though non-toxic by themselves, increase the aggressiveness of the bacteria. In some cases they may act by interfering with phagocytosis, opsonisation or bacteriolysis by normal or immune serum. Various non-pathogenic bacteria, however, may possess similar properties, and the existence of a specialised substance of this type is doubtful.

Capsules and Pathogenicity.—The role of capsules in conferring virulence on bacteria by enabling them to resist destruction by the phagocytes and bactericidal substances in body fluids is demonstrated by making comparative observations on capsulate and non-capsulate bacteria derived from the same strain. In this way, evidence has been obtained that capsulation is important for virulence in the pneumococcus, streptococci of groups A and C, anthrax bacillus, plague bacillus, *Klebsiella pneumoniae* and *Haemophilus influenzae*.

When a non-capsulate mutant bacterium or a decapsulated bacterium is injected into a laboratory animal that is highly susceptible to infection with the capsulate form, the non-capsulate form is found to be non-virulent or, at least, much reduced in degree of virulence. For instance, in experiments in which group C streptococci were injected intraperitoneally in mice, decapsulation of the cocci by the simultaneous injection of hyaluronidase decreased their virulence to the extent that their minimum lethal dose (MLD), *i.e.* the number of cocci that had to be injected to cause fatal infection, was *c.* 10,000-fold greater than that of the capsulate organisms.

Differences in virulence between the capsulate and non-capsulate forms of bacteria appear to be due mainly to differences in ability to resist capture and ingestion by phagocytes. Microscopical examination of smears of peritoneal exudate from infected animals shows that the non-capsulate bacteria are rapidly phagocytosed and, within a few hours, are mostly destroyed, whereas the capsulate bacteria remain free and soon multiply and increase largely in number. Similar differences in susceptibility to phagocytosis can be observed *in vitro* when capsulate and non-capsulate bacteria are added to normal blood and smears examined after the mixture has been incubated for $\frac{1}{2}$–1 hr. The removal of the microcapsular M protein from living group A streptococci by digestion with trypsin has, for instance, been found to increase the susceptibility of the organisms to phagocytosis.

In these cases the phagocytes and bacteria are suspended freely in fluid. If, however, they are present on certain kinds of solid surfaces, *e.g.* on the wall of a lung alveolus or lymphatic vessel, or on a mass of fibrin, phagocytosis of capsulate organisms such as pneumococci (of types other than the heavily capsulate type 3) may take place fairly readily. This *surface phagocytosis* occurs independently of the presence of specific opsonic antibodies and normal serum opsonins. When capsulate bacteria are exposed to specific antibodies and these combine with and coat the surface of the capsule, phagocytes can then capture, ingest and destroy the bacteria even where they are suspended freely in fluid.

It must be emphasised that capsulation is not necessarily sufficient by itself to confer resistance to phagocytosis and the property of virulence. Many harmless saprophytic bacteria, e.g. *Klebsiella aerogenes*, are heavily capsulate, and certain non-virulent strains of plague bacillus and anthrax bacillus are fairly susceptible to phagocytosis although they are capsulate.

BACTERIAL TOXINS

Toxins are defined as the products of bacteria that are injurious to the tissues and in virtue of which disease processes result from bacterial infection. They are classified broadly as:

(1) Extracellular toxins, or *exotoxins*, which diffuse readily from the living bacteria into the surrounding medium.

(2) Intracellular toxins, or *endotoxins*, which are retained within the bacterial cells until they die and disintegrate.

The majority of the pathogens produce endotoxins only, and these are significantly potent in the Gram-negative bacteria. Some, mainly Gram-positive species, develop powerful exotoxins, *e.g.* the tetanus bacillus and other clostridia, the diphtheria bacillus and certain staphylococci and streptococci. Particular pathogenic bacteria may fail to produce toxins in ordinary culture media, but do so when growing in the animal tissues, *e.g.* the anthrax bacillus.

Preparations of *exotoxins* may be obtained by growing the bacteria in a liquid medium and then removing them by centrifugation or by filtration through a bacteria-stopping filter; the toxin remains in the supernatant liquid or filtrate. The exotoxins that have so far been isolated in a purified state, *e.g.* tetanus and diphtheria toxins, have been identified as simple proteins. Exotoxins are generally unstable substances, their toxic effect being readily annulled by chemicals, *e.g.* by formaldehyde, as in conversion to *toxoid*; by free oxygen, *e.g.* oxygen-labile haemolysins, and by heat, *e.g.* diphtheria toxin at 65° C. and *Cl. welchii* alpha toxin at 100° C. A few are more resistant to heat, *e.g.* botulinus toxin and staphylococcal enterotoxin. Some are exceedingly potent, the tetanus and botulinus toxins being the most powerful poisons known and having a lethal dose for man in the order of 0·0001 mg. Some are toxic to tissue cells generally and rapid in action, whilst others have a specialised action on particular tissues (*e.g.* tetanus and botulinus toxins on certain kinds of nerve cells) and produce symptoms of poisoning only after several hours or days following their introduction into the body. Toxins may be designated according to certain of their effects, e.g. *haemolysin* (causing lysis of red blood cells), *leucocidin* (destructive to leucocytes), *necrotoxin* (causing necrosis of tissue). By immunising animals with a preparation of exotoxin, a specific neutralising antibody (*antitoxin*) is developed which can be demonstrated in the blood serum of the immune animals

(p. 119). The mechanisms of action of the exotoxins are with few exceptions unknown. The alpha toxin of *Cl. welchii* has been defined as a lecithinase, or lecithin-splitting enzyme, which apparently acts on the lecithin components in cell membranes, *e.g.* of red blood cells. The toxin of the diphtheria bacillus appears to be the isolated protein moiety of the bacterial cytochrome-*b* enzyme and may act by interfering with synthesis of cytochrome-*b* in the tissues of the host.

Endotoxins are structural components of the bacterial cell and are liberated only on death and disintegration of the cells. In the infected animal this occurs through phagocytosis and bacteriolysis by antimicrobial substances in the body fluids. Endotoxins are not found in bacteria-free supernatants of cultures, unless these have undergone autolysis through ageing. In several species (*e.g.* of *Salmonella*, *Shigella*, *Brucella* and *Neisseria*), the endotoxin has been extracted with solvents (*e.g.* diethylene glycol) and identified as a polymolecular lipid-phospholipid-polysaccharide-protein complex; this may comprise 5–10 per cent. of the dry weight of the cells and corresponds to the O somatic antigen of the virulent "smooth-type" organisms. The toxic action may be demonstrated by injecting animals with such a culture extract or with killed whole cells. The endotoxins of different species all produce more or less similar symptoms, particularly pyrexia, diarrhoea, prostration and visceral haemorrhages. They also have important actions in the production of hypersensitivity reactions of the Shwartzman type (see Chapter 8). Immunisation with endotoxins leads to the formation of antibodies that exert important antibacterial effects, *e.g.* bacteriolysis, but are incapable of neutralising the toxic action. Endotoxins are more stable than exotoxins and can withstand a temperature of 100° C.

In the course of an infective disease the tissues of the body at large may become hypersensitive to specific products of the infecting organism. Such *hypersensitiveness*, or *allergy*, may contribute to the toxic manifestations of the disease, since microbial products that are normally non-toxic may thus become highly toxic and irritant to the tissues. (See Chapter 8).

VIRULENCE OF MICROORGANISMS

Virulence is an important property of microorganisms in relation to their pathogenic action, and is defined as the capacity to invade the tissues, multiply and produce toxic effects. It is estimated by the *minimum lethal dose* (MLD), *i.e.* the smallest dose of the organism (number or weight of cells from a culture) that will kill a particular species of animal. As a result of the varying susceptibility of individual animals to bacteria and their toxins, it is often impossible to state the exact minimum dose, and it is customary to refer to the *average lethal dose* for a number of individual animals (*i.e.* the LD50, or dose giving a 50 per cent. mortality) (see Chapter 52). It must be noted that virulence depends on two factors that may be largely independent of one another: the invasive power or aggressiveness, and the toxigenic or toxin-producing property of the organism. Thus, the tetanus bacillus is highly toxigenic but only weakly aggressive; in contrast, the pneumococcus is markedly aggressive and its toxicity is minimal. The virulence of bacterial strains cannot be fully explained in terms of known toxins and invasive mechanisms; strains which possess the same known components may still vary greatly in virulence.

The virulence of an organism can be either "exalted" or "attenuated" artificially. *Exaltation* of virulence may be produced by passing the strain through a series of individual animals of the same species, inoculating the animals one from another in succession, *i.e* "passage". In this way a mutant strain is selected that has increased virulence for that particular species. *Attenuation* usually results when organisms are cultivated artificially for some time; thus, stock laboratory cultures are usually of low virulence, as compared with recently isolated strains. Similarly, passage through animals of a different species may select mutants having reduced virulence for the original host species.

In many species a loss of virulence is correlated with a change of colony texture from smooth to rough and a corresponding loss of the O somatic antigens. This is the so-called S→R mutation (p. 115).

SOURCES OF INFECTION FOR MAN

The epidemiology of an infective disease depends to an important extent on the nature and distribution of the sources of infection. The term *source* of infection applies to the normal growth habitats of the microbe, *e.g.* sites in the body of the human or animal host. Objects contaminated with live but non-growing microbes may act as, and should be called *vehicles* or *reservoirs* of infections not sources of infection. Human disease may be acquired from the following:

(1) Patients.—Infections due to some microbial species are acquired mainly or exclusively from ill humans with active or manifest infection, *e.g.* pulmonary tuberculosis (human-type bacilli), leprosy, whooping-cough, syphilis, gonorrhoea, measles, smallpox, mumps and influenza. Some cases of the infection may be mild or atypical, and thus not recognised as a source of danger.

(2) Healthy Carriers.—Many pathogenic species are able to produce in certain individuals a limited or subclinical infection that is insufficient to cause the signs and symptoms of illness. Persons having such an inapparent infection are commonly capable of disseminating the causative microbes to other persons; they are then termed "carriers" and constitute an unsuspected and thus especially dangerous source of infection. Some infectious diseases are contracted from carriers as frequently or much more frequently than from patients, *e.g.* streptococcal, staphylococcal, pneumococcal and meningococcal infections, diphtheria, typhoid fever, bacillary dysentery and poliomyelitis. *Convalescent carriers* are persons in whom a limited, localised infection continues for a period of weeks, or months following

clinical recovery from a manifest infection. Other carriers suffer no more than subclinical infection from the time of first acquiring the pathogen; those who acquire it from a patient are termed *contact carriers* and those who acquire it from another carrier are termed *paradoxical carriers*. If carriage persists for more than an arbitrary period of time, *e.g.* one year in the case of typhoid infection, the person is called a *chronic carrier*.

(3) Infected Animals.—Some pathogens that are primarily parasites of a different animal species may in appropriate circumstances spread from the infected animal to man and so cause human disease. Such infections are called *zoonoses*. Infections normally acquired from animals include bovine-type tuberculosis, salmonella food poisoning, bubonic plague, anthrax, brucellosis, leptospiral jaundice, rabies and psittacosis. In most such infections there is rarely any secondary spread from the patient to other persons; an exception is the man-to-man spread of pneumonic plague which may supervene on bubonic plague contracted by men from rodents.

(4) Soil.—A few infective diseases of man are caused by saprophytic microbes derived from the soil, vegetation and similar habitats, *e.g.* tetanus, gas gangrene, maduromycosis and sporotrichosis.

(5) Endogenous.—In the above examples, the source of infection is described as *exogenous*, *i.e.* outside the body of the person becoming infected. In contrast *endogenous* infection may occur in carriers of potentially pathogenic organisms when these previously harmless bacteria invade other surfaces or tissues in the carrier, e.g. *Esch. coli* derived from the bowel may cause infection in the urinary tract and *Staph. aureus* from the nostrils may cause a boil or infection of a wound. The endogenous source of infection is thus the site in the patient's body (*e.g.* the colon or nostrils) where the organism grows harmlessly as a commensal. An infection that is commonly endogenous, as for instance staphylococcal sepsis of skin and wounds, may in certain circumstances become transmissible, as in hospital where conditions may favour cross-infection between patients. Thus the cross-infected patients suffer exogenous infections. Patients with endogenous infections with organisms of low virulence, on the other hand, are not likely to infect others.

MODES OF SPREAD OF INFECTION

Some infections, *e.g.* respiratory and intestinal, can spread from host to host by a variety of mechanisms, whilst others, *e.g.* venereal and arthropod-borne blood infections, are normally transmitted by a single mechanism for which the parasite is specially adapted.

(1) **Respiratory Infections.**—The causative microbes are mainly disseminated into the environment in masses of infected secretion, *e.g.* secretion removed from the nose or mouth on fingers, handkerchief, cups, spoons, etc., or expelled in spitting or blowing the nose; they are also discharged to a less extent in the droplet spray produced by sneezing, coughing and speaking, but hardly at all in normal breathing.

Handkerchiefs, clothing, bedding, floors, furniture and household articles (*fomites*) become contaminated with the secretion and may act as vehicles or reservoirs of infection. The secretion dries and becomes pulverised into dust. When dried in dust, most kinds of respiratory microbes can remain alive for several days, and some even for several months if shielded from direct daylight, *e.g.* tubercle and diphtheria bacilli, streptococci, staphylococci and smallpox virus. Infection may therefore be passed to the recipient by *contact*, either (*a*) direct contact, *i.e.* touching of bodies as in handshaking, kissing and contact of clothing, or (*b*) indirect, or mediate contact, involving an inanimate vehicle of infection, *e.g.* eating utensils, door handles, towels, and other *fomites*; the recipient may finally transfer the microbes with his fingers into his nose or mouth.

Infection may be ***dust-borne*** and occur through inhalation of air-borne infected dust particles. Very large numbers of such particles are liberated into the air from the skin and clothing during normal body movements, from the dried parts of an infected handkerchief during its use, from bedclothes in bedmaking, from the floor when walked on or swept, and from furniture during dusting. The larger infected particles settle within a few minutes on the floor and other exposed surfaces, *e.g.* skin, clothing, wounds, surgical and medical supplies, but the smaller infected particles remain air-borne for up to one or two hours and can be inhaled into the recipient's nose, throat, bronchi or lung alveoli. Air-borne infection is mainly a danger within the room of its origin; spread to other rooms in the same building is usually slight, though it can occur if the ventilating or convectional air currents move in the appropriate direction.

Droplet spray constitutes a third means of spread of respiratory infection. It is probably the least important, except perhaps in the case of the pathogens that are rapidly killed by drying, *e.g.* the meningococcus, whooping-cough bacillus and common cold virus. Sneezing, coughing, speaking and other forceful expiratory activities expel a spray of droplets derived almost exclusively from the saliva of the anterior mouth; this may be infected with small numbers of pathogenic microbes from the nose, throat or lungs. Very many droplets are expelled, but only a few are infected. The *large droplets* (over 0·1 mm. diam.) fly forwards and downwards from the mouth to the distance of a few feet; they reach the floor within a few seconds, or bespatter the surfaces of intervening persons and objects, but probably cannot be inhaled directly. The *small droplets* (under 0·1 mm.) evaporate immediately to become minute solid residues, or "*droplet-nuclei*" (mainly 1–10 μ diam.), which remain air-borne like infected dust particles and may be inhaled into the nose, throat or lungs. It is thought that very few of the droplet-nuclei are likely to be infected with pathogenic microbes, but it is possible that certain virus infections are commonly spread by droplet-nuclei, *e.g.* measles, chickenpox and dog distemper.

(2) **Skin, Wound and Burn Infections.**—These superficial infections may be acquired through contact with infected hands, clothing or other articles, through exposure to sedimentation of infected air-borne dust and through contamination by droplet spray. Pathogenic

streptococci and staphylococci derived from the respiratory tract are important causes of wound and burn infections.

(3) **Venereal Infections.**—The venereal diseases are so-called because they are transmitted almost exclusively by sexual contact. An important reason for this limitation is that the causative organisms, *e.g. Trep. pallidum* and *N. gonorrhoeae,* are extremely susceptible to the lethal effects of drying and the other conditions encountered on potential vehicles whereby infection might be transmitted less directly.

(4) **Alimentary Tract Infections.**—Here, pathogenic microbes are discharged in the faeces of infected persons and are transmitted in various ways leading to their ingestion by the recipient. Most intestinal pathogens are poorly resistant to drying; they tend to die within a period of hours, though rarely may survive on cloth or in dust for several days. They are more likely to be spread by moist vehicles such as water or foods, in which they may survive for up to several weeks (*e.g.* typhoid, dysentery and cholera organisms). (a) *Water-borne infection* occurs through excreta contaminating a supply of water, *e.g.* a river or well, which is used, without purification, for drinking or culinary purposes. Purification of water is effected on a large scale by storage, filtration and chlorination. Small amounts may be treated by boiling or by addition of hypochlorite tablets. (b) *Hand Infection.*—A carrier tends to contaminate his hands with minute traces of faeces and with bacteria that pass through toilet paper; nurses may infect their hands in attending patients and in touching bed-pans. Such persons may handle and contaminate foodstuffs, eating utensils and other vehicles of infection. A recipient may pick up the microbes on his fingers and thus transfer them into his mouth. (c) *Food-borne infection* may occur through a carrier handling the food, through preparation of the food in utensils infected by handling, or washing in infected water, and through flies alighting on the food after feeding on exposed infected faeces. Conditions enabling growth of the bacteria and the production of enterotoxins in the contaminated food, are prerequisites for "bacterial food-poisoning", though not for "food-borne infection".

(5) **Arthropod-borne Blood Infections.**—In several systemic infections the causative microbes are abundantly present in the blood and are spread to other individuals by blood-sucking arthropods such as the mosquito (malaria, yellow fever), flea (plague), louse (epidemic typhus fever, European relapsing fever), tick (Rocky Mountain spotted fever, West African relapsing fever), mite (scrub typhus) and tsetse fly (trypanosomiasis). The parasite is adapted to spread by its particular arthropod vector and is rarely transmitted by other means.

(6) **Laboratory Infection.**—Laboratory workers occasionally become infected from artificial cultures and from infected diagnostic and necropsy materials from patients and experimental animals. Some organisms are especially liable to cause laboratory infections, *e.g.* the brucellae, rickettsiae and *Past. tularensis,* whilst many others require special care, *e.g.* tubercle bacillus, anthrax bacillus, freshly isolated typhoid and dysentery bacilli, pathogenic leptospirae and borreliae, and the psittacosis virus. Especial danger attaches to the pipetting of

infected liquids by mouth, leading to their accidental ingestion; a rubber teat or a mouth-piece with two cotton-wool filters should always be used for pipetting cultures and exudates. Accidental self-inoculation with a syringe and spraying of the conjunctiva when the needle becomes loosened from the syringe during an injection may occur. Many laboratory procedures atomise liquids and so can contaminate the air with infected droplet-nuclei, *e.g.* the expulsion of liquid from a pipette or syringe, the shaking of liquid in an open vessel, the use of mechanical blenders, the centrifugation of tubes bearing traces of liquid on their rim, and the breaking of liquid films as when a wetted stopper or a screw-cap is removed from a bottle or a drop is separated from an inoculating loop. When working with dangerous pathogens such as the tubercle bacillus, it is recommended that all such procedures be carried out within a specially ventilated "protective cabinet" or "inoculation hood" (Williams & Lidwell, 1957).

For further information on the spread of infections, particularly of respiratory infections, see Williams (1960) and Williams *et al.* (1960).

REFERENCES

COHN, Z. A. & HIRSCH, J. G. (1960a). The isolation and properties of specific cytoplasmic granules of rabbit polymorphonuclear leucocytes. *J. exp. Med.*, **112**, 983.

COHN, Z. A. & HIRSCH, J. G. (1960b). The influence of phagocytosis on the intracellular distribution of granule-associated components of polymorphonuclear leucocytes. *J. exp. Med.*, **112**, 1015.

HIRSCH, J. G. & DUBOS, R. J. (1952). The effect of spermine on tubercle bacilli. *J. exp. Med.*, **95**, 191.

PILLEMER, L. (1956). The nature of the properdin system and its interactions with polysaccharide complexes. *Ann. N.Y. Acad. Sci.*, **66**, 233.

ROWLEY, D. (1962). Phagocytosis. *Advanc. Immunol.*, **2**, 241.

SALTON, M. R. J. (1957). The properties of lysozyme and its action on microorganisms. *Bact. Rev.*, **21**, 82.

SKARNES, R. C. & WATSON, D. W. (1957). Antimicrobial factors of normal tissues and fluids. *Bact. Rev.*, **21**, 273.

Symposium on mechanisms of non-specific resistance to infection. (1960). *Bact. Rev.*, **24**, 1.

WILLIAMS, R. E. O. (1960). Intramural spread of bacteria and viruses in human populations. *Ann. Rev. Microbiol.*, **14**, 43.

WILLIAMS, R. E. O., BLOWERS, R., GARROD, L. P. & SHOOTER, R. A. (1960). *Hospital Infections: Causes and Prevention.* London: Lloyd-Luke.

WILLIAMS, R. E. O. & LIDWELL, D. M. (1957). A protective cabinet for handling infective material in the laboratory. *J. clin. Path.*, **10**, 400.

CHAPTER 8

ACQUIRED IMMUNITY

In contrast to natural immunity or non-specific resistance discussed in Chapter 7, acquired immunity is specific in the sense that it protects against one particular pathogen or its toxic products. Acquired immunity may depend on the presence and amount of specific globulin molecules or *antibody* in the blood elicited in response to the stimulus of a foreign protein or other large molecular substance which is called the *antigen*; the antibody to diphtheria toxin is a good example and this is known as *humoral* immunity. Or it may result from an enhanced capacity of particular cells or tissues to counteract infection, and this is called *cellular* immunity. Thus in typhoid fever and brucellosis the fever may go on for weeks or months despite a high content of humoral antibodies, and it is presumably the cellular response that eventually overcomes the clinical infection. This latter form of immunity is often associated with the state of *microbial hypersensitivity* (p. 130) as in tuberculosis. Immunity may be acquired *naturally* or *artificially*; and both forms of immunity may be acquired either *actively*, i.e. the antibodies are produced by the host's tissues, or *passively*, i.e. the antibodies are supplied to the host ready made. Thus, an attack of measles gives immunity to further attacks and this is naturally acquired active immunity. Most infants are immune to measles for the first 4–6 months of life, due to the placental transfer of antibodies from mother to foetus; this is an example of a naturally acquired passive immunity. Troops on active service are given two or more injections of tetanus toxoid (see p. 333) to protect them against the risk of tetanus; this is artificially acquired active immunity. Civilians are often given a dose of tetanus antitoxin following injury, and this is an example of artificially acquired passive immunity. Passive immunity is rapid in onset and immediate if the antiserum is given intravenously, and requiring only a few hours to reach adequate levels if given intramuscularly or subcutaneously. It has a short duration of a few weeks since, being a foreign protein, it is eliminated by the body. Active immunity takes time to develop but persists for months or years and, once acquired, is usually capable of restoration when it has dropped to a low level.

ANTIGENS: BACTERIAL ANTIGENS

Antigens are usually defined in relation to their capacity to elicit a specific immunological response when they gain access to the tissues of some animal species. The response is usually in the shape of the production of specific antibodies (*q.v.*) but in certain instances humoral antibody may not be demonstrable. Instead, the antigen, or some fraction of it, may elicit a tissue response as in the hypersensitivity reactions in tuberculosis: such an antigen may be called an *allergen.*

Again, a fraction of a microorganism may not itself be capable of eliciting an immunological response in the host but may combine specifically with antibody formed to the parent microorganism: the name *hapten* (to grasp) is applied to such substances and the capsular polysaccharide of the pneumococcus is often quoted as an example of a hapten although, in fact, this material is antigenic for some animal species, *e.g.* man and mouse, but not for others, *e.g.* rabbit.

The first requirement for a molecule to be antigenic is that it contains surface chemical groupings which are unfamiliar or foreign to the antibody-producing cells of its new host. Obviously, many potentially antigenic substances are present in the body fluids—plasma proteins, cellular elements—which evoke no antibody response in the parent host but do so when they are injected into another animal species or even one of the same species as may happen with blood transfusions or tissue grafts. The second requirement is that the substance should have a molecular weight (MW) of not less than 5,000–10,000 and, with certain limitations, the larger the molecule the better the antigen. However, certain small molecular chemical substances, such as anti-microbial drugs and even formaldehyde, may act as antigens by becoming attached to host proteins and thus creating a large foreign molecule. In general, proteins such as the albumins and globulins make good antigens and, because of their complex make-up of many amino-acids, constitute an almost endless variety of antigenic substances. Polysaccharides are less efficient antigens and greater molecular weight is needed than in the case of proteins. However, they persist longer in the tissues because they are less readily digested by enzymes and this helps to maintain the antigenic stimulus for longer periods. This prolonged effect may also be obtained by the use of antigen *adjuvants* such as alum or water-in-oil emulsions (a modification of the Freund complete adjuvant, consisting of a suspension of mycobacteria—or fractions thereof—in a mineral oil): the adjuvant probably acts by creating a tissue depot of the injected material from which the antigen is slowly released. Lipids *per se* are not antigenic but a lipid, cardiolipin, can act as a hapten in the complement-fixation test (*q.v.*)—or Wassermann reaction—used in the diagnosis of syphilis.

Antigens have ordinarily a high degree of specificity in the sense that the responding serum-antibody reacts only with its own antigen. This antigenic specificity is related to chemical groupings, known as determinants, which are usually situated at or near the surface of the molecule. Highly specific antigens can be produced artificially by linking a determinant chemical substance, such as sulphanilic acid or picryl groups, to free amino-groups in the protein molecule. No doubt this kind of conjugate explains why patients may develop sensitivity to certain drugs that become attached to the host's proteins.

Bacterial Antigens

The bacterial cell has a chemically complex structure and only the more superficial elements of the intact bacterium, such as cell wall, capsule, flagella, fimbriae, will act as antigens. Among motile bacterial species (*e.g.* typhoid bacillus) two different kinds of antigen, or *agglutinogen* (*i.e.* antigen that stimulates agglutinin production) can be recognised: *flagellar* (contained in the flagella) and *somatic* (in the body of the organism). The flagellar antigen is usually designated by the symbol H and the somatic by O. For these different types of antigen separate agglutinins are likewise produced, also designated H and O, and the agglutinations that result from the interaction of these antigens and agglutinins are described by the same symbols. Differential testing of H and O agglutinins can be carried out by varying the condition of the bacterial suspension. For H agglutination, a flagellate strain of the particular organism must, of course, be used, and if the suspension is treated with formalin an almost pure H reaction is obtained, since formalin-fixed flagella interfere with O agglutination. Treatment of the suspension with ethanol, on the other hand, removes and inactivates the H antigen and an alcoholised suspension is therefore a suitable reagent for testing O agglutination. Another method is to use a non-motile variant of the organism. The H and O antigens differ in thermostability: thus the H antigen is labile at 80°–100° C., whereas the O antigen withstands 100° C. A bacterial suspension that has been kept at 100° C. for about 20 min. yields an almost pure O agglutination.

These aspects of antigenic structure are well illustrated by the salmonella group of bacteria (see Chapter 16 and Table p. 234).

In the case of capsulated organisms, like the pneumococcus, where the capsular material is composed of complex polysaccharides of high molecular weight, antigenic specificity is determined by the chemical composition of the capsule which results in over 70 different pneumococcus serotypes. In the streptococcus family, a microcapsule of protein material similarly shows variation in its chemical make-up to give about 50 different serotypes.

Fimbriae are antigenically distinct from the other surface antigens in the bacterial species with which they are associated; they can evoke antibodies which may cause confusion in the interpretation of agglutination reactions in clinical infections with the salmonella and shigella groups (see p. 245).

S→R Variation.—In laboratory cultures of certain bacterial species, *e.g.* species of *Salmonella* and *Shigella*, two types of colony may be observed: (1) the normal smooth, round and transparent form—S (*smooth*) type, and (2) a rough, irregular and opaque—R (*rough*) form. The S type when suspended in 0·85 per cent. saline forms a stable suspension; the R type tends to auto-agglutinate, though it may remain stable in weaker saline solutions (*e.g.* 0·2 per cent.). These types are antigenically different; thus, an antiserum for S may not agglutinate R, and an antiserum for R may not agglutinate S.

The variation from S to R is associated with a change in the somatic antigen, the variant antigen being designated by the symbol Ø (or R); the H antigen is usually unaltered. Among pathogenic bacteria the S——→R transformation is frequently associated with loss of virulence. Moreover, whilst the antigen characteristic of the S type is often highly specific, the R antigen may exhibit characters common to other, though related, species. It should be noted that changes in the somatic antigens often change markedly the susceptibility of the organism to the action of bacteriophages.

It has been shown that the typhoid bacillus and certain related organisms when freshly isolated possess an additional somatic antigen which is associated with virulence for the mouse. When the organism is continuously cultivated artificially and loses virulence this antigen is no longer present. It has been designated the Vi (virulence) antigen and can be detected by agglutination tests with an appropriate antiserum. It seems likely that various organisms possess analogous *virulence* antigens, and the capsular hapten of the pneumococcus has a somewhat similar role. The coliform group of organisms also carry surface or K antigens which are subdivided into L, A and B antigens (p. 246).

THE NATURE AND PRODUCTION OF ANTIBODIES

Tiselius showed that the plasma proteins are separable by electrophoresis, *i.e* their mobility in an electric field, into four main constituents—albumin, alpha (α), beta (β) and gamma (γ) globulins. The gamma-globulin fraction contains most of the antibodies and has been subdivided into three main classes of globulins: IgG (or γG), IgM (or γM) and IgA (or γA). IgA, thought for some time to be concerned with allergic reactions, now appears to be the predominant globulin of mucous secretions probably acting against microorganisms. An additional globulin IgE (or γE) is now considered more likely to be responsible for allergic reactions (p. 128).

The antibody molecule can be split by means of enzymic and chemical treatment into its various polypeptide chains. This work, initiated by R.R. Porter in London, has shown that the molecule consists of two pairs of polypeptide chains, the so-called heavy and light chains joined by disulphide bonds. The various biological activities of the molecule can be shown to reside in particular parts of these chains, for example the portion of the heavy and light chains which combine with antigen (the antibody-combining site, or Fab portion) is quite separate from the area which is responsible for the antigenic properties of the molecule, i.e. the Fc portion of the heavy chains. The different classes of immunoglobulin can be distinguished by antigenic differences in the Fc portion. Antibodies of different specificity have recently been shown to have different amino acid sequences in the light chains.

To initiate an immune response an antigen is believed to be first taken up by a macrophage which processes the antigen and transfers either an active antigenic fragment associated with RNA or perhaps RNA alone to a lymphocyte which then becomes transformed into an antibody-forming cell. The main γ-globulin antibody has a molecular weight around 160,000 and a sedimentation constant of 7S in the ultracentrifuge. There is also a macroglobulin antibody with molecular weight around 1,000,000 and a sedimentation coefficient of 19S and such antibodies as the somatic salmonella agglutinins, cold agglutinins and some auto-antibodies have the characteristics of this fraction. Once the stimulus to antibody production has been given, there is a logarithmic increase in the amount of antibody in the blood, which must mean that the capacity to manufacture antibodies is a function, not only of the cells originally stimulated, but also of their progeny. The production of antibody, say against the yellow fever virus, may go on for years after the original stimulus. This function could be accomplished by the production and genetic transfer of induced enzymes in a manner analogous to the phenomenon that occurs in bacteria.

The current view on the production of polypeptides is that they are built up from long chains of amino acids, linked together by enzyme action, and held in a monomolecular layer against a film of ribonucleic acid (RNA) which is specially concerned with protein synthesis. There is presumably a template of RNA plus a protein organiser on which the new protein is built up, rather as in the formation of crystals. Only when the polypeptide chain is shed off from the template does it become folded up to assume the characteristic form of globulin or albumin particles. Globulin macromolecules have a half-life of about twenty days, so fresh globulin must be produced continuously.

In explanation of the continuing production of antibodies, it has been postulated that the determinant group in the antigen persists in the tissues of the host for a long time after the introduction of the antigen, and repeatedly makes its imprint on the polypeptide chain so that antibody is produced in the process of folding up of the macromolecule. It is true that some antigens, particularly polysaccharides, may persist in tissues for many months after inoculation, but most of them seem to disappear fairly quickly, so, unless they remain as undetectable determinant fractions, this hypothesis would not fit the facts.

The most recent theory on antibody production is based on *clonal selection*, where the unit is not a single cell but the clone—a family of cells that have multiplied asexually and so have identical genetic constitution. Clonal selection, which is accepted for bacterial cells, has been applied by Burnet (1959) to mammalian cells to explain the facts of acquired immunity and other immunological phenomena (such as immune tolerance, delayed hypersensitivity and the somatic mutation theory of cancer). As regards antibody production, the basic contention is that the capacity to produce specific globulins is a genetic attribute of the cell and that the effect of an antigen is simply to stimulate proliferation of the particular cells concerned with the production of the specific antibody (one of many thousands) which fits that particular antigen. One difficulty with this hypothesis is that more than one specific antibody may be produced by one clone of cells.

Specificity is one of the characteristic features of antibodies. In the case of some bacteria, all strains of the species may be antigenically alike, *e.g.* the whooping-cough bacillus, so that species-specific antibodies are produced. Or there may be antigenic varieties within the species, *e.g.* the pneumococci, which creates subdivisions or *serological types.*

Thus, after an attack of lobar pneumonia due to pneumococcus type 1, antibodies specific to that type develop in the patient's blood and give him resistance against further attacks by type 1 pneumococci but not against other pneumococcal types. This type-specific immunity is also seen in streptococcal infections, in influenza, and presumably in other infectious diseases where there are different antigenic types within the species of the infecting microorganism.

The specificity of antibody depends on the chemical make-up of the corresponding antigen, *e.g.* in the case of the pneumococcus, the chemical composition of the capsular substance determines the type specificity. An organism usually contains more than one antigenic constituent, and for each of these a separate antibody is produced. When related bacterial species have certain antigenic constituents in common, as happens in the salmonella family, an antiserum for one of these species exhibits to a greater or less degree *group action* towards the others.

In some instances, the occurrence of antibodies may have no aetiological significance. In typhus fever a serum-antibody is demonstrable which is specific for a particular type of Proteus, though this organism has no aetiological relationship to the disease (Chapter 39). Antibodies like that present in typhus fever, which appear to be specific for an antigen having no biological relationship to that constituting the immunising stimulus, are designated "heterophile". As originally shown by Forssman, guinea-pig tissues, and also those of certain other species, when injected into a rabbit bring about the production of a heterophile antibody which is haemolytic for sheep red corpuscles. This antibody is generally designated "Forssman antibody".

ACTIVE AND PASSIVE IMMUNITY

The appearance of specific antibody in the blood about the time of clinical recovery, as in lobar pneumonia, the correlation between demonstrable antibody and clinical protection, as in diphtheria, and the experimental demonstration that antibodies can specifically neutralise the infecting pathogen, as in smallpox, are all findings that support the importance of humoral immunity. It should be made clear, however, that certain specific antibodies which appear after a clinical infection may have no protective value. The whole bacterial cell, which is commonly used in vaccines, contains a variety of antigens of which only one or two may be important in protection against infection. These protective (or virulence) antigens are often present on the surface of the bacterial cell wall, as is the case with the capsular polysaccharides of the pneumococcus and the M protein of the streptococcus, but they may also be incorporated in the cell wall itself. On the other hand, certain superficial antigens, *e.g.* the flagella of the typhoid bacillus, seem to play little or no part as protective antigens.

Active Immunity.—When natural infection with a pathogen occurs, specific antibodies are usually demonstrable in the blood stream within a few days to a few weeks after onset. The time of appearance and the concentration, or *titre*, of these antibodies depend on a number of variables including the nature of the pathogen, its distribution in the tissues, the incubation period of the disease and the responsiveness of the host. When immunity is induced artificially, the antibody response will depend on such factors as the nature and the amount of antigen used, the number and sites of injections and the rate at which antigen is dispersed from the site of injection. The time of appearance and amount of demonstrable antibody is best measured by following the response to injections of bacterial *toxoids*, which are toxins detoxicated by treatment with weak formalin without losing their antigenic potency. The first injection of toxoid (or primary stimulus) elicits only a small amount of antitoxin after a latent period of about two weeks. A second injection (secondary stimulus) some weeks later elicits a much greater increase in antibody which reaches its peak about 10 days after the injection and gradually falls over a period of months or years. Thus, two or sometimes three injections of the antigen constitute the primary course, which, if properly performed with good antigens, confers substantial immunity. When over a period of time immunity wanes as illustrated by a low level or absence of demonstrable antitoxin, a small *booster* or reinforcing dose will stimulate a rapid outpouring of antibody which reaches a high level and persists, as a rule, for several years (see Fig. 14).

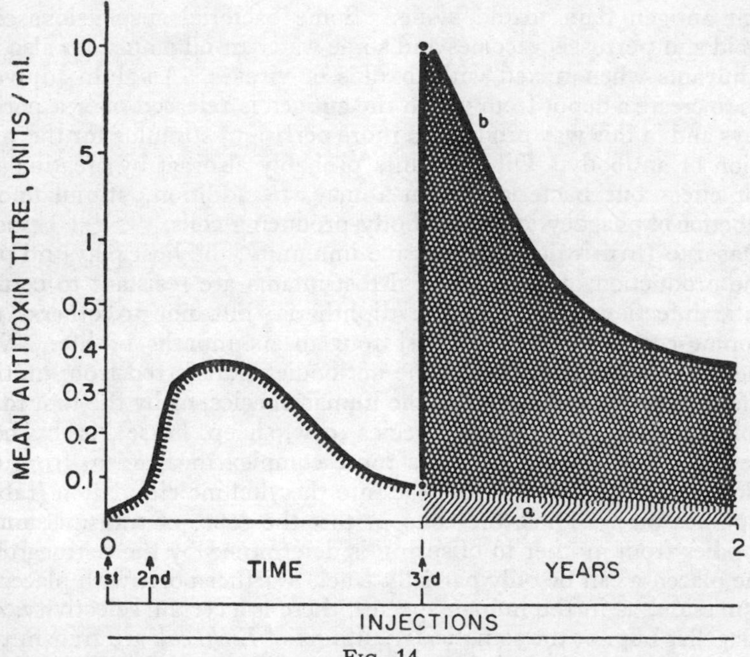

FIG. 14

Antitoxin titres in the serum of subjects receiving either (*a*) two doses of toxoid or (*b*) two doses plus a third dose about one year after first injection.

In bacterial and viral diseases where the infection is not due predominantly to powerful exotoxins, killed suspensions of the microorganism or living attenuated cultures may be used to produce artificial active immunisation and these prophylactic agents are called *vaccines*. In the case of killed vaccines, suspensions of the organism in its virulent phase are inactivated by heat at a temperature around 55°–60° C. or by antiseptics such as formalin, phenol, alcohol, etc., care being taken not to destroy or denature any possibly important antigens by overheating or by too strong concentrations of the antiseptic. Two or more injections of the inactivated vaccine are given, preferably at 4-week or longer intervals; examples are the vaccines against typhoid fever, whooping-cough and poliomyelitis. Sometimes, a purified bacterial fraction, *e.g.* pneumococcus polysaccharide derived from the capsule, can be used as the immunising agent.

Living attenuated bacterial and viral vaccines have been used principally when killed vaccines have proved ineffective. A modified form of the smallpox virus has been used for many years to produce a localised infection, vaccinia, which immunises against smallpox. A living non-virulent culture of the tubercle bacillus, BCG vaccine, is used to give protection against tuberculosis.

When an enhanced response to an antigen is desired in the process of active immunisation, the antigen may be mixed with an *adjuvant*. Thus, bacterial toxoids may be precipitated by or adsorbed on to alum (aluminium hydroxide or phosphate) and this mixture is a much more potent antigen than toxoid alone. Some bacterial suspensions, *e.g.* typhoid and pertussis vaccines and some water-in-oil emulsions also act as adjuvants when mixed with toxoids or viruses. An alum adjuvant helps to create a depot from which the antigen is released over a period of days and in this way produces a more persistent stimulus for the production of antibody. Oil adjuvants probably also act by creating the depot effect but bacterial vaccines may, in addition, stimulate the production of phagocytic and antibody-producing cells.

Passive Immunity.—In passive immunity, the host plays no part in the production of antibodies. Most infants are resistant to certain specific infections, *e.g.* measles, diphtheria, but not to others, *e.g.* whooping-cough, during the first four to six months of life. This immunity is due in large part to the antibodies transferred from mother to offspring—via the placenta in the human species, or by the first milk, or colostrum, in some animal species (cow, sheep, horse), or by both routes (dog and rodents) or by a more complex mechanism from the uterine cavity through the yolk sac into the vitelline circulation (rabbit and guinea-pig). Thus, the concept that the route of transmission of antibodies from mother to offspring is determined by the permeability of the placenta can be only partially true. Furthermore, with placental transmission, as in the human species, there is a certain selectivity, *e.g.* the flagellar but not the somatic agglutinins of *Esch. coli* are transmitted to the infant; "complete" antibodies are held back while "incomplete" pass through and here the size of the molecule may be important. But size is not the only factor since natural diphtheria antitoxin is readily transmitted from mother to foetus whereas the smaller molecule of peptic-digested (refined) antitoxin is not. Another interesting phenomenon, not yet satisfactorily explained, is that the concentration of certain antibodies may be significantly higher in the blood of the newborn infant than in that of the mother.

Gamma-globulin, which contains most of the natural antibody in human serum, may be separated from the other constituents and injected as a prophylactic measure in susceptible persons exposed to measles or infectious hepatitis; or the gamma-globulin of convalescent cases may similarly be used to protect against smallpox, measles or German measles (Chapters 31, 33 and 37). Antibodies to certain bacteria or their toxins may also be produced artificially in animals such as the horse. Repeated injectious are given until a high level of antibody is reached when the animal is bled and the antibody is concentrated by getting rid of the albumin and non-antibody-containing globulin. These concentrated antisera may be used both prophylactically and therapeutically, as in tetanus and diphtheria.

The practical aspects of artificial immunisation are discussed under individual infections and in Chapter 43.

ANTIGEN-ANTIBODY REACTIONS

A variety of methods may be used to demonstrate the presence of a specific antibody to a particular antigen, whether that be toxin, bacterium or some extract of it, or virus. Most of these tests are demonstrated *in vitro*, i.e. in test-tubes or other containers; but some are demonstrable only *in vivo*, i.e. in living animals or in tissue cultures. The tests most commonly used are *neutralisation* of toxin protection (against infection with the living microbe), *precipitation* or *flocculation*, *agglutination* and *complement fixation*; antibodies may also specifically assist in bacteriolysis (lysin) and in phagocytosis (opsonin). Antigen-antibody tests can be used quantitatively to measure the amount of antibody present in a given volume of serum by making a series of increasing dilutions of the serum or antigen or in other ways. The use of different methods for demonstrating antibody does not necessarily mean that several different antibodies are being identified; in most instances it is one antibody that is being demonstrated in different ways. The different classes of immunoglobulin do however vary in their ability to take part in particular serological reactions.

Neutralisation and Protection Tests

If a microbe or its toxin is highly lethal for an experimental animal like the mouse or guinea-pig or, in the case of viruses, for living tissues (chick embryo or tissue culture), the average lethal dose or LD50 (*i.e.* the dose which kills 50 per cent. of the susceptible animals or tissues) is first assayed. Some multiple of this dose, say 10 LD50, is then mixed with different dilutions of the antibody-containing serum and after standing for 30–60 minutes, the mixtures are injected into groups of animals or eggs or tissue cultures. Where animals are used, they should be homogeneous in regard to breed, weight, sex, etc. If a microbe or, more often, a toxin produces characteristic and measurable lesions in the skin of a susceptible animal, series of intradermal tests with different dilutions of serum can be carried out on one animal. Diphtheria antitoxin can be assayed in this way (see p. 181).

In *passive protection* tests the serum in different doses is first injected into the susceptible animal, and after an interval of some hours the animals are "challenged" with a fixed dose, say 10 LD50, of the microbe or toxin. *Active protection* tests are designed to measure the immunising or protective potency of a particular antigen (vaccine or toxoid). The antigen is injected in several dilutions (or sometimes in two or more spaced doses) into groups of animals and, after an interval of 1–3 weeks, the animals are challenged with a fully virulent strain of the organism or of the toxin under test. When assays of a prophylactic agent are first carried out on experimental animals, it is usually essential to compare the laboratory findings with the protective efficiency of the prophylactic in controlled trials on human volunteers. For example, a mouse protection test of whooping-cough vaccine was found to show good correlation with the protection of young children in field trials and has therefore been adopted as the method of assay for standardising the potency of whooping-cough vaccines (see Chapter 52).

Agglutination

Agglutination is the most easily observed effect of an anti-bacterial serum. It differs from precipitation in that particulate rather than soluble antigens are brought together by antibody. If antibody-containing serum is added *in vitro* to a uniform suspension of the particular organism and the mixture is incubated, the bacteria become aggregated in clumps and the suspension appears flocculent or granular, the clumps or floccules being easily visible to the naked eye. The phenomenon is attributed to a specific antibody designated *agglutinin*. IgM antibody is considerably more effective in agglutination than other classes. The agglutinin does not affect the viability of the bacteria. It clumps dead as well as living bacteria. An electrolyte, such as sodium chloride (but not complement: *vide infra*) is necessary for its action, and agglutination tests are usually carried out in a medium of physiological saline. The mechanism of bacterial agglutination has not yet been fully elucidated; it may be due to (*a*) reduction of mutually repellent charges on the bacterial cells after coating with antibody, (*b*) a change in the hydrophilic property of the bacterial suspension to a hydrophobic character or (*c*) linkage of cells together by bivalent antibody molecules. Agglutination tests are applied in the diagnosis of clinical infections and for the identification of species and types of bacteria.

Haemagglutination.—Soluble antigens may be adsorbed on to larger particles, *e.g.* collodion, which then behave as the specific antigen and are agglutinated by the corresponding antibody. Red blood cells, particularly sheep cells and group-O human cells, are frequently used for this form of haemagglutination, which is designated as indirect or conditioned haemagglutination to distinguish it from direct bacterial and viral haemagglutination which does not involve antibody (pp. 7, 73). Polysaccharides are rapidly adsorbed on to red blood cells; proteins rather more slowly. In the latter case, adsorption is facilitated by preliminary treatment of the red cells with dilute tannic acid (1 in 20,000). Any antibody to the red cells that may be present in the serum being tested must, of course, be first removed by absorption with "untreated" red blood cells. This method of agglutination has been used to detect antibodies to the tubercle bacillus, Vi and O typhoid antibodies, virus antibodies, etc.; it usually gives a much higher titre than is obtained by direct bacterial agglutination (see Chapter 54).

Another form of indirect agglutination is the antiglobulin reaction or Coombs test, used in blood grouping to detect weak or incomplete antibody.

Precipitation and Flocculation Tests

When an antigen in solution, *e.g.* a toxin or bacterial extract, is layered on top of serum in a test-tube, a ring of white precipitate will form if the serum contains the specific antibody or precipitin. A quantitative assay can be made by adding increasing dilutions of the antigen to tubes containing a constant amount of antibody until no precipitate forms. If a series of precipitin tests, using a fixed concentration of antibody and varying dilutions of the antigen, are set up in test-tubes, precipitation (sometimes called flocculation) will occur first and in greatest amount in one tube of the series. This is the optimal proportions test of Dean and Webb and indicates the ratio of antigen to antibody where neither is in excess. It is used as a method for assay of diphtheria antitoxin. Precipitation tests are also used for the detection (by extraction) of group-specific and type-specific bacterial antigens as in the classification of the haemolytic streptococcus and in the identification of blood stains in forensic medicine.

In recent years, the occurrence of precipitation reactions in gels of agar or gelatin has been used for assay purposes and also to demonstrate the presence of more than one diffusible antigen in a microbe or toxin. There are several variations in technique for demonstrating precipitation reactions in gels, based on the method of Oudin who layered antigen solutions on top of a column of antiserum-containing agar or gelatin with the subsequent development of a band or bands of precipitation and on the Elek-Ouchterlony methods of allowing antigen and antibody to diffuse towards each other from wells or impregnated filter paper in a plate of agar gel. In this double diffusion technique several hypothetical antigens may be placed in cups around a central well of antiserum and the number of precipitin lines where antigen and antibody are in equivalence will indicate the number of antigens in each solution. Gel diffusion precipitation can be used, not only for quantitative and qualitative assays of antigens and antibodies but also to detect the presence of diffusible toxins in bacterial cultures, *e.g.* in the diphtheria bacillus and the staphylococcus. For further details see Chapter 54.

Complement

Complement is a thermolabile constituent of serum and its formation does not depend on stimulation by an antigen. It acts as a kind of catalyst for a variety of antigen-antibody reactions besides the complement-fixation test. Intensive studies have shown that complement contains at least four distinct components—labelled C_1, C_2, C_3 and C_4—which come into action in a definite sequence in the completion of red cell haemolysis when a suspension of red cells is mixed with the corresponding antibody. C_1, a heat-labile euglobulin, probably an esterase, is first adsorbed to the antigen-antibody mixture in the presence of calcium salts; then the heat-stable C_4 (which can be inactivated by ammonia) becomes attached; next C_2, a heat-labile globulin, is taken up in the presence of magnesium salts and the reaction is completed by the heat-stable C_3, which can be inactivated by treatment of the serum with yeast cell walls (zymosan). These four components are found in different concentrations in the sera of various animal species and complement is reduced or disappears from the serum in the presence of certain diseases such as glomerulonephritis, serum sickness and infective conditions.

Complement-Fixation; Lysin

The *bactericidal action of an immune serum* is due to a specific thermostable antibody (*bacteriolysin* or *bactericidin*) acting along with a normal non-specific constituent of serum (*complement*) which is thermolabile (at 55° C.). The antibody apparently combines firmly with the bacterial antigen and the complement then unites with the combined antigen and antibody. The antibody and complement have no independent combining affinity. It has thus been supposed that the antibody acts by "sensitising" the bacteria to the action of complement, and that the latter is the essential lytic agent.

Thus:

Bacteria + Specific antibody + Complement = Bacterial lysis.

Bacteria + Specific antibody = No lysis (but agglutination).

Bacteria + Complement = No lysis.

It may be noted here that complement is an exceedingly unstable substance and becomes quickly inactivated when it is kept at room temperature.

In vivo bacteriolysis can be demonstrated readily by *Pfeiffer's* reaction: a suspension of cholera vibrios is injected intraperitoneally in a guinea-pig along with an anticholera serum that is devoid of complement as a result of heating (*e.g.* at 55° C. for ½ hr.); if peritoneal fluid is drawn off with a hypodermic syringe at intervals within an hour, it is seen that the vibrios undergo progressive lysis and disappear from the fluid. In this case the animal complement acts along with the antibody of the injected serum.

Haemolysis by a Haemolytic Antiserum is analogous to bacteriolysis —*i.e.* it is due to a specific thermostable antibody acting along with the normal complement. Haemolytic antiserum may be produced by injecting blood cell suspensions of one species of animal, *e.g.* sheep, into another species, *e.g.* rabbit.

Thus:

$$\text{Red Cells} + \begin{array}{c}\text{Specific}\\ \text{antibody}\end{array} + \text{Complement} = \text{Haemolysis.}$$

$$\text{Red Cells} + \begin{array}{c}\text{Specific}\\ \text{antibody}\end{array} \qquad = \text{No lysis.}$$

$$\text{Red Cells} + \text{Complement} \qquad = \text{No lysis.}$$

The phenomenon of haemolysis by serum can be demonstrated *in vitro* with blood suspensions and is easily visible with the naked eye, the blood becoming laked and transparent.

A suspension of red blood corpuscles in isotonic salt solution *plus* the antiserum that has been heated at 55° C. to destroy complement (*i.e.* red cells + specific antibody *only*) serves as an indicator for the presence or absence of complement—*e.g.* in complement-fixation tests —and is spoken of as a *haemolytic system.* Serum haemolysin must not be confused with the haemolysins produced by various bacteria, *e.g.* streptococcal haemolysin, which are "toxins" or enzymes secreted by the bacteria and act directly on the red blood cell.

An immune serum may contain antibodies which, along with antigen, fix or absorb complement; and a *complement-fixing antibody* is therefore spoken of.

Thus:

$$\text{Antigen} + \begin{array}{c}\text{Specific}\\ \text{antibody}\end{array} + \text{Complement.}$$

To test for this effect, the haemolytic system is used as an indicator: on adding the haemolytic system, if complement has been fixed, then no haemolysis will occur.

Complement-fixation tests are employed in diagnosis of bacterial and viral infections and occasionally for the identification of species in the same way as the agglutination reaction. See also the Wassermann Reaction, Chapter 54.

Opsonin

Opsonic action of normal serum. Normal serum usually contains a thermolabile substance called *opsonin* which facilitates phagocytosis. Its action is dependent on the coating of bacteria with plasma protein which changes the surface characters of the bacterial cell and so renders it more susceptible to phagocytosis. This effect may be due to very small quantities of normal antibody acting together with complement which helps to increase the amount of protein deposited on the bacterium.

The increased opsonic action of an antibacterial serum is due to a specific thermostable antibody (*immune opsonin*) which can function independently of complement, though the latter may enhance the effect of the opsonin. The opsonins combine with the bacteria, rendering them susceptible to phagocytosis but without directly affecting their viability. Thus, if a serum is allowed to interact with organisms, which are then separated from it by centrifuging and washing with salt solution, they are still susceptible to phagocytosis by leucocytes though the serum has been removed, and the leucocytes have also been freed from serum. The opsonin is apparently "absorbed" from the serum by the organisms, and bound by them.

The *opsonic index* is a numerical expression of the opsonic power of the serum of a person for a given organism as compared with normal, and has been regarded as significant of the degree of resistance possessed by the person to the particular infection. The index can be estimated according to the following system: a preparation of leucocytes, the bacteria in question and the patient's serum are mixed, and, after a period of incubation, film preparations are made from the mixture and suitably stained; by counting under the microscope the number of bacteria phagocytosed by fifty, or preferably by a larger number of, leucocytes, the average for one leucocyte can be calculated—the *phagocytic index*. A similar experiment is carried out, substituting the pooled serum of two or three normal persons, and the phagocytic index again estimated. The opsonic index is then calculated by dividing the phagocytic index of the serum in question by that of the normal serum. Thus unity is normal, and the opsonic power of the serum is greater or less than normal according as the index is greater or less than unity. It has been shown that the results of counting bacteria in a small number of leucocytes, *e.g.* 50, may not be a statistically accurate representation of the actual number phagocytosed.

CELLULAR IMMUNITY

Although the development of specific humoral antibodies can be demonstrated following a clinical infection with most bacterial and viral pathogens, these antibodies may play an insignificant part in the patient's recovery from the infection. For example, despite the high level of specific antibodies present in the blood of patients with brucellosis by the second or third week of the illness, the clinical infection may continue for 6–12 weeks or longer; and if in this infection or in typhoid fever the illness is terminated early by chemotherapy, relapses of infection are more likely to occur. The lack of correlation between humoral antibodies and immunity is best illustrated from studies in experimental tuberculosis. Immunity to tuberculosis in a susceptible animal like the guinea-pig follows inoculation with living attenuated cultures, *e.g.* BCG vaccine, and, less surely, with killed bacillary suspensions; humoral antibodies similar to those in the immunised animal can be produced by the injections of protein-lipid fractions of the tubercle bacillus without inducing any immunity. Serum from immune guinea-pigs transferred to susceptible animals gives no protection against tuberculous infection. Again, tubercle bacilli in collodion capsules permeable to antibody globulins and planted intraperitoneally in immunised guinea-pigs grow at the same rate as similar cultures in susceptible animals. Thus, all the available evidence indicates that humoral antibodies play little or no part in immunity to tuberculosis.

The evidence regarding a specific cellular immunity is still rather contradictory. Lurie showed that monocytic cells from an immunised guinea-pig when injected into the eye chamber of a rabbit along with living tubercle bacilli prevented the growth of the organisms, whereas normal monocytes failed to do so. Some workers have described similar results with mixtures of "immune" and normal monocytic cells and tubercle bacilli *in vitro*, but their findings need corroboration. Recent observations on patients with hypogammaglobulinaemia have demonstrated the selective importance of humoral and cellular immunity in different infections. Hypogammaglobulinaemia is a sex-linked genetic anomaly seen only in males in which there is an almost complete absence of gamma globulin and humoral antibodies, including the blood iso-agglutinins. Children with this anomaly fail to produce antibody in response to antigenic stimulation and are highly susceptible to acute bacterial and toxic infections, *e.g.* pneumonia, streptococcal infections and diphtheria. On the other hand, the common virus infections including measles, chickenpox and mumps run a normal course and are followed by clinical immunity. The child can also be successfully vaccinated against smallpox and develops hypersensitivity to tuberculin following BCG vaccination (q.v., p. 206). Hypogammaglobulinaemic children therefore seem to develop a cellular immunity to infections with intracellular pathogens such as viruses and the tubercle bacillus, and in such infections, humoral antibody does not seem to be essential for protection or clinical cure.

IMMUNOLOGICAL REACTIONS AS A CAUSE OF DISEASE

In this chapter the immune processes have been so far discussed in relation to their importance in defending the body against infection with microorganisms and their products. There exist however certain states in which the immune mechanism can have results that are disadvantageous to the individual. These states can be divided into two main categories, (1) *Injury to tissues secondary to the combination of antibody with foreign antigenic material.* Here the actual tissue damage is mediated by pharmacologically active "intermediary substances" such as histamine, the release of which is fired off by antigen-antibody combination on or in the cell. Such reactions are known as HYPERSENSITIVITY REACTIONS and include anaphylactic and allergic conditions. (2) *Injury to cells or tissues as a direct result of an immunological reaction directed against such cells or tissues.* Conditions that fall into this category include (i) transfusion reactions, haemolytic disease of the newborn (erythroblastosis foetalis) and graft rejection reactions. In these conditions the immunological reaction is directed against foreign antigens present on the cells or tissues. (ii) Direct injury to the subject's *own* cells either as the result of a breakdown in tolerance to "self antigens" (*i.e.* auto-immune disease) or the damaging effect on cells of antibody directed against a foreign antigen (*e.g.* a drug) that is adsorbed on to such cells.

HYPERSENSITIVITY

Hypersensitivity may be defined as an increased tissue reactivity to specific antigenic stimuli which may be protein or protein-linked substances or certain chemicals. The term *allergy* is frequently used synonymously with hypersensitivity but in this chapter it is used in a more restricted sense. Hypersensitivity may be divided into two main categories, *immediate* and *delayed*, according to the time of appearance of the response. The immediate type of response, which includes *anaphylaxis*, *serum sickness*, *atopy* (or allergy in the restricted sense) and the *Arthus phenomenon*, develops within seconds or minutes after exposure to the antigenic stimulus, is mediated by serum antibodies and is characterized by increased capillary permeability and smooth muscle spasm. The delayed type of response, which includes *microbial hypersensitivity* (*bacterial* or *infection allergy*), *contact dermatitis* and certain forms of *drug allergy*, does not manifest itself until 12–48 hours after the stimulus, is not associated with demonstrable antibodies and is characterised locally by a marked cellular reaction.

In the immediate type of hypersensitivity the reaction is associated with the release of histamine or other substances with somewhat similar pharmacological activities, *e.g.* serotonin (5-hydroxytryptamine), bradykinin and slow-reacting substance (SRS–A). These substances, found mostly in mast cells, are released when there is union between antigen and antibody at the cell surface or intracellularly. Sometimes the reaction is so violent and generalised as to cause death as in anaphylaxis or, if more localised, tissue necrosis as in the Arthus phenomenon.

Anaphylaxis and atopy have certain points in common. The tissue reaction is immediate (within a few minutes) and the hypersensitivity can be passively transferred in the serum. Atopy, however, is of long duration and has a strong hereditary predisposition, whereas anaphylaxis is limited in time and is probably not genetically linked. Microbial hypersensitivity, which is a feature of some of the more chronic infective diseases, is not passively transferable in serum but may be transferred by suspensions or extracts of leucocytes.

Anaphylaxis.—If a guinea-pig is injected subcutaneously with a very small dose of horse serum (*e.g.* 0·0001–0·01 ml.), and after an interval of ten days receives a larger second dose of the same serum (*e.g.* 0·2 ml. intravenously or 5 ml. subcutaneously), it will develop within a few minutes a sudden illness, or *anaphylactic shock*, in which the chief manifestation is suffocation due to spasmodic contraction of unstriped muscle, particularly that of the small bronchi and pulmonary oedema. The serum is non-toxic *per se* when given to an unsensitised animal even in large doses.

Anaphylactic shock is more liable to occur and is more marked when the injection is intravenous, and when a large dose is given, than when the injection is subcutaneous or a small quantity is introduced. Thus, a dose that would produce shock if given at once, when introduced in repeated small fractions may not lead to an anaphylactic shock, and the animal is desensitised in this way. If, after the sensitising injection but before hypersensitivity has developed, a second dose of the substance is given, the animal is protected for a time against a subsequent injection.

Haptens may produce anaphylactic shock in animals specifically sensitised with the complete antigen of which the hapten is a constituent.

Serum anaphylaxis is of practical importance in medicine in relation to serum therapy—for example, when it is necessary to give a second dose of a prophylactic or therapeutic serum after an interval of 10 days or more, and especially by intravenous injection. A single injection of foreign serum may, in certain persons, particularly those with a personal or family history of allergy, produce immediate symptoms of shock. The risk of anaphylactic shock may, in such cases, be obviated by desensitisation with very small doses of serum. Fortunately, the human subject is much less liable to anaphylaxis than are certain animals. Tests for hypersensitivity and the hazards of repeat injections are discussed under tetanus (p. 335).

Serum Sickness or Serum Disease.—It should be noted that after a *single* dose of foreign serum (*e.g.* a therapeutic antiserum prepared in the horse) given for the first time, characteristic symptoms may develop in a proportion of cases. These occur after an interval of eight to twelve days, and may consist of fever, an erythematous or urticarial rash, swelling of lymph glands and joints and albuminuria, and there may be an inflammatory reaction at the site of the injection. Such symptoms may be related to anaphylaxis; thus, at the time when symptoms appear, the antigen (the serum protein injected) may still be present in the system, whilst antibody is beginning to appear in the blood and tissues so that an antigen-antibody reaction may occur *in vivo* as in anaphylactic shock. Fortunately, with the use of smaller doses of refined antisera, serum sickness reactions are now much less common and affect only two to five per cent. of those injected.

Atopy: Allergy.—In certain persons, probably as a result of genetic factors, hypersensitivity may occur towards a considerable variety of substances of protein or non-protein nature, so that when the person is exposed to contact with the substance to which he is sensitive, toxic effects result, *e.g.* coryza, asthma, urticaria, gastro-intestinal disturbance. This form of hypersensitivity has been designated either as atopy, where there is a marked hereditary predisposition, *e.g.* hay fever, asthma, eczema; or allergy, where the genetic factor is much less important and there is almost always a history of contact, *e.g.* certain food allergies. Allergy can be tested for by cutaneous reactions with preparations of the particular allergen, *e.g.* pollen extracts. Also, when the serum of an allergic person is injected into the skin of a non-sensitive person, and after an interval the allergen is injected at the same site, an urticarial wheal results (Prausnitz-Küstner reaction). These localised responses appear and disappear quickly in contrast to the delayed and persistent reactions in microbial hypersensitivity. The sensitising antibodies, called *reagins*, are not detected by precipitation or other conventional in vitro tests.

Arthus Phenomenon.—This is a local hypersensitivity reaction characterised by an acute inflammatory response going on to tissue necrosis following repeated injections of an antigen. It may sometimes be encountered in man, *e.g.* after frequent injections of rabies vaccine.

Microbial Hypersensitivity (INFECTION ALLERGY).—Sensitisation to microbes or their products occurs in a variety of bacterial, viral and fungal infections. This microbial hypersensitivity develops in the course of a naturally acquired or experimentally produced infection and is not usually demonstrable until 1–2 weeks, or sometimes longer, after the onset of infection. It is found in chronic bacterial infections characterised by intracellular parasitism, *e.g.* tuberculosis, leprosy, brucellosis; in certain virus infections, *e.g.* psittacosis, lymphogranuloma venereum; and in both superficial and systemic fungal infections, *e.g* ringworm, histoplasmosis. This infection allergy has been studied particularly in experimental and clinical tuberculosis. The finding, as demonstrated by Koch, that a guinea-pig infected with virulent tubercle bacilli would after an interval of 10 days or more react to the intradermal injection of living or killed tubercle bacilli by a delayed local inflammatory reaction is known as the *Koch phenomenon* and has become the basis of the tuberculin test (p. 199) which is used as evidence of antecedent tuberculous infection. In addition to the local reaction at the site of injection, tuberculin may also elicit focal inflammatory reactions around existing tuberculous lesions and may activate quiescent "healed" foci. These local and focal reactions do not appear until 12–24 hours or longer after the injection of tuberculin and this is known as the *delayed* hypersensitivity reaction. Microbial hypersensitivity, although it cannot be passively transferred in serum as in the Prausnitz-Küstner phenomenon, is transferable experimentally in the cells of an induced peritoneal exudate from a sensitised animal, which suggests that in this form of hypersensitivity the reactive substance or Transfer Factor is closely bound to certain cells. Tuberculin hypersensitivity can be transferred in man with leucocytic extracts.

Contact Dermatitis: Drug Allergy.—Hypersensitivity of the delayed type may occur after prolonged or repeated exposure of the skin or mucous membranes to certain plants and drugs. The skin lesion usually develops from the 6th–18th day after exposure as a moist eczematous dermatitis. The primula and, in America, poison ivy are the plants most commonly incriminated, while the insecticide pyrethrum, derived from a flowering plant, is also an excitant. Drugs like penicillin, streptomycin and the sulphonamides may cause contact dermatitis when used as topical applications; furs containing the hair-dye, paraphenylenediamine, and suspenders containing nickel similarly produce a delayed type dermatitis. Since these substances are not antigenic *per se*, it seems likely that they combine with the host's proteins and indeed many of them have an avidity for animal proteins. Sensitisation can be demonstrated by a patch test with the chemical substance in an oily solvent applied to a non-affected area of the skin. There is, presumably, a predisposing genetic factor in the host.

In addition to the delayed type of drug allergy, acute anaphylactic shock or a symptom resembling serum sickness, *i.e.* immediate type reactions, may occur in patients who have received prolonged or repeated courses of penicillin or certain other drugs. Again, the antigenic stimulus comes from a drug-host-protein conjugate and, fortunately, there is usually some warning of the development of hypersensitivity in the form of localised reactions or skin eruptions, *e.g.* urticaria. But deaths from anaphylaxis have followed injections of penicillin.

Transfusion Reactions, Haemolytic Disease of the Newborn and Graft Rejection

Transfusion Reactions.—Prior to blood transfusions routine examinations include tests to determine the blood group of both the donor and the recipient (the A, B, O and Rhesus blood groups) and a "cross matching" test in which the donor's cells are mixed with the recipient's serum and *vice versa*. Despite careful precautions occasional errors and difficulties can arise as a result of which the transfused individual produces antibodies against a foreign antigen on the transfused cells and develops a transfusion reaction because his antibodies agglutinate or lyse the injected cells with consequent occlusion of vascular channels and interference with renal excretion.

Haemolytic Disease of the Newborn (erythroblastosis foetalis).—This is a disease in which foreign antigens on the red cells of the foetus (usually Rhesus antigens) stimulate antibody production in the mother. Such antibody passing into the foetal circulation damages the red cells and causes a severe haemolytic condition.

Graft Reactions.—It has been known for a long time that tissues can be grafted successfully only between individuals who are genetically identical. Grafts between non-identical individuals, *e.g.* brother and sister who are not identical twins, are not accepted. The immunological rejection process depends upon the foreign nature of certain mucopolysaccharide or lipopolysaccharide antigens derived from cells of the grafted tissue. These antigens differ antigenically in different individuals and are known as ***transplantation antigens***. In a normal individual both humoral and cellular immune reactions develop to these antigens and the graft is rejected.

Direct Injury to Subject's Own Cells

Auto-immune Disease.—The mechanisms underlying reactions to foreign antigens depend on the ability of the ***immunologically competent*** *cells* to recognise and react in response to foreign agents. The body must at the same time possess a built-in mechanism to prevent its reacting immunologically against its own tissues (*self recognition*). This is accounted for in Burnet's Clonal Selection Theory (1959) by postulating the elimination in early life of any clone of cells (formed during the initial development of antibody-forming cells) that are capable of reacting against self. During the early stages of their maturation the antibody-forming cells are considered to be sensitive to contact with antigen (*i.e.* any accessible "self" antigen and even to a foreign antigen introduced at this stage) and to be functionally eliminated by such contact.

It might be expected that under certain circumstances the mechanism of self recognition would fail and result in the formation of antibody to antigens of the individual's own tissues. That this does occur has been clearly shown by the description in recent years of a number of human diseases in which *auto-sensitisation* is part of the disease process. Included in this group of diseases are auto-immune haemolytic anaemia, chronic lymphoid thyroiditis (Hashimoto's disease) and the connective tissue diseases.

Disease due to the Action of Antibody against an Antigen adsorbed on to Cells.—Drug-induced anaemia in which haemolysis of red blood cells occurs is due to the action of antibody on red cells with adsorbed antigen (drug) in the presence of complement. Examples of drugs which have been implicated in this way are quinidine, fuadin, sulphanilamide and sulphapyridine. It is possible that some bacteria and viruses with affinity for the red cell surface may also be concerned with reactions of this kind. Other examples of drug-induced disease have been described in which platelets with adsorbed sedormid, quinine and other drugs are destroyed by the action of antibody against the drug; this results in a condition known as thrombocytopenic purpura. Leucocytes are also sometimes involved in reactions of this type; *e.g.* amidopyrine is known to act as a leucocyte-adsorbed drug and the resultant antibody response leads to a destruction of circulating leucocytes—*granulocytopenia* or *agranulocytosis*—and an increased susceptibility to infection.

Shwartzman Phenomenon

This reaction merits consideration in relation to the general subject of hypersensitivity. It was observed by Shwartzman that, when a culture filtrate of the typhoid bacillus had been injected into the skin of a rabbit (preparatory inoculation) and after 24 hours (but not later than 32 hours) the same filtrate was injected intravenously (provocative inoculation), an intense reaction occurred at the site of the intradermal injection, viz. an area of haemorrhagic inflammation with subsequent necrosis. A general reaction can be induced by giving both inoculations intravenously and is characterised by bilateral cortical kidney necrosis. The reaction is not specific: thus, after the intradermal injection of typhoid bacillus filtrate, or other endotoxin-containing organisms, a coliform bacillus filtrate injected intravenously may excite the reaction. The precise significance of this phenomenon is still somewhat obscure, but it may contribute to the toxaemia of Gram-negative bacterial infections.

For further reading on immunology see books by Raffel (1961), Cruickshank and Weir (1967), and Humphrey and White (1964).

REFERENCES

BURNET, F. M. (1959). *The Clonal Selection Theory of Acquired Immunity.* Cambridge: University Press.

CRUICKSHANK, R. & WEIR, D. M. (1967). *Modern Trends in Immunology, II.* London: Butterworth.

HUMPHREY, J. H. & WHITE, R. G. (1964). *Immunology for Students of Medicine*, 2nd Ed. Oxford: Blackwell Scientific Publications.

RAFFEL, S. (1961). *Immunity*, 2nd Ed. New York: Appleton-Century Crofts.

PART II

PATHOGENIC AND COMMENSAL BACTERIA

CHAPTER 9

STAPHYLOCOCCUS

GRAM-POSITIVE cocci which grow in clusters are ubiquitous and can be isolated from air, dust, water and soil, and human and animal sources. The cocci that grow on solid nutrient media to give relatively large opaque white or coloured colonies with a smooth surface and that ferment glucose aerobically and anaerobically and may liquefy gelatin, belong to the genus *Staphylococcus*. Some of them are saprophytic and may be useful in agricultural processes because of their fermentative activity. Others have become adapted to live as parasites and are found as commensals or pathogens in human beings and animals.

The staphylococci are classified primarily on the basis of coagulase production (p. 137). Coagulase-positive strains, most of which also produce α, β or δ haemolysins, are called *Staphylococcus aureus*; an alternative name preferred by some workers is *Staphylococcus pyogenes*. Coagulase-negative strains are called *Staphylococcus epidermidis*, since they commonly occur on the skin, or *Staphylococcus albus*.

Most strains of coagulase-positive staphylococci grow as colonies with a yellow or orange pigment; hence the name *Staph. aureus*. Colour, however, is subject to variation and a significant minority of pathogenic staphylococci grow as white or creamy colonies; these should be described as white varieties of *Staph. aureus* but are sometimes called *Staph. pyogenes* var. *albus*. Occasionally colonies of coagulase-positive staphylococci have a lemon colour (*Staph. aureus* var. *citreus*). Most strains of *Staph. epidermidis* grow as white colonies and in this book *Staph. albus* will be used as an alternative name for these commensals. Other coagulase-negative staphylococci have growths coloured lemon (citreus), golden (aurianticus) and red (roseus).

Most strains of staphylococci isolated from lesions in man and animals are coagulase-positive but coagulase-negative strains are occasionally associated with infective conditions such as subacute bacterial endocarditis and the secondary sepsis of acne lesions. The greater part of the surface of the healthy human skin yields large numbers of *Staph. epidermidis*, and this organism appears to grow and multiply in the sebaceous and sweat glands and hair follicles. Certain restricted sites on the skin are colonised by *Staph. aureus* in 30–40 per cent. of healthy persons who are, therefore, carriers of the organism. The commonest of these sites is the nasal vestibule (anterior nares). The perineum, groin, axilla and, to a less extent, the umbilicus may also be colonised.

In animals staphylococci occur as commensals of the body surfaces in many species that have been examined, and lesions, though probably less frequent than in man, are similar in character.

Most of the lesions caused by *Staph. aureus* are superficial, *e.g.* boils, styes and wound infections. Less frequently a more extensive infection involving deeper tissues may develop, *e.g.* bronchopneumonia, osteomyelitis and pyaemia; and occasionally septicaemia and death may result from widespread dissemination of the organism from a focus.

Generally speaking, the staphylococci show a marked degree of variation in their biological characters. This is reflected in the variable reaction of many strains to antibiotics and chemotherapeutic agents so that the antibiotic resistance of strains of *Staph. aureus* has become of great epidemiological and therapeutic importance.

STAPHYLOCOCCUS AUREUS

Morphology and Staining.—Gram-positive spherical cocci arranged in irregular clusters, the individual cells being approximately 1 μ in diameter. Single forms and pairs may also be noted. In films made from cultures a certain amount of breaking-up of the clusters occurs and a few short chains may be noted. Long chains are never found.

Cultural Characters.—Aerobe and facultative anaerobe. Temperature range for growth 10°–42° C.; optimum 35°–37° C. Growth occurs in ordinary nutrient media. A uniform turbidity forms in broth cultures. Colonies are circular disks, relatively large after 24 hours' growth with a diameter of 2–4 mm. They are opaque and convex with a shining surface and may be pigmented white (var. *albus*), yellow, golden-yellow or golden (var. *aureus*). Confluent growth appears like "oil-paint".

Staphylococci will grow in the presence of 10–15 per cent. sodium chloride. The salt may be incorporated in media, making them highly selective for *Staph. aureus*, e.g. 10 per cent. salt broth or 7 per cent. salt milk agar (Chapter 47).

On blood agar the colonies are similar to those on agar but somewhat larger. Marked zones of haemolysis appear on sheep or rabbit blood agar, particularly in an atmosphere containing carbon dioxide, but are small or absent on horse blood agar.

On MacConkey's medium colonies are small but show a characteristic colour due to the yellow pigment being tinged pink by the acid change of the neutral red indicator.

Gelatin is liquefied quickly and coagulated serum slowly.

On milk agar the colonies are similar to those on nutrient agar, but the pigment is more rapidly formed, more intense, and different shades of colour are easily recognised. Clearing around the colonies represents digestion of heat-coagulated casein by staphylococcal proteases. These proteolytic effects and also pigmentation are accentuated on heated blood agar.

Nutrient agar containing one per cent. glycerol monoacetate has been used to enhance pigmentation and allow differentiation of *Staph. aureus* into groups showing different kinds of pigmentation. This can be of epidemiological value as strains showing multiple antibiotic resistance and belonging to certain well-known phage-types usually produce yellow colonies, whilst strains of miscellaneous phage-types produce orange and buff colonies (Willis & Turner, 1963).

Another useful indicator medium contains a low concentration (1 in 27,500) of mercuric chloride in a peptone agar base. Strains resistant to this concentration tend to be resistant to antibiotics such as penicillin and the tetracyclines, and include the well-known "hospital" strains of phage groups I and III (Moore, 1960).

Colonies of staphylococci growing on media containing a number of biological fluids such as milk or egg yolk, may be surrounded by zones of opacity or clearing. Many of these are the result of the action of enzymes, *e.g.* proteinases or lipases. As these enzymic activities are usually associated with the coagulase-positive staphylococci, they have been adapted by certain workers in selective media for the isolation of pathogenic staphylococci.

Opacity in Medium containing Egg Yolk.—Many coagulase-positive staphylococci when grown in glucose egg yolk broth give a dense opacity due to lipolytic activity. This effect can be neutralised by staphylococcal antiserum. The reaction is given by a high proportion of human strains but only by a few animal strains. Coagulase-negative strains do not give this reaction (Gillespie and Alder, 1952).

Opacity in media containing plasma or fibrinogen may be due to coagulase, and also other factors such as the β-lysin. Frequently coagulase-negative strains produce opacity. The test may be made more specific for coagulase by incorporating fibrinogen in the medium as follows: Make up a 1·5 per cent. solution of bovine fibrinogen in saline (Messrs. Armour, Hampden Park, Eastbourne, Sussex). Clarify the solution through a filter paper and add a trace of soya-bean inhibitor before filtering through a membrane filter (a Seitz filter removes much of the fibrinogen). Add 4–5 ml. of the filtered, sterile fibrinogen solution to 100 ml. of nutrient agar at 50° C. together with 2–3 ml. of sterile human plasma. Store the plates at 4° C. for up to ten days. Dry plates before use. Colonies of coagulase-positive staphylococci are easily identified by the white halo or ring of opacity which they produce. The soya-bean trypsin inhibitor prevents fibrinolysin from digesting this opacity and producing a zone of clearing.

Viability.—The thermal death point is about 62° C. for half an hour, but some strains are more resistant to heat, withstanding 70° C. for a short time. Laboratory cultures survive for months, and in some cases for years. Freeze-dried cultures in broth or serum survive for many years. Most strains of *Staph. aureus* are resistant to slow drying and may survive for many months in dust in the absence of direct sunlight. Prolonged survival on textile fabrics is a feature of some strains found in hospitals.

Staphylococci are readily killed by most antiseptics and disinfectants at the appropriate concentrations in the absence of serum, pus or albuminous material, *e.g.* they are killed in a few minutes by 2 per cent. phenol and in solutions containing free chlorine—*e.g.* hypochlorite solutions. A concentration of 1 in 500,000 crystal violet is inhibitory to staphylococci, and when incorporated in solid culture media, *e.g.* blood agar, acts as a selective medium for the isolation of streptococci and pneumococci in mixed wound and middle ear infections. Low concentrations of brilliant green (1 in 10,000,000) and other organic dyes are bactericidal. Proflavine and acriflavine maintain their effect in the presence of serum and pus at concentrations of 1 in 100,000, and 1 in 1000 solutions may be safely used in wounds.

Antibiotics.—As a general rule *Staph. aureus* strains are highly sensitive to most of the antibiotics used in therapy. Growth of these strains is prevented by 0·02–0·05 μg./ml. of benzyl penicillin, 0·5–2 μg./ml. of methicillin, 0·5 μg./ml. of streptomycin, 1·5–10 μg./ml. of chloramphenicol, 0·1–1·0 μg./ml. of tetracyclines and 0·25 μg./ml. of erythromycin, dependent to a certain extent on the method of test.

In the hospital environment, and to a less extent in the general community, the proportion of strains isolated from carriers and lesions that are resistant to antibiotics used in therapy has increased, roughly in proportion to the amount of these substances used. Thus in many hospitals today over 80 per cent. of strains isolated are penicillin-resistant; 50 per cent. are resistant to streptomycin; 25-50 per cent. are tetracycline-resistant; and 5–15 per cent. are resistant to chloramphenicol. Among the general community about 20–30 per cent. of strains are penicillin-resistant, and much smaller proportions are resistant to the other antibiotics.

The strains of *Staph. aureus* resistant to benzyl penicillin are resistant because they produce the enzyme penicillinase. Penicillinase-producing strains of staphylococci were originally infrequent but they have been selected and have become widespread as a result of the general use of penicillin. Staphylococci resistant to other antibiotics probably arise by mutation and their spread is favoured by the continued use of these antibiotics. The great majority of strains that are resistant to streptomycin, the tetracyclines, erythromycin and chloramphenicol are also penicillinase producers. A minority of strains are isolated which are resistant to all of these antibiotics, and drug treatment depends on the use of more recently developed antibiotics such as the penicillinase-resistant penicillins, fusidic acid, novobiocin, vancomycin, ristocetin, and kanamycin, against which resistant mutants have not yet appeared in large proportions.

Most strains are sensitive to the polymyxins, neomycin, framycetin and a number of other antibiotics that are frequently used in topical therapeutic preparations and creams to suppress surface carriage of *Staph. aureus*. Some strains are susceptible to the sulphonamides but these drugs have little place in treatment.

Biochemical Reactions.—Various carbohydrates are fermented with acid but no gas production, *e.g.* glucose, lactose, sucrose and mannitol. Most strains from human sources ferment mannitol, and as *Staph. epidermidis* and other coagulase-negative strains rarely ferment this carbohydrate, mannitol fermentation has been used as a test to indicate probable pathogenicity. There is no correlation between mannitol fermentation and coagulase production in animal strains. Nitrates and methylene blue are reduced. Urea is hydrolysed and catalase is produced.

Coagulase.—The production of coagulase is characteristic of *Staph.*

aureus; this substance is almost certainly an enzyme and a precursor of a thrombin-like substance which coagulates blood plasma. The Tube Coagulase Test is a reliable test for coagulase production. Citrated, oxalated or heparinised human or rabbit plasma is diluted 1 in 10 with isotonic saline or other suitable diluent. Place 0·5 ml. of diluted plasma in each of 2 small test-tubes; to one tube add 5 drops of an overnight broth culture or agar culture suspension. Incubate both tubes at 37° C. and examine after one hour and at intervals up to twenty-four hours. A clot after forming may be lysed at a variable rate so that care must be taken to avoid a false negative reading.

Clotting usually occurs within a few hours and indicates that the strain is coagulase-positive. The second tube serves as a control and should show no coagulation. It is advisable to include tubes containing a known coagulase-positive and coagulase-negative strain as controls in any batch of tests.

Slide Coagulase Test.—An alternative technique is to carry out the test on a microscope slide as follows. Divide the slide into two sections with a grease pencil. Place a drop of normal saline on to each area; emulsify a small amount, *e.g.* one or two colonies from an agar plate, of the test strain in each of the two drops to make a smooth suspension. Add a drop of undiluted human or rabbit plasma to one of the drops and stir gently with a wire. Coagulase-positive strains of staphylococci are clumped within 15 sec. because fibrin is precipitated on the cell surfaces, causing them to stick together. The factor causing this is the "clumping factor", or "bound" coagulase, which is attached to the cell and acts directly on the fibrinogen (Duthie, 1954). (The tube test measures "free" coagulase which requires an accessory factor present in the plasma). The second drop is a control to show spontaneous granularity of the strain which if it occurs invalidates the test.

This slide test is fairly reliable, though false positive reactions occasionally occur. Doubtful results are best confirmed by a tube test. A small number of strains give a positive slide test and negative tube test due to the production of "bound" coagulase alone which is not detected by the tube test.

Phosphatase Test.—It has been found that there is a certain degree of correlation between phosphatase and coagulase production in staphylococci. The detection of phosphatase in direct plate cultures has been suggested for the exclusion of non-virulent strains and as a substitute for the coagulase test, *e.g.* in cultures obtained from possible carriers of pathogenic (coagulase-positive) staphylococci. For this purpose an agar medium incorporating phenolphthalein diphosphate is used. Organisms producing phosphatase liberate free phenolphthalein which can then be detected by exposing the plate culture to ammonia vapour, when the growths become bright pink (Barber and Kuper, 1951).

Antigenic Characters.—There are protein antigens common to both pathogenic and non-pathogenic staphylococci, but sera prepared against pathogenic strains do not agglutinate non-pathogenic strains, and the converse is also true.

Agglutination tests using sera prepared against a selection of coagulase-positive strains can be used to distinguish a number of groups or types of *Staph. aureus*. Using simple slide agglutination and agglutinin-absorbed sera, Cowan (1939) recognised three types (I, II and III). Six further types were added by Christie and Keogh. Other systems of classification on the basis of agglutination tests have been described by Hobbs (1948) and Oeding (1952).

The typing of strains by these agglutination techniques has been used in epidemiological studies of outbreaks of staphylococcal infection, but on the whole the information has not been as satisfactory as that obtained by phage typing (p. 67).

Precipitin reactions show that at least two serologically distinct carbohydrates occur in staphylococci, one characteristic of pathogenic strains and the other of non-pathogenic strains.

Pathogenicity.—Although all strains of *Staph. aureus* are potentially pathogenic to man or animals there is evidence of marked difference in virulence. Thus certain strains are associated with the ability to cause sepsis and have "marker characteristics" such as phage type or pattern (*e.g.* type 80), antibiotic-resistance (*e.g.* tetracycline-resistance), resistance to mercury salts, and frequency of appearance in epidemics. Such strains have been termed "epidemic strains", and form a small minority of all strains. In contrast endemic strains which appear only sporadically in outbreaks of infection involving more than one case are usually different in their characters. The characters of the epidemic strains may be contributory to survival outside the body since such survival is important in the perpetuation of the strain, and it has been shown that 'epidemic strains' survive longer on textiles without loss of infectivity.

Strains of *Staph. aureus* isolated from human lesions are actively pathogenic to rabbits; thus a small quantity of culture injected subcutaneously produces a localised abscess, and intravenous inoculation leads to either septicaemia or pyaemia with multiple abscesses in the kidneys, lungs, myocardium or other organs. Mice and guinea-pigs can also be successfully infected, but are less susceptible than rabbits.

Many strains of *Staph. aureus* are strongly toxigenic; they are haemolytic (when mixed with suspensions of red cells), kill and lyse leucocytes (when added to a preparation of leucocytes), produce necrosis of tissue (when injected into the skin), and exert a rapidly lethal effect on intravenous injection. Thus *haemolysin*, *leucocidin*, *leucolysin*, *necrotoxin* and *lethal* toxin activity can be demonstrated in cultures. In addition, certain strains produce *fibrinolysin* and *hyaluronidase* which are distinct from those produced by streptococci. As yet the part played by these toxic factors in natural infections has not been elucidated. The digestion of the clot formed by coagulase is due to a fibrinolytic agent, staphylokinase, which activates a protease, plasmin, present in human and animal plasma.

A considerable number of distinct staphylococcal haemolysins have been described but among those derived from coagulase-positive strains only 3 have as yet received general recognition. These are the α, β and δ haemolysins. Elek (1959) has drawn attention to the production of haemolysin by a number of coagulase-negative strains and for this toxin has suggested the designation ϵ haemolysin. Such strains have been isolated from low-grade infections but their toxin was non-antigenic (McLeod, 1963).

The *α-lysin* produces rapid lysis of rabbit and sheep red cells at 37°C.; the *β-lysin* lyses sheep cells, the effect being progressive at room temperature (*e.g.* after the test mixture of blood suspension and culture filtrate have been removed from the incubator and allowed to stand overnight at room temperature); and *δ-haemolysins* have also been defined and can be demonstrated by testing with human or horse red cells. The α, β and δ lysins are antigenically distinct. The α-haemolysin may be responsible for the necrotic and lethal effects of filtrates referred to above. The α and δ haemolysins seem to be characteristic of strains of human origin and are generally associated with coagulase production. Coagulase-negative strains do not produce them. β-lysin is produced by strains of animal origin, many of which also produce α and δ lysins.

The method most successfully used for obtaining α and β haemolysins is growth for several days in fluid or semi-fluid media exposed to air reinforced in its content of CO_2. The production of β haemolysin is promoted by the presence of magnesium salts in the medium. δ haemolysin is most readily produced by growing the staphylococcus on the upper surface of cellophane sheets lying in contact with the medium. The toxin is obtained after 18 hours' incubation by washing off the growth on the upper surface of the cellophane with saline, centrifuging the organisms and collecting the supernatant fluid.

Certain strains of *Staph. aureus* produce an *enterotoxin* which is different from the other staphylococcal toxins. It is thermostable and can resist boiling for a short period. When ingested this toxin produces a gastritis or gastro-enteritis in man and is a common cause of *food poisoning*. Unfortunately there is no satisfactory in-vitro or animal test for demonstrating this toxin. It is believed that most food poisoning strains belong to phage group III.

Pathogenesis.—*Staphylococcus aureus* is a common commensal of the nasal vestibule, and also of the skin, particularly those areas with apocrine glands, the groin, perineum and axilla. The organisms may be isolated in large numbers from the anterior nares of 30–40 per cent. of the healthy adult population, from the groin and perineum of 10 per cent. and less frequently from other areas. It may also colonise the nasopharynx, though this is more common in babies and young children. In a minority of normal persons quite large numbers of *Staph. aureus* may be isolated from the faeces.

In hospitals the proportion of members of staff whose anterior nares are colonised with *Staph. aureus* is usually higher (50–60 per cent.) than in the general population, and patients in hospital tend to be colonised depending on the length of their stay. Young babies are extremely susceptible to colonisation by the organism, and 80–100 per cent. of infants born in hospital yield large numbers of *Staph. aureus* from the anterior nares and, less frequently, from the throat, umbilicus and faeces on discharge eight to ten days after birth.

Numerous staphylococci are found in the air and dust and on clothing and fomites. A variable proportion of these will be *Staph. aureus*, depending upon the site. Thus the relative and absolute number of this organism is greater in the hospital environment than in the home, and the environment reflects the rate of dissemination of the organism from human sources. *Staph. aureus* is also a commensal of most domestic animals.

Staph. aureus occurs commonly in pyogenic lesions in the human subject. The great majority of these infections are superficial inflammatory lesions with pus formation such as skin pustules, boils, carbuncles, blepharitis, styes, impetigo, and pemphigus neonatorum and "sticky eye" in babies. It is a common cause of wound suppuration and of mastitis in lactating mothers. It may be present in large numbers in the skin lesions of eczema and psoriasis. More serious and deep-seated infections are osteomyelitis, renal carbuncle, peri-renal abscess, bronchopneumonia and localised abscesses. In a minority of cases pyaemia, septicaemia and malignant endocarditis may result from spread from a primary focus.

Cases of food poisoning are frequently due to the *enterotoxin* produced by staphylococci growing in certain articles of food, such as cooked meats, milk and milk-products (cream-cakes, custard, ice-cream), fish and gravies. These foods are most frequently contaminated by food-handlers, although when milk and milk-producers are responsible the staphylococci may have been derived from the milk itself, *e.g.* from an udder lesion in the cow. The production of the toxin depends upon suitable conditions (time, temperature, moisture) for the growth of the organism in the food.

Inflammatory and suppurative lesions similar to those found in the human subject are found in animals, though on the whole they are less frequent, *e.g.* mastitis in most species of domestic animals; pyaemia associated with tick infection in lambs; and septicaemia and arthritis in poultry. In the condition of "botryomycosis" in horses (*Staphylococcus ascoformans*) the cocci are frequently capsulated in the tissues and, especially in chronic lesions, occur in zooglea-like masses or clusters. These aggregates may resemble in naked-eye appearance actinomycotic "granules" (p. 304). In culture, capsules are not seen and the organism resembles *Staph. aureus* in its general characters. A similar staphylococcal infection, sometimes pathologically resembling actinomycosis, may occur in the udders of cattle and pigs.

Epidemiology.—The sources of *Staphylococcus aureus* are persons who are carriers or suffering from lesions. Less important sources are animals and inanimate material in which the organism is capable of growth, *e.g.* contaminated foodstuffs under suitable growth conditions.

Healthy carriers or persons with lesions disseminate the organism over their skin surfaces and impregnate their clothes. The environment is contaminated by direct contact, *e.g.* by direct contact via the hands, or by the distribution of contaminated particles from the skin and clothing which occurs during movement, and in use of the handkerchief. New hosts are infected by direct contact, or indirectly from the contaminated environment.

A proportion of staphylococcal lesions are due to autogenous infection such as occurs when a carrier contracts a lesion due to the same type of staphylococcus as is present in his anterior nares. In other cases the source of the organism is exogenous and cross-infection takes place. Autogenous infections are commonest among the general population; the phage-types of *Staph. aureus* producing these infections are diverse and most of the strains are sensitive to penicillin and other antibiotics. Cross-infection is more common in hospitals; a limited number of types are involved in any one hospital and the majority of these strains are resistant to penicillin and frequently to one or more of the other antibiotics (see Williams *et al.*, 1960).

Laboratory Diagnosis

Examination of Material from Lesions.—This is most conveniently carried out by sampling the pus or exudate with a sterile swab, or if there is sufficient material, collecting it in a screw-cap vial. Blood agar and milk agar are inoculated and a Gram-stained film is prepared. After overnight incubation the plate cultures are examined for colonies morphologically resembling *Staph. aureus.* Representative colonies are examined for coagulase production (and haemolysins if desired).

Subcultures of representative colonies are made in nutrient broth and these may be used to measure antibiotic sensitivity and determine the phage type.

Recognition of Carriers.—Swabs are taken from the anterior nares, perineum or other suspect site and plated on suitable medium such as milk agar. Occasional colonies of *Staph. aureus* probably indicate transient contamination of the surface that has been sampled. A large number of colonies or confluent growth indicates true colonisation characteristic of the carrier. A persistent carrier state may be confirmed by examining three swabs taken at weekly intervals, as the presence of *Staph. aureus* may be intermittent in some persons.

Serological Diagnosis.—Normal serum frequently agglutinates staphylococci in low titre. In staphylococcal infections the titres may be quite high, but the results are too variable to be of diagnostic value. Various other antibacterial antibodies can be demonstrated in the sera of animals immunised with *Staph. aureus*, but their relationship to disease is not clear and little of clinical value can be learnt from their presence in the sera of patients.

Assistance in the diagnosis of suspect cases of deep-seated staphylococcal infections such as bone or kidney disease may be obtained by estimating the serum titre of anti-α haemolysin.

Anti-Staphylolysin test

Requirements.—0·1% gelatin saline.

Standard stock α-haemolysin (obtainable from Burroughs Wellcome) solution is prepared by diluting according to the stated unitage on the bottle, to 20 units per ml. with 0·1% gelatin saline, and may be preserved by the addition of merthiolate. Before the test this is further diluted to 2 units per ml. with gelatin saline.

Red cell suspension—freshly drawn rabbit red cells are washed 3 times, packed and suspended in 0·1% gelatin saline 10% v/v.

Patient's serum is inactivated at 56°C. for 30 min.

Test.—The reagents are added to a series of 3″×½″ test tubes as follows

Tube	1	2	3	4	5	6	7	8	9	10	11	12
0·1% gelatin saline	—	0·5	0·5	0·5	0·5	0·6	0·5	0·5	0·5	0·5	0·5	0·5
Patient's serum	0·5	0·5 MIX	0·5	0·5	0·5	0·4 MIX	0·5	0·5	0·5	0·5	—	—
Haemolysin	0·5	0·5	0·5	0·5	0·5	0·5	0·5	0·5	0·5	—	0·5	—
Equivalent contents of haemolysin	2	4	8	16	32	5	10	20	40	—	—	

The tubes are now shaken and allowed to stand at room temperature for 30 minutes after which 0·1 ml. of the rabbit cell suspension is added to each tube. The tubes are gently shaken and placed in a 37°C. waterbath for 1 hour. Next add 3 ml. of saline to each tube. Centrifuge all tubes and read the degree of haemolysis. The tube showing 50% haemolysis is the end point and the reciprocal of this dilution is expressed as the titre in units per ml. There should be no haemolysis in the serum control (tube 10) or saline (tube 12), and 100 per cent. haemolysis in the haemolysin control (tube 11).

Normal titres range from 0–2 units. A titre of more than 2 units, and especially a rising titre is more significant, but the absence of demonstrable antibody does not exclude staphylococcal disease.

Chemotherapy.—Owing to the variable susceptibility of strains of *Staph. aureus* to antibiotics it is advisable to carry out antibiotic sensitivity tests on the causative organism whenever possible. Guidance as to the best antibiotic to use can be obtained most quickly by the use of the primary sensitivity test (Chapter 53). Benzyl penicillin is effective in the majority of staphylococcal infections in the general population which require antibiotic therapy but infections occurring in hospital are not usually amenable to penicillin therapy. Combinations of antibiotics have been recommended by several workers for the treatment of patients infected with strains resistant to multiple antibiotics. The best combinations can be determined only by laboratory tests.

Prophylaxis.—The prevention of staphylococcal infection depends on (*a*) preventing the dissemination of the organisms from open lesions and dangerous carriers, (*b*) reducing the numbers of the organism in reservoirs in the environment and (*c*) preventing access to susceptible hosts.

(*a*) Staphylococcal lesions must be carefully treated and covered with impervious dressings. In hospital, strict aseptic techniques in dressing lesions and isolation nursing should be carried out wherever possible.

Staphylococci growing at carrier sites, *e.g.* the anterior nares, may be suppressed by applying antibacterial creams containing antibiotics such as neomycin or bacitracin, or antiseptics such as chlorhexidine or hexachlorophene. This eliminates or reduces contamination of the carrier's skin, handkerchief and clothing and reduces dissemination to the environment. Frequent washing of the hands with antiseptic reduces spread by contact.

(*b*) The number of staphylococci in the environmental reservoirs may be controlled by means designed to reduce dust—oiling of floors and blankets, damp dusting and sweeping, the use of vacuum cleaners (fitted with filters), cleaning of surfaces with disinfectants. Surgical theatres can be equipped with efficient air filtration and positive-pressure ventilation systems. Ultra-violet light may be used to reduce bacterial counts in closed environments.

(*c*) Patients known to be susceptible to infection with *Staph. aureus* (*e.g.* cases of influenza, chronic bronchitis) should be nursed away from likely sources of the organism. The administration of antibiotics frequently renders patients more susceptible to colonisation or infection with antibiotic-resistant strains. The use of antitoxin is generally thought to be of little value.

Immunisation.—For the treatment of chronic or recurrent staphylococcal infections, stock and autogenous vaccines have been extensively applied in the past, but with variable success. Staphylococcal toxoid has also been advocated for immunisation in such cases, again with variable results though it has proved useful in the treatment of pustular acne.

Staphylococcus albus (*Staph. epidermidis*)

Morphologically and culturally this organism is similar to *Staphylococcus aureus*. Colonies are porcelain white or creamy in colour. It does not produce coagulase and is best distinguished from *Staph. aureus* var. *albus* in this way.

This organism is much less active than *Staph. aureus* in its liquefaction of gelatin and fermentation of sugars; on blood agar colonies may or may not show zones of haemolysis. Most strains fail to produce any haemolysin.

It occurs as part of the normal flora of the skin. Whilst regarded as non-pathogenic, it has been reported in lesions such as acne pustules, "stitch" abscesses and urinary tract infections, and rarely in more serious lesions, *e.g.* subacute bacterial endocarditis.

Staphylococcus citreus.—A relatively uncommon and mainly saprophytic type of organism; does not liquefy gelatin, is coagulase-negative and is distinguished by its lemon-yellow colour.

Other Gram-Positive Cocci

A great variety of these occur as saprophytes in nature and may be met with often as contaminants of plate cultures, being derived from air and dust. Some resemble staphylococci in morphology, others appear in the form of tetrads or packets of eight (*Sarcina*). Colonies of growth resemble those of the staphylococci and some species are chromogenic, producing coagulase but are non-toxigenic. An example of this group is *Sarcina lutea*, characterised by its yellow growth and widely used in assay of antibiotics, notably the penicillins. Another is *Micrococcus ureae* which is found as a contaminant in urine and converts urea to ammonium carbonate; it is non-chromogenic.

Gaffkya tetragena (Micrococcus tetragenus)

Morphology and Staining.—Gram-positive spherical cocci in tetrads, each cell being about 1 μ in diameter, and capsulated when in tissues.

Cultural Characters.—Aerobe and facultative anaerobe. Optimum temperature 37°C.; grows well on ordinary media and colonies resemble those of *Staph. albus*. Gelatin is not liquefied.

Occurrence.—It is a commensal of the mucosa of the upper respiratory tract and can be isolated from suppurative lesions of the mouth, neck and respiratory tract, *e.g.* dental abscesses, cervical adenitis, pulmonary abscess and rarely endocarditis.

Cultures of *Gaffkya tetragena* are often pathogenic to the mouse, producing a generalised infection. Thus it may sometimes be isolated from mixed cultures by injecting this animal. Rabbits and guinea-pigs show only localised lesions.

BACTERIOPHAGE TYPING

Bacteriophage typing (page 67) may be used like serological typing, for the precise identification of strains of bacteria within a genus or species, *e.g.* Salmonella, Staphylococcus and Pseudomonas, and is of considerable value in the epidemiological study of outbreaks of infection due to these organisms. If the reaction between the phage and corresponding strain of bacterium were specific the interpretation of results would be easy and allow of designation of type according to the active bacteriophage. However most staphylococcus and pseudomonas phages are active against a number of different strains, so that "patterns" of lytic activity are usually observed. These patterns are reproducible within narrow limits and determine the 'phage type' of the particular strain.

Source of the Typing Phages.—Phages isolated from lysogenic strains of *Staph. aureus* are the most suitable for typing and are selected on the basis of the specificity of their host range. A number of staphylococcal phages are recognised internationally as a basic typing set, and these have been numbered accordingly. These phages are grown on susceptible host strains of *Staph. aureus* (propagating strains), which are numbered with the prefix PS, *e.g.* PS 52. Both the basic typing phages and the propagating strains of *Staph. aureus* are obtainable by accredited laboratories from the Cross-infection Reference Laboratory, Colindale. There are four groups of these phages, and patterns of lysis most frequently involve lysis with phages of one group and less frequently phages of different groups are found to lyse one strain of staphylococcus. This is particularly true if the phage filtrates used are relatively dilute (*e.g.* at routine test dilution—RTD *vide infra*). Patterns tend to be wider when undiluted phage filtrates are used.

The phages in each of the groups are shown in the table and the designations of some of the types of staphylococci lysed by them.

Phage Group	Individual Phages	Common phage types of staphylococci
I	29; 52; 52A; 79; 80	29; 52/52A; 52/52A/80/81; 80
II	3A; 3B; 3C; 55; 71	3A/3B/3C; 3C/55, etc.
III	6; 7; 42E; 47; 53; 54; 75; 77; 83A; 84; 85	6/7/47/53/54/75/77 and many others, usually complex
IV	42D	
Unclassified	81; 187	

Medium for Propagation and Typing with Phages.—Digest broth with the addition of 400 mg. of $CaCl_2$ per litre may be used for propagating. For solid media for both propagating and typing digest broth containing 0·7 per cent. powdered agar (i.e. sufficient to give a rather soft gel), is used.

Propagation of Bacteriophages.—Propagating strains of *Staph. aureus* are cultured in nutrient broth from freeze-dried stock preparations. To reduce the chance of contamination and variation occurring in both phage and propagating strain it is best to start the preparation of each batch of phage from freeze-dried stock.

Basically two methods are used to propagate phages. The simpler is the broth propagation method which can be used to obtain suitable titres of the majority of the basic set of typing phages (Blair and Williams, 1961). The propagating strain is grown at 37° C. overnight and added to a nutrient broth to give a final dilution of 1 in 100. Phage is then added to give a dilution equivalent to the RTD (see below). The mixture is then incubated with shaking at 37° C. for 6 hours after which the lysate is centrifuged and the supernatant collected. This supernatant is titrated by decimal dilution and if suitable may be filtered and stored at 4° C.

When higher titres are required, and particularly with phages 29, 42D, 47, 52, 52A, 79, 80 and 187, propagation on solid media is preferable. One method is the freeze-and-thaw method of Williams and Rippon (1952). Petri dishes are poured to a depth of 5 mm. with digest agar. The surface of this medium is inoculated with an overnight broth culture of the propagating strain, using a sterile glass spreader to distribute the minimum number of drops that will give confluent growth. When the culture has been absorbed into the agar, the phage, reconstituted in broth from freeze-dried material, is spread overall save a small segment of the surface of the inoculated medium. This serves as a control area. The plates are then incubated at 30° C. overnight. The concentration of phage particles in the inoculum should be 10–100 times that required to produce confluent lysis of the propagating strain.

Following incubation the control area is examined; this must show no evidence of spontaneous lysogenicity of the propagation strain otherwise the plate must be discarded. If clear, the control area is cut out with a sterile knife and the remaining agar frozen by holding at −60° C. for one hour. After freezing, the agar is allowed to thaw at room temperature, when the agar gel disintegrates with extrusion of fluid. The fluid is separated, centrifuged to remove bacterial cells and debris, and titrated by applying 0·02 ml. drops of decimal dilutions in peptone water to the surface of a digest agar plate previously seeded with the propagation strain. Individual plaques of lysis indicate the activity resulting from single phage particles, thus a plaque count gives the number of phage particles in a preparation. When the plaques are numerous they coalesce into confluent lysis. The highest dilution of a phage preparation producing lysis which is almost confluent is generally referred to as the Routine Test Dilution (RTD).

If the titre is satisfactory (i.e. RTD greater than 1 in 1000) the phage preparation is filtered, preferably through a sintered glass filter ("5/3") to remove remaining bacteria. The sterile filtrate is re-titrated to check on loss of potency during filtration. The identity of the phage is also checked by spotting drops of the undiluted filtrate on plate cultures of a set of indicator strains to confirm that the lytic spectrum (host range) has remained unchanged. Stock, undiluted filtrates of phage are stored at 4° C. and samples are freeze-dried for future propagation.

For typing purposes the phage filtrates are used at their RTD or at RTD ×1000. These dilutions are prepared weekly and stored in the refrigerator.

The Typing Technique.—Either 4–5 hour or overnight nutrient broth cultures of the strains of *Staph. aureus* to be typed are flooded on to the surface of Petri dishes cast with any good nutrient medium to give a total depth of 2–3 mm. of medium, and excess culture is removed. The plates are allowed to dry at room temperature with their lids partly removed, and when absolutely dry, are ready for the application of phage.

The typing phages may be applied manually with fine capillary pipettes delivering approximately 0·01 ml. in which case a grid with a number of squares corresponding to the number of phages in the typing set (approx. 25) is marked on the bottom of the Petri dishes. Drops of the typing phages are applied in a constant order but care must be taken not to touch the plate when applying the filtrates, since any of the test strains may be lysogenic and carry over may result in non-specific lysis.

A more rapid method is to use a machine* which delivers the phages simultaneously via a battery of stout loops to the surface in a fixed and uniform pattern. This obviates the necessity of marking the plates providing an orientation mark has been made, and several hundred plates may be inoculated with phage in an hour.

The inoculated plates are allowed to dry and are incubated at 30°C. overnight, or alternatively at 37°C. for 6 hours. Next day the plates are examined in a good light and each square of the typing grid examined for lysis which may be reported as follows:

+ + + strong reaction—confluent lysis with or without phage resistant growth.
+ + moderate reaction—50 or more plaques
+ weak reaction—up to 50 plaques.

The complete pattern of lysis for each strain is recorded. If no reaction is apparent with any of the phages the strain is reported as non-typable, but may be tested again with stronger preparations of the phages and reactions obtained.

* Obtainable from Messrs Biddulph & Son, Manchester.

REFERENCES

BARBER, M. & KUPER, S. W. A. (1951). Identification of *Staphylococcus pyogenes* by the phosphatase reaction. *J. Path. Bact.*, **63**, 65.

BLAIR, J. E. & WILLIAMS, R. E. O. (1961). Phage typing of staphylococci. *Bull. Wld Hlth Org.*, **24**, 771.

COWAN, S. T. (1939). The classification of staphylococci by slide agglutination. *J. Path. Bact.*, **48**, 169.

DUTHIE, E. S. (1954). Evidence of two forms of staphylococcal coagulase. *J. gen. Microbiol.*, **10**, 427.

ELEK, S. D. (1959). *Staphylococcus Pyogenes and its Relation to Disease.* Edinburgh: Livingstone.

GILLESPIE, W. A. & ALDER, V. G. (1952). Production of opacity in egg-yolk media by coagulase-positive staphylococci. *J. Path. Bact.*, **64**, 187.

HOBBS, B. C. (1948). A study of the serological type differentiation of *Staphylococcus pyogenes*. *J. Hyg. (Lond.)*, **46**, 222.

MCLEOD, J. W. (1963). Thermostable staphylococcal toxin. *J. Path. Bact.*, **86**, 35.

MOORE, B. (1960). A new screen test and selective medium for the rapid detection of epidemic strains of *Staph. aureus*. *Lancet*, **2**, 453.

OEDING, P. (1952). Serological typing of staphylococci. *Acta. Path. microbiol. scand.* Suppl., **93**, 356.

WILLIAMS, R. E. O., BLOWERS, R., GARROD, L. P. & SHOOTER, R. A. (1960). *Hospital Infection.* London: Lloyd-Luke.

WILLIAMS, R. E. O. & RIPPON, J. E. (1952). Bacteriophage typing of *Staphylococcus aureus*. *J. Hyg. (Lond.)*, **50**, 320.

WILLIS, A. T. & TURNER, G. C. (1963). Staphylococci in the hospital environment. *J. Path. Bact.*, **85**, 395.

CHAPTER 10

STREPTOCOCCUS; LACTOBACILLUS

Streptococci are Gram-positive, spherical or oval cells arranged in pairs or chains of varying length; each cell is approximately 1μ in diameter, non-motile, non-sporing and may be capsulate.

Classification of the *Streptococcus* genus presents difficulties. The majority are aerobes or facultative anaerobes, but there are species that are anaerobic or micro-aerophilic. The aerobes may first be divided into those that produce a soluble haemolysin and those that do not. The first of these groups usually produces a clear zone of haemolysis on fresh blood agar—*beta* (β) *haemolytic*—and includes most of the species associated with primary streptococcal infections in man and animals. They can be subdivided into broad groups according to the chemical nature of the carbohydrate (or C antigen) contained in the body of the organism (Lancefield groups). Strains that belong to Lancefield's group A are responsible for over 90 per cent. of human streptococcal infections and they can be further divided into Griffith types according to their surface protein antigens (M, T and R). The non-haemolytic varieties may be divided into two broad categories according to their effect on blood agar or heated blood agar. Those that produce a greenish pigmentation with a narrow zone of partial haemolysis are called *alpha* (α) *haemolytic* or *Streptococcus viridans* and it must be understood that these strains do not produce a soluble haemolysin. Those without effect on the blood-containing medium may be called *non-haemolytic* or *gamma* (γ) type streptococci and include the faecal streptococci (*Streptococcus faecalis*). Whilst most of the Lancefield group A streptococci (*Streptococcus pyogenes*) produce *β-haemolysis*, some variants are non-haemolytic. Conversely, a variant of *Strept. faecalis* (Lancefield group D) may be actively haemolytic on blood agar, although it does not produce a soluble haemolysin.

STREPTOCOCCUS PYOGENES (GROUP-A STREPTOCOCCUS)

Morphology and Staining.—As above.

Cultural Characters.—Aerobe and facultative anaerobe; temperature range, 22°–42° C.; optimum 37° C.; grows on ordinary media but better on serum- or blood-containing media.

Blood agar—colonies are 0·5–1 mm. in diameter after twenty-four hours' incubation; circular, discrete, semi-transparent, low-convex disks, showing β-haemolysis on fresh blood agar plates. Virulent strains isolated from lesions give a matt type of colony, whereas avirulent strains produce glossy colonies; a mucoid colony type is also encountered and corresponds in virulence to the matt type.

Viability.—The thermal death-point is about 54° C. for half an hour.

The organism can survive for days, weeks or months in dust, particularly if protected from daylight; laboratory cultures do not survive for long unless stored at *c.* 3–5° C., preferably in blood broth or cooked-meat medium. Like staphylococci, *Strept. pyogenes* is highly sensitive to the antiseptic dyes, *e.g.* proflavine, but is more resistant than staphylococci to crystal violet; it is sensitive to sulphonamides and to a wide range of antibiotics. It is more sensitive to bacitracin than other haemolytic streptococci and this phenomenon can be used for preliminary grouping.

Biochemical Reactions.—These have, in the past, been extensively used for the differentiation of β-haemolytic streptococci but have largely been replaced by serological procedures; certain reactions can be employed to recognise species within a particular serological group.

Antigenic Characters.—β-haemolytic streptococci can be allocated to one of 15 serological groups (A-Q; no groups designated I or J) based on the group-specific carbohydrate antigens, present as structural components of the cell wall; these can be extracted in soluble form and identified by precipitation reactions with the corresponding antisera. The groups are, in general, related to various animal hosts; the majority of strains from man belong to group A, which is *Strept. pyogenes.*

Group A streptococci also possess one or more additional antigens (M, T, R) of a protein nature. M antigens are type-specific, located at or near the cell-surface whence they can be removed with trypsin without destroying the organism; they resist heating at low pH, *e.g.* pH 2 for thirty minutes at 100° C. M antigens occur in organisms producing matt or mucoid colonies but are absent from glossy, avirulent colonies.

T antigens, so-called because they were originally considered to be type-specific, frequently occur along with M antigens, but they are distributed independently of the latter and are not type-specific. Unlike M antigens, the T antigens resist digestion by proteolytic enzymes and are destroyed by heating at an acid pH; they occur in avirulent as well as in virulent strains and can be detected in intact streptococci by means of agglutinating antisera.

R antigen was long regarded as a unique, type-specific M protein characterising type-28 strains; but a similar, serologically distinct, R antigen occurs in type-3 strains; the importance of R antigens lies in their liability to confuse type identification.

The serological techniques involved in group and type identification of *Strept. pyogenes* are dealt with on pp. 159-161.

Pathogenicity.—Recently isolated cultures are usually pathogenic to rabbits, mice and guinea-pigs, producing local inflammatory and suppurative lesions on subcutaneous inoculation; intravenous injection usually results in septicaemia with the formation of multiple pyaemic abscesses if the animal survives. The pathogenicity of group A streptococci is directly related to the M protein content rather than to specific exotoxins (*vide infra*); the latter cannot be effective until the organism has successfully established itself in the host tissues.

Serum containing M antibodies has a protective effect against infection with the homologous serotype; T and R antigens have no known relationship to virulence and their antibodies have no protective influence in experimental infections.

The virulence of group C streptococci for mice is related to the production of capsules composed of hyaluronic acid; the injection of hyaluronidase protects mice against 1,000–100,000 MLD of such strains, whereas it has very little protective value against experimental infection with group A streptococci. Yet the hyaluronic acid of the capsules of strains belonging to groups A and C is chemically identical, and equally large capsules, composed of this polysaccharide, are formed by streptococci of both groups.

In addition to the cellular constituents mentioned above, *Strept. pyogenes* produces several exotoxins. Two distinct *haemolysins* can be recognised; O-streptolysin which is oxygen-labile but can be reactivated by reducing agents and is produced in serum-free broth; and S-streptolysin, which is not oxygen sensitive and not produced in serum-free broth. These two streptolysins are antigenically distinct and both are toxic to animals; the S-streptolysin is responsible for β-haemolysis occurring on blood agar cultures grown aerobically.

Leucocidal activity can be demonstrated *in vitro* with culture filtrates of *Strept. pyogenes*; streptococcal leucocidin may be identical with the O-streptolysin.

Fibrinolysin (streptokinase) is present in culture filtrates of recently isolated strains and causes rapid lysis of human fibrin *in vitro*.

Hyaluronidase is produced by many strains; this product gives increased permeability of tissues by hydrolysing hyaluronic acid, which forms the cement substance in tissues.

Erythrogenic toxin is so designated because it produces an erythema when injected intradermally in susceptible persons or animals. The role of this toxin in scarlet fever is dealt with below.

Pathogenesis.—*Strept. pyogenes* is the principal aetiologic agent in tonsillitis and scarlet fever and the organisms can be isolated in large numbers from the throat; on recovery, the patient may continue to harbour the organisms for varying periods. A feature of streptococcal infection is its tendency to spread locally to neighbouring tissues, *e.g.* from the throat to the middle ear, or by the lymphatics to regional lymph glands. *Strept. pyogenes* also causes primary skin infections (impetigo, erysipelas) and occurs in infected wounds (cellulitis) and burns, puerperal sepsis, localised abscesses and in suppurative adenitis, otitis media, mastoiditis, arthritis, etc. Healthy individuals may act as carriers of *Strept. pyogenes*, the site of carriage commonly being the throat and less frequently the nose; secondary extensive contamination of the body and clothing of the carrier may occur, particularly if he is a nasal carrier.

Strept. pyogenes is also causally related to acute rheumatism and acute glomerulo-nephritis (*q.v.*).

Scarlet Fever (Scarlatina)

Group A streptococci of any serotype may cause this disease provided that the strain produces erythrogenic toxin and the host lacks immunity to the latter. The site of infection is usually in the upper respiratory tract, most frequently on the tonsils; the terms puerperal and surgical scarlet fever are employed when the primary lesion is in the puerperal uterus or in a wound or burn.

The Dick Test is a biological test which determines the immune status of an individual to erythrogenic toxin; it is performed by injecting intradermally, 0·2 ml. of a standardised preparation of erythrogenic toxin (Dick Test Toxin) in the flexor surface of one forearm and, as a control, a similar volume of the same material previously heated to destroy the erythrogenic toxin (Dick Control Fluid) may be injected into the skin of the other forearm.

In a *positive* (susceptible) reaction, an erythematous area at least 1 cm. in diameter appears at the site of the test toxin injection within six to sixteen hours and begins to fade in the next twenty-four hours; the control fluid injection site shows no response.

Dick testing was employed particularly to test the immune status of nursing and medical attendants in scarlet fever units as a preliminary to active immunisation of positive reactors with erythrogenic toxin. This latter procedure is no longer undertaken and Dick testing is rarely performed.

Schultz-Charlton Reaction.—This reaction is occasionally employed clinically to assist diagnosis in doubtful cases of scarlet fever. It was originally performed with serum from convalescent cases of scarlet fever; such serum, containing erythrogenic antitoxin, when injected intradermally in a patient with a scarlatinal rash causes a local blanching or extinction of the rash within six to eighteen hours. In practice, the test is now performed with antitoxin obtained from animals which have been actively immunised with erythrogenic toxin.

Acute Rheumatism

The aetiologic relationship of group A streptococcal infections to acute rheumatism was first postulated on *clinical* grounds more than sixty years ago. Early attempts to isolate such strains from the blood stream and affected tissues did not succeed, but confirmation of the relationship was obtained from *epidemiologic* studies; further evidence implicating *Strept. pyogenes* has accrued from recent bacteriologic, serologic and chemotherapeutic investigations.

The use of penicillin or other appropriate antimicrobial drug for the prevention of recurrences in rheumatic subjects and the elimination of acute rheumatism as a sequel to streptococcal infections in non-rheumatic individuals has afforded the most convincing evidence of the part played by *Strept. pyogenes* in inciting acute rheumatism.

Acute Glomerulo-nephritis

Unlike other diseases caused by group A streptococci, acute glomerulo-nephritis is associated with only a few specific serotypes, namely 12, 25 and 4; type-12 strains are the commonest of these nephritogenic types, both in sporadic cases and in epidemics of nephritis. Experimental studies indicate that the nephritogenic agent produced by type-12 strains is of a polypeptide nature and when administered intravenously in low dosage to rabbits produces the clinical picture of nephritis; histologic examination of kidney tissue from these animals shows lesions characteristic of the disease (Matheson & Reed, 1959).

Epidemiology

The factors influencing the spread of infection caused by *Strept. pyogenes* are numerous; certain bacterial factors that determine the virulence of a strain have already been mentioned.

Sources of infection are cases of any one of the recognised clinical illnesses caused by *Strept. pyogenes* and also carriers; the modes of spread are probably similar to those of other organisms discharged principally from the upper respiratory tract, namely, direct spread which includes spread by large droplets projected directly from one individual to another (droplet spray) as well as by more intimate associations, airborne spread by dust and indirect spread by fomites (books, toys, etc.).

Carriers are not all equally dangerous to the community; the factors determining the importance of a carrier are: *age*—children are more likely to transmit infection than are adults, probably because they have greater opportunities to infect susceptible contacts at school, etc.; *duration of carriage*—chronic carriers are less commonly the source of new infections than are convalescent carriers; perhaps increasing duration of carriage is associated with reduced M protein production and consequently reduced virulence of the strain ; *location of the organisms*—although nasal carriers of *Strept. pyogenes* are less common than throat carriers, they are much more dangerous because of the large numbers of streptococci they disseminate in the environment.

Factors affecting host susceptibility are: *age*—school-age children experience a high incidence of infection, probably due to increased exposure but perhaps also because they are more susceptible; *pre-existing disease*—patients suffering from virus respiratory infections (measles, influenza, etc.) are particularly liable to secondary streptococcal infections, including scarlet fever; *familial susceptibility*—acute rheumatism is not infrequently seen in particular families; whether this is due to environmental and/or hereditary influences is still not clear. It has been shown that, in comparison with a rheumatic-free group of children, a similar group with rheumatic fever contained a significantly higher proportion of Lewis^{a} secretors (Glynn & Holborow 1952). Prospective studies should reveal whether such individuals, *i.e.* non-secretors of A, B and H blood-group substances, are more prone to acute rheumatism; *previous infection with group A streptococci*—recovery from such infection is accompanied by the formation of M antibodies which are type-specific and long-lasting; re-infection with a strain of identical serotype is unusual.

Laboratory Diagnosis

In taking a throat swab from a suspect case of tonsillitis it is essential that a spatula be employed so that after inspection the affected area can be swabbed accurately and without unnecessary contamination from the buccal cavity; swabbing should not be undertaken within six hours of gargling with antiseptics.

Serum-coated swabs are distinctly advantageous in ensuring the survival of *Strept. pyogenes* (Rubbo & Benjamin, 1951); the swab should be transmitted to the laboratory promptly, and if a delay of twelve or more hours is expected, the swab should be stabbed into a tube of modified Pike medium.

Gram-stained films of throat swabs are of no value in diagnosis, since the commensal streptococcal flora is indistinguishable from *Strept. pyogenes* in such preparations; on the other hand, a direct smear from swabs of burns, pus, etc., is worth making, provided that any conclusions resulting from its examination are regarded as tentative.

As well as attempting isolation of *Strept. pyogenes* from the throat swab, media designed to selectively isolate *C. diphtheriae* may be used and also the preparation and staining of a film to exclude Vincent's angina.

The medium recommended for the isolation of *Strept. pyogenes* is crystal-violet blood agar (CVBA) (blood agar containing a 1 in 500,000 or 1 in 1,000,000 concentration of crystal violet added from a 1 in 10,000 stock solution); plates of this medium should be incubated anaerobically as well as aerobically. A disk impregnated with bacitracin should be placed in the well-inoculum of the plates before incubation to ensure rapid recognition of group A strains (Maxted, 1953).

If group identification of β-haemolytic colonies on the CVBA is not contemplated, then Gram-stained film preparations must be examined to ensure that the organisms are Gram-positive cocci; not dissimilar colonies are given by haemolytic haemophili and certain corynebacteria.

β-haemolytic streptococci of groups other than group A are only occasionally incriminated as human pathogens; such strains belong almost invariably to groups C, G, B and, in the case of urinary tract infections, to group D.

Group C.—Predominantly animal parasites; 4 biochemical types are recognised and that designated *Strept. equisimilis* is most commonly associated with human disease, e.g. it has been found in cases of puerperal infection, and has also been isolated from cases of cellulitis, tonsillitis, wounds and scarlet fever.

Group G.—The majority of strains have been found as commensals in the human subject; its pathogenic role is virtually restricted to puerperal infections; it has been responsible for epidemics of canine tonsillitis.

Group B.—Colonies on blood agar do not produce such marked β-haemolysis as do group A strains. Some strains give α-haemolysis or are non-haemolytic. Most often associated with bovine mastitis it is also encountered as a commensal in the human vagina and throat. It is only rarely pathogenic to the human subject, but has been recorded in a few cases of puerperal infection, including cases of ulcerative endocarditis. Group B streptococci correspond to the organism designated *Strept. agalactiae.*

Group D.—Originally described as β-haemolytic. Such strains were isolated from human faeces and the vagina, and their relationship to the enterococcus was recognised. The group includes strains that are devoid of haemolytic activity; they may be classified according to their biochemical activities as shown in the following table.

Biochemical "types" of Group D streptococci

Type	Sorbitol	Arabinose	Gelatin Liquefaction	Growth at pH 9·6	Haemolysis on Horse-blood Agar
Strept. faecalis var. *faecalis* .	A	–	–	+	–
var. *liquefaciens*	A	–	+	+	–
var. *zymogenes*	A	–	+	+	β
Strept. faecium .	–	A	–	+	α
Strept. durans .	–	–	–	–	α or β
Strept. bovis –	–	A	–	–	α

Key: Fermentation Reaction: A = acid produced; – = no fermentation.

Prophylaxis.—The spread of *Strept. pyogenes* from infected cases can be limited by early penicillin therapy. In semi-closed communities measures aimed at reducing the streptococcal population of the environment, *e.g.* oiling of floors, bed-linen and patients' bed-wear, are successful, but only in certain circumstances is this reduction accompanied by a similar fall in morbidity rates.

In the past, persons at special risk, *e.g.* the staff of infectious disease units who were Dick-positive reactors were actively immunised with erythrogenic toxin; this is no longer advocated, not only because of the multiple injections required and the frequency of their side-effects but also since the protection thus afforded was antitoxic and did not reduce the incidence of infection with *Strept. pyogenes.* Prompt eradication of *Strept. pyogenes* from cases being treated in hospital is the most effective way of controlling infection in nurses and other susceptible contacts (Jersild, 1959).

Chemoprophylaxis with sulphonamides was practised during the Second World War, but the emergence of sulphonamide-resistant strains discouraged such a practice.

Tonsillectomy has no prophylactic value either in reducing *Strept. pyogenes* infections in the upper respiratory tract or in protecting rheumatic subjects against recurrences.

Prevention of Acute Rheumatism.—The prompt and effective treatment of streptococcal sore throat with penicillin eliminates the risk of acute rheumatic sequelae. Therapy should be instituted as soon as the diagnosis has been confirmed and preferably within seven days of onset; penicillin therapy should, however, still be undertaken even if a case does not come under medical care until this period has elapsed.

Sulphonamides should *not* be used in *treatment* of streptococcal infections, since they are bacteriostatic and the organisms are not eradicated. It is essential that adequate blood levels of penicillin should be maintained for seven to ten days, even although the patient has fully recovered from the infection.

It is recommended that persons with a previous history of acute rheumatism should be protected against streptococcal infection by continuous prophylaxis (Report, 1957). Provided that the person is initially free of *Strept. pyogenes*, sulphomanides may be employed in small daily doses. Penicillin, preferably a long-acting preparation given intramuscularly, is a better agent for long-term prophylaxis in such cases. Not only is there 100 per cent. reduction in recurrence rate of acute rheumatism compared with an 85 per cent. reduction in those receiving sulphonamides, but monthly intramuscular administration ensures regular medical supervision and eliminates the possibility of interrupted prophylaxis associated with oral administration. Alternatively, daily doses of oral penicillin (200,000 units) may be given, but control of medication is less certain and a break in prophylaxis need only be brief for the subject to be again at risk.

Community control of streptococcal infection is being undertaken in some areas in the U.S.A. with a view to preventing first attacks of rheumatic fever (Bunn & Bennett, 1955; Phibbs *et al.*, 1958).

Prevention of Acute Glomerulo-nephritis.—From published evidence (Rammelkamp, 1955) it would appear that the prophylactic value of treating the primary streptococcal illness with penicillin is not so dramatic as in the case of rheumatic sequelae; even with adequate dosage of penicillin given in the primary infection the incidence of acute nephritis was reduced by only 60 per cent.

Streptococcus viridans

Morphology and Staining.—Similar to *Strept. pyogenes*; no significance should be attached to length of chains in differentiation.

Cultural Characters.—Essentially similar to *Strept. pyogenes* in cultural requirements.

Blood agar.—Colonies tend to be smaller and more convex than those of *Strept. pyogenes* and produce distinctive changes in blood agar; surrounding the colonies there is a zone of partial haemolysis and greenish discolouration with, often, a thin outer rim of complete lysis, especially in cultures stored in the refrigerator after incubation. The green colouration is best demonstrated on heated blood-agar.

Viability.—Thermal death point is approximately 55° C. for half an hour. Survival in nature and in laboratory cultures is similar to that of *Strept. pyogenes.*

Biochemical Reactions.—These have been studied in an endeavour to differentiate species within the group but with little success. From the medical viewpoint the value of such reactions lies in the differentiation of *Strept. viridans* from pneumococci; the relative rarity with which *Strept. viridans* ferments inulin has been used for such purposes but has been superseded by tests for bile solubility and optochin sensitivity.

Antigenic Characters.—Apart from the fact that strains of *Strept. viridans* do not possess carbohydrate group antigens like β-haemolytic streptococci, little is known of their antigenic structure. Several distinct serotypes have been recognised in strains isolated from healthy mouths and from cases of subacute bacterial endocarditis.

Pathogenesis.—*Strept. viridans* occurs in the throat and mouth secretions of virtually all persons and there leads a commensal existence; in individuals with predisposing cardiac lesions, *e.g.* rheumatic endocarditis and congenital defects, *Strept. viridans is incriminated as the commonest cause of subacute bacterial endocarditis.* This is an endogenous infection, the organisms gaining entry to the blood stream in subjects with poor dental hygiene, particularly during dental therapy even of a conservative nature. In the otherwise healthy individual the streptococci are rapidly eliminated from the blood stream, but in those with heart lesions of a congenital or rheumatic nature the organisms may settle in or on the defective valves. *Strept. viridans* and other non-haemolytic streptococci are commonly found in carious teeth and as the major infecting organism in dental pulp and periapical infections.

Laboratory Diagnosis.—*Strept. viridans* is almost constantly present on blood agar media inoculated from throat swabs and sputum; in such cases it is important to differentiate it from pneumococci. *In the diagnosis of subacute bacterial endocarditis,* repeated blood culture should be undertaken; venepuncture should preferably be performed during pyrexial episodes and the blood inoculated into a good substrate broth medium which may contain saponin to prevent clotting. Growth appears after a few days' incubation, usually as small compact colonies on the surface of the blood layer, provided that the culture bottle is left undisturbed.

Chemotherapy.—Penicillin remains the drug of choice in subacute bacterial endocarditis due to penicillin sensitive strains of *Strept. viridans.* A combination of penicillin and streptomycin has proved effective in infections with penicillin resistant strains of *Strept. viridans* or *Strept. faecalis.*

Prophylaxis.—Individuals with congenital or other valvular cardiac defects should be given penicillin one hour before having any dental attention and such protection continued for at least two days thereafter.

Streptococcus faecalis (Enterococcus)

Morphology and Staining.—Usually oval in shape and occur in pairs or short chains.

Cultural Characters.—Colonies are similar to those of *Strept. pyogenes*, but rarely is any change noted on blood agar media.

MacConkey medium.—Colonies are minute, 0·5–1 mm., and usually magenta-coloured.

Viability.—Withstand exposure to 60° C. for thirty minutes, which kills other streptococci; similarly, *Strept. faecalis* has a much wider growth range, 10°–45° C., and has considerable viability in culture.

Biochemical Reactions.—In contrast to other aerobic streptococci, *Strept. faecalis* is capable of growing on media containing bile salts (*e.g.* MacConkey's) and in the presence of 6·5 per cent. NaCl; fermentation of mannitol with gas production also differentiates enterococci from other streptococci.

Antigenic Characters.—Characteristically belong to sero-group D and biochemical types within the group can be recognised (p. 155).

Pathogenicity.—Lead an essentially commensal existence in the human and animal intestine but are not infrequently incriminated in urinary tract infections, sometimes alone but more often in association with *Esch. coli*, etc. They are also rarely causative organisms in subacute bacterial endocarditis.

Laboratory Diagnosis.—Routine plating of urine specimens on MacConkey's as well as blood agar medium allows ready recognition of *Strept. faecalis*.

Anaerobic Streptococci

Streptococci that can grow only as obligate anaerobes have been recognised for several decades and the pathogenicity of some of these for man is undoubted ; nevertheless, they have attracted relatively little attention and *Peptostreptococcus putridus* is the only well-documented species.

Morphology and Staining.—Gram-positive cocci resembling aerobic streptococci but frequently much smaller (0·5 μ or less) and exhibiting pleomorphism in artificial culture.

Cultural Characters.—After anaerobic incubation for forty-eight hours, colonies on blood agar are smooth, low-convex, approximately 1–2 mm. in diameter; no alteration occurs in the medium. Cultures, *e.g.* in meat broth, usually give off an exceptionally foul odour.

Biochemical Reactions.—Attempts have been made to classify the anaerobic streptococci on the basis of such reactions; provided that a sulphur compound is present (*e.g.* 0·1 per cent. sodium thioglycollate) in the medium, *Pepto. putridus* strains ferment glucose, maltose and fructose with abundant gas production.

Pathogenicity.—It would appear that their normal habitat is the vagina; so far they have not been isolated from the upper respiratory tract, intestinal contents or the skin of healthy persons. *Pepto. putridus* is incriminated in puerperal sepsis, probably as an endogenous infection precipitated by trauma and the presence of necrotic material; it has also been isolated from brain abscess, infected wounds, *e.g.* post-operative synergistic bacterial gangrene and anaerobic streptococcal myositis.

Laboratory Diagnosis.—Strictly anaerobic methods are required if isolation is to be successful. Inoculation of blood agar plates and incubation for forty-eight hours in a McIntosh and Fildes' jar produces colonies as described above; for details of the biochemical reactions of species other than *Pepto. putridus* the papers of Hare *et al.* (1952) and Thomas & Hare (1954) should be consulted.

Chemotherapy.—Strains are sensitive to penicillin which should be employed therapeutically.

Streptococci in Diseases of Domesticated Animals

Streptococci are relatively infrequent in suppurative lesions of sheep and swine, but are not uncommonly associated with mastitis of cattle and with strangles and contagious pleuropneumonia of horses.

Bovine Mastitis

Streptococci are frequently found as the sole organism, especially in chronic mastitis (*Strept. agalactiae*); such streptococci vary in their action on blood agar and may exhibit α- or β-haemolysis or none. They belong to Lancefield group B and identification with group-specific antiserum has replaced fairly extensive biochemical testing.

Another streptococcus occurring in bovine mastitis is designated *Strept. dysgalactiae* and is non-haemolytic; serologically it belongs to group C; biochemical differentiation of *Strept. dysgalactiae* from group C strains associated with other hosts may be undertaken as in the table.

	Lactose	Trehalose	Sorbitol
Strept. dysgalactiae . . .	⊥	⊥	v
Strept. equi (horses) . . .	–	–	–
Strept. equisimilis (human) . .	v	⊥	–
Strept. zooepidemicus (animals) .	⊥	–	⊥

Key: ⊥ = acid produced; v = acid production variable; – = no reaction.

Laboratory Diagnosis of Bovine Mastitis.—Centrifugal deposits from milk samples are plated out on a medium comprising 2 ml. 0·1 per cent. crystal violet, 1 g. aesculin and 50 ml. defibrinated ox-blood in 1 l. of Lemco agar (pH 7·4). Many of the other organisms present in milk are inhibited by the crystal violet and these which are dye-resistant usually produce black colonies in the presence of aesculin and can be readily differentiated from streptococci. Pure cultures of any streptococci isolated are obtained and their serological group determined; if the strain belongs to group C it can be biochemically identified as in the table.

Serologic Identification of β-haemolytic Streptococci

Lancefield Grouping.—Extraction of group-specific polysaccharide can be undertaken by one of the following methods:

(1) *Acid extraction*

The centrifuged deposit from 50 ml. of overnight culture in Todd-Hewitt broth is harvested in a $3 \times \frac{1}{2}$ in. test-tube. The deposit is thoroughly re-suspended in 0·4 ml. of 0·2 *N* HCl. Place tube in a boiling water-bath. After ten minutes' exposure, remove tube from bath and allow to cool. Add 1 drop of 0·02 per cent. phenol red. Neutralise carefully with 0·5 *N* and 0·2 *N* NaOH. The clear supernatant obtained by centrifugation is the extract.

(2) *Formamide extraction*

The centrifuged deposit from 5 ml. of overnight culture in Todd-Hewitt broth is re-suspended in 0·1 ml. of formamide in a $3 \times \frac{1}{2}$ in. test-tube. Place tube in oil-bath at 160° C. for fifteen minutes; centrifuge and discard any deposit. Mix supernatant with 0·25 ml. of acid-alcohol and centrifuge. 0·5 ml. of acetone is added to the new supernatant and the precipitate obtained by further centrifugation is dissolved in 0·4 ml. of saline. Add 1 drop of phenol red and neutralise with 0·2 *N* NaOH.

(3) *Enzyme extraction*

Suspend a loopful of growth from an eighteen-hour blood-agar culture in 0·25 ml. enzyme solution (see below) contained in a flocculation tube. Place tube in 50° C. water-bath. Inspect tube at one, one and a half and two hour periods, and when contents are clear, use as extract.

The enzyme is produced from a *Streptomyces albus*[1] growing in the following medium.

NaCl . . .	5 g.
K_2HPO_4 . .	2 g.
$MgSO_4$, $7H_2O$.	1 g.
$CaCl_2$ . . .	0·04 g.
$FeSO_4$, $7H_2O$.	0·02 g.
$ZnSO_4$, $7H_2O$.	0·01 g.
Yeastrel . .	5 g.
Agar powder . .	11 g.
Distilled water .	1 l.

Place suitable amounts (75-100 ml.) in Roux bottles, sterilise and add aseptically glucose and casmino acids, each in a final concentration of 0·5 per cent. pH should be 7·0–7·4.

(1) Inoculate the surface of above medium by flooding with *Streptomyces albus* glucose-broth culture.

(2) Incubate at 30–37° C. for four to five days.

(3) Place Roux bottles in a −10° C. refrigerator and then allow to thaw out; the fluid expressed on thawing is the enzyme solution.

(4) Adjust pH to 7·5 by adding 1 *N* HCl; filter through a Seitz disk.

(5) Test for potency of the filtrate by adding 0·1 ml. of a heavy suspension of heat-killed group A streptococci to 0·4 ml. of the enzyme preparation. Place in a 50° C. water-bath along with a tube containing a control mixture in which the enzyme has been destroyed by heating. An active preparation will lyse the streptococcal suspension in one-half to one hour.

(6) Stored in the cold with 0·5 per cent. phenol as preservative, the preparation keeps well and is active over a pH range of 5·6–9·6.

The enzyme extraction method (Maxted, 1948) is reliable for streptococci in groups A, C or G; for other groups the acid (Lancefield, 1933) or formamide (Fuller, 1938) methods are preferred, the latter being less likely to give minor cross-reactions occasionally encountered with acid extracts. Group-O polysaccharide is sensitive to formamide so that such extracts do not react with O antiserum. Acid extracts can also be used for identification of type-specific M antigens.

Precipitation Test for Grouping of Strept. pyogenes.—This may be performed in the narrowing neck of small Pasteur pipettes. A small

[1] Obtainable from NCTC, Colindale Avenue, London.

volume of group A antiserum is placed in the pipette and the antigenic extract carefully superimposed. If the extract contains polysaccharide specific for group A, then precipitation will be observed at the interface with the serum within five minutes; reactions appearing after this time should not be regarded as positive. Extracts should also be tested with antisera for groups C and G routinely, and if necessary with other group sera.

In order to conserve serum, tests may be performed in capillary tubes; a ½-in. column of serum is run into the tube, the exterior of which is carefully wiped before an equivalent volume of antigen extract is introduced. The contents are allowed to run well up the tube and the upper end is then occluded with the forefinger until the tube has been placed in a plasticine block. Macroscopic precipitation should be evident within the time limits stated above if the reaction is positive.

Type Identification of Group-A Strains.—All strains should be tested for type both by agglutinating (T) and precipitating (M) antisera, since a smaller percentage of strains will thus be regarded as untypable than when either method is employed alone (Williams & Maxted, 1953).

Slide agglutination test.—The strain is grown in 5 ml. of Todd-Hewitt broth at 28° C. for eighteen to twenty-four hours and the centrifuged deposit thoroughly resuspended in 0·5 ml. of supernatant broth. Provided that the suspension is not granular, 6 loopfuls are placed on a clean glass slide and each then mixed with a small (1 mm.) loopful of pooled antisera and the slide rocked to and fro for one minute. Agglutination may be noted with one of the pooled antisera and fresh loopfuls of suspension should then similarly be tested with all the specific sera comprising that particular pool. Strains may react in more than one type-specific serum, but the pattern of such reactions is epidemiologically significant.

Granular suspensions and those that react with many sera should be treated as follows: Add 1 drop of B.D.H. Universal Indicator and 2 drops of pancreatic extract to the suspension; adjust the pH to 8–8·5 with 0·2 *N* NaOH and place in 37° C. water-bath for one hour, shaking the tubes every fifteen minutes. On re-testing with pooled and specific antisera as above, many such strains will react normally; if results are still unsatisfactory, a further period of fifteen minutes in a 50° C. bath may be tried.

Precipitation test.—Acid extracted antigen prepared for group determination is used. Using the results of slide agglutination as a guide, the extract is tested against the relevant antisera by the capillary tube method. The mixtures are incubated for two hours at 37° C. and results noted; after overnight refrigeration the tubes are again examined.

THE LACTOBACILLI

This genus belongs, as do the streptococci, to the family Lactobacillaceae. The lactobacilli constitute a group of acid-resistant (aciduric), Gram-positive, non-sporing bacilli, which occur in the intestine of mammalian animals and are particularly numerous during the stage of suckling. Thus, in breast-fed infants such organisms may constitute the predominant flora of the intestine, and two main types, *Lacto. acidophilus* and *Lacto. bifidus*, have been recognised and specially studied.

Organisms of this group form one of the main elements of the commensal flora of the human alimentary canal, including the mouth, stomach and intestine, and occur also in the vagina and on the skin. They are found in cow's milk, silage and bran.

Lactobacillus acidophilus

So called because it is able to flourish in a highly acid medium (pH 4·0), it occurs in the faeces, saliva and milk. In morphology it is a relatively large, non-sporing, non-motile, Gram-positive bacillus. The individual organisms vary in length, and may appear even in short coccal forms. Some are about 1 μ broad, but slender forms may be noted, and there is a tendency to chain formation. The organism thus shows considerable pleomorphism. It may be cultivated under aerobic conditions on whey agar at 37° C., but when first isolated it tends to be micro-aerophilic and grows best at a reduced oxygen tension. The colonies are small, and vary in appearance as seen under the low power of the microscope; two main types are described: (1) "feathery", in appearance not unlike a *Cl. tetani* colony (*q.v.*), and (2) rounded with projecting outgrowths ("crab-colony"). A convenient method of obtaining cultures from faeces is to inoculate broth, to which is added 0·5 per cent. of glacial acetic acid; after incubation, subcultures can be made on agar plates under aerobic conditions.

This organism produces acid fermentation of glucose and lactose without gas formation. It also ferments maltose, whereas *Lactobacillus bulgaricus*, a related organism originally isolated from Yoghurt (a fermented milk), has usually no action on maltose. The latter organism cannot grow in the intestine of man. It is a thermophile, the optimum temperature being 45°–62° C.

Closely related organisms are *Bacillus acidophilus odontolyticus* described in association with dental caries, the so-called Boas-Oppler bacillus found in the stomach contents in conditions in which the hydrochloric acid is absent or deficient, and *Döderlein's bacillus*, which is found normally in the vagina.

Dental Caries.—This destructive condition is noted in its earlier stages by discolouration of the enamel of the tooth and loss of translucency; cavity formation follows and at the dentino-enamel junction there is always lateral extension of the process with progressive softening into the dentine.

For many years there have been differing opinions on the part played by bacteria, particularly lactobacilli, in promoting caries; their role has been confused with that of cariogenic foodstuffs, but even with such a diet, caries does not apparently occur in the absence of bacteria. Thus, germ-free rats do not develop caries with a cariogenic diet unless streptococci or lactobacilli are added to the food, when caries develops rapidly in the molar teeth.

Lactobacilli Counts.—It is known that there is a quantitative difference in the number of lactobacilli in the mouths of those prone to caries in comparison with those who are apparently immune. The estimation of lactobacilli is thus of increasing importance in dentistry: the salivary flow is activated by the person chewing a small piece of paraffin wax for ten minutes; saliva is collected in a sterile container as it is produced and the volume made up to 10 ml. with sterile saline. The lactobacillus count is the number of lactobacilli present in 1 ml. of this standard specimen; the sample is serially diluted in broth or peptone water and distributed in 0·1 ml. quantities on a medium selective for lactobacilli, *e.g.* Kulp's tomato peptone agar plates. After three or four days' incubation at 37° C. counts of more than 10^5 lactobacilli per ml. of saliva are often taken as indicative of caries activity. In the same individual, significant reductions in the count are noted when a non-cariogenic diet is taken.

Lactobacillus bifidus (Bacillus bifidus)

This organism derives its name from the apparently bifid appearance described by the original observers. It is found in large numbers in the faeces of breast-fed infants. Its average dimensions are 4 μ by 0·5–0·7 μ, but it displays considerable pleomorphism. The ends are often expanded. Three bacilli together may be arranged like a Y. Though usually Gram-positive, there is a certain amount of variation in its reaction to Gram's staining method.

In primary culture it is a strict anaerobe. Cultures have been obtained at 37° C. in tubes of neutral lactose-broth containing a piece of sterile rabbit kidney, and sealed with a layer of sterile soft petroleum jelly. After several days' growth, subcultures are made on glucose agar plates which are incubated anaerobically. Pure cultures on glucose agar can be obtained from single colonies. The organisms may ultimately become microaerophilic. Glucose, sucrose, maltose and various other sugars are fermented with acid production, but no gas.

REFERENCES

Bunn, W. H. & Bennett, H. N. (1955). Community control of rheumatic fever. *J. Amer. med. Ass.*, **157**, 986.

Fuller, A. T. (1938). The formamide method for the extraction of polysaccharides from harmolytic streptococci. *Brit. J. exp. Path.*, **19**, 130.

Glynn, L. E. & Holborow, E. J. (1952). Conversion of tissue polysaccharides to auto-antigens by Group-A Beta-haemolytic streptococci. *Lancet*, **2**, 449.

Hare, R., Wildy, P., Billett, F. S. & Twort, D. N. (1952). The anaerobic cocci: gas formation, fermentation reactions, sensitivity to antibiotics and sulphonamides. Classification. *J. Hyg.* (*Camb.*)., **50**, 295.

Jersild, T. (1959). In *Rheumatic Fever*, p. 58. Oxford: Blackwell.

Lancefield, R. C. (1933). A serological differentiation of human and other groups of haemolytic streptococci. *J. exp. Med.*, **57**, 571.

Matheson, B. H. & Reed, R. W. (1959). Experimental nephritis due to type specific streptococci. (contains references to earlier work of these and other authors). *J. infect. Dis.*, **104**, 213.

Maxted, W. R. (1948). Preparation of streptococcal extracts for Lancefield grouping. *Lancet*, **2**, 255.

Maxted, W. R. (1953). The use of bacitracin for identifying Group A haemolytic streptococci. *J. clin. Path.*, **6**, 224.

Phibbs, B., Becker, D., Lowe, C. R., Holmes, R., Fowler, R., Scott, O. K., Roberts, K., Watson, W. & Malott, R. (1958). The Casper project—an enforced mass-culture streptococcic control program. *J. Amer. med. Ass.*, **166**, 1133.

RAMMELKAMP, C. H. (1955). Prevention of acute nephritis. *Ann. intern. Med.*, **43**, 511.
REPORT (1957). *Wld Hlth Org. techn. Rep. Ser.*, No. 126.
RUBBO, S. D. & BENJAMIN, M. (1951). Some observations on survival of pathogenic bacteria on cotton-wool swabs. *Brit. med. J.*, **1**, 983.
THOMAS, C. G. A. & HARE, R. (1954). The classification of anaerobic cocci and their isolation in normal human beings and pathological processes. *J. clin. Path.*, **7**, 300.
WILLIAMS, R. E. O. & MAXTED, W. R. (1953). The type classification of *Streptococcus pyogenes*. *Congr. int. Mircobiol. 6th Congr. Rome*, **1**, 46.

CHAPTER 11

PNEUMOCOCCUS
(Diplococcus pneumoniae)

THE causative organism of lobar pneumonia; also incriminated in acute and chronic infections of the respiratory tract, in conjunctivitis, otitis media, meningitis, peritonitis, arthritis, etc.

Morphology and Staining.—Characteristically appears as an oval or lanceolate Gram-positive coccus in pairs with the long axes in line with each other; approximately 1 μ in its long diameter and capsulate. In culture the appearance is less typical, the cocci being more rounded with a tendency to occur in short chains in liquid media; capsules may not be evident except in India-ink films.

Cultural Characters.—Aerobe and facultative anaerobe; temperature range 25°–40° C., optimum 37° C ; grows on ordinary media but best on blood- or serum-enriched media. The addition of glucose (*e.g.* 0·1 per cent.) to culture media promotes growth and similarly cultivation in an atmosphere of 5 per cent. CO_2 is advantageous. It should be noted in the preparation of broth for the cultivation of pneumococci that they may be inhibited by an oxidised constituent of the peptone; this can be prevented by adding the peptone to the medium *before* heating so that it is later subjected to the reducing action of the meat infusion; commercial peptones may also contain metallic impurities which are responsible for inhibitory effects on the growth of the pneumococcus.

Blood agar.—Colonies are small (1 mm. in diameter), semi-transparent and are usually surrounded by a zone of α-haemolysis which may cause confusion with *Strept. viridans*; unlike the latter, the colonies are at first plateau-shaped and later develop elevated margins and concentric ridges—the so-called draughtsman colony. Green pigmentation is more obvious when the organism is growing on heated blood agar.

Viability.—Thermal death point is about 52° C. for fifteen minutes. Ordinary laboratory cultures lose viability rapidly; cultivation in a semi-solid agar containing blood ensures longer survival and for maintenance of culture over long periods, rapid drying *in vacuo* eliminates the need for frequent subculture. Repeated *in vitro* cultivation leads to transformation from the smooth (S) to the rough (R) form, a change associated with loss of capsule formation, type specificity and virulence.

Biochemical Reactions.—Ferments various carbohydrates and differs from the majority of *Strept. viridans* strains by frequently fermenting inulin; such tests may be performed in Hiss's serum water or in the serum agar medium used for testing the biochemical reactions of neisseriae. There are other more specific tests for identification.

Bile Solubility.—Pneumococci are soluble in bile. The test consists of adding 1 part of a sterilised 10 per cent. solution of sodium taurocholate in normal saline to 10 parts of a broth culture. Alternatively, 0·1 ml. of a 10 per cent. solution of sodium desoxycholate may be added to 5 ml. of a broth culture which should not be more acid than pH 6·8; this method gives very satisfactory results, lysis occurring within fifteen minutes at 37° C.

Optochin Sensitivity.—Pneumococci are sensitive to optochin. Disks of filter paper, 8 mm. in diameter, sterilised by dry heat at 160° C. are impregnated with a 1 in 4000 aqueous solution of optochin (ethyl hydrocuprein hydrochloride), each disk containing approximately 0·02 ml. The solution can be sterilised in the autoclave at 121° C. for 30 minutes without appreciable effect on its potency. Organisms are tested by making radial stroke cultures on a blood agar plate, a disk being placed in the centre of the plate; a known sensitive strain is included in each set of tests. Pneumococci are inhibited in a zone of at least 5 mm. from the circumference of the disk, whereas strains of *Strept. viridans* grow up to the disk margin; occasionally a few colonies of pneumococci, resistant to optochin, will be noted in the zone of inhibition.

Antigenic Characters.—At least 77 specific serotypes of pneumococci have been recognised. Type specificity is dependent on chemically specific polysaccharides contained in the capsule of the organism and type identification can be established by means of agglutination tests or by "capsule-swelling" reactions. For the latter technique, a loopful of broth culture or a saline suspension of growth from a blood-agar plate is mixed with a loopful of diagnostic antiserum and the mixture covered with a No. 1 coverslip and examined with an oil-immersion lens, the substage condenser being suitably lowered or the diaphragm reduced in aperture. The "swelling" reaction of the capsules with type-specific antiserum is observed in 1-2 min. A positive reaction consists of the margin of the capsule becoming visible and distinct: there is no enlargement.

Typing sera usually contain methylene-blue so that the capsules remain unstained and present a ground-glass appearance; a set of sera may be purchased from The State Serum Institute, Copenhagen, and comprises 9 pooled sera (A-I) and 44 constituent specific sera; strains are first tested in the pooled sera and then in the type-specific sera comprising the pooled serum with which a reaction is obtained.

Pathogenicity.—Pathologic material containing pneumococci (*e.g.* pneumonic sputum) or a young virulent culture, injected subcutaneously into rabbits or mice, produces a rapidly developing septicaemia and death in one to three days; at necropsy, typical capsulated diplococci are present in large numbers in the heart blood. The virulence for animals may rapidly decrease when the organism is subcultured *in vitro*, due to the emergence of non-capsulate mutant forms which are avirulent and no longer react with type-specific antiserum.

Pathogenesis.—In lobar pneumonia the pneumococcus is present, often in considerable numbers, in the consolidated areas and can easily be detected in the sputum. The organism may reach the lung parenchyma either by inhalation or by the peribronchial lymphatics. Excess mucus secretion, *e.g.* from an antecedent respiratory virus infection, may facilitate the onset of pneumonia. In a proportion of cases the pneumococcus can be demonstrated in the blood by blood culture, and also occurs in the complications of pneumonia, *e.g.* empyema, peri- and endocarditis, meningitis, etc. Pneumococcal meningitis is often associated with middle ear infections or with traumatic or congenital defects in the skull, *e.g.* absence of cribriform plate; such cases tend to suffer recurrent attacks.

Epidemiology.—Lobar pneumonia is a communicable infection occurring particularly in the age range 10–50 years and caused predominantly by certain pneumococcus types (*e.g.* types 1, 2, 3, 5, 7, 14) which seem to be endowed with invasive properties; epidemics of lobar pneumonia have occurred in semi-closed communities (barracks, institutions, factories, etc.). The pneumococcus is essentially a human parasite and sources of infection are cases and carriers; carriers convalescing from lobar pneumonia may continue to harbour the organism for considerable periods, particularly if they are predisposed to chronic catarrhal pharyngitis or nasal sinusitis. Contact carriers, who have never suffered clinically apparent infection, may also become carriers of "epidemic" pneumococci.

Type-distribution studies showed that, in Britain, types 1 and 2 were together responsible for more than 50 per cent. of hospitalised cases of lobar pneumonia and type 3 strains were incriminated in less than 10 per cent. of cases. More recently, there has been an increase of type 3 infections which are more common in elderly patients.

Case-fatality rates in lobar pneumonia show that type 3 is the most virulent and type 2 is more virulent than type 1. At the same time, types 1 and 2 are more invasive than other types, as shown by their prevalence in meningitis and peritonitis.

The modes of spread are similar to those of other organisms excreted from the respiratory tract, e.g. *Strept. pyogenes*; the incidence of lobar pneumonia is at its highest in the spring.

Bronchopneumonia, in which pneumococci are commonly involved as secondary bacterial pathogens, occurs most often at the extremes of life or after primary virus respiratory infections (influenza, measles, etc.). The infecting pneumococci are those types found in the upper respiratory tract (*e.g.* types 6, 19, 23), and this is an endogenous, not a communicable, infection. Infections occur mostly in the winter months and are more common in economically poor communities. High fatality rates in the older age-groups occur in spite of therapeutic advances.

Laboratory Diagnosis

A specimen of sputum is obtained and a mucopurulent portion used to inoculate a blood agar plate; films stained by Gram's method are also prepared and examined to obtain an impression of the predominant bacterial flora. In order to improve the chances of isolating pathogens like the pneumococcus and *H. influenzae* in culture, the sputum may be homogenised by shaking with beads or treatment with pancreatin.

On the blood agar plate, characteristic colonies can be recognised among the other organisms that are frequently present; bile solubility and/or optochin sensitivity tests may be performed as confirmatory procedures.

Mouse Inoculation.—Intraperitoneal injection into mice of sputum or a young broth culture of a supralaryngeal swab is a useful and reliable method for isolating pneumococci when they are scantily present.

The need for serotyping of strains as a preliminary to giving specific therapeutic antiserum disappeared with the introduction of sulphonamide therapy, and type identification is now only performed in epidemiologic investigations.

Chemotherapy.—Most pneumococcal infections are amenable to chemotherapy with sulphonamides, penicillin, tetracyclines. In cases of pneumococcal meningitis, penicillin may be given intrathecally as well as systemically.

Prophylaxis.—The prophylaxis of lobar pneumonia has been attempted by the use of combined vaccines of the prevalent pneumococcus types in circumstances where there is a high incidence of infection, *e.g.* among native labourers in the South African mines, where the results were disappointing, and in Army camps, where more encouraging results have been obtained. In particular, a controlled trial during the Second World War of a combined antigen of purified polysaccharides prepared from four of the main epidemic types (types 1, 2, 5 and 7) indicated that a high degree of protection could be obtained against infection with these types after a single injection of 0·06 mg. of each of the polysaccharides. But lobar pneumonia is a sporadic infection in civilian communities, where prophylactic vaccination would not be a practicable procedure.

Since a large proportion of pneumococcal infections supervene on antecedent virus respiratory infections, measures for the control of these virus infections, *e.g.* prophylactic vaccination against influenza, particularly in elderly persons with chronic chest and heart disease, may help to reduce the morbidity and mortality of secondary pneumonias. Improvements in social and environmental conditions and protection against sudden changes in climate will contribute to the control of bronchopneumonia in young children.

CHAPTER 12

NEISSERIA

Definition.—The Neisseriae are Gram-negative cocci, usually arranged in pairs with long axes parallel: strict parasites, often growing poorly on ordinary culture media. The two principal pathogenic members of the group are *Neisseria meningitidis* and *N. gonorrheae*; *N. meningitidis* is the causal organism of Epidemic Cerebrospinal Meningitis (or Cerebrospinal Fever), sometimes called Spotted Fever because of the frequent presence of a purpuric rash; it may also produce an acute or chronic septicaemia without meningitis. *N. gonorrhoeae* causes gonorrhoea, a venereal infection characterised by urethritis in the male and urethritis and cervicitis in the female; there may be local and metastatic complications.

NEISSERIA MENINGITIDIS
(Meningococcus)

Morphology and Staining.—Oval diplococci with opposed surfaces flattened or concave; sometimes in tetrads; cocci are about 0·8 μ in diameter; the long axes of the cocci in pairs are parallel, not in line as in the case of the pneumococcus; Gram-negative. Morphological capsules are not evident, but when the organisms react with specific antiserum, capsule-like structures become apparent, this effect corresponding to the "capsule-swelling" reaction of the pneumococcus. In cerebrospinal fluid the intracellular position in polymorph leucocytes is characteristic. In culture the usual shape and arrangement seen in the spinal fluid may be lost, and involution forms may be present.

Cultural Characters.—Aerobe; primary cultures are obtained most readily in an atmosphere containing 5 per cent. of carbon dioxide; temperature range is 25°–42° C., and the optimum is about 37° C. Although the meningococcus will grow on good nutrient agar, growth is enhanced by the addition of blood or serum; optimum pH is 7·0–7·4. A specially suitable medium is nutrient agar prepared from a digest broth, and containing 5 per cent. blood added to the melted agar at 90° C.

Colonies on serum agar, after 24 hours, are small, greyish, transparent, circular disks about 1–2 mm. in diameter; after 48 hours, the centre of the colony becomes more opaque and raised, while the periphery remains thin and transparent; the borders may become crenated. While this is the common type of colony, considerable variation in the appearance may be noted.

Colonies on blood agar are like those on serum agar but somewhat larger; they are smooth, grey and semi-transparent; no haemolysis occurs.

Viability.—When first cultured artificially, the meningococcus tends to die quickly in culture, *e.g.* within two or three days, probably due to alkali production. In culture it persists best at incubator temperature on moist egg medium. Alternatively, 1 per cent. agar in digest broth *plus* 20 per cent. serum gives good results. It is killed by heat at 55° C. in five minutes or less. When dried under ordinary atmospheric conditions the meningococcus usually dies within two hours, but cultures can be preserved by rapid drying *in vacuo.* The organism is sensitive to the sulphonamides and most antibiotics.

Biochemical Reactions.—Can be tested by growing on peptone-water-agar slopes containing 5 per cent. serum, 1 per cent. of the particular sugar, and an indicator.

Ferments glucose and maltose with acid production, but has no action on lactose, sucrose or inulin.

Cultures of the meningococcus give the oxidase reaction like those of the gonococcus.

Antigenic Characters.—Gordon and Murray described four serological *types* (I-IV) of the meningococcus, but later, Griffith reduced these to two *groups* (I and II), his group I corresponding with the earlier types I and III, and group II with types II and IV. A more recent classification recognises four main groups, now designated A, B, C and D, of which A corresponds to Griffith's group I, B to the old type II and D to the old type IV. Group C is identified with a group C described by French workers (Branham, 1953).

The majority of cases of cerebrospinal meningitis during epidemics are due to group A, whereas many strains found in the nasopharynx of persons who have not been in contact with cases belong to the other groups. It has been concluded that the latter are of lower pathogenicity than group A.

Pathogenesis.—The meningococcus is actively toxigenic, and potent products have been obtained from cultures. The toxin has been classified as an endotoxin though it is readily diffusible from the organisms, probably as a result of their rapid autolysis in culture.

The natural habitat of the meningococcus is in the nasopharynx or post-nasal space, where it may be found in 5–10 per cent. of healthy persons. When outbreaks of cerebrospinal fever occur, the carrier rates may increase to 50–90 per cent. The route of spread of the meningococcus from the nasopharynx to the meninges is a controversial matter; the organism may either spread directly through the cribriform plate to the subarachnoid space by the perineural sheaths of the olfactory nerve, or it may be blood-borne. In favour of the latter route are the frequent positive blood cultures in the early stages of infection, the purpuric rash in many cases with the isolation of meningococci from the skin lesions, and the occurrence, particularly during epidemics, of meningococcal septicaemia with rash but no clinical meningitis. Rare types of primary meningococcal infection are conjunctivitis and endocarditis, while complications of the typical disease are labyrinthitis, arthritis and teno-synovitis.

In general, it has been found difficult to establish an active infection in laboratory animals by inoculation with cultures. However, intraperitoneal injection in mice of even small doses of the meningococcus *suspended in a solution of gastric mucin* brings about a rapidly fatal general infection.

Epidemiology.—Outbreaks of cerebrospinal fever occur particularly under conditions of overcrowding, *e.g.* among recruits in training camps and in ships and gaols. When cases occur under such circumstances, bacteriological examination usually reveals high nasopharyngeal carrier rates of the epidemic strain among healthy contacts. It has been stated that clinical cases are likely to occur when the carrier rate exceeds 20 per cent., but the case/carrier ratio may vary considerably. Meningeal infection is probably facilitated by fatigue and other factors which lower physical well-being and may be preceded or accompanied by a local nasopharyngitis. Apart from localised outbreaks, the highest attack rate and also the highest case fatality is in infancy. Cases occur most commonly in the spring in the United Kingdom and in other countries with temperate climates. Large-scale epidemics spread over wide areas of East and West Africa during the dry season and end abruptly with the onset of the rains.

Laboratory Diagnosis

Lumbar puncture should be done as soon as meningitis is suspected. In a case of cerebrospinal meningitis the spinal fluid is under pressure and is turbid in appearance due to the large number of pus cells present. In the early stages of infection the organisms are present usually in considerable numbers in the cerebrospinal fluid and can be recognised by microscopic examination. At a later stage they may be scanty and even apparently absent.

In the laboratory the fluid is centrifuged and films are made from the sediment and stained by (*a*) methylene blue (*b*) Gram's method (with Sandiford's counterstain). Cultures should be made on blood or heated blood (chocolate) agar and incubated in an atmosphere of 5–10 per cent. CO_2. Films are made from the resulting growth and stained by Gram's method. The colony characters should be noted and subcultures for biochemical tests are made by picking off single colonies on to sugar-containing serum-agar slopes. The serological group may be identified by agglutination tests with the appropriate antisera.

For quick differential diagnosis which is essential for early effective chemotherapy the microscopic examination is often sufficient—*i.e.* if Gram-negative, intracellular diplococci with the characteristic shape of the meningococcus are observed. However, in the later stages of infection or if sulphonamides have been administered, the organisms may be scanty or undetectable in the centifuged deposit. In such cases the meningococcus may be demonstrated by cultural methods. A method which is sometimes successful is to add an equal volume of glucose broth to the cerebrospinal fluid and incubate the mixture for 18 hours ; thereafter sub-inoculations are made on a solid medium as described above.

In cases of suspected meningococcal septicaemia and also in cases of meningitis, blood cultures should be carried out and subcultures made on blood agar every day for 4–7 days.

Chemotherapy.—Meningococcal infections respond well to treatment with the sulphonamide compounds, which diffuse readily into the CSF and are therefore preferable to any other antimicrobial drug.

Prophylaxis.—The early recognition of a high carrier rate, particularly of the more invasive group A, in a closed or semi-closed community, *e.g.* military recruits in barracks where apparently sporadic cases of meningitis are occurring, may help to prevent an outbreak, since the carriers can be quickly and effectively treated with small doses of sulphonamide, e.g. 1 g. twice a day for 3 days.

If a search is to be made for meningococcal carriers, swabs should not be taken within 12 hours after the application of antiseptics to the throat. The specimen is best obtained by means of a swab with a longer wire-holder than the usual throat swab and with the terminal ¾ in., carrying the cotton-wool pledget, bent through an angle of about forty-five degrees. The swab is enclosed in a stoppered test-tube of sufficient width to admit the bent end.

With the tongue depressed, the swab is passed behind the soft palate, introduced into the nasopharynx and rubbed over the posterior wall.

The swab is spread *at once* over a small area at the edge of a serum- or blood agar plate already prepared and warmed to 37° C., and then successive stroke inoculations are made on the remainder of the plate by means of a wire loop, the loop being charged several times from the area inoculated directly with the swab. The plate must be incubated without delay.

When it is impossible to make an immediate culture, a convenient method of maintaining the viability of the meningococcus for 24 hours or so is to place in the foot of the swab-tube a small amount of blood agar so that the swab, when returned to the tube, is kept in contact with the medium. In the laboratory the swab is used to inoculate a blood-agar plate, and the swab-tube is also incubated. Alternatively, the swab may be placed in Stuart's transport medium.

Cultures should be incubated for 48 hours when suspect colonies are examined by means of Gram-stained films, and subcultures from single colonies made on serum- or blood-agar slopes. The resulting pure cultures are then available for identification by biochemical and serological tests.

NEISSERIA GONORRHOEAE
(Gonococcus)

Morphology and Staining.—Oval diplococci with opposed surfaces flattened or concave. The diameter of the coccus is about 0·8–1 μ: Gram-negative. Morphologically the gonococcus is identical with the meningococcus. In inflammatory exudates the intracellular position of the organism is characteristic and some pus cells appear to be almost filled with diplococci. In culture, involution forms are frequent.

Cultural Characters.—Aerobe; temperature range, 30°–39° C.; optimum about 37° C.; requires blood or serum for growth—*e.g.* agar containing 10 per cent. blood (heated at 55° C.), serum agar prepared from fresh sterile serum or agar containing 10 per cent. hydrocele fluid. Various special media have been recommended, but the above-mentioned serve satisfactorily in the routine cultivation of the organism. The agar should be carefully standardised to pH 7·5.

Most strains grow better in an atmosphere containing carbon dioxide (*e.g.* 5 per cent.) than in ordinary air. Incubation inside a closed jar also helps to maintain a moist surface on the culture medium, which helps the growth of gonococci. The CO_2 may also prevent the development of alkalinity.

Colonies on serum agar are semi-transparent disks about the size of a pin head, tending to remain discrete, circular in outline at first, but later showing a "scalloped" or crenated margin, a raised more opaque centre, and sometimes radial and concentric markings. Papillae may be noted after some days' growth.

In primary cultures, colonies may be slow in developing and growth may not appear for two or three days.

Viability.—The thermal death-point is about 55° C. for 5 minutes. The gonococcus is a strict parasite and tends to die in a few hours when discharged from the body, especially if subjected to cooling and drying. It has been found, however, that under certain conditions, *e.g.* in pus on linen or other fabric, the gonococcus may remain viable for periods up to three days. When first isolated, cultures have a feeble viability, and subcultures should be made every three or four days to maintain the strain. When accustomed to artificial growth, cultures survive longer if kept at 37° C. and in a moist condition, but die at room temperature in two days.

Biochemical Reactions.—With the same sugar-containing media used for meningococcus, the gonococcus ferments glucose but not maltose.

Antigenic Characters.—The gonococcus is not antigenically homogeneous; there are probably two main serological groups with intermediate types. There is an antigenic relationship with the meningococcus.

Pathogenesis.—The gonococcus is a strictly human parasite and all attempts to infect animals from mice to monkeys have failed. Its toxicity to animals is due to an endotoxin like that of the meningococcus.

In the *male* the organism infects the mucosa of the urethra and produces a suppurative inflammation with purulent discharge. The cocci are present in large numbers in the discharge at an early stage, but later diminish, and are then associated with secondary infecting organisms—*e.g.* pyogenic cocci, coliform bacilli, diphtheroid bacilli. Infection may spread backwards to the prostate, seminal vesicles and epididymis or may invade the peri-urethral tissue (producing a peri-urethral abscess and subsequent stricture).

In the adult *female* the urethra and cervix uteri are infected, but rarely the vaginal mucosa. Infection may extend to the vestibular glands, the endometrium and the Fallopian tubes (causing salpingitis) and even the peritoneal cavity may be invaded.

Blood invasion may result from primary gonorrhoeal infections, and arthritis and tenosynovitis may occur as complications. While the gonococcus has on occasion been cultivated from the joint fluid in arthritis, the possibility of gonococcal arthritis being a manifestation of allergy must also be considered. Ulcerative endocarditis has been noted as a rare sequela. Purulent conjunctivitis may sometimes occur as a complication.

In female infants and children the gonococcus may produce a persistent vulvo-vaginitis with involvement sometimes of the rectum. Outbreaks of this infection used to occur in paediatric wards and children's institutions, but are now rare.

In newborn infants gonorrhoeal ophthalmia (acute purulent conjunctivitis) may result from direct infection at birth.

Epidemiology.—Gonorrhoea is a venereal infection spread by sexual intercourse. Incidence, which increased sharply during the Second World War, fell steadily in the post-war years, but is increasing again in Britain, probably related to greater laxity in extra-marital sexual intercourse, an increase in homosexuality and, in certain areas, to the large influx of coloured immigrants. Incidence is about four times more frequent in males than in females, prostitutes and other promiscuous women being the main reservoirs.

Laboratory Diagnosis

Films are made from the discharge. In the *male*: from the urethral discharge; the meatus should be cleansed with sterile gauze soaked in saline solution, and specimens are taken either with a wire loop or directly on slides. In the *female*: from the urethra and cervix uteri, with a wire loop or swab and with the aid of a vaginal speculum.

The films are stained by (*a*) methylene blue and (*b*) Gram's method (with neutral red or Sandiford's stain as the counter-stain), and in the acute stage, both in the male and female, the occurrence of the *characteristic Gram-negative intracellular diplococci* is strongly suggestive of a gonorrhoeal infection, though it must be borne in mind that Gram-negative diplococci other than the gonococcus may occur on the mucous membranes of the genital passages, *e.g.* the commensal species to be described.

In *chronic infections*, particularly in the female, the cocci may be relatively scanty in films and difficult to identify accurately among the secondary infecting organisms. In the male the "morning drop" of secretion from the urethra should be examined, or films made from the centrifuged urinary deposit or the discharge after prostatic massage. In the female the secretion from the cervix uteri should be examined.

The diagnosis must be confirmed by cultivation, the organism being identified by cultural and biochemical characters, and differentiated from non-pathogenic neisseriae by fermentation tests; but where there is a mixed infection isolation of the organism may be technically difficult. Inoculation with material to be cultivated should, if possible, *be made directly from the patient on a suitable medium*, and the culture should be incubated at once. If the material is kept at room temperature for some time before inoculation and incubation, or if it is allowed to dry, the organisms may die and fail to grow on the culture medium.

When it is impracticable to make direct cultures and it is necessary to use a swab for the transport of exudate to the laboratory, a swab on a wooden applicator may be broken into a tube of Stuart's transport medium (p. 781).

It should be remembered that in cases already treated with penicillin it may not be possible to demonstrate the organism in discharges.

The Oxidase Reaction in the Detection of Colonies of the Gonococcus.—Cultures are made on plates of heated blood agar and after two days' incubation, freshly prepared 1 per cent. tetramethyl-*p*-phenylenediamine solution is poured on to the plate so as to cover the surface, and then decanted. The colonies of the gonococcus rapidly develop a purple colour (oxidase reaction). If subcultures are required from the colonies, these should be made immediately because the dye is bactericidal; after five minutes it may not be possible to subcultivate them. This method is specially useful in dealing with heavily contaminated material containing only scanty gonococci (*e.g.* cases of chronic cervicitis). Colonies of non-pathogenic neisseriae also give a positive oxidase reaction, but the purple colour develops more slowly and is less intense.

Serology—The complement-fixation test is applicable for diagnosis of chronic infections and complications and may be of value to the clinician, particularly in the differential diagnosis of such conditions as salpingitis and arthritis. However, positive reactions are much less common since the introduction of the sulphonamides and antibiotics.

Chemotherapy.—Although the sulphonamides were at first very effective chemotherapeutic agents, the development of sulphonamide-resistance, particularly in the Second World War, greatly reduced their value. Penicillin therapy has been applied with conspicuous success, although in recent years there has been evidence of the development of penicillin-resistant strains (Report, 1961). Gonococcal infections are also amenable to treatment with certain other antibiotics, *e.g.* streptomycin and the tetracyclines, though those drugs would be used mainly in penicillin-resistant cases.

Non-specific Urethritis

Much attention has been given in recent years to urethritis, usually of more chronic form, in which the gonococcus cannot be demonstrated, and other agents may be causally concerned. This condition has increased considerably in incidence since separate notification was begun in 1951 (10,794 cases), probably associated with a greater awareness and more accurate diagnosis; 24,472 new cases were reported in the United Kingdom in 1961. The infection differs epidemiologically in certain respects from gonorrhoea and a proportion of cases are probably non-venereal. It may form part of a more generalised disease with arthritis and conjunctivitis as major features (Reiter's syndrome).

Pleuro-pneumonia-like organisms have been most often incriminated and are present in a variable proportion of both male and female cases (and also in cases of prostatitis and cystitis). Although these organisms are also found in a smaller proportion of healthy persons, particularly females, their aetiological relationship to non-specific urethritis is now being accepted. Other possible causative agents are *Trichomonas*, *Haemophilus vaginalis* and other bacteria, fungi and trauma. Attempts to find a virus aetiology for non-specific urethritis have so far been unsuccessful.

THE COMMENSAL GRAM-NEGATIVE DIPLOCOCCI

These organisms occur on various mucous surfaces of the body and are found with great regularity in the mucous secretions of the throat, nose and mouth; they may likewise occur on the genital mucosae. When inflammatory or other pathological conditions affect these mucous membranes, such commensals often flourish in large numbers and constitute a prominent feature of the local bacterial flora. They may possibly act as secondary infecting agents in such conditions, but appear to have little or no intrinsic virulence.

Classification

It should be noted that there is some uncertainty regarding the biological classification of this group of organisms, and the taxonomic significance to be attached to colony characters, pigmentation and fermentation of different carbohydrates is doubtful. The group, however, can be broadly divided into two subgroups: (1) characterised by complete absence of fermentative properties, *e.g.* *N. catarrhalis*, and (2) possessing such properties, *e.g.* *N. flava* and related types (see Table).

Fermentative Reactions of Neisseria Group

	Glucose	*Maltose*	*Lactose*	*Sucrose*
Meningococcus .	⊥	⊥	–	–
Gonococcus . .	⊥	–	–	–
N. catarrhalis .	–	–	–	–
N. flava and related types	⊥	$\underline{\perp}$	–	$\underline{\perp}$

(⊥ = acid; $\underline{\perp}$ = variation in reaction among different types.)

Neisseria catarrhalis

A frequent commensal in the throat and nose and often present in large numbers in catarrhal inflammations of the respiratory tract.

Morphology and Staining.—Practically identical with the meningococcus. In some strains the cocci are relatively large.

Cultural Characters.—Grows on ordinary media without serum and at room temperature; the colonies may be larger than those of the meningococcus, especially when fully grown, and are thicker and more opaque. The colony characters, however, may vary considerably, and both "smooth" and "rough" forms are observed. The organism exhibits no fermentative properties. Cultures when emulsified in saline tend to be auto-agglutinable.

N. catarrhalis is not agglutinated by meningococcus antisera.

Neisseria flava

The morphology of these organisms is like that of *N. catarrhalis* and they grow on ordinary media at room temperature. Cultures develop, after 48 hours, greenish-yellow or greenish-grey colours. Young colonies may simulate closely those of the meningococcus.

Biochemical reactions vary according to the type (see Table).

Neisseria flavescens.—This organism has been described as the causative pathogen in a group of cases of meningitis in America. It resembles the meningococcus in morphology, but on blood agar produces golden-yellow colonies. It does not ferment carbohydrates. It may be biologically related to *N. flava.*

Neisseria mucosa.—Differs from the other members of the group in being definitely capsulate and producing mucoid colonies. This type may represent a variant of one of the other members of the group. Strains corresponding to it have been reported in cases of meningitis.

Neisseria sicca.—Resembles *N. catarrhalis,* but its colonies are markedly dry, tough and adherent to the medium. It seems possible that this organism is not a separate species, but a "rough" variant of some other member of the group.

Organisms of Genus Veillonella

These are of some interest in view of their occurrence as commensals in natural cavities of man and animals, particularly the mouth and alimentary tract. They have not been definitely proved pathogenic though sometimes isolated from cases of appendicitis, pyorrhoea and pulmonary lesions, and regarded as potentially pathogenic.

They are minute Gram-negative cocci about 0·3 μ in diameter and occurring in masses. In cultural characters they are anaerobic and grow best at 37° C. The type species is *Veill. parvula,* whose distinctive characters are: the formation of hydrogen, carbon dioxide, hydrogen sulphide and indole from polypeptides, the fermentation of glucose and certain other sugars, haemolytic action, and the reduction of nitrate to nitrite.

REFERENCES

Branham, S. E. (1953). Serological relationships among meningococci. *Bact. Rev.*, **17**, 175.

Report (1961). Resistance of gonococci to penicillin. *Lancet*, **2**, 226.

CHAPTER 13

CORYNEBACTERIUM

Definition.—Gram-positive rods, arranged in pairs or palisades; often with club-shaped swellings at the poles; generally staining irregularly (metachromatic granules); non-motile (parasitic species), non-sporing, non-capsulated; aerobic, micro-aerophilic or facultative anaerobe; some species produce a powerful exotoxin.

Corynebacterium diphtheriae is the causative organism of diphtheria, which, in its characteristic form, consists of a localised inflammation in the throat with adherent exudate (false membrane) and a toxaemia due to the secretion and dissemination of a highly potent exotoxin. Certain species (*C. pyogenes*, *C. renale*, *C. ovis*, etc.) cause acute or chronic suppurative lesions in various domestic and laboratory animals. *Erysipelothrix* and *Listeria*, which are closely related members of the Corynebacteriaceae family, are primary pathogens in animals but sometimes cause infection in man.

CORYNEBACTERIUM DIPHTHERIAE

Morphology and Staining.—Slender rod-shaped organism, straight or slightly curved; the average size is 3 μ by 0·3 μ, but longer and shorter forms may be noted; the ends are often expanded; it is non-motile and non-sporing. In culture, involution forms may be observed which are pear-shaped, club-shaped or even globular. The bacillus is Gram-positive, though more readily decolourised than many other Gram-positive organisms; stained with methylene blue it shows a "beaded" or "barred" appearance: the latter is characteristic of the *intermedius* type of diphtheria bacillus. By Neisser's method, volutin (metachromatic) granules are characteristic, staining blue-black in contrast with the light-brown coloration of the rest of the organism; the granules are mainly polar in situation. If over-decolourised in the Gram method the granules tend to retain the violet stain, while the rest of the organism is decolourised. These characteristic staining reactions depend on environment; thus, in culture, volutin granules are most pronounced when the bacillus is growing on a serum medium such as Löffler's; by electron microscopy they can be demonstrated as well-defined structures. Appearances also vary among strains, some of which exhibit very short forms with poorly developed granules (*e.g. gravis* type).

By phase contrast microscopy one or more septa can be observed in a single diphtheria bacillus, and the *intermedius* type appears to be multicellular. Branched forms have also been observed.

Cultural Characters.—Aerobe; temperature range, 20°–40° C.; optimum, 37° C.; grows on ordinary nutrient media, but best on serum media.

Colonies on Löffler's serum—at first small, circular, white, opaque disks with regular borders; later the centres become thicker and the borders crenated; they may reach 3–4 mm. in diameter after several days' growth; sometimes the growth on serum shows a distinct yellow tint.

Broth—some strains grow in small white masses, which sediment in the tube and also adhere to the side; surface film of growth may also develop. Other strains produce a uniform growth in broth.

On a medium containing potassium tellurite the diphtheria bacillus reduces the tellurite and yields greyish or black colonies. Potassium tellurite is also selective in certain concentrations for this organism and the allied diphtheroid bacilli.

On blood tellurite media the colonies tend to show distinctive appearances. Three types of colony have been recognised as characteristic of different biological types, designated *C. diphtheriae gravis*, *mitis* and *intermedius*. The designations *gravis* and *mitis* have been applied in virtue of the association of these types with severe and mild forms respectively of the disease. The *gravis* type produces relatively large greyish-black, flat, lustreless colonies exhibiting often a "daisy-head" formation. Growth in broth is granular. The *mitis* type yields a convex, smooth, translucent colony, and growth in broth presents a uniform turbidity. The *intermedius* type is represented by relatively small, black, lustreless colonies with domed centre and flat, irregular margin, like a poached egg.

The colony characters on Hoyle's tellurite medium and blood agar are described later in relation to the diagnosis of diphtheria.

Viability.—In culture, diphtheria bacilli may remain alive for two or more months at room temperature. In the moist condition they are comparatively easily killed by heat (in ten minutes at 60° C.), but when dry survive for much longer periods. Diphtheria bacilli may remain alive and virulent for a considerable period in the dust of premises.

Biochemical Reactions.—Ferments with acid production, glucose, galactose, maltose and dextrin, but not lactose, sucrose or mannitol. (Some strains of proved virulent diphtheria bacilli have been stated to ferment sucrose.) No proteolytic activity.

Gravis strains ferment starch and glycogen, and these reactions are characteristic features of this type. These reactions can be elicited by using Hiss's serum medium made with 0·1 per cent. peptone-water: phenol red may be used as the indicator, the initial pH being 7·6. Acid production also causes clotting of the medium.

Haemolysis.—Strains of the *mitis* type are generally haemolytic when growing in a medium containing ox or rabbit blood; the *intermedius* strains are invariably non-haemolytic; strains of the *gravis* type usually lyse rabbit but not ox blood.

It should be noted that the stability of the biological types of the diphtheria bacillus has been questioned; thus, it is stated that strains undergo variation in colony form and starch fermentation. Strains which do not fit into the three biological types have been isolated from both cases and carriers.

Antigenic Characters.—By agglutination reactions with antisera *gravis* strains have been classified into thirteen types, of which type I has been found to be by far the commonest in Great Britain. Among *intermedius* strains four types have been recognised, and *mitis* strains have been allocated to forty different types, one type being related to a particular *gravis* type.

Diphtheria Toxin

The diphtheria bacillus produces a powerful exotoxin with specialised toxic properties. While the bacillus remains localised at the site of infection, the diffusible toxin is absorbed into the blood stream and leads to the various systemic disturbances of diphtheria (in particular myocardial damage) and to such sequelae as post-diphtheritic paralysis.

It has been observed that diphtheria due to the *gravis* type of bacillus may be of a hypertoxic type and refractory to antitoxin treatment. All strains of the diphtheria bacillus produce the same toxin, but it has been claimed by O'Meara (1940) that two distinct substances, designated A and B, enter into its constitution and that the toxins from different strains may vary in the relative amounts of these constituents. According to O'Meara the A substance is the toxin which is lethal to the guinea-pig; the B substance is not definitely toxic *per se* but acts by promoting the spread of A in the tissues, and if it is formed in sufficient amount renders the latter hypertoxic. O'Meara points out that the avidity of antitoxin depends on its power to neutralise the B substance and that for the production of an avid antitoxin, the toxin used must be rich in the B constituent.

When diphtheria bacilli are grown in suitable fluid media, abundant toxin is produced. The strain used is, however, of considerable importance, for in artificial culture the organism may not adapt itself so readily to toxin production as it does in the human body. A single strain (Park-Williams No. 8) of the *intermedius* type is almost universally used for toxin production on a large scale. The bacilli are removed from the culture by filtration or other means, and the bacteria-free liquid, which contains the exotoxin mixed with the culture medium and other products of bacterial growth, is referred to as *toxin.*

Certain cultural conditions and nutritional ingredients are required for maximal production of diphtheria toxin. It is now possible to produce very potent toxin in a medium containing known amino acids, inorganic salts, maltose, and in addition, certain growth factors (pimelic acid, nicotinic acid and β-alanine). The toxin produced in this type of synthetic medium has been isolated in a purified state; it has the properties of a labile protein with a molecular weight of 15,000 to 72,000 and a lethal dose of 0·0001 mg. for a 250-gram guinea-pig.

The toxin is unstable and its potency diminishes on exposure to air and light. In sealed tubes and in the dark it may remain unaltered for several weeks. The reduction in toxicity is due to the spontaneous conversion of toxin into *toxoid*, which has no pathogenic effect on animals but still retains the power of combining with antitoxin and of stimulating specific antibodies (antitoxin).

The conversion of toxin into toxoid can be carried out most effectively by adding 0·3 per cent. of formalin and incubating the toxin for two or three weeks at 37° C. The change from the toxic into the non-toxic state is assessed by injecting the material into guinea-pigs; when 5 ml. injected subcutaneously or intraperitoneally produce no symptoms, the change is regarded as complete. Toxoid produced through the action of formalin in this way is a valuable immunising agent.

Tests for Toxigenicity.—When organisms morphologically resembling the diphtheria bacillus are found in the throat or nose unassociated with active disease (*i.e.* in carriers), it is important to determine whether they are virulent, *i.e* toxigenic. The virulence test is usually done by the intradermal injection of a pure culture into guinea-pigs as follows.

The primary culture from the nose or throat is plated out on a tellurite medium, and a single colony is subcultured to obtain a pure growth. The fermentative powers of the selected pure growth are tested, and if the organism ferments glucose, but not sucrose, a suspension from a culture on Löffler's serum or serum agar is made in *broth* of such a strength that the fluid is distinctly opalescent (about 5×10^8 bacilli per ml.). Two white guinea-pigs of about 400 grams weight are selected, and the hair is removed from the flanks. The day before the test is carried out, one of the animals—the control guinea-pig—is injected intraperitoneally with 1000 units of diphtheria antitoxin (*vide infra*). For the actual test each guinea-pig is injected intradermally with 0·2 ml. of the suspension of organisms, a 1-ml. syringe and fine-bore needle (26 gauge, $\frac{3}{4}$ in. long) being used. Up to 8–10 different cultures may be tested on each guinea-pig, and the injections should be at least one inch apart. A careful note of the position of the injection of each different culture should be made. The test guinea-pig is now injected with $\frac{1}{50}$th unit of antitoxin per gram of body-weight. The guinea-pigs are examined 24, 48 and 72 hours after inoculation.

Virulent diphtheria bacilli produce in the test animal a well-defined red area about 15 mm. in diameter. After the third or fourth day the colour fades, leaving a necrotic patch with a scab surrounded by growing hair. The control guinea-pig shows no such reaction, the puncture wound caused by the needle being generally the only evidence of injection. If the organism is non-virulent there is no reaction in either the test or control animal. A reaction in both animals shows that the organism is not the diphtheria bacillus, because the products of growth are not neutralised by diphtheria antitoxin, as indicated by the reaction of the control animal.

Rabbits are also suitable for intradermal virulence tests, and some workers have used these animals for the purpose.

Subcutaneous injection of a culture of toxigenic *C. diphtheriae* (or of the toxin) in an unprotected guinea-pig causes death within two to four days with characteristic haemorrhages in the suprarenal glands and blood-stained pleural effusion.

The Gel-precipitin Test.—The production of toxin by a virulent strain of *C. diphtheriae* may be demonstrated by the line of precipitation when toxin meets antitoxin in the agar gel diffusion technique (Elek, 1948; Ouchterlony, 1948). For technical details, see Chapter 54.

Diphtheria Antitoxin.—By immunising horses with toxoid and then with toxin, both in repeated doses, an antitoxin is produced from the tissues and is present often in large amount in the blood; the serum of such animals constitutes *diphtheria antitoxin.* The principles used in the standardisation of diphtheria antitoxin are described in Chapter 52.

Pathogenesis.—The local infection occurs typically in the faucial region in the form of an adherent greyish-white exudate or "false membrane". Infection often begins on one side of the fauces, usually on the tonsils, and gradually extends to involve the whole oropharynx. The bacilli are present in large numbers in the adherent exudate and in the throat secretions. They do not invade the lymphatics to any extent and there is no blood invasion. The diffusible toxin has a marked affinity for heart muscle and death in the severe infections is usually due to acute myocarditis and heart failure. In nasal diphtheria, characterised by crust formation, the organisms can be detected in the blood-stained nasal discharge. Infection of wounds, the conjunctiva, vulva and vagina may occasionally occur. A diphtheritic paronychia is sometimes met with.

The most severe forms of diphtheria are mostly caused by the *gravis* and *intermedius* types. The *mitis* type is usually associated with mild infections except when it involves the larynx and trachea (laryngeal diphtheria), when it may cause severe illness and death by obstruction and anoxia. The relative prevalence of these types varies in different areas and varies also at different times.

Epidemiology.—Before immunisation was introduced on a national scale in this country, the incidence of clinical diphtheria ranged from 50,000 to 60,000 cases annually, with 2500 to 3000 deaths. It is a disease of early childhood with peak incidence around four to six years of age, but when the large-scale immunisation of children has been well developed there is a shift of infection to young adults. Infection is rare in early infancy because of the passive immunity transferred via the placenta from the mother. Infection is spread by close contact, *e.g.* in schools, families and institutions, but the actual mode of transference has not been clearly defined. Spread by contaminated dust and fomites may play a more important part than direct droplet infection. Nasal cases and carriers have long been recognised as particularly dangerous sources of infection and there is evidence that, like heavy nasal carriers of *Strept. pyogenes*, they may disperse very large numbers of diphtheria bacilli in their immediate environment. Persistent throat or combined nose and throat carriers follow clinical infection in 5–10 per cent. of cases and no doubt contribute to the spread of infection. In investigating outbreaks of infection, nose and throat swabs from all contacts should be examined and Schick tests (q.v.) done, so that (*a*) the

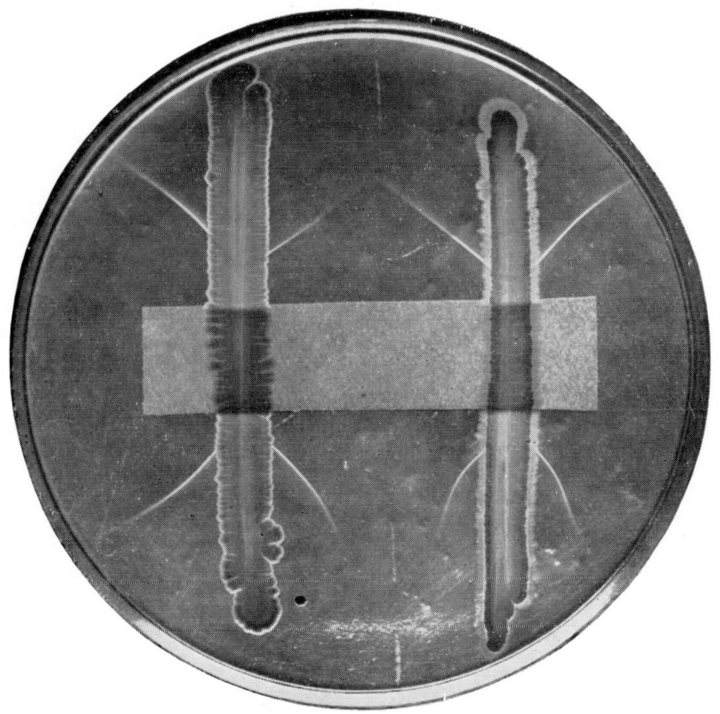

Photograph showing the recognition of toxigenic strains of the diphtheria bacillus by Elek's method. In the centre is the horizontal strip of filter paper containing the antitoxin with the growths of the diphtheria bacillus at right angles to it. The fine white lines showing a positive reaction are well defined.

carriers may be segregated and (*b*) the susceptibles protected by combined active-passive immunisation (see Chap. 43). Carriers as well as cases of diphtheria have become rare in communities subjected to mass immunisation.

Schick Test

When a minute quantity of diphtheria toxin is injected intradermally, a local reaction follows in persons with less than a certain content of antitoxin in the blood. The average amount of antitoxin required to ensure neutralisation of the test dose of toxin is about 1/200 of a unit per ml. of blood, but there may be considerable variation in antitoxin content among non-reactors. This reaction has been extensively applied with a view to gauging immunity or susceptibility to diphtheria. As an indicator of the amount of antitoxin in the blood and of actual resistance or susceptibility to diphtheria its value must be regarded as relative.

For the test a matured and stabilised toxin preparation is chosen, and the selected dose is that amount which is just neutralised by approximately 1/1000 unit of antitoxin. The toxin preparation is diluted with a special buffer solution[1] so that 0·2 ml. contains the test dose. This is injected intradermally in the left forearm, and, as a control, an equal amount of a similar dilution of the same toxin previously heated at 70°–85° C. for thirty minutes is injected intradermally in the right forearm. A positive Schick reaction consists in an area of redness and swelling appearing after one or two days, reaching its maximum about the fourth day, when it measures 1–5 cm. in diameter. It persists for 7–15 days, and on fading shows superficial scaling and a persistent brownish pigmentation. The absence of reaction on either arm *i.e.* "negative Schick reaction" indicates that the toxin has been neutralised, sufficient antitoxin being present in the blood of the individual. A "pseudo-reaction" may occur, *i.e.* an area of redness appearing early (within 6–12 hours), which is less intense and usually disappears in one to three days. If this appears in a Schick-negative person, both forearms show similar reactions; in a positive reactor, the unheated toxin produces a reaction which is more pronounced and more persistent than that due to the heated material. A convenient time to examine results is between the fifth and the seventh days when true reactions are still visible and pseudo-reactions have faded.

Pseudo-reactions are more common in older children and adults, because they have apparently been sensitised by exposure to diphtheria bacilli. Pseudo-reactors are usually immune to diphtheria. Children between six months and eight years of age are generally non-sensitised and rarely suffer from reactions after prophylactic immunisation. However, in older children a preliminary Schick test should be carried out to ascertain whether immunisation is required; pseudo-reactors

[1] A mixture of 57 grams crystal borax, 84 grams boric acid, 99 grams sodium chloride is made; 1·5 grams of this mixture are dissolved in 100 ml. of distilled water. A small amount of human serum (containing no detectable antitoxin) may also be added as a stabiliser

should not receive any diphtheria prophylactic because of the risk of severe reactions and because most of them will be immune.

Laboratory Diagnosis

A specimen of the throat secretion should be obtained. No antiseptics (*e.g.* in form of gargles, etc.) must have been applied within twelve hours. A sterile throat swab should be rubbed over the affected area, or, where there is no definitely localised lesion, over the mucous membrane of the pharynx and tonsils.

Various diagnostic methods for cultivating and identifying the diphtheria bacillus have been advocated. The following procedures may be recommended.

A tube of Löffler's medium is inoculated by rubbing the throat swab over the whole surface of the medium, moistening the swab in the condensation water at the foot of the tube. The tube is incubated for 12–18 hours at 37° C. If an earlier result is urgently required, the culture may be examined after 6–12 hours: if this should be negative, however, the examination must be repeated after 18–24 hours.

The resulting growth is mixed by emulsifying it with a wire loop in the condensation fluid, and from this, films are made and stained by Neisser's or Albert's method.

Films may also be made directly from the swab and stained by the above methods, but only in a small proportion of cases can positive results be obtained in this way, and cultures should always be made as a routine procedure, irrespective of direct examination.

In the case of suspected throat diphtheria, the appearance in cultures of bacilli showing the characteristic morphology and staining reactions (especially the metachromatic granules by Neisser's or Albert's stain) may be regarded as significant in confirming the clinical diagnosis.

It should be noted that in some cases other organisms may overgrow the diphtheria bacillus in culture and lead to an apparently negative result. Moreover, the *gravis* type is often difficult to recognise in early growths, the bacilli being short and thick with absence of metachromatic granules. In mild cases and carriers the bacilli may be scanty and easily missed.

In the case of supposed nasal diphtheria, diphtheria carriers, diphtheria affecting mucous surfaces other than the throat, and wound-diphtheria, the microscopic examination of cultures is not conclusive. The suspected organism must be isolated in pure culture and its virulence or toxigenicity determined as described on p. 181.

The above method cannot be relied on in all cases, and it is essential to cultivate the swab at the same time on a tellurite medium, incubating for 24–28 hours and making a diagnosis by recognition of the characteristic colonies, including the identification of the different colony-types, *gravis*, *mitis* and *intermedius*. (On tellurite media the typical metachromatic granules may not be demonstrable.) The two methods used together serve to check one another. It should be remembered that while tellurite inhibits many other organisms, diphtheroid organisms may grow on it as well as the diphtheria bacillus, and must be carefully differentiated from the latter. Hoyle's tellurite medium may be recommended. Growths are only just visible after twelve hours, but by using a plate-culture microscope colonies of *C. diphtheriae* can often be recognised by certain characters (*vide infra*); at this stage, however, the value of the plate is mainly in attracting attention to the presence of diphtheria bacilli missed on the Löffler's medium. After 18–24 hours the growth is more abundant, the characters of the colonies are more distinct and by the combined use of the two methods a high degree of diagnostic accuracy is attained. When the bacilli are scanty or when nasal or aural swabs are examined, 36–48 hours may be required for the recognition of *C. diphtheriae* colonies, and if there is any doubt at 24 hours, further incubation should be allowed before reporting. The tellurite plate also facilitates the isolation of pure cultures, and when there is difficulty in identifying the diphtheria bacillus by colony characters, and where this organism occurs in a carrier, a pure culture must be obtained and tested for its biochemical reactions and virulence. If, however, the organisms present all the characters of the *gravis* or *intermedius* type, in bacteriological practice in Britain, virulence has been generally assumed without resorting to a toxigenicity test.

As tellurite has some degree of inhibitory effect on the diphtheria bacillus, the swab may be plated on digest agar containing 10 per cent. horse blood, which also helps to clarify a differential diagnosis of sore throat due to *Strept. pyogenes*. The diphtheria bacillus grows well on this medium, and, after incubation overnight, colonies can often be recognised and differentiated from those of other organisms. If no colonies can be recognised, a film is made from the confluent part of the growth on the plate and stained by Albert's method. This gives the same information as the microscopic examination of a Löffler's serum culture.

It must be emphasised here that the responsibility for the diagnosis of diphtheria rests with the clinician. The bacteriologist can merely state whether organisms morphologically resembling the diphtheria bacillus are present in cultures from the specimen submitted to him or whether the growths on a tellurite medium are typical of this organism. Failure to find such organisms does not necessarily exclude diphtheria, nor does their presence prove the disease to be diphtheria. *If the clinician considers a case to be diphtheria it is his duty to administer antitoxin at once*, and continue to do so even if a negative laboratory report is received. The case fatality is directly correlated with the delay in administering antitoxin, and where there is reasonable suspicion that the case may be diphtheria, antitoxin must immediately be used without waiting for a bacteriological report. It is also emphasised that a reliable laboratory report, particularly in cases where there is doubt clinically, cannot be made under 18–24 hours, and at that stage the bacteriologist can report on morphological or cultural appearances only. To prove conclusively the identity and virulence of the organism may necessitate tests extending over several days. In order that the bacteriological report should be as helpful as possible, the utmost care must be taken that a suitable specimen is submitted and precise details as to the nature and source of the material should be furnished.

Allowance being made for the possible limitations of the diagnostic methods described, the results of such examination have undoubtedly proved of the greatest value as an aid to, and confirmation of, the clinical diagnosis.

The Recognition of Colonies of C. diphtheriae on Hoyle's Medium (Wright, 1943)

After 12 *hours' Incubation.*—To the naked eye, growths of the *gravis* and *mitis* types represent a grey "haze" hardly distinguishable from growths of diphtheroid bacilli, though the latter are somewhat blacker and more glistening. Magnified and by reflected light, the colonies are matt and not smooth like those of diphtheroid organisms. The *intermedius* type show very tiny colonies which are strikingly uniform in size and appearance.

After 24–48 *Hours.*—*Gravis type*—seen by daylight, growths are slate-grey with a bluish tinge; individual colonies have a paler border and if well separated attain a diameter of 3 mm. after 36–48 hours. Magnified and by reflected light from an electric bulb, the surface of the colonies has a ground-glass appearance which only indistinctly reflects the image of the bulb; touched with a wire and observed with the plate-culture microscope the colonies are seen to break up very readily; the shape may approximate to the daisy-head formation as originally described, but often the colonies show merely a radial striation sloping from the raised centre to the slightly crenated periphery; sometimes the colonies are convex and circular in outline, with only slight striation and crenation.

Mitis Type—the colour, consistence and size of colonies are similar to those of the *gravis* type and they also show a ground-glass appearance, though more glistening; the colonies, however, are convex and have a perfectly circular outline.

Intermedius Type—the colonies are never larger than 2 mm. and growths are more delicate than those of the other types; magnified and by transmitted light, the colonies are very uniform in size and seem "pricked out" on the surface of the medium; they are blacker than the other types, but are of the same roughness and consistency; they are usually domed and circular with a tendency to crenation, but occasionally the margin is flattened and they show a "poached egg" appearance; after 48 hours they are frequently papillate.

It should be noted that these colonies are sometimes difficult to distinguish from those of certain streptococci growing from throat swabs, but the latter are black or brown and somewhat flatter. A microscopic examination should be made if there is any doubt.

Diphtheroid Bacilli.—Growths are generally more glistening than those of the diphtheria bacillus; magnified and by reflected light, colonies usually have a smooth surface on which the image of the electric bulb is sharply delineated; in colour, they range from black or dark-brown to pale grey or greyish-white; the characteristic slate-grey colour of the *gravis* type of diphtheria bacillus is seldom seen; colonies are sometimes tough or mucoid in consistence, or soft and butyrous.

In examining plates a uniform procedure should be used throughout, since the precise appearance and colour vary with the nature of the illuminant and the angle of the light. Colour is best seen with the naked eye in the confluent parts of the growth. It must also be remembered that variations in batches of medium may influence colony characters; and in diagnostic work it is advantageous to use, for comparison, plates on which known strains of *gravis*, *mitis* and *intermedius* types have been inoculated and grown at the same time as the cultures under examination.

Chemotherapy.—Although diphtheria bacilli are sensitive to penicillin and other antibiotics, these drugs have no direct antagonistic action on diphtheria toxin and cannot be substituted for antitoxin therapy. Penicillin and erythromycin have, however, been used with some success to eliminate diphtheria bacilli from the respiratory tracts of both cases and carriers.

Prophylaxis.—Individuals having little or no antitoxin in the blood stream, *e.g.* as indicated by a positive Schick reaction, may be actively immunised by the injection of one of the following preparations:—

(1) Formol-toxoid (FT): diphtheria toxin rendered non-toxic by formalin. The recommended dosage is three intramuscular or deep subcutaneous injections each of 1·0 ml. at four-weekly intervals. However, recent studies have shown that purified diphtheria toxoid is, *per se*, a poor antigen.

(2) Toxoid-antitoxin floccules (TAF): a suspension of the precipitate of floccules formed when toxoid and antitoxin are mixed in appropriate "neutralising" amounts. Its tendency to cause reactions is slight, and a good immunity follows the injection of three doses, each of 1 ml., given at intervals of four weeks. TAF has been recommended for the immunisation of adolescents and adults.

(3) Alum-precipitated toxoid (APT): a suspension of the washed precipitate produced by the addition of a small amount of aluminium hydroxide to toxoid. The precipitate is relatively insoluble and the toxoid is gradually liberated from the site of injection. Reactions are negligible in children under eight years, but in older children and adults they may be somewhat more severe than with TAF. Two doses, each of 0·5 ml. are given at an interval of four weeks, but this interval may be lengthened, *e.g.* to three or six months without any loss of antibody response to the second dose.

(4) Another alum-containing prophylactic is a suspension of purified toxoid adsorbed on hydrated aluminium phosphate (PTAP) and this preparation is a more potent and more reproducible antigen than APT. However, with alum-adsorbed antigens there is a slight risk of provocation poliomyelitis in susceptible individuals (see Chap. 43).

Whatever prophylactic is used, a subsequent Schick test should be carried out on a sample of the inoculated community to test the immunizing potency of the antigen.

When an outbreak of diphtheria has occurred in a school or institution, the susceptible contacts should, after preliminary Schick-testing, be given passive immunity by the injection of a small dose of antitoxin (500–1000 units) followed by active immunisation, which may be begun immediately or after two weeks.

DIPHTHEROID BACILLI

These are non-toxigenic corynebacteria with little or no pathogenicity.

Corynebacterium hofmannii

A commensal of the throat.

Morphology and Staining.—Compared with the diphtheria bacillus it is shorter (about 2 μ) and may present a somewhat oval shape; stained with Löffler's methylene blue, an unstained bar in the middle of the organism is a frequent character and renders it not unlike a diplococcus. It is strongly Gram-positive; usually no volutin granules are detected by Neisser's or Albert's stains.

Cultural Characters.—Grows aerobically on ordinary media; growths are more abundant than those of the diphtheria bacillus, and the colonies are larger and more opaque. For appearances on one of the tellurite media, see p. 186.

Biochemical Reactions.—No fermentation of glucose or sucrose.

It is non-pathogenic to laboratory animals.

Corynebacterium xerosis

A commensal in the conjunctival sac; it was originally thought to be the cause of xerosis conjunctivae. Closely resembles the diphtheria bacillus, and may show volutin granules.

Can be differentiated from the diphtheria bacillus by its production of acid in sucrose as well as in glucose and by its non-pathogenicity to laboratory animals.

Corynebacterium acnes (*Propionibacterium acnes*)

An organism associated with acne, but its aetiological relationship to the disease is doubtful. It is Gram-positive, rod-shaped, and measures about 1·5 μ by 0·5 μ. It is markedly pleomorphic and frequently shows a beaded appearance: Micro-aerophilic.

Other Diphtheroid Species

Certain of these present a close morphological similarity to the diphtheria bacillus, and may exhibit the characteristic volutin granules by Neisser's staining method, though differing in fermentative reactions, *e.g.* fermenting sucrose. They are mostly non-pathogenic, and have been isolated from the secretions of the nose and nasopharynx, the external ear, conjunctival sac, the skin, lymph glands (apart from disease) and other tissues, pus, wounds, etc.

Barratt has described diphtheroid bacilli in the nasopharynx which tend to resemble *Corynebacterium ovis*, the Preisz-Nocard bacillus (*vide infra*); these organisms liquefy gelatin; they are virulent to guinea-pigs and rats, but diphtheria antitoxin has no protective action against them. Cook and Jebb have reported somewhat similar organisms which ferment starch and might seem to be intermediate between *C. diphtheriae gravis* and *C. ovis* (Cook & Jebb, 1952).

Infections in Animals

The following corynebacteria are common pathogens among domestic animals.

Corynebacterium ovis (*Pseudotuberculosis ovis*)

This, the *Preisz-Nocard bacillus*, is the causative organism of caseous lymphadenitis and pseudotuberculosis in sheep. A similar organism is associated also with ulcerative lymphangitis of horses (*vide infra*).

This organism is allied to *C. diphtheriae* in its biological characters.

Morphology and Staining.—Non-motile, slender rod-shaped organisms 1–3 μ in length by 0·4 μ in breadth. When stained, it shows beading or a barred appearance like other diphtheria-like bacilli, and is Gram-positive. By Neisser's method volutin granules can be demonstrated. Club-shaped forms may be noted.

Cultural Characters.—Growth occurs at 37° C. under both aerobic and anaerobic conditions on ordinary nutrient media.

Agar—growth is at first scanty; the colonies are small, thin, dry and greyish-white in colour, folded and granular and often show concentric rings.

Löffler's medium—colonies are similar to those on agar, but exhibit a yellowish colour; there is no liquefaction.

Broth—a granular growth occurs with sometimes a surface pellicle.

Gelatin—slow liquefaction occurs with most strains.

Glucose, maltose and dextrin are fermented, but usually not sucrose, lactose or mannitol. A haemolysin is produced.

Occurrence.—The associated disease in sheep is chronic and characterised by involvement of lymphatic glands, which are enlarged and caseous. Caseous nodules are seen also in the internal organs, *e.g.* lungs, spleen, liver and kidneys. The organism can be demonstrated in films or sections prepared from the various lesions.

Experimental Inoculation.—Laboratory animals, *e.g.* guinea-pig and rat, are susceptible to experimental infection with cultures. Intravenous injection in the guinea-pig produces a lethal effect within about ten days, and at autopsy caseous areas are noted in internal organs, *e.g.* lungs and liver. Intraperitoneal injection in a male animal leads to involvement of the tunica vaginalis as in the case of experimental glanders. Subcutaneous injection is followed by lymphatic gland involvement, the glands showing the characteristic caseation. In rats, inoculation produces a fatal septicaemia. Sheep are also susceptible to experimental inoculation and die with an intense icterus associated with intravascular haemolysis.

This organism produces an exotoxin resembling, to some extent, that of the diphtheria bacillus, but not neutralisable by diphtheria antitoxin. Guinea-pigs are highly susceptible to this toxin and show at the site of subcutaneous inoculation an inflammatory lesion with oedema and haemorrhage, while the internal organs are congested and often contain small haemorrhages; there is, however, no change in the suprarenals and no pleural effusion.

Diagnosis.—Films are prepared from the lesions and stained by Gram's method, methylene blue and by Ziehl-Neelsen's method (to exclude acid-fast bacilli). Cultures are made, and pure growths from single colonies are investigated as regards cultural characters and experimental pathogenesis.

Similar organisms are found in equine ulcerative lymphangitis (pseudo-farcy), and in pseudo-tuberculosis (caseous lymphadenitis) of bovines

(*Corynebacterium bovis*). These organisms form a group of closely related types. They have frequently been classified as one species—the "*Preisz-Nocard bacillus*". A similar organism (*C. murisepticum*) produces a septicaemic disease in mice.

Corynebacterium pyogenes

An organism associated with suppurative lesions in pigs, cattle and certain other animals. It may occur in mastitis of cattle and sheep.

Morphology and Staining.—Non-motile, rod-shaped organism not usually exceeding 2 μ in length. Shows great pleomorphism. Gram-positive in young cultures. Stained with methylene blue, diphtheroid forms may be seen with deeply stained bands or granules, but volutin granules are not usually observed in preparations stained by Neisser's method.

Cultural Characters.—Aerobe and facultative anaerobe, but some strains grow better under anaerobic conditions. Optimum temperature about 37° C. Generally requires media containing blood or serum. The colonies on serum media are at first minute, but several days' growth may attain a size of 2–3 mm. in diameter. They present no specially characteristic appearances. Inspissated serum, egg medium and gelatin are all liquefied. This organism is haemolytic when growing on blood agar, and a filterable haemolytic toxin demonstrable in suitable culture medium is lethal for mice and rabbits. In milk, acid and clot result in three days and after a time the clot is digested. Glucose, lactose and, in some cases, sucrose but not mannitol are fermented.

A variant type which lacks proteolytic action has been described.

Pathogenesis.—In the natural infection in swine, suppurative lesions may occur in various parts of the body, liver abscesses and arthritis being specially frequent. In cattle, the organism has been found associated with a variety of suppurative lesions, *e.g.* abscesses, pyaemia, pyelitis, mastitis, endometritis.

Rabbits can be infected experimentally; intravenous injection of cultures produces a pyaemic condition with bone and joint lesions. Guinea-pigs are less susceptible.

Corynebacterium renale

This organism has been described in cystitis and in pyelonephritis of cattle. It resembles other Corynebacteria in general characters. It digests milk casein, but has no action on gelatin or coagulated serum and no haemolysin is produced. Litmus milk is rendered alkaline after two or three days' incubation and a deposit is formed with a clear supernatant fluid having the colour of burgundy. Urea is actively converted to ammonia. Glucose is fermented; some strains also ferment laevulose and mannose. Injected intravenously in large doses into mice and rabbits, it may give rise to a fatal pyelonephritis within four weeks, the lesions produced being confined exclusively to the medulla.

Corynebacterium equi

This organism has been reported as the causative organism of pneumonia in foals. It has also been isolated from a number of other animal species as in pyometra in cattle and from suspected tuberculous lesions in the cervical lymph nodes of pigs.

It differs from other members of the diphtheroid group in its profuse viscid growth and the production of a red pigment; there is no haemolysis and no liquefaction of coagulated serum or gelatin. Carbohydrates are not fermented and urea is not hydrolysed. Some workers have found it to be weakly acid-fast and unusually resistant to oxalic acid.

Subcutaneous inoculation produces abscess formation in horses, pigs and goats, but there is no evidence of the formation of a toxin. Intraperitoneal inoculation into guinea-pigs gives rise to peritonitis.

ERYSIPELOTHRIX: LISTERIA

Erysipelothrix and *Listeria*, which are members of the family *Corynebacteriaceae*, have many similar biological characters and some workers would place them in the same species. They are common pathogens of both domestic and wild animals and birds and sometimes produce infection in man.

Erysipelothrix rhusiopathiae

(*Ery. insidiosa*)

The causative organism of Swine Erysipelas.

Morphology and Staining.—Slender, Gram-positive, non-motile rod-shaped organism 1–2 μ by 0·2–0·4 μ, occurring singly and in chains. In culture media, longer and filamentous forms are observed. True branching has been described, and on this account the organism was once classified as an *Actinomycete*.

Cultural Characters.—Growth occurs on ordinary media even at room temperature, though the optimum is about 37° C. The organism shows a tendency to be micro-aerophilic when first isolated, and in agar-shake cultures may grow best just below the surface, but is able to grow under both aerobic and anaerobic conditions. In gelatin-stab culture a line of growth occurs along the wire track with lateral spikes or disks radiating from the central growth. Surface colonies on plates are of two types: one exceedingly minute and dewdrop-like, with a smooth surface; it does not exceed 0·5 mm. in diameter when growing on agar. The other is larger and has a granular appearance. Various carbohydrates are fermented (without gas production), *e.g.* glucose, lactose; sucrose and mannitol are not fermented. Different groups of the organism have been recognised according to their antigenic characters.

Animal Pathogenicity.—Mice, rats, rabbits and pigeons are susceptible to inoculation. Mice and pigeons are specially susceptible, and usually die of an acute septicaemia within four or five days after experimental inoculation. Subcutaneous injection in rabbits produces a spreading inflammation and oedema with a fatal result. Experimental inoculation (with cultures) in swine reproduces the disease as it occurs naturally. The smooth-colony type of culture is the more pathogenic.

Pathogenesis.—In pigs the bacilli can be observed in the characteristic diamond-shaped skin lesion, and in internal organs, *e.g.* lungs, spleen and kidney. In some cases there is a septicaemic condition and the organism is detectable in blood films, particularly in leucocytes. In the chronic form of the disease, in which a "verrucose" endocarditis occurs, the bacilli may be confined to the cardiac lesions.

A similar organism, *Erysipelothrix muriseptica*, is responsible for epizootic septicaemia in mice. It is doubtful whether this organism constitutes a separate species.

Ery. rhusiopathiae may occur in apparently healthy pigs, and has been isolated from the tonsils, intestines and faeces. It has a wide distribution in other animals and in birds. It is also found, apparently as a commensal, on the skin and scales of many fish (particularly members of the perch family).

Cases of human infection with this organism are known as "Erysipeloid" and have a distinctive clinical picture. There is very severe pain and swelling of a finger or part of the hand with a dusky, greyish discoloration of the skin of the affected area. The condition is an occupational hazard for those who handle infected animals or fish; the majority of recorded cases have been in abattoir workers, butchers, fishmongers, laboratory workers and veterinary surgeons. According to Sneath *et al.* (1951) it is seldom possible to recover *Erysipelothrix rhusiopathiae* from swabs, and the most satisfactory method is to obtain a biopsy from the actively growing edge of the lesion and to incubate this for 48 hours in 1 per cent. glucose broth, subculturing on to blood agar.

Laboratory Diagnosis.—For diagnostic purposes an attempt should be made to cultivate the organism from lesions and in acute cases from the blood; inoculation tests should also be carried out in mice or pigeons. An agglutination test is applicable.

Artificial immunisation against the disease in animals is carried out by the injection of killed vaccine in which the organisms are adsorbed on aluminium hydroxide and suspended in an oily base. The organism is sensitive to penicillin, which has largely replaced the use of immune serum for therapeutic purposes.

Listeria monocytogenes

This organism owes its specific name to the fact that infection by it in laboratory animals, *e.g.* rabbits and guinea-pigs, produces a monocytosis in the blood. Although it was originally isolated from these animals it is responsible for disease in a wide variety of hosts, *e.g.* foxes, dogs, gerbils, guinea-pigs and recently in chinchillas imported into this country. In farm animals the disease is mainly an encephalitis, although the organism has been found in foetuses from cases of abortion in cattle and sheep; in rodents and poultry necrotic hepatitis and myocarditis are frequently seen. It is a rare cause of meningo-encephalitis in man and of granulomatosis infantiseptica in the newborn.

Morphology.—It occurs as a Gram-positive straight or slightly curved non-sporing rod, 2–3 μ by 0·5 μ (average), often in pairs, end to end at an acute angle. Sometimes elongated filaments may be observed, particularly in solid medium at room temperature. It is feebly motile at 37° C., but in young broth cultures at 25° C. it is more active and exhibits up to four flagella. Young cultures of the organism are Gram-positive, but after forty-eight hours many are Gram-negative, while in older cultures they may be entirely Gram-negative.

Cultural Characters.—Cultures can be obtained at 37° C. under aerobic conditions on ordinary media, but growth is better on media containing liver extract, blood, serum or glucose. The colonies are at first very small and droplet-like; after a few days' growth they may attain a diameter of 2 mm., being smooth and transparent, though later they may be more opaque. Surface colonies on blood agar are surrounded by a narrow zone of complete haemolysis. Gelatin and Löffler's serum are not liquefied. In stab culture, growth occurs evenly along the length of the stab. A scant colourless growth is obtained on MacConkey's medium, while on tellurite medium the colonies are small, black and glistening, surrounded by a characteristic zone of green colouration. In glucose, maltose and certain other common sugars acid is promptly produced without gas; lactose and sucrose are fermented slowly, but mannitol is not acted on.

Listeria is susceptible *in vitro* to penicillin, streptomycin, the tetracyclines, chloromycetin and erythromycin, but resistant to sulphonamides, bacitracin and polymyxin.

Animal Pathogenicity.—No demonstrable exotoxin or endotoxin is produced. Experimentally, the organism is pathogenic for rabbits, mice and guinea-pigs, but not for rats and pigeons. It gives rise to focal lesions on the chorio-allantoic membrane of chick embryos. It has been suggested that for the primary isolation of *Listeria* from the brains of sheep and cattle, refrigeration of the tissues is essential before inoculation of enriched medium.

Human Infections.—Cases of meningo-encephalitis in man have been described, characterised by a suppurative meningitis with mostly a mononuclear or polymorphonuclear exudate in the CSF and a monocytosis. There is no confirmation of the claim that *Listeria* is causally related to infectious mononucleosis.

An intra-uterine infection, characterised by extensive focal necrosis especially of liver and spleen, known as granulomatosis infantiseptica has been described by Continental workers. It causes a high mortality in the affected foetus or newborn child.

REFERENCES

Cook, G. T. & Jebb, W. H. H. (1952). Starch-fermenting, gelatin-liquefying corynebacteria and their differentiation from *C. diphtheriae gravis*. *J. Clin. Path.*, **5**, 161.

Elek, S. D. (1948). The recognition of toxicogenic bacterial strains *in vitro*. *Brit. med. J.*, **1**, 493.

O'Meara, R. A. Q. (1940). *C. diphtheriae* and the composition of its toxin in relation to the severity of diphtheria. *J. Path. Bact.*, **51**, 317.

Ouchterlony, O. (1948). *In vitro* method for testing toxin-producing capacity of diphtheria bacteria. *Acta path. microbiol. scand.*, **25**, 186.

Sneath, P. H. A., Abbott, J. D. & Cunliffe, A. C. (1951). Bacteriology of erysipeloid. *Brit. med. J.*, **2**.

Wright, H. A. (1943). Laboratory diagnosis of diphtheria: note on some present-day methods. *Edin. med. J.*, **50**, 737.

CHAPTER 14

MYCOBACTERIUM

Definition.—Slender rods occurring mostly in pairs or small clumps; tendency to clubbing and even true branching; difficult to stain because of waxy constituents, but once stained resist decolourisation with acid (acid-fast); non-motile, non-capsulated, non-sporing; very slow growth; aerobic; some species have not been cultivated on artificial media.

Pathogenic species affect man, mammals, birds and reptiles and are widely distributed throughout the world. The pathogenic members of *Mycobacterium tuberculosis* which merit particular attention here are the *human* and *bovine* strains; the *avian* strain very rarely affects man and more often pigs; the *murine* strain affects voles and has been used as a prophylactic vaccine in man. *Myco. leprae* is the cause of leprosy, which today occurs mostly in tropical and sub-tropical countries. *Myco. johnei* causes a chronic enteritis in cattle and sheep.

Mycobacteria characteristically produce chronic granulomatous lesions, which, in the case of tuberculosis, break down by caseation. The most common lesion is pulmonary tuberculosis. Leprosy occurs in either a mild tuberculoid form or the more severe lepromatous nodular disease; it is a very chronic infection.

MYCOBACTERIUM TUBERCULOSIS

Human Type

Morphology.—Slender, straight or slightly curved rod-shaped organisms, 2·5–3·5 μ by 0·3 μ, with rounded, pointed or sometimes expanded ends. In the tissues they may occur singly, or in pairs often forming an obtuse angle, or in small bundles of parallel bacilli. The organism is non-motile and non-sporing, though it possesses considerable powers of resistance to drying. In old cultures, individual cells may grow into long filaments and show branching.

Staining.—The tubercle bacillus is more difficult to stain than other bacteria. A strong dye with a mordant is required (*e.g.* carbol fuchsin), and either prolonged staining or the application of heat. It may stain uniformly or show marked beading. When stained it resists decolourisation with 20–25 per cent. sulphuric or nitric acid, and also with alcohol, and is therefore described as "acid- and alcohol-fast". The tubercle bacillus is Gram-positive but this character can be demonstrated only with difficulty.

Cultural Characters.—Aerobe; temperature range, 30°–41° C.; optimum, 37°–38° C.

Does not grow on ordinary media. Primary growths may be obtained on blood or serum media, or preferably on a medium containing whole egg or egg-yolk. In subculture, growths may result on ordinary media (agar, broth, potato) with 5–6 per cent. glycerol added.

Growth is slow—10–14 days at the earliest and as late as 6–8 weeks after primary inoculation.

A most convenient medium for artificial culture in ordinary laboratory work is one of the glycerol-egg media, *e.g.* Löwenstein-Jensen, to which a low concentration of an inhibitory dye, malachite green, is added to prevent growth of contaminants; the growth is luxuriant and presents the following appearance: dry, irregular, tough and tenacious, wrinkled or mamillated, at first white, later buff-coloured.

If a fragment of inoculum is floated on the surface of glycerol broth, growth spreads on the surface of the medium as a white wrinkled pellicle.

Fairly rapid submerged growth can be obtained in a fluid medium designed by Dubos containing casein hydrolysate, bovine serum-albumin, asparagine and certain salts along with a surface-active water-soluble lipid commercially known as "Tween 80", which is a polyoxyethylene sorbitan mono-oleate. This medium can be solidified and used for surface growths by incorporating agar.

Biochemical reactions are not ordinarily used in the identification or classification of tubercle bacilli. Antigenic analysis has shown that there are four main serological groups—mammalian (human, bovine and murine), avian, reptilian and saprophytic.

Viability.—The thermal death-point is 60° C. for 15–20 min. While many individual bacilli die when desiccated, a proportion survive for several weeks or months, if protected from daylight. The organism is relatively resistant to injurious chemical substances; it can survive in putrefying material, and in sputum may resist 5 per cent. phenol for several hours. It is highly susceptible to sunlight and ultra-violet radiation, and ordinary daylight, even through glass, has a lethal effect. *Myco. tuberculosis* is sensitive to streptomycin, viomycin and cycloserine among the antibiotics and to para-amino-salicylic acid (PAS), isonicotinic acid hydrazide (isoniazid), thiosemicarbazone, ethionamide and pyrazinamide among chemotherapeutic agents.

Animal Pathogenicity.—The guinea-pig is highly susceptible to experimental infection. If injected subcutaneously with the bacilli either in pathological material or in culture, after a few days a local swelling results consisting of tubercle nodules, which become confluent, undergo caseation and may finally ulcerate. The neighbouring lymph glands become involved by spread of the bacilli along lymphatic channels and, later, lymph glands in other parts of the body are affected. The animal begins to lose weight and dies in six weeks to three months. At autopsy, a generalised tuberculosis is noted; lymph glands show characteristic tuberculous lesions; the spleen is enlarged and contains greyish-white tuberculous nodules or larger caseous lesions; the liver presents a similar condition. The lungs and the kidneys, however, may show relatively slight lesions or be practically free from tuberculous nodules.

If the animal is killed four or five weeks after injection, secondary tuberculous nodules may be present only in the spleen and on the peritoneum. Smears must always be made from one or more of the lesions and stained by the Ziehl-Neelsen method to demonstrate acid-fast bacilli. Cultures should also be made.

Isoniazid-sensitive tubercle bacilli from Indian patients in the Madras area have been shown to be on average less virulent for the guinea-pig than strains from British patients: the less virulent strains have a greater sensitivity to hydrogen peroxide (see Mitchison *et al.* 1960, 1963).

Mice are much less susceptible to experimental tuberculosis than are guinea-pigs but after intraperitoneal or intravenous (or intracerebral) inoculation they develop progressive or chronic lesions according to the dose and virulence of the strain.

The human type of tubercle bacillus, apart from its occurrence in human disease, has been found also in natural tuberculosis of monkeys, cattle, pigs and dogs.

Bovine Type

Morphology and Staining reactions are practically identical with those of the human type.

Cultural Characters.—As compared with the human type, growth is less luxuriant, and the bovine type is described as "dysgonic" (the human type being referred to as "eugonic"), On egg medium it forms a thin, white, smooth, slightly moist, granular and easily broken-up growth. The difference between the human and bovine types is accentuated by using a glycerol-egg medium. Glycerol favours the growth of the human type, but has no such effect on the bovine variety.

Animal Pathogenicity.—The bovine type is more virulent to cattle and other domestic animals than the human type. In the ox it produces a fatal tuberculosis, whereas the human type causes only a localised lesion which heals spontaneously.

The difference between the two types can be elicited by injecting a rabbit *intravenously* with an emulsion in saline of 0·01–0·1 mg. (dry wt.) of a culture on solid medium. The bovine type produces an acute generalised tuberculosis, and the animals usually die within three to six weeks; in the case of the human type the animals survive, or die only after several months, with lesions confined usually to the lungs and kidneys.

The differentiation may also be made by injecting 10 mg. of culture *subcutaneously* in the rabbit; the bovine type leads to a general tuberculosis, which is fatal usually within ten weeks, whereas the human type produces only a local lesion.

It is to be noted that strains which deviate in their characters from the standard human and bovine types may be met with. Thus, strains isolated from lupus are frequently of attenuated virulence for laboratory animals.

The bovine type of tubercle bacillus, in addition to its association with tuberculosis of cattle, is the commonest variety found in tuberculosis of most other domesticated animals (*e.g.* pigs, horses, cats and dogs), but infection of domesticated animals with the human strain may also occur.

Pathogenesis.—The most common form of primary infection with the tubercle bacillus is a pulmonary lesion, known as the primary complex or Ghon focus. The organisms are inhaled in very small particles (not more than 5 μ in diameter) into the terminal bronchioles or alveoli, and the primary lesion may occur in any part of the lungs. From it, the organisms are carried by lymphatic drainage to the regional mediastinal glands in which there may be progressive enlargement and involvement, followed by caseation and later calcification. More generalised infection may follow spread of the organism either by the blood-stream or the bronchi, resulting respectively in miliary or bronchopneumonic tuberculosis, usually with lesions in other organs besides the lungs, *e.g.* brain and meninges (tuberculous meningitis), spleen, liver. Primary infection may also occur via the intestine with involvement of the mesenteric glands or via the tonsils with secondary cervical adenitis, usually from ingestion of infected milk. These forms of tuberculosis have become much rarer now that most milk supplies are pasteurised and bovine tuberculosis is virtually eradicated from Britain. From studies during the Second World War about a quarter of the cases of cervical adenitis in children under ten years of age were at that time caused by the human type and about three-quarters of the cases of meningeal and bone and joint tuberculosis were also due to the human type. Primary infection of the skin (lupus vulgaris) is now a rare condition; infection via skin lesions sometimes occurs from handling infected materials (laboratory workers and veterinarians) while intracutaneous BCG vaccination may produce a form of primary complex with local skin lesion and an associated adenitis.

While tuberculous meningitis occurs characteristically as a complication of the primary lung infection in very young children, it may also develop, *e.g.* in older children and young adults, as an apparently primary infection. In such cases, as in many instances of renal and bone and joint tuberculosis, there has presumably been an early "seeding" of tubercle bacilli, blood-borne from the primary lesion in the lung or elsewhere, which has lain latent until some factor has encouraged fresh activity. Sometimes, too, an active lesion in one area may help to reactivate a latent infection in another organ or tissue.

The post-primary (or adult) form of pulmonary infection is the most common form of clinical tuberculosis in which one or more lung lesions progress to caseation and cavitation and, involving the bronchial tree, create a case of open tuberculosis. This clinical lesion occurs characteristically in young adults and is often due to a fresh exogenous infection; in older people pulmonary tuberculosis is more likely to be a reactivation of an earlier healed primary or secondary lesion. Tuberculous ulcerations in the larynx and intestine when they occur are usually sequelae of pulmonary tuberculosis spread by infected sputum; similarly secondary infections of ureter, bladder, epididymis may follow renal tuberculosis.

Epidemiology.—Tuberculosis has a world-wide distribution and today probably takes precedence over malaria as *the* most important global contributor to death and disability among the specific infections. Yet, the mortality from tuberculosis has been falling dramatically in the more developed countries due to effective chemotherapy, so that deaths in Britain have been reduced by over 80 per cent. during the decade 1950-60. The decrease has been most marked in children and young adults as illustrated by the Scottish data for 1950 and 1960 (Fig. 15). Morbidity rates, as indicated by notifications, are also showing a decline but lagging behind the dramatic fall in mortality. When intensive case finding is carried out, as in the Scottish mass radiography survey in 1957–58, notifications will show a temporary increase (Fig. 16). A useful indicator of the amount of infection in a community is given by the incidence of tuberculin positive reactors in a particular age group. In Scotland the proportion of positive reactors in children aged 13–14 years has fallen from 48 per cent. in 1953 to 19 per cent. in 1962 (MacGregor, 1962).

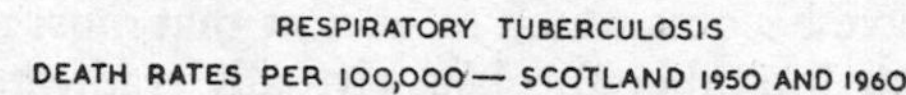

RESPIRATORY TUBERCULOSIS
DEATH RATES PER 100,000— SCOTLAND 1950 AND 1960

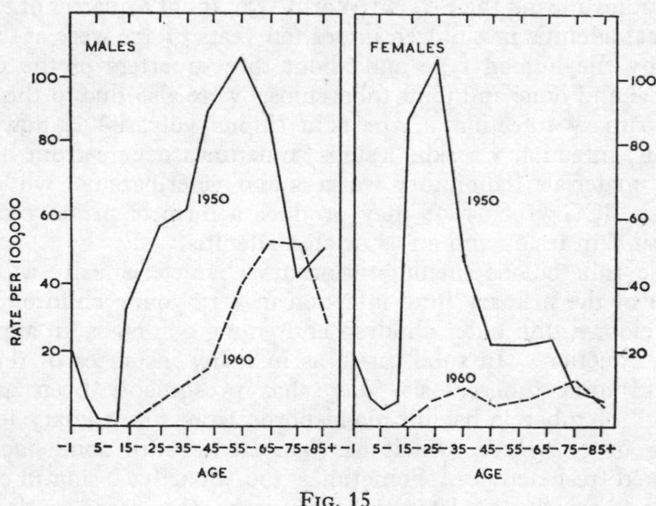

Fig. 15

With the control of bovine tuberculosis which in earlier years accounted for 5–10 per cent. of all deaths from tuberculosis and about a quarter of the cases of childhood tuberculosis, infection is nowadays predominantly due to the human type of *Myco. tuberculosis* and is spread mostly from open cases of pulmonary tuberculosis. The organism is expectorated in sputum and expelled in droplets during coughing and speaking and there have been instances of explosive outbreaks of tuberculosis in school children and others exposed to an infective teacher or singer. But since very small droplets that can be inhaled directly from the infective patient are less likely to carry tubercle bacilli than larger droplets or sputum, infection may occur more often indirectly from dried dust particles than directly from moist droplets or droplet nuclei. Tubercle bacilli survive slow drying for days or weeks if protected from the bactericidal daylight or sunlight so that the spread of infection from infected case to susceptible contacts by contaminated dust or fomites would be facilitated in overcrowded, badly lit rooms or buildings. Primary infection may occur at any age; if it occurs in early life (0–3 years) it is often associated with signs or symptoms of disease, *e.g.* hilar tuberculosis or the more serious systemic infections. At school age (5–15 years) infection usually occurs in an inapparent form, but in adolescents and young adults is again more likely to result in clinical disease.

Infection occurs earlier and is more likely to result in clinical disease among susceptibles living in close contact with open cases, but many personal and environmental factors may contribute to overt tuberculosis, *e.g.* age, malnutrition, other respiratory disease, hormonal dysfunction, pregnancy, stress, genetic constitution, etc.

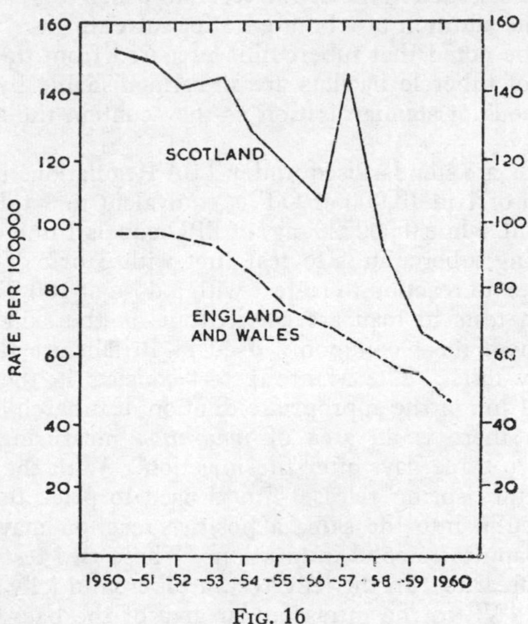

FIG. 16

Workers exposed to the inhalation of dusts containing silica have a high incidence of tuberculosis. Nurses, medical students, doctors and workers in pathological laboratories are more exposed and tend to have a higher than average rate of infection.

The Tuberculin Test

Koch made the original observation that when a live or a killed culture of tubercle bacilli was injected subcutaneously into a guinea-pig infected some weeks earlier with tubercle bacilli (resulting in a slowly progressive disease), there rapidly developed a local inflammatory lesion followed by necrosis and ulceration. This has been called the *Koch phenomenon*, and Koch went on to show that the same phenomenon could be elicited with an extract containing the specific protein of the tubercle bacilli, which he called *tuberculin*. The tuberculin reaction is due to the development of tissue hypersensitivity—or bacterial allergy—and is used in man and animals to find if they have or have had tuberculosis in an active or latent form.

Tuberculin was originally obtained from a six-week-old culture in glycerol-broth, evaporated to one-tenth of its volume, sterilised by heat and filtered (Old Tuberculin—OT). Various other methods have since been employed in its preparation. The specific tuberculo-protein can now be separated from other constituents and products of culture in a synthetic medium and then purified. This Purified Protein Derivative (PPD) is preferable to Old Tuberculin as it is constant in composition and potency, and there is an absence of non-specific substances. It is issued in the dry state, from which it is easy to prepare dilutions by the addition of a borate buffer solvent.

It should be noted that tuberculins prepared from the human and bovine types of tubercle bacillus are indistinguishable by the usually accepted methods of standardisation as they contain the same specific substance.

Tuberculins are standardised under TSA Regulations in such a way that a dilution of 1 in 10,000 of OT is equivalent to 1 tuberculin unit (TU) per 0·1 ml. while 0·000028 mg. of PPD equals 1 unit. A common practice in using tuberculin is to test first with 3 or 5 TU and if the individual gives no reaction to re-test with a dose of 100 TU.

Tuberculin tests in man are carried out on the skin by different techniques; those most commonly used in Britain are the Mantoux, Heaf and jelly tests. The Mantoux test consists in the intradermal injection of 0·1 ml. of the appropriate dilution of tuberculin; the test is positive when there is an area of *induration* measuring 5 mm. in diameter two to three days after the injection. With the Heaf test, a multiple puncture spring release gun is used to prick the previously applied tuberculin into the skin; a positive reaction may range from 4–6 discrete papules to solid induration. These two tests are usually done on the forearm. In the jelly test, a tuberculin jelly is applied in the form of a "V" in the intrascapular area of the back and covered with plaster; with it, but not with the other two tests, a control test is used.

In a recent comparison (Report, 1958) of these three and the Von Pirquet scarification test, in which such factors as sensitivity, reproducibility, ease of performance and consistency were compared, only the Mantoux and Heaf tests were shown to be acceptable for large-scale epidemiological investigations: in general, the Heaf was preferred to the Mantoux test (Report, 1959). The tuberculin test may be used: (*a*) epidemiologically to determine the incidence of tuberculous infection in a community. In a large-scale Medical Research Council survey in England and Wales in 1949-50 to cover the age-period 5–20 years, there was a steadily increasing proportion of positive reactors from around 15 per cent. in the 5-year-olds to 33 per cent. in the 14-year-olds and 70 per cent. in those aged 20 years. Among young children, the incidence was highest in rural areas (especially in counties with much bovine tuberculosis) and was higher in industrial urban than in non-industrial urban areas. There is evidence of a steady reduction in the incidence of positive reactors in recent years; (*b*) diagnostically in young children with suspected clinical infection. A positive reaction in a young child may also be useful for case-finding among the family contacts; (*c*) in immunisation campaigns in order to separate the positive and negative reactors and to assess the response to vaccination by sample testing afterwards.

The Tuberculin Test in Cattle.—The tuberculin reactions have been utilised in the recognition of tuberculosis in cattle, and are of great importance in testing milk cows. Thus, in England *tuberculin-tested milk*, and in Scotland *certified milk* and *tuberculin-tested milk*, must be obtained from tuberculin-tested animals which give no reaction. Until recently the test in cattle has usually been carried out in this country by the double intradermal method, but today the *single intradermal comparative test* is preferred. PPD tuberculins are used, doses of 0·1 ml. being injected intradermally in the neck. Two sites are chosen, the upper one for the avian tuberculin and the lower site (5 in. below) for the mammalian tuberculin: the skin thickness in the area is measured. The test is read at the seventy-second hour, the skin thickness being again measured and the reaction examined for evidence of oedema. Any swelling showing oedema or an increase of 4 mm. or more in skin thickness should be regarded as positive. The interpretation of this test depends on the presence or absence in the herd of non-specific infections such as Johne's disease or so-called skin tuberculosis that may sensitise the animals to tuberculin. In cases where the comparison between the reactions to the two tuberculins proves inconclusive, the animals concerned should be isolated and re-tested not earlier than thirty days following completion of the herd test.

By the systematic use of the tuberculin test for the detection of infection in cattle and the elimination of positive reactors, bovine tuberculosis has been virtually eradicated from Britain since 1962.

Laboratory Diagnosis

Tubercle bacilli are most numerous in lesions showing rapid caseation, *e.g.* adult-type pulmonary tuberculosis. In miliary tuberculosis they appear to be relatively scanty. In chronic closed lesions few tubercle bacilli are observed, and they may not be detectable microscopically though demonstrable by animal inoculation, *e.g.* in the pus from a tuberculous abscess.

Direct Microscopic Examination.—Sputum: a film is prepared from a purulent portion of the sputum and stained by the Ziehl-Neelsen method. The use of the $\frac{1}{7}$-in. oil immersion objective is particularly recommended. The oil is dropped on the film, and the dipper of the oil-bottle should never touch the film, otherwise acid-fast bacilli may be transferred to the oil container. After each examination the front of the objective should be wiped free from oil. The bacilli may be more easily recognised, particularly when they are scanty, by using a blue-green screen, Wratten H (No. 45), in front of a high-intensity illuminant. The bacilli and debris appear black, while if the counterstain is malachite green the background of cells now almost disappears, rendering the bacilli more easily recognised. In case of doubt the screen can be removed, and the organisms verified with the $\frac{1}{12}$-in objective. A prolonged examination may be necessary in some cases where the bacilli are relatively scanty; a negative result by no means excludes tuberculosis, since some 50,000 tubercle bacilli must be present in 1·0 ml. sputum for a positive microscopic finding.

Fluorescence Microscopy, after staining with auramine, may be substituted for ordinary microscopy with Ziehl-Neelsen stained films.

In suspected cases of pulmonary tuberculosis with no obvious sputum, stomach contents obtained by gastric lavage should be examined, or coughing may be induced by passing a swab on to the posterior pharynx, the expectoration on it being then used to prepare a film for microscopic examination.

Urine, pleural and peritoneal fluids are centrifuged, films are made from the deposit and stained by the Ziehl-Neelsen method. As tubercle bacilli are often scantily present in these fluids, the deposit from 50–100 ml. should be used for both direct microscopic examination and for culture; or the cultural method recommended by Ives and McCormick (1956) may be used, *i.e.* 100 ml. of pleural fluid is added directly to 100 ml. of double strength Sula liquid medium.

With all urinary specimens it is essential to treat the film with alcohol (two minutes) after decolourisation with acid in the Ziehl-Neelsen process, in order to exclude smegma bacilli. In examining urine it is advisable to obtain the sediment from a 24 hours' specimen because of intermittency of excretions. Alternatively three consecutive morning specimens may be examined.

Cerebrospinal fluid is allowed to stand in a stoppered tube for an hour or longer, when a "spider-web" coagulum usually forms in the fluid. The clot is carefully transferred to a slide, the preparation is dried, fixed by heat and stained by the Ziehl-Neelsen method. In the absence of clotting the fluid is centrifuged and the deposit examined in the usual way.

In suspected cases of intestinal tuberculosis, Ziehl-Neelsen stained films of faeces may be examined either directly or after concentration with 4 per cent. sodium hydroxide but a positive finding is not necessarily diagnostic since saprophytic acid-fast bacilli may be present.

In the case of tissues, sections are stained by the Ziehl-Neelsen method.

Cultivation of the Tubercle Bacillus from Pathological Material.—If the tubercle bacilli are likely to be present in pure culture in the material, two screw-capped bottles containing slopes of egg medium can be inoculated directly. If other organisms are present, *e.g.* in sputum or urine, one of the procedures described below must be used in order to destroy the contaminating bacteria and homogenise the specimen; in this case the centrifuge tubes, water or other fluid used for washing the sediment, etc., must be sterile.

Great care must be taken in the handling of tuberculosis material and during manipulations the use of a special hood or a separate room is recommended.

(*a*) Petroff's method (modified).—Sputum is mixed thoroughly with an equal volume of 4 per cent. sodium hydroxide and placed in the incubator at 37° C. for 30 min., the container being shaken every five minutes. The mixture is centrifuged at 3000 r.p.m. for 30 minutes and the supernatant fluid poured off. The deposit is neutralised with 8 per cent. hydrochloric acid, which is added drop by drop, the reaction of the mixture being tested by adding a drop of phenol red solution to the tube. The deposit is examined microscopically and is then inoculated on Löwenstein-Jensen medium. Solidified Dubos medium or some modification of it can also be used. Numerous other liquid, semi-solid and solid media for the primary cultivation of tubercle bacilli have been described; it is advisable to use a medium which experience has proved to give constantly good results with a minimum of contaminations.

(*b*) Nassau's modification of Jungmann and Gruschka's method. Prepare the following solutions:

Solution A.

Ferrous sulphate	20 g.
Sulphuric acid 20 per cent.v/v.	100 ml.

Solution B.

Hydrogen peroxide	0·3 per cent. (1 vol.)

Solution A can be made up in bulk and keeps indefinitely. Solution B must be made up fresh on each occasion from a standard pharmacopoeal 6 per cent. w/v solution kept in the dark. For use place 2 ml. of sputum in a universal container. Add 1·2 ml. solution A and 1·2 ml. solution B. Shake the container for thirty seconds and allow to stand on the bench for twenty minutes, shaking at intervals. Centrifuge at 3000 r.p.m. for thirty minutes and discard the supernatant fluid. Fill the container to the shoulder with 5 per cent. sterile sodium citrate, shake vigorously, and again centrifuge. Decant the supernatant fluid and inoculate the deposit on two slopes of Löwenstein-Jensen medium.

Alternative reagents used for the "pre-treatment" of sputum or other contaminated specimens to be cultured for tubercle bacilli include a saturated solution of trisodium phosphate (12–24 hours), quaternary ammonium compounds and mucolytic enzymes or a combination of the latter two substances (Saxholm, 1958)

In examining primary cultures derived from sputum, urine, stomach washings, etc. the possibility must be borne in mind of *saprophytic* acid-fast bacilli (*vide infra*) being present. Since these organisms sometimes yield growths not unlike that of the tubercle bacillus, careful scrutiny of the culture should be made as regards colonial morphology, pigmentation, etc. Subcultures should be made on nutrient agar and incubated at room temperature as well as 37° C. since saprophytic mycobacteria grow quickly over a wide range of temperature. If there is any doubt further tests including animal pathogenicity tests should be carried out (see also Anonymous Mycobacteria, p. 207).

Micro-Culture.—Methods have been devised for cultivating tubercle bacilli directly from sputum by smearing the specimen thickly on glass slides, *e.g.* microscopic slides divided longitudinally in two, treating them with some agent to destroy organisms other than tubercle bacilli, *e.g.* 6 per cent. sulphuric acid for twenty minutes, and then washing thoroughly with sterile distilled water, and finally placing the slides in a suitable fluid medium, *e.g.* citrated human blood lysed in an equal volume of 1 per cent. saponin (Pryce, 1941). After incubation for about a week the slides are stained by the Ziehl-Neelsen method and young colonies of the tubercle bacillus can be seen by microscopic examination first with the low-power and then the oil-immersion lens. This method has also been used in testing resistance to chemotherapeutic drugs.

Guinea-pig Inoculation.—In laboratory diagnosis, where tubercle bacilli cannot be detected in specimens by microscopic examination, guinea-pig inoculation in addition to direct cultivation may be used, as one or other (or both) of these procedures often yields postive results when microscopic examination is negative. With most materials, culture gives at least as high a proportion of positive results as guinea-pig inoculation and has the advantages that a positive finding can be reported earlier and the culture is immediately available for sensitivity tests. In suspected renal tuberculosis, on the other hand, guinea-pig inoculation of microscopically negative urinary deposits seems to be more often positive than culture.

The usual method of carrying out the guinea-pig inoculation test is to inject material subcutaneously in the flank or intramuscularly in the thigh of two guinea-pigs, one of which is killed at four weeks and the other at eight weeks. The result of the guinea-pig test can sometimes be expedited by intradermal inoculation, 0·4 ml. of the material being injected into the shaved abdominal skin. If the specimen is tuberculous, a nodule appears in seven to twenty-one days; this is incised, and films of the lesion are examined for tubercle bacilli.

Laryngeal Swab; Gastric Lavage

Where sputum is absent or, if present, is being swallowed, material for culture may be obtained either by the laryngeal swab or by stomach wash-out.

The laryngeal swab consists of a piece of nickel or "Nichrome" wire 9 in. long and $\frac{1}{16}$ in. in diameter, bent at an angle of 120° an inch and a half from the end. Cotton-wool is wrapped round this end of the wire, which has been flattened and spirally twisted to hold the cotton-wool firmly. Each swab is placed in a boiling-tube (7 × 1 in). the open end of which is plugged with cotton-wool. The tubes with swabs in position are sterilised in the autoclave. Immediately before use the swab is moistened with sterile distilled water.

The swab may be passed into the larynx either with the guidance of a laryngeal mirror, or blindly. For both methods the patient is seated and supplied with a piece of gauze with which to hold his tongue fully protruded. The operator, if using a mirror, sits opposite the patient and with the aid of the mirror guides the tip of the swab over the epiglottis into the larynx. Without a mirror the operator stands at the side of the patient and passes the swab through the mouth backwards and downwards strictly in the mid-line; the manoeuvre is facilitated by asking the patient to take panting breaths. Reflex cough usually develops as the swab enters the larynx, and absence of cough suggests that the swab has not entered the larynx. Two consecutive swabs should be taken from each patient.

In the laboratory sufficient 10 per cent. H_2SO_4 (v/v) is added to the boiling-tube to cover the cotton-wool on the swab. After five minutes in acid the swab is removed, excess of fluid is expressed on the side of the tube, and the swab is transferred for a further five minutes to a second boiling-tube containing a similar amount of 2 per cent. NaOH. The swab is again drained of excess fluid and is rubbed over the surface of a slope of Löwenstein-Jensen medium. The inoculated medium is incubated at 37° C. for six to eight weeks and examined at weekly intervals.

An alternative procedure is to immerse the swab in a saturated solution of trisodium phosphate and incubate at 37° C. overnight. The swab is then removed and the fluid centrifuged at 3000 r.p.m. for 20 min. The supernatant is decanted and the deposit is inoculated on to two Löwenstein-Jensen slopes.

It is inadvisable to leave a long delay between the collection of the swabs and inoculation on to culture medium.

Fasting stomach contents may be aspirated with a Ryle tube in the morning after a period of coughing and swallowing. The material should be despatched to the laboratory as quickly as possible, or if there is likely to be a long delay, the contents should be neutralised with caustic soda. The deposit is homogenised by either the modified Petroff or the modified Jungmann method (*vide supra*) and inoculated on two slopes of Löwenstein-Jensen medium. Patients prefer the laryngeal swab to gastric lavage, which, however, may give at least as high a proportion of positive results. Neither of these methods will give as good results as scanty expectoration.

Serology.—Serological tests for specific antibodies following tuberculous infection have not proved of much diagnostic value. The complement-fixation test becomes positive in a high proportion of established cases but is usually negative in early or suspected cases. Middlebrook and Dubos (1948) described a haemagglutination test which depends on the agglutinating effect of patients' serum on sheep or group-O human red blood cells sensitised with an extract of tubercle bacilli. The red cells are sensitised with an antigenic extract of the tubercle bacillus or with commercial "Old Tuberculin"; the cells are then mixed with varying dilutions of patient's serum, from which any heterophile antibody has been removed by absorption; if specific antibody is present, the cells are agglutinated and the degree of the reaction is indicated by the highest dilution of serum producing agglutination.

This test has received a good deal of study and clinical trial, but its practical value in the diagnosis of clinical tuberculosis is doubtful because of its lack of both specificity and sensitivity (Hilson and Elek, 1951).

Chemotherapy.—Although the tubercle bacillus is sensitive to an increasing range of antimicrobial drugs, clinical experience has shown that the most effective and least toxic chemotherapeutic substances in tuberculosis are streptomycin, para-amino-salicylic acid (PAS) and isonicotinic acid hydrazide (Isoniazid). Because resistant variants of the tubercle bacillus may appear within two to three months after commencing treatment with any *one* of these drugs, it is essential that (*a*) a combination of two—or three—antimicrobial drugs be used from the onset of treatment in cases of tuberculosis in order to minimise this risk and (*b*) every effort must be made to culture and test the sensitivity of infecting strains as early as possible, since resistant mutants in a strain that is already resistant to one of a pair of drugs being used will soon emerge to the other.[1] Strains that are highly resistant to Isoniazid usually show a decrease in virulence for the guinea-pig but not necessarily for man (see Mitchison, 1963).

Prophylaxis.—Killed vaccines of the tubercle bacillus give little or no protection against tuberculosis. In 1921, two French workers, Calmette and Guérin, introduced a living vaccine prepared from a bovine strain that had been cultured for many years on a bile-potato medium. This Bacille Calmette Guérin (BCG) vaccine was at first given orally, but following Scandinavian practice is now given mostly by intradermal injection. Its value in the prophylaxis of tuberculosis has been much disputed, but in recent years controlled trials in different countries and with different communities and age-groups have demonstrated conclusively that BCG vaccination may give protection of the order of 80 per cent. against clinical infection. Thus, in large-scale trials among school-leavers (14 years of age) in industrial areas in England, the incidence of clinical disease was reduced by approximately 80 per cent. in the vaccinated groups during a follow-up period of eight to ten years (Report, 1963). In a study among North American Indians (0–20 years old) a similar degree of protection persisted for some ten years after vaccination (Aronson *et al.*, 1958).

Fresh liquid vaccine deteriorates on storage and it is recommended that it be used within fourteen days of preparation. It loses viability quickly in warm atmospheres (30° C.) or if exposed to light; this reduces its usefulness in tropical and sub-tropical countries. Another disadvantage is that tests for safety and potency cannot be completed before the liquid vaccine is released for use. To overcome these difficulties, freeze-dried vaccines have been developed and clinical trials with a British freeze-dried vaccine reconstituted immediately before use have shown that it is comparable in potency with the Danish liquid vaccine. Laboratory estimates of potency depend on the direct relationship that has been demonstrated between protection and the degree of post-vaccination tuberculin sensitivity in the guinea-pig.

[1] Technical details about drug-sensitivity tests for tubercle bacilli are given in Chapter 53.

The degree of sensitivity required is defined by the Therapeutic Substances Act (TSA) Regulations. For the freeze-dried vaccine, the tuberculin sensitivity produced in children is tested for each batch at the BCG Control Centre in the Oxford Region.

The dose of BCG vaccine is a single intracutaneous injection of 0·1 ml. containing 0·05 to 0·1 mg. moist weight of the constituent bacilli (=1–2 million viable organisms). A small inflammatory lesion develops at the site of inoculation and usually goes on to superficial ulceration after some weeks. Adenitis of the regional lymph nodes may follow in infants (rarely in older children). Occasionally an erysipeloid lesion (lupus) may occur, particularly if vaccination has been done by multiple puncture. Except in the case of babies 0–3 months old, all children must first be tuberculin tested and only the negative reactors given vaccine.

Oral vaccination with repeated large doses is practised in some countries, but there have been very few properly controlled trials to substantiate claims for the protective value of the oral vaccine.

Mycobacteria of Ulcerative Lesions in the Human Subject.—Ulcerative lesions of the skin have been reported in Australia and Sweden from which mycobacteria, clearly distinguishable from the tubercle bacillus, have been isolated. The Australian strains, *Myco. ulcerans*, were found to be pathogenic to mice and rats but not guinea-pigs. In culture the optimum temperature was 33° C. (MacCullum *et al.*, 1948). The infections described in Sweden were derived from swimming pools, and the strains of mycobacteria isolated, *Myco. balnei*, were highly pathogenic to mice; in guinea-pigs they were only slightly pathogenic; in rabbits inoculation of the skin produced ulcers similar to the human lesions. The Swedish strains grew at 31° C. but not at 37° C. (Linell and Norden, 1954).

Anonymous Mycobacteria

Acid-fast bacilli which cannot be identified as either human or bovine tubercle bacilli and which may be associated with human disease have attracted considerable attention in recent years and have been given the name *anonymous* or *atypical mycobacteria*.

These mycobacteria are divisible into a number of groups according to their morphology, colonial texture, production of pigment in the presence of light (photochromogens) or in the dark (scotochromogens), rapidity of growth and growth at different temperatures (25° = psychrophiles; 37° = mesophiles; 42° = thermophiles), production of catalase, resistance to certain anti-tuberculous drugs, *e.g.* thiosemicarbazone, Isoniazid and PAS, and the Niacin test (Gilani & Selkon, 1958). On the basis of such tests, Marks and Richards (1962) have expanded the original four groups of Runyon to seven provisional groups of which group I (the photochromogens) are most commonly associated with respiratory disease, group II (the scotochromogens) are found in neck abscesses or are clinically insignificant, group IV is very similar to *Myco. avium*, and group VII is found in association with cases of pneumoconiosis, *e.g.* in Wales.

In a series of 2916 strains of mycobacteria isolated from sputum in eight different areas of England and Wales, 71 *anonymous* mycobacteria (2·5 per cent.) were identified by *in vitro* screening cultural tests on Löwenstein-Jensen medium as follows:

(1) A plain slope for incubation for 4 weeks at 37° C. in light equivalent to a 25-watt lamp at 30 to 60 cm. distance.
(2) A slope containing p-acetamido-benzaldehyde thiosemicarbazone, 10 μg./ml., for incubation for 4 weeks at 37° C. in the dark.
(3) A slope containing p-aminosalicylic acid (PAS), 1 μg./ml., for incubation as (2).
(4) A plain slope for incubation for up to 4 weeks at 25° C. in the dark.

Screening tests were read daily for three days and then weekly for four weeks. Of these strains, 40 (1·4 per cent.) of which 27 were photochromogens, were regarded as associated with clinical disease (PHLS Report, 1962). When repeated isolation suggests that an anonymous strain may be acting as a pathogen, it is advisable before a final diagnosis to inoculate one guinea-pig with a primary culture and another directly with a decontaminated specimen to ensure that tubercle bacilli are not being masked.

Saprophytic and Commensal Mycobacteria.—Non-pathogenic acid-fast bacilli may be found in milk, butter, manure, water, grass (e.g. *Mycobacterium phlei*) and the smegma of man and animals. They are similar in morphology to the tubercle bacillus, but their growth on culture medium is rapid; they develop on ordinary media and at room temperature (though the optimum may be 37° C.), producing an abundant dry or slightly moist growth which is irregular, coarsely granular and sometimes wrinkled; most strains are definitely pigmented—yellow, pink or brown.

Acid-fast bacilli have been frequently demonstrated in the deposits from the interior of laboratory taps. This possibility must be borne in mind in using tap water for preparing films and staining solutions. It has also been pointed out that such organisms may be present on bark and rubber corks and rubber washers such as are used with specimen containers.

Mycobacterium smegmatis (*Smegma bacillus*).—This is a commensal organism found in smegma and sometimes on the skin. It conforms in biological characters to the saprophytic types described above. As it may occur in specimens of urine, it has to be differentiated carefully from the tubercle bacillus. It is generally shorter and thicker than the latter, and shows greater variation in size and shape. The smegma bacillus is acid-fast, but in urinary deposits is often decolourised by alcohol, which has no effect on the tubercle bacillus. It is also less resistant to antiformin than the tubercle bacillus.

Mycobacterium avium (*Avian tubercle bacillus*).—The causative organism of tuberculosis in birds. Its morphology and staining reactions are the same as those of the other types of tubercle bacilli. Its optimum temperature is 40°–43° C., and on glycerol agar the growth is more rapid in development, moister, more homogeneous and more luxuriant than that of the mammalian types, the culture presenting a somewhat creamy appearance. Individual colonies are large, raised, hemispherical, with a smooth shiny surface and a yellow or brownish-yellow colour.

It is highly virulent to fowls, which are resistant to the mammalian tubercle bacilli. For testing purposes, 0·001 mg. of culture is injected intravenously or the bacilli are administered by feeding. The guinea-pig, which is highly susceptible to the human and bovine types, is resistant to the avian bacillus. The rabbit shows a moderate degree of susceptibility.

This type of tubercle bacillus also occurs in pigs, and has been reported in other domesticated mammals, including cattle. Human tuberculosis due to the avian type has been recorded, but is an extreme rarity.

Mycobacterium tuberculosis var. **muris.**—This organism (*Vole tubercle bacillus*) has been found in a tubercle-like disease of voles, which is fairly widespread. Morphologically the bacilli are longer and thinner than the typical tubercle bacillus and often somewhat curved. Growth on egg medium is very slow and is not enhanced by the presence of glycerol. Antigenically the organism is similar to the human and bovine types. Inoculated experimentally in voles it produces typical tuberculosis, but in guinea-pigs, rabbits and calves is of low virulence, moderate doses producing only a local lesion. The vole tubercle bacillus is practically non-pathogenic to man. Inoculation of the organism in guinea-pigs and calves brings about immunity to virulent tubercle bacilli; and it has been used as a vaccine as an alternative to BCG.

Mycobacterium piscium.—Acid-fast bacilli resembling the tubercle bacillus have been isolated from fish and other cold-blooded animals, *e.g.* frogs, turtles, etc., and have been regarded as aetiologically associated with a tubercle-like disease in such animals. These organisms grow best at 25° C. and flourish even at 15° C. In cultural characters they correspond to the avian type (*vide supra*). They are not pathogenic to mammals or birds, but produce lesions on experimental inoculation in frogs, fish, etc.

Mycobacterium leprae

The causative organism of Leprosy.

Morphology and Staining.—A straight or slightly curved slender bacillus, about the same size as the tubercle bacillus, with pointed, rounded or club-shaped ends; so far as is known it is non-motile and non-sporing. Like the tubercle bacillus it requires, as a rule, a strong stain, and is acid-fast, though not to the same degree; it may stain uniformly, but usually shows marked beading, which may be coarser than that of the tubercle bacillus; it is Gram-positive, and can be stained fairly readily by the ordinary Gram's method (*cf.* tubercle bacillus).

Cultivation.—A great many attempts have been made by various workers to cultivate this organism; the majority have been unsuccessful, and though successful results have been claimed and cultures of acid-fast bacilli have apparently been isolated from leprous lesions, it is doubtful whether these strains represent the true leprosy bacillus. Some success in culturing the organism of rat leprosy on tissue cultures has recently been claimed.

Pathogenesis—Leprosy is an infective granuloma, developing as

(1) the *lepromatous* or *nodular* type, in which granulomatous nodules (lepromata) form in the skin, mucous membranes and various organs (*e.g.* lungs, liver, spleen, testes), or (2) the *tuberculoid* type, where the granulation tissue infiltrates certain nerves and leads to motor and sensory paralysis, with characteristic trophic changes (*e.g.* anaesthetic skin areas—maculae). Both types of the disease may occur in the same patient.

The organisms are found in the granulomatous lesions, being particularly numerous in the nodular form. They are distributed intracellularly for the most part, parallel bacilli occurring in bundles which may completely fill up cells. They may be found also in the tissue spaces, in the walls of small vessels, in lymph glands and in the secretions of the nose, throat and mouth, due to the fact that the mucosal lesions ulcerate readily and discharge bacilli into the mucous secretions.

The bacilli are present in the nerve granulomata, but are less numerous than in the nodular lesions. The organisms do not occur in the maculae which are essentially trophic and not primarily leprous lesions.

Laboratory Diagnosis.—Films are made from any ulcerated nodule on the skin, or a non-ulcerated nodule can be punctured with a needle and squeezed till lymph exudes, from which films are made. Films can be prepared also from a scraping of an excised piece of tissue, or sections may be prepared as for histological examination. A convenient method is to remove, with curved scissors, a piece of skin (about 2 mm. deep) overlying a nodule, and prepare films from the deep surface.

Films should be made in all cases from the nasal mucosa or secretion, as diagnostic information may be obtained in this way even when lesions are not present in the skin.

The films or sections are stained by the Ziehl-Neelsen method, substituting 5 per cent. sulphuric acid for 20 per cent. The presence of the characteristic acid-fast bacilli, especially when they occur in large numbers and are situated inside cells, is generally diagnostic.

When the lungs are affected the bacilli may be demonstrated in the sputum, but require to be differentiated from the tubercle bacillus by differential Ziehl-Neelsen staining and by animal inoculation; the leprosy bacilli do not produce any pathogenic effects in laboratory animals.

Mycobacterium lepraemurium.—The organism of "rat leprosy" which presents some pathological similarity to human leprosy, is an acid-fast bacillus related to, but not identical with, the leprosy bacillus. This disease of rats is transmissible experimentally to animals of the same species, but not readily to other species, though transmission to the hamster has been recorded. It should be noted that human leprosy cannot be transmitted to rats.

Mycobacterium johnei

(*Bacillus of Johne's Disease*)

The causative organism of a chronic enteritis of cattle, and a similar disease of sheep; sometimes called *Myco. paratuberculosis.*

Morphology and Staining.—A Gram-positive, acid-fast and alcohol-fast bacillus like the tubercle bacillus, but more readily stained by the Ziehl-Neelsen method. It is often comparatively short (1 to 2 μ), but cannot be distinguished microscopically from the tubercle bacillus. It stains uniformly, though the longer forms may stain irregularly.

Cultural Characters.—Has proved difficult to cultivate artificially. Growths can be obtained on glycerol-egg medium containing 1 per cent. killed *Myco. tuberculosis* or other acid-fast bacilli, e.g. *Myco. phlei* or extracts of these organisms (Taylor, 1950). The organism requires a growth factor which is synthesised by other members of the acid-fast group; this factor is also present in certain vegetable tissues and in some fungi. It is very stable and can be partially replaced by vitamin K. Primary growths develop very slowly and four weeks may elapse before they are definitely visible. The optimum temperature is about 38° C. After continued cultivation in this way, subcultures may be obtained on egg media without the addition of another acid-fast organism or its products. Cultures resemble those of the tubercle bacillus.

Animal Pathogenicity.—The disease is transmissible experimentally to calves and young goats, the incubation period being several months. Lambs can also be successfully infected. Laboratory animals are mostly refractory although in recent years mice and young rabbits have been artificially infected with the production of lesions, containing the bacilli, in the intestines, mesenteric lymph nodes, liver and spleen.

Pathogenesis.—The lesions are of a granulomatous nature and lead to corrugated thickening of the mucosa of the intestine; the small bowel is primarily affected. The bacilli are present in large numbers, usually packed inside the cells of the lesions (as in leprosy).

The disease in sheep may be caused by either of two types; the classical *Myco. johnei* as isolated from cattle, or a variant which has proved more difficult to grow artificially and produces an orange-coloured pigment. The disease has also been reported in goats, horses, deer, gnu, antelope, camels, and a llama.

Laboratory Diagnosis.—At autopsy, the characteristic acid-fast bacilli may be demonstrated in the mucous membrane of the bowel by the appropriate staining methods and cultivated from this tissue after treatment with antiformin or oxalic acid.

During life, the organism may be observed in the faeces; microscopically, groups of small acid-alcohol-fast bacilli may generally be regarded as diagnostic. Tuberculosis may be excluded by the inoculation of material containing the acid-fast bacilli into laboratory animals.

An allergic skin reaction evoked by "Johnin", a preparation (from cultures) analogous to tuberculin, has been utilised in diagnosis, but its diagnostic specificity is doubtful. Tuberculin prepared from the avian type of tubercle bacillus yields a similar reaction.

The Johne bacillus, in common with other pathogenic mycobacteria, is capable of stimulating the production of complement-fixing antibodies which can be demonstrated in the blood serum of cattle. The value of the complement fixation test for the diagnosis of Johne's disease in tuberculosis-free herds has been under investigation for a number of years and today a negative complement-fixation reaction is one of the requirements for the importation of cattle to a number of countries.

REFERENCES

Aronson, J. D., Aronson, C. F. & Taylor, H. C. (1958). A twenty-year appraisal of BCG vaccination in the control of tuberculosis. *Arch. intern. med.*, **101** (5), 881.

Gilani, S. & Selkon, J. B. (1958). The niacin test for differentiating human tubercle bacilli from other mycobacteria. *Tubercle*, **39**, 396.

Hilson, G. R. F. & Elek, S. D. (1951). The haemagglutination reaction in tuberculosis. *J. clin. Path.*, **4**, 158.

Ives, J. C. J. & McCormick, W. (1956). A modification of Sula's method for the cultivation of tubercle bacilli from pleural fluid. *J. clin. Path.*, **9**, 177.

Linell, F. & Norden, A. (1954). *Mycobacterium balnei*; new acid-fast bacillus occurring in swimming pools and capable of producing skin lesions in humans. *Acta tuberc. scand.* (Supl. 33), pp. 1-84.

MacCullum, P., Tolhurst, J. C., Buckle, G. & Sissons, H. A. (1948). A new mycobacterial infection in man. *J. Path. Bact.*, **60**, 93.

Macgregor, I. M. (1962). Eradication of tuberculosis: where we stand in Scotland. *Hlth. Bull. (Edinb.)*, **20**, 20.

Marks, J. & Richards, M. (1962). Classification of the anonymous mycobacteria as a guide to their significance. *Mth. Bull., Minist. Hlth. Lab. Serv.* **21**, 200.

Middlebrook, G. & Dubos, R. J. (1948). Specific serum agglutination of erythrocytes sensitized with extracts of tubercle bacilli. *J. exp. Med.*, **88**, 521.

Mitchison, D. A., Wallace, J. G., Bhatia, A. L., Selkon, J. B., Subbaiah, T. V. & Lancaster, M. C. (1960). A comparison of the virulence in guinea-pigs of South Indian and British tubercle bacilli. *Tubercle*, **41**, 1.

Mitchison, D. A., Selkon, J. B. & Lloyd, Janet (1963). Virulence in the guinea-pig, susceptibility to hydrogen peroxide, and catalase activity of isoniazid-sensitive tubercle bacilli from South Indian and British patients. *J. Path. Bact.*, **86**, 377.

Mitchison, D. A. (1963). The epidemiology of tubercle bacilli. *The Scientific Basis of Medicine Annual Reviews*, p. 319. The Athlone Press. University of London.

Pryce, D. M. (1941). Sputum film cultures of tubercle bacilli : a method for the early observation of growth. *J. Path. Bact.*, **53**, 327.

Report (1958). A single tuberculin test for epidemiological use : comparison of four tests. *Tubercle*, **39**, 76.

Report (1959). A single tuberculin test for epidemiological use : a comparison of the Mantoux and Heaf tests. *Tubercle*, **40**, 317.

Report (1962). Anonymous mycobacteria in England and Wales. 1.—Prevalence and methods of identification. P.H.L.S. *Tubercle*, **43**, 432.

Report (1963). BCG and vole bacillus vaccines in the prevention of tuberculosis in adolescence and early adult life. *Brit. med. J.*, **1**, 973.

Saxholm, R. (1958). *An Experimental Investigation of Methods for the Cultivation of Mycobacterium tuberculosis from Sputum.* Oslo: Oslo: Univ. Press.

Taylor, A. Wilson (1950). Observations on the isolation of *Mycobacterium johnei* in primary culture. *J. Path. Bact.*, **62**, 647.

CHAPTER 15

HAEMOPHILUS. BORDETELLA

Haemophilus influenzae (Pfeiffer's influenza bacillus) was originally described as the causal organism of epidemic influenza and has been designated *haemophilic* in virtue of its inability to grow on culture medium without the addition of whole blood or certain growth-promoting substances present in blood. These growth factors, however, are not restricted to blood, but are present also in certain vegetable tissues. The Koch-Weeks bacillus, a common cause of acute conjunctivitis, shows the same growth requirements as *Haemophilus influenzae*, and may appropriately be grouped with it. The bacillus of whooping-cough has also been placed in the *haemophilic* group, but its growth requirements are different from those of the influenza bacillus and it has now been given the generic name of *Bordetella*. If the term *haemophilic* is used in a broad sense to designate organisms which require blood for their growth it would embrace a number of heterogeneous species, and the generic term *Haemophilus* is therefore restricted to those organisms which are dependent on one or both of the growth factors required by *Haemophilus influenzae*.

Haemophilus influenzae

This organism is commonly found in the throats of healthy people and is associated with both acute and chronic infections of the respiratory tract. In its *smooth* phase, it may cause pyogenic meningitis and acute laryngo-tracheitis.

Morphology and Staining.—A very small Gram-negative slender bacillus, usually about 1·5 μ by 0·3 μ, occurring singly or in pairs; non-motile; non-sporing; capsulated types occur. Oval coccobacillary forms are noted, and in culture there is marked pleomorphism; some strains, *e.g.* those present in meningitis, may show elongated, curved, threadlike forms.

The counter-staining in the Gram's stain is improved if carbol-fuchsin 1 in 20 is used and applied for 5 minutes.

Cultural Characters.—Aerobe. Optimum temperature about 37° C. Does not grow on ordinary media, but can be cultivated in the presence of blood—*e.g.* on blood agar or preferably heated blood agar.

It has been shown that two growth-promoting constituents present in blood are necessary for the cultivation of *H. influenzae*. One of these, termed the X factor, is thermostable and resists autoclaving at 120° C. This factor is haematin and is supposed to act in virtue of its being required for the synthesis of catalase, which is necessary for the aerobic growth of the organism. It has been found that the X factor can be dispensed with under anaerobic conditions. The other factor, designated V, is more easily destroyed by heat. It has been identified as coenzyme I or II which is essential as a hydrogen acceptor in the oxidation-reduction processes of the organism.

It is noteworthy that *H. influenzae* grows better in symbiosis with staphylococci, due to the fact that these organisms synthesise the V factor. Thus, in a mixed culture, colonies of the influenza bacillus are bigger in the neighbourhood of staphylococcal colonies: this appearance has been described as *satellitism*.

Blood agar: very small, transparent, droplet-like colonies which tend to remain discrete. Optimum growth occurs in media in which the contents of the red blood cells are liberated either by heat, *e.g.* chocolate agar, Levinthal's medium, or by peptic digestion, *e.g.* Fildes' medium. Smooth capsulated strains have rather larger mucoid colonies with a characteristic iridescence which is best seen on translucent media (Levinthal or Fildes).

Glucose and various other carbohydrates are fermented. Indole is produced by some strains.

Certain strains have been found to differ from the typical form in producing a well-marked zone of haemolysis on blood agar (*H. haemolyticus*). These may be coarser in microscopic appearance and tend to develop elongated threads. Most of these haemolytic strains require both X and V factors for growth.

Some non-haemolytic strains are independent of the X factor and require only the V substance; these strains have been designated *H. para-influenzae*. Strains of this type have been described in some cases of subacute bacterial endocarditis.

An organism originally isolated from a purulent condition of the preputial sac in a dog (*H. canis haemoglobinophilus*) resembles *H. influenzae* in general characters, but requires only the X factor for its growth.

H. suis has been found in an influenza-like disease of pigs associated with a filterable virus. It differs from *H. influenzae* in the lack of fermentative action.

Antigenic Characters.—Pittman has classified recently isolated smooth capsulated forms of *H. influenzae* into six serological types (labelled *a* to *f*) based on the specific soluble substance (polysugar phosphates) as capsular constituent. Organisms isolated from meningitis or acute laryngo-tracheitis belong predominantly to type *b*. In culture the smooth organism readily undergoes transformation to the rough form which lacks such specific substance, and, under these conditions, strains assume considerable serological diversity. Change of type can be effected by the action of DNA of one type on rough strains of another type; this phenomenon is similar to that first described for pneumococcus types (p. 92).

Animal Pathogenicity.—*H. influenzae* is not naturally pathogenic for laboratory animals. Mice may be infected by intraperitoneal injection of strains suspended in mucin. Capsulated, but not non-capsulated strains, resist the bactericidal action of normal rabbit blood.

Pathogenesis.—Rough strains of *H. influenzae* are found in a varying proportion (30–80 per cent.) of normal throats. They are opportunists, or potential pathogens, like the pneumococci found in the upper respiratory tract, in that they are associated with infection (sinusitis, bronchitis, bronchopneumonia) when the respiratory tract is less resistant to bacterial invasion, *e.g.* following a primary virus infection or at the extremes of life. The name "influenza bacillus" was given to this organism when it was found in many of the influenzal pneumonias in the pandemic of 1889–90. It was again associated with severe influenzal infections in the 1918–19 pandemic, but other pathogens (pneumococci, streptococci and staphylococci) were also commonly found; by that time it was becoming accepted that these bacteria were secondary invaders, although it was not until 1933 that the virus aetiology of influenza was established.

Besides its importance as a secondary pathogen in acute respiratory infections, *H. influenzae* is the organism most commonly found in cases of chronic bronchitis and bronchiectasis. Its causal relationship to these chronic infections is not clear, but it may be noted that clinical improvement following long-term chemotherapy in these conditions is usually accompanied by a marked reduction in the numbers of *H. influenzae* in the sputum. Antibodies to *H. influenzae* are commonly found in the blood of cases of chronic bronchitis.

As already mentioned, the smooth capsulated *H. influenzae*, particularly type *b*, may be the primary pathogen in two clinical syndromes —pyogenic meningitis and acute laryngo-tracheitis. These infections occur most commonly in young children (meningitis, 0–3 years; laryngo-tracheitis, 2–5 years) and are usually accompanied by blood-stream invasion. The age distribution seems to be related to the absence of a bactericidal activity of the blood against *H. influenzae* in the age-range 2 months–3½ years (Fothergill & Wright, 1933). There is no association with epidemics of influenza.

Laboratory Diagnosis.—Cultivation from sputum is best carried out on heated (chocolate) blood agar or on Levinthal's or Fildes' medium. Rough strains are mostly resistant to penicillin, which may be incorporated in the medium to inhibit Gram-positive bacteria. In smears from the deposit of cerebrospinal fluid from a case of meningitis, small clumps of fine, pleomorphic, Gram-negative bacilli can be seen; blood culture is usually positive. The iridescent colonies of these capsulated strains are best demonstrated on translucent media. The type may be identified by slide-agglutination with the specific antisera.

Chemotherapy.—Although smooth strains of *H. influenzae* are sensitive to penicillin as well as to streptomycin and the tetracylines, the drugs of choice for the treatment of *H. influenzae* meningitis are chloramphenicol and a sulphonamide in combination, since both drugs, given orally, diffuse readily into the cerebrospinal fluid. Good results have been reported from the use of small maintenance doses of the tetracyclines in the control of acute episodes of respiratory infection in patients with chronic bronchitis.

Haemophilus aegyptius

(*Koch-Weeks Bacillus*)

Associated with an acute and often infectious form of conjunctivitis.

Morphology and Staining.—Short, slender, Gram-negative rods about 1–1·5 μ in length and similar to *H. influenzae*; intracellular position in polymorph leucocytes of the inflammatory exudate is characteristic.

Cultural Characters.—Does not grow on ordinary media but like *H. influenzae* can be cultivated on media containing blood; in its growth requirements and general cultural characters it is very similar to the influenza bacillus.

Haemophilus ducreyi

(*Bacillus of Ducrey*)

Associated with Chancroid or Soft Sore.

Morphology and Staining.—A Gram-negative, rod-shaped organism 1·5 μ by 0·4 μ; occurs in pairs and chains; present in the exudate from the sore, in the tissue lesion and in the secondary buboes; it is non-motile and non-sporing.

Cultural Characters.—This organism has proved difficult to cultivate artificially, and appears to be a strict parasite. It requires the X growth factor of blood, but not the V factor. Primary cultures can be obtained from the sore by inoculating directly tubes containing coagulated rabbit blood. These are prepared by distributing fresh rabbit blood, withdrawn from an ear vein or by cardiac puncture, in amounts of 1–2 ml. in small test-tubes. The tubes are sloped and, when the blood has clotted, are heated at 55° C. for five minutes. The inoculum is introduced into the serum which has separated from the clot. After growth in these, the organism can be isolated on blood-agar plates. This method has been used for diagnostic purposes.

Ducrey's bacillus has also been cultivated directly by inoculating the surface of agar containing 20–30 per cent. of defibrinated rabbit blood sloped in wide tubes with a large surface exposed to air, the cultures being incubated at 35° C.

Pure cultures can be obtained by puncturing a bubo with a syringe, drawing up some of the pus, and with this, inoculating tubes of coagulated blood or blood agar.

Strains are all agglutinated by a specific antiserum.

An allergic skin reaction, produced by the intracutaneous injection of killed culture, has been utilised for diagnosis and has been regarded as specific.

Moraxella lacunata

(*Morax-Axenfeld bacillus*)

Associated with subacute or chronic conjunctivitis: believed by some workers to be a secondary bacterial pathogen following a primary virus infection.

Morphology and Staining.—Gram-negative, rod-shaped organism measuring about 2 μ by 1 μ, in pairs end to end; non-motile.

Cultural Characters.—Aerobe; requires blood or serum for growth; optimum temperature is about 37° C., and no growth occurs at room temperature; on coagulated serum, *e.g.* Loeffler's serum, growth produces liquefaction, and colonies develop "pits" or "lacunae" on the surface of the medium.

Moraxella liquefaciens is morphologically similar to the bacillus of Morax, but grows well on ordinary nutrient media at 20°–30° C. It liquefies coagulated serum, but, unlike the other, grows in gelatin at 22° C. and liquefies it. It is associated with conjunctivitis in which there may be primary involvement of the cornea.

Other organisms found in conjunctivitis are: the gonococcus, pneumococcus, meningococcus, staphylococci, streptococci and *Ps. pyocyanea* which may cause a very severe infection. *Staphylococcus albus* and diphtheroid bacilli, e.g. *C. xerosis* (*q.v.*), are frequent normal inhabitants of the conjunctival sac.

BORDETELLA

The principal pathogen in this genus, the whooping-cough bacillus, has until recently been included in the genus *Haemophilus*, because it required blood for its primary isolation. However, this organism is closely related antigenically to two other bacterial species, *parapertussis* and *bronchiseptica*, which are less fastidious in their growth requirements and should not be called *haemophilic.* A separate name for this genus seemed to be justified and *Bordetella* has been adopted, in recognition of Bordet, who first described the whooping-cough bacillus.

Bordetella pertussis

This is the causative organism of whooping-cough, one of the commonest childhood specific fevers, affecting the respiratory tract and characterised by spasmodic coughing often followed by a forced inspiration, or whoop, at the end of the paroxysm.

Morphology and Staining.—A small, oval, Gram-negative coccobacillus, more uniform in size and shape than *H. influenzae*; definite bacillary forms occur and become more numerous in rough cultures; non-motile; non-sporing; capsules are demonstrable in young cultures. In culture films, the organisms tend to form loose clumps with clearer spaces between, giving a "thumb-print" distribution.

Cultural Characters: Aerobe. It is usually first cultivated on media containing a large proportion of fresh blood; in subculture, however, growth may be obtained on media containing serum but without blood corpuscles or haemoglobin, and it is independent of the X and V factors required by the influenza bacillus. Catalase and a substance, *e.g.* albumin or charcoal, which will absorb toxic products (possibly unsaturated fatty acids) are essential for growth. For primary culture the special medium of Bordet and Gengou or a modification of this should be employed. On this medium, growth occurs slowly (two or three days) as small raised discrete colonies which are highly refractile to light, resembling a bisected pearl or a mercury drop. The colonies are cohesive and may be picked off entire. Stroke subcultures have been likened to "streaks of aluminium paint".

Semi-synthetic liquid media for large-scale growth for vaccines have been described (Cohen & Wheeler, 1946).

Viability.—Bord. pertussis differs from the influenza bacillus in its continued viability at low temperatures (0°–10° C.). It is killed by heat at 55° C. for half an hour. It is sensitive to the tetracylines and chloramphenicol and relatively resistant to penicillin.

The organism has no fermentative properties.

Antigenic Characters.— Recently isolated strains appear to be related in antigenic characters and react with the same agglutinating and complement-fixing antisera. Agglutination with absorbed, single factor sera distinguishes three types of strains, type 1, 2, type 1, 2, 3, and type 1, 3, according to their content of antigens 1, 2 and 3.

A number of distinguishable antigenic fractions have been isolated from *Bord. pertussis*, *e.g.* agglutinogen, haemagglutinin, protective antigen and toxin. This last component is only liberated after bacterial disruption, *e.g.* by freezing and thawing or ultrasonic disintegration.

Animal Pathogenicity.—Intranasal inoculation of *Bord. pertussis* cultures in mice anaesthetised with ether produces an interstitial pneumonia which may be fatal. Mice are also highly susceptible to intracerebral injection of virulent strains. A condition similar to clinical whooping-cough has been produced in monkeys by introduction of cultures into the respiratory tract.

Pathogenesis.—Whooping-cough is predominantly an infection of the respiratory mucosa, running a protracted course of four to eight weeks after an incubation period of 7–14 days: convulsions, bronchopneumonia, lung-collapse and bronchiectasis are possible complications. The organisms can be demonstrated on the epithelial surfaces in the bronchioles and presumably this surface infection is responsible for the paroxysmal coughing and the bronchial spasm that are outstanding features of the disease. The organisms are expelled in droplets during coughing or in scanty viscid sputum, and are most readily demonstrable in the first two or three weeks of infection. Lymphocytosis (total white blood cells: 15,000–30,000 and a relative lymphocytosis of 70–80 per cent.) is a characteristic feature of this disease.

Epidemiology.—Whooping-cough affects some 70 per cent. of children in unvaccinated urban communities. It is more common and more severe in females than in males. It is an infection of early childhood since there seems to be little or no passive protection by antibodies from the mother. The early infections are the most severe, so that in Britain nearly all the deaths from whooping-cough occur in the first year of life. Infection is most commonly spread by direct droplet spray and requires close contact ; the attack rate among susceptible children exposed at home is 80–90 per cent. Regularly recurring cycles of epidemic prevalence occur at two-yearly or longer intervals.

Laboratory Diagnosis

For detecting and isolating the organism the "cough-plate" method may be used: a plate of the Bordet-Gengou medium is held about 4 in.

in front of the mouth of the patient while coughing; the plate is thus inoculated directly with the expelled droplets. After three days' incubation the "pearly" colonies of *Bord. pertussis* can frequently be recognised without difficulty, and identified by microscopic, cultural and serological methods.

While the cough-plate method has proved of practical value n the recognition of early cases of pertussis, it is more applicable in hospital cases than in general medical practice. A specimen for bacteriological diagnosis can be obtained more conveniently by using a pernasal swab. For this purpose, a fine pledget of cotton wool is mounted on a long flexible wire and the swab is passed into the post-nasal space through the nose. Alternatively, an ordinary throat swab bent at the end is passed through the mouth and behind the soft palate so as to collect secretion from the nasopharynx. A plate of the Bordet-Gengou medium is inoculated by smearing a section of the plate directly with the swab and then distributing the inoculum from this area on the remainder of the surface with an inoculating wire. To prevent overgrowth of the plate by other organisms and to render colonies of *Bord. pertussis* more easily detectable, penicillin solution is added to the plate and spread evenly over the surface (6 units per 12 ml. of medium in a 4-in. plate). Pernasal swabs usually give more profuse and less contaminated cultures than swabs passed through the mouth.

A total and differential white cell count can give useful confirmatory evidence of infection.

Serology.—Both agglutination and complement-fixation tests have been applied. Such reactions are more likely to be positive from the third week onwards when the organisms are less easily isolated, and may be useful in confirming the diagnosis in atypical cases. Fresh living suspensions of the organism should be used for the agglutination reaction which is a more sensitive diagnostic test than the complement-fixation reaction (Evans & Maitland, 1939).

Chemotherapy.—The tetracyclines and chloramphenicol have been used in the treatment of pertussis and, though *in vitro* the specific organism is sensitive to these antibiotics, clinical response (reduction in number and severity of paroxysms) is largely limited to cases treated in the early stages of infection.

Prophylaxis.—Although whooping-cough vaccines have been used for many years, it is only recently that carefully controlled trials (Report, 1959) have shown that certain pertussis vaccines can give a high degree of protection against whooping-cough. Vaccines, made from strains of *Bord. pertussis* in the smooth phase, grown on defined media and killed by merthiolate or formalin-merthiolate, are given in three doses (each of 2×10^{10} M. organisms) at monthly intervals. Because of the severity of whooping-cough in infancy, it is recommended that vaccination be carried out between two and six months of age. With a good vaccine, the attack rate in home exposures may be less than 10 per cent. compared with 80–90 per cent. in the unvaccinated. Protection may be expected to last for at least two to three years. When whooping-cough occurs in a vaccinated child, the attack is usually milder and of shorter duration than in unprotected children (see Chap. 43).

Bordetella parapertussis

This organism is related antigenically to *Bord. pertussis* but produces a milder form of whooping-cough which is apparently not common in this country. It differs from *Bord. pertussis* in its more rapid growth so that the "pearly" colonies are well developed after two days' incubation on Bordet-Gengou medium. The underlying medium becomes greeny-black due to the production of a brown pigment. It actively produces catalase and on subculture grows readily on ordinary culture media. *Bord. parapertussis* can be specifically identified by agglutination with an absorbed antiserum.

Bordetella bronchiseptica

This organism was originally described in canine distemper and has been considered to have relationships to the *Brucella* group. It is, however, related in its antigenic characters and its toxin to *Bord. pertussis*, but differs from this organism in its motility and in possessing peritrichous flagella. It can grow on ordinary media without blood. In canine distemper it represents a secondary infection, but is frequently responsible for a bronchopneumonic condition in rodents; it may be found in snuffles of rabbits.

REFERENCES

Cohen, S. M. & Wheeler, W. M. (1946). Pertussis vaccine prepared with phase I cultures grown in fluid medium. *Amer. J. publ. Hlth*, **36**, 371.

Evans, D. G. & Maitland, H. B. (1939). Agglutination as diagnostic test for whooping cough. *J. Path. Bact.*, **48**, 468.

Fothergill, L. D. & Wright, J. (1933). Influenzal meningitis; relation of age incidence to bactericidal power of blood against causal organism. *J. Immunol.*, **24**, 273.

Report (1959). Vaccination against whooping-cough. *Brit. med. J.*, **1**, 994.

CHAPTER 16

SALMONELLA

THE family Enterobacteriaceae is composed of numerous inter-related bacteria all of which are Gram-negative rods, either motile with peritrichous flagella or non-motile. They are non-sporing and grow on ordinary media; all ferment glucose rapidly with or without gas production and reduce nitrates to nitrites. Many species are intestinal pathogens or commensals, whilst a few are saprophytic and found in soil and water.

A classification of the Enterobacteriaceae is essential for diagnostic and epidemiologic purposes, and several groups or genera are recognised within the family. Each genus is made up of biochemically similar strains which are antigenically related; it must be noted, however, that the biochemical interrelationships of the family do not allow all strains to be assigned to one or another genus, and intermediate strains are frequently encountered. With this proviso, and recognising that there are intergeneric relationships among typical strains of the several genera, the family can be divided into the following groups: *Salmonella*, *Arizona*, *Shigella*, *Escherichia*, *Citrobacter*, *Klebsiella*, *Cloaca*, *Hafnia*, *Proteus* and *Providencia*. In the present chapter, only *Salmonella* and *Arizona* species will be considered.

THE GENUS SALMONELLA

About 1000 serotypes are included in this genus; *Salmonella typhi* or the typhoid bacillus was the first member to be described and is the causative organism of typhoid fever. The improvements in environmental sanitation and a better knowledge of the epidemiology of the disease led to dramatic reduction in morbidity; this has been followed more recently by a marked reduction in fatality rates effected by chloramphenicol therapy.

Paratyphoid fever is clinically similar to typhoid fever and in Britain is caused almost exclusively by *Salmonella paratyphi B* (the paratyphoid B bacillus); the other aetiologic agents of paratyphoid fever are *Salmonella paratyphi A* and *Salmonella paratyphi C*, but these are rarely encountered in this country. The term "enteric fever" includes typhoid and the paratyphoid fevers; in addition to their clinical similarity, the gross pathology is the same irrespective of the infecting organism and the distinction depends on bacteriological investigation.

SALMONELLA TYPHI

(S. typhosa)

Morphology and Staining.—A Gram-negative, non-sporing bacillus, about 2–4 μ by 0·5 μ, actively motile with numerous long peritrichous flagella; does not possess a capsule. Most strains are fimbriate.

Cultural Characters.—Aerobe and facultative anaerobe; temperature range, 15°–41° C., optimum, 37° C. Grows well on ordinary media.

Colonies on Agar—moderately large, thick, greyish-white, moist, circular disks, dome-shaped and smooth; the opacity and size vary with different strains. Stock laboratory cultures may show a mixture of these smooth colonies with rough colonies which in the extreme are irregular, dull, effuse and dry.

Colonies on MacConkey's Medium.—Similar to above and "pale" or colourless, since *S. typhi* does not ferment lactose.

Desoxycholate-citrate Medium.—Colonies also "pale" or colourless.

Viability.—The thermal death-point is about 56° C. The majority of individual bacilli die within a few hours when subjected to drying. In water the bacilli gradually die, but may survive for some time; thus, in sewage-polluted sea- and fresh-water, viable bacilli have been found after four weeks. In soil, survival may occasionally occur for six weeks or longer; in culture, the organism survives for long periods, *e.g.* several months. Although *S. typhi* is sensitive to several antibiotics *in vitro*, chloramphenicol is the only satisfactory drug in therapy.

Biochemical Reactions.—Glucose and mannitol are fermented without gas production; lactose and sucrose are not fermented, nor is indole produced. By extending biochemical testing to other substrates (particularly organic acids) it is possible to differentiate *S. typhi* from the paratyphoid bacilli ; biochemical subtypes of *S. typhi* can be recognised using arabinose and xylose as substrates and such subtypes are epidemiologically significant, *e.g.* strains usually ferment xylose promptly, but some split xylose late or not at all; similarly arabinose is rarely fermented and then only late.

Antigenic Characters.—The serum of animals immunised with *S. typhi* contains agglutinating antibodies which are specific for the characteristic antigens, somatic (O) and flagellar (H), of the organism, and agglutination reactions are therefore employed in the identification of this species; these are more conveniently considered in relation to other Salmonella types.

Vi Antigen and Agglutinin.—Freshly isolated strains of *S. typhi* possess a somatic antigen designated "Vi", occurring as a surface antigen; such strains are more virulent for mice than strains lacking the Vi antigen. The Vi antigen renders the organism relatively inagglutinable by an O antiserum, and serological identification with the latter must be made with a fresh saline suspension of *S. typhi* which has been boiled for one hour and washed by centrifugation. In addition, an unheated suspension should be tested with Vi agglutinating antiserum, which is obtained by immunising animals with an alcohol-acetone treated saline suspension of *S. typhi* known to contain the Vi antigen; after harvesting the serum, H and O agglutinins are absorbed from it with a strain possessing H and O antigens but devoid of the Vi component. Alternatively, an unabsorbed serum made from a Vi-containing Ballerup culture may be used.

Conversely, for the detection of Vi agglutinin in serum (*e.g.* in a carrier of *S. typhi*), a Vi-containing suspension of *S. typhi* must be employed.[1] The diagnostic application of the Vi Widal reaction is dealt with on p. 229.

Animal Pathogenicity.—In common with other members of the genus, *S. typhi* is primarily an intestinal parasite. It shows a strong host specificity for man; *S. typhi* does not appear to infect animals under natural conditions, and ordinary laboratory animals, *e.g.* rabbit, rat, mouse and guinea-pig, when dosed orally with *S. typhi* do not suffer any harmful result unless massive doses are employed, and even then the illness is quite unlike that of typhoid fever. When adequate doses are administered to mice by the intraperitoneal or intravenous route, death results, but this is probably toxaemic; with non-lethal doses the disease in mice shows little or no tendency to spread by contact from mouse to mouse in distinction to the epizootic spread following the introduction of *Salmonella typhimurium.*

Pathogenesis.—Infection is by ingestion; from the small intestine the organisms pass via the lymphatics to the mesenteric glands, whence after a period of multiplication they invade the blood stream via the thoracic duct; the liver, gall-bladder, spleen, kidney and bone-marrow become infected during this bacteriaemic phase in the first seven to ten days of the disease. From the gall-bladder a further invasion of the intestine results, and lymphoid tissue—Peyer's patches and lymphoid follicles—are particularly involved in an acute inflammatory reaction and infiltration with mononuclear cells, followed by necrosis, sloughing and the formation of characteristic typhoid ulcers. Haemorrhage of varying degree may occur and, less frequently, perforation through a necrotic Peyer's patch may complicate the illness.

S. typhi is present in large numbers in the inflamed tissue in the ulcers and is found in the intestinal contents and the dejecta; it may localise in the kidney and appear in the urine, sometimes producing a marked bacilluria. The bacillus is found in other lesions occurring as complications or sequelae of typhoid fever—*e.g.* acute suppurative periosteitis and osteitis, abscess of the kidney, acute cholecystitis, bronchopneumonia, empyema, ulcerative endocarditis.

In 2–5 per cent. of convalescents, the typhoid bacillus persists in the body, sometimes for an indefinite period. In such chronic carriers, the bacilli are most commonly present in the gall-bladder or rarely in the urinary tract and are excreted in the faeces or urine.

Epidemiology.—The sources of infection are patients suffering from the disease, including the mild and ambulatory forms, and carriers. Typhoid fever is predominantly a water-borne infection and so, in communities where adequate treatment of water supplies is undertaken and where a water-carriage system of sewage disposal is operating, the recognised case of typhoid fever is unlikely to act as a focus of epidemic spread since he should be admitted to hospital and nursed with aseptic precautions.

[1] Such a suspension and other diagnostic suspensions and antisera are obtainable from The Standards Laboratory for Serological Reagents, Central Public Health Laboratory, Colindale, London, N.W.9.

Carriers of *S. typhi* are a more likely source of infection in a community with well developed environmental services. Bacilli present on the hands of the carrier can be transferred to many vehicles; a carrier engaged in dairy work may contaminate milk, which can serve as culture medium and a likely mode of spread (Bradley, 1943) but there is no evidence that *S. typhi* causes bovine infection. Similarly carriers engaged in food-handling either in preparation or distribution of foodstuffs have been incriminated as sources in epidemic outbreaks. Shell-fish harvested from sewage-polluted sea-water, and vegetables, salads and water-cress contaminated with human excreta have all been noted as vehicles of infection.

In materially less favoured countries the absence of community services results in low sanitary standards and greater opportunities for epidemic spread in water supplies or foods contaminated by cases and carriers; in these circumstances also, flies may transmit the bacilli from excreta to foodstuffs.

Bacteriophage Typing of S. typhi.—For epidemiological purposes a method has been elaborated of differentiating Vi strains into types by means of an anti-Vi phage which, on serial cultivation with one of these types, acquires an increased activity to strains of this type. Thus, type-specific phages can be obtained which, in certain dilutions, act selectively. According to their sensitivity to particular phages and groups of phages, 80 different phage-types are recognised. In this way, freshly isolated strains possessing Vi antigen can be classified and the method has proved valuable in epidemiologic studies of typhoid fever, *e.g.* in correlating cases and in tracing the source of an outbreak and the mode of spread. The technique of phage-typing defies summary treatment and reference should be made to published work (Anderson & Williams, 1956).

Vi-phage typing is carried out by the Director of the International Reference Laboratory for Enteric Phage Typing, Central Public Health Laboratory, Colindale, London, to whom cultures should be sent.

SALMONELLA PARATYPHI A (S. paratyphi)
SALMONELLA PARATYPHI B (S. schottmülleri)
SALMONELLA PARATYPHI C (S. hirschfeldii)

These are the causal organisms of paratyphoid fever which is essentially similar to typhoid fever but clinically is milder and of shorter duration. In their morphology and general cultural characters the paratyphoid bacilli are identical with *S. typhi*, but they can be differentiated from the latter by their ability to produce gas in fermentation reactions, and the following table exemplifies this feature and also the differentiation of the paratyphoid bacilli one from the other.

However, as with all members of the genus *Salmonella*, the ultimate identification of type depends on serological examination.

Antigenic Characters.—These bacilli possess different antigens and agglutinating antisera for known strains are used for the identification of the respective types. This is dealt with on pp. 227-28.

	Glucose	Mannitol	Xylose	*d*-tartrate	Mucate
S. typhi	⊥	⊥	V	⊥	V
S. paratyphi A	+	+	–	–	–
„ *B*	+	+	+	–	+
„ *C*	+	+	+	+	–

Keys: ⊥ = acid, no gas; + = acid and gas; V = variable reaction; – = no reaction.

Pathogenesis.—The mode of infection and the distribution of the paratyphoid bacilli in the body of an infected person or carrier are the same as in the case of *S. typhi*.

Epidemiology.—The sources of paratyphoid infections are human cases and carriers, but there is evidence that, in comparison with *S. typhi*, many more paratyphoid bacilli require to be ingested before infection results. Hence water-borne spread of paratyphoid fever is rare and most episodes result from the ingestion of foodstuffs with peak incidence in the summer months like the salmonella food-poisoning infections (Savage, 1956).

Bacteriophage Typing of S. paratyphi B.—Phage-typing of this organism is used for epidemiologic purposes. More than 40 distinct types, subtypes and variations can be recognised. Cultures for phage typing should be sent to the Enteric Reference Laboratory, Colindale.

Laboratory Diagnosis

The bacteriologic diagnosis depends on (1) the isolation from the body, and the identification, of the causative organism, or (2) the demonstration of its presence in the body by the Widal agglutination reaction which is based on the occurrence of specific agglutinins to the organism in the serum of the infected person.

Blood Culture.—In the early stages of the illness, blood culture is the most conclusive diagnostic method, and should be employed in all suspected cases during the first seven to ten days, and in relapses (where a bacteriological diagnosis has not previously been established). The use of blood culture bottles containing bile-salts (0·5 per cent. sodium taurocholate) is recommended; the technique of inoculation and laboratory procedure is referred to in Chapter 48. Another method of isolating the bacilli from the blood stream has been advocated (Thomas, Watson & Hewstone, 1954); blood obtained by venepuncture is distributed in 5 ml. quantities to Universal containers and allowed to clot when the separated serum is aseptically removed. To each bottle is added 15 ml. of 0·5 per cent. bile-salt broth containing 100 units per ml. of streptokinase; the latter causes rapid lysis of the clot with release of any organisms present. Incubation and further examination is performed as for blood culture.

The probability of demonstrating the causative organism in the blood lessens as the disease progresses. If the result is positive, the strain is isolated in pure culture, and identified by morphological, cultural and biochemical characters and by testing it with agglutinating antisera (O and H).

Faeces.—S. typhi and the paratyphoid bacilli can be isolated from the faeces throughout the illness, but are most frequent during the second and third weeks. Repeated examination of the faeces may be required before isolation is successful.

If there is likely to be a delay of some hours before specimens of faeces for culture reach the laboratory, 2 volumes of 30 per cent. neutral glycerol in buffered 0·6 per cent. sodium chloride solution should be added to 1 volume of the faeces and thoroughly mixed with it. This prevents other intestinal organisms from overgrowing the salmonella bacilli. The glycerol solution is apt to become acid on storage and is then unsuitable for use; as a safeguard the solution may be tinted with phenol red, and if there is a change to yellow the fluid should be discarded.

Direct Plating of Faeces.—A medium is required which will differentiate colonies of typhoid-paratyphoid bacilli from those of the normal bowel flora; in the past, MacConkey's bile-salt neutral red lactose agar has been extensively used for this purpose, but more recently has been superseded by other selective media which are inhibitory to the normal flora, *e.g.* deoxycholate-citrate agar (DCA), which, like MacConkey's medium, also contains lactose and neutral red. On both of these media salmonella colonies are "pale" as compared with the pink colonies of most of the commensal bowel organisms. Pale colonies from DCA should be subcultured by plating out on MacConkey's medium to prove their freedom from contamination with inhibited lactose-fermenting *E. coli* bacteria, before further tests are done.

It is essential that the surface of such media should be sufficiently dry before inoculation, otherwise a confluent growth may result instead of separate colonies.

After 18–24 hours' incubation the colonies are usually sufficiently large for subinoculating those that are considered likely to be salmonellae. The plates may also be incubated for longer periods if no suspicious colonies are noted after 24 hours. The colonies of *S. typhi* and the paratyphoid bacilli present a pale or colourless appearance, but other intestinal organisms may produce not dissimilar colonies; several colonies are therefore subcultured on agar slopes, using a straight wire for transfer from the diagnostic plate. The pure cultures isolated are tested and identified as indicated under blood culture (*vide supra*).

Wilson and Blair's bismuth-sulphite medium may also be used with advantage for direct plating and should always be employed in the attempted isolation of *S. typhi*, since it is the most reliable medium so far devised for this purpose. It is recommended that the inoculum be distributed over two plates of this medium; furthermore, it is advisable to incubate for 48 hours before discarding, since, although *S. typhi* will usually appear within 24 hours, *S. paratyphi B* frequently requires the longer incubation period before colonies are recognisable.

Enrichment Methods.—These have proved invaluable for isolating salmonellae when present in small numbers in faeces, as in convalescent cases, or in the detection of carriers. Fluid media are used, incorporating substances which inhibit the commensal flora, while allowing the pathogenic bacilli to flourish. Tetrathionate broth and selenite F broth are widely used; these are liberally inoculated with faecal suspension at the same time as direct plating and are subcultured to DCA medium after incubation for 12–18 hours. In this way an enriched culture of enteric fever bacilli is obtained and sometimes an almost pure growth.

In the examination of faeces from cases of enteric fever the best results are obtained by employing two or three different methods simultaneously. This gives a higher percentage of positive results than when one method only is used. Thus it is recommended that routine inoculation of DCA and Wilson and Blair plates and of both enrichment media should be undertaken in the attempted isolation of enteric fever bacilli.

Urine.—The bacilli may also be isolated from urine. The specimen is centrifuged, several loopfuls of the deposit being used to inoculate the recommended media. In enteric fever there appear to be transient bacilluric periods, and daily examinations for a week of the morning urine are of particular value where the isolation of the causative organism is aimed at and where other methods have been unsuccessful. In carrier detection and in determining the site of carriage, it should be remembered that even small quantities of the urine from a urinary carrier mixing with his stool may lead to the patient being regarded as both a urinary and faecal carrier; care in collecting specimens will eliminate such errors.

Bile.—By means of a duodenal tube, bile may be aspirated and cultured in an attempt to isolate the bacilli. This technique is of value in the later stages of the illness and in carrier detection.

Widal Reaction.—The reaction becomes definitely manifest usually about the 7th to 10th day. Occasionally it is earlier in development (*e.g.* 5th day), but may be delayed. A negative result at an early stage of the illness therefore may be inconclusive. It is customary to test the patient's serum against standard H and O suspensions (in parallel) of each enteric fever organism likely to be encountered—*e.g.* in Britain, *S. typhi* and *S. paratyphi B*. As a rule, both O and H agglutinins are developed, but in some cases only one of these agglutinins is detected, particularly in the early stages of the illness.

The Widal reaction, tested quantitatively, is also progressive up to a certain point, *i.e.* the titre of the reaction rises from the time of the first appearance of agglutinins in the serum and reaches its maximum about the end of the third week. A "rising titre", on repeated testing, is therefore highly significant.

For determining the type of infection, H agglutination is more reliable than the O reaction, since the enteric organisms have some O antigenic components in common (table, p. 234); thus in a typhoid infection, O agglutination may sometimes be pronounced with the test suspension of *S. paratyphi B* as well as that of *S. typhi* (O antigen 12), while in a paratyphoid B infection, marked O agglutination may also occur with both test suspensions. However, the presence of O agglutinins usually reflects *recent* infection and both H and O agglutinins should be tested for routinely.

In interpreting the result of a Widal test, certain additional facts must be kept in mind:

(1) Normal serum may agglutinate the test suspensions in low dilutions, and no diagnostic significance can be attached to such reactions. In Britain, the usual limits of such normal agglutination of Standard Suspensions[1] are *S. typhi* and *S. paratyphi B*, H 1 in 30, 0, 1 in 50, and *S. paratyphi A*, O and H, 1 in 10. The level of "normal agglutinins" to these organisms varies in degree in different communities and different countries. If agglutination occurs only in low dilutions within the possible range of normal agglutination, the test should be repeated as later results may show higher titres and are therefore more conclusive.

In this regard, it should be noted that, where clot culture is practised for isolation of enteric bacilli early in the disease, the serum withdrawn from the specimen can be used for Widal testing and the results used as a base-line against which tests with subsequent specimens can be assessed.

(2) Non-specific antigens, such as fimbrial antigens, may be present in test suspensions and react with an agglutinin in human sera. This may cause a fallacy in the Widal test unless the suspensions employed are known to be free from such antigens (p. 247).

(3) Persons inoculated with typhoid-paratyphoid vaccine (TAB) also show specific agglutinins in their sera, and this may complicate the interpretation of the Widal reaction in such persons. In previously vaccinated cases a definitely rising titre for any one of the organisms has been regarded as significant from the diagnostic viewpoint; however, non-specific factors, such as a non-enteric febrile condition, may cause an increase of agglutinins already present as a result of vaccination, and enteric infection by one organism may lead to an increased agglutination titre for the others (anamnestic reactions).

It has been claimed that in such persons, several months after vaccination, the agglutinins are mainly of the H type, whereas in infected subjects both O and H agglutinins can be demonstrated. Thus, in the application of the Widal reaction in vaccinated persons, the results may be of doubtful significance, but if over six months have passed since the date of vaccination and if the O agglutination titre is

[1] Standard Suspensions and Diagnostic Antisera are obtainable from The Standards Laboratory for Serological Reagents, Central Public Health Laboratory, Colindale, London. The provision of such reagents ensures that results are comparable among laboratories using them.

higher than 1 in 100 and rises on repeated testing, such a result may be considered significant.

The bacteriologist should be informed of the clinical history and any TAB vaccinations; with this liaison, the physician can in turn receive an evaluation of the Widal result rather than a formal statement of reaction titres.

Diagnosis of Enteric Carriers

The proof that a person is a carrier depends on the isolation of *S. typhi* or one of the paratyphoid bacilli from the faeces or urine, and in view of the intermittency of excretion at least 6 consecutive examinations of such specimens should be made before the result is declared negative. The methods employed are as described above; since the bacilli are likely to be most numerous in the bile and in the contents of the small intestine, examination of aspirated bile is valuable or alternatively the subject should be given 3 grains of calomel followed by a saline purgative, and after catharsis the second, or preferably the third stool is examined.

In a considerable proportion of carriers, the Widal reaction is positive, and the test is of some value as a preliminary screening procedure provided that the subject's experience of TAB vaccination is known. A negative Widal reaction does not, of course, exclude the carrier state. If the subject's serum is tested with a Vi-containing strain of *S. typhi*, the presence of Vi agglutinin can be detected and a positive test has considerable value in recognising carriers of *S. typhi*. Thus in suspected typhoid carriers a titre of 1 in 10 is regarded as significant; however, individuals to whom TAB vaccine has been given may possess Vi agglutinins.

Chemotherapy.—In spite of contrary evidence from animal experiment, none of the sulphonamides is of value in treating cases of enteric fever nor in the sterilisation of chronic carriers. Chloramphenicol, in adequate doses, leads to rapid clinical cure, but has also resulted in an increase in the relapse-rate on discontinuing therapy; second attacks of enteric fever have also been reported.

Prophylaxis.—*S. typhi* and the paratyphoid bacilli are never parasitic on hosts other than man; therefore preventive measures against the spread of enteric fever are more readily undertaken and attended with greater success than in diseases in which host specificity is less strict.

General preventive measures include the following:

(1) The institution and maintenance of safe water supplies and water-borne sewage disposal systems.

(2) The supervision of personnel engaged in water-works, dairy-farms and in the food industry; and their instruction in the elementary epidemiology of enteric infections and in good standards of personal hygiene. Many Health Authorities insist on "screening" tests for chronic enteric carriers among water-works employees. Such tests might be extended to certain categories of food-handlers.

(3) Protection of foodstuffs from flies and the storage of food in refrigerators.

(4) Bacteriologic control of imported foods, *e.g.* eggs, desiccated coconut and tinned meats.

Specific preventive measures:

(1) Adequate nursing of cases and the maintenance of an Enteric Register for each community, in which is listed all known chronic carriers; the phage-type of *S. typhi* or *S. paratyphi B* which carriers are excreting should be noted in the Register, since this information may be invaluable in the investigation of future outbreaks.

(2) The control of known carriers in relation to their employment; carriers may be cured by surgical measures, *e.g.* cholecystectomy, or by antibiotic therapy, *e.g.* massive dosage of ampicillin (Christie, 1964; Whitby, 1964).

(3) The administration of TAB vaccine to individuals at special risk, *e.g.* (*a*) troops and other persons travelling into or residing in areas where the standard of sanitation is low or where enteric fevers are common; (*b*) laboratory workers handling specimens or live suspensions; (*c*) individuals residing with known chronic carriers.

TAB vaccine is prepared from selected smooth cultures of *S. typhi*, *S. paratyphi A* and *B* according to the method described in Chapter 46. The vaccine is usually sterilised at 60° C. (thirty minutes) and 0·5 per cent. phenol added as a preservative; it is standardised to contain 1000 million *S. typhi* and 750 million each of *S. paratyphi A* and *B* per ml. The first immunising dose of 0·5 ml. is followed not less than ten days later by a second dose of 1 ml., both administered subcutaneously; for those continually at risk, a booster dose (0·5 ml. or 0·2 ml. intracutaneously) should be given biennially. *S. paratyphi C* may be incorporated in the vaccine (750 million bacilli per ml.) which is then designated "TABC".

The prophylactic value of TAB vaccination was regarded as well established although the vital field trials had not been undertaken. It had been assumed from experimental studies on mice that the full immunising potency of typhoid vaccine depends on the use of virulent strains containing adequate O and Vi antigen, but sterilisation by heat and preservation with phenol tend to destroy the Vi antigen. To preserve this antigen Felix and his team advocated a less severe treatment for the vaccine cultures by killing with 75 per cent. alcohol and preservation with 25 per cent. alcohol; this alcoholised vaccine stimulates the formation of Vi antibody in a substantial proportion of vaccinated subjects.

The comparative efficacy of the two types of vaccine has recently been the subject of strictly controlled field trials in Yugoslavia under the auspices of the World Health Organisation. The results indicate that phenolised typhoid vaccine is superior to the alcoholised vaccine, since it gave a 70 per cent. protection rate; the alcoholised preparation appeared to be little better than a control vaccine prepared against *Shigella flexneri*, which theoretically should have no protective value in typhoid fever. These trials, and also the use of an acetone-killed vaccine are considered in Chapter 43.

ORGANISMS OF BACTERIAL ENTERITIS OR FOOD POISONING

In addition to the enteric fever organisms, about 1000 salmonella serotypes have been recognised and these are associated with cases of food poisoning in which the illness takes the form of an acute gastro-enteritis. These serotypes are identical with the paratyphoid bacilli not only morphologically and in cultural characteristics but also in their general biochemical activities; extended biochemical tests, with a wide range of substrates, are of some value in differentiation, but only antigenic analysis with type-specific sera allows each member of the genus to be identified with certainty.

Pathogenesis.—Different types vary to some extent in their invasiveness. It should be noted that unlike the typhoid-paratyphoid bacilli, these Salmonella serotypes are frequently encountered enzootically in nature and also readily infect laboratory animals when intentionally administered.

In cases of salmonella food poisoning, the organisms multiply in, and are ordinarily confined to, the intestine but in some cases bacteraemia and septicaemia may occur. Cholecystitis may also result and meningitis has been recorded not infrequently as a result of infection; persons with sickle-cell anaemia appear to be more liable to salmonella infections of bone than individuals free of this condition (Hendrickse & Collard, 1960).

Epidemiology.—Unlike typhoid fever, in which human cases and carriers are the sole source of infection, salmonella food poisoning usually originates from animal sources. Domestic animals such as cows, sheep and pigs may be infected clinically or subclinically; in apparently healthy cattle a carrier rate of 1 per cent. has been found. Hobbs & Wilson (1959) have shown an increase in the carrier state as animals are moved from farm, through market to abattoir, and it is thought that the carrier state proceeds to frank infection and septicaemia during transit when the animal is deprived of food and water; similar findings have been made in sheep. The source of epizootic salmonella infection is variable, but feeding-stuffs have been incriminated (Report, 1959) and the maintenance of such infections enzootically is readily explained by the finding that *S. typhimurium* remains viable in water, pasture and faeces commonly for four weeks and sometimes as long as twenty-eight weeks.

After meat has been marketed, whether or not it is already infected with salmonellae, it can be contaminated at all stages of preparation before being consumed; in this regard it is reported that the frequency of salmonella isolations from sausages offered for retail is ten times greater than from the gut of the healthy animals from which the sausage meat was obtained (Report, 1959). The handling of contaminated meat along with clean produce may result in the latter becoming contaminated; if, on purchase, meat and meat products are free of salmonellae, they may still become contaminated in the final stages of preparation at home, in canteens, school-meal kitchens and the like, if any individual involved in cooking or serving the meal is excreting salmonellae either as a carrier or as an ambulant case of infection. Cooking is not always a safe means of destroying salmonellae in foodstuffs (Miller & Ramsden, 1955). The food rarely shows any obvious sign of bacterial contamination.

In addition to meat, cow's milk and milk products may be a source of infection; furthermore, epizootic salmonella infections in rats, mice and other rodents allow such animals to infect foodstuffs with their excreta. The use of *Salmonella enteritidis* as a rodent poison for eradication purposes carries the risk that this organism may sometimes be transmitted to man in this way.

Birds, particularly hens, ducks and turkeys, suffer from salmonella infection and their carcasses may be a source of infection to man; likewise duck and hen eggs may be the source, the egg being infected either during formation in the oviduct, as in the case of the duck, or by the organisms passing through the shell from cloacal discharges in the nesting-box. Contamination through the shell is most likely to occur immediately after laying whilst the egg is still warm and moist externally. During the cooling period bacteria may readily be sucked in through pores in the shell (Haines & Moran 1940).

Unless infected eggs are used for preparation of custards or other communally consumed products, infection is restricted to the individual consumer and such single case infections will rarely attract attention. The pooling of eggs, either as raw whole egg for the baking industry or as spray-dried powder for home use as well as for manufacturing concerns, allows contamination of otherwise clean material with a minority of infected eggs. Circumstantial evidence of the importance of such bulk material in promoting epidemic salmonella infections has occurred simultaneously with the appearance of serotypes which were rarely or never encountered prior to importation of such material; such a circumstance followed the introduction of dried egg powder from the U.S.A. during the early years of the last war and the extensive importation of frozen egg and dried egg albumin from China and other countries in more recent years.

The majority of epidemics investigated bacteriologically are caused by one of the following: *S. typhimurium*, *S. enteritidis*, *S. thompson*, *S. newport*, or *S. dublin*.

S. typhimurium alone accounts for more than 70 per cent. of these outbreaks, and phage-typing of strains has been useful in detecting the source of infection. The biochemical and antigenic similarity to *S. paratyphi B* emphasises the need for accurate serological identification in the genus.

S. enteritidis is the next most frequently encountered in food poisoning outbreaks. This serological entity can be subdivided into four biochemical types, and these types are epidemiologically significant. Similarly, three biochemical types can be recognised of the serotype *S. dublin*.

Laboratory Diagnosis

Faeces and other specimens are dealt with as in the diagnosis of enteric fevers. Blood culture rarely yields positive results and should be carried out only in cases where fever persists or recovery is delayed.

In convalescence, the serum of patients agglutinates the homologous organism, but the agglutination test is not applicable during the acute stage as the agglutinins take some days to make their appearance in the blood. The test may be applied retrospectively in convalescent cases in which either the diagnosis has been delayed or from which no salmonella has been isolated during the acute phase; thus, gaps in the chain of epidemiologic findings may be filled by such evidence.

The bacteriological examination of suspected food-stuffs, if available, should be carried out as in Chapter 55. It must be emphasised that in the investigation of food poisoning outbreaks, the bacteriologist is one of a team including clinician, epidemiologist and others; only by close co-operation will such investigations be carried to a successful conclusion.

Prophylaxis.—The various procedures are tabulated below, and for a detailed account of these reference should be made to a textbook of hygiene.

(1) Supervision of the health of animals on farms with the segregation and disposal of infected members of a herd.

(2) Adequate meat inspection at abattoirs.

(3) Maintenance of all premises in a clean state, combined with rodent-proofing and anti-fly measures.

(4) Adequate cooking and subsequent cold storage of food which is not consumed immediately after preparation.

(5) Supervision of the health of food-handlers and their education in methods of preventing contamination of foodstuffs.

Identification of Salmonella Serotypes

When a lactose non-fermenting bacillus presenting the general characters of the genus has been isolated, its precise identification may involve a considerable amount of detailed testing, and such work has tended to become highly specialised and beyond the scope of the smaller laboratories. The following description outlines the procedures adopted and their underlying principles. (See also Kauffmann, 1954.)

The presence or absence of motility of the strain under investigation is noted by inoculating a tube of semi-solid agar. A set of sugars is inoculated for fermentation reactions. Christensen's urea medium is also inoculated to exclude organisms of the genus Proteus. As a preliminary to testing the strain in an extended range of biochemical tests it is recommended that composite sugar media be employed (see Chapter 47). Other biochemical reactions which may be tested are the fermentation of xylose, arabinose, trehalose, inositol and rhamnose and the utilisation of *d*-tartrate, *l*-tartrate, *i*-tartrate, citrate and mucate.

Determination of O Group.—As will be seen from the table (p. 234), the identification of the O antigen provides a means of placing any member of the genus in one of a number of groups designated A–I. Inspection of the O-antigenic formulae exemplified in this table will show that all members of a particular group possess an O-antigen factor which is common throughout the group and not shared with other groups, *e.g.* Group A—O antigen 2, Group B—O antigen 4, etc. This is designated the determining antigen, and, correspondingly, diagnostic sera which have been absorbed to remove all antibodies except that for the group-specific antigen are designated as "Factor 2" serum, "Factor 4" serum, etc.

Some Representatives of the genus Salmonella
(Kauffmann-White Classification)

Group	Type	Somatic antigens	Flagellar antigens	
			Phase 1	Phase 2
A	*S. paratyphi A*	1, 2, 12	a	–
B	*S. paratyphi B*	1, 4, 5, 12	b	1, 2
	S. typhimurium	1, 4, 5, 12	i	1, 2
	S. stanley	4, 5, 12	d	1, 2
	S. heidelberg	1, 4, 5, 12	r	1, 2
	S. abortus-equi	4, 12	–	e, n, x
	S. abortus-ovis	4, 12	c	1, 6
C_1	*S. paratyphi C*	6, 7, Vi	c	1, 5
	S. cholerae-suis	6, 7	c	1, 5
	S. thompson	6, 7	k	1, 5
	S. bareilly	6, 7	y	1, 5
C_2	*S. newport*	6, 8	e, h	1, 2
	S. bovis-morbificans	6, 8	r	1, 5
D	*S. typhi*	9, 12, Vi	d	–
	S. dublin	1, 9, 12	g, p	–
	S. enteritidis	1, 9, 12	g, m	–
	S. gallinarum[1]	1, 9, 12	(non-flagellate)	
E_1	*S. anatum*	3, 10	e, h	1, 6
	S. meleagridis	3, 10	e, h	l, w
	S. london	3, 10	l, v	1, 6
E_4	*S. senftenberg*	1, 3, 19	g, s, t	–
F	*S. aberdeen*	11	i	1, 2
G	*S. poona*	13, 22	z	1, 6

[1] *S. pullorum* is serologically identical.

Confirmation that the organism is a member of the genus is obtained by slide agglutination tests with polyvalent O serum, and Vi serum. If agglutination occurs only in Vi serum, the culture should be heated in saline at 100° C. for one hour and centrifuged, and a fresh saline suspension of the heated deposit should be retested with polyvalent O serum. In either event, the culture suspension should now be tested with the absorbed "Factor" sera in one of which agglutination will be noted and further testing restricted to identifying the specific type within this particular O group. Cultures which are initially agglutinated by the Vi serum should be in group C if they are *S. paratyphi C* and in group D if they are *S. typhi*. On occasion, a rough culture of *S. typhi* is isolated which does not agglutinate with group D serum after heating and it is essential to determine biochemically whether a culture, which in the live state agglutinates in Vi serum but after heating is inagglutinable in group C, group D and Vi serum, is in fact a rough culture of *S. typhi*.

Determination of Type.—Before proceeding to type the organism by identifying its H-antigen structure, it is necessary to determine whether the culture (if diphasic) is in the specific or non-specific phase. An H-agglutinating serum prepared against the non-specific, monophasic variety of *S. cholerae-suis* is a convenient reagent for this purpose. If a formalised suspension of the unknown organism is agglutinated in large floccules to any extent by this serum, it is in the non-specific phase, and an effort must be made to secure a specific-phase subculture of it before further identification is attempted.

The Craigie tube is a convenient method for obtaining the specific form of a salmonella organism: 5 ml. amounts of nutrient agar (0·2 per cent. agar) are placed in stoppered $6 \times \frac{1}{2}$ in. test-tubes with a small inner tube open at both ends and with the upper end projecting well above the agar; the medium is sterilised, cooled to 50° C. and then 0·5 ml. of a 1 in 5 dilution of the non-specific phase serum (filtered to ensure sterility) is added to one tube (1 in 25) and 1 ml. of it to another tube (1 in 50). The medium is allowed to solidify in the upright position. The agar *inside* the inner tube is inoculated by the stab-method with non-specific, group-phase culture. The specific forms can then be separated by incubating and subculturing from the agar *outside* the inner tube. The best results are obtained by employing the shortest period of incubation, *e.g.* from early forenoon to evening or from late evening to early morning. When the specific phases has been obtained, formolised suspensions are used in agglutination reactions with pure specific-phase H sera prepared against the salmonella types in the group to which the already determined O antigen belongs. In many cases the evidence thus obtained, in association with the bio-

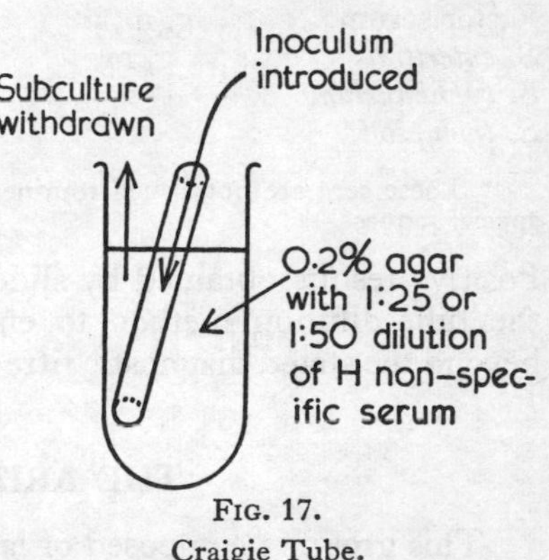

FIG. 17.
Craigie Tube.

chemical reactions, will serve to identify the unknown strain if it is one of the usual types of Salmonellae.

The set of Standard agglutinating sera recommended is as follows:

O antisera:

S. typhi Vi.

Polyvalent O serum containing factors 1–13, 19 and 22.

Factor sera—

2*	for Salmonella O group	A
4	” ” ”	B
7	” ” ”	C_1
8	” ” ”	C_2
9	” ” ”	D
3, 10	” ” ”	E_1 & $_2$
19*	” ” ”	E_4
11*	” ” ”	F
13, 22	” ” ”	G

H antisera:

Polyvalent Salmonella serum, composite H specific and non-specific.

Salmonella H phase-2 polyvalent serum (H factors 1–7).

Specific H sera:

	Antigens		*Antigens*
S. paratyphi A .	a	Factor serum	l, v, w
S. paratyphi B .	b	*S. bovis-morbificans** .	r
*S. paratyphi C** .	c	*S. bareilly** . . .	y
S. typhi . .	d	*S. poona** . . .	z
S. newport . .	e, h	*S. glostrup** . . .	z_{10}
Factor serum .	g. m, p		
S. enteritidis .	g, m	*S. cerro**	z_4, z_{23}
S. typhimurium .	i		
S. thompson . .	k	*S. tennessee** . . .	z_{29}

* These sera are not issued routinely by the Standards Laboratory, but only on special request.

Positive results obtained by slide agglutination must be confirmed by the tube-dilution method to ensure that agglutination occurs at or beyond the stated diagnostic titre of the particular antiserum employed.

THE ARIZONA GROUP

This group is composed of lactose-fermenting organisms which are closely linked, biochemically and antigenically, to the genus *Salmonella*. The first member of the group was isolated from reptiles and described in 1939.

These organisms, most frequently associated with reptiles, have also been isolated from fowls, mammals and man, but have so far attracted little attention in Britain although it is recognised that they can produce severe and fatal human infections.

In their morphology and staining reactions, and in their general cultural characteristics, members of the group are indistinguishable from salmonellae. With the exception of one serotype, these organisms ferment lactose with gas production; so prompt is this activity that many isolates produce pink colonies on the primary DCA plate after overnight incubation; with others, lactose-fermentation may be delayed for three to five days, and occasional strains show no activity until after two or three weeks' growth. Their constant ability to liquefy gelatin is also in contrast to salmonellae, in which gelatinase production occurs only rarely; conversely, their failure to ferment dulcitol further distinguishes Arizona strains from the vast majority of salmonellae. Their biochemical similarity implies that Arizona strains may be mistakenly identified as salmonellae, the more so since antigenic overlapping between the two is extensive as regards both H and O antigens; diagnostic salmonella sera can be used as substitutes for many of the Arizona antisera (Edwards & Ewing, 1962).

At least 32 sero-groups of Arizona are recognised on the basis of different O antigens; most of these groups contain two or more serotypes identifiable by flagellar antigens which, as in the genus *Salmonella*, may occur in two phases: 180 serotypes are at present recognised and these are epidemiologically significant.

The error in identifying a culture as a salmonella rather than as an Arizona strain is of no great importance since, in man, the organisms produce similar clinical syndromes and can be regarded as very similar from the epidemiologic point of view and for prophylactic measures.

A more significant error is the rejection of an organism as "non-pathogenic" on the basis of prompt lactose-fermentation on primary diagnostic media. At present, our knowledge of the distribution of Arizona serotypes in man is elementary but of their pathogenicity there can be no doubt.

REFERENCES

Anderson, E. S. & Williams, R. E. O. (1956). Bacteriophage typing of enteric pathogens and staphylococci and its use in epidemiology: A review. *J. clin. Path.*, **9**, 94.

Bradley, W. H. (1943). An epidemiological study of Bact. typhosum type D 4. *Brit. med. J.*, **1**, 438.

Christie, A. B. (1964). Treatment of typhoid carriers with ampicillin. *Brit. med. J.*, **1**, 1609.

Edwards, P. R. & Ewing, W. H. (1962). *Identification of Enterobacteriaceae*, 2nd ed. Minneapolis: Burgess.

Haines, R. B. & Moran, T. (1940). Porosity of, and bacterial invasion through, the shell of the hen's egg. *J. Hyg.* (*Camb.*), **40**, 453.

Hendrickse, R. G. & Collard, P. (1960). Salmonella osteitis in Nigerian children. *Lancet*, **1**, 80.

Hobbs, B. C. & Wilson, J. G. (1959). Contamination of wholesale meat supplies with salmonellae and heat-resistant *Clostridium welchii*. *Mth. Bull. Minist. Hlth Lab. Serv.*, **18**, 198.

Kauffmann, F. (1954). *Enterobacteriaceae*. Copenhagen: Munksgaard.

Miller, A. A. & Ramsden, F. (1955). Contamination of meat pies by salmonella in relation to baking and handling procedures. *J. appl. Bact.*, **18**, 565.

Report (1959). Salmonella organisms in animal feeding stuffs and fertilisers. *Mth. Bull. Minist. Hlth Lab. Serv.*, **18**, 26.

Savage, W. G. (1956). Problems of Salmonella food poisoning. *Brit. med. J.*, **2**, 317.

Thomas, J. V., Watson, K. C. & Hewstone, A. S. (1954). The use of streptokinase bile salt broth for clot cultures in the diagnosis of enteric fever. *J. clin. Path.*, **7**, 50.

Whitby, J. M. F. (1964). Ampicillin in treatment of *Salmonella typhi* carriers. *Lancet*, **2**, 71.

CHAPTER 17

SHIGELLA

THE members of this genus are the causative organisms of acute bacillary dysentery, a disease which is widespread throughout the world and which has become increasingly common in Britain in the last thirty years. The severity of the illness is, to some extent, related to the particular group or species incriminated; the *Shigella dysenteriae* group is most commonly associated with the classical syndrome of sudden onset of abdominal pain, tenesmus, pyrexia and prostration, with the passage of frequent stools which rapidly lose their faecal nature and become composed of blood and mucus. The illness associated with *Shigella sonnei* infection may be confined to the passage of a few loose motions and is frequently so mild that the individual continues at work or school. The stool is seldom much altered except in consistency, some blood and mucus being frequently present with it, but rarely as the sole constituents.

Two other groups—*Shigella flexneri* and *Shigella boydii*—are encountered as causative agents in bacillary dysentery. The illness associated with members of these groups tends to be more severe than with *Sh. sonnei*.

Morphology and Staining.—Identical with *S. typhi* except that they do not possess flagella and are non-motile. Fimbriae occur only in *Sh. flexneri* types.

Cultural Characters.—Resemble the genus *Salmonella* with the exception that *Sh. sonnei* is a late fermenter of lactose—thus, colonies of the latter on MacConkey or DCA media become pink when incubation is prolonged beyond 18–24 hours.

Viability.—The thermal death-point is about 55° C. for 1 hr.; within the genus, *Sh. sonnei* is more resistant to adverse environmental factors than are the other members.

Biochemical Reactions.—The 4 groups within the genus *Shigella* display the activities shown in the table.

Group	Glucose	Lactose	Mannitol	Indole	No. of serotypes
A. *Sh. dysenteriae*	⊥	–	–	v	10
B. *Sh. flexneri*	⊥	–	⊥	v	6
C. *Sh. boydii*	⊥	–	⊥	v	15
D. *Sh. sonnei*	⊥	(⊥)	⊥	–	1

Key: ⊥ = acid, no gas; ( ) = delayed reaction; v = variable in different types.

The members of group A differ from those in other groups by constantly failing to ferment mannitol; groups B and C comprise species which are biochemically similar to each other whereas group D strains are late fermenters of lactose and never produce indole. With the exception of certain strains of *Sh. flexneri* type 6, dysentery bacilli are anaerogenic.

The practical classification of shigellae into mannitol-fermenting and mannitol non-fermenting strains is retained, notwithstanding the fact that various exceptions have been recognised; indeed, the relative rarity of *Sh. flexneri* strains which do not ferment mannitol gives the latter feature value as an epidemiologic marker. This circumstance is best exemplified by the biochemical sub-division of the serologically homogeneous *Sh. flexneri* type 6 as in the table.

Biochemical Variety	Glucose	Mannitol	Dulcitol
No. 88	⊥	⊥	−
No. 88	⊥	⊥	(⊥)
Manchester	+	+	(+)
Newcastle	+	−	(+)

Key: + = acid and gas; ⊥ = acid only; ( ) = delayed reaction.

Within the Flexner group, mannitol non-fermenting strains are also found in serotypes 1, 2, 3 and 4, but only in type 4 are they as common as such variants in type 6; mannitol non-fermenting strains of *Sh. flexneri* type 4 were previously designated *Sh. rabaulensis* and *Sh. rio*.

The inclusion of dulcitol as a substrate in biochemical subdivision of type 6 strains allows strains designated No. 88 to be divided into two bio-types; one-third of such strains do not ferment dulcitol, whereas the others produce acid in this substrate after two to four days' incubation.

Antigenic Characters.—Group A strains can be recognised as one of at least 10 specific serotypes by agglutination tests with type-specific antisera. These types do not show significant intra- or inter-group sharing of antigens; unabsorbed sera can thus be used in type identification.

Group B strains: 6 serotypes are recognised—these are significantly interrelated by possession of a common group antigen (group antigen 1). Each serotype, when freshly isolated, also possesses a type-specific component (type antigens I, II, III, etc.) as originally shown by Boyd (1938). These findings have been confirmed and types 1, 2 and 4 are each divided into two subtypes on the basis of minor group antigens, e.g. *Sh. flexneri* 1*a* possesses the type-specific antigen I as does type 1*b*, strains designated subtype 1*a* do not possess the minor group antigen 6, whereas subtype 1*b* strains constantly contain this minor antigenic factor. Group B strains tend to lose their type-specific component although retaining their group antigens; thus, two variants, X and Y, of *Sh. flexneri* are also recognised. Diagnostic sera for determining the type of a strain must be absorbed to remove group agglutinins.

Group C strains: The 15 recognised serotypes comprising this group are biochemically indistinguishable from group B strains, but are serologically distinct from the latter, since they do not possess the *Sh flexneri* group antigen 1; however, some serotypes in group C show significant serological relationships with other group C strains as well as with certain types of *Sp. flexneri*, and it is essential that (with the exception of *Sh. boydii* types 2, 3, 7 and 8) diagnostic antisera should be absorbed to remove agglutinins which react non-specifically.

Group D strains: Smooth cultures of *Sh. sonnei* are serologically distinct from other shigellae; the study of smooth-rough (S-R) variation of *Sh. sonnei* has revealed that each form is antigenically distinct and that the recognised relationship with *Sh. boydii* type 6 strains is solely a function of the R form. *Sh. sonnei* strains cannot be subdivided into types by serological methods; attempts have been made to type or characterise strains by other methods (pp. 241-242).

Animal Pathogenicity.—Cultures of dysentery bacilli are generally non-pathogenic when introduced orally in laboratory animals. Intravenous injection produces a haemorrhagic enteritis and, if the animal survives, muscular paralysis may result. These effects are particularly marked in the case of *Sh. dysenteriae* type 1 (*Sh. shigae*), which forms a potent, diffusible toxin. Apart from man, only monkeys and chimpanzees suffer naturally from bacillary dysentery (Rewell, 1949).

Pathogenesis.—Infection occurs by ingestion; it is probable that the infecting dose is of a much lower order than for salmonellae (except *S. typhi*). After reaching the large intestine the shigellae multiply locally with resultant inflammation of the mucosa which may, in severe cases, progress to ulcer formation and sloughing of large areas of mucous membrane. The cellular response is characteristically by polymorphonuclear leucocytes and these are readily noted on microscopic examination of the dejecta. Dysentery bacilli rarely invade other tissues and bacteraemia has only occasionally been reported.

On clinical recovery, the patients may continue to excrete the organisms in their stools for a few weeks and some patients may become persistent carriers. It is worth noting that persons carrying *Sh. dysenteriae* serotypes excrete these organisms persistently compared with carriers of *Sh. flexneri* and *Sh. sonnei* in whom intermittent excretion is more common, *i.e.* the organisms may be isolated from the faeces for two or three days consecutively and then disappear only to reappear after some days or weeks. When comparing earlier studies on carrier rates in bacillary dysentery with more recent reports, it should be remembered that the introduction of more selective media, *e.g.* DCA, ensures the isolation of shigellae when these are present in such small numbers that otherwise they would not be detected.

Epidemiology.—Sources of infection are human cases and carriers; the mild nature of Sonne infections, often amounting to little more than a social inconvenience, allows infected patients to remain ambulant with a greatly increased opportunity for disseminating the organisms compared with the person who is confined to bed. The role of the healthy convalescent and symptomless carrier as a source of infection has been the subject of much debate; provided that such persons are passing formed stools, they are much less important in the spread of the disease than cases with fluid or loose stools.

In Britain, bacillary dysentery is endemic with epidemic waves occurring in the early part of the year and, to a less extent, in late autumn. This contrasts with experience in tropical and sub-tropical countries where the disease is most prevalent during the warmer months. The lack of modern sanitation has been invoked to explain the frequency of epidemics in certain countries, and certainly the construction of elementary toilet facilities, *e.g.* bored-hole latrines, has reduced the incidence in such circumstances; by contrast, in Britain, we have seen the almost unrelenting increase in bacillary dysentery in the last thirty years during which time environmental hygiene has been well above the standard obtained in materially less-favoured communities. Similarly, the spread of organisms by flies from faeces to food, although a potential danger in less satisfactory circumstances, must rarely be important in our community, where the peak incidence of the disease occurs during the months of the year when house flies are uncommon. Dysentery bacilli, being excreted in the faeces, may be transmitted to food through the soiled hands of a case or carrier, or they may pass from such sources to other individuals via inanimate objects such as door-handles, toilet chains and seats, pencils and crockery. A comparative study (Hutchinson, 1956) of the dissemination of *Sh. sonnei* by cases revealed that contamination was heaviest in the immediate vicinity of the toilet pedestal, that the organisms passed through toilet paper on to fingers and that they could be recovered from fingers at least three hours after these had been contaminated.

In summary, there is sufficient evidence to confirm that, in Britain at least, bacillary dysentery is a hand-to-mouth infection depending for its spread on poor personal hygiene rather than on low standards of community services, although sanitary arrangements in many schools leave much to be desired. Whilst bacillary dysentery is uncommon in the first year of life, the majority of cases occur in the under-5 age-group; in recent years, the increasing incidence in the 5–9 years group has drawn attention to the role of primary schools in promoting the spread of dysentery. Males are more frequently infected than females, except in the 15–45 years group, when the intimacy of contact between mother and sick child ensures that women are more exposed to infection, and suffer more commonly, than men.

Serological and colicine typing.—Serological identification of specific types within groups A-C has been valuable in tracing the source of epidemics due to these types. The predominance of *Sh. sonnei* as the principal infecting agent in Britain in the last 20–30 years has stimulated the search for some means of characterising this serologically homogeneous species for epidemiologic purposes. The sub-division of *Sh. sonnei* strains on their ability to ferment xylose has been employed in tracing infection (Tee, 1952), but is of limited value since only two types can thus be identified. Phage-typing of *Sh. sonnei* has similarly been undertaken (Tee, 1955), but instability of type and the predominance of one phage-type did not encourage its use.

The ability of Sonne strains to produce various specific colicines[1] has been employed recently for epidemiologic purposes and encouraging results have been obtained. Our experience of colicine typing is entirely in agreement with the published accounts. The method recommended (Gillies, 1964) is based on that of Abbott and Shannon (1958).

Media :

1. For colicine production. Tryptone Soya (TS) Agar (Oxoid) is reconstituted according to the manufacturer's instructions and horse blood is added to give a final concentration of 2·5 per cent. The medium is dispensed in Petri dishes.
2. For cultivation of Indicator Strains. Infusion broth is used for this purpose.

Technique:

The strain to be tested is inoculated by a single diametrical streak on TS agar and the plate incubated at 35° C. for twenty-four hours. The growth is then removed with the edge of a glass slide and 2–3 ml. of chloroform are poured on to the base of the plate and the medium-containing portion replaced. After ten to fifteen minutes' exposure to the chloroform vapour, the residual liquid chloroform is decanted and the plate exposed to air for a further ten to fifteen minutes; thereafter the indicator (passive) strains are seeded on to the plate at right angles to the original growth line. Incubation at 37° C. for eight to twelve hours reveals various patterns of inhibition of the indicator strains by the colicines in the medium; at least 17 colicine-types of *Sh. sonnei* can thus be identified, and these appear to be stable.

Laboratory Diagnosis

The collection of faecal specimens and their transmission to the laboratory demands the same care as for specimens from cases of enteric fever. Specimens obtained by rectal swabbing are less reliable than faeces unless they have been taken expertly and cultured while still moist. The use of serum-coated rectal swabs enhances their value, but, in general, the use of rectal swabs should be restricted to the investigation of outbreaks in institutions where laboratory facilities are immediately available. A further disadvantage of swab specimens is that they prohibit macro- and microscopic examination of the stool, which can be helpful in the differential diagnosis of aetiologies in acute

[1] Colicines (bacteriocines) are naturally occurring antibiotic substances elaborated by many members of the family *Enterobacteriaceae*. The colicine activity of a strain is often directed against members of another genus, although usually such activity is most marked against strains of the same genus as that of the producing strain. See: Fredericq. P. (1949), *Rev. Belg. Path*, **19**, Suppl. 4.

diarrhoea; the onus of collecting faeces can be placed on the patient or his relatives.

Microscopic Examination.—A wet film preparation of a saline suspension of faeces or a mucoid portion of the specimen will usually reveal an abundant and characteristic cellular exudate. The cells present are mostly polymorph leucocytes with a varying number of red blood cells, and in the early stages numerous epithelial cells. In addition to these, macrophages are frequently a characteristic feature of the exudate; the leucocytes, as a rule, show marked degeneration.

Cultivation.—If the faeces are formed it is essential that they be emulsified in saline prior to plating out on DCA and inoculating a selenite enrichment broth; the latter is subcultured on to a fresh plate of DCA medium after incubation for 18–24 hours. If mucus is present in the specimen, it should be employed as an inoculum. Colonies of dysentery bacilli are pale or colourless after primary incubation on DCA, and at least three such colonies should be selected for further investigation. Tubes of the following media are inoculated: (1) peptone water; (2) glucose, lactose, sucrose, and mannitol peptone water with phenol red or Andrade's indicator and Durham tube, and these are incubated for 12–24 hours. The peptone water is examined after six to seven hours for motility of the organisms. Alternatively, tests may be made using composite media which obviate the need for making a hanging-drop preparation to study motility and are otherwise as satisfactory as the first method (Gillies, 1956).

Cultures with the biochemical characteristics of one or other of the Shigella groups must have their identity confirmed by serological investigation. If the strain is mannitol non-fermenting, it should be tested for agglutination with the individual type-specific sera comprising group A. If the strain ferments mannitol, then it may be a member of groups B-D and should be tested with polyvalent sera for *flexneri* and *boydii* serotypes and with a Sonne antiserum; in the case of positive reactions with one or other of the polyvalent sera, the strain is further tested with the type-specific sera within the particular group. Positive results obtained by slide agglutination must be confirmed by the tube-dilution method to ensure that agglutination occurs at or beyond the stated diagnostic titre of the particular antiserum employed.

Slide agglutination tests with colonies picked directly from diagnostic plates may be used for making early presumptive verbal reports before undertaking confirmatory biochemical and serological investigations.

Agglutination Tests with Patient's Serum.—Such tests do not have the same value as the Widal reaction in the enteric fevers, since, even in cases from which the causative organism has been isolated, the patients' serum frequently shows no increased level of specific antibody compared with sera from healthy individuals; furthermore, the presence of certain natural antibodies in human sera may give non-specific agglutination of the test suspensions.

The following sera are available from the Standards Laboratory for Serological Reagents:

Group A. Individual specific sera for types 1–7.*
Group B. Polyvalent serum.
Individual sera for types 2, 3, 6 and X variant.
Individual sera for types 1, 4, 5 and Y variant.*
Group C. Polyvalent Boyd I (types 1–6).*
Polyvalent Boyd II (types 7–11).*
Individual sera for types 1–11.*
Group D. S-R Sonne serum.
Phase I (S) serum.*
Phase II (R) serum.*

* Available only on special request.

Chemotherapy.—The value of sulphonamides in treating Sonne dysentery has diminished since, in Britain, the majority of strains are now resistant to these agents. Streptomycin in adequate dosage gives satisfactory clinical and bacteriological cure, but inadequate dosage or too brief a treatment period allows *Sh. sonnei* to develop resistance *in vivo*. The tetracyclines or chloramphenicol should be reserved for such cases; area laboratories can usefully check the sensitivity of Sonne strains and advise practitioners regarding the emergence of strains resistant to one or other therapeutic agent.

Prophylaxis.—The epidemiology of bacillary dysentery in temperate climates implies that improvement in personal hygiene, particularly hand-washing after defaecation and before handling foodstuffs, would achieve much in the prevention of spread. Children must be trained in such elementary procedures, and adequate facilities must be provided in schools and other communal centres. The adaptation of existing hand-operated toilet-flushing systems to foot-operated mechanisms and the installation of similar mechanisms for manipulating toilet seats would eliminate the handling of structures which act as vehicles of infection. The replacement of roller-towels with disposable paper-towels or continuous-feed roller systems will encourage hand-washing, but these and wash-basins must be in the same annexe as the toilet otherwise the handling of intervening doors will defeat their purpose.

Sulphonamides have been administered prophylactically in closed community outbreaks, but with little advantage; in many reports of such "trials" no mention is made of whether the epidemic strain was tested for sensitivity to the drug. Since the majority of Sonne strains are resistant to sulphonamides, it is not surprising that their employment in prophylaxis has rarely been successful.

In areas where toilet facilities are primitive or non-existent, either the provision of bored-hole latrines or chemical toilets will reduce the likelihood of insect-borne modes of spread and mechanical and chemical fly-control techniques may be applied to domestic and other premises.

Specific vaccines have no prophylactic value.

Antigenic Relationships in Enterobacteriaceae

The serological identification of enterobacteria depends mainly upon specific agglutination reactions involving group or type-specific somatic (O) and flagellar (H) antigens, *e.g.* in salmonellae.

However, certain other kinds of surface antigen may be present; some are associated with morphological features of the bacteria, *e.g.* capsular or envelope K antigens of Kauffmann (1954) (L, A, B and Vi types) and fimbrial antigens (Gillies & Duguid, 1958) whilst others, such as the α antigen of Stamp and Stone (1944) and the β antigen of Mushin (1949), are not characterised morphologically. Such antigens may cause difficulties in serological identification of the bacteria either by covering and masking the O antigen so that the bacilli are inagglutinable by O antibodies or by producing non-specific cross reactions because of their presence in otherwise unrelated organisms.

Fimbrial antigens.—These are borne on fimbriae and have been found in *Esch. coli*, *Sh. flexneri*, *Cl. cloacae*, *Klebsiella* species, *Salmonellae*, *Proteus* and *Ps. pyocyanea* (Duguid & Gillies, 1957; Duguid, 1959). In many species fimbriation is a variable state; serial aerobic cultivation in fluid media selects a fimbriate mutant while the non-fimbriate mutant is selected by serial cultivation on nutrient agar plates. Fimbriae can be demonstrated only by the electron-microscope but their presence is associated with haemagglutinating activity and their absence with lack of such activity, so that the demonstration of direct bacterial haemagglutination (often specifically inhibited by 2 per cent. D-mannose) affords evidence of fimbriation.

Many *Esch. coli* strains remain partially fimbriate on agar and their fimbrial antigens may give rise to non-specific reactions; K antigens occurring in such strains have some general resemblances to fimbrial antigens in thermolability, anatomical location and liability to mask the O antigen and confer relative somatic inagglutinability.

The main differences between the three types of K antigen are:

L antigens do not combine with L antibodies after heating at 100° C. for one hour, whereas A and B antigens retain agglutinin-binding capacity after such treatment.

Strains possessing L or B antigens become O agglutinable after heating at 100° C. for one hour, but those with A antigens remain inagglutinable in somatic antisera after heating at 100° C. for two and a half hours.

The antigenicity of the L type is destroyed by heating at 100° C. for one hour and that of the A antigens is only reduced.

There are particular differences between L, A and B antigens on the one hand, and fimbrial antigens on the other; these are shown in the table (see page 246).

The rapid, loosely floccular nature of fimbrial agglutination renders it liable to confusion with flagellar agglutination in species such as *Esch. coli*; it may be distinguished from the latter by treating the bacilli either with 0·005 *N* HCl (Duncan, 1935) or with 50 per cent. ethyl alcohol, since fimbriae resist such reagents, whereas flagella are destroyed by them.

Fimbrial antigens differ from α antigen which does not react with natural agglutinins in normal human sera, and from β antigen which has not been detected in fimbriate genera, such as *Salmonella*, yet occurs in some non-fimbriate species, e.g. *Sh. boydii* type 6; furthermore, α and β antigens are not subject to predictable variation in appearance and disappearance under different cultural conditions.

The X salmonella antigens (Topley & Ayrton, 1924) are very similar to fimbrial antigens in thermolability, type of agglutination, variability in differing cultural conditions and in occurring as precipitinogens in the supernatants of cultures heated at 100° C.

Activity and Stability of Superficial Antigens of Enterobacteria (which may mask the O antigen)

Treatment of bacilli		L	A	B	H	F
Living or 0·5 per cent. formalin	1.	+	+	+	+	+
	2.	+	+	+	+	+
60° C. /1 hr.	1.	$\perp$	+	+	+	+
	2.	$\underline{\perp}$	+	+	+	+
100° C./1 hr.	1.	−	+	−	−	−
	2.	−	+	+	−	−
50 per cent. alcohol, 20 hr./37° C.	1.	−	+	+	−	$\perp$
	2.	$\underline{\perp}$	..	+	$\underline{\perp}$	..

Key: L.A.B. = K antigens; H = flagellar antigens; F = fimbrial antigens.
1. Agglutinability
2. Agglutinin-binding } of washed bacilli.

+ = unaffected;
$\perp$ = reduced;
$\underline{\perp}$ = almost eliminated;
− = abolished;
.. = not tested.

Difficulties in Diagnostic Serology caused by Fimbrial Antigens.—In homologous antiserum containing O and fimbrial agglutinins, the agglutination of fimbriate bacilli is mainly due to fimbrial antibodies; somatic agglutination reactions are obscured, since fimbrial agglutination occurs more rapidly and is loosely floccular.

Among the shigellae, fimbriae frequently occur but only in *Sh. flexneri* serotypes 1a, 2a, 2b, 3, 4a, 4b, 5, X and Y; the fimbrial antigens in these types are identical, irrespective of O serotype. It is important, therefore, when undertaking identification of the O serotype of a *Sh. flexneri* isolate, to avoid fimbrial agglutination. This can be ensured by using bacillary suspensions that are devoid of fimbriae, either by serial aerobic cultivation on well-dried agar plates to select non-fimbriate phase bacilli or by defimbriating the suspension by heating at 100° C. followed by centrifugation to harvest the defimbriated cells.

In normal diagnostic laboratory practice, it is unlikely that such difficulties will be encountered, since the procedures of isolation on solid media and subcultivation on agar prior to serological testing usually ensure that *Sh. flexneri* is in the non-fimbriate phase.

An additional safeguard would be the use of diagnostic typing sera free from immune and natural fimbrial antibodies; such sera could be prepared by absorption with a fimbriate culture of *Sh. flexneri* of heterologous O serotype. However, the use of such sera alone would not completely answer the problem, since in non-fimbrial sera fimbriation of test suspensions masks somatic agglutination to a greater or less degree.

Suspensions used for the preparation of diagnostic *Sh. flexneri* antisera in rabbits must be non-fimbriate; even then, since the majority of rabbits possess *Esch. coli* fimbrial antibodies which may cross-react with those of *Sh. flexneri*, agglutinating sera may contain fimbrial antibodies. Tests on pre-immunisation bleedings will allow selection of animals whose sera do not contain fimbrial antibodies; alternatively, the fimbrial antibodies may be absorbed with a fimbriate strain of heterologous O serotype. Sera containing fimbrial antibodies for *Sh. flexneri* do not react with fimbriate strains of Salmonella, Proteus or Cloaca.

Another circumstance in which fimbriae and fimbrial antibodies can cause confusion is in Widal testing of human sera. Fimbrial antibodies have been noted in the sera of healthy persons and such sera have been found to react non-specifically in tests with diagnostic suspensions of salmonellae if the latter are fimbriate; such anomalous serological findings are unrelated to the patient's condition. The use of standard agglutinable suspensions which are non-fimbriate or at most not more than poorly fimbriate, will prevent the occurrence of such non-specific reactions; salmonellae subcultured from agar to broth and incubated for six hours show maximum flagellation and minimal fimbriation. The source of fimbrial antibodies in healthy persons may be from the commensal *Esch. coli* in the gut or as a result of past infections with fimbriate *Sh. flexneri* or salmonellae. The presence of fimbriae in some TAB suspensions may explain the presence of antibodies in individuals receiving injections of TAB vaccines.

In addition to direct examination of suspensions by electron-microscopy, two other methods of controlling production are available; namely, testing for agglutinability with pure fimbrial antiserum and, also, a simple haemagglutination test for the presence of fimbriae.

REFERENCES

Abbott, J. D. & Shannon, R. (1958). A method for typing *Shigella sonnei*, using colicine production as a marker. *J. clin. Path.*, **11**, 71.

Boyd, J. S. K. (1938). The antigenic structure of the mannitol-fermenting group of dysentery bacilli (contains reference to his earlier studies). *J. Hyg.* (*Camb.*), **38**, 477.

Duguid, J. P. (1959). Fimbriae and adhesive properties in klebsiella strains. *J. gen. Microbiol.*, **21**, 271.

Duguid, J. P. & Gillies, R. R. (1957). Fimbriae and adhesive properties in dysentery bacilli. *J. Path. Bact.*, **74**, 397.

Duncan, J. T. (1935). Inactivation of the "H" antigen by dilute mineral acid. *Brit. J. exp. Path.*, **16**, 405.

Gillies, R. R. (1956). An evaluation of two composite media for preliminary identification of Shigella and Salmonella. *J. clin. Path.*, **9**, 368.

Gillies, R. R. (1964). Colicine production as an epidemiological marker of *Shigella sonnei*. *J. Hyg. (Camb.)*, **62**, 1.

Gillies, R. R. & Duguid, J. P. (1958). The fimbrial antigens of *Shigella flexneri*. *J. Hyg. (Camb.)*, **56**, 303.

Hutchinson, R. I. (1956). Some observations on the method of spread of Sonne dysentery. *Mth. Bull. Minist. Hlth Lab. Serv.*, **15**, 110.

Kauffmann, F. (1954). *Enterobacteriaceae*. Copenhagen: Munksgaard.

Mushin, R. (1949). A new antigenic relationship among faecal bacilli due to a common β antigen. *J. Hyg. (Camb.)*, **47**, 227.

Rewell, R. E. (1949). Outbreak of *Shigella schmitzii* infection in men and apes. *Lancet*, **1**, 220.

Stamp, Lord & Stone, D. M. (1944). An agglutinogen common to certain strains of lactose and non-lactose-fermenting coliform bacilli. *J. Hyg. (Camb.)*, **43**, 266.

Tee, G. H. (1952). Xylose fermentation by *Shigella sonnei*. *Mth. Bull. Minist. Hlth Lab. Serv.*, **11**, 68.

Tee, G. H. (1955). Bacteriophage typing of *Shigella sonnei* and its limitations in epidemiological investigations. *J. Hyg. (Camb.)*, **53**, 54.

Topley, W. W. C. & Ayrton, J. (1924). Further investigations into the biological characteristics of *B. enteritidis (aertrycke)*. *J. Hyg. (Camb.)*, **23**, 198).

CHAPTER 18

ESCHERICHIA COLI; PROTEUS

THE members of the Enterobacteriaceae to be considered in this and the following chapter have been the subject of much dispute in so far as their classification is concerned. That used here is given in the table.

Group or Genus	Features						
	Gas from Glucose	Motility	Indole	Gelatin liq.	V.-P.	M.-R.	Citrate
Escherichia	+	+	+	−	−	+	−
Alkalescens-Dispar	−	−	+	−	−	+	−
Citrobacter	+	+	−	−	−	+	+
Klebsiella	+	−	−	−	+	−	+
Cloaca	+	+	−	+	+	−	+
Hafnia*	+	+	−	−	+	−	+

* Results when tests are performed at 20° C. (see p. 259).

ESCHERICHIA COLI

Morphology and Staining.—Identical with salmonella species; most strains are flagellate and fimbriate and a few capsulate.

Cultural Characters.—Generally similar to salmonella species although on nutrient agar, colonies are relatively larger and more opaque than the latter.

MacConkey's medium.—Colonies are rose-pink on account of lactose fermentation. Strains of *Esch. coli* grow poorly, if at all, on DCA medium on which they also produce pink, but smaller and opaque colonies.

Biochemical Reactions.—These have been referred to in the table, and it will be noted that members of the genus *Escherichia* bear a close resemblance to those in the *Alkalescens-Dispar* (A-D) group except that the latter are never motile and never produce gas in fermentation reactions; the two groups are also closely related serologically.

Antigenic Characters.—In addition to O and H antigens, the majority of commonly encountered *Esch. coli* strains possess K antigens. The term K antigen describes collectively a group of antigens designated L, A or B on the basis of physical characteristics; these are somatic antigens which occur as envelopes or capsules and prevent O agglutination of living strains by their homologous O antisera. The serological classification of *Esch. coli* has only been established since the discovery of the K antigens and their recognition as the cause of irregularities and discrepancies in earlier attempts at serotyping members of this genus. The pathogenicity of many strains of *Esch. coli* is related to the possession of K antigens.

Pathogenesis.—*Esch. coli* strains predominate among the aerobic commensal organisms present in the healthy gut. Serological studies have shown that the types present are not only numerous at any one examination but that over a period of time the coli types fluctuate: some types persist over relatively long periods of time, whereas others are quite transient (Wallick & Stuart, 1943; Sears *et al.*, 1950).

These organisms are also incriminated as pathogens. They are found most frequently in pyogenic infections of the urinary tract (pyelitis, cystitis, etc.) either in pure culture or mixed with faecal streptococci; they also occur in appendix abscess, peritonitis, cholecystitis, septic wounds and bed-sores.

Serotype distribution studies (Vahlne, 1945) reveal that strains isolated from pathological material usually belong to a relatively few O-groups and the majority are O-inagglutinable due almost invariably to the possession of L antigens; by contrast, strains isolated from healthy faeces are distributed over many more O-groups and only a minority are O-inagglutinable, and this is due to the presence of L antigen in only 50 per cent. of such strains.

In contrast to the finding of numerous O-groups of *Esch. coli* present in a specimen of healthy faeces, testing of numerous colonies from the urine in a case of cystitis usually reveals that they are all of the same O-group; such serological homogeneity, although to a less degree, is noted also in peritonitis and cases of appendix abscess. The infections mentioned above are of an endogenous nature and the aetiologic role of *Esch. coli* had long been accepted before adequate techniques of serotyping had been introduced.

The suspicion that *Esch. coli* might also be capable of causing gastro-enteritis particularly in infancy has only been confirmed as a result of recent serologic evidence. The pathogenic role of certain coli types in infantile gastro-enteritis was first emphasised by Bray (1945); this strain is now known as *Esch. coli* O 111 and in common with other enteropathogenic types (*e.g.* O 26, O 55, O 119 and O 128) it possesses a B type of K antigen. The antigenic analysis of these types is discussed on pp. 245-46.

In the veterinary field also, *Esch. coli* is a recognised pathogen; careful and protracted studies in Sweden (Wramby, 1948) revealed that in calves dying from "coli-septicaemia", compared with healthy calves, the differences in type distribution and the relative frequencies of O-inagglutinable strains were analogous to those in similar studies in man (*vide supra*).

Esch. coli is associated with the condition of white scours in calves; enteritis in piglets, mastitis in cows, uterine infections in bitches and occasional abortion in ewes can also be attributed to these organisms. Hjarre's disease—a granulomatous condition resembling tuberculosis and occurring in poultry may be caused by certain types of *Esch. coli.*

Epidemiology.—The essentially endogenous nature of many infections caused by *Esch. coli* has already been mentioned; however, exogenous infection of the urinary tract may occur, the organisms being introduced during diagnostic or therapeutic catheterisation. In such instances the instruments may have been inadequately sterilised or insufficient care taken in the pre-operative cleansing of the patient or the operator.

In gastro-enteritis, the majority of reported epidemics have occurred among infants under 18 months of age; that the pathogenicity of such *Esch. coli* strains is not necessarily so restricted is shown by reports of enteritis in adult hospital patients (McNaught & Stevenson, 1953) and of experimentally induced infections in adult volunteers (Ferguson & June, 1952; June *et al.*, 1953), whose sera showed the presence of specific antibodies after recovery.

Artificially fed babies are much more likely to be infected than those fed naturally; the sources of infection in babies are both cases and carriers of the infection and spread may occur by contaminated fomites. Contamination of the milk bottle or introduction of the organisms into the milk feed during its preparation will ensure ingestion and if the feed has been prepared some hours before, the original inoculum will have the opportunity to multiply to a greater or less extent depending on the conditions of storage.

Laboratory Diagnosis

In film preparations from pus, urinary sediment, etc., stained by Gram's method, *Esch. coli* can be recognised as Gram-negative bacilli but indistinguishable from any other member of the Enterobacteriaceae. Specimens are plated on to blood-agar and MacConkey's medium; on the latter, *Esch. coli* yields pink, lactose-fermenting colonies, and if confirmation of its identity is required then the reactions listed in the table (p. 249) must be tested.

Identification of gastro-enteritis-producing strains.—Specimens of faeces submitted from cases of diarrhoea will also be examined for salmonellae and shigellae; since *Esch. coli* usually do not grow on the highly selective DCA medium it is essential that the less inhibitory differential MacConkey's medium should also be inoculated. A blood-agar plate should also be inoculated lightly with faeces since, on occasion, growth appears on this medium when the enteropathogenic *Esch. coli* strain cannot be identified on the parallel MacConkey's plate; further, it is easier to avoid contaminants when subculturing from the blood-agar medium.

After incubation for 18–24 hours, the blood-agar and MacConkey media are examined for colonies of *Esch. coli*; *since colonies of enteropathogenic strains do not differ in appearance either among themselves or from other coli strains* it is essential that at least 10 colonies be subjected to serological testing. Slide tests are performed with a fragment of each colony against a polyvalent antiserum. If agglutination is noted, then further tests are made with the individual type-specific sera; when living, freshly isolated strains are tested in OB antisera, agglutination in the specific serum occurs rapidly.

Sera available from the Standards Laboratory are as follows:

Polyvalent *Esch. coli* serum containing factors O 26, O 55, O 111, O 119, O 127, O 128, and their related B agglutinins. Type specific sera: O 26: B 6; O 55: B 5; O 111: B 4; O 119: B 14; O 127: B 8; O 128: B 12.

A modified MacConkey agar medium (Rappaport & Henig, 1952) in which sorbitol is substituted for lactose, has been used for the differentiation of serotypes O 55: B 5, and O 111: B 4, since it was considered that fresh isolates of these serotypes did not ferment sorbitol and therefore gave pale colonies on this medium whereas many other *Esch. coli* types fermented sorbitol and yielded red colonies; this distinction is by no means complete, and the only circumstance in which such a medium should be employed (in addition to the usual media) is in the search for further cases and carriers in an outbreak where the epidemic strain has been characterised fully and is a sorbitol non-fermenting strain.

Chemotherapy.—Since there is much variation in the sensitivity of *Esch. coli* strains to the commonly employed agents, chemotherapy should whenever possible be guided by an in vitro assessment of the sensitivity of the particular strain. It should be noted that the presence of pathological changes *e.g.* renal stone, bladder diverticulum, hypertrophied prostate, may prevent the eradication of *Esch. coli* from the urinary tract even although the infection is treated with a chemotherapeutic agent to which the strain is highly sensitive.

Prophylaxis.—The prevention of infection by *Esch. coli* in wounds, etc., and in exogenously acquired urinary infections depends upon the provision of properly sterilised dressings and instruments, thorough debridement of wounds and preparation of patients and attendants before operation or wound-dressing.

The measures taken to prevent the spread of gastro-enteritis are those applicable in other types of bowel infection. The preparation of feeds and cleansing and sterilisation of feeding-bottles demands constant care and attention (Report, 1953); the mother must be instructed in personal cleanliness and urged to wash her hands before preparing a feed. Whenever possible, each feed should be prepared immediately before it is required, and if storage of prepared feeds is unavoidable the container should be carefully wrapped to prevent accidental contamination and unnecessary handling. Some form of terminal heat-treatment of feeds for babies in hospital is to be recommended.

PROTEUS

Members of the genus *Proteus* are widely distributed throughout man's environment and can be detected in sewage, soil and on garden vegetables. They are found in the faeces of higher animals and man, and may be present in large numbers following bowel infections; their relationship to various disease processes is dealt with later.

Morphology and Staining.—Gram-negative bacilli; 1·5–3 μ by 0·5 μ (average) but displaying pleomorphism; motile with numerous peritrichous flagella; non-sporing and non-capsulate. Most strains are fimbriate.

Cultural Characters.—Aerobe and facultative anaerobe; grows well at 37° C. on ordinary media. A strong seminal odour is often noticeable. Characteristically, discrete colonies are seen only in the earliest stages of incubation, thereafter a thin film of growth extends round the colony and rapidly spreads all over the available surface of the medium; during this spreading or swarming phase, the bacilli are characteristically long and slender and these are replaced by short forms when the surface of the medium has been covered.

Swarming tends to occur in successive waves so that ultimately a plate inoculated at one central point shows a series of concentric rings of thick growth between which there are smooth translucent areas of spreading growth. Swarming is associated with active motility although its cause is not clearly established; non-motile variants do not spread.

Biochemical Reactions.—All members of the genus ferment glucose but have no action on lactose; four biochemical types can be recognised as indicated in the table.

Substrate	*Pr. vulgaris*	*Pr. mirabilis*	*Pr. morganii*	*Pr. rettgeri*
Mannitol	−	−	−	⊥ or +
Maltose	+	−	−	−
Gelatin	+	+	−	−
Indole	+	−	+	+
Citrate	−	−	−	+

Key: Fermentation reactions; + = acid and gas; ⊥ = acid only; − = negative
Other reactions: + = liquefaction of gelatin, production of indole or growth in citrate medium.

It should be noted that, with the exception of *Pr. rettgeri*, all species usually produce gas; strains of *Pr. rettgeri* are frequently anaerogenic.

The ability of proteus strains to decompose urea rapidly has been used as a test to differentiate them from other enterobacteriaceae; urease activity is also displayed by most klebsiella strains and by some strains of escherichia and citrobacter species. Whilst the absence of urease activity in salmonellae and shigellae allows their distinction from Proteus for diagnostic purposes, a more useful and more specific test is the ability of proteus to transform phenylalanine to phenylpyruvic acid; no other members of the family *Enterobacteriaceae* possess such activity (Henriksen, 1950).

The phenylpyruvic acid (PPA) reaction. This is performed as follows:

To 0·5 ml. of a dense suspension (10^{11} organisms per ml.) of organisms add 0·5 ml. of 0·2 per cent. DL-phenylalanine in saline; add 1 drop of 0·01 per cent. phenol red and make alkaline with 0·1 M Na_2CO_3. Shake vigorously and incubate the tube in an almost horizontal position; after four hours add 10 per cent.

H_2SO_4 until the colour changes from yellow to pink. Add sufficient $(NH_4)_2 SO_4$ to saturate the solution and then 5 drops of half-saturated $FeNH_4(SO_4)_2$. Shake thoroughly and read the results after one minute. Positive reactions are designated + to + + +, depending on the intensity of green colouration developing in the fluid.

Antigenic Characters.—A diagnostic antigenic schema for *Pr. vulgaris* and *Pr. mirabilis* has been established and comprises 49 O groups, which can be subdivided on the basis of H antigens to allow 119 serotypes to be recognised. Similarly 57 serotypes of *Pr. morganii* and 45 serotypes of *Pr. rettgeri* have been recognised.

Much attention has been given to the agglutination of certain proteus types by the blood serum of cases of typhus fever. This reaction is employed as a diagnostic test (Weil-Felix reaction); the *Proteus* strain X 19 which is employed in the reaction is biochemically *Pr. vulgaris* and the reaction is dependent on the specific O antigen present in this strain, which has no aetiological relationship to the disease. The Weil-Felix reaction is explained on the basis of a common antigen shared by *Proteus X* 19 and the rickettsiae of typhus fever (p. 490).

Another proteus type designated XK (biochemically *Pr. mirabilis*) is agglutinated by the serum of patients suffering from the disease "Scrub typhus", occurring in South-east Asia and the Far East. A diagnostic agglutination test similar to the Weil-Felix reaction is based on this antigenic relationship.

Occurrence.—The majority of strains isolated from pathological specimens and human faeces are biochemically typical of *Pr. mirabilis.* The specific relationship of *Pr. morganii* to summer diarrhoea of infants is still in doubt, but it is recognised that, along with other proteus species, this organism is often a concomitant of shigellae, making its appearance in the stools as the case improves and the dysentery bacilli become scanty. Secondary infection of wounds, bed-sores, etc., is probably endogenous in origin; although such a source may account for cases of cystitis in which proteus is incriminated, there are many instances in which exogenous infection takes place following diagnostic or therapeutic instrumentation.

Laboratory Diagnosis

The spreading growth of proteus strains on media such as blood-agar is sufficient for identification in routine diagnostic work; the disadvantage of this characteristic is that other organisms when present may be completely overgrown by the spreading growth and their subcultivation for purposes of identification and antibiotic sensitivity testing delayed. Swarming may be inhibited by several methods; discrete colonies of proteus can be obtained on a blood-agar medium by increasing the agar concentration to 4 per cent.; similarly, inhibition of swarming may be obtained by incorporating chloral hydrate (1 in 500), sodium azide (1 in 5000) or one of the sulphonamide drugs (Holman, 1957). Desoxycholate-citrate agar inhibits swarming and, provided that the other organisms present are capable of growing on this medium, its use in allowing separation from *Proteus* species is valuable.

If necessary, the biochemical type of a proteus strain can be determined as indicated in the table (p. 253).

Chemotherapy.—Proteus infections, *e.g.* of the urinary tract, may respond to treatment with chloramphenicol, streptomycin and the tetracyclines; chemotherapy should whenever possible be guided by in vitro sensitivity tests, since strains vary markedly. As in the case of *Esch. coli* infections, structural or pathological abnormalities impede the eradication of organisms and in many instances, although the original infecting organism is eradicated, there is often replacement with some other species.

Providencia (*Proteus inconstans*)

These Gram-negative, motile bacilli are closely allied to the genus *Proteus*; they alone among the *Enterobacteriaceae* share with *Proteus* species the ability to deaminate phenylalanine although only rarely do Providence strains decompose urea, and they never exhibit spreading on ordinary agar. They occur in normal faeces and in urinary tract infections. Providence cultures may be allocated to one of two biochemical groups depending on their ability to produce gas from glucose and their action on substrates such as adonitol and inositol.

For details of biochemical and serological characteristics of this group the publication of Ewing *et al.* (1954) should be consulted.

REFERENCES

BRAY, J. (1945). Isolation of antigenically homogeneous strains of *Bact. coli neapolitanum* from summer diarrhoea of infants. *J. Path. Bact.*, **57**, 239.

EWING, W. H., TANNER, K. E. & DENNARD, D. A. (1954). The Providence group: an intermediate group of enteric bacteria. *J. infect. Dis.*, **94**, 134.

FERGUSON, W. W. & JUNE, R. C. (1952). Experiments on feeding adult volunteers with *Escherichia coli* 111, B4, a coliform organism associated with infant diarrhoea. *Amer. J. Hyg.*, **55**, 155.

HENRIKSEN, S. D. (1950). A comparison of the phenyl-pyruvic acid reaction and the urease test in the differentiation of Proteus from other enteric organisms. *J. Bact.*, **60**, 225.

HOLMAN, R. A. (1957). The use of sulphonamides to inhibit the swarming of *Proteus*. *J. Path. Bact.*, **73**, 91.

JUNE, R. C., FERGUSON, W. W. & WORFEL, M. T. (1953). Experiments on feeding adult volunteers with *Escherichia coli* 55, B5, a coliform organism associated with infant diarrhoea. *Amer. J. Hyg.*, **57**, 222.

MCNAUGHT, W. & STEVENSON, J. S. (1953). Coliform diarrhoea in adult hospital patients. *Brit. med. J.*, **2**, 182.

RAPPAPORT, F. & HENIG, E. (1952). Media for the isolation and identification of pathogenic *Escherichia coli* (serotypes O 111 and O 55). *J. clin. Path.*, **5**, 361.

REPORT (1953). The cleaning and sterilisation of infant feeding bottles and teats. *Mth. Bull. Minist. Hlth Lab. Serv.*, **12**, 214.

SEARS, H. J., BROWNLEE, I. & UCHIYAMA, J. K. (1950). Persistence of individual strains of *Escherichia coli* in the intestinal tract of man. *J. Bact.*, **59**, 293.

VAHLNE, G. (1945). *Serological Typing of the Colon Bacteria.* Lund, Gleerupska Univ. Bokhandeln.

WALLICK, H. & STUART, C. A. (1943). Antigenic relationships of *Escherichis coli* isolated from one individual. *J. Bact.*, **45**, 121.

WRAMBY, G. (1948). *Investigations into the Antigenic Structure of Bact. coli Isolated from Calves.* Uppsala: Appelbergs Boktryckericktielbolag.

CHAPTER 19

OTHER ENTEROBACTERIACEAE

The Alkalescens-Dispar Group

In Chapter 16 it was stated that, although a classification of Enterobacteriaceae was essential for practical purposes of diagnosis and epidemiological studies, the biochemical and serological interrelationships of members of the family do not allow all cultures to be assigned to one or other genus. The close relationship of many Arizona strains to Salmonella is paralleled in the case of the Alkalescens-Dispar (A-D) group whose members bear close resemblances, both biochemical and serological, to Escherichia ; apart from their lack of flagella and motility and their failure to produce gas in fermentation reactions, strains of the A-D group behave very similarly to Escherichia strains.

It has been shown also that the O antigens of the A-D group are either identical with or bear strong relationships to Escherichia O antigens (Frantzen, 1951); similar findings have been made with regard to the K antigens in the two groups.

Because of this very close similarity it has been recommended that any future cultures with the characters of the A-D group should be classified as anaerogenic *Esch. coli*; thus the A-D group will not be extended beyond its present limits.

The first description of these organisms was in 1918 (Andrewes, 1918) and their relationship to cases of bacillary dysentery was mooted; both Alkalescens (lactose non-fermenting or late fermenting) and Dispar (lactose-fermenting) strains occur in normal faeces and their presence in cases of enteritis (in which recognised bacterial pathogens cannot be found) is regarded as incidental.

Citrobacter freundii (Escherichia freundii) (including the Bethesda-Ballerup group)

Members of this group can utilise citrate and produce H_2S; a further feature distinguishing them from *Esch. coli* is their ability to grow in Moeller's KCN medium. Indeed the Citrobacter group are much more closely allied, biochemically, with Salmonella and Arizona, although the inability of the latter group to grow in KCN medium is a valuable differential feature. Although certain members have been suspected of causing enteric infections, their aetiologic relationship remains to be established. At present the importance of *Cit. freundii* species lies in the fact that many indole negative strains attack lactose slowly, if at all, so that their colonies resemble those of salmonellae and shigellae. Their motility, however, rapidly resolves any confusion with shigella strains, but many bear a close resemblance to salmonellae on biochemical testing; these are the members which comprise the

Bethesda-Ballerup group and they have been studied more intensively than other *Cit. freundii* species which attack lactose promptly.

False-positive reports of salmonella isolations and the delay in issuing negative reports attending the establishment of identity of lactose non-fermenting *Cit. freundii* strains can be eliminated by using the KCN test; salmonellae fail to grow in this medium whilst *Cit. freundii* cultures flourish.

Certain extra-generic relationships are recognised with O antigens of Salmonella and Arizona serotypes, but these need not occasion any great difficulty in identification; reference to Kauffmann's (1954) monograph should be made regarding the serological characteristics of these organisms. The fact that the Vi antigen of *S. typhi* is identical with that of a Ballerup strain has already been noted.

The Genus Klebsiella

Members of this genus conform to the definition of the family Enterobacteriaceae and are, without exception, non-motile. They differ from the groups already described in this chapter by generally giving a positive Voges-Proskauer reaction and a negative methyl-red reaction. The genus includes strains of parasitic and saprophytic origin, some of which are given species designation while others are characterised solely by their antigenic formulae.

Klebsiella aerogenes (*Aerobacter aerogenes*)

Morphology and Staining.—Gram-negative bacillus varying greatly in size—1–4 μ by 0·5–1 μ. Non-motile and non-sporing. Most strains are fimbriate. Capsulate both in the tissues and in artificial culture and produce an abundance of extracellular slime so that their colonies are mucoid or viscid.

Cultural characteristics.—Colonies are large, raised and viscid; on MacConkey's medium the majority of colonies are pink due to fermentation of lactose.

Biochemical reactions.—In addition to the characters listed on p. 249, strains usually produce gas in lactose and sucrose. Characteristically, strains hydrolyse urea but not with the rapidity or intensity displayed by Proteus strains; their lack of motility and inability to deaminate phenylalanine serve to differentiate them from Proteus. A detailed account of biochemical reactions can be found in the publication by Edwards and Ewing (1962).

Antigenic characteristics.—All smooth forms of *Kl. aerogenes* possess O antigens; in addition, capsulate, non-mucoid smooth forms possess a K antigen; non-capsulate, mucoid forms possess an M antigen, and mucoid and capsulate forms possess both an M and K antigen in addition to an O antigen. Similarly, rough forms may possess only R antigens, or in addition one or other or both M and K antigens. It has been shown that in any one strain, the M and K antigens are identical (Edwards and Fife, 1952; Wilkinson, Duguid and Edmunds, 1954); the frequent presence of these antigens and their masking of O and R somatic antigens dictates the use of capsular antisera in typing procedures. By this method the genus can be divided into at least 72 serotypes.

Occurrence.—The majority of isolations are from saprophytic sources such as water supplies. The commonest site in man from which klebsiella strains are isolated and fulfill a pathogenic role is in urinary tract infections; such strains are usually of capsular types 8, 9 and 10. Other strains occur as commensals in the intestinal tract of approximately 5 per cent. of healthy persons.

Four other species, *Kl. pneumoniae*, *Kl. edwardsii*, *Kl. rhinoscleromatis* and *Kl. ozaenae*, which are chiefly associated with respiratory-tract infections, may be distinguished biochemically from *Kl. aerogenes* (Cowan, Steel, Shaw & Duguid, 1960).

Klebsiella pneumoniae (*Friedländer's bacillus*)

This species is responsible for a small proportion (less than 1 per cent.) of bacterial pneumonias ; its importance lies in the high fatality (50 per cent. or more) among cases in which it occurs.

Kl. pneumoniae strains belong to serotype 3, ferment dulcitol, are fimbriate, and give negative Voges-Proskauer and positive methyl-red reactions.

Klebsiella edwardsii

This species belongs to serotypes 1 and 2, and differs from *Kl. pneumoniae* in being non-fimbriate and in failing to ferment dulcitol.

Klebsiella rhinoscleromatis

Cultures of this species belong to serotype 3. They are non-fimbriate and contrast biochemically with *Kl. aerogenes* in being anaerogenic, failing to ferment lactose, giving a negative V-P and positive M-R reaction and not utilising citrate. *Kl. rhinoscleromatis* is associated with a chronic granuloma, rhinoscleroma, which is prevalent in south-eastern Europe; the bacilli are situated intracellularly in the lesions which occur in the mucous membrane of the nose, throat and mouth.

Klebsiella ozaenae

Such strains are not confined to cases of ozaena so that its causal relationship to the condition is in doubt. Biochemically, *Kl. ozaenae* strains are intermediate between the *Klebsiella* species described above; they belong to capsule types 4, 5 and 6 and are mostly non-fimbriate.

Species	Glucose	Lactose	Dulcitol	V-P	M-R	Citrate
Kl. aerogenes	+	+	− or +	+	−	+
Kl. pneumoniae	+	+	+	−	+	+
Kl. edwardsii	+	late +	−	+	+	+
Kl. rhinoscleromatis	+	−	−	−	+	−
Kl. ozaenae	+	late +	−	−	+	+ or −

The Genus Cloaca

Consequent to the incorporation of *Aero. aerogenes* in the genus *Klebsiella* it was necessary to define the position of strains previously designated *Aerobacter cloacae*. This has been accomplished by resurrecting the genus *Cloaca*, of which *Cloaca cloacae* is the type species.

Members of this genus are microscopically indistinguishable from other Enterobacteriaceae; they are seldom capsulate and frequently motile, flagellate and fimbriate, and their ability to liquefy gelatin is a further characteristic assisting the differentiation from Klebsiella species.

More definitive studies, both biochemical and serological, are required to clarify interrelationships with other genera of Enterobacteriaceae. Members of the genus *Cloaca* are widely distributed in nature and are commonly encountered in water and grasses; they are occasionally isolated in small numbers from normal faeces but are not regarded as pathogenic for man or animals.

The Genus Hafnia

Members of this genus are probably non-pathogenic for man; their interest to medical bacteriologists lies in their ubiquity and similarity to other lactose non-fermenting Enterobacteriaceae. The temperature at which biochemical tests are performed with *Hafnia* strains has a marked effect on the results; tests of motility and for V-P and M-R reactions as well as various fermentation reactions are variable when performed at 37° C. whereas if these are carried out at 20–22° C. the results for any one test are uniform.

In addition to the reactions noted in the table (p. 249), it should be noted that *Hafnia* cultures invariably ferment glucose and mannitol with accompanying acid and gas production, give a positive KCN result but do not hydrolyze urea.

REFERENCES

ANDREWES, F. W. (1918). Dysentery bacilli: the differentiation of the true dysentery bacilli from allied species. *Lancet*, **1**, 560.

COWAN, S. T., STEEL, K. J., SHAW, CONSTANCE & DUGUID, J. P. (1960). A classification of the klebsiella group. *J. gen. Microbiol.*, **23**, 601.

EDWARDS, P. R. & EWING, W. H. (1962). *Identification of Enterobacteriaceae*, 2nd Ed., Minneapolis: Burgess.

EDWARDS, P. R. & FIFE, M. A. (1952). Capsule types of *Klebsiella*. *J. infect. Dis.* **91**, 92.

FRANTZEN, E. (1951). *Biochemical and serological studies of the Akalescens—Dispar, Group*, Copenhagen: Munksgaard.

KAUFFMANN, F. (1954). *Enterobacteriaceae*. 2nd Ed., Copenhagen: Einer Munksgaard.

WILKINSON, J. F., DUGUID, J. P. & EDMUNDS, P. N. (1954). The distribution of polysaccharide production in *Aerobacter* and *Escherichia* strains and its relation to antigenic character. *J. gen. Microbiol.*, **11**, 59.

CHAPTER 20

PSEUDOMONAS: LOEFFLERELLA

PSEUDOMONAS

THE genus *Pseudomonas* comprises more than 140 species but only one, *Pseudomonas pyocyanea*, is pathogenic to man. The other species are either saprophytic in water and soil or are pathogenic for plants or less commonly for animals.

Pseudomonas pyocyanea

(*Ps. aeruginosa*)

Morphology and Staining.—A Gram-negative, non-sporing bacillus, measuring 1·5 μ by 0·5 μ, actively motile by virtue of polar flagella which rarely number more than three; many strains are monotrichous; non-capsulate; some strains are fimbriate.

Cultural characters.—Essentially aerobic but a few strains grow, although poorly, under anaerobic conditions. Temperature range, 5°–43° C.; optimum 37° C. Grows on ordinary media, producing a musty odour like trimethylamine.

Colonies on Agar.—Stroke inoculation produces an abundant, moist greenish-blue fluorescent growth; the pigments (pyocyanin and fluorescin), on which the colour depends, also diffuse through the medium and are most abundantly produced at room temperature. Individual colonies are large, low-convex, with an irregular spreading edge which is translucent compared with the dark, greyish centre. Colonies on MacConkey's medium—similar to growth on agar; colonies are pale since lactose is not fermented. Some strains give a brown pigmented growth when a third pigment, pyorubrin, is produced; a minority of strains appear to be incapable of any pigment production.

Biochemical Reactions.—Acid is produced oxidatively from glucose; none of the other commonly employed sugars is utilised by *Ps. pyocyanea*. Gelatin is rapidly liquefied by the majority of strains: growth occurs in inorganic media with citrate as the sole carbon source. Indole and H_2S are not produced and the Voges-Proskauer and methyl-red reactions are negative. In contrast with other common Gram-negative rods, *Ps. pyocyanea* gives a positive oxidase reaction; this fact can be used as a rapid identification test particularly in those strains which do not produce the characteristic pigments (Kovacs, 1956; Gaby & Hadley, 1957).

Antigenic characters.—Difficulty in differentiating between flagellar and somatic antigens has delayed the introduction of serotyping as a method of dividing the species for epidemiologic purposes; phage typing may be of value in recognising "types" of *Ps. pyocyanea* (Gould & McLeod, 1960). More recently a method of typing dependent on pyocine production, analogous to colicine typing of *Sh. sonnei*, has been found reliable in epidemiologic studies (Gillies & Govan, 1966).

Pathogenesis.—*Ps. pyocyanea* is frequently present, although in small numbers, in the normal intestinal flora of men and animals and thus can be isolated from sewage. It is also found on healthy human skin. As a pathogen it is usually associated with pyogenic cocci or with a member of the family *Enterobacteriaceae*. It is sometimes incriminated in urinary tract infections and is introduced by catheterisation or other diagnostic or therapeutic instrumentation; it is commonly found in infected wounds and burns and in chronic otitis media. Acute purulent meningitis may follow accidental introduction of the organism during lumbar puncture or after cranial injury.

Infection is usually localised but in infants or debilitated persons it may invade the blood stream and give rise to fatal generalised infection; this risk is greater in persons receiving antineoplastic drugs or in radiation therapy.

Animal pathogenicity.—Subcutaneous injection in rabbits, guinea-pigs and mice produces fever and local abscess formation. Death is associated with the intravenous injection of large doses in these animals.

Chemotherapy.—This organism has vied with members of the genus Proteus in its resistance to antimicrobial agents; some strains are sensitive to streptomycin and chloramphenicol; however the polymyxins seem at present to be the agents of choice. Colistin methane sulphonate ("Colomycin") is particularly effective (McMillan *et al.*, 1962).

LOEFFLERELLA

The genus *Loefflerella* comprises for medical purposes two species, *Loefflerella mallei* and *Loefflerella pseudomallei*; both species are essentially parasitic on animals and only occasionally pathogenic to man.

Loefflerella mallei

(*Actinobacillus mallei*)

The causal organism of glanders, a disease of equines which has been eradicated from Britain but still occurs in Eastern Europe and various parts of Asia. In horses, two types of lesion occur and are named "glanders" proper and "farcy". In glanders, nodule formation starts in the nasal septum and adjacent parts and is attended by profuse catarrhal discharge; ultimately, the nodules break down and give rise to irregular ulcerations. The term "farcy" is applied to the affection of superficial lymph vessels and glands seen especially when infection has occurred through the skin, frequently via abrasions from the rubbing of the harness; the lymph vessels become irregularly thickened and corded and are spoken of as "farcy pipes". The disease may occur in man as a result of direct inoculation of a skin abrasion or wound by discharges from an infected animal.

Morphology and Staining.—A slender, straight or slightly curved bacillus with rounded ends, 1·5–4 μ by 0·4 μ. Pleomorphic and involution forms occur in old cultures. Gram-negative, non-motile and non-sporing. In the tissues it often stains irregularly with a beaded appearance.

Cultural Characters.—Aerobic and facultatively anaerobic; temperature range 20°–44° C. with an optimum of 37° C. Grows on ordinary media containing serum or blood; colonies are approximately 1 mm. in diameter after 24–48 hr., white in colour, semi-transparent and later became more opaque and yellowish. Colonies are often viscid. Difficult to isolate in primary culture although adjustment of culture media to a slightly acid reaction (pH 6·6) enhances growth.

Pathogenesis and Epidemiology.—Glanders is an infective granuloma with a marked tendency to suppuration. It is essentially a disease of horses, asses and mules, and is only occasionally transmitted to man, usually by direct infection from an animal source. Under natural conditions the usual mode of transmission appears to be ingestion but infection by inhalation can also occur. Carnivora in captivity may become infected from feeding on the carcases of infected animals.

In acute and subacute glanders in animals, ulcerating nodules occur in the nasal mucosa and later in the lungs and internal organs. The bacilli are present in considerable numbers in all lesions, situated for the most part extracellularly. Latent infections are not infrequent in animals and have also been observed in the human subject.

In human glanders, the infection usually originates in the skin (e.g. wound, abrasion, etc.), more rarely in the mucosa of the mouth or nose. The bacilli are found in the local inflammatory lesion and spread via the lymphatics, producing an acute lymphangitis. Ultimately a pyaemic condition results with secondary foci in which the bacilli are numerous.

Experimental Inoculation.—Guinea-pigs are markedly susceptible, and after subcutaneous injection die in a week or two with generalised lesions, as in acute animal glanders. If a male guinea-pig is inoculated intraperitoneally, the tunica vaginalis is rapidly invaded, and, externally, swelling of the testis is noted (Straus reaction).

Laboratory Diagnosis.—Films are prepared from the pus, discharge from sores, etc., or from nodules in internal organs, found at post-mortem examination; these are stained with methylene blue and by Gram's method. The appearance of beaded Gram-negative organisms corresponding to the glanders bacillus is suggestive.

Cultures are made on a Löffler serum slope and on blood agar; if a mixed growth results, pure cultures are obtained from single colonies.

In all cases the nature of the infection must be confirmed by animal inoculation. A male guinea-pig is injected intraperitoneally with the pathological material or the isolated culture; in two to three days an enlargement of the testis results, and the animal subsequently dies, showing the lesion of acute glanders. If the inoculum contains a large number of other organisms, it may be introduced by subcutaneous injection. The organism can then be recovered from the enlarged regional glands and tested further by intraperitoneal injection of pure cultures.

Agglutination and complement-fixation tests can also be used in the diagnosis of glanders in horses.

Mallein is a preparation from the glanders bacillus analogous to tuberculin; when inoculated into the skin or subcutaneously a positive delayed reaction has proved to be of value in the diagnosis of infection, particularly in horses.

Loefflerella pseudomallei

(*Bacillus whitmori*; *Pseudomonas pseudomallei*)

This is the causative organism of Melioidosis—a glanders-like disease occurring in Indo-China, India, Malaysia and parts of the East Indies; a few cases have also been described in the United States. The disease occurs as an epizootic among rodents; rats seem to be the most important source of the infection in man, and the contamination of food with their excreta may be an important method of transmission. Experimentally the disease can be transmitted by the rat-flea.

The organism is similar to the glanders bacillus but is motile and grows well in gelatin at 20° C., liquefying the medium. The flagella are polar and 1–4 in number. Growth on agar may be mucoid or dry and corrugated, and on potato a brown coloured growth similar to that of *Loeff. mallei* is produced. Other distinguishing features are that *Loeff. pseudomallei* is oxidase positive, grows on MacConkey's medium and does not produce H_2S. Susceptible animals such as the guinea-pig and white rat may be infected experimentally, and a Straus reaction occurs in the male animal similar to that produced by *Loeff. mallei*. *Loeff. pseudomallei* is serologically distinct from *Loeff. mallei*. The organism is resistant to high concentrations of penicillin, streptomycin, chlortetracycline and chloramphenicol.

Ordinarily the disease develops in man as an acute pulmonary infection followed by blood-spread to the viscera, the development of miliary abscesses and death. There are relatively few cases of chronic melioidosis described, and most of these have survived what was probably an acute phase of the disease. Other cases are pyaemic with cutaneous eruptions which may last for two to three months before death.

REFERENCES

Gaby, W. L. & Hadley, C. (1957.) Practical laboratory test for the identification of *Pseudomonas aeruginosa*. *J. Bact.*, **74**, 356.

Gillies, R. R. & Govan, J. R. W. (1966). Typing of *Pseudomonas pyocyanea* by pyocine production. *J. Path. Bact.*, **91**, 339.

Gould, J. C. & McLeod, J. W. (1960). A study of the use of agglutinating sera and phage lysis in the classification of strains of *Pseudomonas aeruginosa*. *J. Path. Bact.*, **79**, 295.

Kovacs, N. (1956). Identification of *Pseudomonas pyocyanea* by the Oxidase Reaction. *Nature* (Lond.), **178**, 703.

McMillan, M., Price, T. M. L., MacLaren, D. M. & Scott, G. W. (1962). *Pseudomonas pyocyanea* infection treated with colistin methane sulphonate. *Lancet*, **2**, 737.

CHAPTER 21

CHOLERA VIBRIO AND ALLIED ORGANISMS

VIBRIO CHOLERAE (V. COMMA)

Vibrio cholerae, or the comma bacillus, is the causative organism of Asiatic Cholera, a disease now more restricted in incidence and distribution than formerly whereas infection with the El Tor variant is becoming widespread in Asian countries. It is characterised by an acute gastroenteritis of sudden onset and often running a rapid and fatal course, the patient becoming acutely dehydrated, acidotic and shocked within a few hours.

Morphology and Staining.—Curved or "comma-shaped" rod (vibrio) with rounded or slightly pointed ends, about 1·5–3 μ by 0·5 μ. In stained mucous flakes where the rods lie parallel, they have been likened to fish in a stream. The vibrio is actively motile, and the movement is of a "darting" type due to a single long terminal flagellum. In liquid cultures the vibrios occur singly, in pairs, or in chains end to end with the curves alternating, *i.e.* presenting a somewhat spiral arrangement. "S" forms and spirals representing elongated undivided single cells may be noted. Involution occurs readily, especially in culture, and globular, club-shaped or irregular forms may be observed. *V. cholerae* is Gram-negative and non-sporing.

When the organism has been growing in artificial culture for a time, the morphology becomes less typical and the curvature of the vibrios is less pronounced.

Cultural Characters.—Aerobe; slight growth also occurs under anaerobic conditions. Temperature range, 16°–40° C.; optimum, 37° C. Grows on ordinary media. An acid reaction is inhibitory, but abundant growth occurs on alkaline media; the optimum pH is about 8·2.

Colonies on agar (12-24 hours): moist, translucent, regular disks, 1–2 mm. in diameter, showing a characteristic bluish colour in transmitted light. Colonial variants include opaque, mucoid colonies, ring colonies, and rugose colonies with dry, corrugated appearance. S–R dissociation is not readily detected from colonial morphology alone.

Gelatin stab—at first there is a white line of growth along the track of the inoculating wire; then liquefaction occurs at the top and spreads downwards in funnel-shaped form.

Coagulated serum is liquefied.

Viability.—*V. cholerae* is killed at 56°C. within 30 min. It dies within two or three hours when subjected to drying. In stagnant water with an alkaline reaction the organism may survive for a considerable period, *e.g.* 5–10 days or longer, but it probably does not multiply to any extent in such waters. It is sensitive to sulphonamides, streptomycin, chloramphenicol and the tetracyclines.

Biochemical Reactions.—The fermentative reactions after 18-20 hours incubation are as follows:—

Glucose	*Lactose*	*Dulcitol*	*Sucrose*	*Mannitol*	*Maltose*	*Mannose*	*Arabinose*
⊥	–	–	⊥	⊥	⊥	⊥	–

(⊥ = acid; no gas)

Cholera-red reaction—this depends on the production of indole *and nitrites* and can be elicited by adding a few drops of sulphuric acid to a 24 hours' peptone water culture. A reddish-pink colour develops, due to the formation of nitroso-indole.

Haemolysis—the classical *V. cholerae* does not lyse sheep or goat red blood cells and thus differs from many other vibrios, including the El Tor vibrio, which also give a strong Voges-Proskauer reaction. Nonhaemolytic vibrios may, however, produce a greenish clearing in blood-agar media, due probably to a chemical alteration of the haemoglobin.

The original test for haemolysin (the Greig test) was carried out by using mixtures of 72–hour alkaline broth cultures and 5 per cent. washed goat erythrocytes incubated for 2 hours at 37°C and the result read after standing overnight in the refrigerator. Because of discrepant results with various modifications of the original test, Feeley and Pittman (1963) have recommended the following procedure in order to obtain more uniformity:—

0·5 ml. of a 24-hour heart infusion broth (commercial dehydrated medium, pH 7·4) culture (grown at 35° C. in a 16 mm. × 150 mm. tube containing 10 ml. of medium) is mixed with 0·5 ml. of 1 per cent. washed sheep cells. The mixture is incubated for two hours at 35°–37° C. and held overnight at 4° C., after which it is read for the presence of haemolysis.

Antigenic Characters.—For practical purposes the cholera vibrio may be regarded as a homogeneous species, and unknown strains can be identified by testing their agglutination reaction with an antiserum for a known *V. cholerae*.

The organism possesses both H and O antigens. The H antigen may be shared with certain other vibrios, though these organisms are distinct as regards their O antigens and are sometimes called non-agglutinating vibrios. This serological difference is best demonstrated with bacterial suspensions made up in plain saline solution (without formalin). The El Tor strains (p. 269) possess the same H and O antigens as the classical cholera vibrio.

Within the serological subgroup represented by the classical *V. cholerae* and with a common O antigen, serological types can be recognised, distinguished by agglutinin-absorption tests with O antisera; this difference depends on a subsidiary O antigenic component characteristic of the type. Two such types have been recognised and designated according to the names of standard strains "Inaba" and "Ogawa". It is possible that a third type, "Hikojima", also exists, possessing the characteristic components of both the above-mentioned types.

Transformation of a *V. cholerae* strain to the "rough" form is associated with loss of the specific O antigen.

Pathogenesis.—Typical cholera is an acute disease of sudden onset characterised by profuse watery diarrhoea, vomiting, muscular cramps and extreme collapse.

The vibrios multiply freely in the lumen of the small intestine and are present in large numbers in the intestinal contents and dejecta. The stools contain many white flakes consisting mostly of mucus and some epithelial cells—the "rice water" stool. The organism does not penetrate deeply in the bowel wall and practically never invades the blood stream. The gall-bladder may be infected.

The older concept that the profuse diarrhoea was related to a transudate of fluid through a denuded intestinal mucosa does not seem to be tenable since (*a*) biopsies of the bowel epithelium of affected patients show an intact mucosa; (*b*) the bacteria-free cholera stools contain less than 0·1 gm. of protein per 100 ml. of fluid, whereas a transudate would contain 20 times that amount; and (*c*) when iodine-tagged polyvinyl pyrrolidone (PVP) was injected intravenously in cholera patients there was no greater PVP content in their stools than in those of control cases.

Studies by Phillips and others (see Phillips, 1963) on the pathophysiology of cholera indicate that the fluid loss is isotonic and that there is excess loss of bicarbonate and potassium so that rehydration should be effected by intravenous normal saline and bicarbonate solutions (added separately) in the ratio of 3: 1. It has been postulated that the excess loss of fluid from the bowel is due to a metabolite of the cholera vibrio which acts as an inhibitor of the transport of sodium ions by the intestinal mucosal cells—the so-called "sodium pump." A thermolabile inhibitor has been demonstrated in cholera stools.

Experimental infection with *V. cholerae* may be produced in baby rabbits (10-12 days old) following either oral adminstration or injection of a small dose into the lumen of the small bowel. Profuse diarrhoea with dehydration and death follows a short incubation period of 12-18 hours (Dutta and Habbu, 1955).

Injection of a culture of *V. cholerae* into isolated loops of the small bowel in adult rabbits or guinea-pigs causes a rapid outpouring of fluid into the loop followed by haemorrhagic necrosis of the bowel epithelium (De and Chatterjee, 1953).

Epidemiology.—The Bengal basin, with the deltas of the Ganges and Brahmaputra rivers, is nowadays the principal area where cholera exists endemically throughout the year.

During the nineteenth century, pandemics of cholera spread east and west from this endemic area and involved many countries in Asia, Europe, Africa and America. In the present century there has been a steady contraction in the affected area until only India and East Pakistan have had annual epidemics, although outbreaks have occurred in recent years in Egypt (1947), Thailand (1958-59) and Nepal (1958). Then, in 1961, cholera due to the El Tor vibrio, which had been confined to endemic foci in the Celebes, began to spread to other parts of Indonesia and in the past few years outbreaks have occurred in Hong Kong,

Macao, the Philippines, Korea, S.E. Asia and the Middle East. Clinically, infection due to the El Tor vibrio is indistinguishable from cholera due to *V. cholerae*; epidemiologically, although outbreaks may be less explosive, it has similarities in its attack on under-nourished people living under insanitary conditions; the same quarantine regulations and control measures are applicable.

In the Bengal basin the maintenance of endemic foci of classical cholera probably depends on case-to-case infection in an insanitary environment. The infection flares up and becomes epidemic in the early spring, reaching a peak in Bengal in April–May just before the monsoon season. Spread of infection is probably facilitated by the large water-storage tanks which are used as laundry, bathing pool, etc. as well as water-supply. The alkaline reaction of these tanks favours survival of *V. cholerae.* Extension of cholera inland from the endemic area depends on human movement and large outbreaks have been associated with fairs and religious festivals. Contamination of water supplies by cases is the greatest single source of epidemic spread, but case-to-case infection by contamination of fomites, food, etc., presumably occurs. Transient carriage during convalescence may continue for one to three weeks or longer and symptomless contact carriers occur but chronic carriers are very rare.

Bacteriophage typing.—Recently Mukerjee (1963b) has introduced a system of classifying *V. cholerae* strains into five types (1–5) according to their susceptibility to four groups (I–IV) of freshly isolated choleraphages. This typing method has obvious epidemiological uses in tracing the epidemic spread of cholera; unfortunately, most of the strains of *V. cholerae* in West Bengal belong to only two types (1 and 3).

Laboratory Diagnosis

In a wet preparation of the liquid stool, examined under dark-ground illumination, the vibrios may be seen darting about like a "swarm of gnats." They are quickly immobilised by the addition of the specific antiserum and with this technique, a rapid diagnosis can be made in over 80 per cent of the acute cases (Benenson, personal communication).

Where there may be delay in the transmission of stools to a laboratory for examination, a preserving fluid has been found valuable in maintaining the viability of the vibrio and preventing overgrowth by other organisms.

Preserving Fluid.—Prepare the stock solution as follows:—Dissolve 12·405 grams boric acid and 14·912 grams potassium chloride in 800 ml. hot distilled water; after cooling make up the volume to a litre with distilled water. To 250 ml. of this stock add 133·5 ml. 0·2 *M* sodium hydroxide, make up the volume with distilled water to a litre, and add 200 grams dried sea-salt (*vide infra*). Filter the solution through paper, distribute in 10 ml. amounts in screw-capped bottles and autoclave. The final pH should be 9·2. Emulsify 1 to 3 grams of the stool in 10 ml. of the preserving fluid. The following mixture may be substituted for sea-salt: NaCl 27 grams, KCl 1 gram, $MgCl_2,6H_2O$ 3 grams, $MgSO_4,7H_2O$ 1·75 grams.

Cultural Methods.—(*a*) A plate of tellurite-gelatin-agar (Monsur's medium, Chapter 47) is inoculated directly from the stool, and incubated for 18–24 hours. This medium is highly selective for vibrios, inhibiting the growth of most other intestinal bacteria. Alkaline nutrient agar (pH 8·2) may also be used and gives successful results.

(*b*) At the same time a tube of peptone water is inoculated with a mucus flake from the stool, or, in the case of a fluid faecal stool, with a large loopful of the specimen. The peptone water used contains 1 per cent. peptone with 0·5 per cent. sodium chloride, standardised to pH 9·0. The tube is incubated for six to eight hours. Within this time vibrios, if present, grow freely and at the surface of the medium, and even outgrow other intestinal bacteria.

The peptone water culture is examined by means of a stained film made from a drop of the surface layer of the culture: a large loopful is placed on a slide and, without spreading, slowly dried at room temperature; the film is then fixed by heat, and washed in a stream of water to remove the dried peptone particles which stain deeply and obscure the organisms; the preparation is stained with dilute carbol fuchsin for one minute and examined microscopically. At the same time a hanging-drop preparation may be examined; at the edge of the drop, vibrios are easily detected by their characteristic morphology and darting motility. If vibros are present, a sub-inoculation is made on the selective culture medium. If no vibrios are detected, a sub-inoculation is made into a second peptone water tube; this tube is incubated for six to eight hours, and film from it is then examined as in the case of the primary culture. If no vibrios are detectable in the second peptone water culture the result may be regarded as negative.

Pure cultures are tested for the fermentation of lactose, sucrose, mannose and arabinose, the VP reaction and haemolysis. Finally, a specific O-antiserum is used for the agglutination test. An otherwise typical strain that does not agglutinate in the specific serum should be tested with an antiserum for rough vibrios. Inaba and Ogawa types are diagnosed by absorbed monospecific sera. Differentiation from the El Tor vibrio depends on haemolysin production, VP reaction, phage sensitivity and other tests (*vide infra*).

Isolation of Vibrio cholerae from Water.—100 ml. of a sterile alkaline (pH 9·0) 10 per cent. solution of peptone containing 5 per cent. sodium chloride are added to 900 ml. of the water specimen, which is then distributed in sterile stoppered flasks or bottles. These are incubated, and sub-inoculations are made (from the surface growths) on a selective medium after 24 and 48 hours, as in the method described for the isolation of *V. cholerae.* A larger quantity of water may be tested by filtering it through a Seitz disk or membrane filter and by using the disk as the inoculum for a peptone water culture.

Prophylaxis.—Cholera vaccine has been used in the prophylaxis of the disease. The vaccine may be prepared from a 24-hour culture on nutrient agar, the bacterial suspension being killed by heat and standardised to 8000 million organisms/ml. Two doses each of 1·0 ml. are given at an interval of 1 to 4 weeks; protection is believed to last for four to six months. The establishment and maintenance of purified water supplies which are free from the risk of contamination by cases or carriers eliminates the greatest single mode of spread of this disease. As a temporary expedient, wells and storage tanks may be treated with hypochlorite or other chlorine derivative. In the absence of a safe supply, all water for personal and culinary use must be boiled. Mineral waters and ice supplies must be carefully supervised. The rapid elimination of vibrios from the stools of cases treated with a suitable antimicrobial drug *e.g.* tetracycline reduces the duration of infectivity and such treatment may help to diminish community spread.

El Tor Vibrio

The El Tor vibrio was first isolated from unaffected pilgrims returning from Mecca and although it resembles *V. cholerae* in its cultural, biochemical and serological characters, it was originally regarded as a non-pathogenic variant because it was detected frequently in water and, like other water vibrios, gives a positive Voges-Proskauer reaction. Then it became known that localised outbreaks of cholera due to an organism of the El Tor type were occurring in Celebes and when infection began to spread more widely the pathogenicity of this vibrio was accepted. Its main differences from *V. cholerae* are (1) the production of haemolysin although this property may be inapparent on primary cultures and persistently non-haemolytic variants do occur; (2) all strains are resistant to most cholera phages and in particular to cholera phage IV to which classical *V. cholerae* is always susceptible (Mukerjee, 1963a); (3) El Tor strains always agglutinate fowl cells whereas freshly isolated *V. cholerae* does not; (4) El Tor strains give a positive V-P reaction. Other reported differences like suspension instability are not absolute.

Other Vibrios

Certain species of Gram-negative vibrio have been described in diseases of animals, e.g. *V. fetus*, *V. jejuni*, *V. coli* and *V. metchnikovi*.

V. fetus occurs in abortion of sheep and cattle, and can be isolated from the placenta and also from the foetus. The organism varies in length, the short forms being comma-shaped, the longer individuals exhibiting two to four coils. It is relatively slender and shows a flagellum at one or both ends. This organism is micro-aerophilic and has been cultivated on agar slopes in sealed tubes containing in the condensation water a few drops of sterile defibrinated horse blood. When first cultivated growth may only develop between the agar and the wall of the tube; after repeated subculturing a surface growth is obtained.

Under natural conditions cattle are infected during insemination; on the other hand, sheep are most probably infected from contaminated food and water supplies. Diagnosis depends on the isolation of the organism from the stomach contents of the aborted foetus or from uterine exudates. Non-pathogenic strains resembling *V. fetus* have been isolated from bovine genitalia, e.g. *Vibrio bubulus*; such strains are not to be confused with *V. fetus*, since unlike the latter they do not form catalase, they produce H_2S and are strict anaerobes.

Chemotherapy.—Streptomycin, chloramphenicol and the tetracyclines are of value and may also be used in the treatment and storage of bull semen.

V. jejuni has been described in an infectious diarrhoea ("winter dysentery") of cows in America. It is a Gram-negative vibrio with a flagellum at one or both poles and, although similar to *V. fetus* in other respects, it is serologically distinct.

V. coli, an organism closely resembling *V. fetus*, is causally related to a form of dysentery in young pigs.

V. metchnikovi was first isolated from a septicaemic disease of fowls. It resembles closely *V. cholerae* in general biological characters, but differs serologically, and in its high virulence for guinea-pigs, pigeons and fowls: a minute amount of culture introduced intramuscularly or into a cutaneous wound produces in these animals a rapidly fatal septicaemia.

Various other vibrios have also been described. These are mostly water forms. In certain parts of India, vibrios are regularly present in unprotected wells and rivers. These may present some similarity to the cholera vibrio but are serologically distinct and they occur in areas where cholera is not endemic. Many of them correspond to the vibrios described in paracholera though such water vibrios are apparently non-pathogenic. Certain water vibrios exhibit in culture marked phosphorescence, e.g. *V. phosphorescens*. Vibrios have been isolated from a variety of other sources, *e.g.* from sputum (*V. sputigenus*), from cheese (*V. tyrogenus*), from intestinal contents in "Cholera nostras" (*V. proteus*—Finkler and Prior's spirillum), and from infections in fish.

SPIRILLUM MINUS

A causative organism of rat-bite fever. Though often described as a spirochaete, this organism conforms in its biological characters to those of a spirillum, and the name *Spirillum minus* is generally used.

It is a short spiral organism about 2–5 μ in length and relatively broad, with regular short coils numbering one for each micron of the length of the organism. Longer forms up to 10 μ may also be observed. This organism is very actively motile, showing darting movements like those of a vibrio. Movement is due to terminal flagella, which are variable in number—from one to seven at each pole. In moving, the organism itself remains rigid and shows no undulation. It can be demonstrated easily by dark-ground illumination in fresh preparations, in which its active movement is seen and its flagella are also observed. It is most readily stained by a Romanowsky stain (*e.g.* Leishman's), but can also be stained by the ordinary aniline dyes. The organism has probably never been cultivated successfully.

In rat-bite fever the spirillum may be demonstrated in the local lesion, the regional lymph glands, and even in the blood, either by direct microscopic methods (*vide supra*) or by animal inoculation. Guinea-pigs, white rats and mice are susceptible to infection: the spirilla appear in the peripheral blood and can be detected by dark-ground illumination. Guinea-pigs develop a progressive disease and die of the infection. The intra-peritoneal inoculation of human infective material in mice is followed by no sign of disease; spirilla appear in the blood after five to fourteen days, but always in very small numbers. If the spirillum cannot be detected microscopically in the local lesion, or if the original bite-wound has healed, an enlarged lymphatic gland may be punctured by means of a hypodermic syringe; "gland juice" is aspirated, and investigated by direct methods or animal inoculation.

Spirillum minus occurs naturally in wild rats and certain other wild rodents, producing a blood infection. Conditions similar to rat-bite fever have also been reported following the bites of cats and ferrets.

Pathogenesis.—It should be noted that at least two different specific infections may result from rat-bite and may be designated clinically "rat-bite fever", the condition due to *Spirillum minus* (described above) and that produced by *Streptobacillus moniliformis* (p. 292). The former presents a highly characteristic clinical syndrome: a relapsing febrile illness with a local inflammatory lesion, enlargement of regional lymph glands and a macular skin eruption, all these lesions fluctuating in parallel with the temperature. *Spirillum minus* has been demonstrated by direct examination in the local lesion and glands, and even in the blood of cases. Infection by *Streptobacillus moniliformis* is likewise an acute or subacute febrile condition and may be associated with a skin eruption (*e.g.* erythema multiforme), but involvement of joints, even resembling the polyarthritis of acute rheumatism, is a feature of this illness. It seems likely that the two conditions have been confused with one another in the past.

Spirillum minus infections respond to treatment with the tetracyclines and penicillin.

REFERENCES

DE, S. N. & CHATTERJEE, D. N. (1953). An experimental study of the mechanism of action of *Vibrio cholerae* on the intestinal mucous membrane. *J. Path. Bact.* **66**, 559.

DUTTA, N. K. & HABBU, M. K. (1955). Experimental cholera in infant rabbits: a method for chemotherapeutic investigation. *Brit. J. Pharmacol.*, **10**, 153.

FEELEY, J. C. & PITTMAN, M. (1963). Studies on the haemolytic activity of El Tor vibrios. *Bull. Wld. Hlth. Org.*, **28**, 347.

MUKERJEE, S. (1963a). The bacteriophage-susceptibility test in differentiating *Vibrio cholerae* and *Vibrio el tor*. *Bull. Wld. Hlth. Org.*, **28**, 333.

(1963b). Bacteriophage typing of cholera. *Ibid.*, 337.

PHILLIPS, R. A. (1963). The patho-physiology of cholera. *Bull. Wld. Hlth. Org.*, **28**, 297.

CHAPTER 22

PASTEURELLA

The genus *Pasteurella* constitutes a group of closely related, biochemically inactive, Gram-negative rods showing bipolar staining. Members of the genus are associated with plague in man and acute and chronic systemic infections in a wide variety of animals and birds. One of the first members to be studied was the bacillus of fowl cholera which Pasteur used in his early work on immunity.

PASTEURELLA PESTIS

This is the organism of Oriental Plague, which has been one of the major pestilences of the world, with rats as the main reservoir and the flea as the intermediary between rodent and man. Typically, the severe forms of illness (*Pestis major*) occur either as *bubonic* plague or as *pneumonic* plague. In these cases there is a sudden onset with high fever, great prostration and varying degrees of delirium, with usually an associated septicaemia. There is also an ambulatory form (*Pestis minor*) in which the patient is only mildly pyrexial, with some lymphadenitis and a vesicle or pustule at the site of the flea bite.

Morphology and Staining.—In its most characteristic form this organism is a short, oval bacillus with rounded ends—*i.e.* coccobacillary —about 1·5 μ by 0·7 μ, occurring singly and in pairs. In the tissues a typical capsule may be observed; in cultures grown at 37° C. capsular material can be demonstrated by means of India ink preparations, but it is not well-defined.

The organism is Gram-negative, and when stained with a weak stain (*e.g.* methylene blue) shows characteristic bipolar staining which is an important feature in identification.

In culture the plague bacillus is less typical. Longer forms are frequent, and polar staining is less obvious. Pleomorphism is marked especially in old cultures, and involution or degeneration forms are particularly noticeable. These are markedly enlarged, stain faintly and include globular, pear-shaped, elongated or irregular forms. In fact, the microscopic picture of an old culture often suggests that of a yeast or mould. Involution in culture can be hastened by the presence of 3 per cent. sodium chloride, and this has sometimes been utilised in identifying the organism.

In fluid culture the bacilli tend to be arranged in chains.

The organism is non-motile and non-sporing.

Cultural Characters.—*P. pestis* grows aerobically and anaerobically on ordinary culture medium. The optimum temperature of the plague bacillus, unlike most other pathogens, is below 37° C., and primary cultures grow best at 27° C. The minimum temperature is about 14° C.

The plague bacillus is somewhat sensitive to free oxygen and growth may not develop under aerobic conditions if the inoculum is small; this inhibition can be avoided by the addition of blood or sodium sulphite to the medium or by the exclusion of air.

Colonies on agar are at first very small, transparent, white, circular disks (1 mm. or less), later becoming larger (3-4 mm.) and opaque; they are not specially characteristic.

In older cultures some of the colonies may have outgrown the others and become more opaque. This gives the appearance of a mixed growth.

In broth, growth consists of a granular deposit at the foot and on the side of the tube, not unlike that of a streptococcus. If cultured in a flask of broth with drops of sterile oil on the surface, and provided the flask is not subjected to shaking or movement, a characteristic growth develops, consisting of "stalactites" hanging down into the fluid from the oil drops.

Viability.—The thermal death point is about 55° C. for 15 minutes. The organism dies quickly when subjected to drying. Laboratory cultures remain viable for months if kept moist and at low temperatures.

The risk of laboratory infection of staff handling pathological material and cultures is considerable, and all manipulations should be carried out with the utmost care.

Biochemical Reactions.—

Glucose	*Lactose*	*Dulcitol*	*Sucrose*	*Mannitol*
⊥	–	–	–	⊥

(⊥ = acid; no gas)

Indole is not produced.

Milk medium is unaltered: *P. pestis* does not liquefy gelatin.

The organism grows on a bile-salt medium such as MacConkey's (cf. other members of the Pasteurella group).

Antigenic Characters.—It has been shown that *P. pestis* contains two types of antigen, one somatic and heat-stable, the other heat-labile at 100° C. and associated with the capsule which is formed in cultures growing at 37° C. The capsular antigen may be of importance in relation to the immunising properties of *P. pestis* vaccines; thus, a killed vaccine prepared from cultures grown at 37° C., in which capsular material is well developed, has greater immunising properties in mice than one from cultures grown at lower temperatures, *e.g.* 25°–30° C., as in the preparation of the Haffkine plague vaccine which has been extensively used in India. On the other hand, the somatic or "residue" antigen is important in the protection of guinea-pigs. A non-toxic complex of antigenic fractions can be prepared which immunises both mice and guinea-pigs (Keppie, Cocking & Smith, 1958) and may prove useful as a protective vaccine against plague. Strains of *P. pestis* are serologically homogeneous.

Animal Pathogenicity.—The bacillus is pathogenic to monkeys, rats, guinea-pigs and other rodents, and plague is essentially an epizootic disease among wild rats and certain other rodent animals. A guinea-pig or white rat injected subcutaneously with a recently isolated culture dies in a few days, and at autopsy a marked local inflammatory condition is noted, with necrosis and oedema; the related lymph glands are also involved ; the spleen is enlarged and congested and often shows small greyish-white areas in its substance; there is also septicaemia. The characteristic bacilli can be seen in large numbers in films from the local lesion, lymph glands, spleen pulp and heart blood. A similar condition is found in rats dying of epizootic plague (*vide infra*).

Marked local and general toxic effects can be produced in animals by injection of dead cultures, but a true exotoxin is not produced. The "toxin" can be released by lysis of the bacterial cells and from it a toxoid can be prepared; its relationship to the pathogenicity of the plague bacillus is doubtful.

Pathogenesis.—In *bubonic plague* the bacilli are inoculated by a bite from an infected rat flea (see below) and there is an incubation period of 2–8 days. The organisms may then be present in relatively small numbers in the blood stream but they are largely localised in the regional lymph glands (usually the inguinal group as the leg is most commonly the site of inoculation) where they give rise to progressive swelling of the lymph glands and periglandular tissue. The resultant mass is referred to as the primary bubo. There is intense inflammation, and plague bacilli are initially present in large numbers in the bubo. Secondary buboes may develop in other lymph nodes. Haemorrhages occur in the bubo and there is subsequent necrosis, with reduction in the number of plague organisms locally present until they may disappear. If the case is septicaemic, however, the bacilli gain access in large numbers to the blood stream and an intense septicaemia precedes death in fatal cases. In primary septicaemic plague there is insufficient time for marked involvement of lymph nodes. *Post mortem* the organisms are found in the spleen.

In *pneumonic plague* there is a pulmonary focus of infection with a fulminating haemorrhagic bronchopneumonia. The bacilli are present in the bronchopneumonic areas in the lung and they occur in large numbers in the sputum which is highly infectious in this form of the disease.

Epidemiology.—Plague is epizootic in rats and certain other rodents. The infection is spread by rat fleas (e.g. *Xenopsylla cheopis*). The occurrence of bubonic plague in man is due to transmission of the infection from rats by the rat flea. The mechanism of transmission is briefly as follows: the flea sucks blood (containing plague bacilli) from an infected animal; the bacilli multiply in the stomach and proventriculus, which may become blocked with bacillary masses; when the insect again bites and sucks blood, regurgitation takes place from the blocked proventriculus into the bite wound, and so inoculation results.

The time during which the bacilli survive in a flea and the insect remains infective depends on temperature and humidity. A temperature of about 50° F. (10° C.) and a high degree of humidity have been found to be the most suitable conditions. A temperature over 80° F. (27° C.) is unfavourable.

Pneumonic plague is communicated from person to person by

infected droplets from the respiratory passages. This form of the disease may be initiated from cases of bubonic plague in which the organisms localise in the lung and produce a pneumonic lesion.

Laboratory Diagnosis

Bubonic Plague.—The bubo is punctured with a hypodermic syringe and exudate withdrawn. From this material films are made and stained with methylene blue and by Gram's method. The appearance of the characteristic bacilli showing bipolar staining is highly suggestive.

Cultures are also made on blood agar, and single colonies are subcultured. The resulting growths are then available for further investigation.

Some of the exudate should also, if possible, be injected subcutaneously into a guinea-pig or white rat. If plague bacilli are present, the inoculated animal will die, showing at autopsy the appearances described above.

The cultures obtained may be tested as regards biochemical reactions, involution on 3 per cent. salt agar, chain formation in broth, and stalactite growth. The cultures can also be used for further animal inoculation experiments.

Pneumonic Plague.—The bacilli can be detected microscopically in the sputum, and for identification should be isolated in pure culture as in dealing with material from bubonic plague.

In carrying out animal inoculation with sputum, other virulent organisms may be present (*e.g.* pneumococcus); instead of injecting subcutaneously, successful inoculation with the plague bacillus can be effected by applying the material to the nasal mucosa, or to a shaved area of skin.

In septicaemic plague, the bacillus can be demonstrated and isolated by blood culture.

There may be racial prejudices against obtaining material for laboratory examination *post mortem*. If excision of buboes, liver, spleen, bone-marrow or lung tissue is not allowed, samples may be obtained for culture or animal inoculation by needle puncture (Pollitzer, 1954).

Chemotherapy.—Tetracyclines have given spectacular results even in pneumonic plague, which, if untreated, is invariably fatal. Chloramphenicol, streptomycin and sulphonamides have also been found effective. Irrespective of the agent employed, therapy must be instituted early in the disease and continued for at least ten days if relapses are to be avoided.

Prophylaxis

Plague vaccines have been widely used for prophylactic purposes. The preparation known as Haffkine's vaccine is a heat-killed culture of *P. pestis* grown for 4 weeks at 27° C. in digest broth. Phenol, 0·5 per cent., is added as a preservative. Two doses of 1·0 and 2·0 ml. are injected subcutaneously at an interval of seven to ten days. The protective value of this and other killed vaccines is in doubt.

Living non-virulent cultures have also been employed as vaccines and seem to give a good degree of protection.

Rodent control on an organised and permanent basis combined with flea destruction will do much to eliminate epizootic conditions. The need for personal protection of medical and nursing personnel, particularly those caring for cases of pneumonic plague, is vital and entails the wearing of protective clothing, masks, etc. Such persons may be given immediate temporary protection with anti-plague serum.

Diagnosis of Plague Infection in Wild Rats

At autopsy the following appearances are noted:—enlargement of lymphatic glands, with periglandular inflammation and oedema, most frequently in the cervical glands owing to the fact that the neck is the common harbourage of fleas; serous effusion in the pleural cavity; enlargement of the spleen, which may show small white areas in the pulp; congestion and a mottled appearance of the liver; congestion and haemorrhage under the skin and in the internal organs.

Films are prepared from the heart blood, the glands and spleen, and stained by Gram's method and with methylene blue. Cultures should also be made, and the isolation of the organism attempted by the usual methods. Guinea-pigs should be inoculated subcutaneously with an emulsion of the splenic tissue. In rats found dead of plague it may be difficult to demonstrate the bacilli microscopically or to isolate them in culture. Carcases in a state of decomposition may be heavily contaminated with other organisms which render the microscopic examination confusing and isolation difficult. Inoculation of a white rat or guinea-pig, by smearing the nasal mucous membrane or a shaved area of skin with material from the lesions, should be carried out. Differentiation of *P. pestis* and *P. pseudotuberculosis* is important.

OTHER ORGANISMS OF PASTEURELLA GROUP

The plague bacillus is only one species in a biological group, *Pasteurella*, which includes at least three species of veterinary importance, namely *Pasteurella multocida* (syn. *P. septica*), *Pasteurella haemolytica* and *Pasteurella pseudotuberculosis*. These organisms and *P. pestis* are all similar in morphology and staining reactions, but they differ in certain features including their parasitism and virulence to different animal species.

Pasteurella multocida (*Pasteurella septica*)

Strains of this organism have been generally named in the past according to the animal from which they have been isolated (*P. boviseptica*, *P. oviseptica*,

P. aviseptica, etc.), but they are now regarded as members of the same species, *P. multocida*, differing in their parasitic adaptations to particular hosts.

P. multocida causes haemorrhagic septicaemia, transit fever and mastitis in cattle; pneumonia with septicaemia in pigs; septicaemia and snuffles in rabbits; fowl cholera and septicaemia in poultry. Characteristic bipolar staining is exhibited by the organisms which are present in the blood and tissues. *P. multocida* differs from other members of the genus in certain cultural and biochemical details (see table, p. 278).

Antigenic Characters.—Strains from different sources can be divided into five types by cross-protection tests (Hudson, 1959).

Pathogenicity.—There are conflicting reports regarding possible relationships between colony type, nature of colony fluorescence and type of encapsulation of *P. multocida* strains and their virulence. The organism may be carried by apparently normal cattle, sheep, swine, dogs, cats and rats. It may also occur in the upper respiratory tract of healthy persons associated with animals. *P. multocida* freshly isolated from haemorrhagic septicaemia in cattle is usually highly pathogenic for mice and rabbits but not so for ducks and chickens. Fowl cholera strains are equally pathogenic for mice, rabbits, ducks and fowls.

Cases of human infection by *P. multocida* occur, especially in septic wounds following cat or dog bites (Allott *et al.*, 1944; Coghlan, 1958).

Pasteurella haemolytica

This organism, which may occur in longer and filamentous forms on culture, causes narrow zones of haemolysis when grown on ox- or sheep-blood agar, but the production of wide outer zones of partial haemolysis in addition to the typical narrow zone of complete haemolysis has been reported when strains are grown on agar plates containing blood of young lambs (Smith, 1962). *P. haemolytica* occurs in the upper respiratory tract of healthy animals and is generally regarded as a secondary or opportunist invader when associated with serious disease in animals. It has been isolated from pneumonic lungs of cattle and sheep and it may produce a form of septicaemia in lambs. In contrast with *P. multocida*, *P. haemolytica* is virtually non-pathogenic for rodents.

Urease-producing organisms otherwise resembling *P. haemolytica* have been isolated from human sputum (Jones, 1962).

Pasteurella pseudotuberculosis

This is the causative organism of pseudotuberculosis in guinea-pigs, turkeys, rats, rabbits and other animals. The organism has also been isolated from birds. It might be confused with *P. pestis* if isolated from wild rats, but can be distinguished by its motility when growing at 22° C. *P. pseudotuberculosis* is very similar to *P. pestis* in many respects, however, and differentiation may not always be straightforward (Wilson & Miles, 1955).

Antigenic Characters.—Five different serological types of *P. pseudotuberculosis* have been recognised by agglutination reactions (types I-V). The organism possesses three antigenic constituents: a flagellar, a type-specific somatic, and a common somatic antigen. The common somatic antigen, which is shared by all five types, is the same as the somatic antigen of *P. pestis*. There is also an antigenic relationship between *P. pseudotuberculosis* type II and IV and certain salmonellae of groups B and D respectively.

The following table shows how *P. pestis*, *P. septica*, *P. haemolytica* and *P. pseudotuberculosis* may be differentiated:

	Motility at 18°–22° C.	Maltose	Indole	Growth on Bile-salt Medium
P. pestis . . .	−	⊥	−	+
P. septica . . .	−	−	+	−
P. haemolytica . .	−	⊥	−	−
P. pseudotuberculosis .	+	⊥	−	+

⊥ = acid; no gas.

In freshly isolated culture *P. pestis* can be differentiated from *P. pseudotuberculosis* and other *Pasteurella* organisms by adding very small inocula (from dilutions of the culture) to rabbit-blood agar and incubating at 37° C.; *P. pseudotuberculosis* grows well in 24 hours while *P. pestis* develops slowly at this temperature, small colonies appearing only after 48 hours as the optimum temperature for *P. pestis* when freshly isolated is 27° C.

Pathogenicity.—Pseudotuberculosis in the guinea-pig is associated with yellowish caseous foci in the liver, spleen and mesenteric lymph nodes. The natural infection is thought to occur by ingestion and is usually chronic. Pseudotuberculosis may be introduced into guinea-pig colonies via green food contaminated with the excreta of infected wood pigeons (Paterson & Cook, 1963).

Human infection with *P. pseudotuberculosis* has been generally regarded as rare. A few cases of a septicaemic typhoid-like illness have been recorded. A more benign infection involving the mesenteric lymph nodes is apparently more common and may be mistaken for acute appendicitis (Mair *et al.*, 1960).

PASTEURELLA TULARENSIS

This organism is classified by some workers with the *Brucella* family because of its growth requirements, its biochemical behaviour and its serological relationship with that group. It is also, like the *Brucella*, highly pathogenic for laboratory workers handling cultures of the organism. However, in its ecology as an animal and human parasite and its possible transmission by insects, it comes closer to the *Pasteurella* group and is included in this family in Bergey's classification.

The organism is a small Gram-negative cocco-bacillus not usually exceeding 0·7 μ in length and 0·2 μ in width, with a tendency to pleomorphism in artificial culture. It stains best with dilute carbol-fuchsin and shows bipolar staining. It is present in large numbers as a capsulated organism in the spleen and liver of infected animals. Its occurrence in large numbers inside cells in these organs has suggested that it may multiply as an intracellular parasite. *P. tularensis* cannot be cultivated on ordinary media. Cultures can be obtained, however, on a medium consisting of pure egg-yolk, on blood agar or serum agar containing a piece of sterile rabbit spleen, and on horse-serum agar containing 0·1 per cent. cystine and 1 per cent. glucose.

In the Western States of America it produces a plague-like disease (tularaemia) in wild rodents (*e.g.* rabbits, hares, ground-squirrels, etc.). The lesions are not unlike those found in plague-infected animals, and this infection has to be considered, therefore, in the diagnosis of plague in animals. The disease has also been observed in Japan, U.S.S.R., Yugoslavia, Norway and certain other parts of Europe. Various rodents and other wild animals may be infected.

This infection is transmissible to man as a result of handling infected animals (*e.g.* rabbits and hares) or laboratory cultures. A prolonged febrile illness results, sometimes with glandular lesions and ulcers of the skin. The serum of infected persons agglutinates the organism. It may be noted that the serum of cases with *Brucella* infections may contain agglutinins for *P. tularensis*. For diagnostic purposes guinea-pigs or mice may be inoculated with exudate from the glands or ulcers.

Infection is also spread by ticks and other biting arthropods, and *P. tularensis* has been cultivated from ticks. The disease is sometimes apparently water-borne; thus, water-rats may be infected and contaminate water by their excreta.

The tetracyclines can be used in the treatment of the infection.

REFERENCES

ALLOTT, E. N., CRUICKSHANK, R., CYRLAS-WILLIAMS, R., GLASS, V., MEYER, I. H., STRAKER, E. A. & TEE, G. (1944). Infection of cat-bite and dog-bite wounds with *Pasteurella septica*. *J. Path. Bact.*, **56**, 411.

COGHLAN, J. D. (1958). Isolation of *Pasteurella multocida* from human peritoneal pus and a study of its relationship to other strains of the same species. *J. Path. Bact.*, **76**, 45.

HUDSON, J. R. (1959). *Infectious Diseases of Animals*; *Diseases due to Bacteria*, ed. Stableforth, A. W. & Galloway, I. A., p. 413. London : Butterworth.

JONES, D. M. (1962). A Pasteurella-like organism from the human respiratory tract. *J. Path. Bact.*, **83**, 143.

KEPPIE, J., COCKING, E. C. & SMITH, H. (1958). A non-toxic complex from *Pasteurella pestis* which immunises both guinea-pigs and mice. *Lancet*, **1**, 246.

MAIR, N. S., MAIR, H. J., STIRK, E. M. & CORSON, J. G. (1960). Three cases of acute mesenteric lymphadenitis due to *Pasteurella pseudotuberculosis*. *J. Clin. Path.*, **13**, 432.

PATERSON, J. S. & COOK, R. (1963). A method for the recovery of *Pasteurella pseudotuberculosis* from faeces. *J. Path. Bact.*, **85**, 241.

POLLITZER, R. (1954). *Plague*, p. 231. Geneva : World Health Organization.

SMITH, G. R. (1962). An unusual haemolytic effect produced by *Pasteurella haemolytica*. *J. Path. Bact.*, **83**, 501.

WILSON, G. S. & MILES, A. A. (1955). In *Topley & Wilson's Principles of Bacteriology & Immunity*, 4th ed., Vol. **1**, p. 887. London : Arnold.

CHAPTER 23

BRUCELLA

THE genus *Brucella* consists of a group of small Gram-negative bacteria which are essentially pathogens of animals, notably goats, sheep, cattle and pigs. In cattle the infection frequently results in outbreaks of abortion (contagious abortion). They also cause brucellosis (undulant fever, Malta fever) in man through his accidental contact with the discharges of infected animals or through the consumption of their milk or milk products. Three different species are recognised which though identical in morphology and staining reaction differ in their host predilection, in certain cultural characteristics and in the amount of the two antigens which are common to all three. They are *Br. abortus* which occurs mainly in cattle, *Br. melitensis* in goats and sheep and *Br. suis* in pigs. In addition to the three main species there are some atypical *Brucella* whose characteristics differ from the normal and a number of types within each species are now recognised. The host-parasite relationship is not absolute and both man and the domestic animals are susceptible to infection by all three species. There is evidence that in some European countries hares and other rodents act as important sources of *Br. suis* infection to livestock, especially to swine, and dogs may sometimes be responsible for spreading infection in herds of sheep (Biberstein & Cameron, 1961).

Brucellae are able to grow intracellularly and tend to localise in lymphatic tissue, liver, spleen, bone-marrow and other parts of the reticulo-endothelial system. The presence of *erythritol*, a substance which stimulates the growth of virulent brucella strains may account for the predilection of these organisms for placental tissue of goats, sheep, cattle and pigs causing a placentitis leading to abortion of pregnant animals. Human placental material on the other hand does not contain erythritol and human abortion due to brucellosis is thought to be rare (Williams, Keppie & Smith, 1962).

Each of the three species is pathogenic to man. The infection may remain latent or cause a variety of symptoms, the intensity of which varies from severe to subclinical. The most characteristic manifestation in the acute phase is an intermittent fever (undulant fever). Of the three species, *Br. melitensis* appears to be the most virulent. It tends to cause undulant fever more frequently than the other two. Acute infection by all three species may progress to the chronic state as the organisms become intracellular. This condition, one of hypersensitivity, may affect many parts of the body and last for many years.

Morphology and Staining.—Gram-negative cocco-bacilli, usually appearing as round or oval forms about 0·4 μ in diameter. Definite bacillary forms (1–2 μ in length) may be observed. The organisms occur singly, in pairs, or even short chains. They are non-motile and non-sporing. Small capsules are sometimes present.

Cultural Characters.—Aerobic; optimum temperature, 37° C. The brucellae grow best on media enriched with animal protein such as serum or liver extract (p. 767). Colonies on agar in primary growth may not appear for two or three days; they are small smooth transparent disks without special characters, about 1 mm. in diameter but increasing in size to 2–3 mm.

Gelatin stab—a delicate line of growth along the track of the inoculating wire, with little or no surface growth. No liquefaction occurs. Potato medium—after several days a characteristic chocolate-brown growth is produced.

Viability.—A temperature of 60° C. destroys brucellae in ten minutes and they are readily killed in milk by pasteurisation. They are moderately sensitive to acid and tend to die out within a few days in fresh cheese undergoing lactic acid fermentation. They may survive for a number of days in butter made from infected milk. The organisms are very sensitive to direct sunlight, but if protected from it they may persist in dust or soil for two to three months and in dead foetal material for even longer periods. They are susceptible to sulphonamides, streptomycin, the tetracyclines and chloramphenicol.

Biochemical Reactions.—Although carbohydrates are utilised, brucellae produce insufficient acid or gas to be demonstrable by the ordinary methods.

Animal Pathogenicity.—Laboratory animals may be experimentally infected, the guinea-pig being the most susceptible to small inocula. The infection is not usually progressive and the guinea-pig normally recovers spontaneously although infection by *Br. melitensis* may be fatal. If the animal is killed after six or eight weeks the lymph nodes in the region of the site of inoculation are often found to be swollen, the spleen may be greatly enlarged and engorged and necrotic areas are seen in the liver and spleen from which the organisms may be cultured. Agglutinating antibodies are detectable in the serum.

Differential Tests for Brucella

The three main types of *Brucella* differ in certain characteristics which form the basis for their classification. These are as follows: (1) carbon dioxide requirement; (2) production of hydrogen sulphide; (3) sensitivity to certain dyes; (4) urease activity.

1. Carbon Dioxide Requirement.—When cultivation is attempted directly from the animal body, *Br. abortus* requires an atmosphere containing 5–10 per cent. of carbon dioxide. This can be obtained by placing the inoculated tubes or plates in an air-tight jar or tin and generating carbon dioxide within the container (p. 802). After continued culture the organism may be grown in the ordinary atmosphere. On the other hand *Br. melitensis* and *Br. suis* can be grown without the addition of carbon dioxide even in primary culture. *Br. melitensis* may benefit from the gas, but some strains of *Br. suis* may be inhibited by it. Bang originally cultivated *Br. abortus* by preparing shake cultures in tubes of serum agar, the colonies developing best in a zone just below the surface of the medium. This is due to the fact that in

this zone the partial pressure of carbon dioxide is at an optimum for the growth of the organism and the conditions are still aerobic. The reason for the effect of carbon dioxide in promoting growth of *Br. abortus* is not fully understood.

2. Production of Hydrogen Sulphide.—Both *Br. abortus* and American strains of *Br. suis* form hydrogen sulphide (the latter more markedly and for a longer period). This can be detected with lead acetate paper (filter paper soaked in 10 per cent. lead acetate solution is dried, cut into strips 8 cm. by 0·5 cm., and stored in a stoppered tube ready for use). One strip is inserted into a tube containing a serum dextrose agar slope culture and held in place with the cotton-wool stopper. The paper is examined daily and renewed as soon as it becomes blackened. *Br. melitensis* and Danish strains of *Br. suis* do not produce H_2S.

3. Inhibition by Dyes.—*Br. melitensis*, *abortus* and *suis* have been differentiated by means of media containing 1 in 25,000 basic fuchsin and 1 in 50,000 thionin respectively. *Br. melitensis* is not inhibited to any extent by these dyes, *Br. abortus* is typically inhibited by thionin, not by fuchsin, whereas *Br. suis* is inhibited by fuchsin but not by thionin (see Table, p. 283). Methyl violet, 1 in 50,000, and pyronin, 1 in 100,000 give results similar to those with basic fuchsin (see table).

These dye-sensitivity tests can be carried out in the following ways:

A. Cruickshank's method. This method is useful in laboratories where an occasional strain is examined.

Sterilised strips of filter paper (6 by 0·5 cm.) are impregnated with the dye solutions, dried and stored for future use; the following concentrations have been found satisfactory: thionin 1 in 600, basic fuchsin 1 in 200. The strips are placed in parallel on the surface of a plate of liver-infusion agar and then covered by pouring the same medium (melted) over them to form an additional layer. Stroke inoculations from cultures of the strains to be tested are made at right angles to the strips. After incubation in 5–10 per cent. carbon dioxide for two to three days the results can be determined as follows: if the organism resists the dye it grows across the strip; if sensitive, growth is inhibited for some distance (up to 10 mm.) from the strip.

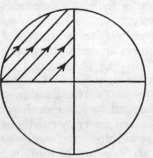

B. Huddleson's Method recommended by the FAO/WHO Brucellosis Centre, Weybridge, England.—Useful for frequent examinations or research purposes.

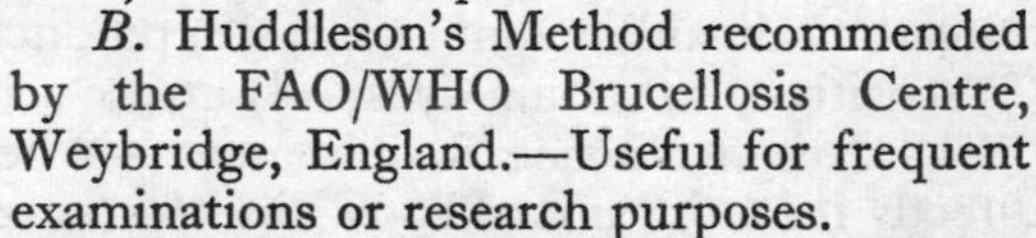

Fig. 18

Each dye is added to serum dextrose agar at 50° C. to give a final concentration in each case as follows: basic fuchsin 1 in 25,000; thionin 1 in 50,000; methyl violet 1 in 50,000 pyronin 1 in 100,000. The two latter dyes may be useful but are not normally used.

Each dye-agar mixture is poured into a Petri dish and allowed to solidify. Suspensions of the unknown strains in the smooth phase are inoculated on to a quarter of each plate, five strokes being made, commencing from the edge and working inwards without recharging the loop so that the smallest inoculum is made nearest the centre (see Fig. 18). Known strains are included as controls. By using five inocula of different sizes there is less likelihood of unsatisfactory results deriving from an inoculum which is either too large or too small. The plates are incubated in an atmosphere of 10 per cent. CO_2 for five days.

4. Urease Activity.—Another useful differential test, though one of limited value unless correlated with other tests is afforded by the urease activity of *Br. abortus* and *Br. suis*. One ml. of a buffered 5 per cent. urea solution (pH4) containing phenol red as an indicator is inoculated with a loopful of a 48-hr. culture of the unknown strain grown on a solid medium. The tubes are incubated at 37° C. in a water bath and readings made after 15 min., 30 min., 1 hr. and hourly thereafter until a pink colour develops indicating a positive result. In general *Br. abortus* requires 2 hr. or more for the pink colour to develop whereas *Br. suis* gives a positive result in 15–30 min. *Br. melitensis* on the other hand gives variable results sometimes resembling *Br. abortus* and sometimes *Br. suis*.

	CO_2 requirement	H_2S production (days)					Growth in presence of		Methyl violet 1:50,000	Urease activity demonstrable within (min.)
		1	2	3	4	5	Basic fuchsin 1:25,000	Thionin 1:50,000		
Br. melitensis	−	− (or slight)					+	+	+	variable
Br. abortus	+	+	+	+	−	−	+	−	+	120 or more
Br. suis (American strains)	−	++	++	++	+	+	−	+	−	15–30

Danish strains of *Br. suis* are similar to the American strains but do not produce H_2S.

Antigenic Characters.—Br. melitensis, abortus and *suis* show a very close biological relationship. Direct agglutination tests with antisera fail to distinguish between them. Agglutinin-absorption tests, however, elicit a difference between *Br. melitensis* on the one hand and *Br. abortus* and *Br. suis* on the other; but the two latter cannot be distinguished serologically. This difference in antigenic constitution is quantitative rather than qualitative. Thus, the three species possess two similar antigenic constituents A and M though in different proportions, one constituent being dominant in *Br. melitensis* (M), while the other predominates in *Br. abortus* and *Br. suis* (A).

For the practical identification of the two serological types of *Brucella*, agglutinating sera absorbed with the heterologous organisms respectively are used, the absorbing dose being adjusted according to the titre of the serum so that the minor agglutinin is removed without substantially altering the major agglutinin. These absorbed sera are monospecific and agglutinate only strains in which the particular antigen is dominant (Hamilton & Hardy, 1950).

Variation.—While typical, virulent brucellae produce colonies that are smooth and transparent, growth on laboratory media results in mutation to a rough type of colony with a corresponding loss of virulence; mucoid colonies may also appear. The organisms also change antigenically so that they are no longer readily agglutinated by homologous sera. Rough variants are recognised by their ability to agglutinate in 1 in 1000 acriflavine solution (shown by the slide-agglutination test). It has been suggested that the susceptibility or resistance of an individual animal may be determined by the presence or absence of factors in the serum which suppress rough variants thus favouring the more virulent smooth types. Resistant individuals do not have this serum factor and the smooth to rough (avirulent) mutation readily occurs (Jawetz, Melnick & Adelberg, 1962).

Epidemiology.—In the Mediterranean littoral and islands, a considerable proportion of goats are infected with *Br. melitensis* and most of the infected animals excrete the organisms in the milk, in the vaginal mucus and in the urine, thereby disseminating the infection. Certain types of sheep are susceptible to *Br. melitensis* and in France, the Middle East and the U.S.S.R. these animals also constitute reservoirs of infection. Cattle too may carry the organism. In those countries cases of brucellosis occur mostly in the rural population, among persons who come into contact with infected animals and their carcases or drink unpasteurised milk or consume freshly made butter and cheese prepared from infected milk. Infection of cattle in Great Britain by strains resembling *Br. melitensis* in some respects have been reported. These strains are now known to belong to a type of *Br. abortus* (Type 5).

Br. abortus which causes brucellosis mainly in cattle in many parts of the world is responsible for human infection through contact with infected animal discharges or through consumption of infected milk. The disease occurs mostly in farming communities and among veterinarians and butchers, and in these circumstances where it is mainly an occupational disease the incidence is highest in adult males. Although *Br. abortus* may occur in a considerable proportion of samples of unpasteurised market milk, the incidence of human brucellosis due to thc consumption of milk appears to be relatively low. Latent infections may however occur and subclinical infections remain unrecognised. In Great Britain *Br. abortus* is the only type responsible for human brucellosis as far as is known. In spite of fairly widespread vaccination of cattle, which has reduced the incidence of clinical abortion, the infection is still endemic and milk is a major source of infection. Since the disease is now no longer predominantly an occupational one, women and children feature more in the total number of diagnosed cases than previously.

Human brucellosis due to *Br. suis* is almost entirely an occupational infection arising through contact with infected pigs or pig meat. It is more limited in its distribution, occurring mainly in America although outbreaks have been reported from other pig-rearing countries. It tends to be more virulent for the human subject than *Br. abortus*, but strains isolated from animals in Denmark are avirulent for man.

The brucellae enter the body through abraded skin surfaces, through the mucous membranes of the alimentary and respiratory tracts and sometimes through the conjunctiva. Farmers and veterinarians may readily become infected through inhalation of dried infected animal secretions. The organisms enter the blood stream by way of the regional lymphatics and subsequently localise in various parts of the reticulo-endothelial system where they multiply intracellularly producing granulomatous nodules. Surviving organisms within these granulomata may cause relapses and a chronic hypersensitive condition. Infection among laboratory workers handling cultures of *Brucella* is not uncommon; it may occur through inhalation or via the conjunctiva or abraded skin.

Laboratory Diagnosis in Man

Blood cultures should be carried out repeatedly on all suspected cases but are not likely to be positive in more than 30–50 per cent. of cases. It is not necessary to limit the tests to the febrile phase and at least 10 ml. of blood should be withdrawn as the organisms may be relatively scanty. In the case of *Br. melitensis* the organisms may sometimes be isolated from the urine. Blood cultures should be carried out in duplicate in glucose-serum broth, one of each pair being incubated in 10 per cent. carbon dioxide. Subcultures on to solid media are made every few days and characteristic colonies looked for. The broth cultures should be retained for as long as six weeks before they are discarded as negative. *Br. melitensis* and *Br. suis* are more readily isolated in this way than *Br. abortus*. Castaneda's method for blood culture may be more successful.

Castaneda's Method of Blood-culture in Brucella Infection.—Three per cent. melted agar is allowed to set on one of the narrow sides of a 120 ml. flat rectangular bottle with a perforated screw cap; 20 ml. broth are then added. 5 ml. of blood are mixed with the broth and the mixture is allowed to flow over the agar. Carbon dioxide is introduced by a needle through the perforation in the cap to yield a 10 per cent. concentration. The bottle is incubated in the upright position, and the agar surface is examined daily for colonies; if no colonies are seen in 48 hours the blood broth is allowed to flow gently over the agar by suitably tilting the bottle, which is again incubated in the upright position. If *Brucella* is present in the blood, colonies can usually be observed within a week.

A positive agglutination reaction may be elicited after seven to ten days from the onset of the illness. Serum dilutions from 1 in 10 to 1 in 1280 or more should be tested against carefully standardised antigens obtained from FAO/WHO brucellosis centres. (WHO, 1958). Tests are incubated at 37° C. for 24 hours and recorded as follows:

+ + + + (complete agglutination and sedimentation, *i.e* 100 per cent. or water clear).

+ + + (about 75 per cent. clearing or nearly complete agglutination and sedimentation).

+ + (about 50 per cent. clearing and marked sedimentation).

+ (about 25 per cent. clearing and distinct sedimentation).

A more dilute antigen suspension as used by the Public Health Laboratories in England gives agglutination titres of a somewhat higher level than the standard antigen referred to above. The results of tests with the two antigens are otherwise comparable.

In the acute stage of the disease the serum agglutinating antibodies rise to give titres of well over 1000 before beginning to fall again. Since prozones may occur in the agglutination test with high-titre sera, it is advisable to make a range of serum dilutions sufficiently high (*e.g.* to over 1000) in order to avoid false-negative readings. Both agglutinating and complement-fixing antibodies are present in the acute stage, the former being mainly associated with the high molecular weight gamma-globulin fraction of the serum (IgM, 19S) and the latter with the low molecular weight (IgG, 7S) immuno-globulin (see page 116).

As the disease progresses from the acute to the chronic form and the organisms become localised intracellularly in various parts of the body the IgM antibodies decrease, so that the agglutination titre falls to a low level and may finally be absent even when the patient is still ill. The complete absence of agglutination therefore does not rule out the possibility of infection. As long as infection continues, IgG antibodies are present in the serum and these may be detected by complement-fixation tests using as antigen the same brucella suspension as is used in the agglutination test, diluted to a level that is shown by titration with a known positive serum to be optimum and not anticomplementary.

Another method of detecting non-agglutinating brucella antibodies is by using an anti-human globulin serum as in the Coombs test for rhesus antibody (Wilson & Merrifield, 1951). This results in the agglutination of the brucella suspension already sensitised by the IgG antibodies in the patient's serum (Kerr *et al.*, 1966).

It should be noted that sera from a proportion (about 1-2 per cent.) of the normal population agglutinate brucellae in low dilutions. The percentage is higher in rural than in urban areas. This may be due either to a latent or to a past infection. In latent infection the complement-fixation test is likely to be positive whereas in past infection it is negative. Agglutinins for brucella organisms may be present in the serum of persons who have been immunised against cholera. Other non-specific agglutination reactions may be due to the use of suspensions of rough strains of brucellae. After recovery from brucellosis the antibody level falls slowly sometimes taking many months to reach low levels.

Reference to the following table may be of help in interpreting the results of the three main diagnostic tests:

Type of brucellosis	Agglutination test	Complement-fixation test	Anti-human globulin test
Acute	positive	positive	...
Chronic	weak or negative	positive	positive
Past infection	weak or negative	negative	weak or negative

Skin Test.—The intradermal injection of a killed suspension of brucellae or of a purified extract "Brucellin" may elicit a delayed tuberculin-like allergic reaction (minimum diameter 5 mm. induration) which may mean past or present infection. The test should be used with caution since a more violent reaction with generalised symptoms may occur in persons who are still actively infected.

Chemotherapy.—Brucella infections respond best to a combination of streptomycin and tetracycline, continued for a period of two to three weeks. Successful results by combined therapy with streptomycin and sulphonamides have also been claimed. Intensive therapy in the acute stage of the disease is advisable to prevent the infection progressing to the chronic stage, which is less likely to respond to treatment.

Laboratory Diagnosis in Animals

The agglutination test on the serum of supposedly infected animals using standardised brucella suspensions has been used in diagnosis. Results in which 50 per cent. agglutination occurs in dilutions of 1 in 40 or over are generally regarded as evidence of infection.

The *milk ring test* (MRT) is a very sensitive means of detecting agglutinins in milk samples. The technique is given in detail in Chapter 55 (p. 985).

Since a positive reaction may occur in the milk of cows vaccinated in adult life with the avirulent strain of *Br. abortus* S19, positive milk ring tests should be confirmed as being the result of infection either by culturing the organism directly from the cream or by inoculating guinea-pigs with cream and the deposit after centrifuging the milk. A convenient confirmatory test is the *whey-agglutination* test which is rarely affected by vaccination of cattle prior to breeding age. The technique of this test is given in Chapter 55 (p. 986).

In animals that have aborted, the organism can be demonstrated microscopically in the uterine discharge[1] shortly after calving and also in the stomach contents of the foetus, and can be cultivated by the methods referred to above. Inoculation of a guinea-pig may be resorted to for demonstrating and isolating the organism; the inoculated animal is killed after 6 weeks, cultures are made from the spleen and the blood serum agglutinin titre is determined. The inoculation test is also utilised for demonstrating the organism in milk.

Immunisation.—Certain attenuated strains of *Br. abortus*, *e.g.* S19, used in the living state as vaccines have been shown to produce a degree of immunity against brucellosis and are applied practically in controlling abortion of cattle. In view of the fact that vaccination in adult life may

[1] A useful differential stain for the demonstration of *Br. abortus* in infected material is as follows: Dilute carbol-fuchsin (1 in 10) is allowed to act, without heating, for fifteen minutes. The slide is then decolourised with ½ per cent. acetic acid solution for fifteen seconds, washed thoroughly and counterstained with Löffler's alkaline methylene blue for one minute. This staining method may also be used for demonstrating the elementary bodies of *enzootic abortion* of ewes in smears from the diseased cotyledons and chorion.

result in serum antibodies which confuse any subsequent serological tests it should be restricted to about the sixth month of calfhood. In the majority of animals serum antibodies do not then persist, although the animals are protected against brucellosis through five pregnancies. Although it protects against abortion, vaccination does not always prevent infection, and localisation of brucellae in the mammary glands may result in an infected milk supply even from herds that have been vaccinated.

Other Types of Brucella

Strains of *Brucella* which differ in some of their characteristics from the normal species pattern may be identified as biotypes of one or other of the three main species by means of oxidative metabolic, phage-susceptibility and other tests. The rates of oxygen uptake by brucella cultures on eight amino-acids and four carbohydrate substrates have been determined and shown to form a different pattern for each of the three species. By this means strains may be identified as belonging not only to one or other of the three species but also to biotypes within the species. There are three types of *Br. melitensis*, nine of *Br. abortus* and three of *Br. suis*, type 1 in each case being the normal (prototype) of the species. The phage-susceptibility test is performed with a standard reference phage known as Tbilisi (Tb) at two dilutions, RTD (routine test dilution) and 10,000×RTD (these phage preparations may be obtained from the Central Veterinary Laboratory, Weybridge, Surrey, England). Since the oxidative metabolic tests are highly specialised and time consuming, it is recommmended that aytpical brucella strains should first be identified as far as possible using the conventional tests and phage-typing and should then be sent to an active brucellosis centre for final identification. A table showing the main characteristics of the various biotypes of *Brucella* and their reactions to four of the metabolic tests is given in the WHO fourth report on brucellosis (1964) and is reproduced in a modified form in the appendix.

A species of *Brucella* known as *Br. ovis* is mainly responsible for epididymitis of rams and may also cause abortion of pregnant ewes. It occurs in Australia and New Zealand (Buddle & Boyes, 1935) and in Czechoslovakia, Roumania and parts of the U.S.A. and Africa (WHO, 1964). It requires carbon dioxide for primary isolation, it produces little or no H_2S, has weak urease activity and has a dye sensitivity similar to that of *Br. suis* although it is not inhibited by basic fuchsin to the same extent. It has only been observed in the non-smooth phase and has no antigenic relationship with smooth brucella of other species although it has common antigens with rough brucella variants. Strains of *Brucella* isolated from reindeer in the U.S.S.R. have been named *Br. rangiferi tarandi*. Similar strains have been isolated from Eskimos and caribou in Canada and Alaska. They do not require CO_2 for growth and do not produce H_2S. Antigenically they resemble melitensis rather than abortus but are lysed by phage at 10,000×RTD. In oxidative metabolic tests they give results similar to *Br. suis* type 3.

REFERENCES

Biberstein, E. L. & Cameron, H. S. (1961). The family brucellaceae in veterinary research. *Ann. Rev. Microbiol.*, **15**, 93.

Buddle, M. B. & Boyes, B. W. (1953). A brucella mutant causing genital diseases of sheep in New Zealand. *Aust. vet. J.*, **29**, 145.

Hamilton, A. V. & Hardy, A. V. (1950). The brucella ring test. Its potential value in the control of brucellosis. *Amer. J. publ. Hlth*, **40**, 321.

Jawetz, E., Melnick, J. L. & Adelberg, E. A. (1962). *Review of Medical Microbiology*, 5th ed. p. 180. Berlin : Lange.

Kerr, W. R., Coghlan, Joyce D., Payne, D. J. H. & Robertson, L. (1966). The laboratory diagnosis of chronic brucellosis. *Lancet*, 2, 1181.

Williams, A. E., Keppie, J. & Smith, H. (1962). The clinical bases of the virulence of *Brucella abortus*. *J. exp. Path.*, **43**, 530.

Wilson, M. M. & Merrifield, E. V. O. (1951). The antiglobulin (Coombs) test in brucellosis. *Lancet*, 2, 913.

World Health Organisation. Expert committee on brucellosis.
(1958). *Wld Hlth Org. techn Rep. Ser.* No. 148.
(1964). *Wld Hlth Org. techn Rep. Ser.* No. 289.

CHAPTER 24

BACTEROIDACEAE: DONOVANIA

THE family *Bacteroidaceae* comprises five genera of medical importance. Three are simple rod-shaped cells, rarely pleomorphic and all strictly anaerobic: of these, *Bacteroides* and *Fusobacterium* are greater than 0·3 μ in diameter, the former having rounded ends and the latter pointed ends: *Dialister* has a diameter of 0·15 μ or less.

The remaining two genera of the family are highly pleomorphic rods: *Sphaerophorus* is strictly anaerobic whereas *Streptobacillus* is facultatively anaerobic.

BACTEROIDES

There are 30 species in the genus *Bacteroides* and the majority have been found as commensals or pathogens in the mammalian intestinal tract. All species are Gram-negative, 2–3 μ by 0·4–0·8 μ, non-sporing and usually non-capsulate and non-motile.

Bacteroides fragilis

This, the type species of the genus, is non-motile and non-capsulate, often showing bipolar staining: strict anaerobe; optimum temperature 37° C. but growth is scanty and the colonies small, greyish and irregular in outline. Gelatin is not liquefied and various carbohydrates are attacked without the evolution of gas. This species has been found in appendicitis, urinary tract infections and septicaemias in man; some strains produce subcutaneous abscesses when injected into guinea-pigs, rabbits or mice. All strains are resistant to penicillin and sensitive to the tetracyclines.

Fusobacterium

There are six members of this genus but only one, *Fusobacterium fusiforme* is of proven pathogenicity for man. It is a concomitant of *Borrelia vincentii* in Vincent's angina and in other necrotic inflammatory conditions, e.g. gingivitis, stomatitis. Characteristically *Fusobacterium fusiforme* is a large (5–14 μ by 1 μ) non-motile, cigar-shaped bacillus; the centre of the bacillus often stains less deeply than the main body. It is strictly anaerobic and grows only on enriched media, e.g. serum agar, and even then grows poorly; after 36 hr. incubation colonies are only 1–2 mm. in diameter, high convex and with a regular edge. Isolation is very difficult owing to the admixture of large numbers of other organisms present in pathogenic material from the buccal cavity.

Dialister

Both members of this genus have been found in the respiratory tract usually in cases suffering from influenza. *Dialister pneumosintes* and *Dialister granuliformans* are microscopically identical; very short rods not more than 1 μ by 0·5 μ—frequently smaller. Gram-negative, non-capsulate, non-motile and non-sporing. Colonies on agar and blood agar are minute, transparent and have an entire edge; the optimum temperature is 37° C. and although both species prefer anaerobic conditions, *Dial. granuliformans* is less strictly anaerobic.

Neither produces indole but *Dial. granuliformans* produces acid from glucose, sucrose and mannitol while *Dial. pneumosintes* utilises only the first of these substrates. Both species are pathogenic for rabbits and intratracheal inoculation may give rise to fever, sometimes conjunctivitis and a mononuclear leucopenia.

Sphaerophorus necrophorus (*Fusiformis necrophorus*)

This is the type-species of the genus Sphaerophorus which comprises 18 species; all but one (*Sphaerophorus bullosus*) are non-motile. All members are Gram-negative, straight or slightly curved rods and are markedly pleomorphic. They are anaerobic and found variously as commensals in the mammalian intestinal tract; some are recognised pathogens. *Sphaer. necrophorus* is responsible for diphtheritic and necrotic lesions ("necrobacillosis") in various animals, e.g. gangrenous dermatitis of equines, calf diphtheria, foot rot of sheep, necrotic stomatitis of pigs, lung abscesses in various domesticated animals, labial necrosis of rabbits.

Morphological and Cultural Characters.—The organism is extremely pleomorphic and may appear in the form of elongated slender filaments varying in length, sometimes measuring 80 to 100 μ. Branching has occasionally been described. The filaments are Gram-negative and show a characteristic beaded appearance when stained by the ordinary strain. In addition to the filamentous form, the organism may be seen as small Gram-negative bacilli. Growth is obtained at an optimum temperature of 34°–36° C. on serum agar under strictly anaerobic conditions. The colonies are small, white, opaque disks with projecting wavy filaments. Cultures yield a characteristic "cheese-like" odour, especially in a milk medium. Indole is formed. Gelatin is not liquefied. A thermostable necrotising endotoxin is produced.

For diagnostic purposes stained films made from the edges of the necrotic tissue are examined.

Direct cultivation is difficult owing to the large numbers of other organisms present in the lesions. Pure cultures can be obtained readily by inoculating rabbits or mice with the necrotic tissue and isolating the organism on serum-agar from the inoculated animal at autopsy: death usually occurs in 1–2 weeks.

Pathogenesis.—Human infections with this type of organism are probably commoner than was at one time realised. Localised lesions in the skin and subcutaneous tissues are found particularly in workers who are obliged to handle infected animals; veterinary surgeons, meat inspectors, laboratory technicians and butchers are liable to this infection, especially when there are small abrasions of the skin on their hands. Ulceration of the throat, often after tonsillectomy, and purulent gingivitis after dental extractions, are also manifestations of the infection. A larger and more important group of cases occur following abortion and less frequently after normal childbirth; puerperal fever due to suppuration in the genital tract or a suppurative thrombophlebitis results. After surgical operations on the abdomen these organisms may cause peritonitis and are sometimes associated with sloughing of the edges of the incision. Occasionally appendicitis and urinary infection are associated with the organism. Another important group of cases suffer from empyema with or without lung abscess formation. In severe infections with *Sphaer. necrophorus* and also with members of the *Bacteroides* group, septicaemia or pyaemia may follow a suppurative thrombophlebitis. Bacterial endocarditis has been reported and widespread abscess formation, osteomyelitis, purulent meningitis and suppurative arthritis may occur. The organism is sensitive to penicillin, moderately sensitive to chloramphenicol and relatively resistant to streptomycin.

Streptobacillus moniliformis

This organism occurs as a normal inhabitant in the nasopharynx of wild and laboratory rats and is the cause of a spontaneous disease of mice characterised by multiple arthritis often involving the joints of the feet and leading to swellings of the feet and legs. It is also the cause of a proportion of cases of "rat-bite fever" in man. Although the organism is usually introduced through a bite, this history cannot always be obtained; in some cases the infection seems to be acquired by the ingestion of contaminated food. A group of cases in America, characterised by fever, multiple arthritis and an erythematous eruption (Haverhill Fever), was shown to be associated with the organism which was swallowed in contaminated milk.

Morphology and Staining.—The organism is a Gram-negative, pleomorphic bacterium, occurring as short rod-shaped forms (1–3 μ by 0·3–0·4 μ) or as elongated filaments which are either undivided or consist of chained bacilli. They may show characteristic fusiform, oval or spherical enlargements sometimes projecting laterally from the filaments; non-capsulate and non-motile.

Cultural Characteristics.—Growth can be obtained in the presence of blood, serum or ascitic fluid, and a high proportion of blood or serum is required in the medium. Löffler's serum serves well for cultivation. The colonies are small (1 mm.). Viability in culture is feeble and cultures die in 2–4 days.

On solid media, after 2–3 days' incubation, raised granular colonies 1–5 mm. in diameter develop. Adjacent to these, and best seen with the plate microscope, a variable number of minute colonies 0·1–0·2 mm. in diameter may be seen; they grow into the depths of the medium and can only be transferred by excising a small portion of the agar. These small colonies breed true on subculture and constitute the "L forms" or "L phase" of the organism's growth; they consist mainly of very small coccoid or coccobacillary elements but larger and bizarre forms may be present.

"L" organisms are extremely resistant to penicillin, while the streptobacilli are very sensitive to this antibiotic. However, both forms have identical fermentative properties and one antigen is common to them. L forms lack an antigen present in the streptobacillus and they have little or no virulence for laboratory animals. It is now generally accepted that L forms are variants of *Streptobacillus moniliformis* in which there is a defective mechanism of cell wall formation. It should be noted that L phase variation occurs spontaneously to a greater or lesser extent with all strains of *Streptobacillus moniliformis*. In other bacteria where L phase dissociation is recognised, abnormal cultural conditions are required to induce the production of L-type colonies.

In morphology and mode of reproduction L phase organisms have many similarities to the pleuropneumonia-like organisms (mycoplasma).

Mice are susceptible to experimental inoculation and develop either a rapidly fatal generalised infection without focal lesions or a more slowly progressive disease with swelling of the feet and multiple inflammatory lesions of joints.

Laboratory Diagnosis.—In the human infection the organism has been isolated by blood culture, and from joint fluid in cases with arthritis. In fluid culture, colonies of the organism take the form of "fluff balls" situated on the surface of the sedimented blood cells.

It should be noted that another type of rat-bite fever (Soduku) is caused by *Spirillum minus* and clinically may be indistinguishable from that caused by *Streptobacillus moniliformis* (see p. 270).

Donovania granulomatis

(*Calymmatobacterium granulomatis*)

This organism, whose biological relationships are still doubtful, is responsible for a chronic granulomatous disease ("granuloma venereum") observed in tropical and subtropical countries. The initial lesion is on the genitalia. In the mononuclear cells of the lesions the organism is seen as a small Gram-negative pleomorphic bacillus (1 to 2 μ in length). It may show polar staining and appears to be capsulate. Extracellular forms are also observed. The organism has proved difficult to cultivate on the usual bacteriological media, but cultures have been readily obtained in the yolk sac of the chick embryo; after adaptation, growth can be obtained on enriched artificial media. Laboratory animals are not susceptible to inoculation, but the disease has been reproduced in man by inoculation with yolk sac cultures. The organism is not filterable. Sterilised cultures yield an allergic skin reaction in infected persons, and give a complement-fixation reaction with patient's serum. A capsular material has also been found to fix complement with sera from patients with the disease. The organism has morphological resemblances to *Klebsiella* and cross-reacts serologically with *Klebsiella rhinoscleromatis*.

It should be noted that this infection is quite different from lymphogranuloma inguinale—and should not be confused with the latter disease (see p. 481).

CHAPTER 25

THE ANTHRAX BACILLUS

LARGE straight Gram-positive rods occurring in chains which grow aerobically and form heat-resistant spores belong to the genus *Bacillus*. The Gram-positive property of strains is variable. The spores are ubiquitous and are extremely common in dust so that a large proportion of bacteria contaminating cultures belong to this group. These organisms exist as saprophytes in soil, water, air and on vegetation—e.g. *Bacillus mycoides* and *Bacillus subtilis*. *Bacillus anthracis*, the causative organism of anthrax in man and animals is the only pathogen of the group, though very occasionally species such as *B. subtilis* have been isolated from the tissues in terminal disease.

Anthrax is primarily an infectious disease of domestic herbivores; in them it occurs in various forms from a fulminating septicaemia to a subacute or chronic fever with localising pustular lesions. Man contracts the disease sporadically by coming into contact with infected animals or contaminated animal products. Anthrax is uncommon in the United Kingdom and North America but is relatively common in many other parts of the world.

BACILLUS ANTHRACIS

Morphology.—A non-motile, straight, sporing bacillus, rectangular in shape and of relatively large size—4–8 μ by 1–1·5 μ. The bacilli tend to be arranged in chains end to end (streptobacilli), but may occur singly and in pairs. In blood and tissue they exhibit a distinct capsule when suitably stained. Unlike the capsules of the pneumococcus and some other bacteria which are of polysaccharide nature, the capsule of the anthrax bacillus contains a polypeptide of D-glutamic acid. The spore, when fully developed, can be seen as a refractile oval structure, central in position and of the same cross-diameter as that of the bacillus. Sporulation occurs readily when the organism is discharged from the body of an infected animal, and spores are a morphological feature of the bacilli when growing in artificial culture, but sporulation does not occur in the tissues. After the spore is fully formed, the residual protoplasm of the bacillus disintegrates and the spore becomes a free structure. The spore represents a highly resistant phase of the organism, and can survive under conditions which would be unfavourable to the vegetative form. When replaced in favourable conditions, the envelope of the spore ruptures at one pole and the vegetative phase is reproduced.

Staining.—The organism in the tissues is strongly Gram-positive. In films prepared from cultures the staining reaction of individual bacilli is variable; older cells and the vegetative remnants of sporulating cells may be Gram-negative. The spore is unstained by the ordinary methods, but can be stained differentially by special methods.

Methylene-blue reaction of McFadyean.—This staining reaction has been utilised in veterinary work for the recognition of anthrax bacilli in blood films. The films are made in the usual way on slides, dried and passed rapidly three times through the flame; they are then stained with polychrome methylene blue for a few seconds, washed and dried. Between the bacteria an amorphous purplish material is noted, representing the disintegrated capsules of the organisms; this appearance is characteristic of the anthrax bacillus.

Cultural Characters.—Aerobe and facultative anaerobe; temperature range, 12°–45° C.; optimum, 35° C.; grows on all ordinary media; aerobic conditions are necessary for sporulation, for which the optimum temperature is 25°–30° C. Germination of spores takes place under both aerobic and anaerobic conditions. Rapid germination occurs in the presence of certain amino acids such as adenosine, *l*-alanine and *l*-tyrosine.

Colonies on agar—white, granular, circular disks (about 3 mm. in diameter after twenty-four hours' growth) which, under the low power of the microscope, show a wavy margin, often likened to locks of hair, and presenting the "medusa-head" appearance. The colony is one continuous convoluted thread of bacilli in chain formation.

Agar stroke—thick, white, opaque, somewhat dry, friable growth with irregular edges, showing the same microscopic characters as the colonies. To the naked eye this growth presents a ground-glass appearance.

Gelatin stab—a line of growth along the wire puncture from which fine lateral spikes radiate, longest towards the top. This is the so-called "inverted fir-tree growth"; liquefaction occurs later, starting at the top of the growth.

Coagulated serum is partially liquefied.

Broth—growth develops as white flakes which sediment, and sometimes shows pellicle formation.

On blood agar the anthrax bacillus is only slightly haemolytic as compared with the saprophytic members of the genus, which are markedly lytic.

Variation.—Capsule formation is subject to variation, and when the capsule is absent or imperfectly developed the colonies tend to be moist and slimy and may be devoid of the characteristic wreathed margins. This is well seen in cultures which have been attenuated in virulence by growth at temperatures above the optimum, *e.g.* 42°–43° C., as in Pasteur's method of attenuating the organism for prophylactic vaccination.

The typical colony, as described above, is of the "rough" form; the variant is small, "smooth" and without the characteristic wreathed appearance, while the bacilli in this type of colony are arranged in bundles, not in a convoluted chain. Virulence is associated with the "rough" form, the "smooth" variant being relatively avirulent.

Viability.—The vegetative cells are as susceptible as other non-sporing bacteria. The thermal death-point is about 60° C. for half an hour. The spore is highly resistant to chemical and physical changes in the environment, though there is a marked strain variation in this respect. The spores of many strains will resist dry heat at 140° C. for one to three hours and 100° C. moist heat (steam or boiling) for five to ten minutes. Five per cent. phenol requires several weeks to kill the spores, but 1 in 1000 mercuric chloride destroys them in thirty minutes and 4 per cent. potassium permanganate in fifteen minutes. For the disinfection of wool a 2 per cent. formaldehyde solution can be used and allowed to act for twenty minutes at 39°–40° C. Animal hair and bristles can also be disinfected of anthrax spores by six hours' treatment with 0·25 per cent. formaldehyde solution at 60° C., and such treatment does not affect the colour and texture of the material.

It should be noted that the usual heat fixation and staining of microscopic preparations from cultures of the anthrax bacillus may not affect the viability of the spores, and laboratory infection from handling such material has been recorded. The fixation of films by 1: 1000 mercuric chloride for five minutes has been claimed to kill the spores and does not interfere with the staining reactions.

Spore germination and the vegetative growth of most strains is inhibited by penicillin (0·1 μg./ml. or less), streptomycin (0·5–2 μg./ml.), the tetracyclines (0·1–0·5 μg./ml.), erythromycin (1 μg./ml), chloramphenicol (2·5–10 μg./ml.) and sulphonamides, in *in vitro* tests.

Biochemical Reactions—Glucose, sucrose, maltose, trehalose and dextrin are fermented with acid but no gas production. Nitrates are reduced to nitrites.

Antigenic Structure.—Three distinct antigenic components have been recognised, a somatic protein, a capsular polypeptide and a somatic polysaccharide.

The protein somatic antigen (protective antigen) stimulates immunity in most animals and it can be shown to be present in the oedema fluid of anthrax lesions. The protective antigen is difficult to assay. The usual in-vitro tests are unreliable and detection by assessment of its immunising activity in experimental animals is tedious and not very sensitive. A better in-vivo method is now available based on the following procedure. Protective antigen neutralises the antitoxic activity of anthrax antiserum and if anthrax "toxin" is subsequently added the final toxic activity of the system can be measured by a skin test in the rabbit. On agar-diffusion plates a line of precipitation occurs which correlates with the immunising activity of preparations containing the antigen and this is a useful in-vitro method.

The capsular polypeptide is composed mainly of D-glutamic acid, and this substance is found only in virulent strains. Antisera prepared by inoculating animals with encapsulated organisms react with the isolated polypeptide which by itself is not an antigen (hapten). Capsular antibody is not protective. Polypeptides of related chemical and immunological nature are found in other members of the group. The capsular polypeptide of *B. subtilis* for example contains L-glutamic acid as well as the D- form.

The somatic polysaccharide is combined with a peptide moiety containing $\alpha\epsilon$-diaminopimelic acid to form a complex included in the cell wall of the organism. By itself the isolated polysaccharide acts as a hapten and will react with antisera produced against the whole bacillus—*e.g.* in precipitin reactions. This antigen does not seem to be associated with the virulence of the organism.

Additional antigens are undoubtedly present, but as yet are uncharacterised.

Pathogenesis.—All mammals are susceptible, though to a varying degree. Some cold-blooded animals can also be infected. Guinea-pigs and mice are highly susceptible to experimental inoculation. If a guinea-pig is injected subcutaneously with pathological material containing the bacilli, or cultures, the animal dies, usually within two days, showing a marked inflammatory lesion at the site of inoculation and extensive gelatinous oedema in the subcutaneous tissues. Large numbers of the bacilli are present in the local lesion. The animal exhibits a profound septicaemia and the anthrax bacilli are present in large numbers in the heart blood and in the capillaries of the internal organs. They are specially numerous in the spleen, which is enlarged and soft, and in the kidneys. With virulent strains the LD50 by the subcutaneous route is of the order of five bacteria or less.

Experimental production of anthrax by inhalation of contaminated aerosols has also been studied. Spores deposited on the alveolar walls are taken up by phagocytes and carried to the tracheo-bronchial glands. Infection spreads via the lymphatics to the general circulation. The LD50 is about 20,000 organisms if the particle size of the aerosols is less than 5 μ, since the smaller particles are more likely to penetrate in the air-stream to the alveolar walls, but is much higher if the particles are larger.

Infection of some species of animal may be produced by the oral route with a relatively large number of spores (*e.g.* 10^{8-9}), but guinea-pigs are resistant to infection by this route.

The pathogenesis of anthrax was obscure for many years. No lethal exo- or endo-toxins could be found in artificial cultures of the organism and it was believed that death was due to the massive terminal septicaemia; the bacilli were thought to block the capillaries and exhaust the tissues of essential nutrients and oxygen. The absolute number of organisms, however, is not all important because after a certain stage of the disease control of the septicaemia with antibiotics will not prevent death and partially immunised animals die with greatly reduced numbers of bacilli in their blood. It is now recognised that the virulence of *B. anthracis* is determined by at least two unconnected factors—an extracellular toxin and the capsular polypeptide (Smith, 1960). The toxin, lethal to experimental animals on intravenous injection and evoking extensive oedema when injected intradermally, produces oligaemic shock in infected animals and it is now recognised that this is the cause of death. It was first detected in the sterile plasma of guinea-pigs dying of anthrax, but it has now been produced *in vitro* and consists of at least three practically non-toxic components which act synergistically (Stanley & Smith, 1961).

The anthrax bacillus produces an epizootic disease in herbivorous animals, particularly among sheep and cattle, but no species is completely immune. The condition is usually septicaemic in nature, and *post mortem* the bacilli are found in large numbers in the heart blood and internal organs, especially the spleen, which is enlarged and soft (splenic fever). Subacute and chronic disease also occurs in animals as do localising pustules which are analogous to the malignant pustule in man. In animals the portal of entry is the mouth and intestinal tract, the spores being ingested with coarse vegetation which probably predisposes to trauma of the mucosa.

The spores germinate at the site of entry and the vegetative cells produce "toxins" leading to the formation of gelatinous oedema and haemorrhage. In the susceptible animal the bacilli resist phagocytosis and reach the lymphatics and thence the blood stream. Before death the bacilli multiply freely in the blood and tissues. In the resistant animal there is a more profuse leucocyte response with phagocytosis and decapsulation of the organism.

In man infection is acquired from animal sources, usually through damaged skin or mucous membranes, or more rarely by inhalation of spores into the lungs. Infection thus occurs most commonly through the skin in persons such as farmers and veterinarians handling infected animals, or among dock workers, factory workers and farmers from handling carcases and hides, animal hair and bristles, shaving-brushes, feeding-stuffs, bone-meal, etc. The resulting lesion is usually described as a *malignant pustule*. This starts as a papule and becomes a blister within 12–48 hours and then a pustule with an increasing area of inflammation depending upon the resistance of the host. Coagulation necrosis of the centre results in the formation of a dark-coloured *eschar* which is later surrounded by a ring of vesicles containing serous or sero-sanguineous fluid, and outside this is an area of oedema and induration which may become very extensive.

Infection may result from inhalation of spores carried in dust or filaments of wool from infected animals, as in the wool factories—"wool-sorter's disease". The organisms settle in the lower part of the trachea or in a large bronchus, and an intense inflammatory lesion results, with haemorrhage, oedema, spread to the thoracic glands, involvement of the lungs, and effusion into the pericardial and pleural cavities; the organisms are present in considerable numbers in the lesions; a septicaemic condition or a haemorrhagic meningitis may supervene.

Infection may occur by the intestinal route, but this is relatively uncommon except in primitive societies using infected animals for food in which outbreaks with a high mortality may occur.

Epidemiology.—Anthrax is primarily a disease of animals, and man is only secondarily infected. The world incidence of human anthrax was estimated in 1958 at between 20,000 and 100,000 cases annually.

In the terminal stages of the disease in animals the bacilli are present in very large numbers in faeces, urine and saliva, and these may contaminate ground and pasture and be ingested directly by other animals, though direct spread of this type is rare. Pasturage may also be contaminated from the carcases of dead animals. The vegetative cells rapidly sporulate and the spores remain viable for many years, constituting foci of soil contamination. The spores are ingested by cattle and sheep, pass the stomach and invade the small-intestine mucosa of the new hosts which serve to perpetuate the disease. In the United Kingdom the disease is sporadic amongst cattle and is commonest in the winter months when it can usually be traced to imported feeding-stuffs that have been contaminated with anthrax spores, especially bone-meal imported from areas where animal anthrax is common, *e.g.* the Far East (Jamieson & Green, 1955).

In countries where the disease is relatively rare in animals, industrial anthrax from contamination with imported materials is the commonest form of infection in man. In general, the infectivity of the anthrax bacillus for man is not of a very high order and when a case of anthrax occurs in an industrial establishment, spores of the bacillus are often widely distributed and in large numbers in the environment. In 1958 Liverpool Docks handled over 6000 tons of dry hides and when discharged from the ships one-quarter of the hides were found to be contaminated with anthrax spores (Semple & Hobday, 1959). Nevertheless, anthrax is very rare amongst the hide handlers, only 6 cases having been recognised in 5 years. Cutaneous anthrax is by far the commonest human lesion. In the 17 years up to 1960, 109 cases of human anthrax were reported in New York State and in all but two instances the patient suffered from malignant pustule (Miller, 1961). Pulmonary anthrax, common in Great Britain and Germany as wool sorters or rag pickers disease in the nineteenth century, is now rare and the 1957 outbreak in New Hampshire is claimed to be the first in the twentieth century (Brachman *et al.*, 1960). In this small epidemic there were 5 cases (4 fatal) of inhalation anthrax during a 10-week period in a mill processing imported goat hair. During handling there was an excessive amount of dust and the air contained large numbers of anthrax spores.

Laboratory Diagnosis

Malignant Pustule.—Films are made from the exudate and stained by Gram's method; the finding of bacilli morphologically like *B. anthracis* is suggestive but not conclusive. If there are unbroken vesicles round the lesion, fluid from these should be examined.

Successive-stroke inoculations should be made on an agar plate. The resulting colonies are recognised by examining them with the low power of the microscope, and films are made and stained by Gram's method. Spores are noted in cultures.

In all cases the identity of the suspected organism must be confirmed by inoculation of a guinea-pig or mouse with exudate from the lesion, or with the isolated culture. A small dose of culture is sufficient to produce a lethal effect. The occurrence of the bacilli in the heart blood and in the spleen in considerable numbers, and the other post-mortem appearances described above, are diagnostic. In carrying out the post-mortem examination every precaution should be observed. If exudate used for inoculation contains other organisms, it is advisable to inoculate it on a scarified area of skin in preference to subcutaneous injection.

Diagnosis of Anthrax in Domestic Animals (*post-mortem*).—The usual form of post-mortem examination must not be made, in order to prevent any distribution of sporing bacilli from the carcase. In the body no sporulation occurs, but spores are readily formed when the bacilli are exposed to air. Films of blood taken from a superficial vein in the ear are prepared, and stained by Gram's method and by McFadyean's methylene-blue method (*vide supra*). The finding of characteristic bacilli in the blood giving the methylene-blue reaction is diagnostic. In pigs and horses the bacilli may not be detectable in the blood. If necessary, the organism can be cultivated and identified by the procedure described above, a specimen of blood from the ear being used for the investigation.

Isolation of Bacillus Anthracis from Heavily Contaminated Material.—If the material (*e.g.* hair, hide, tissue, bone-meal) is heavily contaminated, shake a portion with water and allow it to stand for three to four hours with occasional shaking. Squeeze or tease the material and heat the supernatant fluid to 70° C. for ten minutes. Add different volumes (0·2 ml.–2·0 ml.) of this fluid to melted agar, pour plates and incubate at 37° C. for 12–15 hours. It is essential to examine the plates early. Examine for deep colonies which have a typical filamentous appearance sometimes likened to knotted string. A rich culture medium is essential and plates should not be too crowded with colonies. Confirmation is obtained by inoculation subcutaneously in the mouse or guinea-pig.

For direct isolation by animal inoculation centrifuge 50 ml. (or more) of the heat-treated fluid described above at high speed (3000 r.p.m.) for fifteen minutes. Discard the supernatant and inoculate the residue intramuscularly into a guinea-pig which has been passively immunised 24 hours previously with *Cl. welchii* antitoxin 1000 units, *Cl. septicum* antitoxin 500 units, *Cl. oedematiens* antitoxin 1000 units and tetanus antitoxin 500 units; or a polyvalent gas-gangrene serum with added tetanus antitoxin. Death due to anthrax occurs in two to three days. Death from gas-gangrene (usually due to *Cl. septicum* or *Cl. bifermentans*) occurs earlier. In the latter cases aerobic cultures from the local lesion and spleen should be made as they may yield *B. anthracis*. The minimum infecting dose is 30–50 spores.

Precipitin Test.—This test was first used by Ascoli in the recognition of anthrax infection in organs and tissues from suspected carcases, and may be applicable even in the case of putrefied material. It depends on the occurrence of a specific precipitin in the serum of an artificially immunised animal. Immune sera, however, vary in their precipitin content, and for the test a serum with known precipitating properties must be selected. About 2 grams of the tisssue are boiled for five minutes with 5 ml. of normal saline, to which acetic acid has been added in the proportion of 1: 1000. The fluid is cooled and then filtered through paper. 0·5 ml. of the serum is placed in a narrow tube and the filtrate is carefully run on to the top. The development within fifteen minutes of a white ring of precipitate at the junction of the two fluids denotes a positive result.

Chemotherapy.—Most antibiotics to which the anthrax bacillus is sensitive in in-vitro tests have been used sucessfully in the treatment of anthrax in man. Chemotherapeutic agents have no effect upon the "toxins" already produced, therefore it is important to institute therapy as soon as possible.

The serum of artificially immunised animals, *e.g.* Sclavo's serum, has been used in the treatment of human anthrax combined with anti-bacterial drugs. Doses of 50–100 ml. given intravenously, and repeated daily if necessary in severe cases, have been recommended.

In animals, treatment is not often possible as most cases are not diagnosed till moribund or dead. Penicillin in large doses and chlortetracycline should be given combined with immune serum.

Prophylaxis and Control.—In outbreaks of animal anthrax, affected animals must be promptly diagnosed and isolated. Carcases must be disposed of by deep burial in quicklime or cremation to limit sporulation of the organism from the tissues and spread to pasturage and other animals. The limitation of the import of animal hides and hair to a single port (Liverpool), where facilities for mechanical handling and disinfection are available ("Duckering"), has done much to reduce the danger of anthrax in the United Kingdom (see Anthrax Order, 1938).

The eradication of anthrax in animals can be assisted by active immunisation procedures and numerous vaccines have been used. Active immunity can be induced by immunisation with either live attenuated bacilli, live spores or the somatic protein (protective) antigen. Vaccines of live bacilli which have been grown at 42°–43° C. were first introduced by Pasteur in 1881, but it has always proved difficult to regulate the degree of attenuation of these vaccines. Live spore vaccines (*e.g.* the "Sterne" strain) prepared from the non-encapsulated avirulent bacilli were originally employed in South Africa. Protection is produced by one dose and these vaccines, more stable and much safer than the Pasteurian vaccines, have now been used on a large scale. In Russia, where 2·7 million farm animals have been immunised with spore vaccines, the incidence of accidental death from its use was about 1 in 100,000. The spore vaccines, however, are not generally considered safe enough for man. Preparations of protective antigen are effective non-living immunising agents whereas the capsular polypeptide is not immunogenic. Protective antigen is present in extracts of anthrax lesions and it is elaborated when *B. anthracis* is grown, under rather critical conditions, in serum-containing or certain chemically defined media (Belton & Strange, 1954; Wright *et al.*, 1962). There is a strong serological connection between this antigen and the anthrax toxin. Alum-precipitated protective antigen is very safe, but the immunity produced does not last as long as that following immunisation with a spore vaccine. It has been used (Brachman *et al.*, 1962) in the United States to immunise workers handling raw imported goat hair; six injections of antigen were given over a 19-month period followed by an annual booster dose. Reactions were regarded as negligible and the vaccine was considered effective in protecting against cutaneous anthrax. Recent work (Klein *et al.*, 1962) using guinea-pigs suggests that there is a great increase in protection when immunisation with protective antigen is supplemented by an injection of a live spore vaccine.

THE AEROBIC GRAM-POSITIVE SPORING BACILLI BIOLOGICALLY ALLIED TO BACILLUS ANTHRACIS

These organisms are saprophytes, and represent a large number of different species. They are found in soil, water, dust and air. Being ubiquitous, they are frequent contaminants of culture medium in the laboratory, and bacteriological workers should be acquainted with their general biological characters.

Classical types representative of this group are *B. subtilis* (the "Hay bacillus"), *B. mycoides*, *B. mesentericus*, *B. megaterium* and *B. cereus*. The type-species is *B. subtilis*, and for convenience these organisms are sometimes spoken of as the "*B. subtilis group*". For the detailed differential features of the various species, reference can be made to *Bergey's Manual of Determinative Bacteriology* (7th edition). The general characters of the commoner types met with in laboratory work may be summarised as follows, and for general purposes it is unnecessary to identify a particular species.

Morphology and Staining.—Certain large-cell types tend to resemble the anthrax bacillus, e.g. *B. mesentericus*. Others, e.g. *B. cereus*, *B. mycoides* and *B. megaterium*, are shorter with rounded ends, and several motile species with peritrichous flagella are met with, e.g. *B. subtilis*. The spore is central or excentric, e.g. *B. subtilis*, *B. mycoides*, subterminal or terminal. It may be relatively small, not exceeding 0·8 μ, e.g. *B. mesentericus*, or large, up to 1·8 μ, e.g. *B. megaterium*.

Cultural Characters.—The optimum temperature is usually low, *e.g.* about 20° C., but certain types grow best between 30° and 37° C. and some are thermophilic, with their optimum temperature at 55° C.; they are characteristically aerobes, but, usually, also facultative anaerobes; abundant growth occurs on all the ordinary culture media. The appearance of the growth varies considerably among different types. *B. subtilis* produces a white, glistening, adherent, somewhat membranous growth, which tends to spread, and somewhat similar growths are seen among other species. Certain types produce colonies and growths practically similar to *B. anthracis*, with the same "medusa-head" appearance, e.g. "*B. anthracoides*". The colonies of *B. mycoides* are at first similar to those of the anthrax bacillus, but are easily differentiated by their feathery appearance, due to long projecting and branching threads radiating out from the central growth. The growths may be dry, gummy or moist, and white, greyish-white, yellowish or brown. Certain species producing a black pigment have been described. On potato, characteristic cultural appearances may be noted, e.g. *B. mesentericus* develops a thick wrinkled or folded layer of growth which assumes a brownish colour. Pellicle formation in broth is a frequent character. Generally, gelatin is liquefied and proteolytic action is well developed. Some types ferment carbohydrates. Starch may be hydrolysed.

McGaughey and Chu (1948) have shown that of the group of aerobic sporing bacilli only *B. mycoides*, *B. cereus*, and to a less extent *B. anthracis*, are capable of splitting the lecithin of egg-yolk incorporated in a culture medium. This reaction, which is due to an enzyme, phospholipinase, separates them quite sharply from *B. subtilis* and other members of the group. *B. cereus* is commonly found in heat-treated milk and it may be identified by culture on an egg-yolk-agar plate.

These organisms are usually non-pathogenic on experimental inoculation into laboratory animals.

Bacillus anthracoides.—This designation has been applied to a type of organism of the above group, which in morphological and cultural characters closely resembles *B. anthracis* and may exhibit the "medusa-head" colonies characteristic of the latter. Under certain conditions this organism might at first be confused with the anthrax bacillus. It can be differentiated, however, by its motility. Colonies on blood agar are usually haemolytic (*cf.* anthrax bacillus). It should be noted that if a large dose of culture of this type of organism is injected into a guinea-pig or mouse, a local inflammatory lesion with oedema may be produced, followed by septicaemia and death. The organism can be detected in the heart blood and internal organs, though *in small number* (*cf.* anthrax). In blood or tissues it does not exhibit the McFadyean methylene-blue reaction.

REFERENCES

Belton, F. C. & Strange, R. E. (1954). Studies on a protective antigen produced *in vitro* from *Bacillus anthracis*: medium and methods of production. *Brit. J. exp. Path.*, **35**, 144.

Brachman, P. S., Gold, H., Plotkin, S. A., Fekety, F. R., Werrin, M. & Ingraham, N. R. (1962). Field evaluation of a human anthrax vaccine. *Amer. J. publ. Hlth*, **52**, 632.

Brachman, P. S., Plotkin, S. A., Bumford, F. H. & Atchison, M. M. (1960). An epidemic of inhalation anthrax: The first in the twentieth century. II. Epidemiology. *Amer. J. Hyg.*, **72**, 6.

Jamieson, W. M. & Green, D. M. (1955). Anthrax and bone-meal fertiliser. *Lancet*, **1**, 560.

Klein, F., De Armon, I. A., Lincoln, R. E., Mahlandt, B. G. & Fernelius, A. L. (1962). Immunological studies of Anthrax. II. Levels of immunity against *Bacillus anthracis* obtained with protective antigen and live vaccine. *J. Immunol.*, **88**, 15.

McGaughey, C. A. & Chu, H. P. (1948). The egg-yolk reaction of aerobic sporing bacilli. *J. gen. Microbiol.*, **2**, 334.

Miller, J. K. (1961). Human anthrax in New York State. *N.Y. St. J. Med.*, **61**, 2046.

Semple, A. B. & Hobday, T. L. (1959). Control of anthrax. *Lancet*, **2**, 507.

Smith, H. (1960). Studies on organisms grown *in vivo* to reveal the bases of microbial pathogenicity. *Ann. N. Y. Acad. Sci.*, **88**, 1213.

Stanley, J. L. & Smith, H. (1961). Purification of Factor I and recognition of a third factor of the anthrax toxin. *J. gen. Microbiol.*, **26**, 49.

Wright, G. G., Puziss, M. & Neely, W. B. (1962). Studies on immunity in anthrax IX. Effect of variations in cultural conditions on elaboration of protective antigen by strains of *B. anthracis*. *J. Bact.*, **83**, 515.

CHAPTER 26

ACTINOMYCES: NOCARDIA: ACTINOBACILLUS

ACTINOMYCES is a genus of anaerobic or micro-aerophilic, non-acid-fast organisms within the family *Actinomycetaceae.* This genus is parasitic on man and animals. By contrast the other genus of the family, *Nocardia*, is comprised of members which are obligate aerobes, some of which are acid-fast and the majority are saprophytic although a few are facultatively parasitic on man and certain animals. The family *Streptomycetaceae* bears certain resemblances to the *Actinomycetaceae* and within the former, the genus *Streptomyces*, which is entirely saprophytic has a particular medical significance, *viz.* some species produce antibiotics of recognised therapeutic importance, e.g. *Streptomyces griseus* produces streptomycin.

ACTINOMYCES

There are three species within this genus; *Actinomyces israelii* which is primarily commensal and occasionally pathogenic in man, *Actinomyces bovis* which fulfills a similar role in bovines and *Actinomyces baudetii*, the causal organism of actinomycosis in dogs and cats.

Actinomyces israelii

Morphology.—In morbid tissues the organism forms colonies which are recognisable to the naked eye and are referred to as sulphur granules; in early infections these are white and semi-transparent but develop a yellow colour and eventually become dark brown if the infection is not recognised for some time. Microscopically *Actino. israelii* comprises a mycelium or felted mass of branching filaments which are 1 μ thick; centrally the filaments are irregularly interlaced but at the periphery of the colony the filaments tend to be arranged radially. The mycelium shows true dichotomous branching but undergoes fragmentation very rapidly so that extensive branching is rare.

Around the actinomyces colony, particularly in animal tissues, pyriform or club-shaped structures develop; originally these were thought to result from swelling of the sheath at the extremities of the peripheral radial filaments. It is more likely that the clubs represent lipoid material deposited from the host tissues around the invading filaments. In human lesions club formation is less frequent than in animals; in tissue sections the clubs are noted to lie radially with their wide-end outwards and form a complete ring around the colony (ray fungus). In animal lesions the clubs may constitute the main morphological feature of older colonies owing to degeneration of the mycelial elements which become fused into structureless material in the centre of the colony. In *in vitro* culture the microscopic appearances are usually quite different from the tissue forms; the typical mycelium is incomplete and although some branching filaments are seen the main feature is of short bacillary forms closely resembling diphtheroid bacilli.

Staining.—The filaments are Gram-positive. The clubs usually stain Gram-negatively, but are acid-fast and can be stained differentially by Ziehl-Neelsen's method, using 1 per cent. in place of 20 per cent. H_2SO_4 for decolourisation.

Cultural Characters.—Anaerobic or micro-aerophilic conditions are required for growth which is also favoured by an increased concentration of carbon dioxide. The optimum temperature for growth is 37° C. and growth does not occur at temperatures much below the optimum. Although growth will occur on nutrient agar it is enhanced if blood agar, glucose agar or 5 per cent. serum agar is employed.

Colonies are raised, nodular, cream-coloured and opaque; they show considerable polymorphism but in all cases are firmly adherent to the medium.

A shake culture in a tube of nutrient agar reveals a characteristic distribution of the colonies, which are most numerous in a zone 10–20 mm. below the surface, where there is only a trace of free oxygen present and an optimal concentration of carbon dioxide.

Biochemical Reactions.—These are essentially restricted to saccharolytic anaerogenic activities against a wide range of substrates. The species is non-haemolytic, non-proteolytic and soluble pigments are not produced on protein media; neither are insoluble pigments produced by growth.

Antigenic Characteristics.—Strains are antigenically homogeneous and quite distinct from strains of *Actino. bovis*.

Animal Pathogenicity.—Circumscribed tumour-like granulomatous lesions containing colonies of the organism have been produced by experimental inoculation of rabbits and guinea-pigs; however, experimental inoculation does not always give rise to such lesions and when they do occur they are neither extensive nor fatal.

Pathogenesis.—*Actino. israelii* occurs as a commensal in the human mouth and can be isolated from tonsils and carious teeth in 5 per cent. of otherwise healthy individuals (Sullivan & Goldsworthy, 1940).

Actinomycosis in man is essentially an infection of the cervico-facial region (65 per cent. of cases) with abdominal infections (19 per cent.) the next most common; other sites, *e.g.* thorax, skin are also involved. In human cases the lesions usually show a suppurative tendency and secondary infection with pyogenic cocci is common. The commonest avenue of infection is through the mucosa of the mouth or throat and frequently the lesion is related to a carious tooth or tooth extraction; the initial infectivity of the organism is probably low and tissue invasion may occur only when some additional factor, *e.g.* trauma, is applied.

Metastatic lesions are liable to occur by blood-stream spread, *e.g.* to the kidney, lung or brain or to the liver from a primary intestinal lesion, *e.g.* in the appendix.

Epidemiology.—At one time it was thought that infection might be from grain, since fragments of the latter were occasionally found in relation to the primary lesion. However *Actino. israelii* is a strict parasite and incapable of a saprophytic existence; hence human actinomycosis is now regarded as endogenous in origin.

There are still some puzzling features in the incidence of the disease; males are more commonly affected than females (3 : 1) and although cases occur at all ages, most fall in the 20–29 yr. group with the 10–19 yr. group a close second. Between them these two decades account for more than half the incidence.

Although there is no relationship with bovine actinomycosis, male agricultural workers are more liable to suffer infection with *Actino. israelii* than men in other occupations (Porter, 1953).

In addition to the trauma caused by grain in probably inciting infection in the buccal mucosa, it has long been recognised that dental extractions may precipitate infection; similarly appendicectomy is often associated with the onset of abdominal infection. External trauma, accidental or intentional, has also been noted to precede the onset of the disease.

Laboratory Diagnosis

If the pus from an actinomycotic lesion is spread out in a thin layer in a Petri dish or on a microscope slide, the characteristic colonies or granules can be recognised with the naked eye. For microscopic examination the granules in a drop of pus are crushed between two slides. In this way films can be prepared and then stained by Gram's method.

The granules can easily be separated by shaking up the pus with water in a test-tube, allowing them to sediment and collecting them in a capillary pipette. They are then deposited on a slide and films made by crushing. Preparations obtained in this way are more satisfactory than those made directly from pus in which the granules may be relatively scanty.

Microscopic demonstration of Gram-positive branching filaments arranged in the form of a mycelium is generally sufficient for clinical diagnosis.

In tissue lesions the colonies can be recognised by preparing histological sections and staining by Gram's method, and, in the case of animal lesions, by the modified Ziehl-Neelsen method described above.

To cultivate the organism it is essential that actual granules should be used for inoculating the medium. For this purpose the pus is mixed with sterile water, the granules are allowed to sediment or deposited by centrifuging and then removed with a pipette; this is repeated two or three times so that the granules are thoroughly washed. This procedure is particularly necessary when there is mixed infection. Two blood-agar plates are inoculated with the separated granules. One is incubated aerobically, the other anaerobically. Tubes of melted agar containing 5 per cent. serum may also be inoculated as shake cultures to demonstrate micro-aerophilic growth.

Actinomyces bovis

Morphologically similar to *Actino. israelii*; in culture, colonies are smoother and softer in consistency and do not adhere to the medium. *Actino. bovis* is more tolerant of oxygen. There is no serological relation between the two species.

Actino. bovis is commonly found in and around the mouths of healthy cattle and is responsible for local lesions, *e.g.* lumpy jaw; like infection in man, bovine actinomycosis may spread metastatically by the blood stream.

Actinomyces baudetii

This species was at one time thought to be identical with *Actino. israelii*. Morphologically they are distinctive in that the club formation associated with *Actino. baudetii* absorbs basic stains and not acid stains. The organism is micro-aerophilic, grows slowly with the production of dull, whitish colonies about the size of a pin-head after 4–5 days incubation.

Actino. baudetii has been isolated from actinomycotic lesions in dogs and cats; it is not pathogenic for man or cattle.

NOCARDIA

Apart from the typical actinomycoses, granulomatous and suppurative conditions occur in animals and man, resulting from infection with mycelial organisms of the genus *Nocardia*. There are more than 40 species in the genus but the majority are saprophytic; they differ from members of the genus *Actinomyces* in being obligate aerobes, frequently chromogenic and often acid-fast.

Nocardia asteroides (*Actinomyces asteroides*; *Eppinger's Streptothrix*)

Originally isolated from a brain abscess. The filaments are relatively broad (1 μ in diameter) and very readily break up in culture into bacillary forms. They stain Gram-positively and are slightly acid-fast. This organism can be cultivated aerobically on ordinary media as a friable, white, dry, wrinkled or nodular growth, which later becomes pigmented (yellow or pink).

Nocardia farcinica (*Actinomyces farcinicus or nocardii*)

The organism of bovine "farcy", in which superficial lymph glands become swollen and ulcerate through the skin.

The organism shows mycelium formation, but in culture it readily fragments into shorter bacillary and oval forms. A feature of the organism is the beaded, irregular appearance of the filaments when stained by Gram's stain. It is Gram-positive; some strains are strongly acid- and alcohol-fast whilst others are completely decolourised. It grows aerobically at 37° C. on ordinary media, producing raised irregular greyish-white colonies after 2–3 weeks. On Löwenstein's medium, however, small yellow colonies appear after 4–5 days' incubation.

Guinea-pigs are susceptible to experimental inoculation and develop nodular or tubercle-like lesions. In cattle, subcutaneous injection leads to a localised abscess which breaks through the skin and produces a chronic ulcerated lesion. Rabbits are not susceptible to inoculation.

Nocardia madurae

One of the causal organisms of mycetoma (madura foot) which is an infective granuloma usually localised to the tissues of the foot. The condition is restricted to certain tropical or sub-tropical countries.

In the tissue lesion and the pus, granules are noted as in actinomycosis and are usually pale yellow in colour; morphologically *Noc. madurae* resembles *Actinomyces* microscopically. Colonies are round and shiny, early growth is white but changes to yellow and eventually pink but pigment production is irregular and unpredictable. Other species isolated from cases of mycetoma include *Noc. transvalensis*, *Noc. africana* and *Noc. pelletieri.* It should be noted that in some cases of madura foot, the infection is caused by true fungi such as *Madurella.*

ACTINOBACILLUS

There are four members of the genus *Actinobacillus* all of which are pathogenic for various animals and one of which, *A. actinomycetemcomitans* is found in human cases of actinomycosis either alone or more usually along with *Actino. israelii.* Actinobacilli are small, Gram-negative, non-motile rods which rarely grow into filaments. They are aerobic and facultatively anaerobic although preferring micro-aerophilic conditions for primary isolation.

Actinobacillus lignieresii

The cause of slowly developing granulomata especially in the soft tissues of the lower jaw and neck in cattle; lesions also develop in the tongue muscles —so-called "woody-tongue" disease. Unlike actinomycosis, there is little tendency to invade bones and spread is usually lymphatic.

Strains of *Actino. lignieresii* identical with those isolated from pathological material have been isolated from bovine ruminal contents and from the tongues of normal cattle (Phillips 1961; 1964) and it would appear that infection is endogenous in origin.

REFERENCES

Phillips, J. E. (1961). The commensal role of *Actinobacillus lignieresi. J. Path. Bact.*, **82**, 205.

Phillips, J. E. (1964). Commensal actinobacilli from the bovine tongue. *J. Path. Bact.*, **87**, 442.

Porter, I. A. (1953). Actinomycosis in Scotland. *Brit. med. J.*, **2**, 1084.

Sullivan, H. R. & Goldsworthy, N. E. (1940). Comparative study of anaerobic strains of *Actinomyces* from clinically normal mouths and from actinomycotic lesions. *J. Path. Bact.*, **51**, 253.

CHAPTER 27

CLOSTRIDIUM

I: THE GAS-GANGRENE GROUP

THE genus *Clostridium* comprises the Gram-positive spore-bearing anaerobic bacilli. Most species of this genus are saprophytes that normally grow in soil, water and decomposing plant and animal matter, playing an important part in the process of putrefaction. Some are commensal inhabitants of the animal or human intestine, and a few species produce disease. The latter include: *Cl. welchii*, *Cl. septicum* and *Cl. oedematiens*, the causes of gas gangrene and other infections; *Clostridium tetani*, the cause of tetanus; and *Cl. botulinum*, the cause of botulism. With only a few exceptions, the bacteria producing powerful exotoxins belong to this genus.

The bacilli are typically large, straight or slightly curved rods, 3–8 μ by 0·6–1 μ, with slightly rounded ends. Pleomorphism is common and a pure culture may contain many forms, including filaments, citron, spindle-shaped and club forms. Some members of this group tend to lose their Gram-positive reaction early in culture, especially in broth culture, and may then appear Gram-negative. All produce spores but vary widely in their readiness to do so. Information regarding the shape of the spore and its position in the bacillus is of use in classification. *Cl. welchii* and the type species *Cl. butyricum* are the only capsulate members.

Almost all members of the genus are motile, but *Cl. welchii* is an important exception. Some motile species do not show active motility under the relatively aerobic conditions of the usual wet-film preparations. These may be examined in tissue fluid preparations following animal inoculation. A semi-solid nutrient-agar medium for the demonstration of motility is recommended. Stab cultures in this medium, freshly prepared with 1 per cent. glucose added to enhance anaerobiosis, should be examined frequently before excessive gas production invalidates the test. It should be noted that a non-motile species (e.g. *Cl. welchii*) may show lateral spikes of growth along "faults" extending from the stab line, but the appearance is not likely to be confused with the diffuse growth of a truly motile species.

The clostridia are biochemically active, frequently possessing both saccharolytic (carbohydrate-decomposing) and proteolytic (protein-decomposing) properties. In general, one or other of these activities is predominant in any one species, and two groups are thus recognised:

The Saccharolytic Organisms are characterised by their rapid and vigorous growth in carbohydrate media with the production of acid and abundant gas. Saccharolytic species ferment glucose and may, in addition, be usefully examined for fermentation of lactose, maltose, sucrose and salicin. In routine sugar fermentation tests a small iron nail may be conveniently included in each tube. The nail should not project above the level of the fluid medium. The indicator dyes in such tests become reduced and may be irreversibly decolourised so that it is advisable to add a little fresh indicator to the tests when recording the results or to check their final reaction by spot tests on a tile with bromothymol blue indicator. When grown in cooked-meat broth, saccharolytic clostridia rapidly produce acid and gas but do not digest the meat; the cultures may have a slightly sour smell and the meat is often reddened. Gas production is not necessarily indicative of sugar fermentation, as proteolysis may be accompanied by evolution of gas bubbles.

The Proteolytic Group digest protein and liquefy gelatin and coagulated serum. Cultures in meat medium cause blackening of the meat, decomposing it and reducing it in volume with the formation of foul-smelling products.

Cl. welchii, *Cl. septicum*, *Cl. tertium* and *Cl. fallax* are examples of predominantly saccharolytic clostridia. *Cl. sporogenes*, *Cl. histolyticum* and *Cl. tetani* are proteolytic or predominantly so. There is, however, no hard and fast line of demarcation between the two groups. Thus, *Cl. welchii* has slight proteolytic activity, and *Cl. sporogenes* some saccharolytic properties.

Morphological and biochemical variations within strains of the same species, and indeed within subcultures of the same strain, render identification of the clostridia difficult. Whenever possible, the identity of a toxigenic species should be confirmed by specific toxin neutralisation tests, though it should be borne in mind that non-toxigenic strains of toxin-producing species occur.

Strains may be preserved by freeze-drying or by storage in various media. Cooked-meat broth containing chalk and minced cooked egg-white is a useful preservation medium. Germination of spores is sporadic, especially following heat-resistance tests, and this is considered to be due to fatty acids in the subculture medium. The inhibitory effect may be reduced by incorporating a little soluble starch or serum in the medium when subcultures are made from preservation media or from heat-resistance tests.

GAS GANGRENE

Several members of the genus *Clostridium* are associated with rapidly spreading oedema, necrosis and gangrene of the tissues, and gas production, occurring as a complication of wound infection in man. The main source of these organisms is animal and human excreta. They were responsible for the gas gangrene which was so prevalent among the armies in Europe during the war of 1914-18 and, though much less frequent, was met with in the war of 1939-45. Of more than two hundred war cases of gas gangrene infected with a single *Clostridium* species, recorded in 1918 and 1943, *Cl. welchii* occurred in more than 30 per cent., *Cl. oedematiens* in 5–17 per cent., *Cl. bifermentans* (*sordellii*),

Cl. histolyticum and *Cl. fallax* each in less than 1 per cent. In 42–60 per cent. of wounds in these two series, more than one species of *Clostridium* were involved. Data obtained in the two wars indicate that *Cl. welchii* occurred most frequently (about 60 per cent. of all cases) in gas gangrene, while *Cl. oedematiens* and *Cl. septicum* occurred in about 20–40 per cent. and 10–20 per cent. of cases respectively. The other clostridia mentioned occurred much less frequently.

The infection usually results from the contamination of a wound with soil (particularly that of manured and cultivated land), dirty clothing, street dust, etc., but may also be derived from the skin, especially in areas of the body that may be contaminated with intestinal organisms. Impairment of the normal blood supply of tissue, and the presence of devitalised or dead tissue, blood clot, foreign bodies or coincident pyogenic infection, are factors which promote the occurrence of gas gangrene in a wound. The predisposing factors later discussed in detail with regard to tetanus (p. 331) are equally applicable in the case of gas gangrene. It is particularly important that there should be no delay in treating wounds. In puerperal cases, and especially in cases of septic abortion, the organisms may gain access via the perineum to necrotic or devitalised tissues and set up a dangerous infection. It should be remembered, however, that a clostridial infection may also be located in subcutaneous tissue where there has been extravasation of blood or an accumulation of tissue fluids. Infection occurs, frequently in less severe form, in association with ischaemic conditions of the extremities, for example in diabetic gangrene. Other less severe forms of clostridial infection may occur without the typical toxaemia, such wounds having a foul odour and showing evidence of gas formation. Moreover, potentially pathogenic anaerobes may be cultivated from a wound that never shows any signs of gas gangrene. MacLennan (1943) has classified anaerobic infections on clinical grounds and he recognises (*a*) simple contamination of a wound with clostridia; (*b*) anaerobic cellulitis, in which muscle is not involved; and (*c*) anaerobic myositis, which includes clostridial gas gangrene but may also be caused by anaerobic streptococci. *Cl. welchii* may also be involved in infections occurring as a result of extension of the organism from the alimentary tract, as in cases of appendicitis or intestinal obstruction.

In wounds there is practically always a mixed infection, so that simple plating alone is frequently inadequate for diagnostic purposes. It must be emphasised that the separation and cultivation of anaerobes is more difficult than is the case with aerobes, but this is partly due to the fact that techniques for the isolation of anaerobes are not so well developed at present. While alternate culture on plates and in fluid media may sometimes be necessary before a pure culture is obtained, *direct* culture on selective agar media can yield more information regarding the importance of infection by any one pathogen. An account is given on p. 321 of the methods in general use for isolating and identifying the more important anaerobes, with particular reference to cases of gas gangrene.

CLOSTRIDIUM WELCHII
(Cl. perfringens)

This is the organism most commonly associated with gas gangrene. There are five types designated A to E and distinguished by the various combinations of toxins they produce. The classical *Cl. welchii* of *gas gangrene* belongs to type A. The other types are more commonly associated with disease in animals.

Morphology and Staining.—A relatively large Gram-positive bacillus, about 4–6 μ by 1 μ, with square or rounded ends, occurring singly or in pairs, and always capsulate when seen in the tissues. In sugar media the bacilli are shorter, while in protein media they tend to become filamentous. The bacilli are non-motile. Spores are formed, but only in the absence of fermentable carbohydrates and abundantly only on special media such as Ellner medium. They are typically oval, subterminal and not bulging, but many bizarre forms are seen. Sporulation in Ellner medium is very variable, even when different cultures of the same strain of *Cl. welchii* are studied (Cash & Collee, 1962).

Cultural Characters.—Obligatory anaerobe. Optimum temperature about 37°C. Grows best on carbohydrate-containing media, *e.g.* glucose agar or glucose-blood agar.

Surface colonies are large, round, smooth, regular and slightly opaque disks. Other types of colonies are observed, including one having a raised opaque centre and a flat transparent border which is radially striated. Rough flat colonies with an irregular edge resembling a vine-leaf also occur. On horse-blood agar the colonies are usually surrounded by a variable zone of complete haemolysis, and a wider zone of incomplete haemolysis may occasionally develop.

A variant occasionally produces very mucoid broth cultures and this yields tenacious colonies on blood agar.

Biochemical Reactions.—In litmus milk medium, acid, clot and gas production result; the gas breaks up the clot, producing the "stormy clot" reaction that is produced by almost all strains of *Cl. welchii* but is not specific for this organism. The culture has a sour, butyric-acid odour.

Cl. welchii is actively saccharolytic and ferments, with gas production, glucose, lactose, sucrose, maltose, starch, and, in the case of some strains, salicin, glycerol and inulin. Mannitol and dulcitol are not fermented.

Gelatin is liquefied. Coagulated serum is usually not liquefied. In cooked-meat medium the meat is reddened and no digestion occurs.

Viability.—*Cl. welchii* spores resist the action of the routinely used antiseptics and disinfectants. The spores of classical type A strains of *Cl. welchii* are only moderately heat-resistant and will not survive boiling for more than a few minutes. The spores of food-poisoning strains and certain type C strains, however, are markedly heat-resistant and may survive boiling for several hours.

Toxins.—The types of *Cl. welchii* differ in the combinations of various toxic and enzymic factors that they produce. Several of these factors have haemolytic, lethal or necrotising properties and others have enzymatic activity against biological substrates. The differences are indicated in detail in the following Table adapted from the work of

THE MAJOR LETHAL TOXINS AND MINOR LETHAL OR NON-LETHAL FACTORS PRODUCED BY THE VARIOUS TYPES OF *Cl. welchii* (after Brooks, Sterne & Warrack, 1957.)

Type	Occurrence	Major Lethal Toxins				Minor Lethal or Non-Lethal Factors							
		α	β	ε	ι	γ	δ	η	θ	κ	λ	μ	ν
A	Gas gangrene. Puerperal infection : Septicaemia.	+ + +	−	−	−	−	−	(+)	+ −	+ −	−	+ −	+ −
	Food-poisoning.	+ + +	−	−	−	−	−	−	(+)	+ −	−	+ −	+ +
B	Lamb dysentery.	+ + +	+ + +	+ +	−	+ +	(+)	−	+ +	−	+ + +	+ + +	+ +
C	" Struck " in sheep.	+ + +	+ + +	−	−	+ +	+ + +	−	+ + +	+ + +	−	−	+ −
	Enteritis in other animals.	+ + +	+ + +	−	−	?	−	−	+ + +	+ + +	−	−	+ −
	Enteritis necroticans in man.	+ + +	+ +	−	−	+ +	−	−	−	−	−	−	+ + +
D	Enterotoxaemia of sheep and pulpy kidney disease.	+ + +	−	+ + +	−	−	−	−	+ +	+ +	+ +	+ −	+ −
E	Doubtful pathogen of sheep and cattle.	+ + +	−	−	+ + +	−	−	−	+ +	+ +	+ +	(+)	+ −

+ + + = produced by all strains. + + = produced by most strains. + − = produced by some strains.
(+) = produced by very few strains. +++ = large amounts.

Brooks, Sterne and Warrack (1957). It is evident that the types of *Cl. welchii* can be differentiated on the basis of their production of the four major lethal toxins. Type A strains produce alpha toxin; type B strains typically produce alpha, beta and epsilon toxins; type C strains produce alpha and beta toxins; type D strains produce alpha and epsilon toxins; and type E strains produce alpha and iota toxins.

Antitoxin to the types of *Cl. welchii* commonly encountered in disease will neutralise the major lethal antigens of these types as follows:

Type A antitoxin neutralises only the homologous toxin.
Type B antitoxin neutralises the toxins of types A, B, C and D.
Type C antitoxin neutralises the toxins of types A and C.
Type D antitoxin neutralises the toxins of types A and D.

The neutralisation tests may be performed by intracutaneous or intravenous injection of guinea-pigs or mice respectively, with mixtures of toxin and antitoxin. Epsilon and iota toxins do not occur in fully active form in cultures and these prototoxins require to be activated by trypsinisation of samples of the culture filtrates prior to neutralisation tests. A combination of *in vivo* and *in vitro* tests has been recommended for the routine typing of *Cl. welchii* (Oakley & Warrack, 1953).

Intracutaneous Serum Neutralisation Tests in Guinea-pigs.—The following procedure has been developed at the Wellcome Research Laboratories, Beckenham, England, and is recommended:

Aliquots (0·5 ml.) of bacteria-free filtrate from a 5-hr. cooked-meat broth culture are made up to 0·8 ml. quantities by adding nutrient broth and 0·1 ml. volumes of specific antisera as indicated below (see Table). A similar set of mixtures is prepared after activation of any epsilon and iota prototoxins and destruction of any beta toxin present, by treatment of the crude filtrate with 0·005 per cent. (w/v) crystalline trypsin for 1 hr. at 37° C. The filtrate-antitoxin mixtures are held at room temperature for 30 min., and 0·2 ml. of each is then injected into the skin of a depilated albino guinea-pig. Reactions are read at 24 and 48 hr. Death of the guinea-pig is occasionally due to excess epsilon toxin and this necessitates repetition with filtrate diluted (1 in 5 or 1 in 10) with broth. The alpha toxin produces a spreading yellowish necrotic lesion on intracutaneous injection. The beta toxin produces a purplish necrotic lesion. Epsilon toxin causes a whitish necrotic lesion with occasional patches of small purplish haemorrhages, and iota toxin produces a circular area of purplish white necrosis vaguely outlined with purple.

Intravenous Serum Neutralisation Tests in Mice.—Two 0·3 ml. volumes of each mixture prepared as for the intracutaneous tests are injected intravenously into pairs of mice which are subsequently observed for 3 days. The presence or absence of the major lethal antigens is indicated by death or survival of the appropriate mice.

Alpha Toxin.—Produced by all types of *Cl. welchii* but notably by type A strains, this is the most important of the lethal toxins of the organism and is considered to be the main cause of the profound toxaemia associated with gas gangrene in man. The alpha toxin is lethal

TOXIN-ANTITOXIN MIXTURES EMPLOYED IN NEUTRALISATION TESTS FOR THE TYPING OF *Cl. welchii* [1]

Substance Tested	Mixture Number	Type-Specific Antiserum added (0.1 ml. volumes)	Sterile Broth added (ml.)	Reactions with *Cl. welchii type* A	B	C	D	E
Untreated Filtrate	1	—	0·3	+	+	+	+	+
	2	A	0·2	—	+	+	—*	(±)
	3	A & C	0·1	—	—*	—	—*	(±)
	4	A, C & D	—	—	—	—	—	(±)
Trypsin-treated Filtrate	5	—	0·3	(±)	+	—*	+	+
	6	A	0·2	—	+	—*	+	+
	7	A & D	0·1	—	—*	—*	—	+
	8	A, C & D	—	—	—	—	—	+
	(9†	A & E	0·1	—	+	—*	+	—)
		Toxins identified		alpha	beta & epsilon	beta	epsilon	iota

† Often omitted as iota toxin seldom encountered
— = no reaction (intracutaneous test); survival (intravenous test)
+ = necrotic lesion (intracutaneous test); death (intravenous test)
(±) = variable result
—* = nearly always negative either because epsilon is in inactive prototoxin form, or beta toxin is destroyed by trypsin

[1] Table amended and reproduced by courtesy of Wellcome Research Laboratories.

for laboratory animals and it is necrotising on intradermal inoculation. It is relatively heat stable, being only 50 per cent. inactivated after five minutes at 100°C. The toxin is an enzyme, lecithinase C. In the presence of free Ca or Mg ions it can split lipoprotein complexes in serum or egg-yolk preparations with resulting opalescence. The reaction can be inhibited by specific antitoxin.

It appears that the lecithinase also attacks phospholipid constituents of the red blood cells of various animals, and the alpha toxin is thereby haemolytic for the red cells of most species with the exception of the horse and the goat. The clear zones of haemolysis typically seen around colonies of classical type A strains of *Cl. welchii* grown on horse blood agar are produced by the theta toxin and not by the alpha toxin. With the red cells of the sheep in particular the alpha toxin provides an example of a "hot-cold" lysin.

Alpha toxin activity may thus be assayed by several methods, including turbidity tests using egg-yolk emulsion (lecitho-vitellin, L.V.) or human serum as indicator, and sheep red cell lysis tests incorporating antisera to other haemolytic toxins which may be produced by *Cl. welchii*.

Nagler's Reaction.—Several clostridia are able to produce opalescence in both human serum and egg-yolk media, due to the production of lecithinases which cause visible precipitates in these media. The reaction was first demonstrated with the alpha toxin of *Cl. welchii* and is specifically neutralised by *Cl. welchii* alpha antitoxin (but the serologically related lecithinase of *Cl. bifermentans* is also inhibited).

This reaction has also been utilised for the rapid detection of *Cl. welchii* in direct plate culture, and allows a serologically controlled identification of the organisms to be made within 20 hours of inoculating the plate from the wound exudate (Hayward, 1943). A plate of nutrient agar containing 20 per cent. of human serum and 5 per cent. of Fildes' peptic digest of sheep blood is prepared and dried. On one half of the plate (which is appropriately marked) two or three drops of standard *Cl. welchii* antitoxin are spread and allowed to dry. The whole plate is then inoculated from the wound swab. On the section containing no antitoxin, *Cl. welchii* colonies show a surrounding zone of opacity, *i.e.* the Nagler reaction, while colonies of the organism on the remainder of the plate show no change. The use of egg-yolk, 5 per cent., in place of serum is recommended. Further developments of this type of medium have included the incorporation of neomycin sulphate to inhibit aerobic sporing organisms and coliforms (Lowbury & Lilly, 1955); lactose and neutral red to indicate lactose-fermenting organisms, and milk as an indicator of proteolysis (Willis & Hobbs, 1959). Results of culture on Willis and Hobbs' complex medium can be variable and are occasionally confusing. For this reason, a simpler selective medium such as that of Lowbury and Lilly is preferred for routine use.

Beta Toxin.—Types B and C produce this toxin, which is lethal and necrotising. Intradermal inoculation in the guinea-pig produces a purple-tinged necrotic area which is almost circular in the case of type C filtrates but, with type B filtrates, is more extensive and irregular in shape due to the associated hyaluronidase produced by type B strains.

Epsilon Toxin.—This is produced by type B and D strains as a prototoxin which is thereafter activated by proteolytic enzymes. It is lethal and necrotising and its activity is largely dependent upon the presence of an activating enzyme and an alkaline environment. Filtrates may be trypsinised before assay.

Iota Toxin.—Only type E strains produce this toxin, which is also lethal and necrotising and, like epsilon toxin, is formed as a prototoxin which is then activated by proteolytic enzymes.

Theta Toxin.—This is an oxygen-labile haemolysin which may be related to streptolysin O. It is produced by most strains of *Cl. welchii*, types A-E; it is not produced by typical food-poisoning strains or by strains associated with enteritis necroticans in man. It lyses the red cells of the horse, ox, sheep and rabbit, but is virtually inactive against mouse erythrocytes. Many animal sera inhibit theta toxin and, while this may be due to contained antibodies, it is known that tissue lipids and cholesterol inactivate it. Theta toxin is adsorbed on to meat particles so that strains assayed for theta production must be grown in medium free of meat particles. Culture supernatants (unfiltered, as the toxin is oxygen-sensitive) are then titrated for haemolysing activity against horse red cells in the presence of alpha antitoxin and under reducing conditions.

Theta toxin is also a lethal toxin.

Gamma toxin is a minor lethal toxin.

Delta toxin is lethal. It is haemolytic for the red cells of even-toed ungulates (sheep, goats, pigs, cattle).

Eta toxin is said to be an insignificant lethal toxin.

Kappa toxin is a collagenase which attacks native collagen as well as hide powder and gelatin. It may be this toxin which causes the softening of muscle connective tissue associated with gas gangrene.

Lambda toxin is a proteinase and gelatinase. It will decompose hide powder, but it does not attack native collagen.

Mu toxin is a hyaluronidase.

Nu toxin is a deoxyribonuclease.

Other Enzymes.—*Cl. welchii* cultures have been shown to possess other enzymatic properties. Enzymes are produced, particularly by some type B strains, which destroy blood-group substances. The organism also renders red blood cells inagglutinable by the myxoviruses (Chap. 33), probably by destroying virus receptors at the red cell surface. This is thought to be due to a receptor-destroying enzyme (neuraminidase) similar to that of *Vibrio cholerae. Cl. welchii* renders red blood cells panagglutinable by exposing their T antigens so that they lose their specificity and react with any of the ABO antisera. A diffusible haemagglutinin elaborated by *Cl. welchii* causes agglutination of the red blood cells of man and most animals. It is produced by some strains after prolonged artificial subculture, but it is not produced by freshly isolated strains. It has been claimed that virulent strains of *Cl. welchii* produce an aggressin which has been named " bursting factor ". This agent has not yet been adequately characterised.

Animal Pathogenicity.—The virulence varies greatly with different strains. Some are markedly pathogenic to guinea-pigs by subcutaneous or intramuscular injection of 1 ml. of a 24-hour culture in cooked-meat broth into the thigh, and the animal may die within 24 hours. A control animal may be protected by a prior injection of *Cl. welchii* antitoxin, *e.g.* 300–500 units. At autopsy, a spreading inflammatory oedema with gelatinous exudate and gas production is noted in the subcutaneous tissue; necrosis occurs in the underlying muscles which are sodden, friable and pink. Organisms from cultures washed with saline solution to free them from toxin and other soluble products are practically non-pathogenic. The products of growth of the bacillus increase its aggressiveness and, as toxin production occurs during early growth, young cultures should be used. The pathogenicity of a strain may be further enhanced by incorporating an equal amount of a sterile 5 per cent. solution of calcium chloride in the inoculum immediately before injection. Pigeons are exceedingly susceptible to experimental inoculation of *Cl. welchii.*

Occurrence.—Apart from its pathological relationships, *Cl. welchii* occurs normally in the large intestine of man and animals; its frequency in the human intestine approaches 100 per cent. It may invade the blood *ante mortem* and, multiplying in internal organs after death, produces the small gas cavities sometimes noted (*e.g.* in the liver) at *post-mortem* examinations.

Apart from wound infections, it may occur in uterine infections (*e.g.* septic abortion) and occasionally gains access to the blood stream from this site, producing intravascular haemolysis with subsequent oliguria or anuria. *Cl. welchii* also occurs in infections of the intestinal tract when these extend locally or generally.

Cl. welchii Food-poisoning

Strains of *Cl. welchii*, conforming in most respects to type A but producing non-haemolytic or feebly haemolytic colonies on horse-blood agar, are associated with a mild form of food-poisoning (Hobbs *et al.*, 1953). Spores of these strains are markedly heat-resistant, surviving boiling for several hours. Non-haemolytic strains of *Cl. welchii* occur frequently in human faeces (Collee, Knowlden & Hobbs, 1961), but carrier rates for "*typical food-poisoning strains*", i.e. non-haemolytic on horse-blood agar and producing spores that resist boiling in cooked-meat broth for one hour, range from 2·2 per cent. in the general population to 20–30 per cent. in hospital personnel and patients. Food-poisoning strains of *Cl. welchii* are thus widely distributed, occurring in the faeces of healthy man and animals. The vehicle of infection is usually a pre-cooked meat food that has been allowed to stand at a temperature conducive to the multiplication of *Cl. welchii*. While the heat-resistance of spores of food-poisoning strains ensures their survival in cooked foods and presumably accounts for the association of these potentially heat-resistant strains with most of the reported outbreaks of *Cl. welchii* food-poisoning, similar trouble can be caused by classical heat-sensitive β-haemolytic strains which may gain access to food during the cooling period under conditions suitable for their subsequent multiplication (McKillop, 1959), but it may be that these were not type A strains (see Warrack, 1963). The mechanism of *Cl. welchii* food-poisoning is not fully understood. Ingestion of large numbers of the viable organisms in contaminated food appears to be necessary (Dische & Elek, 1957). Typical symptoms are abdominal cramps beginning about 8–12 hours after ingestion, followed by diarrhoea. Fever and vomiting are not typically encountered. The condition is usually transient and symptoms normally subside within 24–48 hours.

The Bacteriological Diagnosis of Cl. welchii Food-poisoning.—This involves the isolation of typical food-poisoning strains from faeces of patients and those at risk and from the suspected food. (1) Isolation of these strains from *faeces* is facilitated by their being present in spore form. A portion of faeces is carefully emulsified by coating a swab with the faecal specimen and stirring this into a tube of cooked-meat broth. The inoculated tube is then held in a steamer at 100° C. for an hour, cooled and incubated overnight at 37° C. If heat-resistant *Cl. welchii* is present, a virtually pure culture will frequently be obtained by this simple procedure and pure subcultures can readily be obtained on solid media. If large particles of faeces are initially inoculated into the tube, however, many organisms are protected from the heat and survive to produce a very mixed culture including non-sporing organisms. Even when a pure culture of *Cl. welchii* is obtained, the result is of no quantitative significance; direct plating procedures on selective media (see below) are of value in this respect. (2) Isolation of typical food-poisoning strains from *food* by selective heating is rarely successful because spores of *Cl. welchii* are not normally abundant in food. The vegetative organisms are recovered by selective culture methods. Weighed samples of the suspected food should ideally be macerated and suspended in broth. Measured volumes are then pipetted on to selective media such as Lowbury and Lilly's medium, or an egg-yolk agar medium containing 70μg. of neomycin sulphate per ml., or horse-blood agar containing this concentration of neomycin. Suspected colonies are counted and further identified. Typical strains show lack of true haemolytic activity on horse-blood agar because, although they produce lecithinase which may cause zones of doubtful haemolysis, they do not produce theta toxin which is the cause of the complete β-haemolysis typical of the colonies of classical strains grown on horse-blood agar. In order to demonstrate the heat-resistance of food-poisoning strains, it is necessary to produce sporing cultures, *e.g.* in Ellner medium. Samples of sporing culture deposits are then held in cooked-meat broth at 100° C. for an hour, cooled and thereafter incubated. As many strains do not produce spores readily, this is often a laborious task. Final identification of the serological type of a typical food-poisoning strain is done by slide agglutination tests of colonies taken from blood-agar cultures and tested against a range of 13 agglutinating antisera prepared against different food-poisoning strains (Hobbs' types).[1] Untypable strains are not infrequently encountered.

It should be noted that the above methods are those in current use for the detection of typical food-poisoning strains of *Cl. welchii*, but they automatically exclude heat-sensitive strains. If large numbers of classical strains of β-haemolytic *Cl. welchii* are isolated from suspected food by quantitative methods, this finding should not be dismissed solely because the organism does not conform to the criteria of typical food-poisoning strains. On the other hand, the isolation of large numbers of classical β-haemolytic strains of *Cl. welchii* from *faeces* is of no significance as regards *Cl. welchii* food-poisoning. Warrack (1963) made a plea for more general typing of *Cl. welchii*, particularly in investigations of food-poisoning caused by this organism.

A sub-group of *Cl. welchii*, type C, has been reported as the cause of a condition occurring in Germany affecting man and named *enteritis necroticans*. The spores of these strains, originally referred to as *Cl. welchii* type F, are markedly heat-resistant.

Infections in Animals.—Type B strains cause *lamb dysentery*. The disease is characterised by an enteritis, occurring within the first week of life, and death is due to toxaemia as a result of absorption of the toxins produced. Antitoxic serum has been utilised with great success in the prophylaxis of the disease, the lambs being injected as soon after birth as possible. Ewes may also be immunised during pregnancy with toxoid or with a formolised culture, a second dose being given 14 days before lambing. The antibodies produced

[1] Dr. Betty C. Hobbs, Director, Food Hygiene Laboratory, Central Public Health Laboratory, Colindale Avenue, London.

by such immunisation are conveyed to the lamb in the colostrum. A similar disease occurs in foals.

Cl. welchii, type C, is associated with an enterotoxaemic disease of sheep known in Kent as "*struck*" and occurring also in Wales. Enterotoxaemias associated with *Cl. welchii* type C have been reported in lambs and calves in U.S.A. and in piglets in England.

A similar disease of sheep, *infectious enterotoxaemia*, is due to *Cl. welchii*, type D. This is a sporadic disease which is well known in Great Britain and has been reported in Australia and America. *Pulpy kidney disease* is also due to *Cl. welchii*, type D, and this is predominantly an acute and fatal disease of young lambs (three to eight weeks old), though older sheep may be affected. The disease is usually associated with overeating or high-level feeding, and is characterised by sub-endocardial haemorrhages with excess pericardial fluid. Appropriate methods of active or passive immunisation may be carried out against these diseases, as in the case of lamb dysentery. Type E strains cause enterotoxaemia of calves.

CLOSTRIDIUM SEPTICUM
(Vibrion septique)

Morphology and Staining.—Moderately large bacillus, with rounded ends, about 3–10 μ by 0·6–1 μ. Motile, with peritrichous flagella. Tends to grow also in the form of long curved filaments. In the tissues it develops into large, swollen, Gram-positive "citron bodies". Spores are readily formed and are oval, central or subterminal, and "bulging". *Cl. septicum* stains Gram-positively as a rule, but degenerate forms are Gram-negative.

Cultural Characters.—Obligatory anaerobe. Optimum temperature, 37° C. Capable of growing on ordinary media. Glucose promotes growth.

Surface colonies are irregular, transparent, droplet-like colonies, later becoming greyish and opaque, with projecting radiations somewhat like those of *Cl. tetani*. On blood agar haemolysis is observed.

Agar stab.—A white line of growth with short, lateral processes.

Biochemical Reactions.—Litmus milk medium—slight acid is formed, and the milk is slowly clotted, but often the change is slight.

Various sugars are fermented, *e.g.* glucose, lactose, maltose and salicin, but not mannitol. Sucrose is not usually fermented.

Gelatin is liquefied. Coagulated serum is not liquefied. In cooked-meat medium the meat is reddened and not digested.

Antigenic Characters.—Agglutinations involving somatic antigens distinguish four groups which can be further subdivided on the basis of H antigens. There is considerable antigenic cross-relationship to *Cl. chauvoei*.

An exotoxin with lethal and haemolytic properties, the alpha toxin, can be demonstrated in cultures, and a specific antitoxin can be obtained by immunising animals. The beta toxin is a deoxyribonuclease, the gamma toxin is a hyaluronidase, and the delta toxin is an oxygen-labile haemolysin. A fibrinolysin has also been reported. Dafaalla and Soltys

(1951) considered that a haemagglutinin produced by *Cl. septicum* is non-diffusible, but see Gadalla & Collee (1967).

Animal Pathogenicity.—Subcutaneous injection of cultures in laboratory animals produces a spreading inflammatory oedema, with slight gas formation in the tissues. The organisms invade the blood and the animal dies within a day or two. Smears from the liver show long filamentous forms and also citron bodies.

Occurrence.—*Cl. septicum* is associated with gas gangrene in man. It is responsible for *braxy* in sheep (see below) and for *malignant oedema* following wound infection in cattle and sheep. Gas gangrene due to *Cl. septicum* is quite common in pigs. The organism may also be the cause of some cases of blackleg in cattle and sheep.

Epidemiology.—The primary habitat is the soil. Areas with large numbers of spores of *Cl. septicum* appear to be associated with a higher incidence of *Cl. septicum* infections in man and animals than less heavily infected areas.

Laboratory Diagnosis.—The microscopic appearances, cultural characteristics and the results of pathogenicity tests in guinea-pigs allow of initial identification. Differentiation from *Cl. chauvoei* may present difficulties and is discussed later (p. 326).

Braxy is an acute fatal disease of yearling sheep characterised by a haemorrhagic inflammatory lesion of the abomasum. The disease is invariably associated with a *Cl. septicum* infection, and although it has not been reproduced experimentally the successful prophylaxis achieved with a formolised culture vaccine suggests that *Cl. septicum* is the organism responsible. The organism is thought to invade the mucous membrane of the abomasum, under conditions of stress, when it multiplies rapidly and gives rise to rapid death from a toxaemia. Braxy appears in the late autumn or winter and is almost entirely confined to lambs born in the previous spring which are outwintered on hill grazings or old lowland pastures. The disease does not occur if the flock is moved to new pastures on arable farms.

CLOSTRIDIUM OEDEMATIENS
(Clostridium novyi)

This Gram-positive bacillus resembles *Cl. welchii* in morphology, but is somewhat larger and more pleomorphic. It possesses peritrichous flagella, but its motility is not active and is inhibited in the presence of oxygen. The spores are oval, central or sub-terminal.

Cultural Characters.—Surface colonies are transparent, flat, irregular and tend to fuse, forming a spreading film of growth. Cultures on blood agar produce slight haemolysis. Very small motile "daughter colonies" may move on the surface of the medium and break away from the edge of a large parent colony. Colonies on heated blood agar may produce a green halo and colonies on heated blood agar with benzidine become black after exposure to air for an hour or so. Some strains of *Cl. oedematiens* will not readily grow on the surface of solid media such as blood agar, especially if the medium is not freshly prepared. The addition of fresh brain infusion to the medium is recommended by Smith (1955). Primary isolation of such strains may only be accomplished by resorting to deep shake cultures in which colonies appear as small, irregular, "woolly" or "snow-flake"-like balls of growth.

Litmus milk medium—late clotting may occur without digestion.

The organism is actively saccharolytic and ferments certain sugars including glucose and maltose.

Gelatin is liquefied. Coagulated serum is not digested. In cooked-meat medium the meat is reddened but not digested.

Type A strains produce a pearly layer or iridescent film on egg-yolk media; this is presumably caused by the epsilon toxin, a lipase, produced only by type A strains.

Antigenic Characters.—Four different serological types, A, B, C and D, have been defined and these differ in the distribution of various soluble antigens.

Virulence.—Culture filtrates are highly toxic and possess haemolytic and lecithinase activity in addition to necrotising and lethal properties. The organism produces a natural infection in a wide range of animals. Type C strains are thought to be non-toxigenic.

Pathogenesis.—*Cl. oedematiens* is associated with a markedly toxic form of gas gangrene in man. The organism causes gangrenous infections in animals, *e.g.* "Big head" in rams in Australia. It also causes "Black disease" among sheep in Australia and New Zealand. This condition, which has been observed in Scotland, is activated apparently by the invasion of the liver fluke. A fatal necrotic hepatitis supervenes. Type D strains (*Cl. haemolyticum*) produce red-water disease (infectious icterohaemoglobinuria) in cattle.

Prophylaxis.—Recommended procedures for the prevention of Black disease in Great Britain include fluke eradication and the use of an alum-precipitated vaccine in late summer.

Laboratory Diagnosis of Gas Gangrene

The bacteriological diagnosis of gas gangrene is usually combined with a general bacteriological examination of the infected wound with which this condition is associated. It is convenient here to give special reference to the recognition of the anaerobic bacilli.

Specimens of exudate should be taken from the wound, particularly from the deeper parts and from parts where the infection seems to be most pronounced. These may be obtained in capillary tubes, but sterile swabs (similar to throat swabs), rubbed over the wound surface and soaked in the exudate, serve well for the purpose.

Two swabs should be taken from the wound, one of which is used for film preparations, the other for culture. If there are sloughs or necrotic tissue present in the wound, small pieces should be placed in a sterile screw-capped bottle and used for microscopic examination and culture.

Microscopical Examination.—Films are made in the usual way and stained by Gram's method. If gas gangrene is present, Gram-positive bacilli may predominate, although *Cl. oedematiens* may appear to be relatively scanty in the wound exudate, even in an active infection. Thick, rectangular, Gram-positive bacilli suggest the presence of *Cl. welchii*, *Cl. fallax* or *Cl. bifermentans*; "citron bodies", boat- or leaf-shaped pleomorphic bacilli with irrregular staining may indicate *Cl. septicum*; slender bacilli with round terminal spores suggest *Cl. tetani* or *Cl. tetanomorphum*; *Cl. oedematiens* occurs in the form of large bacilli with oval subterminal spores.

Cultures.—In addition to the media routinely inoculated for the detection of aerobes, the following media should be inoculated: (*a*) blood-agar plate to be incubated anaerobically; the surface should be well dried before inoculation to prevent spreading of colonies of certain anaerobes. If the agar content of a solid medium such as blood agar is increased to 4·5–6·0 per cent., depending upon the brand of agar used and the other constituents of the medium, the spreading tendency of organisms is inhibited. Although the concentrated agar does not prevent the growth of any species, colonies tend to be smaller and morphologically atypical. (*b*) Plate of Lowbury and Lilly's medium or a good nutrient agar containing egg-yolk (5 per cent., v/v) and neomycin sulphate (70–100 μg. per ml.). (*c*) Two tubes or bottles of cooked-meat medium; after inoculation, one is heated for 30 min. at 65° C. to kill non-sporing organisms; for the cultivation of *Cl. oedematiens* it has been recommended that a third tube or bottle should be inoculated with a broth emulsion of exudate or tissue which has been heated for 5-10 min. at 100° C.

The anaerobic plates are examined after 24 and 48 hours' incubation. It must be remembered that these may yield growths of various facultative anaerobes as well as the strict anaerobes. Comparison of the aerobic and anaerobic plates affords some indication of the presence of strictly anaerobic organisms in the wound exudate, but any suspected anaerobe must later be tested in subculture to ensure that it is unable to grow under aerobic conditions. (It may be noted that *Cl. tertium* and *Cl. histolyticum* can grow to some extent under aerobic conditions.) The colony characters of suspected anaerobes on the blood-agar plate are carefully studied with the naked eye and plate-culture microscope, and films are made and stained by Gram's method; this may give some preliminary information as to the type of anaerobe. Each type present must be isolated in pure culture for further examination, *e.g.* fermentation tests and animal inoculation. A table of differential characters is given on pp. 338 and 339. The lactose egg-yolk milk-agar medium developed by Willis and Hobbs is useful for the preliminary examination of pure cultures of clostridia but results tend to vary with different batches of this medium. It indicates lactose-fermenting colonies; lecithinase-producing colonies produce a marked zone of opalescence extending beyond the colony (Nagler effect); and zones of clearing develop around proteolytic colonies. Opalescence restricted to the medium underlying a colony and associated with an overlying iridescent "pearly-layer" appears to indicate lipase activity.

In the cooked-meat medium both aerobes and anaerobes flourish, but this growth is useful for later subculture should the plate cultures fail to yield successful isolation of organisms present in the wound. Film preparations also yield further information as to the morphological types of organisms growing in it.

Additional Methods.—Anaerobes may be isolated in deep agar-shake cultures. Four or five serial decimal dilutions of the exudate are prepared in broth, and each of these is used to inoculate melted agar kept at 45° C., which is then allowed to solidify in tubes. Following incubation, one of the dilutions will show colonies sufficiently separate to allow of single-colony subculture by means of a capillary pipette, after cutting the tube transversely. A convenient, alternative method is to take up the melted agar after inoculation in sterile capillary pipettes stoppered with cotton-wool, the capillary ends being then sealed and the pipettes incubated horizontally.

Certain reducing agents may be used for rendering fluid media anaerobic in the bacteriological examination of wounds, etc.—ascorbic acid (0·1 per cent.), sodium thioglycollate (0·1 per cent.), reduced iron and iron strips, and these may be adopted advantageously in routine work with the anaerobic organisms.

Prophylaxis of Gas Gangrene.—A polyvalent serum is available for prophylactic use and for treatment of cases in which the causal organism has not been determined. The prophylactic dose, given intramuscularly (or in urgent cases intravenously), is 10,000 international units *Cl. welchii* antitoxin, 5000 units *Cl. septicum* antitoxin and 10,000 units *Cl. oedematiens* antitoxin. The therapeutic dose, given intravenously, should be at least three times the prophylactic dose, and the administration should be repeated as necessary. Monovalent sera are also available for the treatment of cases after the causal organism has been identified. Reactions to antitoxin administered intravenously may be severe and precautions should be taken (p. 336).

Chemotherapy.—Much work on the antibiotic sensitivities of numerous clostridia isolated from wounds suggests that the order of activity of the common antibiotics is, in general, tetracyclines > penicillin > chloramphenicol (Garrod, 1958). However, many factors must be considered in the antibiotic treatment of clostridial infections in addition to *in vitro* proof of antibiotic sensitivity (MacLennan, 1962). Adequate clinical evidence is lacking, but in the treatment of gas gangrene, penicillin is widely used and may be administered together with a tetracycline. There is no evidence of antagonism. *Prophylactic* administration of penicillin (400,000 units each of potassium and procaine penicillin, repeated at intervals of six hours) in cases of serious, contaminated wounds, has largely replaced the prophylactic use of gas-gangrene antisera. The use of an antibiotic in this manner must never preclude prompt and adequate wound toilet. MacLennan recommended that severe wounds considered liable to gas gangrene demand intravenous gas gangrene antiserum in addition to meticulous débridement plus local and parenteral penicillin.

CLOSTRIDIUM SPOROGENES

This Gram-positive motile bacillus is very widely distributed in nature and is generally regarded as a harmless saprophyte. It is about the same size as *Cl. welchii*, but more slender. Gram-negative forms are frequent in older cultures. It forms oval central or subterminal spores which may be highly resistant so that the organism is frequently encountered in mixed cultures in the laboratory, even after preliminary heating of these cultures to select heat-resistant pathogens. Its spores may survive boiling for periods of 15 min. up to 6 hr.

Cultural Characters.—Surface colonies may present a "medusa-head" appearance (cf. *B. anthracis*) if the plate is dry. Young colonies may be small, circular, raised and slightly opaque, but these soon produce outgrowths and the spreading margin of the colony becomes irregular with feathery outgrowths. On horse-blood agar the colonies are haemolytic, irregular and transparent with some central opacity where the colonies are raised. Shake colonies show as "woolly" balls of growth. A stab culture develops, like that of *Cl. tetani*, with lateral spikes.

The organism decomposes protein, producing amino-acids, ammonia, sulphuretted hydrogen, etc., and cultures have an exceedingly putrid odour.

Milk—the casein is precipitated and digested.

Gelatin and coagulated serum are liquefied.

Meat medium—the meat is blackened and digested

Acid and gas are produced from some sugars, including glucose and maltose. Lactose and sucrose are not fermented.

Occurrence.—*Cl. sporogenes* is a ubiquitous saprophyte and also occurs in the intestine of man and animals. It is frequently isolated from wound exudates in association with accepted pathogens. While its presence may accelerate an established anaerobic infection by enhancing local conditions, it is not regarded as a pathogen in its own right.

In pure culture it is virtually non-pathogenic to laboratory animals.

Clostridium histolyticum resembles *Cl. sporogenes* and is actively proteolytic but non-saccharolytic. It is not a strict anaerobe. In meat medium, digestion occurs with the formation of white, crystalline masses consisting of tyrosine. When cultures are injected into animals, *in vivo* digestion of the tissues results. This organism is pathogenic and produces an exotoxin. It may be associated with gas gangrene in man.

Clostridium bifermentans.—Some workers consider this species distinct from *Cl. sordellii*, but the names are virtually synonymous. The latter title is frequently reserved for pathogenic strains (see Table, p. 338). The organism produces spores readily and abundantly and these are usually oval and central or subterminal. The name *bifermentans* refers to the organism's ability to decompose both sugars and proteins. It does not ferment lactose (cf. *Cl. welchii*). A lecithinase is produced which is serologically related to the alpha toxin of *Cl. welchii*. Pathogenic strains also produce a lethal toxin and are occasionally associated with wound infections in man and disease in animals.

Clostridium fallax resembles *Cl. welchii* in some respects, and has sometimes been mistaken for it (hence the name "fallax"). It is, however, shorter and more slender. The spores are usually subterminal. In milk, the organism produces clotting and gas formation, but these changes take place slowly (as compared with *Cl. welchii*). It does not liquefy either gelatin or coagulated serum, and is non-proteolytic. It possesses saccharolytic properties. An exotoxin is formed, and when freshly isolated the organism is pathogenic on experimental inoculation in animals.

Clostridium tertium.—This organism tends to be long and slender. It is weakly motile. The spores are terminal and, when fully developed, oval in shape. It is not a strict anaerobe. The organism shows active saccharolytic properties. In milk, acid is formed with gas production and slow clotting. Meat is reddened, but not digested. Neither gelatin nor coagulated serum is liquefied. Its pathogenicity is doubtful, but when present in wounds, it may give rise to gas production. No exotoxin is produced.

CLOSTRIDIUM CHAUVOEI
(Clostridium feseri)

This is the causative organism of most cases of quarter evil (blackleg, or symptomatic anthrax) in cattle and sheep, a disease characterised by a swollen and emphysematous condition of the subcutaneous tissues and muscles. The infection frequently affects the fore- and hind-quarters, which become dark or almost black in colour.

Morphology.—Resembles closely *Cl. septicum.* Individual organisms tend to occur singly or in pairs, and not in long filaments. "Citron bodies" may be seen in the tissues. The bacilli are motile, with numerous peritrichous flagella. Spores are usually central or subterminal in position, elliptical in shape, and are broader than the bacillus.

Cultural Characters.—Strict anaerobe ; optimum temperature, 37° C., but grows at room temperature. Grows poorly on ordinary medium and a blood or meat medium is preferable. Liver infusion aids growth.

Cl. chauvoei ferments glucose, lactose, sucrose, maltose, but not mannitol, salicin or inulin.

Antigenic Characters.—A somatic antigen is common to all strains.

Flagellar antigens distinguish two groups. Cross-reactions with *Cl. septicum* occur.

A lethal exotoxin is obtained in glucose-broth cultures, especially if calcium carbonate is added to neutralise the acid produced. Culture-filtrates are also haemolytic.

Occurrence and Pathogenicity.—The disease occurs in cattle and sheep. *Cl. chauvoei* infection has also been reported in pigs and in fresh-water fish. The organism is pathogenic for guinea-pigs and mice, these animals dying 24-36 hours after experimental inoculation. It has been supposed that the natural disease results from infection of a wound by the spores which may be present in the soil of infected pastures. In cattle, infection usually takes place through the ingestion of spores with the fodder or drinking-water, and although the distribution of the lesions suggests a focus of infection in the musculature, the disease is seldom associated with a history of wounding. In sheep, on the other hand, most cases arise from wound infection (shearing, castration, docking, vaccination, and dog bites) and also in connection with parturition.

Laboratory Diagnosis.—*Cl. septicum* may also be responsible for a condition similar to blackleg.

In the differentiation of *Cl. septicum* and *Cl. chauvoei*, stress has been laid on the morphological elements seen in infected guinea-pigs : *Cl. chauvoei* exhibits " citron " and club-shaped forms, but no elongated filaments are observed on the peritoneal surface of the liver of inoculated animals, as in the case of *Cl. septicum*. *Cl. chauvoei* ferments sucrose but not salicin; *Cl. septicum* ferments salicin but not sucrose. The two organisms, however, are closely related. Specific antisera have now been conjugated to different fluorescent dyes at the Wellcome Research Laboratories. Direct microscopic examination of tissue smears stained by these conjugates and illuminated by ultraviolet light allows prompt differentiation between *Cl. septicum* and *Cl. chauvoei* infections (Batty & Walker, 1963).

Prophylaxis.—A formolised whole culture of *Cl. chauvoei* in broth has been used as a vaccine with successful results. An antitoxic serum has been used for therapeutic purposes.

REFERENCES

Batty, I. & Walker, P. D. (1963). Differentiation of *Clostridium septicum* and *Clostridium chauvoei* by the use of fluorescent labelled antibodies. *J. Path. Bact.*, **85**, 517.

Brooks, M. E., Sterne, M. & Warrack, G. H. (1957). A re-assessment of the criteria used for type differentiation of *Cl. perfringens*. *J. Path. Bact.*, **74**, 185.

Cash, J. D. & Collee, J. G. (1962). Sporulation and the development of resistance in sporing cultures of *Clostridium welchii*. *J. appl. Bact.*, **25**, 225.

Collee, J. G., Knowlden, J. A. & Hobbs, B. C. (1961). Studies on the growth, sporulation and carriage of *Clostridium welchii* with special reference to food poisoning strains. *J. appl. Bact.*, **24**, 326.

Dafaalla, E. N. & Soltys, M. A. (1951). Studies on agglutination of red cells by clostridia. I. *Cl. septique*. *Brit. J. exp. Path.*, **32**, 510.

Dische, F. E. & Elek, S. D. (1957). Experimental food-poisoning by *Clostridium welchii*. *Lancet*, **2**, 71.

Gadalla, M. S. A. & Collee, J. G. (1967). The nature and properties of the haemagglutinin of *Clostridium septicum*. *J. Path. Bact.*, **93**, 255.

Garrod, L. P. (1958). The chemoprophylaxis of gas gangrene. *J. R. Army M. Cps.*, **104**, 209.

Hayward, N. J. (1943). The rapid identification of *Cl. welchii* by Nagler tests in plate cultures. *J. Path. Bact.*, **55**, 285.

Hobbs, B. C., Smith, M. E., Oakley, C. L., Warrack, G. H. & Cruickshank, J. C. (1953). *Clostridium welchii* food-poisoning. *J. Hyg.* (*Lond.*), **51**, 75.

Lowbury, E. J. L. & Lilly, H. A. (1955). A selective plate medium for *Cl. welchii*. *J. Path. Bact.*, **70**, 105.

McKillop, E. J. (1959). Bacterial contamination of hospital food, with special reference to *Cl. welchii* food-poisoning. *J. Hyg.* (*Lond.*), **57**, 31.

MacLennan, J. D. (1943). Anaerobic infections of war wounds in the Middle East. *Lancet*, **2**, 63, 94, 123.

MacLennan, J. D. (1962). The histotoxic clostridial infections of man. *Bact. Rev.*, **26**, 177.

Oakley, C. L. & Warrack, G. H. (1953). Routine typing of *Cl. welchii*. *J. Hyg.* (*Lond.*), **51**, 102.

Smith, L. de S. (1955). *Introduction to the Pathogenic Anaerobes*. Chicago, Ill., University of Chicago Press.

Warrack, G. H. (1963). Some observations on the typing of *Clostridium perfringens*. *Bull. Off. int. Epiz.*, **59**, 1393.

Willis, A. T. & Hobbs, G. (1959). Some new media for the isolation and identification of clostridia. *J. Path. Bact.*, **77**, 511.

CHAPTER 28

CLOSTRIDIUM

II. THE ORGANISMS OF TETANUS AND BOTULISM

TETANUS

TETANUS occurs in man and animals when a wound is infected with *Cl. tetani* under conditions that allow the organism to multiply and produce toxin. Absorption of the toxin leads to hyperexcitability of voluntary musculature. The disease is thus characterised by increased muscle tonus and exaggerated muscular responses to trivial stimuli. Trismus occurs when the muscles of the jaw are affected and, as this is quite frequently an early sign of tetanus in man, the disease is sometimes called lockjaw.

CLOSTRIDIUM TETANI

The causative organism of tetanus in man and animals.

Morphology.—A straight, slender, rod-shaped organism, 2–5 μ by 0·4–0·5 μ, with rounded ends; shorter forms and longer filaments are also noted; motile, with numerous long peritrichous flagella. Movement is not markedly active. The spores, early in development, may produce an oval and subterminal enlargement. The fully developed spore is characteristically terminal and spherical, two to four times the diameter of the bacillus, producing the drum-stick appearance which is a striking morphological feature of the organism. Strains vary in their tendency to produce spores. If sporing forms are scanty in normal culture media, the strain may be encouraged to produce spores by stab subculture in a tube of horse-flesh digest agar with 1 per cent. glucose, incubated for two to three days.

Staining.—Gram-positive, but there is considerable variation and Gram-negative forms are frequently encountered, especially in broth cultures. Only the periphery of the mature spore is stained by the Gram counterstain.

Cultural Characters.—An obligatory anaerobe; temperature range 14°–43° C.; optimum, 37° C.; grows on ordinary nutrient media but is more readily grown in cooked-meat medium or in Fildes' peptic blood broth.

On solid media, surface colonies of the normal motile type of tetanus bacillus are characterised by their long branching projections. After 48–72 hours' incubation the central part of the colony, which rarely grows more than 1 mm. in diameter, becomes slightly raised and has a ground-glass appearance, while the edge shows a delicately filamentous appearance. A fine spreading growth may thus extend over the entire surface of the medium and the spreading film of growth may not be apparent on cursory examination. On blood agar, haemolysis is evident in the region of initial confluent growth and may develop below individual colonies, but frequently does not appear below the spreading growth in young cultures.

Non-motile variants may produce quite isolated colonies lacking the characteristic feathery processes.

Agar Stab Culture.—No growth occurs on the surface; a white line of growth appears along the track of the inoculating wire but stops short of the surface, and lateral spikes, which are longest in the deeper part of the tube, develop from the central growth.

Biochemical Reactions.—Nutrient gelatin is slowly liquefied. Coagulated serum is slowly rendered more transparent and softened only. Litmus milk medium may show no coagulation or there may be delayed clotting. Cooked-meat medium shows slight digestion and blackening of the meat. Some gas is evolved due to breakdown of amino-acids, but no carbohydrates are fermented by typical strains of *Cl. tetani.* Cultures have an unpleasant slightly pungent odour.

Viability.—The spores may be highly resistant to adverse conditions, but the degree of resistance varies. Many strains are killed by exposure to boiling water for 5–15 min., but rarer, more resistant strains require boiling for up to three hours before being killed. They may resist dry heat at 150° C. for one hour, 5 per cent. phenol or 1 in 1000 perchloride of mercury for up to two weeks or more. Iodine 1 per cent. in watery solution and hydrogen peroxide (10 volumes) are said to kill them within a few hours.

Antigenic Characters.—Ten types are distinguishable by agglutination tests involving flagellar H antigens. Type VI consists of non-flagellate strains. All types produce the same neurotoxin, and toxigenic and non-toxigenic strains may belong to the same type.

Toxin.—The exotoxin, of which the neurotoxic component *tetanospasmin* is the essential pathogenic constituent, develops in broth cultures after 5–14 days' growth at 35° C., the optimum time varying with the strain. Toxin yields from *Cl. tetani* cultures vary from strain to strain and also depend upon the culture medium used. One of the most satisfactory media is that of Mueller and Miller (1954).

Tetanolysin is another constituent and this causes lysis of red blood corpuscles. It is oxygen-labile. *Tetanospasmin* has been separated as a pure crystalline protein with an estimated lethal dose for the mouse of 0·0000001 mg. Tetanus toxin is thus an extremely powerful poison, second in potency only to the exotoxin of *Cl. botulinum.*

When tetanus toxin is injected into guinea-pigs or mice, the animals die within a day or two with the typical signs of tetanus. In animals, tetanic spasms may start in the muscles related to the site of injection ("local tetanus"). Experimental findings indicate that the toxin reaches the central nervous system by passing along the motor nerves, being absorbed probably by the motor end-plates and spreading up the spaces between the nerve fibres (Wright *et al.*, 1950). It seems to act as an excitant to the motor cells in the anterior horn of the spinal cord and may then diffuse to involve the whole central nervous system. The toxin may also interfere with the normal inhibition of motor impulses exercised by the upper motor neurone over the lower, producing early increase in tonus and tonic spasms localised initially to the musculature controlled by the spinal segment involved. This affords an explanation of local tetanus but the actual mode of action of tetanus toxin is not known. Whereas the toxin of *Cl. botulinum* produces visceral symptoms and signs, tetanus toxin does not appear to do so directly (Wright, 1955). Dysphagia and urinary retention observed in clinical tetanus can be attributed to paralysis of associated skeletal muscles. Certain strains of *Cl. tetani* produce a factor that enhances the lethal action of tetanospasmin for rabbits and this factor may facilitate access of the toxin to its susceptible cell substrate. Consideration of the specific affinity of the toxins of *Cl. tetani* and *Cl. botulinum* for nervous tissue, the relatively small amount of these toxins required to produce death, and the lag period between intoxication and its manifestation, has given rise to the theory that both of these toxins may act through interference with vital enzyme systems. A disorganisation of the normal metabolism of choline in nerve cells with a resultant impairment of the availability of acetyl choline has been postulated, but the different symptomatology of tetanus and botulism has not been explained.

Antitoxin.—Tetanus antitoxin, often called antitetanus serum or ATS, can be obtained by immunising horses with toxoid. This serum is of value in the prophylaxis of tetanus, given immediately after wounding. Its use as a curative agent after the development of tetanus is less effective than the corresponding antitoxin treatment of diphtheria. Tetanus antitoxin is standardised in Great Britain in terms of the *International Unit* (*1950*) by comparison with a preserved standard serum.

Occurrence.—The tetanus bacillus occurs in the intestine of man and animals, but there is considerable variation in the frequency with which it is reported to have been isolated from their faeces. Tenbroeck and Bauer (1922) isolated *Cl. tetani* from 34·7 per cent. of stools from 78 individuals in Peking. Kerrin (1929) examined more than 300 human stools in Scotland and none yielded *Cl. tetani*. The wide divergence in these figures may be partly related to the different ways of life of the communities investigated. The use of human faeces (night-soil) as fertiliser in the fields of China, whose population lives in more intimate contact with the soil, will play a part in the re-distribution of the bacillus.

It is uncertain whether this organism flourishes as a saprophyte in the soil or is derived entirely from the animal intestine. It is especially prevalent in manured soil, and, for this reason, a wound through skin which may be contaminated with soil or manure deserves special attention. Whether derived from the soil or the faeces, however, tetanus spores occur very widely; they are commonly present, for instance, in street dust and may be present in the dust and plaster in hospitals and houses, on clothing and on articles of common use.

Pathogenesis.—Tetanus is usually the result of contamination of a wound with *Cl. tetani* spores. The source of the infection may be soil dirty clothing or dust, but spores may also be derived from the skin—especially in areas of the body that may be contaminated with intestinal organisms. Spores of *Cl. tetani* and other anaerobes may be embedded in surgical catgut (prepared from sheep's intestine), and this has been the source of infection in some post-operative cases of tetanus. The sterility of surgical catgut is rigorously controlled in this country.

If washed spores alone are injected into an animal they fail to germinate, are phagocytosed and do not give rise to tetanus. It has been shown that the germination of spores of *Cl. tetani* is dependent on the reduced oxygen tension occurring in devitalised tissue and non-viable material in the wound. Infection, when it occurs, remains strictly localised in the wound and the tetanic condition is due to the effects of a potent diffusible exotoxin on the nervous system. Certain conditions favour the germination of the spores and the multiplication of the organisms in the tissues, *e.g.* deep puncture wounds; wounds accompanied by compression injury associated with devitalised tissues; necrotic tissue and effused blood; wounds contaminated with soil, the ionised calcium salts and silicic acid in which cause tissue necrosis; wounds containing foreign bodies such as pieces of clothing and shrapnel; infection by other organisms, such as pyogenic cocci and *Cl. welchii*. Thus, in war casualties, infection tends to occur when there are deep lacerated wounds caused by shrapnel which may carry in fragments of muddy clothing and particles of earth. Spores are then introduced under most favourable conditions for the development of the organism. Similar wounds may be sustained in civil life, notably as a result of gunshot injuries or following accidents on the roads and on farms. It should be borne in mind, however, that cases of tetanus have been reported, especially in children, in which the infection apparently derived from a superficial abrasion, a contaminated splinter or a minor thorn-prick. *Cl. tetani* infection may also occur in the uterus, as in cases of septic abortion. *Tetanus neonatorum* follows infection of the umbilical wound of newborn infants. Cases of post-operative tetanus have been recorded due to imperfectly sterilised catgut, dressings or glove-powder, and some cases of post-operative tetanus have been attributed to dust-borne infection of the wound at operation.

Laboratory Diagnosis

Films may be made from the wound exudate and stained by Gram's method; the appearance of "drum-stick" bacilli is suggestive evidence of the presence of *Cl. tetani*, but it is not conclusive as other organisms having terminal spores, which are morphologically indistinguishable from *Cl. tetani*, may be present. Moreover, it is often impossible to detect the tetanus bacilli in wounds by microscopic examination.

Direct plating on blood agar incubated anaerobically is often the best method of detecting *Cl. tetani*. The production of tetanus in mice by subcutaneous injection of an anaerobic fluid culture prepared from the wound may also be attempted but this technique is limited by the fact that some strains of *Cl. tetani* from cases of human tetanus are non-pathogenic to mice. The injection, *e.g.* 0·2 ml. of a five- to ten-day cooked-meat broth culture, is made into the tissues to the right of the base of the animal's tail. Within a day or so in a positive test there may be stiffness of the tail and the hind limbs. The right hind leg is subsequently paralysed and the tail and spine of the animal tend to curve to the right. Thereafter, more generalised muscular involvement becomes increasingly evident, and tetanic convulsions may be elicited by trivial stimuli. Control animals are each protected with a dose of tetanus antitoxin, *e.g.* 500 units, injected subcutaneously or intraperitoneally one hour prior to inoculation of the culture.

While significant results may thus sometimes be obtained with impure or mixed cultures from the wound, it is desirable that the tetanus bacillus, if possible, should be obtained in pure culture so that it can be identified by its biological characters and its specific toxicity. In Fildes' method, which exploits the tendency of *Cl. tetani* colonies to spread and extend beyond the growth of other bacteria, the material is incubated anaerobically in 5 per cent. peptic-blood broth for two to four days at 37° C. The culture is then heated at 65° C. for 30 min. to kill spreading non-sporing organisms such as *Proteus*. The condensation water of a peptic-blood agar slope is then inoculated from the heated culture, and the tube is incubated anaerobically. After 24–48 hours the edge of the culture is examined with a hand lens, when a growth of tetanus bacilli is seen as a mass of very fine filaments. Subcultures from the marginal growth frequently yield pure cultures of *Cl. tetani.* (It is advantageous to keep the blood-agar tubes prior to inoculation until the surface of the medium is dry at the top.)

This method of isolation will not be successful if a non-motile type VI strain is involved, and it is advisable to employ additional methods. It is also recommended, when possible, to vary the degree of preliminary heating of portions of the specimen under investigation. Thus, tissue from the wound may be ground up with sand under sterile conditions. After direct plating on blood agar for anaerobic incubation, one-quarter of this material may be extracted and used for direct animal inoculation. The remaining three-quarters is dispensed into six universal containers of freshly prepared cooked-meat medium. Two of these are heated at 80° C. for 10 min., two at 70° C. for 30 min. and two are not heated. After several days' incubation at 37° C., subcultures from these may be made to blood agar, into shake cultures and into the condensation water of Fildes' peptic-blood-agar slopes as already described.

An antitoxin-controlled plate haemolysin test for the presumptive identification of *Cl. tetani* involves the use of fresh blood agar plates half-smeared with tetanus antitoxin (Lowbury & Lilly, 1958). *Cl. tetani* produces haemolysis which is inhibited by the antiserum. While there are several objections to this technique (see Willis, 1960), the method is convenient for the provisional screening of large numbers of strains. Confirmation by mouse inoculation is recommended.

The Prevention of Tetanus

Prompt and adequate wound toilet and proper surgical débridement of wounds are essential steps in the prevention of tetanus as there is an increased risk that tetanus spores may germinate in a wound if there is delay in cleansing or if sepsis develops. Clean superficial wounds that receive prompt attention may not require specific protection against tetanus and it is unreasonable to insist that every small prick or abrasion demands protection with antibiotic or antitoxin. Moreover, some surgeons consider that patients receiving thorough and prompt wound treatment, plus antibiotic treatment when indicated until healing is advanced, do not require tetanus antitoxin in addition (see Ministry of Health Memo., 1964). Specific prophylaxis is indicated in the case of deep wounds, puncture or stab wounds, ragged lacerations, wounds associated with bruising and devitalised tissue, and animal bite wounds. It is also advisable to regard all open wounds in children, farm workers and road-accident cases as potentially infected with spores of *Cl. tetani* and requiring protection.

The method of prophylaxis depends upon the state of immunity of the patient. While some degree of latent immunity is conferred even after only one injection of toxoid, for practical purposes it is wise to differentiate clearly between those likely to have a definite immunity and those who may not be immune. A patient may be regarded as *immune* for six months following the first two injections, or for five years following three injections (or a booster injection) of a planned course of tetanus toxoid (p. 336). Tetanus antitoxin should not be given to immune patients, but their active immunity should be enhanced by giving 0·5 ml. of tetanus toxoid intramuscularly at the time of injury.

A patient is considered *non-immune* if he has never had an injection of tetanus toxoid or if he has had only one such injection. If more than six months have elapsed after a course of two injections, or more than five years after a full primary course of three injections (or a booster injection) of tetanus toxoid, he may be regarded as non-immune; but recent evidence suggests that these time limits may be extended. He is non-immune if more than one week has elapsed since a previous injection of tetanus antitoxin. He should be considered non-immune if there is any doubt about his immunisation history.

Passive immunisation.—Tetanus antitoxin is given to the *non-immune* patient to provide passive protection. This is usually but not invariably effective. There may be untoward reactions (q.v.). In some non-immune patients antitoxin may be contra-indicated, or antitoxin may not be considered a sufficient protection. In such cases, the prophylactic use of an antibiotic is reasonable (see below). The usual prophylactic dose of antitoxin is 1500 units given by intramuscular or subcutaneous injection as soon as possible after injury. The dose is not reduced for a child. The injection may be repeated at weekly intervals as long as the risk of tetanus persists. Larger initial doses, *e.g.* 3000 to 10,000 units, may be given when the wound is a severe one. Antitoxin is never given intravenously as a prophylactic measure.

Combined active-passive immunisation.—It is desirable that patients receiving passive protection with antitoxin should also be actively immunised against tetanus with toxoid, because, apart from involving the risk of anaphylaxis, a second dose of antitoxin tends to be more rapidly eliminated than the initial dose and the passive protection afforded on the second occasion is reduced. Purified tetanus toxoid adsorbed on aluminium hydroxide is a powerful antigen released over a period of days and the use of this preparation of toxoid overcomes previous objections to the concurrent administration of tetanus antitoxin for immediate protection and tetanus toxoid for active immunisation (Smith *et al.*, 1963). Thus, with the precautions outlined above, an injured non-immune patient may receive from separate syringes, 1500 units of tetanus antitoxin intramuscularly in one arm and 0·5 ml. of the adsorbed toxoid preparation in the other. Active immunisation is therefore started at an opportune moment and the patient is advised to have a second injection of 0·5 ml. of adsorbed toxoid 6–12 weeks later.

Antibiotic protection.—Although the prophylactic administration of antibiotics to all cases of open wounds is not recommended, there is justification for the prophylactic administration of an antibiotic such as penicillin to a patient with a previous history of a severe immediate reaction to horse serum, in which case antitoxin is withheld. In the case of a deep contaminated wound or an open wound associated with much devitalised tissue antibiotic protection should be given in addition to antitoxin because pyogenic infection is likely to occur in such wounds and this favours the development of tetanus. Penicillin may be given at the time of injury and dosage maintained (either by repeated administration or by the use of a long-acting preparation such as benzathine penicillin) until healing is established. As in gas gangrene, this additional safeguard cannot take the place of prompt and adequate surgical wound toilet and it can be criticised on the grounds that strains of *Cl. tetani* vary in their sensitivity to penicillin, that access of antibiotic to the infected area may be impaired, and that penicillinase-producing organisms may also be present. Nevertheless, the prompt administration of antibiotics can prevent the development of tetanus in animals inoculated with spores of *Cl. tetani*. The use of a tetracycline for this purpose may be theoretically safer than penicillin. There is good evidence that the combination of a prolonged course of antibiotic plus active immunisation with adsorbed toxoid at the time of injury may prevent tetanus spores germinating until active immunity has developed (Smith, 1964).

The following diagram, slightly amended from that proposed originally by Lowbury, Batten and London (1961), illustrates a realistic approach to the integration of antibiotic prophylaxis with the other measures discussed above. The recent articles by Laurence, Evans and Smith (1966) and Rubbo (1966) should be consulted.

Active immunisation.—Many authorities consider that all persons should be actively immunised against tetanus in infancy and their immunity maintained by booster doses of toxoid at intervals of five to

A GUIDE TO THE INTEGRATION OF PROCEDURES WHICH MAY BE ADOPTED FOR THE PREVENTION OF TETANUS IN INJURED PERSONS (after Lowbury, Batten & London, 1961.)

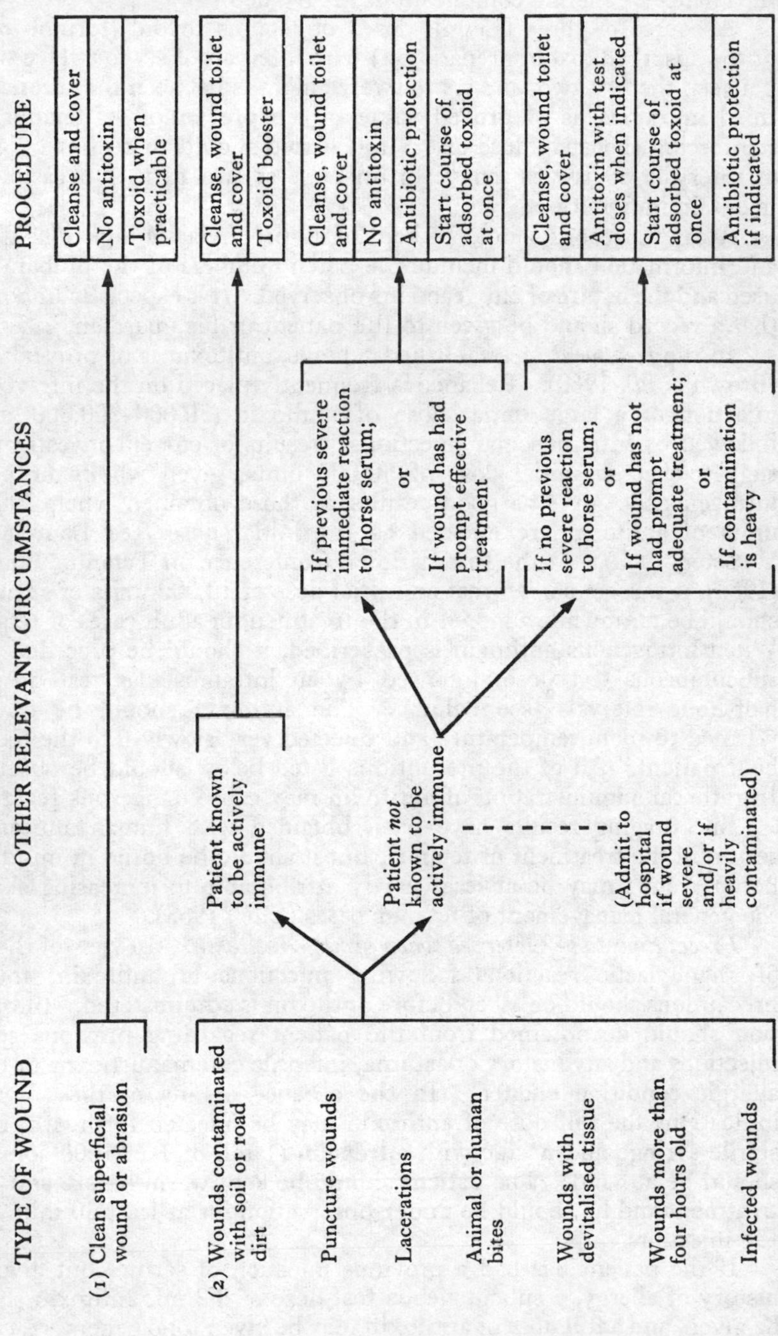

ten years. This is of particular value in the case of allergic patients, since the necessity of serum prophylaxis in the event of wounding, and the chance of allergic complications, is avoided.

A course of three 0·5 ml. doses of tetanus toxoid (formol-toxoid or the adsorbed toxoid preparation) with intervals of six to twelve weeks between the first two, and six to twelve months between the second and third injections, is of proved value in the prevention of tetanus. A reinforcing (booster) dose of 0·5 ml. toxoid should thereafter be given at intervals of five to ten years on at least two further occasions to maintain immunity.

A careful record should be kept of all prophylactic injections given, and information should include the batch numbers of the preparations used and the nature of any reactions observed. It is especially important that a record should be given to the patient or his guardian.

In the *treatment* of established tetanus, antitoxin is of proven value (Brown *et al.*, 1960). Reliance is frequently placed on the intravenous injection of a large initial dose of antitoxin (30,000–200,000 units) followed by intramuscular injections; results of current investigations suggest that an initial dose of 50,000 units, given wholly or partly intravenously, gives as good results as those obtained when 200,000 units of antitoxin are injected as the initial dose (see Laurence & Webster, 1963). At the International Conference on Tetanus, Bombay (1963), it was concluded that an initial dose of 10,000 units of antitoxin should be meanwhile adopted in the treatment of adult cases of tetanus. When intravenous antitoxin is prescribed, it should be preceded by a subcutaneous test dose, followed by an intramuscular test dose, at half-hour intervals (see below). The antitoxin should be diluted, warmed to room temperature and injected very slowly into the recumbent patient. All of the precautions listed below should be observed. Intrathecal administration of antitoxin may cause dangerous reactions.

Encouraging results have been obtained with human antitetanus serum in the treatment of tetanus, but it should be borne in mind that better results may be at least partly attributable to increasing skill in the general management of tetanus cases (Ellis, 1963).

Precautions to be Observed when giving Antitoxin.—In view of the risk of anaphylactic reactions following injections of antitoxin, routine precautions should be taken before antitoxin is administered. Information should be obtained from the patient regarding previous serum injections and any history of asthma, infantile eczema, urticaria or other allergic condition elicited. In the absence of any of these contra-indications the full dose of antitoxin may be injected forthwith, but a sterile syringe and needle with adrenalin (1 ml. of 1 in 1000 solution) should be at hand. The patient should be kept warm before and after treatment and he should be under observation for at least 30 min. after the injection.

If the patient has had a previous injection of serum, but gives no history of allergy, a subcutaneous test dose of 0·2 ml. antitoxin should be given, and a full dose of antitoxin may be given if no general reactions have occurred after 30 min. If the patient gives a history of allergy, the initial test dose should be 0·2 ml. of a 1 in 10 dilution of antitoxin subcutaneously. If no general symptoms develop within 30 min., this may be followed by 0·2 ml. of undiluted antitoxin subcutaneously. The full dose may be given if there are no general reactions after a further 30 min.

Chemotherapy.—A course of systemic penicillin or tetracycline therapy should be given in cases of established tetanus. There may be some justification for the local instillation of antibiotic into the wounded area after adequate débridement. Antibiotics may also be required to control complications such as pneumonia.

Tetanus in Animals.—Many animals are susceptible to tetanus, young animals being more susceptible than adults. The horse is particularly susceptible. Infection may be acquired in lambs, calves, pigs and goats after castration or docking, especially if these operations are performed under dirty conditions. Young colts may develop tetanus following umbilical infection. In cows, tetanus is usually associated with parturition, especially after retention of the placenta. Carnivores are rarely affected and birds are almost completely resistant to the natural disease, although an occasional case has been described in geese and in a turkey. The guinea-pig and the mouse are susceptible to tetanus toxin, and mice are extensively used in the laboratory investigation of *Cl. tetani.*

The blood of most cattle contains neutralising antibodies, with small amounts in sheep and goats, which may account for the comparative rareness of tetanus in ruminants. The blood of horses, dogs, cats, pigs and humans does not normally contain antitoxin. Birds and other naturally resistant animals have no antibodies in their blood, so that their immunity cannot be attributed to the presence of neutralising antibodies similar to those found in artificially immunised animals.

CLOSTRIDIUM BOTULINUM

Botulism is a fatal form of food poisoning characterised by pronounced toxic effects mainly on the parasympathetic system—*e.g.* oculomotor paralysis, pharyngeal paralysis, aphonia, etc. It is not a common disease in this country, only four incidents having been recorded since the Loch Maree tragedy in 1922 when eight victims died after eating duck paste infected with *Cl. botulinum.* Six main types of *Cl. botulinum* have been differentiated on the basis of their antigenically distinct toxins and designated A, B, C, D, E and F. Types A, B and E are most frequently associated with botulism in the human subject, but types C, D and F have also caused disease in man.

Morphology and Staining.—A sporing bacillus with rounded ends, about 4–6 μ by 0·9–1·2 μ, occurring singly and in pairs. Spores are oval, subterminal and slightly "bulging". The bacilli are motile with peritrichous flagella, and stain Gram-positively unless degenerate.

Cultural Characters.—Strict anaerobe. The optimum temperature has been variously stated; earlier workers found growth occurred best at 20°–30° C.; more recent observations indicate that the optimum is about 35° C. Grows on ordinary media; meat medium yields abundant growth.

SOME DIFFERENTIAL CHARACTERS OF CLOSTRIDIA

	Morphology in culture*	Colonies on Blood-agar	Cooked meat medium	Milk medium	Liquefaction of coagulated serum	Fermentation of					Pathogenicity to guinea-pigs and mice
						Glucose	Lactose	Sucrose	Maltose	Salicin	
Cl. tetani	Slender bacilli with round terminal spores	Transparent, with long feathery spreading projections; usually haemolytic	*Slight* digestion, blackening and pungent odour	Unaltered	− (but may be softened)	−	−	−	−	−	+ (tetanus produced)
Cl. tetanomorphum	Resembles *Cl. tetani*; round terminal spores	Small and transparent, with irregular outline	Gas; no digestion; no putrefactive odour	Unaltered	− (but may be softened)	+	−	−	+	−	−
Cl. welchii	Large, thick, often rectangular bacilli; spores usually absent	Large, circular, with regular outline; haemolytic	Gas, no digestion, meat reddened	Acid, gas, rapid clotting; "stormy-clot"	−	+	+	+	+	(−/+)	+
Cl. septicum	Large bacilli with central or subterminal spores†	Transparent, irregular, with spreading projections; usually haemolytic	Gas, no digestion, meat reddened	Acid, gas, slow clotting	−	+	+	−	+	+	+
Cl. oedematiens	Like *Cl. welchii* but somewhat larger and more pleomorphic; central or subterminal spores (not numerous)	Transparent, flat, tend to fuse and form spreading film; usually haemolytic	Gas, no digestion, meat reddened	Sometimes slow clotting	−	+	−	−	+	−	+
Cl. histolyticum	Filamentous in old cultures or if grown aerobically; spores large, oval and subterminal	Irregular, round, opaque, greyish-white colonies; haemolytic	Digestion of meat with evolution of H_2S; white crystals deposited late	Acid, gas; casein precipitated and digested	+	−	−	−	−	−	+

Cl. bifermentans[1]	Usually numerous sporing forms, often in chains; spores large, oval, central or sub-terminal	Round, crenated, irregular; usually haemolytic	Gas, digestion, blackening and putrefactive odour whitish mucoid deposit	Acid, gas, digestion	+	+	−	−	+	$(\pm)$	$(\mp)$
Cl. botulinum	Large pleomorphic bacilli; oval spores, usually subterminal	Large irregular colonies with raised opaque centre; usually haemolytic	Gas; types vary in proteolytic activity (*see* text)	Casein precipitated and digested by some types; others produce no digestion	$(\pm)$	+	$(\mp)$	$(\mp)$	+	$(\mp)$	+
Cl. sporogenes	Somewhat slender bacilli; central or subterminal spores	Usually irregular colonies with feathery projections; haemolytic young colonies small, circular, opaque.	Gas, digestion, blackening and putrefactive odour	Acid, clot, digestion, later alkaline	+	+	−	−	+	$(\mp)$	−

See also table of characters of anaerobic bacilli in *Medical Research Council War Memorandum No.* 2, Revised Second Edition, 1943.

* All these organisms are Gram-positive, but Gram-negative forms are seen in older cultures; they are all motile, with peritrichous flagella, except *Cl. welchii*, but motility is not pronounced and has to be observed while the organisms remain in an anaerobic environment, *e.g.* withdrawn from a young anaerobic culture into sealed capillary tubes.

† Morphological forms seen in tissues are referred to in the text (*vide supra*).

\+ Under fermentation signifies acid and gas production.

Double symbols in brackets signify variability in reaction among strains.

[1] For a discussion of the differentiation between *Cl. bifermentans* and *Cl. sordellii*, see Willis, A. T. (1960).

For full details of the biological and other characters of the various members of the group, one of the larger works on bacteriology should be consulted.

Surface colonies—large, greyish, irregular, semi-transparent, with a central "nucleus" and a reticular or fimbriate border; haemolytic on horse-blood agar. The semi-transparent colonies of toxigenic *Cl. botulinum* ("TOX" colonies) may be differentiated from opaque colonies containing sporing organisms. Toxigenic strains are said to revert to non-toxigenic opaque sporing ("OS") colonial mutants (Dolman, 1957; Dolman & Murakami, 1961).

Agar stab—a white line of growth, stopping short of the surface, with short lateral spikes or radiations; gas production is marked, especially in glucose-agar.

Gelatin is liquefied.

Coagulated serum is slowly liquefied, milk-casein is digested and meat is digested and usually blackened by toxigenic type A, B, and F strains; other strains of A, B and F and types C, D and E are generally non-proteolytic (but see Dolman, 1957).

The organism ferments glucose and maltose; type A also frequently ferments salicin and glycerol; type B ferments glycerol but not salicin; type C does not act on either of these substances.

All types produce lecithinase.

Viability.—Spores of some strains of *Cl. botulinum* withstand moist heat at 100° C. for several hours. They are destroyed at 120° C. (moist heat) usually within 5 min. Insufficient heating in the process of preserving foods is an important factor in the causation of this form of poisoning, and great care is taken in canning factories to ensure that sufficient heating is achieved in all parts of the can contents.

Antigenic Characters.—In culture media and in contaminated foods, *Cl. botulinum* produces a powerful exotoxin which is responsible for the pathogenic effects in the disease. This toxin is destroyed when exposed to a temperature of 80° C. for 30–40 min.

The toxin of type A has been isolated as a pure crystalline protein and quantitatively is probably the most potent toxic substance in nature, the estimated lethal dose for mice being 0·000000033 mg. In spite of its potency, the action of the toxin is slow and victims or experimental animals may die many days after receiving a lethal dose. The different types of the bacillus produce toxins that are immunologically different and neutralisable only by the appropriate antitoxin; thus, antitoxin produced from toxin A does not neutralise toxin B, and *vice versa*. Type C has been subdivided into two subtypes, C_α and C_β; C_α antitoxin neutralises C_α and C_β toxins, while C_β antitoxin fails to neutralise C_α toxin.

Diffusible haemagglutinins have been described in culture filtrates of *Cl. botulinum*.

Antitoxin can be prepared by immunising animals with toxoid preparations, and it is used therapeutically. In general, a bivalent serum containing antitoxins to the A and B types of toxin is employed, but its efficacy in the treatment of established botulism is doubtful.

Animal Pathogenicity.—Laboratory animals are susceptible to experimental inoculation and feeding with cultures. The resulting condition resembles the human disease in its symptomatology, the guinea-pig showing difficulty in breathing, flaccid paralysis of the abdominal muscles and salivation following intraperitoneal injection; at autopsy, marked congestion of the internal organs, extensive thrombosis and haemorrhages are noted.

Pathogenesis.—*Cl. botulinum* is a saprophytic organism and is widely distributed. Its natural habitat is soil, even virgin and forest soil. It may be found in vegetables, fruits, leaves, mouldy hay, ensilage and animal manure.

Botulism has been found to originate from a considerable variety of preserved foods—*e.g.* ham, sausage, canned meats and vegetables, etc. Type E strains occur in fish (see Dolman & Chang, 1953). Foods responsible for botulism do not always exhibit signs of spoilage. Botulism is thought to be due mainly to absorption from the intestine of toxin preformed by the bacilli in the food, but there may be some formation of toxin by the organisms after ingestion.

In cases of botulism the bacillus may sometimes be demonstrated in the stomach contents and faeces, and *post mortem* in the intestinal contents and in the liver and spleen. It can also be isolated from the food responsible for the outbreak.

Rare cases of wound infection by *Cl. botulinum*, resulting in the characteristic signs and symptoms of botulism, have been recorded.

Botulism also occurs in such animals as horses, cattle, sheep and poultry due to feeding on material in which the organism has been growing. Type C_α is responsible for a paralytic disease of chickens and botulism of ducks. Type C_β is responsible for forage poisoning in horses and cattle; lamziekte of cattle in South Africa is due to type D and results from eating the bones of decomposed carcases on the veldt. Limberneck of chickens is caused by types A and B. The ingestion of the larvae of carrion flies harbouring the organism is frequently responsible for botulism in birds. Sporadic outbreaks of botulism have been reported in mink in America, Scandinavia and England.

Laboratory Diagnosis.—As botulism is essentially a food intoxication, the suspected food should be examined bacteriologically. It may occasionally be possible to demonstrate the presence of toxin in the patient's blood or in *post-mortem* material, *e.g.* blood, liver, by direct animal inoculation.

Gram-stained films of the food may first be examined for sporing bacilli. The food is then macerated in sterile salt solution and an extract cleared by centrifugation. This may be sterilised by filtration prior to animal inoculation. The extract is then injected intraperitoneally into guinea-pigs in 2 ml. amounts. Injections of heated extract (ten minutes at 100° C.) should be made in a group of control animals, and unheated extract plus the different type antitoxins, if available, may be inoculated into a third group. No deaths should occur in the second group if a specific botulinum toxin is involved and this may be indicated by the third group of tests.

Cl. botulinum may be isolated in pure culture from the food by preliminary heating of various samples at 65°–80° C. for thirty minutes to eliminate non-sporing bacteria. Cultures may then be made under anaerobic conditions on solid media, including a selective medium such as Willis and Hobbs' medium, and in cooked-meat broth. Subsequent identification of *Cl. botulinum* is based upon its biological characters and its toxigenicity. Culture filtrates may be prepared from five- to ten-day cooked-meat broth cultures and tested for toxicity by animal inoculation tests as described above. Faeces and vomit from a case of botulism may be similarly investigated for the causative organism.

Prophylaxis.—Home-canning of foodstuffs should be avoided and home preservation of meat and vegetables is not advisable. Acid fruits may be bottled safely in the home, heating at only 100° C., since a low *p*H is inhibitory to the development of *Cl. botulinum.* A prophylactic dose of antitoxin (10 ml.) should be given intramuscularly to all asymptomatic persons who have eaten food suspected of causing botulism. Active immunity in man can be produced by the injection of three doses of mixed toxoid (types A and B) at two-month intervals, but the incidence of the disease under normal conditions does not justify this procedure. Similar immunisation of animals against the predominant type may be economically worth while and has been carried out in Australia on a small scale.

REFERENCES

Brown, A., Mohamed, S. D., Montgomery, R. D., Armitage, P. & Laurence, D. R. (1960). Value of a large dose of antitoxin in clinical tetanus. *Lancet*, **2**, 227.

Dolman, C. E. (1957). Recent observations on type E botulism. *Canad. J. publ. Hlth.*, **48**, 187.

Dolman, C. E. & Chang, H. (1953). The epidemiology and pathogenesis of type E and fish-borne botulism. *Canad. J. publ. Hlth.*, **44**, 231.

Dolman, C. E. & Murakami, L. (1961). *Clostridium botulinum* type F with recent observations on other types. *J. infect. Dis.*, **109**, 107.

Ellis, M. (1963). Human antitetanus serum in the treatment of tetanus. *Brit. med. J.*, **1**, 1123.

Kerrin, J. C. (1929). The distribution of *B. tetani* in the intestines of animals. *Brit. J. exp. Path*, **10**, 370.

Laurence, D. R. & Webster, R. A. (1963). Pathologic physiology, pharmacology, and therapeutics of tetanus. *Clin. Pharmacol. Ther.*, **4**, 36.

Laurence, D. R., Evans, D. G. & Smith, J. W. G. (1966). Prevention of tetanus in the wounded. *Brit. med. J.*, **1**, 33.

Lowbury, E. J. L., Batten, R. L. & London, P. S. (1961). Correspondence: Antitetanus immunization. *Brit. med. J.*, **2**, 1783.

Lowbury, E. J. L. & Lilly, H. A. (1958). Contamination of operating-theatre air with *Cl. tetani*. *Brit. med. J.*, **2**, 1334.

Ministry of Health Memo. (1964). Protection against tetanus. *Brit. med. J.*, **2**, 243.

Mueller, J. H. & Miller, P. A. (1954). Variable factors influencing the production of tetanus toxin. *J. Bact.*, **67**, 271.

Rubbo, S. D. (1966). New approaches to tetanus prophylaxis. *Lancet*, **2**, 449.

Smith, J. W. G., Evans, D. G., Jones, D. A., Gear, M. W. L., Cunliffe, A. C., & Barr, M. (1963). Simultaneous active and passive immunization against tetanus. *Brit. med. J.*, **1**, 237.

Smith, J. W. G. (1964). Correspondence: Tetanus prophylaxis. *Brit. med. J.*, **1**, 373.

Tenbroeck, C. & Bauer, J. H. (1922). The tetanus bacillus as an intestinal saprophyte in man. *J. exp. Med.*, **36**, 261.

Willis, A. T. (1960). *Anaerobic Bacteriology in Clinical Medicine*, pp. 59 and 80. London: Butterworth.

Wright, G. P. (1955). In *Mechanisms of Microbial Pathogenicity*, ed. Howie, J. W. & O'Hea, A. J., p. 78. Cambridge University Press.

Wright, E. A., Morgan, R. S. & Wright, G. P. (1950). Tetanus intoxication of the brain stem in rabbits. *J. Path. Bact.*, **62**, 569.

CHAPTER 29

SPIROCHAETES

THE pathogenic and commensal spirochaetes are slender flexuous spirals 4–16 μ in length and 0·1–0·6 μ thick. They are composed of regular tight coils or of loose irregular spirals of varying amplitude. As a group these organisms are more highly organised than other bacteria, for in addition to a cell wall and cytoplasm they contain from one to twelve long filaments applied to their bodies and it is to these structures that they owe their shape and in all probability their elasticity and characteristic movements. Some cells are only visible by dark-ground microscopy, many can be cultivated and the majority are parasitic in vertebrates. The three genera, *Treponema*, *Borrelia* and *Leptospira*, together constitute the family *Treponemataceae*.

TREPONEMA PALLIDUM

Syphilis is an infectious venereal disease caused by *Tr. pallidum*. Clinically the disease includes a sore on the genitalia which is followed by generalisation of the infection with protean clinical manifestations.

Morphology.—An exceedingly delicate, spiral filament 6–14 μ (average 10 μ) by 0·13 μ, with six to twelve coils which are comparatively small, sharp and regular. The length of the coils is about 1 μ and the depth 1–1·5 μ. The ends are pointed and tapering. The organism is feebly refractile, and in the unstained condition requires dark-ground illumination for its demonstration.

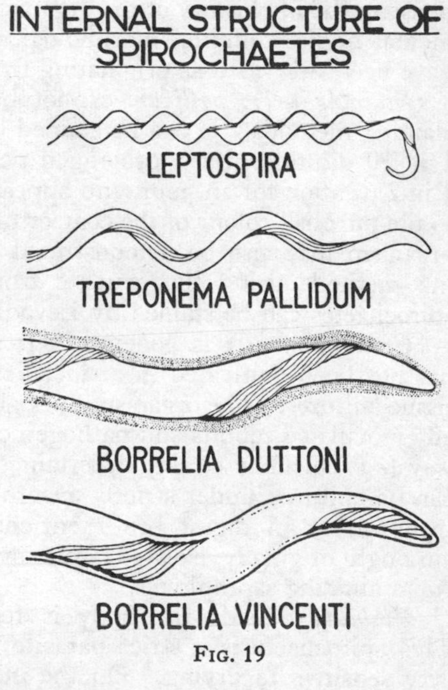

In electron micrographs *Treponema pallidum* is seen to be covered by an outer periplast which covers the whole organism. When this periplast is removed by digestion with pepsin or trypsin four fine filaments about 10 mμ in diameter are seen twisted around the organism and conforming to its coils. Fracture of these filaments results in the disappearance of the organism's coils; the filaments may then be spread out on the supporting film, in which situation they

INTERNAL STRUCTURE OF SPIROCHAETES

LEPTOSPIRA

TREPONEMA PALLIDUM

BORRELIA DUTTONI

BORRELIA VINCENTI

FIG. 19

were mistaken by earlier workers for true flagella. *Tr. pallidum* is therefore not flagellate (Swain, 1955). The nature of the fibrils twisted around its protoplasm is uncertain, but it seems likely that they are contractile and concerned in the maintenance of the characteristic shape and motility of the organism.

In addition to the typical form, as described, some variation in morphology may be observed: the number of coils to the unit of length may be more or less than normal, the filament may be thicker than normal in whole or part and the coils may be shallower and less regular than usual.

The spirochaete shows rotatory corkscrew-like motility and also movements of flexion. The coils remain relatively rigid, but there may be some expansion and contraction. Angulation, with the organism bending almost to 90° towards its centre is highly characteristic. Its progression is relatively slow as compared with many of the motile bacteria.

The organism divides by transverse binary fission. There is good evidence for the existence of a more complicated life cycle of reproduction in the case of cultivated non-pathogenic strains of treponemes such as the Reiter spirochaete, in which a granular, filterable phase has been described. Division into four and even more fragments has also been described. Some observers have claimed that granules or bud-like structures may be split off, remaining attached by pedicles or stalks before final separation. This budded form has also been regarded as a phase in the life history of the organism, and various supposed developmental bodies differing morphologically from the normal spirochaete have been described as originating from such structures.

Staining.—Tr. pallidum cannot be demonstrated by the ordinary staining methods. It can be stained by Giemsa's solution applied in a 1 in 10 dilution over a prolonged period (twenty-four hours) or in a 1 in 2 dilution for an hour, and appears faint pink in colour in contrast to the purplish colour of the coarser non-pathogenic spirochaetes. The organism may also be demonstrated by Fontana's silver or the India ink methods using the exudate from the chancre. In tissues, the spirochaetes can be stained by Levaditi's silver impregnation method.

Cultivation.—It is generally agreed that pathogenic *Tr. pallidum* has not been cultivated in artificial media or in embryonated eggs or tissue cultures. The organism does grow in the testicles of experimentally inoculated rabbits and pathogenic strains can be maintained in this way (*e.g.* Nichol's strain). Certain other strains (*e.g.* Reiter's strain) can be cultured under strictly anaerobic conditions in Smith-Noguchi medium, or in digest broth enriched with serum. These strains, although originally isolated from syphilitic lesions, may have been contaminating saprophytes.

Viability outside the body is feeble under ordinary conditions. This spirochaete is a strict parasite; it dies rapidly in water and is very sensitive to drying. On the other hand it has been found that *Tr. pallidum* can retain its viability and virulence in necropsy material for some time at ordinary temperatures, and in serum kept in sealed capillary tubes it remains motile for several days. It is readily killed by heat (even at 41·5° C. in an hour) and dies out more slowly (in two to three days) if kept at 0°–4° C. *Tr. pallidum* remains viable in tissue slices of rabbit testis for long periods at temperatures of −55° to −65° C.

Animal Pathogenicity.—Monkeys have been infected experimentally by inoculation of a scarified area on the eyebrows and genitals, or by implanting tissue from a syphilitic lesion under the epidermis. The anthropoid apes are the most susceptible, and lesions typical of primary and secondary syphilis may result in these animals. Rabbits can also be infected in some cases by inoculation in certain sites: inoculation into the anterior chamber of the eye produces keratitis and iritis; intratesticular injection leads to a syphilitic orchitis; and inoculation of the skin of the scrotum may set up a chancre-like sore. Metastatic lesions may succeed the primary infection.

Inoculation of mice produces no lesions, and though infection takes place it is symptomless and apparently latent.

Pathogenesis.—After exposure to infection there is an incubation period of four to six weeks before the appearance of the initial sore of primary syphilis. This lesion shows first as a small red papule usually on the genitalia; it gradually enlarges, becomes indurated and necroses in the centre to leave an ulcer; simultaneously there develops a marked generalised lymphadenopathy which is most obvious in the inguinal region. Spirochaetes are present in large numbers in the primary chancre and in the exudate from it. As the sore heals, the organisms become less numerous and may not be demonstrable in the exudate, but at this stage it may be possible to find them in fluid obtained by lymph gland puncture.

In the secondary stage which develops six to twelve weeks after the appearance of the primary chancre, the spirochaetes invade the blood stream and are widely disseminated throughout the body. The clinical manifestations may include those of fever, a generalised roseolar skin rash, mucous patches in the mouth and condylomata of the anus and vulva. The severity of these lesions is extremely variable and those of minor extent may heal and disappear without their presence being noticed.

In the tertiary stage the spirochaetes become localised producing low grade inflammatory lesions in the cardiovascular and central nervous systems and in chronic granulomata (gummata) in the skin, bone and internal organs. Often this process continues for long periods and several years may pass before any clinical sign or symptom is apparent. Thus tabes dorsalis and meningo-vascular syphilis may only be detected 5–15 years after the appearance of the primary chancre. In this stage *Tr. pallidum* can only be demonstrated in the lesions with difficulty although it can be observed by suitable staining methods in the periphery of gummata, in arterial lesions, and in the cerebral cortex in general paralysis of the insane.

In congenital syphilis, spirochaetes are found in certain internal organs, *e.g.* liver, often in very large numbers. They are present also in the skin lesions, the blood, and the mucosa of the intestine and bladder, and have been demonstrated in the placenta.

Epidemiology.—Most cases of syphilis are contracted during sexual intercourse. Rarely, however, other forms of direct contact may facilitate the spread of the disease as is witnessed by primary lesions on the hands of venereologists, the lips after kissing, and the skin of the abdominal wall. The open lesions of the primary and secondary stages of syphilis discharge many millions of spirochaetes. The organisms are so sensitive to the adverse influence of conditions outside the human body that they seldom survive on fomites long enough to transfer infection.

During the Second World War the incidence of syphilis increased and reached its peak in 1946 (23,878 cases in England and Wales). With the introduction of penicillin therapy there was a dramatic decline in the years that followed and a more gradual fall in the decade 1951-61 (from 8,432 to 4,442 clinic cases in England and Wales). During this time clinical cases of gonorrhoea increased from 18,064 to 37,107 and there is some evidence of an increase in the incidence of infectious syphilis in the past few years (BMA Report, 1964).

Each case of syphilis is a potential source of a small outbreak of the disease and 10–20 cases may be traced to a single individual. Control of the disease depends on early diagnosis, case and contact tracing, effective chemotherapy of cases to reduce infectivity, sex education and other social measures. No protective vaccines exist.

Chemotherapy.—Penicillin is highly effective in the treatment of syphilis but the results obtained depend on the stage and nature of the disease. Broad spectrum antibiotics such as the tetracyclines are almost as effective as penicillin.

Laboratory Diagnosis

The clinical diagnosis of syphilis is confirmed in the laboratory by finding *Tr. pallidum* in the exudates from the lesions or in the tissues and by demonstrating antibodies in the serum.

THE EXAMINATION OF SYPHILITIC EXUDATES.—There is a serious risk of infection to the person who collects specimens from patients with primary or secondary syphilis and it is important to wear rubber gloves and to exercise great care in handling the lesions. The sore is first cleansed carefully with a gauze swab soaked in warm normal saline and the margins are gently scraped so that superficial epithelium is abraded. Gentle pressure is applied to the base of the chancre until serum exudes from its surface; if this serum is blood-stained it should be wiped away and the process repeated until a clear fluid is obtained. Excessive numbers of red blood cells in the specimen must be avoided as they tend to obscure the spirochaetes. Wet films are now made on thin glass slides, covered with a thin coverslip and examined under the dark ground microscope. If the examination has to be made in a laboratory at some distance some of the exudate should be taken up into several capillary tubes, both ends of which are then sealed in a flame. Do not store in the refrigerator or the incubator.

If a local antiseptic has been applied to the sore spirochaetes may not be found until a wet dressing of gauze soaked in sterile normal saline has been applied to the sore for 24–48 hours. When antisyphilitic treatment (*e.g.* penicillin), has been used before the examination the likelihood of a successful microscopic diagnosis is greatly diminished.

If a primary sore is healing the macroscopic examination of the exudate is often negative. At this stage, however, the spirochaetes may be found in the fluid aspirated with a syringe from enlarged inguinal lymph glands. Before reliance can be placed on negative findings, the microscopical examination must be repeated on at least three occasions at daily intervals.

The observation of living motile spirochaetes under *the dark ground microscope* is the most satisfactory method and in experienced hands provides a rapid and reliable diagnosis. *Tr. pallidum* is recognised by its slender spiral structure, characteristic slow movements, and angulation. It must be carefully distinguished from the many other spirochaetes which can be found in ulcerating sores (e.g. *Tr. calligyrum*). If no dark ground microscope is available a wet film of the exudate mixed with India ink may be examined or Fontana's staining method can be used.

In the secondary stage spirochaetes can be demonstrated in the serous exudate obtained from the skin eruption by scarifying and "cupping" with test tubes. The spirochaetes are also present in large numbers in the mucous patches in the mouth and in condylomata about the vulva and anus. Specimens from these situations, however, may contain large numbers of non-pathogenic spirochaetes which may be morphologically identical with *Tr. pallidum* and great caution is required in reporting the observations.

Serological Methods.—Three distinct antibodies appear in the serum after a syphilitic infection. The first is known as a "reagin" and reacts with an antigen composed of an alcoholic extract of heart muscle to which cholesterol and lecithin have been added; it can be demonstrated either by complement fixation as in the Wassermann reaction or by flocculation as in the Kahn or similar tests. Reactions which demonstrate the presence of the "reagin" are known as the standard tests for syphilis (STS) or as conventional tests. A second antibody reacts with a protein component found in the spirochaetal bodies of a non-pathogenic strain of *Tr. pallidum* and can be demonstrated in the Reiter Protein Complement Fixation Test (RPCF). The third antibody reacts directly with a pathogenic strain of *Tr. pallidum* and can be demonstrated in the Treponema Immobilisation and Fluorescent Treponemal Antibody tests (TPI and FTA).

Standard Tests for Syphilis (STS).—*The Wassermann Reaction* (WR), usually becomes weakly positive at the second or third week after the appearance of the primary sore; the degree of positivity increases and the test is markedly positive by the sixth week; in the secondary stage it is always strongly positive. Occasionally, however, a positive reaction is slow to develop and if, at first, a negative result is obtained it is essential to repeat the test on two or more occasions before excluding syphilis. A negative reaction in a case of suspected secondary syphilis is highly significant in excluding syphilitic infection but in supposed tertiary or latent cases the negative finding does not exclude the disease. Thus in 20–30 per cent. of cases of tabes dorsalis and in about 10 per cent. of cases of meningo-vascular syphilis the test is negative.

In cases of tertiary syphilis the reaction should be carried out on the cerebrospinal fluid as well as on the blood. The cerebrospinal fluid gives a positive reaction in virtually all cases of general paresis, and in most cases of tabes dorsalis at some stage, although during remissions it may be negative; in meningo-vascular syphilis about one half of the cases give a positive reaction.

Flocculation Tests such as the Kahn or VDRL tests are often used for screening tests on sera because they are quick and simple to carry out. The results of these reactions, however, do not always run parallel with those of the Wassermann Reaction and to obtain the maximum amount of information both tests must be carried out in parallel. In general flocculation tests are more sensitive but less specific than the Wassermann reaction. Repeated positive tests with both methods give a reliable indication of syphilis. Furthermore one reaction acts as a check on the other and although a positive finding with one test in the presence of a negative finding with the other may be diagnostic of syphilis, such a discrepancy indicates the need for repeated serological testing and the employment of more specific reactions with spirochaetal antigens (*vide infra*).

The Wassermann and flocculation reactions are constantly positive in yaws, bejel and pinta that are diseases caused by spirochaetes very closely related to *Tr. pallidum*. In tropical and subtropical regions the serological differentiation of these diseases from syphilis may be a matter of great difficulty.

Biologic False Positive Reactions.—Since the lipoidal antigen used in the Wassermann and flocculation tests is non-specific in nature it is not surprising that false positive reactions occur in a considerable number of conditions quite unrelated to syphilis. Although such false positive reactions cause difficulties in interpretation they do not occur with sufficient frequency to detract from the general diagnostic value of the tests. The highest incidence of these reactions is in malaria (4–10 per cent.), leprosy (especially the nodular type), collagen diseases such as lupus erythematosus and periarteritis nodosa, infectious mononucleosis, measles and rubella. They have been occasionally reported in almost all febrile diseases and occur regularly in a small proportion of cases of relapsing fever, leptospirosis, scarlatina, pneumonia of bacterial or viral origin, typhus, lymphogranuloma venereum, infectious hepatitis, varicella and trypanosomiasis. In addition they may be found after blood donation, smallpox vaccination, the administration of tetanus toxoid or therapeutic injections of serum. During pregnancy weakly positive reactions may occur but they gradually diminish and disappear after the birth of the child.

Biological false positive tests often take the form of a positive Kahn test associated with a negative Wassermann reaction, but latent or treated syphilis may also present this finding. In such circumstances the *Kahn verification test* is often helpful in distinguishing true syphilitic from non-specific reactions. A positive STS in association with a negative Kahn verification test is almost always non-specific.

Treponemal Antibody Tests.—*The Reiter Protein Complement-Fixation* (*RPCF*) *Test* employs as an antigen a protein extract obtained by the ammonium sulphate precipitation of a suspension of non-pathogenic spirochaetes obtained from cultures of the Reiter's strain of *Tr. pallidum* (D'Alessandro & Dardanoni, 1953). Sequeira (1959), Wilkinson & Johnston (1959) and Foster, Nicol & Stone (1958) are all in agreement that the RPCF Test is more sensitive and more specific than the standard tests for syphilis. There has not yet been sufficient time for a full evaluation of this test, but in general it would appear that it agrees closely but not completely with the TPI test. In primary untreated syphilis as well as in the later stages the RPCF test has a sensitivity equal to the STS. The incidence of positive findings in sera giving biologically false positive STS is markedly reduced but a small proportion of non-specific positive and false negative reactions do occur (Bekker, 1962). Since the RPCF test is no more difficult to carry out than the Wassermann reaction and as the antigen is available commercially (Organon Laboratories), it is very suitable for routine serological work.

The Treponema Pallidum Immobilisation (*TPI*) *Test* depends on the observation of immobilisation of living spirochaetes when they are incubated with syphilitic sera. Dilutions of the serum to be tested are mixed with a suspension of motile *Tr. pallidum* (Nichol's strain) which are maintained in the laboratory by the intra-testicular inoculation of rabbits. An appropriate amount of fresh complement is added and after incubation the test is read by determining, under the dark ground microscope, the proportion of treponemes which have been immobilised. This proportion is then compared with a similar estimate of the spirochaetes immobilised by normal and known positive control sera (Nelson & Mayer, 1949; Wilkinson & Johnston, 1959). The test is complicated to perform, expensive in animals and reagents, and is very time consuming. It is not suitable for use as a routine test and is reserved for specially selected cases.

The TPI test is generally accepted as being almost completely specific and a positive finding is a reliable indication of syphilitic infection. The sensitivity of the test, however, is not so great as that of the STS and negative findings may be obtained in untreated cases of primary and early secondary syphilis and also in congenital syphilis (Sequeira & Wilkinson, 1955; Wilkinson & Sequeira, 1955). The main value of the test is in latent and tertiary syphilis and in clarifying those problems which arise when discrepancies occur in the STS, *e.g.* biological false positive reactions. The TPI test remains positive for long periods even after the STS have become negative and thus it is of little value in following the effects of treatment. Since the TPI test has the highest specificity of all the tests for syphilitic antibodies it is used as a reference in assessing the value of other tests.

The Fluorescent Treponemal Antibody (*FTA*) *Test* offers an alternative to the TPI test and is simpler and easier to carry out. The antigen used is a suspension of treponemes of the Nichol's strain of *Tr. pallidum* which remains stable for several months at refrigerator temperature. The antibody with which this antigen unites would appear to be identical with that reacting in the TPI test. Smears of the antigen are treated with dilutions of the patient's serum, stained with a fluorescein labelled antiserum to human gamma-globulin and then examined in the fluorescent microscope (Wilkinson, 1961). Preliminary reports suggest that this test has a high level of sensitivity and specificity and also indicate that it gives positive findings in the early stages of primary syphilis. In late untreated cases the FTA test remains positive for prolonged periods in the same manner as the TPI test (Deacon, Freeman, & Harris, 1960).

The FTA test has a number of economic and technical advantages over the TPI test. The time required to carry out the test is short and the results can be read after 30 min. incubation at 37° C. The standard antigen is stable and retains its potency for months, only minimal amounts of glassware are needed and the only other reagents required are a phosphate buffered saline diluent pH 7·3–7·4 and a 2 per cent. solution of Tween 80.

In routine diagnostic work a combination of serological methods must be used. Two tests for the reagin antibody are required; one of high sensitivity such as the VDRL or Kahn Test and one of normal sensitivity such as the WR. In addition a third test for an unrelated treponemal antibody is needed and for this the RPCF test is recommended as convenient, inexpensive, highly sensitive, and very specific; alternatively, where microscopical facilities exist the FTA can be used with excellent results. When discrepancies are found the TPI test is the final reference test for the differentiation of syphilitic from biologic false positive reactions.

Non-venereal Syphilis

Although syphilis is a venereal disease, conditions with closely similar clinical manifestations occur in circumstances when it seems scarcely possible that infection was transmitted during sexual intercourse. One such condition is *Bejel*, which is found in Bedouin Arabs in Syria and Iraq. Bejel occurs predominantly in young children who show mucous patches and other lesions of secondary syphilis without as a rule having any primary lesion. It is thought that the infection is transmitted by close personal contact or by contaminated drinking vessels or other utensils; in some cases the child has been infected from a primary chancre on the nipple of the nursing mother. Meningo-vascular lesions may occur as late manifestations but involvement of the central nervous system is rare.

Closely similar diseases which are sometimes referred to as endemic syphilis have been reported in Bosnia, West Africa, Southern Rhodesia and in India. Except for the mode of transmission and the epidemiological findings endemic syphilis does not differ essentially from venereal syphilis and the laboratory diagnosis and treatment of both diseases is the same.

TREPONEMA PERTENUE

This spirochaete is the cause of *Yaws* (*Framboesia*) a chronic disease which is virtually limited to humid tropical areas. The primary lesion, which is practically always extra-genital, takes the form of a painless yellowish-red papule which slowly erodes and becomes an ulcerated discharging granuloma. This "mother yaw" is followed six weeks to three months later by generalised secondary superficial lesions of similar appearances situated on the limbs, neck and at muco-cutaneous junctions on the face and genitalia. The later manifestations of yaws include destructive lesions of bone in about 15 per cent. of cases, but cardiovascular and neurological complications are rare. Treponemata abound in the exudates from the lesion and the infection is transmitted by direct personal contact, the spirochaetes entering the new host through small skin abrasions. Flies may play a part as vectors of infections and *Hippolates pallipes* has been observed to feed on the open lesions; *Tr. pertenue* persists in the proventriculus of the insect for upwards of seven hours and is regurgitated when the fly feeds again.

Tr. pertenue is indistinguishable from *Tr. pallidum* in morphology, motility, staining properties, ability to provoke reagin and treponemal antibodies, and in its susceptibility to arsenical drugs and antibiotics. Thus the diagnostic procedures and treatment are the same as those used in syphilis. A long-acting penicillin is the drug of choice and a dramatic response follows its use.

Treponema Carateum (Tr. herrejoni)

This spirochaete is the cause of *Pinta*, a disease of dark-skinned races in the West Indies, Central and South America and in some parts of the Pacific. The primary lesion, which is extra-genital and non-ulcerating, appears as an erythematous, scaly patch about one centimetre in diameter assuming later a psoriatic or licheniform appearance. It is followed after about five months by secondary lesions of a similar nature which later become characteristically depigmented and hyperkeratotic. Progressive hyperpigmentation of some areas follows to give a third stage of the illness characterised by multicoloured lesions. Involvement of the cardiovascular and central nervous systems occurs late in the disease. *Tr. carateum* can be demonstrated in the skin lesions and in the lymphatic glands. Transmission is not venereal and usually occurs by direct contact. Like yaws, pinta may be spread by the fly *Hippolates pallipes*.

Tr. carateum is morphologically indistinguishable from *Tr. pallidum* which it resembles closely in many other respects. Immunologically, however, there may be some difference because patients with pinta can contract syphilis and syphilitic subjects have been successfully infected experimentally with pinta. The methods for the laboratory diagnosis and treatment of pinta are the same as those used for yaws and syphilis.

OTHER TREPONEMATA

Treponema calligyrum (or *gracile*).—This organism may occur in the secretions of the genitals, and morphologically resembles *Tr. pallidum*. Its differentiation from the latter is therefore of practical importance in syphilis diagnosis. It is not usually found if care has been taken to obtain serum from below the surface of the chancre. It is thicker than *Tr. pallidum* and its spirals are shallower; by the dark-ground illumination method it appears "glistening", whereas *Tr. pallidum* is "dead white"; it stains more readily than *Tr. pallidum* by Giemsa's method.

Treponema genitalis, which is very similar to *Tr. pallidum*, has also been described as a commensal on the genital mucosa.

Treponema microdentium.—This organism flourishes in carious teeth, and may be found in the secretion between the teeth. It closely resembles *Tr. pallidum* in morphology, but is shorter (3–10 μ), and the coils are shallower. It is more easily stained by the ordinary methods than *Tr. pallidum*.

Treponema mucosum.—Similar to *Tr. microdentium* in morphology, but is stated to have the property of producing a mucin-like substance.

Treponema macrodentium.—Occurs in the mouth like *Tr. microdentium*. It bears some resemblance to *Tr. pallidum*, but is larger and thicker, with larger and less regular coils, usually two to eight in number. Its motility is also more active. It is more easily stained than *Tr. pallidum* and is coloured blue by Giemsa's method.

Treponema cuniculi.—Associated with an infectious disease of rabbits, which usually takes the form of a chronic local and superficial infection of the genitals. The spirochaetes can be demonstrated in the exudate from the lesions and in tissue sections. They are morphologically identical with *Tr. pallidum*.

BORRELIAE

These are large, motile, refractile spirochaetes (about 10–30 μ by 0·3–0·7 μ) with irregular wide and open coils, which are relatively few in number. They are easily stained by the ordinary methods, and are Gram-negative. Some occur as commensals on various mucous membranes, *e.g.* mouth, and in gangrenous and ulcerative conditions on the surface of the body, the mouth and throat and the genitals. *Borrelia buccalis* is found in the healthy mouth; it is sluggishly motile with wavy serpentine movements. *Borrelia refringens* occurs on the normal mucous membranes of the genital and anal regions. It is actively motile with lashing and rotating movements; under the dark field microscope it is refractile and appears brighter than other spirochaetes. This type of organism may also be found in the surface exudate of a syphilitic sore, and has to be differentiated morphologically from the *Tr. pallidum*. Other *Borreliae* are pathogenic and cause relapsing fever in man and the disease of fowls known as "spirochaetosis".

BORRELIA VINCENTII

Borrelia vincentii is generally associated with a large fusiform bacillus —*Fusobacterium fusiforme*—and large numbers of both these organisms can be found in a variety of mouth lesions and ulcerative and necrotic processes elsewhere in the body. They are constantly observed in the exudates of the pseudomembranous ulcers on the pharynx and tonsils in Vincent's angina and in the inflamed gum margins in acute ulcerative gingivitis; they are also occasionally found in the lesions of acute balanitis, lung abscess, bronchiectasis, and in chronic ulceration of the skin especially in tropical countries.

Morphology and Staining.—Borr. vincentii is 7–18 μ long and 0·2–0·6 μ wide. There are three to eight loose, open coils varying greatly in amplitude and the organism is actively motile with coarse lashing movements. It resembles *Borr. refringens*, but is sometimes described as smaller and more delicate. The spirochaetes are Gram-negative and stain readily with dilute carbol fuchsin, methyl violet, and with Giemsa's and Leishman's stains. Under the electron microscope *Borr. vincentii* is seen to have a clear-cut wall within which some ten axial filaments are twisted spirally around the protoplasm of the body of the spirochaete (see fig. 19).

Cultivation.—Borr. vincentii is an obligate anaerobe. It can be cultivated in sealed tubes containing digest broth enriched with ascitic fluid; it grows abundantly in mixed primary cultures but is extremely difficult to maintain in pure culture.

Pathogenesis. *Borr. vincentii* and its concomitant fusiform bacillus form a symbiotic combination that is found in small numbers inhabiting the healthy gum, but the numbers may increase enormously when the resistance of the local tissues is reduced. Thus infection with these organisms is superimposed when the superficial tissue is damaged by trauma, deficiencies of vitamins such as ascorbic acid or niacin, infection with the virus of herpes simplex, infectious mononucleosis, or bacterial invasion by haemolytic streptococci or diphtheria bacilli. In agranulocytosis and leukaemia the infection is often seen as a complication. It is probable that these microorganisms are secondary invaders rather than primary pathogens.

Epidemiology.—The source of infection is the patient's own mouth and the disease is not contagious but sporadic. Epidemics of the infection have, however, been reported in children and young adults.

During the First World War the condition was so common in soldiers that it was known as "Trench Mouth". Poor nutrition and poor dental hygiene are factors which are thought to facilitate infection and the transmission of a virus (*e.g.* herpes simplex) in a susceptible population may also play a part.

Laboratory Diagnosis.—Smears are made directly from the ulcerative lesions in the mouth or from swabs and are stained with dilute carbol fuchsin. A clinical diagnosis of Vincent's infection would be confirmed when very large numbers of both the spirochaetes and the typically barred fusiform bacilli are seen together with the many pus cells which indicate the presence of an active inflammatory process. Cultural procedures are not satisfactory for diagnosis of the infection but are necessary because other pathogenic organisms such as haemolytic streptococci or diphtheria bacilli may also be present.

Chemotherapy.—Vincent's organisms are highly sensitive to penicillin which is the drug of choice. The organisms are also sensitive to tetracyclines.

BORRELIA RECURRENTIS (OBERMEIERI)

The causative organism of European Relapsing Fever.

Morphology and Staining.—This organism is a spiral filament, cylindrical or flattened, with tapering ends, varying in length, as a rule, from 10 to 20 μ, and about 0·3–0·5 μ broad, with about five to seven fairly regular coils 0·9–1·7 μ in amplitude. Active motility of a rotatory or oscillating type is noted in fresh preparations. Multiplication is by transverse fission. The structure of the organism as it is seen under the electron microscope is that of a bundle of some twelve filaments twisted spirally around the spirochaetal body external to the cell wall. These filaments are similar to those seen in *Tr. pallidum* and are probably concerned in the contractile movements of the organism. They are rather easily displaced during the manipulations of staining and may resemble flagella, for which at one time they were mistaken. The whole spirochaete is covered by a layer of slime-like material to a thickness of about 0·08 μ.

This spirochaete stains readily with Romanowsky stains (*e.g.* Leishman's), and may exhibit uniform staining or beading. It can be stained also with carbol fuchsin, and is Gram-negative. In fresh preparations of blood it can be seen with the ordinary microscope, but dark-ground or preferably phase-contrast illumination is more suitable for its demonstration in the living state. Silver impregnation methods may also be used for demonstrating the spirochaete in films or tissues.

Cultivation.—Artificial cultures were first obtained anaerobically in Smith-Noguchi medium, citrated blood containing spirochaetes from an infected animal, *e.g.* a white rat, being used as the inoculum.

Cultures have also been obtained in the following media, but the organism does not readily adapt itself to artificial growth in the laboratory: (1) horse serum diluted with 2 parts of saline solution, and with 1 ml. of broth, containing 10 per cent. peptone, added to 10 ml. of the diluted serum; for subcultures, a drop of rabbit blood is also added; the medium is covered with a paraffin seal; (2) 20 per cent. rabbit serum with 80 per cent. Hartley's broth in tubes to each of which 1 g. of coagulated egg albumin is added; petroleum jelly is superimposed and the cultures are incubated at 30° C.; (3) egg albumin is placed in a test-tube and coagulated by heat in the form of a slope; 5 ml. of horse serum diluted 1: 10 or rabbit serum diluted 1: 5 are then added, the serum having previously been heated at 58°–60° C. for one hour; the medium is covered with sterile petroleum jelly; before an inoculation is made, a drop of fresh rabbit or human blood is added. The spirochaetes may also be grown in the chick embryo. The inoculum is introduced into the allantoic cavity of 17–18 day embryos and on hatching large numbers of spirochaetes can be found in the chick's blood (Oag, 1940).

Pathogenesis.—The organism is present in the peripheral blood during the pyrexial stage of the illness, and can be detected in blood films. When defervescence occurs it disappears from the blood, but may still be present in considerable numbers in the spleen, where it is phagocytosed by large mononuclear cells.

It is transmitted from person to person by the body louse, *Pediculus humanus* var. *corporis*. After this insect has sucked blood from the infected individual the organisms are demonstrable in the stomach for a day, and then disappear. They reappear after about six days in the body cavity, become widespread throughout the body of the insect and are transmitted to the eggs. Infection results either through the contamination of the bite-wound with the infective excreta of the louse, or by crushing of the infected lice with the fingers in the act of scratching and by the simultaneous inoculation of the abrasions. Monkeys, white mice and white rats can be infected experimentally by subcutaneous injection of blood from a case of relapsing fever. The guinea-pig is not susceptible.

Chemotherapy.—Borr. recurrentis is sensitive to penicillin and also to the tetracyclines.

Borrelia duttonii

The organism of West Africa Relapsing Fever (African tick fever).

This organism is morphologically similar to *Borr. obermeieri*, but represents a separate species. Granules with the staining reactions of chromatin have also been observed in the spirochaete; these apparently separate from the spirochaete, and have been regarded as a phase in the life history of the organism. There is electron microscopical evidence that these granules contain coiled-up spirochaetes. It seems probable that they are formed under adverse physical conditions and that they represent a resting phase rather than a stage in reproduction. Such granules have been noted in the Malpighian tubules of infective ticks.

Borr. duttonii is transmitted by ticks (*Ornithodorus moubata* and other species). After taking a blood meal a tick may remain infective for as long as five years. The spirochaetes are transmitted transovarially to succeeding generations of ticks. Man is infected in most cases from contamination of the bite wound by infective excreta of the tick, but occasionally the bite itself or particularly the bite of the larva may also transfer the spirochaetes. The main mammalian reservoir of infection is small rodents but pigs, porcupines, opossums and armadillos may also harbour the spirochaetes.

Borr. duttonii is pathogenic to monkeys and certain laboratory animals (*e.g.* rat, mouse). It possesses a greater virulence for monkeys and other animals than *Borr. recurrentis*. Like *Borr. recurrentis*, *Borr. duttonii* is sensitive to penicillin and the tetracyclines.

Other Relapsing Fever Spirochaetes.—The originally described spirochaete of North American relapsing fever resembles *Borr. recurrentis*, but has been regarded as a separate species on the basis of immunity reactions. It has been designated *Borrelia novyi*. It is louse-borne.

The organism of Indian relapsing fever also corresponds in its biology and pathogenesis to *Borr. recurrentis*. It has been named *Borrelia carteri*, but it is doubtful if the Indian strains can be differentiated from the European. This infection is also louse-borne.

Various specific names have been given to relapsing fever spirochaetes in different parts of the world, but it is questionable whether all these biological designations are justified.

Louse-borne spirochaetal relapsing fever, similar to the Indian form, occurs in various parts of Asia, but in Central Asia tick-borne relapsing fever is also present.

The common form of relapsing fever in North Africa is louse-borne. In tropical Africa the prevalent type is tick-borne (African tick fever, *vide supra*), though louse-borne infections occur in West Africa.

In the United States, Central and South America both louse-borne and tick-borne forms of the disease have been observed.

Immunity to the Relapsing Fever Spirochaetes.—Recovery from an attack is associated with the appearance of agglutinating and lytic antibodies in the blood serum (Stein 1944), and in this way the general infection is temporarily checked, though spirochaetes may still persist in the internal organs. It would appear that the relapse is due to antigenic variation in the surviving spirochaetes. The variant strain, uninfluenced by the antibodies produced towards the parent organisms, is able to flourish and re-infect the blood. Multiple relapses, as in African relapsing fever, are apparently due to repeated antigenic variation. In Indian relapsing fever in which there are usually two attacks only, the relapse-strain transmitted experimentally to animals reverts to the serological characters of the original strain after producing a first attack in the animal.

Laboratory Diagnosis

During the pyrexial phases, the spirochaetes can frequently be demonstrated in the blood, but not during apyrexial intervals.

Thin or thick blood films are made as in malaria diagnosis, and stained by Leishman's method.

Some workers prefer to stain the films with dilute carbol fuchsin.

If a drop of blood is mounted on a slide under a cover-slip and examined with the oil-immersion lens, the spirochaetes may be detected in the unstained condition and show active movement. A more satisfactory method of demonstrating them, however, is by dark-ground, or phase-contrast illumination.

If spirochaetes are not detectable, inoculation intraperitoneally of white mice with 1·0–2·0 ml. blood drawn from a vein may reveal the infection, the organisms appearing in considerable numbers in the blood of the animals. A drop of blood from the tail of the inoculated animal is examined daily for a considerable period. An inoculum of 0·2 ml. of blood into the chorio-allantoic sac of the chick embryo may also be used.

Lice taken from a case can be examined for spirochaetes by keeping them in a test-tube for a day, then placing them in drops of distilled water on slides and piercing them with a needle so that the haemocele fluid becomes mixed with the water, which is then examined microscopically by dark-ground illumination. The spirochaetes can also be demonstrated in ticks by examining stained films from the stomach contents.

Borrelia theileri

This spirochaete is responsible for a blood infection occurring in cattle, sheep and horses in Africa. The disease is of a comparatively mild type. The organism appears as a spiral filament, 10–30 μ by 0·25–0·3 μ, and is actively motile when seen in fresh preparations of blood. It is transmitted by a tick (*Margaropus decoloratus*).

Borrelia anserina

This organism is the cause of "fowl spirochaetosis" a septicaemic disease with a high mortality. Geese, ducks, turkeys and other poultry may also be affected. The disease occurs in the Middle East, the Sudan and other parts of Africa and in North and South America. *Borr. anserina* can be seen in the blood of the infected bird both in unstained preparations and in films stained by a Romanowsky stain or dilute carbol fuchsin. It is a motile spiral organism, 10–20 μ in length by 0·3 μ in breadth, and exhibits several coils. Artificial cultures have been obtained in Smith-Noguchi medium. The disease is transmitted by ticks, e.g. *Argas persicus*, and a granular phase has been described analogous to that observed in the case of *Borr. duttonii* (*vide supra*). By experimental inoculation various species of birds may be infected, but mammals are not susceptible. Birds at the height of infection can be cured by the use of penicillin.

REFERENCES

D'ALESSANDRO, G. & DARDANONI, L. (1953). Isolation and purification of the protein antigen of the Reiter treponeme. *Amer. J. Syph.*, **37**, 137.

BEKKER, J. H. (1962). Limitations of the Reiter protein complement-fixation (R.P.C.F.) test. *Brit. J. vener. Dis.*, **38**, 131.

B.M.A. Report (1964). *Venereal Disease in Young People.* London: British Medical Association.

DEACON, W. E., FREEMAN, E. M. & HARRIS, A. (1960). Fluorescent treponemal antibody test. Method based on quantitation. F.T.A. 200. *Proc. Soc. exp. Biol.* (N.Y.), **103**, 827.

FOSTER, W. D., NICOL, C. S. & STONE, A. H. (1958). Reiter's protein complement fixation test. Report of a trial in 1000 unselected cases. *Brit. J. vener. Dis.*, **34**, 196.

NELSON, R. A. & MAYER, M. M. (1949). Immobilisation of *Treponema pallidum* in vitro by antibody produced in syphilitic infection. *J. exp. Med.*, **89**, 369.

OAG, R. K. (1940). The comparative susceptibility of the chick embryo and the chick to infection with *Borrelia duttoni*. *J. Path. Bact.*, **51**, 127.

SEQUEIRA, P. J. L. & WILKINSON, A. E. (1955). Studies on the reproducibility and specificity of the treponemal immobilisation test. *Brit. J. vener. Dis.*, **31**, 134.

SEQUEIRA, P. J. L. (1959). An examination of the treponemal Wassermann reaction and Reiter protein complement-fixation text. *Brit. J. vener. Dis.*, **35**, 139.

STEIN, G. J. (1944). The serological diagnosis of relapsing fever. *J. exp. Med.*, **79**, 115.

SWAIN, R. H. A. (1955). Electron microscopic studies of the morphology of pathogenic spirochaetes. *J. Path. Bact.*, **69**, 117.

WILKINSON, A. E. (1961). Fluorescent treponemal antibody test. *Brit. J. vener. Dis.*, **37**, 59.

WILKINSON, A. E. & JOHNSTON, N. A. (1959). Results of parallel tests with the Reiter protein complement-fixation test, the treponemal immobilisation test, and the treponemal Wassermann reaction on 1,046 sera. *Brit. J. vener. Dis.*, **35**, 175.

WILKINSON, A. E. & SEQUEIRA, P. J. L. (1955). Studies on the treponemal immobilisation test. *Brit. J. vener. Dis.*, **31**, 143.

CHAPTER 30

SPIROCHAETES (*continued*)

Leptospira

THE genus *Leptospira* consists of a group of spirochaetal organisms some of which cause leptospirosis in man and animals. It includes both saprophytic and parasitic members. The saprophytes derived from water are known collectively as *Leptospira biflexa*. They are distinguished from parasitic leptospires by their inability to infect animals and by the ease with which they can be grown in simple media without the addition of serum. The parasitic members include all the known pathogenic leptospires of man and animals. They are indistinguishable from one another morphologically and culturally and any differences in their pathogenicity, geographical distribution and animal host predilection are not sufficiently constant to form the basis for classifying them into further species. Antigenic differences however exist and on this basis a large number of serotypes have been identified and named. Classically the infection in man occurs as a haemorrhagic jaundice (Weil's Disease), but a febrile anicteric syndrome is common and benign meningitis may be the most prominent feature. Serological tests have also shown that infection may occur without any obvious symptoms of disease being produced. These subclinical cases are mostly found in certain occupational groups where the risk of infection is high—*vide infra*.

Morphology and Staining.—Leptospires are about 7–14 μ long by 0·1 μ broad. The coils are very numerous and so small and closely set together that they are difficult to demonstrate in stained preparations, though quite obvious by dark-ground illumination. In addition to these "elementary" spirals, larger "secondary" coils may be seen, especially in stained films. Hooked ends are a characteristic morphological feature. Leptospires have a single, straight and somewhat rigid central axistyle around which is wound the cytoplasm of the spirochaete, the whole being contained within a clearly defined cell wall. Active movement is observed in fresh preparations examined with the dark-ground microscope. The movement is mainly rotary but the organisms are also seen to glide rapidly across the field with either end foremost, occasionally bending and straightening again into the rigid form so characteristic of the genus.

The organisms can be stained by Giemsa's solution and by the silver impregnation methods of Levaditi and Fontana (q.v.).

Cultivation.—Leptospires are readily cultured in fluid media but the parasitic members require the addition of animal serum. Rabbit serum is usually employed but guinea-pig, sheep and cattle sera may be equally satisfactory provided no natural antibodies are present (it is advisable to test serum for the presence of leptospiral antibodies before incorporating it in the medium). For the primary isolation of leptospires and for maintaining stock cultures of the various serotypes for serological work, Stuart's and Korthof's liquid media are recommended. A semi-solid medium such as Dinger's modification of Noguchi's medium is useful for maintaining stock cultures. It has the advantage of evaporating less rapidly than fluid media and is thought to maintain the virulence of the organisms longer, since subculturing need not be done so frequently. Solid culture media on which single colonies of leptospires may develop have been devised by Cox and Larson (1957) and by Kirschner and Graham (1959) but culture on solid media is not readily obtained. Leptospires grow best between 28° C. and 32° C. For primary isolation from animal tissues incubation at 37° C. may be advantageous. The culture is transferred to the lower temperature when growth is established.

Viability.—Unlike the saprophytic leptospires it is unlikely that the pathogenic serotypes multiply much outside the animal body although they may survive for many days if the external conditions are favourable. They require moisture for their survival and since they are particularly susceptible to acid, they seldom remain viable for long in localities where the pH of the water is less than 6·8. Salt water has a deleterious effect. They die out rapidly in acid urine, in sewage and in badly polluted water. They are susceptible to heat: 10 min. at 50° C. or 10 sec. at 60° C. kills them. They may survive for a time in infected animal tissue provided it is kept at a low temperature; thus guinea-pig liver has remained infective for up to 26 days at 4° C. and for 100 days at −20° C. They are rapidly dissolved by bile and by trypsin. The organisms in culture and in experimental animals are moderately sensitive to penicillin, streptomycin and the tetracyclines and these antibiotics may have value as therapeutic agents in man if given early in the infection.

Pathogenesis.—Most types of pathogenic leptospires are carried by various species of wild rodents (although in some cases, other animals, *e.g.* dogs and pigs, appear to act as the natural animal hosts). Each serotype has apparently a host of predilection, e.g. *L. icterohaemorrhagiae* is carried by the brown rat (*Rattus norvegicus*) and *L. hebdomadis* (the cause of seven-day fever of field workers in the Far East) by the field mouse (*Microtus montebelloi*). The leptospire is usually well adapted to its host. It localises in the kidneys where it colonises the convoluted tubules without apparently causing any harmful effects. Periodically leptospires are shed in large numbers in the urine and in this medium may be transferred to other susceptible animals and to man. The organisms probably penetrate the skin and mucous membranes through cuts and abrasions. Certain occupations predispose to infection, *e.g.* workers in wet coal mines, sewage workers, fish handlers, etc. are particularly liable to infection by *L. icterohaemorrhagiae* since the conditions in which they work frequently encourage rat infestation, while moist conditions allow the leptospires to survive for a time outside the animal body.

Leptospiral infection may follow bathing or accidental total immersion in stagnant ponds, canals or rivers polluted by rodents and in these cases the organisms may penetrate the mucous membranes of the eyes and nasopharynx. Instances of infection through the consumption of contaminated food and water have also been reported.

Agricultural workers especially those engaged in work in the fields, *e.g.* rice-field workers, sugar-cane cutters, etc., are particularly liable to infection derived from the urine of rodents; in fact, this group of workers provides the highest proportion of all cases.

Laboratory Diagnosis

Because of variability in the severity of the infection and the frequent absence of jaundice, leptospirosis should always be considered in cases of undiagnosed pyrexia when the patient is likely to have been exposed to infection either through the conditions of his work or from some other cause (*vide supra*).

When attempting a laboratory diagnosis of suspected leptospirosis, the following points should be borne in mind:—(*a*) During the first week of illness, leptospires are present in the blood, but leptospiraemia is rare after the eighth day. (*b*) Leptospires may be present in the urine during the second week of the illness and continue to be excreted intermittently for 4 to 6 weeks after the onset (infrequently for longer periods). They are more readily detected during the second and third weeks than later. Since leptospires are very sensitive to acid urine and may be lysed by antibodies present in the urine, the urine should be examined immediately after being voided. (*c*) Antibodies may generally be detected in the blood serum towards the end of the first week (although their production is occasionally delayed for longer periods) and increase in amount during the second and third weeks, after which they begin to decline. Residual amounts, however, may remain for many years after an infection. It is advisable to examine a specimen of serum during the early days of the illness and at 4 to 5 day intervals thereafter in order to demonstrate a rise in titre. This is necessary to eliminate the possibility that the reaction may be due to residual antibodies. Paradoxical reactions in which the titres of heterologous antibodies may at first exceed those of the homologous ones are also clarified in this way.

(1) EXAMINATION OF BLOOD (a) *Dark-ground Microscopy*.—During the first week leptospires may be detected by dark-ground microscopic examination of untreated blood. Only a small percentage of cases of leptospiraemia are likely to be detected in this way, but the technique of differential centrifugation of Ruys (Wolff, 1954) may enhance the chances of seeing the organisms and thereby make an early diagnosis possible. This is done on a blood specimen to which a buffered anti-coagulant (pH 8) has been added. (1 ml. of 1 per cent. solution of sodium oxalate in buffer to 10 ml. blood or 1 ml. of 1 per cent. "liquoid" in sterile saline to 5 ml. blood. These are preferable to sodium citrate which may have a deleterious effect on leptospires). The blood is centrifuged at 500 r.p.m. for 15 min. A drop of plasma is examined by dark-ground microscopy (guinea-pigs may be inoculated with the sediment). If negative the plasma is centrifuged at 1,0000 r.p.m. for

20 minutes and the sediment examined microscopically. (b) *Cultivation.* Bijou bottles containing 3 ml. fluid culture medium are inoculated with 3 or 4 drops of the patient's whole blood, great care being paid to aseptic technique (leptospires will not usually grow in the presence of contaminants). Alternatively, the deposit after differential centrifugation (*vide supra*) may be re-suspended in 2·0 ml. phosphate buffered saline (pH 8·1) and a few drops of it used to inoculate 4 to 6 bottles of culture medium. Daily culturing of the blood during the first few days of the infection considerably enhances the chances of isolating the organisms. (c) *Animal Inoculation.*—Laboratory animals, usually guinea-pigs and hamsters, are inoculated intraperitoneally with whole blood during the first few days of the illness. Three days after inoculation and daily thereafter peritoneal fluid is withdrawn with a finely drawn-out Pasteur pipette introduced into the lower part of the abdomen while the animal is held in an upright position with stretched hind legs. As soon as leptospires are detected microscopically in the peritoneal fluid where they tend to localise during the early stages of infection, blood is withdrawn by cardiac pucture and a few drops introduced into several bottles of culture medium. Guinea-pigs are very susceptible to *L. icterohaemorrhagiae*, whereas the golden hamster (*Cricetus auratus*) is more susceptible than the guinea-pig to *L. canicola.* The animals should be used when about 6 weeks old, since older animals may be more resistant. In typical cases, the inoculated animals die in 8 to 12 days with jaundice, haemorrhages in the lungs, under the serous membranes and in the muscles.

(2) Examination of Urine.—During the second and third weeks and sometimes for longer periods leptospires may be present in the urine. They may be seen by dark-ground examination of the sediment after centrifuging a portion of the urine at 3,000 r.p.m. for 10 minutes. Direct culture of urine is not usually successful because of contaminating organisms, but they may be demonstrated by the inoculation of two young guinea-pigs intraperitoneally with 2 ml. of freshly voided urine and the subsequent culture of the animals' blood (*vide supra*).

(3) Identification of Newly Isolated Strains.—With a suspension of the organism and its homologous antiserum prepared by immunising a rabbit with a living culture an attempt can be made to identify a newly isolated strain as far as possible by comparing it with stock serotypes and antisera by agglutination and agglutinin-absorption tests. The procedure of identification may be a lengthy one and require the use of stock antigens and antisera not available in the average diagnostic laboratory. In such cases, or whenever there is doubt about the identity of a newly isolated strain, it is recommended that help should be sought from one of the WHO/FAO Leptospirosis reference laboratories. For the addresses of these laboratories see WHO Report (1959).

(4) Serological Diagnosis.—Two methods are described below for carrying out a diagnostic serological investigation of the patient's serum.

(a) *Agglutination-Lysis Test.*—The following technique is based on the standard procedure used in laboratories throughout the world and first developed by Schuffner (see Wolff, 1954).

For the test well-grown cultures of leptospires in Korthof's or Stuart's media are used. They should be from 7 to 10 days old and uniform in suspension. Separate tests are set up against each serotype likely to be responsible for the case under investigation. Dilutions of the patient's serum are made by the dropping method either in tubes or in depressions in porcelain plates. The procedure is summarised as follows:

Tube No.	(1)	(2)	(3)	(4)	(5)	(6)	
First row:							
Saline	8	9	9				drops
Serum	2	1, from (1)	1, from (2)				drops
Dilution of serum	1/5	1/50	1/500				
Second row:							
Culture	3	3	3	3	3	3	drops
Saline		2		2		2	drops
Serum 1/500					3	1	drops
Serum 1/50			3	1			drops
Serum 1/5	3	1					drops
Final dilution:	1/10	1/30	1/100	1/300	1/1000	1/3000	

The mixtures are incubated at 32° C. (or 37° C.) for 3 hours and allowed to stand at room temperature for 1 hour before being read. Alternatively, if specimens are received late in the day the test mixtures are kept in the refrigerator (4° C.) overnight and read the following morning. Place a drop from each tube on a slide and examine with a 16 mm. objective using dark-ground illumination. Wolff advocates the use of water instead of immersion oil between the condenser and the slide. It gives quite adequate illumination and is much cleaner than oil. It is not necessary to place a cover-slip over the drop and if each drop is quickly examined consecutively a large number may be included on one slide. Both agglutinating and lytic reactions are observed by this test. Agglutination is more obvious in the lower dilutions and lysis in the higher. Lysis is indicated by a reduction in the number of live leptospires present in the serum-antigen mixture when compared with a non-serum control.

(b) *Agglutination Test* (*Broom*).—This involves essentially the same technique as the agglutination-lysis test except that the cultures are killed by adding formalin to give a final concentration of 0·2 per cent. The formalin should be neutralised with magnesium carbonate, since any traces of formic acid will cause non-specific agglutination. The serum-antigen mixtures are kept in the refrigerator overnight (not incubated) before being examined for agglutination. Lysis does not occur. Killed antigens are more convenient and safe for routine work and stock suspensions of various serotypes may be stored until required. They have the disadvantage of tending to be unstable and liable to clump spontaneously. Titres of agglutination are slightly lower than those attained with living cultures.

Diagnostic Titres.—Since many serotypes are related serologically (e.g. *L. canicola* and *L. icterohaemorrhagiae* have common antigens) there may be a certain amount of cross-reaction between the strains used in one test. Titres of 300 and 1000 for a particular strain may be significant (they may rise to 30,000 or higher). Bearing in mind the possibility of non-specific agglutination and residual antibodies (*vide supra*) the significance of a single positive titre must remain in doubt unless a rising titre can be demonstrated.

A control must be included in both methods.

Other serological tests may also be employed. A rapid macroscopic-slide test has been devised by Galton *et al.* (1958) and is being used in some laboratories as a screening test. In the *erythrocyte sensitisation test* (Chang and McComb, 1954), human red blood cells are treated with an ethanol extract of leptospires and are rendered agglutinable by serum antibodies. In the *sensitised erythrocyte lysis test* (Sharp, 1958), the addition of complement to this system causes the lysis of sensitised cells. Both these tests are genus specific, their main value lying in the rapid screening of human sera for evidence of antibodies resulting from leptospiroses of all kinds.

Complement-fixation tests have also been used. In most of these the antigens used have proved to be type-specific in their reactions although Sturdza and Elian (1960) report successful results from a genus specific antigen prepared by adding sodium merthiolate in a concentration of 10,000 to a 8–10 day-old culture of the saprophytic *L. biflexa* (strain Patoc).

5. Examination of Rats and other Rodents for Leptospiral Infection.—Carcases of rats dead for even a few hours are unsatisfactory for examination. Whenever possible the live animal should be sent to the laboratory. It is then possible to anaesthetise the animal and to obtain blood by cardiac puncture for examination by the methods described. Indirect evidence of infection can be obtained by the agglutination test with serum. Even low titres, 1 in 100 or less may indicate infection. The kidneys should also be examined by both cultivation and animal inoculation methods.

In screening rats and other rodents for leptospiral infection satisfactory results have been obtained by inoculating culture media with small particles of kidney tissue punched out with a sterile Pasteur pipette after the surface of the kidney has been seared with a red-hot scalpel blade.

6. Examination of Water for Pathogenic Leptospires.—This can be done by immersing a shaved and scarified area of skin of a young guinea-pig in the water for an hour at 30° C. Infection takes place through the skin with the resulting characteristic condition as described above.

Pathogenic Leptospires

Over 80 different pathogenic serotypes and subserotypes have been identified, many of which are associated with disease in man. They tend to differ in the degree of their pathogenicity to man and animal and in their natural hosts, but the only reliable method of classifying them is on the basis of their serological differences demonstrated by agglutination and agglutinin-absorption tests.

In Great Britain only two serotypes of leptospires have so far been isolated from human infections, viz. *icterohaemorrhagiae* and *canicola*, but it has been ascertained that field mice, voles and hedgehogs are carriers of other serotypes, viz. *ballum*, strains related to *saxkoebing* and *bratislava* which are known to be pathogenic for man in other parts of the world (Broom and Coghlan, 1958, 1960)

The following exemplify the various pathogenic serotypes which have been recognised in different parts of the world.

L. icterohaemorrhagiae.—This organism is one of the more virulent forms of Leptospira. It is the most frequent cause of classical Weil's disease (haemorrhagic jaundice) although milder conditions may result. It is carried by species of rats (notably *R. norvegicus*) and other rodents in all parts of the world and human cases arise under conditions where rats abound. Two biotypes exist one having an antigenic structure AB represented by strain *Wijnberg*, the other the incomplete biotype A by strain *Kantorowicz*; both strains having been isolated from human cases of Weil's disease in Amsterdam.

L. canicola.—This serotype is closely related antigenically to *icterohaemorrhagiae* but may be distinguished from it by serological tests. It is the cause of so-called "canicola fever" in man and of a common infection of dogs characterised by nephritis often chronic in nature and rather inconstantly by a variable degree of jaundice. The leptospires are excreted in large numbers and may invade through abrasions in the skin of people whose hands become contaminated with dog urine. Jackals and pigs may also harbour the organism, and piggery workers have contracted the infection through handling infected pigs (Coghlan, Norval & Seiler, 1957).

Canicola fever in man is one of the milder forms of leptospirosis, in which meningeal symptoms predominate. Jaundice is only occasionally produced and then only in a slight degree. As with most forms of leptospirosis, renal involvement is a common feature, but the symptoms vary considerably in their intensity. The disease is rarely fatal.

L. hebdomadis.—This organism is responsible for "Seven-day fever" of the East, which is a non-icteric febrile illness with meningitis. It is carried by a field-mouse (*Microtus montebelloi*) and consequently, field workers are liable to the infection through becoming contaminated with infected mouse urine.

L. autumnalis.—This organism has been found associated with a disease in Japan called Akiyami or harvest sickness clinically indistinguishable from "Seven-day fever". *L. autumnalis* can be distinguished from *L. hebdomadis* by its high infectivity to guinea-pigs, in which it produces typical haemorrhagic jaundice. It is carried by certain species of field-mice and rats. "Fort Bragg fever", which occurred among troops in North Carolina, U.S.A., was found by serological tests to have been caused by a closely related organism.

L. grippotyphosa has been described as the cause of "Swamp fever" of Europe and certain parts of Asia, Africa, Israel and U.S.A. It usually attacks agricultural workers and produces a relatively mild illness resembling canicola fever with a low mortality rate. Various species of voles carry the organism. In the U.S.S.R. and Israel, cattle have been seriously affected.

L. pyrogenes produces a febrile illness with or without jaundice and varying in its severity. It occurs among field workers in Indonesia and other parts of the Far East. Certain species of rats appear to act as reservoirs of infection.

L. australis and *zanoni* (previously referred to as *australis* A and B respectively).—These organisms are causal agents of "Cane fever" in North Queensland. Sugar-cane workers are mainly affected, but *zanoni* may also infect urban dwellers. The illness is comparatively mild but convalescence is protracted. Lymphadenitis is a common feature. Certain species of rat are the carriers of the organism.

L. pomona (syn. *suis*).—This organism was first isolated from cases of "Seven-day fever" among dairy farmers in North Queensland. It was later found to be the cause of "Swineherds' " disease in Switzerland. Pigs act as the reservoir hosts and usually suffer little effect; cattle are susceptible, especially calves and pregnant cows. In the U.S.A. the infection causes a heavy yearly loss of cattle due to jaundice and haemoglobinuria of calves and abortion of cows and pigs. The organism has been isolated in many parts of the world from human and animal sources. Certain species of field-mice may also act as carrier hosts.

L. bataviae.—This organism causes leptospirosis of rice-field workers in Italy, where the field-mouse (*Micromys minutus sorcinus*) is the reservoir host. The disease in that part of the world is comparatively mild and jaundice is rare. In S.E. Asia, however, where the chief carrier host is the brown rat (*R. norvegicus*) cases are much more severe, jaundice is common and death may occur.

L. sejroe was first observed in human infection in the island of Sejroe (Denmark). It has also been recorded in other parts of Europe. The disease is relatively mild. Certain rodents are carriers of the organism, and related strains have been isolated from rodents in Great Britain.

REFERENCES

BROOM, J. C. & COGHLAN, J. D. (1958). Leptospira ballum in small rodents in Scotland. *Lancet*, **2**, 1041.

BROOM, J. C. & COGHLAN, J. D. (1960). Leptospira bratislava isolated from a hedgehog in Scotland. *Lancet*, **1**, 1326.

CHANG, R. S. & MCCOMB, D. E. (1954). Erythrocyte sensitizing substances from five strains of Leptospirae. *Amer. J. trop. Med. Hyg.*, **3**, 481.

COGHLAN, J. D., NORVAL, J. & SEILER, H. E. (1957). Canicola fever in man through contact with infected pigs. *Brit. med. J.*, **1**, 257.

COX, C. D. & LARSON, A. A. (1957). Colonial growth of leptospirae. *J. Bact.*, **73** 4, 587.

GALTON, M. M., POWERS, D. K., HALL, A. D. & CORNELL, R. G. (1958). A rapid macroscopic-slide screening test for serodiagnosis of leptospirosis. *Amer. J. vet. Res.*, **19**, 71, 505.

KIRSCHNER, L. & GRAHAM, L. (1959). Growth purification and maintenance of Leptospira on solid media. *Brit. J. exp. Path.*, **40**, 57.

SHARP, C. F. (1958). Laboratory diagnosis of leptospirosis with the sensitized-erythrocyte lysis test. *J. Path. Bact.*, **76**, 349.

STURDZA & ELIAN (1960). Comparative study of different strains of L. biflexa as antigen for the complement fixation test in leptospirosis. *Arch. Roum. Path. exp.*, **20**, 1.

WOLFF, J. W. (1954). *The Laboratory Diagnosis of Leptospirosis*. Springfield: Thomas.

WORLD HEALTH ORGANISATION (1959). Joint WHO/FAO. Expert committee on zoonoses. 2nd report. *Wld. Hlth. Org. tech. Rep. Ser.* No. 180.

PART III

VIRUSES AND OTHER MICROORGANISMS

CHAPTER 31

THE POX VIRUSES

THE characteristic feature of the diseases caused by the pox group of viruses is the formation of papules, vesicles and pustules in the skin; generalised manifestations of illness may be very severe or entirely absent. In man these viruses cause smallpox, alastrim, vaccinia, and molluscum contagiosum. In animals they give rise to cow-pox, swine-pox, monkey-pox, mouse-pox (ectromelia) and to similar diseases in all domestic animals except the dog and cat. Myxomatosis in rabbits is the result of infection with a virus which has many of the characters of a pox virus. Avian pox viruses cause fowl-pox and similar infections in turkeys, pigeons, canaries and a wide variety of other birds. In avian pox diseases the lesions tend to be proliferative rather than pustular with the formation of multiple tumour-like masses.

Pox viruses are within the size range 200×300 mμ to 264×332 mμ and are large enough to be visible with the light microscope. They have a predilection for infecting epithelial cells, in which they produce characteristic eosinophilic intracytoplasmic inclusions. The great majority of pox viruses can be cultivated in the chorio-allantoic membrane of chick embryo, where they give rise to pock-like lesions which are easily recognised with the naked eye. Under natural conditions, however, most of these viruses are restricted to a single host, although notable exceptions are the cow-pox and vaccinia viruses which can infect man, cattle and a number of other animals. Animal pock-producing viruses are closely related antigenically to each other, but are distinct from the avian pox viruses.

SMALLPOX AND VACCINIA

Smallpox virus (Poxvirus variolae) and vaccinia virus (Poxvirus officinalis)

Morphology and Staining.—The particles of both viruses are 200–300 mμ in diameter as seen by dark-ground microscopy or in stained preparations and are roughly spherical in shape. They can be stained with aniline dyes, as in Gutstein's or Paschen's methods but not by Castaneda's method. When dried films of purified virus preparations are examined electron-microscopically, the appearance is that of brick-shaped particles measuring 210×260 mμ, in which the central area is a mass of material especially opaque to the electron beam. This brick-shaped appearance, however, may be an artefact because in ultra-thin sections of infected cells the virus particles are oval in shape and have a multi-layered covering membrane. In preparations stained negatively with phospho-tungstic acid the virions appear to be cylindrical with convex ends. Internally a central disk-like structure, a "nucleoid", is seen together with hollow tubular structures 7–9 mμ in diameter (Westwood *et al.*, 1964). The latter give a striking appearance and are wound from side to side of the particle into a criss-cross pattern. It has not yet been possible to determine the nature of these strands nor to decide whether they are multiple or whether the appearances are those of a single continuous strand. The vaccinia virus contains DNA and is thought also to contain phospholipids, neutral fat, carbohydrate, flavin and biotin in proportions similar to those of bacteria and mammalian cells.

Host Range.—The host range of the smallpox virus is limited to the primates; apart from man, monkeys are the only animals susceptible to natural infection. Other animals are only slightly susceptible, and of these the rabbit is sometimes used in Paul's test for the smallpox virus; here the virus is inoculated into the scarified cornea and produces a keratitis. Intracytoplasmic inclusions (Guarnieri bodies) in epithelial cells are characteristic of infection with variola and vaccinia viruses; they are round or oval, eosinophilic and there may be one or more in an infected cell. Guarnieri bodies consist of masses of elementary bodies set in a matrix. The vaccinia virus has a much wider host range than the variola virus; calves, rabbits and sheep are all used regularly for the propagation of the virus for vaccine lymph, and monkeys, mice, rats, hamsters and guinea-pigs can also be infected, though they are rather less susceptible.

Both viruses grow well on the chorio-allantoic membrane of the ten-day-old chick embryo, each producing its own characteristic pocks. The variola virus gives rise to white circular plaques of epithelial hyperplasia which are visible to the naked eye 48 hours after inoculation and reach 1–2 mm. in diameter in 72 hours; these lesions are uniform in size and often lie near the blood vessels of the membrane. The virus of alastrim grows less vigorously in the chick embryo than the variola major virus and is more sensitive to increases of heat (Dumbell, Bedson, and Rossier, 1961). Vaccinia virus pocks are generally much larger and more variable in size than those of the variola virus; after incubation for 72 hours the majority are 4–5 mm. in diameter with a definite yellowish colouration. Small seedling pocks beside the larger pocks of vaccinia are characteristic. The pox viruses can be differentiated by the maximum temperature of incubation at which they are able to produce pox on the allantoic membrane of 12-day chick embryos. Bedson and Dumbell (1961) estimated these "ceiling temperatures" for alastrim as 37·5 °C., variola major 38·5 °C., ectromelia and monkey-pox 39 °C., cow-pox 40° C., and rabbit-pox and vaccinia 40·5–41° C., and found there was no correlation between these temperatures and the thermal stabilities of the viruses at 55° C. *in vitro*. A useful distinguishing character is that the variola virus will multiply and produce pocks at 38·5° C., whereas the alastrim virus will not multiply or produce any lesions at this temperature. In general the higher the ceiling temperature of a virus the greater is its virulence for the chick embryo.

Vaccinia virus grows readily in many types of tissue culture; minced tissue suspensions of the Maitland type, explants in plasma clot of chick embryo, and rabbit kidney tissues are all highly susceptible. In monolayer cultures of trypsinised human or monkey kidney, or in human amnion or HeLa cells the vaccinia virus produces a marked cytopathic effect within 48 hr. of inoculation. In suitably prepared monolayer cultures of monkey kidney or other cells the virus gives rise to plaques.

Viability.—Variola virus is very stable and survives in exudates from cases for many months; living virus has been recovered from crusts kept at room temperature for over a year. It can be preserved in sealed ampoules at 4° C. for many months and indefinitely by freeze drying. Vaccinia virus in calf lymph stored in the dark at −10° C. retains its activity for at least three months. Between 0° C. and 10° C. vaccine lymph retains its potency for at least 14 days, but at temperatures above 10° C. its activity may be lost after seven days. Freeze dried vaccine kept under an atmosphere of nitrogen at 37° C. and 45° C. maintains its activity for two years and at 4° C. indefinitely. The virus is destroyed by moist heat at 60° C. in ten min., but in the dry state can resist 100° C. for five to ten min. Both viruses withstand 10 per cent. phenol at 4° C. for several weeks, but at 37° C. are killed by it within 24 hr. Ultra-violet light, X-rays and gamma rays are rapidly lethal; 0·01 per cent. potassium permanganate and 50 per cent. ethyl or methyl alcohol and acetone kill the virus within one hour. A pH value of 3 destroys the virus within an hour.

Antigenic Characters.—It is very difficult to distinguish the three viruses of variola major, alastrim and vaccinia by serological methods because they all share major common antigenic components. Purified suspensions of variola and vaccinia viruses can be shown to contain two antigens; one, the LS antigen, dissociates from the elementary bodies on standing at refrigerator temperature; the other, the nucleoprotein (NP) antigen, is associated with the virus particles themselves. The LS antigen is a loose combination of the L and S components in an elongated protein molecule which is known to have a molecular weight of about 240,000. Thc L component is inactivated by heat at 60° C., but the S component is stable at 90° C. or above. Antibodies to the LS antigen precipitate and also fix complement with their homologous antigens, but they do not protect an animal from the effects of the vaccinia virus nor will they neutralise the virus in laboratory tests. The NP antigen can be extracted from elementary bodies with dilute alkali; it is known to contain 6·0 per cent. desoxyribonucleic acid and is a serologically specific component of the vaccinia virus. A soluble protective antigen shared by the vaccinia and rabbit-pox viruses has been described by Appleyard, Zwartouw, and Westwood (1964); it combines with the neutralising antibody in hyperimmune sera and has a molecular weight of 100,000–200,000. It is developed during the early stages of the reproductive cycle of the virus, is smaller than the virus itself but is too large to be dialysable. The relationship of this protective or "serum-blocking" antigen to the NP antigen or the haemagglutinin is not yet decided.

Haemagglutination.—Preparations of the vaccinia and variola viruses agglutinate the red blood cells of mammals, but erythrocytes from only about 60 per cent. of fowls are sensitive to the virus. The haemagglutinin is smaller than the virus particle and can be separated from it by centrifugation; it is 65 mμ in diameter and is mainly composed of lipoprotein. When the haemagglutinin is removed from virus preparations there is no loss of infectivity. The haemagglutinin is heat stable and able to withstand boiling for ten minutes; it is distinct from the virus particles and from the LS and NP antigens. Antibodies to the haemagglutinin are developed after smallpox and after vaccination; they are not related to either neutralising or LS antibodies.

Pathogenesis.—Smallpox virus enters the body through the upper respiratory tract; it first infects the mucosal cells and soon afterwards is thought to reach the regional lymph nodes. At this stage the patient is not infectious and it is improbable that there is an open lesion in the respiratory mucosa. A transient viraemia may follow with the infection of reticulo-endothelial cells throughout the whole body; multiplication of the virus in these cells leads to a second and more intense viraemia which heralds the onset of the clinical illness. The virus can be isolated from the blood in a proportion of cases of smallpox, but the phase of viraemia is short-lived and by the end of the second day of the fever the virus can no longer be detected. During the first three or four days of the fever the virus multiplies in the epithelial cells of the skin; focal lesions are formed which give rise to the rash, and macules appear in typical centrifugal distribution and progress to papular, vesicular and pustular stages. Smears made from the early papular lesions show very large numbers of elementary bodies and in the later stages crusts from the pustules still contain virus.

Classical smallpox (*variola major*) has a case mortality which varies from 5 per cent. in patients with a discrete rash to 40 per cent. in fulminating cases with a confluent rash. *Variola minor* (*alastrim*) is much less severe than variola major at all stages of the illness, the rash is less profuse, the fever of shorter duration and the fatality rate is below 1 per cent. Variola minor may be indistinguishable from a mild case of variola major in a well vaccinated person. In other vaccinated contacts the infection may give rise only to fever and symptoms similar to those of the pre-eruptive phase without progressing further, a condition known as *variola sine eruptione*.

Epidemiology.—The origin of infection in smallpox is a patient suffering from the disease. Infected particles may be inhaled directly by the susceptible contact. The virus may also be transmitted indirectly by clothing, bed-linen, utensils or dust, and there have been many occasions when workers in hospital laundries have contracted the infection from contaminated bed-linen. Patients are not infective during the incubation period of the disease, but from the time of the first appearance of the rash until all crusts disappear they may be a source of the virus. The clinical picture of variola may be considerably modified by previous vaccination and persons who develop only minor symptoms of the disease provide a dangerous source of infection.

Variola major is endemic in India, Pakistan, Burma, the Middle East, Latin America and parts of Africa. In Britain the disease is no longer endemic and outbreaks, when they have occurred, have been traced to importation of the infection from abroad. Although smallpox is a highly infectious disease it has not so great an epidemic potential as measles or chickenpox. When the disease has been introduced from abroad into Britain, extensive epidemics have not occurred and spread has usually been limited to close contacts of cases. A full description of the epidemiology and clinical aspects of smallpox is given by Dixon (1962).

Laboratory Diagnosis

Often there is great urgency in confirming the clinical diagnosis of smallpox. The collection of the necessary specimens is described elsewhere (see p. 575; also the Ministry of Health Memorandum 1963). A quick presumptive diagnosis can be made in about 60 per cent. of cases by the direct microscopic examination of smears from the skin lesions. These smears should be taken from papules or vesicles but *not* from pustules because leucocytic granules and debris are indistinguishable from the virus. The films are stained preferably by Gutstein's alkaline methyl violet stain (see Chapter 45) and in cases of smallpox large numbers of elementary bodies uniform in size and about 0·3 μ in diameter can be recognised. In chickenpox elementary bodies are usually scanty or absent but multinucleate giant cells are often present indicating that the infection is varicella. A report on this finding can be given within two hours of the specimen reaching the laboratory. Smears may also be examined by the indirect immune fluorescence technique which Murray (1963) has developed.

Preparations of the exudate stained with phosphotungstic acid and examined electronmicroscopically give rapid and accurate identifications of the virus (Christie *et al*, 1966).

The presence of the virus can be detected rapidly in material from the skin lesions by preparing suspensions of vesicle fluid or crusts and using them as antigens with a high titre antivaccinal serum in complement fixation (Craigie and Wishart, 1936), or agar gel diffusion precipitin reactions (Dumbell and Nizamuddin, 1959). The results of these tests are available in 6–24 hr. The complement-fixation test gives a positive reaction in over 90 per cent. of cases of smallpox, but does not distinguish between the vaccinia and variola viruses.

The virus can be isolated from the skin lesions or from the blood in the pre-eruptive phase of the illness. A suspension of vesicle fluid or ground-up crusts or serum from the blood is inoculated on to the chorio-allantoic membrane of ten- to twelve-day-old chick embryos; after 48 hr. small white pocks are present and by 72 hr. they are 2 mm. in diameter and identifiable as specific smallpox lesions. This procedure detects the virus in over 90 per cent. of cases of smallpox and has replaced the older method of inoculating the rabbit's cornea (Paul's test) which is not sufficiently reliable for routine use.

The three methods described should be used in combination so that the tests may serve to check each other. The combined use of these tests also helps to overcome the occasional difficulties which may arise from anticomplementary activity by the crust-suspension or the appearance of non-specific lesions on the chorio-allantoic membrane. The results of the tests provide a very sensitive indication of the presence of the variola virus and give reliable confirmation or exclusion of the clinical diagnosis.

Antibodies in patients' sera can be titrated by their power to neutralise the capacity of the vaccinia virus to form pocks on the chorio-allantois (Boulter 1957). Another method employs complement fixation with an antigen prepared from vaccinial lesions in the rabbits' skin. Antibodies do not appear in the serum in smallpox until the eighth day of the disease, and the test is seldom of diagnostic value. As 30–40 per cent. of persons vaccinated within six to twelve months give a positive result, the test is only of value in a limited number of cases.

Vaccination may provide a useful diagnostic procedure because less than 10 per cent. of cases can be successfully vaccinated on the first day of the rash in smallpox, and none after the sixth day.

Prophylaxis.—When a case of smallpox is diagnosed the patient must be removed to a hospital or unit specially reserved for variola cases and, after admission, strict isolation precautions must be observed. The patient's clothing, bedding, personal possessions and his house should be disinfected with steam or formaldehyde vapour. All persons who could possibly have been in contact with the patient or his possessions during the feverish phase of his illness must be traced and placed under supervision for sixteen days.

The source of the infection must be sought and the chain of contacts followed back to the first notified case. In this work the results of laboratory tests may often be of great value in the diagnosis of doubtful cases.

Close contacts of smallpox patients should be vaccinated as soon as possible, but this measure may only be effective if used within two to three days of exposure. There is evidence to suggest that gamma-globulin prepared from hyperimmune serum in a dose of 1·5 g. affords some protection and it may be used to supplement vaccination of close contacts (Pierce *et al.*, 1958).

Recently, Bauer *et al.* (1963) have reported strikingly successful results from the prophylactic oral use of the drug N-methylisatin β-thiosemicarbazone (also known as "Marboran" or "Compound 33T57").

VACCINATION

The practice of vaccination stems from 1798, when Jenner inoculated a boy on the arm with the exudate which he obtained from a cow-pox lesion on the hand of a dairy-maid. When two months later the boy was inoculated with material from a case of smallpox no illness resulted and there was no local lesion. This simple and safe measure for protection against so serious an illness was soon taken into general use all over Europe. At first arm-to-arm vaccination was practised, but this was replaced by the inoculation of vaccinia lymph obtained from the skin of calves infected with the virus. The strains of vaccinia at present used in vaccine lymph manufacture are avirulent mutants of obscure parentage but date from this time.

The Preparation of Vaccine Lymph.—Vaccinia virus for vaccination is usually obtained by inoculating the shaved skin of a calf with pustular material from the skin of a rabbit similarly inoculated. The seed virus is maintained by the alternate inoculation of calves and rabbits, a procedure which is thought to hold its virulence at a constant level. First the skin of the belly and flanks of the calf is carefully shaved and then washed thoroughly three times with soap and water; this is followed by treatment with 70 per cent. alcohol and a final wash with sterile distilled water. The area of skin to be vaccinated is then scarified with a multiple needle scarifier. The seed virus is next rubbed into the scarified area. To reduce bacterial contamination the area is treated with an antibiotic ointment and covered with a tight bandage. After an incubation period of five to seven days, and when well developed vesicular lesions are present, the animal is exsanguinated and killed. The vaccinated area of the skin is washed gently with soap and water three times, sprayed with penicillin and streptomycin, and then washed again with sterile distilled water. The contents of the vesicles are harvested with curettes and after weighing are stored at −20 to −60° C. This crude pulp is further treated by homogenisation in a mechanical blender and is diluted four to ten fold in glycerol saline or phosphate buffer solution. The glycerol concentration used varies with different manufacturers from 40 to 80 per cent. but it is now recognised that glycerol in high concentration tends to impair the stability of the virus and thus 40–50 per cent. glycerol is generally recommended (Dostal, 1962).

The bacterial content of the preparation is usually further reduced by the addition of 0·4 per cent. phenol and incubation for several hours at 22° C. Bacterial counts are made from the lymph from time to time and when the number of viable bacteria is reduced to a certain figure prescribed by the Therapeutic Substances Act, the material is passed for issue provided that it is free from haemolytic streptococci, clostridia and other pathogenic bacteria, and conforms to the standard of potency. It is necessary to store the lymph in the dark at temperature below −10° C. to maintain its potency. Details of the requirements for smallpox vaccines are to be found in W.H.O. Technical Report (1959).

A modification of the method adopted at the Lister Institute employs the propagation of the virus in the shaved skin of the flank of sheep. The lymph produced in the lesions is homogenised with two parts of one per cent. phenol and held for 48 hr. at 22° C.; this generally lowers the bacterial count to the requirement of the Therapeutic Substances Act though if necessary the treatment can be prolonged for a further 24 hours; after this glycerol is added at a concentration of 40 per cent. and the lymph is stored at −10° C. (McClean, 1949).

The potency of smallpox vaccines of this type declines at temperatures above 10° C. and may be entirely lost after seven days. To overcome this difficulty and to facilitate transport over long distances in hot climates Collier (1955) devised an improved method of preservation in which the lymph is suspended in five per cent. bacteriological peptone in distilled water and adjusted to pH 7·4, then freeze dried. Vaccines prepared by this method have been shown to retain full potency, in that they gave 100 per cent. successful vaccination rates after storage for periods of 32 and 64 weeks at both 37° C. and 45° C. (Cockburn *et al.*, 1957).

Egg Vaccines.—Smallpox vaccine can also be prepared by cultivating the vaccinia virus on the chorio-allantois of chick embryos, a procedure which has the considerable advantage that it can be carried out under sterile bacteriological conditions. Because the virus tends to lose some of its immunising potency on repeated subculture in the egg, the seed virus used is obtained from calf lymph. The virus is extracted from the infected allantoic membranes and is suspended in saline; no glycerol is added but the required viscosity is obtained by including 0·35 per cent. agar. Tests of potency and sterility are similar to those required for calf lymph. Although the efficiency of egg vaccines has not yet been assessed in extensive controlled trials they appear to offer considerable promise. In Sweden an egg vaccine is used for public vaccination and 95–97 per cent. of successful "takes" on primary vaccination has been claimed (Dostal, 1962).

Tissue Culture Vaccine.—Bovine and chick embryonic tissues have been used for the propagation of the vaccinia virus for smallpox vaccine production (Wesslén, 1955; Kaplan & Micklem, 1961). The stability and potency of these vaccines are still in the process of development. In a comparative trial of a vaccine prepared from vaccinia virus propagated in chick embryo fibroblasts with the conventional vaccine, Shaw and Kaplan (1964) reported that the tissue culture vaccine produced fewer successful primary takes and fewer successful re-vaccinations. The vesicles and the size of the lesion with this tissue culture vaccine were smaller than with the conventional vaccine.

Technique of Vaccination.—The multiple-pressure method is recommended. The skin is first cleansed with soap and water and allowed to dry. A drop of lymph is then placed at the site of inoculation and with the side of a Hagedorn needle held parallel to the skin multiple "pressures" are made to the skin through the lymph (figs. 20 and 21)). In this way the inoculum is forced into the deeper layers of the epidermis. The area inoculated may be only one-eighth of an inch in diameter. The number of "pressures" varies from ten to thirty, *e.g.* thirty for primary vaccination of infants, ten for primary vaccination of children of school-age. This procedure involves less risk of septic infection and less severe reactions than may occur with the older scarification cross-hatched method (Parish, 1952). The method also has the advantage that it gives a higher success rate than the scratch method in persons previously vaccinated (Bourke & Clarke, 1963).

Alternatively a single scratch $\frac{1}{4}$ in. in length may be made through the drop of lymph. Care should be taken to avoid any bleeding. No dressing is required until four to five days after vaccination, and the lymph should simply be allowed to dry *in situ*.

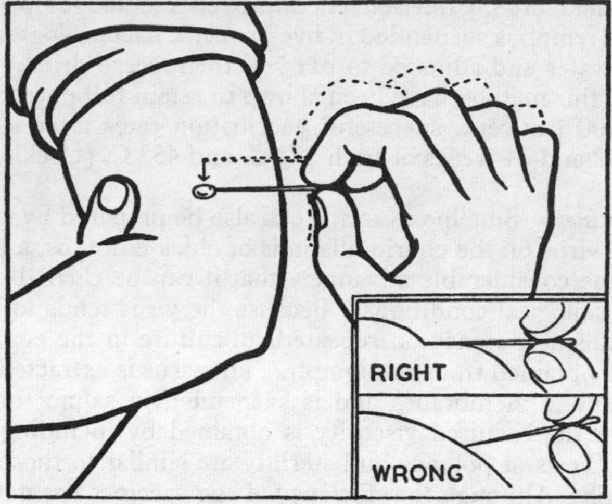

FIG. 20

The multiple pressure method of vaccination against smallpox. Notice the up and down motion of the needle and the angle at which it should be held.

Reproduced by permission of the Controller of Her Majesty's Stationery Office from Memo on Vaccination against Smallpox. Minist. of Health (1948). London: H.M. Stationery Office.

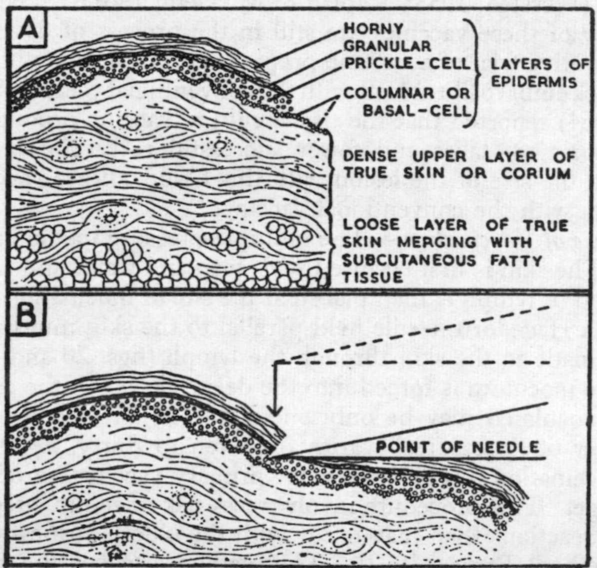

FIG. 21

The multiple pressure method of vaccination against smallpox. Diagram of a section of the skin of the arm. The motion of the needle and its final position penetrating only as far as the basal cell layer.

Reproduced by permission of the Controller of Her Majesty's Stationery Office from Memo on Vaccination against Smallpox. Minist. of Health (1948). London: H.M. Stationery Office.

In a person lacking immunity a papule forms at the site of inoculation in three to four days and this becomes vesicular in five to six days; in eight to ten days the vesicle becomes pustular with a zone of surrounding inflammation; finally the pustule heals with the formation of a crust which is desquamated about the twenty-first day, leaving a depressed scar. In persons who have been recently vaccinated and possess a satisfactory immunity, there may be no reaction, or a papule may appear more rapidly than in the non-immune subject and resolve without the development of a vesicle. (Such reaction, however, cannot be accepted in all cases as indicating an effective immunity.) In those who have been previously vaccinated but have lost their original degree of immunity, an accelerated "vaccinoid" reaction is noted: a papule appears quickly, becoming vesicular and pustular more quickly than in the completely non-immune person.

Before a vaccination can be regarded as successful it is essential that the stage of vesiculation should have been reached. Primary vaccination in children should be carried out in the second year of life. It should not be done on a child with eczema or other skin lesions. There is a rather greater risk of generalised vaccinia and of neurological complications following vaccination in infancy (0–1 years) than in children 1–4 years old. Revaccination in non-epidemic countries should be done at regular intervals of five to seven years, for example on entering school and again on leaving, as well as in circumstances when there is a risk of exposure to smallpox. A certificate on a special internationally accepted form showing vaccination in the previous three years is required for entry into many countries. Between the ages of 5 and 18 years primary vaccination carries a risk of post-vaccinal encephalitis (*vide infra*); the incidence varies from 1 in 8000 to 1 in 70,000 vaccinations with a case mortality of up to 50 per cent. For this reason the primary vaccination of young adolescents should only be carried out when there is a grave risk of variola or if they are entering the medical or nursing professions.

Vaccination provides a powerful defence against the risk of contracting smallpox and is an effective protection against the risk of dying if the disease is contracted. Immunity can be demonstrated eight to nine days after vaccination and antibodies reach their peak within two to three weeks. Protection lasts for a variable period according to the individual; in general five to seven years pass before a primary type revaccination is successful. Experience has shown that case mortality in smallpox is four times greater in unvaccinated than in vaccinated persons.

Complications of Vaccination.—Septic infection at the site of vaccination may be caused by the introduction of pathogenic bacteria either at the time of vaccination or later when the vaccinial lesion has developed. *Generalised vaccinia* is a rare complication characterised by the appearance of discrete vaccinial lesions in crops over the surface of the body; the condition has an incidence of 1 in 100,000 vaccinations and a case mortality of 30–40 per cent. *Vaccinia gangrenosa* is another very rare complication. It is characterised by areas of deep ulceration and necrosis which extend gradually to involve large areas of skin and subcutaneous tissue. Like generalised vaccinia this condition may be associated with hypogammaglobulinaemia. Treatment may involve the use of antivaccinial gammaglobulin in large doses; the drug N-methylisatin β-thiosemicarbazone has been tried but with little success.

Persons with chronic skin diseases and especially young children with eczema are prone to develop widespread vaccinial lesions—*Eczema vaccinatum*—the result of implantation of the vaccine virus on the open skin lesion. *Eczema vaccinatum* is very similar to *Eczema herpeticum* (Kaposi's disease or varicelliform eruption) in which herpes simplex is a causal virus.

Postvaccinial Encephalitis.—Within a fortnight of vaccination an acute disseminated encephalomyelitis may supervene in a very small percentage of cases, mostly older children who have not been vaccinated as infants. A disease identical in its clinical and histological characters has been recorded following certain infective diseases, such as smallpox and measles, and occasionally in non-exanthematous cases.

Clinically there is paralysis, at first flaccid and later spastic, while meningeal symptoms are frequently noted in children. Histologically the outstanding characteristic is the demyelination of the areas round the blood vessels.

It was originally thought that the encephalitis might be due to the vaccinia virus affecting the central nervous tissue, but it is now considered that post-vaccinial encephalitis may be a different disease, due possibly to a separate virus or toxic agent, activated by the vaccinial lesion. It has also been suggested that the condition is due to allergy, with resultant vascular thromboses which produce the characteristic areas of demyelination round the blood vessels.

Chemotherapy.—Vaccinial lesions of the skin *e.g.* accidental implantations, have been treated successfully by the topical application of interferon or 5-iodo-2′ deoxyuridine.

MOLLUSCUM CONTAGIOSUM

The lesions of this disease are small copper-coloured warty papules on the trunk, buttocks, arms and face. It is spread by direct contact or by contaminated fomites. In the epithelial cells very large inclusion bodies, mainly acidophilic in their staining reaction, can be observed. The inclusions may reach 20–30 μ in diameter and crowd the host cell nucleus to one side, eventually filling the whole cell. When material from the lesions is crushed, some of the inclusions are burst open and from them large numbers of elementary bodies escape. These virus particles have the size, internal structure and morphology of the vaccinia virus. The infection has been transmitted with filtrates to human subjects. The virus produces a cytopathic effect in tissue cultures of human cells but does not multiply readily.

COW-POX VIRUS

In cow-pox the eruption appears on the teats as small papules which later give rise to vesicles and pustules. The cows themselves are not seriously affected and no generalised symptoms occur. Friction during the milking process generally causes the lesions to break and raw tender areas are formed. Crusting follows and the dried scabs fall off in about ten days, leaving an unscarred surface. This disease was first described by Jenner, who realised that the infection could be transferred to the hands of milkers with vesicle formation. In man the lesions may occur in the interdigital clefts, or the back of the hands and also on the fore-arms and face. The lesions resemble those that follow primary vaccination, although they may be more indurated and the vesicle fluid is often blood-stained.

Properties of the Cow-pox Virus (*Poxvirus bovis*).—In size, morphology and resistance to heat and chemical agents the cow-pox virus is identical with the vaccinia virus. It can be distinguished from vaccinia virus by the characteristic red haemorrhagic pocks to which it gives rise in cultures on the chorio-allantoic membrane of the chick embryo. The intracytoplasmic inclusions of the cow-pox virus are much larger than the Guarnieri bodies of vaccinia and have a denser matrix; they have also a tendency to distort the shape of the host cell. Serological studies indicate that there is a quantitative difference in the minor antigenic components of the two viruses.

Other Animal Pox Diseases

Sheep-pox can be an extremely serious disease when it occurs in epizootics and has a case mortality varying from 5 to 50 per cent. The virus is quite unrelated antigenically to any other members of the pox group. Goats also may be infected.

Swine-pox is clinically similar to cow-pox and sheep-pox. The disease may be severe in form with a case mortality of about 20 per cent. or, as in Britain, mild with ill-defined pock-like lesions, mainly in young pigs. The milder form, however, may be due to infection with the cow-pox virus. The swine-pox virus from the severe disease is not related to other pox viruses.

Infectious Ectromelia of Mice.—This virus disease occurs in a chronic or acute form. In the chronic disease one foot becomes oedematous with serous exudation on the surface and crusting; later necrosis and sloughing results and spread may take place to another foot or the tail. In the acute disease necrotic lesions occur in the liver and other viscera. In the epithelial cells of the skin and intestine large acidophilic cytoplasmic inclusions are found, and elementary bodies about 260–300 mμ in diameter have also been demonstrated in lesions by ordinary microscopic examination of suitably stained preparations. The virus can be cultivated in the chorio-allantoic membrane and produces pocks similar to those of vaccinia. A serological relationship exists between the virus and the variola-vaccinia viruses. Epizootics of ectromelia in mouse colonies can usually be prevented or controlled by vaccinating the tails of the susceptible animals with vaccinia lymph.

The ectromelia virus has been studied extensively by Fenner (1948), who used it as a model to elucidate the pathogenesis and epidemiology of pox diseases.

Avian Pox Viruses

These viruses affect many different species of birds, including the domestic fowl, canary, pigeon, turkey, sparrow and magpie. The viruses are adapted to their own hosts and when transferred to birds of different species cause only minor signs of disease. The canary-pox and fowl-pox viruses have been more thoroughly investigated than the remainder.

The Properties of the Fowl-pox Virus.—In morphology, size, cultural characters and in resistance to physical and chemical agents the fowl-pox virus is closely similar to the vaccinia virus. In the infected bird the virus gives rise to large spherical inclusions (Bollinger bodies) in the epithelial cells of the cornified layer of the skin. These inclusions are highly characteristic of fowl-pox; they are eosinophilic and larger than the nuclei, which are often displaced by them and pushed to the side of the cells. Within the Bollinger bodies there are many elementary bodies of the virus.

The fowl-pox virus can be cultivated on the chorio-allantoic membrane of the developing chick embryo. Fowls can be immunised against fowl-pox by inoculation with the pigeon-pox virus, which has a low pathogenicity for the fowl.

Contagious Pustular Dermatitis of Sheep (Orf)

The manifestations of this disease are pustules on the lips and round the mouth and on the mucosa of the mouth, the cornea, the feet and legs and other parts of the sheep's body. The infection is transmissible experimentally in lambs by inoculation of the skin with filtrates from the pustules. Human infections with the virus are sometimes seen as granulomata on the hands of those who handle diseased animals, their skins, or their carcases. The causative virus has the same size and morphology as the vaccinia virus, but little is yet known of its other characters. It has not been cultivated in the chick embryo but has been grown successfully in tissue cultures of human amnion. The only susceptible natural host at present available is the lamb. The disease has been controlled under field conditions by means of a living vaccine consisting of finely ground fully virulent scabs suspended in a 1 per cent. concentration in glycerol saline.

Myxomatosis

Myxomatosis is a highly infectious and almost invariably fatal disease of rabbits; it is characterised by mucopurulent discharges from the eyes, nose and genital openings and by the presence of tumour-like masses of tissue involving the head, neck and many other parts of the body. The disease was originally endemic in Brazil and affected only the native wild rabbit (*Sylvilagus brasiliensis*) in which it was manifested as a single localised tumour of the skin. It is spread amongst the animals by the bites of mosquitoes and fleas, but there is no evidence that the virus ever multiplies in the body of the vector. Myxomatosis has now spread over the whole of the North and South American continents and has been introduced into Europe and Australia. The European rabbit (*Lepus europeus*) is highly susceptible to the infection, and sweeping epizootics during the last ten years have decimated the rabbit populations of Australia and Great Britain.

Properties of the Virus.—Morphologically the virus is identical with the vaccinia virus and electron-microscopical examination shows that it measures $290 \times 230 \times 75$ mμ. It is related antigenically to the rabbit fibroma virus of Shope.

Host Range and Cultivation.—The only susceptible animal is the rabbit and all other animals including the hare, monkeys and man are resistant. The virus can be cultivated in the developing chick embryo and produces pocks on the chorio-allantoic membrane. The virus will also grow in the brains of newborn mice and a variety of mammalian cells in tissue culture.

Myxomatosis is mechanically transferred from the skin of the infected animal to the susceptible rabbit by the mosquito, whose mouth parts are contaminated with the virus. In Great Britain the main vector is not a mosquito but the rabbit flea. The viraemia which follows infection is not of direct importance in providing a source of the virus for the arthropod vectors, but, of course, is the means whereby the disease is spread throughout the rabbit's body. Tumourous masses with a rubbery consistency are found in the lymph nodes of the head and neck and throughout the body and the spleen is enlarged. Sections of myxomatous tissue show large stellate cells embedded in a homogeneous mucinous material. Haemorrhages and inflammatory changes are present and in the epithelial cells are large acidophilic inclusions which resemble the Bollinger bodies of fowl-pox.

The complex subjects of the mechanisms of transmission of myxomatosis in Australia and Europe and of the emergence of genetically resistant rabbits have been reviewed by Fenner (1959).

In wild rabbits myxomatosis is virtually an uncontrollable disease. Domestic rabbit and laboratory stocks can be protected by insect-proofing of their breeding quarters. Vaccination of the animals with the related rabbit fibroma virus (Shope) offers a high but not absolute degree of protection.

REFERENCES

Appleyard, G., Zwartouw, H. T. & Westwood, J. C. N. (1964). A protective antigen from the pox viruses. *Brit. J. exp. Path.*, **45**, 150.

Bauer, D. J., St. Vincent, L., Kempe, A. C., & Downie, A. W. (1963). Prophylactic treatment of smallpox contacts with N-methylisatin β-thiosemicarbazone. *Lancet*, **2**, 494.

Bedson, H. S. & Dumbell, K. R. (1961). The effect of temperature on the growth of pox viruses in the chick embryo. *J. Hyg.* (*Lond.*), **59**, 457.

Boulter, E. A. (1957). The titration of vaccinial neutralising antibody on chorio-allantoic membranes. *J. Hyg.* (*Lond.*), **55**, 502.

Bourke, G. J. & Clarke, N. (1963). Smallpox vaccination success rates of scratch and multiple pressure techniques. *Brit. med. J.*, **1**, 281.

Christie, W. G., Donnelly, J. D., Fothergill, R., Ker, F. L., Millar, E. L. M., Flewett, T. H., Bedson, H. S., & Cruickshank, J. G. (1966). Variola minor: A preliminary report from the Birmingham hospital region. *Lancet*, **1**, 1311.

Cockburn, W. C., Cross, R. M., Downie, A. W., Dumbell, K. R., Kaplan C., McClean, D. & Payne, A. M-M. (1957). Laboratory and vaccination studies with dried smallpox vaccines. *Bull. Wld. Hlth. Org.*, **16**, 63.

Collier, L. H. (1955). The development of a stable smallpox vaccine. *J. Hyg.* (*Lond.*), **53**, 76.

Craigie, J. & Wishart, F. O. (1936). Complement fixation reaction in variola. *Canad. publ. Hlth. J.*, **27**, 351.

Dixon, C. W. (1962). *Smallpox*. London: Churchill.

Dostal, V. (1962). Advances in the production of smallpox vaccine. *Prog. med. Virol*, **4**, 259.

Dumbell, K. R., Bedson, H. S. & Rossier, E. (1961). The laboratory differentiation between variola major and variola minor. *Bull. Wld. Hlth. Org.*, **25**, 73.

Dumbell, K. R. & Nizamuddin (1959). An agar-gel precipitation test for the laboratory diagnosis of smallpox. *Lancet*, **1**, 916.

Fenner, F. (1948). The pathogenesis of acute exanthems. *Lancet*, **2**, 915.

Fenner, F. (1959). Myxomatosis. *Brit. med. Bull.*, **15**, 240.

Jenner, E. (1798). An enquiry into the causes and effects of the variolae vacciniae, a disease discovered in some of the western counties of England, particularly Gloucestershire and known by the name of the Cow Pox. Reprinted in *Milestones in Microbiology* Ed. Brock, T. D. (1961). London: Prentice-Hall.

Kaplan, C. & Micklem, L. R. (1961). A method for preparing smallpox vaccine on a large scale in cultured cells. *J. Hyg.* (*Lond.*), **59**, 171.

McClean, D. (1949). "Purification" of vaccine lymph. *Lancet*, **2**, 476.

Medical Memorandum. Ministry of Health and Scottish Home and Health Department (1963). Diagnosis of smallpox. Edinburgh: H.M.S.O.

MURRAY, H. G. S. (1963). The diagnosis of smallpox by immunofluorescence. *Lancet*, **1**, 847.

PARISH, H. J. (1952). *Bacterial and Virus Diseases*. Edinburgh: Livingstone.

PIERCE, E. R., MELVILLE, F. S., DOWNIE, A. W. & DUCKWORTH, M. J. (1958). Anti-vaccinial gamma-globulin in smallpox prophylaxis. *Lancet*, **2**, 635.

SHAW, A. & KAPLAN, C. (1964). A field trial of tissue culture smallpox vaccine (1964). *Mth. Bull. Minist. Hlth. Pub. Lab. Serv.*, **23**, 2.

WESSLÉN, T. (1955). The production of smallpox vaccine in tissue culture of bovine embryonic skin. *Arch. ges. Virusforsch*, **6**, 430.

WESTWOOD, J. C. N., HARRIS, W. J., ZWARTOUW, H. T., TITMUSS, D. H. J. & APPLEYARD, G. (1964). Studies on the structure of vaccinia virus. *J. gen. Microbiol.*, **34**, 67.

WORLD HEALTH ORGANISATION (1959). Requirements for smallpox vaccines. (Requirements for biological substances No. 5.) *Wld. Hlth. Org. tech. Rep. Ser.* No. 180.

CHAPTER 32

HERPESVIRUSES

THIS group contains five related viruses; they are *Herpesvirus hominis*, the cause of herpes simplex in man, *Herpesvirus simiae*, or virus B of monkeys, *Herpesvirus suis* the cause of pseudorabies in cattle and pigs (Aujeszky's disease), *Herpesvirus cuniculi* or Virus III of rabbits, and *Herpesvirus varicellae*, the cause of chicken-pox. The first three in this list are related antigenically to each other.

All the members of the group have a similar fine structure when viewed with negative staining in the electron microscope. The core of the viruses is DNA, and is contained within a capsid composed of 162 capsomeres arranged to form an icosohedron. The capsomeres are hollow prisms $12 \times 9{\cdot}5$ mμ in diameter with a central hole about 4 mμ across; twelve of the prisms, placed at the corners, are pentagonal in outline and the remaining 150 are hexagonal and located on the edges or faces of the icosohedron (see Fig. 22). The mature virions seen in the cytoplasm of the host cells are enclosed by a double membrane. The diameter is 100–180 mμ.

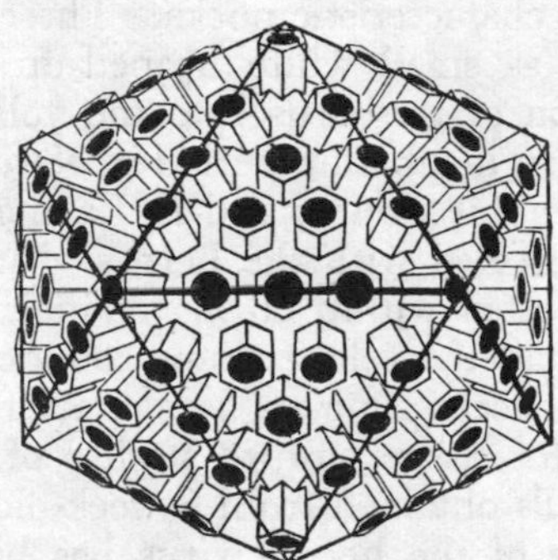

FIG. 22

A diagram of the capsid of a herpesvirus to show the icosohedral symmetry and the hollow capsomeres. (After Horne; 1963). Reprinted with permission. Copyright © 1963 by *Scientific American*, Inc. all rights reserved.

All the viruses grow in tissue cultures and most also in the chick embryo. It is characteristic of this group that they multiply within the nucleus of the host cell producing changes which are sometimes visible as eosinophilic intranuclear inclusions (Cowdry Type A).

Herpesvirus hominis

The most common form of infection with this virus is that of *Herpes simplex*, a vesicular eruption at the mucocutaneous borders around the lips and nose. The lesions somewhat resemble those of *Herpes zoster* both clinically and histologically, and in the past there has been some confusion between the terms *Herpes simplex* and *Herpes zoster*. For clarity it is perhaps better to use the prefix *Herpes* only for *Herpes simplex* and to omit it in "Zoster" infections because the two conditions are caused by two distinct viruses.

Properties of the Virus.—The herpes simplex virus has a diameter of 100–180 mμ. The morphology and fine structure are described above.

Cultivation and Host Range.—A wide range of laboratory animals are susceptible; they include rabbits, guinea-pigs, rats, mice and hamsters. The reactions produced depend upon the route of inoculation. When introduced into the scarified cornea of the rabbit, keratoconjunctivitis results between twelve hours and seven days after inoculation. The conjunctiva and nictitating membrane become intensely inflamed and a mucopurulent discharge develops. After intracerebral inoculation there is encephalitis with fever, convulsions and muscle weakness. Death is the usual termination. A similar encephalitis follows the intracorneal inoculation of certain neurotropic strains. Suckling mice 1–3 days old are particularly susceptible to intraperitoneal and intracerebral inoculation with the virus. Many strains produce an inflammatory reaction when injected into the skin of the pads of the guinea-pig or intracutaneously in the rabbit.

The fertile hen's egg is susceptible to infection, and inoculation of the virus on to the chorio-allantoic membrane of 11–13-day-old chick embryos gives rise to characteristic pocks. These lesions appear 24–48 hr. after inoculation as small white heaped-up plaques 1–2 mm. in diameter. Inoculation of the virus into the yolk-sac or amnion may kill the embryo after an incubation period of 48 to 72 hours.

Human amnion, rabbit kidney, and HeLa and HEp2 cells in tissue culture are readily infected with the herpes virus and a typical cytopathic effect is seen often within 20 hr. of inoculation. Cytoplasmic granulation appears and the cells become rounded and ballooned; the formation of multinucleate syncytia is characteristic of some strains. The cells of choice for tissue culture studies of the herpes virus are trypsinised kidney cells obtained from 6-week-old rabbits.

Reproductive cycle of the herpes virus has been studied in HeLa cells. The particles are slowly adsorbed to the surface of the host cells over a period of two or three hours and there follows an eclipse phase lasting at least nine hours. By the twelfth hour it is possible to detect, with the electron microscope, virus particles 30–40 mμ in diameter in the nucleus. These particles gradually enlarge to a diameter of 70–100 mμ and acquire a single covering membrane, whilst progressive changes in the nucleus incorporate them in an eosinophilic inclusion body which fills the whole nucleus. By 15 hr. the particles begin to leave the nucleus and as they pass through the nuclear membrane they seem to acquire a second covering membrane. They then pass on through the cytoplasm and are liberated through breaches in the cell wall as the fully mature elementary bodies, 120–130 mμ in diameter and covered by a double membrane. The first infective virus is liberated about 15 hr. after infection and by 26 hr. many mature particles can be seen on the cell surface. The release of the virus is by a slow leak rather than by rupture of the cell.

Viability.—In infected egg membranes the virus is somewhat unstable; activity is lost after 20 hr. at 30° C. and after five hr. at 37° C. Exposure for 30 min. at 50–52° C. inactivates the virus. The virus has a half-life of 1½ hr. at 37° C., and 3¾ hr. at 30–31° C. If egg-yolk, 10 per cent. normal rabbit serum, or 1·0 per cent. skim milk is included in the suspending fluid, the virus may, however, be preserved in the frozen state for many months. In whole animal tissues in 50 per cent. glycerol saline at 4° C. the virus remains virulent for years. Herpes virus is killed by moist heat at 52° C. in 30 min., but it may survive dry heat at 90° C. for the same period. It is inactivated by ether, 0·5 per cent. formaldehyde and 1 per cent. phenol, but is more resistant than non-sporing bacteria to 1·0 per cent. gentian violet.

Antigenic Characters.—Antibodies in serum can be estimated by complement-fixation or neutralisation methods. Antigens for these tests can be made from infected tissue cultures (*e.g.* HeLa cells showing maximal cytopathic effect), infected choriollantoic membranes showing confluent lesions, or the brains of 5–7 day old mice inoculated intracerebrally by the virus. A plaque reduction counting technique can be employed in neutralisation tests but for this purpose a virus strain known to give macro-plaques is required. Complement-fixation is associated with a soluble antigen smaller in size and separate from the virus itself. Individuals subject to recurrent attacks have as a rule high titres of antibodies to the virus but those who are free from the infection often have no antibody in the serum.

Strains of herpes simplex do not form one single antigenically homologus group and it is possible to distinguish, on the basis of neutralisation curves, two subtypes (Plummer, 1964). The herpes simplex virus is neutralised by Virus B (*Herpesvirus simiae*) antiserum but the reverse of this does not hold. Sabin (1934) showed that there are serological cross-reactions between the herpes simplex, virus B, and pseudorabies viruses.

Pathogenesis.—Infections with the herpes virus are extremely common and very variable in their clinical manifestations. There are two forms of herpetic disease; (1) primary infections of susceptible persons who have no circulating antibodies and (2) recurrent localised disease in patients who are partially immune. Primary infections are common early in life and probably take place soon after the child has lost its maternal antibodies; in many of the cases the disease is subclinical but in the remainder aphthous stomatitis or various other clinical manifestations occur. Serological surveys have shown that many more adults have circulating antibodies than can be accounted for by a history of clinical infection.

Recurrent Herpetic Infections.—The commonest is *Herpes simplex* (*Herpes labialis* or *Herpes febrilis*). Reddish papules appear at mucocutaneous junctions and quickly vesiculate. They are especially common around the lips and nostrils. When fully developed thin-walled vesicles are closely grouped on an erythematous base; later the lesions become pustular, crust over and some finally heal without a scar. After healing the infection commonly remains latent for long periods and the lesions recur often at precisely the same site, and at frequent intervals. They seem to be provoked by such non-specific stimuli as cold, exposure to sunlight, menstruation, a variety of common bacterial and viral infections (*e.g.* lobar pneumonia) and artificial fever.

Herpetic kerato-conjunctivitis may take many forms, varying from superficial punctate keratitis to marginal keratitis, multiple corneal erosions, dendritic ulcer or diskiform keratitis. The lesions are frequently characterised by recurrences and relapses and the resulting corneal opacities are a serious hazard to sight. American authors have stated that these lesions are a common cause of blindness. These manifestations may be preceded by primary herpetic infection of the eye which begins with an acute follicular conjunctivitis and swelling of the eyelids with vesicle formation.

Primary Herpetic Infections occur in persons lacking any immunity and take the form of acute local inflammatory reactions which appear after an incubation period of four to seven days. They include:

(a) *Aphthous stomatitis*, or acute herpetic gingivo-stomatitis, which is the commonest type of primary infection with the herpes virus. The condition is usually seen in children 1–3 years old and is characterised by fever with red swollen gums and a vesicular eruption on the oral mucous membranes. Submaxillary and cervical lymphadenopathy is very common.

(b) *Genital herpes*.—Typical herpetic lesions may occur as a primary infection on the genitalia. In infants the virus may give rise to a severe rash in the napkin area or to a vulvo-vaginitis. Primary infection also occurs later in life and inflamed vesicular areas are seen on the genitalia of young adults of both sexes. The infection in some instances is spread during sexual intercourse.

(c) *Eczema herpeticum* (*Kaposi's varicelliform eruption*) is a primary manifestation of infection with the herpes virus in a patient already suffering from eczema. The condition is characterised by vesicles widespread over the eczematous skin and is very severe, especially in children under the age of 1 year.

(d) *Herpetic whitlow* is a lesion localised on the fingers and is found not infrequently in nurses and doctors. The virus is probably inoculated through small skin abrasions during handling instruments or endotracheal catheters that have been contaminated with oropharygeal secretions. An individual with a herpetic whitlow may readily spread the virus to patients or other persons.

(e) *Meningo-encephalitis* may occur either as a benign form of aseptic meningitis or as a severe type of encephalitis with destructive lesions involving the ganglionic nerve cells mainly in the cerebral cortex. The latter is more common when primary infection occurs in young adults. The virus is present in the cerebrospinal fluid.

(f) *Disseminated herpes*.—A fatal generalised form of the disease has been described occurring principally in premature infants. There is high fever, jaundice, and encephalitis. Necrotic lesions are found at autopsy in the liver, spleen, brain, kidney, and suprarenal glands.

Epidemiology.—The herpes simplex virus like the measles virus is very widely distributed in man. Commonly more than 60 per cent. of persons over the age of thirty years have been infected by the herpes virus. Overcrowding increases the incidence markedly and the percentage of persons with herpetic antibodies is markedly higher in urban communities than in the country (MacCallum, 1959).

Infection is transmitted in many cases by direct touch with hands as when the mother or nurses handle a new born baby, or in kissing or sexual intercourse. Most herpetic infections are, however, acquired in infancy. Fomites such as towels, soap, cutlery, china, or drinking vessels may also spread the infection. The source of the virus is a case or a carrier who is excreting the virus in the secretions from his oropharynx, eyes or genitalia.

Specific antibodies are present during the first few months of life in the serum of children born to herpetic mothers and young babies seldom develop herpetic infection. Primary infection occurs most commonly in infants between the ages of one and five years. In an unknown proportion, possibly high, these primary infections are subclinical in nature. In apparently healthy children in one series, studied by Buddingh *et al* (1953), there was a salivary carrier rate of 20 per cent. among children aged seven months to two years but by the age of 20 only 2·5 per cent. still carried the virus. The commonest acute manifestation is aphthous stomatitis and children excrete the virus in the saliva and faeces for several weeks after clinical infection. Primary infection in adults, *e.g.* genital herpes, is less common.

Laboratory Diagnosis

The virus may be isolated from the vesicle fluid from lesions on the skin or mucous membranes and may also be found in the throat, saliva and faeces. Material should be inoculated into suitable hosts of which the chorio-allantoic membrane of 12-day-old chick embryo and 2-day-old suckling mice are recommended (*vide supra*). Primary cultures of the kidney cells of young rabbits and also human amnion are very sensitive to the virus. Of continuous lines, HEp2 and particularly the rabbit kidney GRK cells are useful. On primary isolation the viruses produce a general rounding of the cells in the monolayer which is seen two to six days after inoculation; giant cells and syncytia are not formed in early passages. One or occasionally two blind passages may be required before the virus can be detected. The lesions developed in these hosts should be examined histologically for intranuclear inclusions and the virus identified by neutralisation tests with specific antiserum.

Antibodies in the patient's serum may be measured in complement-fixation reactions and in neutralisation tests. The presence of antibody in the serum of an adult, however, is of doubtful significance because 60–90 per cent. of people have antibodies continually present in their serum.

Chemotherapy.—There is evidence that 5-iodo-2′ deoxyuridine instilled into the eye at 1–2 hourly intervals, has a therapeutic effect in cases of herpetic kerato-conjunctivitis (Kaufman *et al.*, 1962). The virus, however, has been known to develop resistance to the drug.

Herpesvirus simiae (Virus B)

Virus B has achieved in monkeys the same state of successful parasitism that obtains in man with the herpes virus. Two per cent. of rhesus monkeys carry the virus in a latent form. Virus B is thus a natural parasite of monkeys.

The morphology and physico-chemical characters of the virus are closely similar to those of *Herpesvirus hominis*. Virus B grows readily in tissue cultures of human, monkey and rabbit tissues and also on the chorio-allantoic membrane of the chick embryo. The virus has a close antigenic relationship to the herpes simplex virus and a remote one to the pseudorabies virus. An antiserum to virus B neutralises the herpes simplex virus as well as it does virus B but an antiherpes simplex serum has but little power to neutralise virus B.

Pathogenesis.—Human infections with this virus are almost invariably fatal but are fortunately infrequent. The virus is introduced through the bite of an infected monkey; vesicles develop at the site of the bite after an interval of about three days and on about the seventh day the virus reaches the central nervous system by way of the peripheral nerves. An ascending paralysis follows with involvement of the respiratory centres and death.

In monkeys infection is characterised by vesicular lesions on the lips and tongue and an aphthous stomatitis. Subclinical infection is common and spread is by direct contact. Many apparently healthy monkeys excrete the virus in the saliva but not as far as is known in faeces or urine. Overcrowding greatly facilitates the spread of infection and in one colony 75 per cent. of the monkeys were found to be infected. One per cent. of pools of infected monkey kidney tissue cultures used for the preparation of poliomyelitis vaccines have been found to be contaminated with virus B and steps are now required to eliminate this risk.

Infection with this virus presents a hazard to laboratory workers who handle monkeys or who use their tissues in cultural work. Bites and wounds require prompt disinfection and it has been suggested that an inactivated vaccine should be developed to protect laboratory workers.

Herpesvirus suis (Pseudorabies Virus)

Pseudorabies or Aujeszky's disease affects the central nervous system, causes paralysis, and occurs in dogs, cattle, horses, pigs, sheep, rats and certain other animals. It is rapidly fatal in all these species except the adult pig. In pigs the disease closely resembles Teschen or Talfan disease (see p. 442). An important point of differentiation from rabies is that the animals suffer from intense itching of the hindquarters, a symptom that has led to the condition being known as the "mad itch". It also differs in that the animals are not aggressive. The virus is not strictly neurotropic, for it may be demonstrated in the oedematous subcutaneous tissue in the local skin lesion and in the lungs. It is not found in the saliva. Histologically the virus causes severe and widespread neural damage and characteristic intranuclear inclusions have been described in the most severely affected neurons. Antigenically it is distinct from the virus of rabies with which it has no relationship whatever. The pseudorabies virus contains DNA and is similar in size and fine structure to *Herpesvirus hominis*. The virus survives 30–46 days in hay at atmospheric temperatures. The virus grows on the chorio-allantoic membrane of the chick embryo where it produces white plaques or haemorrhages and death of the embryo by the fourth day. It will also grow in the yolk sac. When inoculated on to monolayers of chick fibroblasts, pig kidney, or guinea-pig, rabbit, or dog tissues a cytopathic effect is produced and plaques are produced. Rabbits are highly susceptible to the infection. Guinea-pigs, rats and mice are more resistant. Neutralisation tests indicate that there may be antigenic components of this virus that are shared with the herpes simplex virus and virus B. The principal natural reservoir of the virus is the adult pig, but the rat is also latently infected. There is evidence that the disease may spread from rats to pigs and from pigs to cattle. The virus of Aujeszky's disease has been isolated from cattle, pigs, cats and rats in Northern Ireland. It can be cultivated in the chorio-allantoic membrane of the chick embryo, where it produces white pocks after four to five days' incubation and also by tissue culture methods. Many strains cause a haemorrhagic encephalitis and death of the embryo.

CHICKENPOX AND ZOSTER

These two diseases differ greatly in their clinical manifestations but there can be little doubt that they are caused by a single virus.

Chickenpox (varicella) is a mild and extremely infectious disease occurring principally in young children. Papules which rapidly become vesicles appear on the first day of the illness; they occur in successive crops and spread from the face and scalp to the trunk and limbs but do not involve the hands or feet.

In zoster a very similar vesicular eruption is confined to an area of skin corresponding to the distribution of a sensory nerve. These lesions may be very painful and are usually unilateral; the most frequent sites are the trunk and an area on one side of the face supplied by one of the divisions of the trigeminal nerve. Zoster is a sporadic condition in adults and seldom occurs in children. It is not highly infectious.

Properties of the Virus.—Elementary bodies are abundant in vesicle fluid collected within 12 hr. of the appearance of the chickenpox lesion; by 24 hr., however, they have become very scanty. They can be demonstrated by the staining methods used for the smallpox virus. The mature virions are rounded and variable in size, their average diameter is 200 mμ. When first detectable in ultra-thin sections of infected cells they appear as bodies 30–40 mμ in diameter, covered by a thin membrane but by the time they have reached the cytoplasm they have increased in size to 150–200 mμ and have acquired a second and thicker covering membrane. Mature virus stained negatively by phosphotungstic acid is seen to have a cubical symmetry identical with that of *Herpesvirus hominis*; the capsid takes the form of an icosohedron with 162 hollow capsomeres (Almeida, Howatson and Williams, 1962).

Cultivation.—The virus in vesicle fluid from cases of chickenpox and also from zoster can be cultivated in a variety of cells of human origin and in some from monkeys. The virus will multiply in growing explants of human prepuce or in human embryonic skin-muscle in plasma clots (Weller, Witton and Bell, 1958). Trypsinised cultures of human amnion cells have been used successfully for the isolation of the virus from vesicle fluid, and monkey kidney and HeLa cells support the growth of virus strains in infected fluids from tissue culture (Taylor-Robinson, 1959).

The cytopathic effect in all types of tissue cultures is characteristic and is identical whether the inoculum is obtained from chickenpox or zoster material. Foci of infection appear and enlarge slowly as contiguous cells are infected; these lesions are first seen six or seven days after inoculation and reach their maximum in about three weeks. Characteristic acidophilic inclusions develop within the nuclei of the cells at the centre of the lesion and later syncytial cytoplasmic masses are formed. The supernatant fluid from tissue culture usually contains very little infective virus since elementary bodies are retained within the host cells. To propagate the virus it is necessary to detach infected cells from the glass and to transfer them to fresh cultures. Infective virus can be released from infected cells by ultrasonic disintegration.

Laboratory animals and the chick embryo are not susceptible to infection with the virus and the only susceptible host (apart from tissue cultures) is man. When vesicle fluid from a case of zoster was inoculated experimentally into the skin of young susceptible children a local lesion at the site of inoculation appeared nine to twelve days later. One of 17 such children developed a generalised rash on the 14th day. Contacts of the inoculated children developed chickenpox after the usual incubation period. It has been repeatedly observed that natural infection of children with chickenpox may follow contact with a patient with zoster and it is established that varicella contracted in this way is epidemiologically and immunologically typical. In contrast, the reverse process, when the adult develops zoster after contact with children with chickenpox, is thought to occur only very rarely.

Viability.—The virus survives for only a few days in tissue culture suspensions but can be preserved for many months at $-70°$ C. It is inactivated in 30 min. at 60° C.

Antigenic Characters.—Vesicle fluid or extracts of crust from chickenpox or zoster behave identically in the presence of sera from convalescents from either disease. There is no difference between the two in agglutination tests nor in complement-fixation reactions (Taylor-Robinson and Downie, 1959). In precipitin tests using the Ouchterlony technique no difference can be detected between the antigens of zoster and varicella or in the antibodies in the sera (Taylor-Robinson and Rondle, 1959). The virus is unrelated to the virus of herpes simplex.

Pathogenesis.—It is thought that chickenpox is contracted by inhaling infected particles and that the virus enters the body through the respiratory mucosa. The rash is presumed to be caused by the localisation of the virus in the skin from the blood stream; a viraemic phase is postulated at or just before the onset of the illness. The incubation period is twelve to sixteen days. Histologically the vesicles in chickenpox and zoster are identical. The lower layer of the epidermis is ballooned and there is degeneration of the epidermal cells with the formation of multinucleate giant cells. In the cells at the base of the lesions there are eosinophilic intranuclear inclusions similar to those seen in infected tissue culture cells.

Zoster has, as a rule, a prodromal period of three or four days of fever and malaise before the appearance of the skin eruption. At this time there is commonly pain and tenderness over an area of skin supplied by nerves from one of the dorsal nerve roots. In this area papules appear and rapidly become vesicles; during the succeeding days the vesicle fluid becomes cloudy, and then after rupture of the vesicles the lesions dry up and healing slowly follows. The lesions are unilateral and may be very painful; in some cases especially when the trigeminal nerve is involved there may be residual paralysis. In 2–3 per cent. of cases there is a generalised rash. In some cases there may be a meningeal reaction with an increased number of mononuclear cells in the cerebrospinal fluid. Encephalitis is a rare complication.

The site of infection in zoster is in the dorsal root ganglion where there is an acute inflammatory reaction; a monocytic inflammatory exudate is seen with haemorrhage and necrosis of the ganglion cells. Degenerative changes follow, passing down the nerve fibres to reach the skin and in some cases centrally to reach the posterior column where they involve the anterior horn cells and give rise to paralysis.

The incubation period in zoster is difficult to determine; it is shorter than in varicella and estimates range from three to seven days and up to seven to fourteen days.

Laboratory Diagnosis.—In chickenpox there is seldom any need for laboratory help in diagnosis unless the possibility of smallpox has to be considered. Confluent chickenpox in a young adult may resemble smallpox very closely, and in such patients specimens must be collected and examined by the methods described for smallpox on p. 372. In direct smears from the skin lesions elementary bodies may be seen, but they appear smaller than the variola virus and are much less numerous. The presence of multinucleate giant cells in Giemsa stained films is highly suggestive of chickenpox. Vesicle fluid and extracts of crusts from patients with zoster and varicella fail to fix complement when mixed with anti-vaccinial serum.

The virus in material from either disease may be identified in complement-fixation reactions with antisera from convalescent cases of chickenpox and zoster. Antibodies in the serum can be measured in complement-fixation and neutralisation tests using as antigen vesicle fluid or tissue culture fluids.

Epidemiology.—Chickenpox is a highly contagious disease of childhood. Its maximum incidence is between the ages of two and six years, but it is not uncommon in the first year of life. About 20 per cent. of cases may occur in adult life. The disease has a seasonal prevalence in the winter and spring; the case mortality is negligible.

Zoster is a sporadic disease uncommon in children. The disease is not highly infectious and there is no prevalence at any particular season. The mode of infection in zoster is unknown. Contacts with zoster do not usually develop zoster themselves, but are more liable to suffer from chickenpox.

The Relationship of Zoster to Chickenpox.—The pathogenesis of these two diseases and laboratory studies of the viruses isolated from them leave little doubt that they are different responses to infection with the same virus. It has been shown that high antibody titres are present in zoster in the early stages after the onset of the infection and that in chickenpox such levels are not attained until late in convalescence. This, together with the shorter incubation period of zoster, has led to the suggestion that zoster is the manifestation of infection in the partially immune subject. Thus varicella may represent dissemination of the virus in the blood stream of the susceptible person, whereas zoster represents the invasion of nerve pathways in a patient who has a small measure of immunity remaining from a childhood infection. Alternatively, zoster may represent the reactivation of a latent virus dormant for many years in the patient's tissues. There is, however, little evidence to indicate in which tissue the latent virus lies.

Infectious Laryngo-Tracheitis

This is a highly contagious respiratory infection of domestic fowls, turkeys and pheasants. The incubation period is less than 48 hours, and after entering the flock infection does not stop until almost every bird has been attacked. The symptoms are those of cough and severe dyspnoea due to respiratory obstruction. The principal pathological lesion is a thick blood-streaked inflammatory exudate over the surface of the larynx and trachea. Intranuclear inclusions are found in infected epithelial cells in the trachea.

The virus of infectious laryngo-tracheitis is 45–85 mμ in diameter. Filamentous forms are described. Under the electron microscope negatively stained particles have an appearance resembling the virus of herpes simplex (q.v.). It can be propagated on the chorio-allantoic membrane of the developing chick embryo, where it produces white pocks. The virus can be cultivated in minced chick tissue cultures of the Maitland type and also in monolayers of chick cells. The virus survives at room temperature for periods up to 90 days but it is readily inactivated by heat at 55°–75° C. and by the usual antiseptics. No haemagglutinating activity has been described. The relationship of this virus to other respiratory viruses is not determined.

Recovered birds may carry the virus for as long as two years and thus form the reservoir from which new outbreaks are derived.

Control of the disease usually necessitates the complete eradication of infected flocks and the vigorous disinfection of contaminated premises. In some countries vaccination is practised; an unattenuated strain is used for the purpose and is introduced by painting on the cloaca.

REFERENCES

ALMEIDA, J. D., HOWATSON, A. F. & WILLIAMS, M. G. (1962). Morphology of varicella (Chickenpox) virus. *Virology*, **16**, 353.

BUDDINGH, C. J., SCHRUM, D. I., LANIER, J. C. & GUIDRY, D. J. (1953). Studies of the natural history of herpes simplex infections. *Pediatrics (N.Y.)*, **11**, 595.

HORNE, R. W. (1963). The structure of viruses. *Sci. Amer.*, **208**, 48.
KAUFMAN, H. E., NESBURN, A. B. & MALONEY, E. D. (1962). IDU therapy of herpes simplex. *Arch. Aphthal.*, **67**, 583.
MACCALLUM, F. O. (1959). Generalised herpes simplex in the neonatal period. *Acta virol.*, **3**, 17.
PLUMMER, G. (1964). Serological comparison of herpes viruses. *Brit. J. exp. Path.*, **45**, 135.
SABIN, A. B. (1934). The immunological relationships of pseudo-rabies. *Brit. J. exp. Path.*, **15**, 372.
TAYLOR-ROBINSON, D. (1959). Chickenpox and herpes zoster. Tissue culture studies. *Brit. J. exp. Path.*, **40**, 521.
TAYLOR-ROBINSON, D. & DOWNIE, A. W. (1959). Chickenpox and herpes zoster. Complement-fixation studies. *Brit. J. exp. Path.*, **40**, 398.
TAYLOR-ROBINSON, D. & RONDLE, C. J. M. (1959). Chickenpox and herpes zoster. Ouchterlony precipitation studies. *Brit. J. exp. Path.*, **40**, 517.
WELLER, T. H., WITTON, H. M. & BELL, E. J. (1958). The aetiologic agents of varicella and herpes zoster. *J. exp. Med.*, **108**, 843.

CHAPTER 33

MYXOVIRUSES; ADENOVIRUSES; OTHER RESPIRATORY VIRUSES

THE infections discussed in this chapter are common maladies which make up the bulk of the respiratory diseases occurring every winter. They vary in severity from a simple cold to a feverish and prostrating attack of influenza, or to severe bronchitis and bronchopneumonia. Although the pharynx, larynx and the upper air passages are most frequently involved, the conjunctiva and salivary glands may also be affected. Most of these diseases are highly infectious and many commonly occur in epidemics. Our knowledge of their aetiology is far from complete, but two main groups of viruses, the Myxoviruses and the Adenoviruses, are responsible for a considerable proportion of respiratory illnesses. In addition, the common cold viruses, the ECHO viruses, and a number of other viruses also cause respiratory infections. Influenza is the name of an acute febrile infectious respiratory disease of man commonly encountered in epidemic form.

MYXOVIRUSES

The myxoviruses cause respiratory diseases in man, animals and poultry. They derive their name from the affinity they possess for the mucus present in the respiratory tract and elsewhere. They vary in size from 60–200 mμ (more usually 80–150 mμ) and are spherical or filamentous in shape. They contain a core of RNA with protein capsomeres arranged along its coils, and have a lipid-containing covering membrane which makes the viruses sensitive to 20 per cent. ether. Many members of the group, though not all of them, possess an enzyme which causes the agglutination of erythrocytes.

Two kinds of myxoviruses can be distinguished (Waterson, 1962). The first group contains the true influenza viruses A, B and C., the viruses of swine, duck and horse influenza, and also the virus of fowl plague. The second group includes the mumps, Newcastle, parainfluenza 1, 2, 3 and 4, simian myxovirus SV5, and perhaps the measles, canine distemper, and rinderpest viruses. This second group differs from the first in that its members are larger and more variable in size, possess haemolysins as well as haemagglutinins, and lack filamentous forms. The internal RNA of this group takes the form of a filament about 18 mμ in diameter and contrasts with the slender structure 9 mμ in diameter found in the true influenza viruses.

Myxovirus influenzae A, B and C

Morphology.—In infected allantoic fluid the virions are roughly spherical and mostly 80 to 120 mμ in diameter. Filamentous forms of about this diameter and up to several microns in length are often present in strains of virus A recently isolated from man; they can be demonstrated by dark-ground microscopy and in stained preparations. Under the electron microscope the virion is seen to consist of a hollow helically arranged nucleoprotein structure, about 800 mμ in length and 9·0 mμ in diameter, twisted and wound upon itself to form a centrally disposed mass, the whole being covered by an outer membrane 7–10 mμ thick. Protruding from the surface of the virion are rod-like projections (the haemagglutinins) which are about 8–10 mμ long with a centre to centre spacing of about 8·0 mμ.

Host Range and Cultivation.—The ferret is the most susceptible animal; after intranasal inoculation it develops fever and a nasal discharge due to inflammation of the ciliated epithelium over the turbinate bones. Ferrets recover quickly from the infection and develop high titres of antiviral antibodies in their serum. Mice are less susceptible, but with repeated "blind passage" by intranasal inoculation under ether anaesthesia, strains of the virus can be adapted to give rise regularly to pulmonary consolidation.

The developing chick embryo at the age of thirteen days provides in its trachea and lung buds, cells which are highly susceptible to small doses of the myxoviruses. Although free growth of the virus takes place, the embryos do not die from the infection and no obvious lesions can be detected. The eggs, after inoculation, should be incubated for 48–72 hr. at 35° C. The presence of the virus is detected by the demonstration of haemagglutinating activity in the embryonic fluids. Once adapted to the amniotic cavity, influenza viruses A and B can be transferred to the allantoic cavity where a rapidly growing mutant emerges to outgrow the original virus inoculum. The original, or "O", virus grows better in the amniotic than the allantoic cavity and its variation to the derivative, or "D" phase, is accompanied by altered haemagglutination properties (see p. 400). Influenza virus C grows only in the amniotic cavity.

Influenza viruses can also be grown in tissue culture monolayers prepared from chick or human embryonic tissues, human amnion cells or monkey kidney cells at 32° C. Their cytopathic effect may not be obvious and they are detected by the demonstration of haemagglutinating activity in the tissue culture fluids or of the adsorption of guinea-pig erythrocytes to the surface of the monolayers (haemadsorption) (Vogel & Shelokov, 1957).

Haemagglutination.—Virus is adsorbed to receptor areas on the red-cell surface and agglutination of erythrocytes results from the elementary bodies acting as bridges which join adjacent cells. Bivalent cations (*e.g.* Ca) must be present in the suspending fluid for the reaction to take place. After prolonged contact at room temperature the virus is released, or *eluted* from the red cells. The eluted virus is unaltered and remains capable of agglutinating fresh red cells. The treated red cells, however, are permanently altered and can no longer be agglutinated by the same virus although they still may be agglutinated by some other kinds of viruses. Myxoviruses have a varying ability to remove or destroy receptors from red cells and some, which are placed low on the so-called "receptor gradient", remove receptors not only for themselves but for all other viruses placed higher on the gradient. The order of viruses on the receptor gradient starting with those with the weakest action on red cell receptors is: mumps, Newcastle, influenza A (MEL strain), influenza B (Lee), influenza A (Swine), influenza B (Mil). A series of events similar to the virus reaction with red cells occurs with the cells of the respiratory tract. The receptor destroying reaction is enzymic in nature, and the cell surface receptor is a neuraminic acid-containing mucopolysaccharide which is attacked specifically by the virus enzyme (neuraminidase).

The Virus Growth Cycle.—Infection of the cell begins when the virus particle becomes attached to the receptor area on its surface; for a short time the attachment is loose, but it soon becomes irreversible and either the whole or part of the particle passes through the cell wall to enter the cytoplasm. Once within the cell, the virus loses its identity for a period of two or three hours and cannot be detected by infectivity experiments or by haemagglutination or complement-fixation reactions. This stage of the reproductive cycle is known as the "eclipse phase" and it is thought that at this time the virus particle has broken down to components, each of which multiplies separately. Fluorescent antibody staining and isotope studies suggest that replication of viral nucleoprotein takes place in or very close to the nucleus.

Three or four hours after infection of the cell, the newly formed viral nucleoprotein becomes antigenically active and can fix complement in the presence of antiserum. The antibodies developed against this antigen are group-specific; *i.e.* they can react not only with the original infecting strain but also with all members of the same group.

The properties of this complement-fixing or soluble antigen can be studied when cells are broken open by rapid freezing and thawing a few hours after infection. The antigen is found to consist of small protein particles 12 mμ in diameter, *i.e.* about one-tenth the original size of the virus of the elementary body. They have a molecular weight of approximately 600,000, and contain 5·3 per cent. ribonucleic acid; they are non-infective and non-haemagglutinating. On account of its small size the antigen is usually referred to as the *soluble* antigen, a term which is to be preferred since other constituents developed later in the influenza virus particle are also able to fix complement. Antibodies against the soluble antigen are induced during infection, but not by the inoculation of inactivated virus; they are not protective and do not neutralise live virus.

Following the formation of the soluble antigen, the haemagglutinin which is synthesised separately, appears in the cells; it is not infective and is considered to be a mucoprotein which contributes about 13 per cent. of the weight of the mature particle. In the haemagglutinin resides the enzymatic activity of the virus which gives it a special affinity for the host cell. The assembly of the mature infective particle can be seen in ultra-thin sections of cells under the electron microscope. The process takes place at the periphery of the cell cytoplasm with the active participation of the cell wall through which the particles are extruded taking on a coating of lipid material as they go. The latent period elapsing before the liberation of new virus is four to eight hours. The extrusion of the virus continues over a period lasting some 36 hours without apparent damage to the cell. A single infected cell releases between 60 and 120 mature infective particles. With some virus strains, filaments rather than spherical elementary bodies emerge and this process may be a stage in the reproductive cycle modified so that normal segmentation does not occur. Filamentous virus has normal haemagglutinating and antigenic properties, but may not be fully infective.

Structure of the virion.—The particles are roughly spherical and 80–100 mμ in diameter. They are covered by a surface envelope 7–10 mμ thick through which protrude rod-like projections 8–10 mμ long spaced regularly at intervals of 7–10 mμ (see Fig. 23). When the

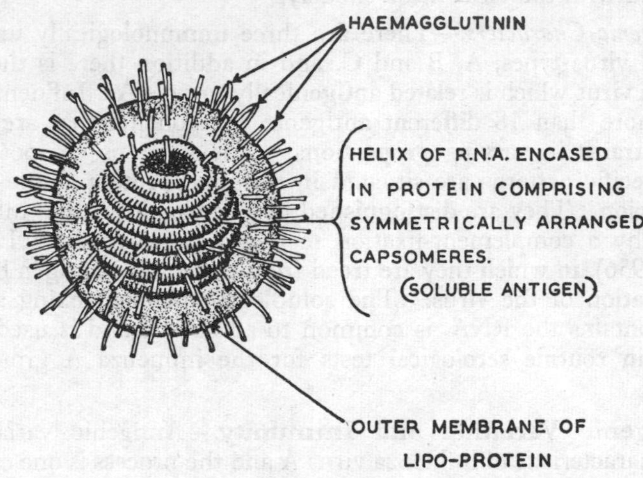

FIG. 23

Diagram to indicate present views on the structure of the influenza virus. (Horne, R. W. (1963). Modified with permission. Copyright © 1963 by *Scientific American*, Inc. all rights reserved.

virion is disrupted by ether treatment the internal RNA core is revealed as a long, slender, hollow, filament about 9–10 mμ in diameter. From its herring-bone appearance it seems that protein capsomeres are combined at intervals along the spirals of the RNA. This long strand is coiled and tightly packed within the envelope of the complete virus particle (Horne & Wildy, 1963).

Viability.—The influenza virus withstands slow drying at room temperature on articles such as blankets and glass; it has been demonstrated in dust after an interval as long as two weeks. When contained in allantoic fluid, or in infected tissues immersed in glycerol saline it will survive for several weeks at refrigerator temperature. It can be preserved for long periods at −70° C. and remains viable indefinitely after freeze drying.

Exposure to heat for 30 min. at 56° C. is sufficient to inactivate most strains; the few which survive this treatment are killed by a ninety-minute exposure at the same temperature. These viruses are also inactivated by 20 per cent. ether in the cold, phenol, formalin in a concentration of 1 in 5000, salts of heavy metals, detergents, soaps, and many other chemicals. Iodine in the form of vapour or as a solution is particularly effective. Propylene glycol vapour is active against the virus present in airborne droplets.

Toxicity.—Influenza virus elementary bodies are toxic to such laboratory animals as mice and rabbits. After the intravenous inoculation of highly purified virus preparations the animals may die in 18–48 hours with gastro-intestinal haemorrhages and necrotic lesions in the spleen and liver. Immunised animals do not suffer these effects when inoculated with the virus intravenously.

Antigenic Characters.—There are three immunologically unrelated influenza virus types, A, B and C, and in addition there is the swine influenza virus which is related antigenically to type A. Influenza virus A has more than 18 different antigenic components that are shared by the strains in varying proportions. The antigens composing the strain-specific patterns are situated in the mucoprotein at the surface of the virion. They are distinguished by haemagglutination inhibition tests or by a complement-fixation technique developed by Lief and Henle (1956), in which they are freed from the soluble antigen by ether disintegration of the virus. The soluble complement-fixing antigen, which contains the RNA, is common to all strains and is used as the antigen in routine serological tests for the influenza A group as a whole.

Antigenic Variation and Immunity.—Antigenic variation is highly characteristic of influenza virus A and the process is one of a continuing evolution of new subtypes which replace the older strains from which they are derived, possibly as a result of the selective action of host antibodies. Many different antigenic patterns emerge by mutation and selection, some antigens advancing to a dominant position and others receding into the background. Strains isolated at the beginning of an epidemic usually have an antigenic structure differing appreciably from that of previous strains. These changes in the antigenic mosaic occur constantly in the course of endemic and epidemic infection in man and can also be induced deliberately in the laboratory. Major mutation with the emergence of completely new dominant antigens is very infrequent and has probably only occurred at intervals of 30 to 40 years. When it happens, the new strain is highly infectious and world-wide epidemics (pandemics) are thought to have been due to the spread of what is in effect a new virus in a highly susceptible population. The disastrous pandemic of 1918-19 in which ten million people died and the pandemic of Asian influenza in 1957-58 were caused by new mutants of type A virus.

Major epidemics of influenza involving whole countries or large parts of a continent are more frequent events and occur at intervals of four or five years. Since 1932, when the first human strain of the influenza virus was isolated, characteristic strains from each epidemic have been collected and compared, using strain-specific absorbed sera in haemagglutination inhibition tests. According to Burnet (1960) these virus strains have shown an immunological drift with the successive emergence of seven new antigenic patterns. Thus the original strain of the 1932 epidemic (labelled the WS strain) was replaced in 1934 by an antigenically different strain which was isolated in Puerto Rico (PR8) strain. During the following years the PR8 strain was replaced by a succession of new types. In 1946 in Australia another new strain known as CAM emerged and proved to be the precursor of yet another change in the antigenic make-up of current influenza viruses. This CAM strain proved to have such slight relationships to previous standard strains that it was classified as a subgroup of influenza A and designated as A prime (A1) virus. The A1 virus and variants of it replaced the A strains and remained dominant throughout the world until the Asian virus appeared in 1957. This latter possessed a new major antigen and differed so much from the A1 strains that it is designated A2. Since 1962 the A2 viruses have shown a progressively increasing shift in antigenic structure (Pereira *et al.* 1964).

The antigenic drift of the influenza virus is reflected in the immunity of the general population. As the individual grows older he experiences an increasing number of epidemics of influenza. With each infection by a new type of virus he acquires in his serum a new specific antibody. Thus in the early years of life the antibody spectrum is narrow, but gradually broadens as age increases. The serum of a person of mature years will often neutralise any of the known standard viruses of previous years, although, of course, that individual will be susceptible to infection with the new virus which appears in the next epidemic. It is these factors which make it difficult to produce an efficient prophylactic vaccine against influenza.

Antigenic variation in type B virus occurs in the same manner as in type A, but the changes are less pronounced and occur more gradually. Type B does not cause the large epidemics that characterise type A; typically it is associated with endemic disease and small epidemics in institutions. It has, however, been recognised as the cause of considerable localised epidemics involving a whole large city. Type C virus appears to exist as a single stable antigenic type.

P–Q–R Variation.—Influenza viruses may vary in the avidity with which they combine with antibody and are neutralised by it. Their behaviour in haemagglutination inhibition tests with convalescent ferret antisera has led to their classification into P, Q and R phases. P phase virus has a high avidity for antibody and is inhibited to a high titre by its homologous antiserum only. Q phase virus is poorly neutralised, even by its own homologous serum, and R phase virus is inhibited to high titre not only by homologous antiserum but by antisera to heterologous but related strains. Freshly isolated strains are commonly in the

P phase, but the Q phase is not infrequently encountered. The identification of a strain in the Q phase is difficult using the haemagglutination inhibition method but is more easily achieved by a neutralisation test in monkey kidney tissue cultures using the haemadsorption technique (Pereira, 1958).

Type A strains also show considerable differences in their sensitivity to non-specific inhibitors such as serum mucopolysaccharides. Highly sensitive strains have a greater avidity for antibody (P phase) and are therefore preferred as antigens in haemagglutination inhibition tests.

O→D Variation.—Yet another type of variation on the part of the influenza virus occurs in the laboratory soon after its primary isolation. Some two to five days after the inoculation into the amniotic cavity of throat washings from a case of influenza the amniotic fluid develops the power to agglutinate red blood cells. With rare exceptions the virus at this stage can agglutinate guinea-pig or human Group O cells but not fowl erythrocytes. If, however, the fluid is passed by the allantoic route to another set of embryos the infected fluid of this second passage will agglutinate fowl cells to almost or quite the same titre as guinea-pig cells. This change in agglutinative power is the result of mutation which occurs at a rate of about 1 in 10,000 as the virus grows in the allantoic membrane and is referred to as *O→D* variation.

Laboratory Diagnosis.—Virus isolation can be carried out by inoculating throat washings or material from throat swabs into the amniotic cavity of the developing chick embryo or tissue cultures (p. 395 and see also Chapter 57).

Serological tests can be performed with the complement-fixation test and the haemagglutination inhibition test (Chapter 54).

Epidemiology.—The influenza virus is disseminated by the patient in infected secretions from the nose and mouth, and perhaps, in droplets expelled in sneezing. Infection probably occurs by inhalation of infected airborne particles; these may be dust particles derived from the discharged secretions or, possibly, droplet nuclei.

Patients are probably infectious for a short time before the onset and for a few days thereafter. Healthy carriers occur and may disseminate the infection, but it is not known how important a part they play.

The periodicity of outbreaks of influenza is characteristic, and in general there would appear to be a pandemic at roughly forty-year intervals with major epidemics of type A infection at about five-year intervals; endemic foci of infection with type B may occur yearly and at three- to six-year intervals moderate epidemics of type B infections are recognised. The epidemiological picture is complicated by the existence of upper respiratory infections due to other viruses such as the para-influenza viruses and the adenoviruses which also occur in epidemic form. Epidemics of virus influenza occur with an abrupt rise in the incidence of cases and a very rapid spread over an irregularly defined region. The course and extent of an epidemic is controlled partly by the nature and antigenic novelty of the prevailing virus and partly by the pre-existing immune state of the community. The cold weather in early spring and increased overcrowding are factors which facilitate the spread of the virus. In major epidemics it has been possible to trace the virus from point to point along travel routes and to record the advance of the epidemic from place to place and country to country.

The age distribution of influenza shows the highest incidence in the age-group 5–15 years, a sharp decline in the 15–20 age-group, a rise between the ages of 20 and 30, and thereafter a downward trend to a low level in older people.

Attack rates in epidemic influenza are high and incidence rates of 20–40 per cent. have often been noted. The disease is rarely fatal, but there is a marked feverish reaction with inflammation of the bronchial mucosa. Some cases, however, are complicated by bacterial pneumonia, and in these the outcome may be rapidly fatal. The invasion of virus-damaged tissue by *Staphylococcus aureus* is followed by the formation of multiple abscesses and severe tissue destruction with necrosis of the trachea, bronchi and bronchioles. Fulminating staphylococcal pneumonia is the cause of many influenzal deaths, especially in the elderly. Secondary invasion with pneumococci, *H. influenzae* or haemolytic streptococci is also associated with influenzal pneumonia. It was this complication which was responsible for the very high mortality in the 1918–19 pandemic.

Immunity to influenza is generally believed to be short-lived and in experiments with type B virus human volunteers could be reinfected with the same strain four months after recovery from this first infection. However, epidemiological evidence suggests that immunity to the natural infection may last for three to four years (Pickles, Burnet and McArthur, 1947).

Influenza virus type C does not cause epidemics but gives rise to widespread subclinical infections.

Prophylaxis.—As influenza has an incubation period of only one or two days, control measures such as isolation and quarantine are scarcely applicable. Intensive efforts have been made to develop vaccines to protect key personnel such as medical and nursing staffs and public service employees. Egg-cultivated vaccines containing formol-inactivated strains with or without adjuvants (alum, oil emulsions) have been under extensive trial and have yielded results which appear to be disappointing. However, there are considerable difficulties in the interpretation of the results of trials of influenza vaccines because the position is blurred by infections with other respiratory viruses. On some occasions, as in the case of the Asian strain, it has been possible to prepare a vaccine containing the current strain and to administer one or two doses of it before the epidemic reached the community. In such circumstances, the attack rate was reduced to about one-third of that in control groups (M.R.C. Report 1958). Polyvalent vaccines prepared from a mixture of strains of types A and B known to contain all the major antigenic groupings have been used with good effect. At present a vaccine containing A2/Singapore/1/57, A2/England1/61,

B/England/939/59 and B/Tai/4/62 is used. Provided that a vaccine contains the right strains and is given at the right time it should protect 50 to 70 per cent. of the recipients. The possibility of enhancing the antigenic effect of these vaccines by the use of mineral oil adjuvants is under investigation and recently published results are encouraging.

Swine Influenza Virus.—This virus is associated with sudden epizootics of acute respiratory disease in pigs. By itself the virus causes only mild symptoms in the animals, but when combined with infection with *Haemophilus suis* it causes a severe disease. During non-epizootic periods the virus is maintained in earthworms and lungworms. The sequence of events is that lungworms living in the bronchi of pigs ingest the virus, which then is carried throughout the life cycle of the parasite. Larvae from the lungs are coughed up, and swallowed and finally reach the ground in the faeces excreted by the animal. Here they are ingested by earthworms, in which they persist for long periods. When such earthworms are eaten by pigs, no ill effects result, but if the animals are also given an intramuscular injection of *H. suis*, or stressed by exposure to cold, they develop typical swine influenza.

The swine influenza virus has the general properties of myxoviruses and is related antigenically to type A virus. Since swine influenza was first noticed as a disease in 1918, when the pandemic of human influenza was rife, it has been suggested that both diseases were caused by the same agent. Support for this theory is given by the fact that many people of the generation who experienced the 1918-19 pandemic still possess neutralising antibodies for the swine influenza virus, while those born after 1923 have no antibodies for the strain.

Para-influenza Viruses

These viruses are associated with febrile respiratory disease early in life. They appear to be ubiquitous causing endemic infections throughout the year. The commonest clinical syndrome is fever with mild respiratory symptoms and pharyngitis but the viruses are also an important cause of croup (acute laryngo-tracheo-bronchitis) and of acute tracheitis and bronchiolitis. Repeated infections with this group of viruses is probably common and antibody surveys indicate the presence of antibodies to para-influenza viruses in a large percentage of children by the time they reach school age.

Para-influenza viruses have many of the general characters of myxoviruses; for instance, they possess the same neuraminidase as the influenza viruses A and B and are thus able to cause the agglutination of mammalian and avian erythrocytes, and they are also ether sensitive. They grow well in primary cultures of monkey kidney and human embryonic, amnion and HeLa cells, but poorly or not at all in the chick embryo. Because they produce only minimal cytopathic effects their presence is detected by the ability of infected cells to adsorb erythrocytes to their surface (haemadsorption). When first isolated the viruses were known as "haemadsorbing (HA)" viruses.

The viruses differ from the influenza viruses in their somewhat larger size (90–180 mμ) and in their ability to lyse as well as agglutinate red blood-cells. They share antigens with the mumps and Newcastle viruses (Cook *et al.*, 1959) and form with them a subgroup of the myxoviruses—the "multiform viruses".

Myxovirus para-influenzae 1.—This group includes the haemadsorption virus type 2, or HA2 virus (Chanock *et al.*, 1958) and the Sendai virus which is also known as the Japanese haemagglutinating virus or influenza D. The HA2 virus has been isolated frequently from cases of croup in young children, minor respiratory illness, bronchitis, and bronchopneumonia. The Sendai virus was originally isolated in mice from cases of pneumonitis in new-born children but its endemicity in stocks of laboratory mice makes it difficult to assess the significance of this finding. The Sendai virus is closely related antigenically to the HA2 virus but differs from it in that it multiplies readily in the allantoic membranes of the chick embryo. The Sendai virus itself has never been isolated in Great Britain.

Myxovirus para-influenzae 2, or the croup associated (CA) virus has been isolated from minor respiratory illnesses and bronchopneumonia and from cases of croup. It may not, however, be as commonly associated with croup as the para-influenza 1 virus. This virus has no cytopathic effect on tissue cultures but is detected by its agglutination of chick (and to a lesser extent of human group O) erythrocytes. Adsorption and agglutination occur at 4° C. and the virus elutes rapidly at 37° C. Antigenically this virus is related to the mumps virus but not to other myxoviruses. It is probably identical with an indigenous monkey myxovirus known as SV5; as many as 30 per cent. of some batches of uninoculated monkey kidney tissue cultures have been found to carry this virus.

Myxovirus para-influenzae 3 or haemadsorption type I (HA1) is associated, like the foregoing para-influenza viruses, with respiratory illnesses and with croup and bronchopneumonia. It has also been found in the nasal secretions of cattle in transit and suffering from a respiratory illness known as "shipping fever". Unlike other para-influenza viruses, para-influenza 3 may produce a cytopathic effect seen as giant cell plaques in tissue cultures of human amnion cells growing under an agar overlay.

Myxovirus para-influenzae 4 (M-25 strain) has recently been isolated from cases of mild respiratory illness. It has no cytopathic effect; does not grow in eggs, and is recognised only by the use of the haemadsorption method.

Laboratory Diagnosis.—Primary isolation of para-influenza viruses in the chick embryo may be difficult or impossible and tissue culture methods are preferred. Cultures of monkey kidney cells are the most useful for this purpose but primary human amnion, human embryonic kidney, HeLa, or HEp2 cells are all satisfactory. The cytopathic effect produced is often minimal and may be absent; the viruses are detected by haemadsorption or haemagglutination. Serologically the diagnosis is confirmed by the observation of rising titres of antibodies in paired sera using neutralisation, complement-fixation, or haemadsorption or haemagglutination inhibition tests. Because of the antigenic sharing between these viruses and the mumps virus the results of these tests may be difficult to interpret. Parallel tests should always be carried out with the mumps S and V antigens for comparison.

Mumps Virus

Mumps is an acute contagious disease whose most constant and characteristic feature is a large painful swelling of one or both parotid glands. The disease is one of great antiquity and was one of the first infections to be recognised, for it was accurately described by Hippocrates in the fifth century B.C. The name is derived from the mumbling speech which is the result of the pain on moving the jaws. Usually there is a constitutional reaction and not infrequently other glands as well as the parotids are involved.

Properties of the Mumps Virus (*Myxovirus parotitidis*).—The size of the elementary bodies varies from 80 to 240 mμ in diameter (Ghosh Ray and Swain, 1954). Filaments have not been described.

Cultivation.—The virus grows rather slowly in the amniotic and allantoic cavity of the chick embryo. Six to eight day embryos are used and should be incubated for five days at 35° C. After two or three amniotic passages, most strains can be transferred to the allantoic cavity where they adapt themselves and grow very readily. A few strains, however, remain incapable of being transferred in this way. When inoculated directly into the opening of the parotid duct in monkeys the virus causes typical clinical mumps; the parotid glands contain much virus and emulsions of them can be used as complement-fixing or skin testing antigens.

The mumps virus agglutinates fowl, human and other red blood cells, fixes complement in the presence of specific antibody, and elicits a delayed allergic reaction in the skin of persons who have previously been infected. Like the Newcastle virus it causes the lysis of erythrocytes. Infective particles can be concentrated by centrifugation at 20,000 r.p.m. for 20 min. but the particles of the complement-fixing antigen require 30,000 r.p.m. for 60 min.

Viability.—Infectivity is rapidly lost at room temperature. The virus is well preserved in skimmed milk at −50° C. or −70 °C. or by freeze drying. The haemagglutinin, haemolysin and infective properties are destroyed by heat at 56° C. for 20 min. The complement-fixing and allergic skin antigens withstand 65° C. for an hour. Exposure to 0·2 per cent. formalin at 4° C. for 24 hr. and intense ultra-violet light irradiation for 0·28 sec. destroy the infectivity of the virus without impairing the haemagglutinin or complement-fixing antigens. Ether treatment at 4° C. completely destroys infectivity. The virus is most stable between pH 5·8 and pH 8·0.

Antigenic Characters.—The mumps virus is a single antigenic entity distinct from other myxoviruses; it is not subject to variation and there are no marked differences between the strains. There are two components of the virus which are capable of fixing complement, the V or viral antigen and the S or soluble antigen. The V antigen is associated with the virus elementary body and the S antigen, which is analogous to the soluble antigen of the influenza virus, is a smaller particle extracted from cells in the early stages of infection.

Pathogenesis.—The incubation period of mumps is one of the longest, 18–21 days. The common manifestations are fever with unilateral or bilateral parotitis. The virus is excreted in the saliva for about three days after the onset and transmission is by the inhalation of infected particles or by fomites contaminated with saliva. Patients are thought to be infectious for about three days before the onset and to remain so for about six days thereafter. In young children convalescence is uneventful and recovery is complete in about ten days. In about 30 per cent. of cases infected with the virus the disease is inapparent. After the virus has been inhaled it multiplies locally in the oropharynx during the incubation period and after an interval reaches the bloodstream to be disseminated to distant organs. Although the virus may reach the parotid and submaxillary glands by direct spread from the mouth, infection of the testes, central nervous system, pancreas, thyroid gland, ovary, and breasts, is almost certainly blood-borne.

In males over the age of 13 years mumps may be complicated by orchitis which appears some four to seven days after the onset of parotitis. Up to 20 per cent. of male cases are affected. In almost every case of mumps there seems to be some involvement of the central nervous system with an increase in the lymphocytes in the cerebrospinal fluid. Occasionally the condition proceeds to a frank meningoencephalitis which presents four to seven days after the onset of parotitis; in these cases the mumps virus can be isolated from the cerebrospinal fluid. Rather uncommonly mumps meningoencephalitis may occur without any sign of involvement of the salivary glands and is indistinguishable clinically from aseptic meningitis caused by other viruses such as those of the ECHO and Coxsackie groups. In many cases submaxillary gland involvement is encountered, but pancreatitis, oophoritis, and thyroiditis are rare complications. Mastitis may occur in up to 15 per cent. of females infected.

Epidemiology.—Mumps is world-wide in its distribution, and the only reservoir of infection is man. The disease is predominantly one of children aged five to fifteen years, but adults who have escaped infection in childhood are often attacked. The disease is probably transmitted by the same mechanisms as those in respiratory tract infections. Epidemics of mumps are not uncommon in young soldiers in army camps. Although mumps is one of the common diseases of childhood, it is not apparently as highly infectious as measles. Amongst adults the history of a clinical mumps infection is obtained in about 60 per cent. of people, whereas 90 per cent. have had measles.

Laboratory Diagnosis

Virus isolation is carried out by inoculating saliva or cerebrospinal fluid into fertile eggs. Saliva can conveniently be collected by placing dental cotton-wool rolls over the openings of the parotid ducts and leaving them in the mouth for about twenty minutes. The rolls are then removed and placed in screw-capped vials containing Hanks' balanced salt solution with added antibiotics. The containers should be transported to the laboratory frozen at $-70°$ C. in insulated boxes containing solid carbon dioxide. On arrival at the laboratory, the saliva is expressed from the rolls, added to the transport fluid and clarified in the centrifuge at 2000 r.p.m. for ten minutes. The supernatant is inoculated into the amniotic cavity of eight 11-day-old chick embryos; the eggs are then incubated for five days at 35° C. The virus may be detected in the amniotic fluid by the haemagglutination of fowl red blood cells and its final identification is established serologically with specific antiserum in complement-fixation or haemagglutination inhibition tests. The primary isolation of the virus is sometimes a matter of difficulty because saliva may have toxic properties for the chick embryo, and because only a small proportion of inoculated eggs show evidence of infection.

Serological Tests.—Antibody rises can be detected in paired acute and convalescent sera. The complement-fixation test using both soluble and viral antigens is recommended. Antibodies to the S antigen develop early and are present in significant amounts within two or three days of the onset of the infection and they may reach their peak titre before the appearance of antibody to the V antigen. Antibodies to the V antigen appear on the eighth or ninth day of the disease, reach their maximum by the end of a month and thereafter decline very slowly (Ghosh Ray and Swain, 1953). Subsequently the anti-S antibodies disappear relatively rapidly and are seldom detectable nine months later. Antibodies to the V antigen persist for several years at very low, barely detectable levels. The haemagglutination-inhibiting antibody is similar in its duration to the anti-V antibody. The skin test for mumps is of little practical value in diagnosis because the hypersensitive state is not developed until three to four weeks after the onset.

Prophylaxis.—Gamma globulin ***prepared from mumps couvalescent serum*** may be of value in conferring passive immunity to exposed persons and if given immediately after the onset of parotitis reduces the incidence of orchitis. Gamma globulin from normal adults contains only traces of specific antibody and has little protective value.

Vaccines prepared from egg-grown strains inactivated by formalin or ultra-violet light have been used with some success in reducing the incidence of mumps in army camps and in adults exposed to infection. Although antibody formation is stimulated by the vaccine, booster doses are needed after six to nine months to maintain the antibody level. A living attenuated egg-adapted strain of mumps has also been used and is sprayed into the mouth; antibody production reaches the same proportions as with the inactivated vaccine. No clinical case of mumps has been reported as a result of the use of the live vaccine, and this method is at present on trial for prevention of the infection.

Newcastle Disease Virus

Newcastle disease (a form of fowl pest) is an extremely infectious epizootic condition of domestic poultry. Fowls, turkeys, pheasants, guinea-fowl as well as many other avian species are affected. Cormorants may suffer inapparent infections and act as a source of infection for poultry in coastal regions. The disease has a world-wide distribution and constitutes a major economic hazard. In Europe the infection is characterised by hyperpyrexia, severe diarrhoea, and a thick mucopurulent nasal discharge. The incubation period is three to ten days. The mortality rate is 90–95 per cent. In America the disease is milder, having a mortality of 5–50 per cent.; signs of tremor, incoordination and wing and leg paralysis predominate.

The disease can be transmitted experimentally to susceptible poultry by the inoculation of discharges from infected animals and also with blood and tissues, *e.g.* spleen and bone-marrow.

The Newcastle virus which causes this disease has been named *Myxovirus multiforme*. The elementary body is roughly spherical with a diameter varying from 80 to 200 mμ (average 115 mμ). Filamentous forms occur, but are found only infrequently. The strains grow readily in the fertile hen's egg and kill the embryo with haemorrhagic lesions in 48 hours. In HeLa cell monolayer tissue cultures they produce a characteristic cytopathic effect with syncytium formation. The virus agglutinates red blood cells from fowls and a variety of mammalian species and elutes from them rather rapidly and often incompletely at room temperature; in high concentrations it has marked powers of haemolysis. The virus is immunologically distinct from other myxoviruses, although there are minor relationships between it and the mumps, Sendai and para-influenza viruses in complement-fixation tests. All strains are closely similar to each other in antigenic structure and there is little or no tendency to variation. Laboratory diagnosis may be accomplished by isolation of the virus in fertile hen's eggs and also by demonstration of specific antibodies in the blood by means of a haemagglutination inhibition test.

Occasionally the Newcastle disease virus causes inflammation of the conjunctiva in man due to an accidental infection in the laboratory or during the handling of the virus. There is a severe conjunctivitis which may be accompanied by a painful swelling of the pre-auricular gland and, more rarely, by a severe generalised influenzal type of illness.

A vaccine containing a living attenuated egg-adapted strain of the Newcastle virus has been developed for poultry flocks and is given by intranasal instillation. In England, however, a β propriolactone-inactivated vaccine is now in general use.

Fowl Plague Virus

This is a highly contagious infection of chickens, turkeys, pheasants and some wild birds. The disease is rapidly fatal; and nearly 99 per cent. of infected birds die within 24–36 hours of the onset. The incubation period is three to five days. A mucopurulent nasal discharge and oedema of the head and neck are the usual signs and at autopsy small petechial haemorrhages are present in the serous membranes. There is histological evidence of a diffuse encephalitis.

Properties of the Fowl Plague Virus (*Myxovirus pestis-galli*).—The size of the elementary bodies varies from 80–120 mμ and filamentous forms which may be up to 6 μ in length, are common. The virus grows readily in all the tissues of the developing hen's egg and kills the embryo in about 36 hours. Intranuclear lesions, probably inclusions, have been described in the tissues. The virus is readily adsorbed to fowl red blood cells and causes their agglutination. The virus shares the group complement-fixing antigen of the influenza A virus. Minor serological differences between strains have been found in haemagglutination-inhibition tests. The blood of infected birds contains the virus in high concentrations and can be used to transfer the infection experimentally.

Respiratory Syncytial Virus

The respiratory syncytial virus was originally isolated from a cold-like illness in a colony of captive chimpanzees and was known for a time as the chimpanzees coryza associated (CCA) virus. It was however soon realised that it was also associated with human infection especially in young children.

Properties of the Virus.—The virions are 90–120 mμ in diameter and resemble the myxoviruses morphologically. There is a central coiled filament enclosed by an outer membrane. Since 5-fluoro-uracil inhibits the growth of the virus it probably has RNA as its nucleic acid. There has been no report of haemagglutination or haemadsorption activity by the virus.

Cultivation.—The virus does not grow in the chick embryo and it has no effect on mice, guinea-pigs, or rabbits. It grows rather slowly in continuous lines of human cancer cells such as HEp2, KB, HeLa, and also the Chang liver cells, but not so readily in primary kidney tissue cultures. One satisfactory method for the cultivation of the virus is to use monolayers of HEp2 cells grown in medium 199 with 10 per cent. calf serum added; when ready for inoculation the monolayers are gently washed with medium 199 to rinse away the calf serum; for a maintenance medium during virus growth medium 199 is supplemented with 5 per cent. chicken serum. The sodium bicarbonate content is increased by adding 4 per cent. of the stock 1·4 per cent. sodium bicarbonate solution; incubation is at 36° C.

The virus grows in the cytoplasm of the host cells where it may produce small eosinophilic inclusions. It produces an obvious cytopathic effect which becomes apparent three to seven days after inoculation with the occurrence of giant cells and syncytia. Infectivity titres are usually low and are seldom above 10^{-5}. Plaques are formed in HEp2 monolayers.

Viability.—The virus survives quick freezing at $-70°$ C. but at higher temperatures its infectivity may rapidly be lost. Specimens such as throat swabs should not be refrigerated but should be treated with antibiotics and introduced into suitable tissue cultures with a minimal delay. The virus is destroyed at pH 3·0.

Antigenic Characters.—A complement fixing antigen is produced and is contained in a particle smaller than the virion itself. Complement-fixation and neutralising tests can be used for diagnostic purposes.

Pathogenesis.—The virus causes colds and minor upper respiratory tract infections with cough in adults but in children especially in infants aged 6–12 months the lower respiratory tract is often involved and bronchitis, bronchiolitis and bronchopneumonia occur (Holzel *et al.*, 1963). Young children aged one to two years may suffer from croup, "virus pneumonia" or from mild cold-like illnesses.

Epidemiology.—Infection with the respiratory syncytial virus appears to be common in the population of this country and Hambling (1964) has found that 66 per cent. of all persons over the age of five years possess both complement fixing and neutralising antibodies in the serum and that over the age of 15 years 93 per cent. have neutralising antibodies. The lowest incidence of antibodies was in the age group six months to one year. Young children under the age of seven months seem to show a relatively poor serological response after infection; some 20 per cent. develop a rising titre of complement fixing antibodies and 45 per cent. neutralising antibodies. It is a characteristic of this virus that it causes localised foci of infection which may be limited to one particular area or community. Infection occurs for brief periods in the winter months with long intervals between the outbreaks.

THE MEASLES, CANINE DISTEMPER, RINDERPEST TRIAD

These three viruses are grouped together because of similarities in a number of their properties. Morphologically they have the helical symmetry and general appearances of the para-influenza viruses and are likely to be classified as members of Waterson's second group of myxoviruses (see p. 394). In their pathogenicity they are characterised by a sharp generalised illness with a viraemic phase and the complications of bronchopneumonia and encephalitis. There is a considerable volume of evidence that the three viruses share some common antigenic material in varying proportions.

MEASLES

Measles is probably the most infectious of all the common fevers. The clinical diagnosis of the disease is usually not a difficult matter because a characteristic macular rash develops after a prodromal period of fever with catarrhal symptoms, conjunctivitis and the appearance of Koplik's spots on the buccal mucosa. The incubation period is 10–14 days and the rash often appears 14 days after exposure.

Properties of the Virus.—The diameter of the virus in filtration experiments is 140 mμ. The central core is composed of helices 16 mμ in diameter with subunits arranged with a 4·5 mμ periodicity. The virion is covered by an outer membrane on which there are radially disposed projections. The nucleic acid of this virus is probably RNA because growth is inhibited by 5-fluoro-uracil. In these respects the measles virus resembles the para-influenza and respiratory syncytial viruses.

Cultivation.—The virus can be isolated from the blood or throat washings of a patient during the first 24 hours after the onset of fever. For this purpose primary cultures of human amnion or chorion cells or a continuous line of amnion cells provide the most suitable susceptible tissue culture cells. Monkey kidney cells are less satisfactory.

Once established in tissue cultures, the measles virus will grow in a wide range of primate tissue cultures. Human kidney obtained at operation or at autopsy and human embryonic lung or kidney all provide highly susceptible cells. The virus also grows in continuous lines of cells derived from human normal tissues such as heart, kidney, amnion and bone marrow, as well as in lines of carcinoma cells such as HeLa, KB, and HEp2. Monolayer cultures of dog, and bovine kidney are also susceptible. In monolayers of monkey kidney cells and of some strains of HeLa cells small plaques are produced.

The cytopathic effect of the measles virus is characteristic, with the formation of large multinucleate giant cells and syncytial masses in which many vacuoles give a lacework appearance. After continued passage of the virus in human amnion cells the nature of the cytopathic effect alters, and in addition to giant cells, increasing numbers of refractile stellate cells appear. Variation of the constituents of the culture medium may modify the cytopathic lesions. With glutamine deficiency, for example, more giant cells are formed, but when the glutamine is restored the number of giant cells is diminished and the appearance of the cytopathic effect is delayed, while the virus yield is increased. The most constant feature of cells infected with measles virus is the late appearance of Cowdry type A eosinophilic intranuclear inclusions. Multiple intra-cytoplasmic inclusions also occur. Grown in monolayers of *patas* monkey kidney cells the virus produces countable microplaques.

Measles can be reproduced in rhesus monkeys by the parenteral inoculation of blood or catarrhal secretions from patients or infected tissue culture fluids. The disease is usually mild and about one-third of the inoculated animals develop fever, conjunctivitis and a macular rash. Many monkeys imported for experimental use harbour a virus, the Monkey-Intra-Nuclear Inclusion Agent (MINIA), which is indistinguishable from the measles virus. This infection is usually inapparent and is acquired soon after the animals are captured. These circumstances make the majority of monkeys unreliable as experimental animals for measles and the presence of MINIA in cultures of their kidney cells may give rise to considerable difficulties. No mammals other than monkeys have been infected successfully with the measles virus. Some strains of the virus have been adapted to the amniotic cavity or choriollantoic membrane of the chick embryo after their primary isolation in tissue culture.

Viability.—The virus survives over two weeks at 4° C. or 22° C., and for many months in the frozen state in the temperature range −15° to −79° C. Freeze drying preserves the virus well, though with some loss of infectivity. Formaldehyde in a concentration of 0·025 per cent. at 37° C. for four days brings about complete loss of infectivity without alteration of the complement-fixing activity. The virus is ether sensitive. Below pH 4·5 the virus is inactivated but it is stable within the range pH 5·5–9 for 3 hours at 0° C.

Haemagglutination.—Concentrated preparations of the measles virus agglutinate rhesus monkey red blood cells at 37° C. The haemagglutinin does not elute spontaneously and is not related to the neuraminadase of the myxoviruses. Haemagglutination-inhibition may be used as a method for the estimation of serum antibodies.

Antigenic Characters.—Measles virus strains are uniform antigenically. A complement-fixing antigen is present in infected tissue culture fluids; it can be separated from elementary bodies by centrifugation and has a particle size of 7–13 mμ.

The measles virus is related antigenically to the virus of canine distemper. It is neutralised specifically by the serum of ferrets recovered from distemper, but not by normal ferret serum. Conversely, ferrets immunised by the measles virus are partially protected when challenged with distemper virus.

Pathogenesis.—Young children in the prodromal phase, when the catarrhal symptoms are prominent, are the main source of the measles virus. They discharge infected particles which are inhaled by the new victim and the virus reaches the respiratory tract, where it grows silently for some days in lymphoid tissue. When multiplication has continued to the point when many infected cells break open, the virus floods into the circulation and causes the prodromal illness. During the following two or three days the virus is localised in the skin and there produces the rash. This viraemia is quenched when antibodies appear in the blood.

It is of interest that multinucleate giant cells (Warthin-Finkeldy cells) similar to those occurring in tissue cultures can be found in the organs of persons who have died during an attack of measles. It is probable that the giant cells begin to be formed about seven days before the appearancc of the rash.

Measles is most infectious in the two or three days before the appearance of the rash; thereafter infectivity rapidly wanes and after a few days is lost.

Epidemiology.—Measles is endemic throughout most countries of the world. The disease has a characteristic tendency to epidemicity every second year so that in Great Britain and North America there are "measles years" which alternate with years in which only a few cases are encountered.

The greatest incidence in measles is in the age group 1-5 years, and by the age of 20 years 90 per cent. of persons have had an attack of the disease. After the first six months of life passively acquired maternal immunity disappears and susceptibility is universal. Only about 1 per cent. of these susceptibles fail to contract measles on their first close contact with it. Although measles is usually benign in young children it may cause severe or even fatal illnesses in infants under the age of one year or in elderly people. Secondary invasion with such pathogenic bacteria as haemolytic streptococci, staphylococci and *H. influenzae* cause the complications of bronchopneumonia or otitis media. Another serious complication of measles is encephalomyelitis developing two to six days after the rash; the features of this condition may resemble those of aseptic meningitis but there is an average case fatality of 15 per cent. Encephalitis occurs in about 1 in 1000 cases of measles, is commoner in girls than boys, and is more frequent in the 5–9 years age-group than in younger children. Miller (1964) gives an analysis of the frequency of the complications in measles.

When measles is introduced into an area where previously it was not endemic, a sweeping epidemic of great severity follows amongst a virgin population of highly susceptible persons. In these circumstances there is a high incidence of complications and the case mortality is increased. Epidemics of this type have occurred in isolated communities, especially on islands; one particularly severe outbreak occurred in Greenland in 1951. When the infection was first introduced into the Fiji Islands in 1875, it carried off 20–25 per cent. of the entire population.

Laboratory Diagnosis

The simplest method is to stain smears of the nasal secretions by Giemsa's method and to search for the typical giant cells. The virus can be isolated from throat swabs or washings taken during the 48 hr. before and after the onset of the rash. It has also been recovered from the blood, and urine in the prodromal period. After antibiotic treatment the materials are inoculated into grown monolayers of monkey kidney or human kidney cells. The cytopathic effect and giant cell formation may begin to appear after 48–72 hr. but not infrequently is not detected for as long as 10–16 days. Subsequently the virus may be propagated in primary human amnion or HEp2 cells with greater yields.

Serum antibodies appear a few days after the onset of the rash, reach a peak about 10 days later and decline slowly thereafter, but a detectable level remains indefinitely. Antibodies are most conveniently estimated by the complement-fixation method but neutralisation and haemagglutination-inhibition techniques can also be employed.

Prophylaxis.—Measles is so infectious and susceptibility to it so high that there is no point in isolating cases to stop the spread of the infection in the population. Hospital patients with measles, however, should be isolated to protect them from the risk of cross-infection with pathogenic bacteria, and to stop the spread of infection to patients ill with other diseases.

Passive immunity can be conferred on contacts by the subcutaneous inoculation of convalescent or adult serum, or gamma globulin prepared from them. The protective effect is complete if an adequate dose is given within five days of exposure; after this time the disease may not be prevented, but its severity is usually modified and the risk of complications reduced. The use of gamma globulin prepared from pooled normal adult sera is effective; the dose is 15 mg. per pound body weight.

Vaccines.—Two types have been subjected to controlled trials. The first contains virus grown in tissue culture and inactivated by formalin; even after a series of three subcutaneous inoculations its antigenic potency is not sufficient to give full protection. The second type contains living measles virus attenuated by much repeated egg passage. A single subcutaneous injection of this vaccine stimulates the production of specific antibodies in 97·5 per cent. of recipients and confers a full measure of protection. This vaccine however suffers from the disadvantage that a proportion of the recipients develop a generalised feverish reaction lasting about 48 hr. and 11 per cent. of the children develop a rash.

Canine Distemper

Distemper is a highly infectious disease which causes more deaths and permanent disability in young dogs than any other infection.

Properties of the virus.—The diameter is 115–160 mμ. In negatively stained preparations helices 15–17 mμ in diameter form the core and the general appearances are the same as those of the measles virus.

Cultivation.—The virus can be isolated from the blood and discharges of infected animals during the acute phase and can also be recovered from the urine and faeces. It is present in the lungs of fatal cases in large amounts and also in the spleen, liver, brain and other tissues. For primary isolation the materials are inoculated on to monolayers of dog or ferret kidney cells in which a cytopathic effect with giant cells and syncytium formation occurs. Intra-cytoplasmic but not intra-nuclear inclusions are formed.

The disease can be transmitted with filtrates of infected materials to dogs, and ferrets which are highly susceptible. The virus has been adapted to grow in suckling mice and suckling hamsters.

Some strains of the distemper virus have been adapted to growth in the chick embryo either in the yolk-sac or on the chorio-allantoic membrane where greyish white lesions are produced.

Viability.—The virus is reasonably stable at room temperature but above 32° C. it rapidly loses its infectivity. It survives for months at −10° C. and indefinitely at −76° C. or after freeze drying. The virus is ether sensitive and is inactivated by 0·1 per cent. formaldehyde in a few hours.

Antigenic Characters.—Antibodies to the distemper virus can be demonstrated by neutralisation tests in tissue cultures and eggs, by complement-fixation and by precipitation in agar gel. The serum of patients recovered from measles has antibodies to the distemper virus and that of dogs recovered from distemper has antibodies for the measles virus. Cross immunity against the heterologous virus however is often only partial and in some instances, *e.g.* with egg-propagated viruses, may be of minor degree or lacking.

Pathogenesis.—After an incubation period of four days the common manifestations are fever, coryza and mucopurulent discharges from the eyes and nose. Bronchopneumonia is a frequent complication and inflammation of the gastric and intestinal mucosa is not uncommon. In their pathogenesis there are many resemblances between canine distemper and measles. Other animals such as ferrets, silver foxes and mink together with wolves and some small rodents are also susceptible to distemper.

The virus is present in the blood and discharges of infected animals during the acute phase and has also been recovered from the urine and faeces. The disease can be transmitted with filtrates of these materials to dogs and ferrets by subcutaneous inoculation. In the ferret the incubation period is nine to eleven days. Intra-cytoplasmic eosinophilic inclusions are characteristically present; they are found principally in the epithelial cells of the respiratory tract and the urinary tract, particularly in those of the bladder.

They can, however, be found in many other situations. Intra-nuclear inclusions may also be present.

Active immunisation of dogs can be carried out with a vaccine containing a living attenuated strain of the distemper virus cultivated in eggs. This vaccine has to a large extent replaced other methods of immunisation in which living virus was combined with a protective dose of hyper-immune serum or with the previous use of a killed vaccine.

Hard pad disease in its initial stages is indistinguishable from distemper. There is fever, conjunctivitis and diarrhoea, followed by a painful hyperkeratosis of the pads of the feet and the nose. Later, nervous symptoms appear, followed by convulsions, and death occurs four to six weeks after the onset. The condition is due to a virus which is closely related to the distemper virus, being infective to ferrets after an incubation period of 23 days (cf. distemper).

Rinderpest

Rinderpest or cattle plague is an acute and highly infectious disease, especially of cattle, but also of all ruminants and swine.

Properties of the virus.—Morphologically the virus resembles the measles virus but is more pleomorphic with diameters ranging from 120 to 300 mμ. There is an internal helix 17·5 mμ in diameter and a covering membrane.

Cultivation.—The virus can be cultivated in tissue culture monolayers of the kidneys or testes of calf, sheep, pig and hamster. Multinucleate syncytial masses are formed containing Cowdry type B inclusions in the nuclei and in the cytoplasm. Some strains have been adapted to grow in the yolk sac or the chorio-allantoic membrane of the chick embryo. Strains have been adapted to grow in goats and rabbits for vaccine production.

Viability.—The virus in dried secretions outside the body does not survive more than 48 hr. and is easily inactivated by heat, ultra-violet light, putrefactive changes and the usual disinfectants of which strong alkalis are the best. The virus in lymph nodes and spleen survives well at $-17°$ C. to $-20°$ C. and is preserved indefinitely by freeze drying. For preservation the optimum is pH 7·0. The virus is ether sensitive.

Antigenic Characters.—Antigenically the virus is stable and there are no confirmed reports to suggest a multiplicity of types. Antibodies to rinderpest can be demonstrated by neutralisation tests in tissue cultures or susceptible animals. Agar-gel diffusion methods show that the virus in infective tissue has two antigens, one heat labile and the other heat stable. This method is useful for detecting the presence of the virus in infected tissues—*e.g.* lymph nodes. Sera from rinderpest infected animals neutralise the distemper virus in dogs and have some power to neutralise the measles virus in tissue cultures. The distemper virus will confer some immunity against rinderpest in cattle and during measles, antibodies active against the rinderpest virus may develop.

Pathogenesis.—Rinderpest is characterised by fever, severe haemorrhagic catarrh from the mucous membranes of the nose and eyes, and by a profuse diarrhoea followed by weakness and exhaustion. The incubation period is three to eight days and the affected animals usually die four to seven days after the onset. Oedema, haemorrhagic ulceration of the intestine, with inflammation of the Peyer's patches are characteristic post-mortem findings. Pneumonia is found in many cases. Cattle, goats, sheep, pigs and many species of wild game suffer the natural infection. Regular passage of strains adapted to grow in laboratory animals such as the rabbit or guinea-pig, or in the chick embryo, may result in the emergence of a mutant with enhanced virulence for the new host but with diminished virulence for cattle. Vaccine strains have been developed in this way.

Epidemiology.—Rinderpest is endemic in all parts of Asia and Africa (South Africa is now free) and is the cause of much economic loss. The disease is spread by direct contact between infected and susceptible animals. The exact route of transfer of the infection is not established, but is thought to be through contaminated food and drinking water. Biting arthropods have not been incriminated as vectors.

Because rinderpest is endemic in many parts of Africa and Asia, there is always a risk that the infection may be conveyed to new areas. The movement of herds and the importation of beasts from distant areas has often introduced the virus into a susceptible animal community with the result that a devastating epizootic has broken out.

Control.—The disease has been excluded from Great Britain, most of Europe, and from North and South America by a rigid embargo on the importation of animals or meat from enzootic areas. In countries where rinderpest is enzootic, the principal means of control is prophylactic vaccination.

Several vaccines containing live attentuated strains of the rinderpest virus have been developed and their use is rapidly followed by an effective immunity which lasts from one to two years. These vaccines have been prepared from goat-adapted, rabbit-adapted, and egg-adapted virus strains. A vaccine containing live virus propagated in tissue culture is at present on trial.

Live vaccines have the advantage that they rapidly induce resistance by virtue of the interference phenomenon and they have been effective in the field in checking an outbreak. Care, however, is needed in selecting the type of vaccine to be used because some of the strains are of sufficient virulence to cause severe reactions and some mortality in certain breeds of cattle. Milder strains, on the other hand, may induce only a short-lived immunity. The goat-adapted (caprinised) virus should not be used on stocks of European cattle, which are usually highly susceptible to rinderpest. It is used successfully on indigenous cattle in Africa and confers an immunity lasting four to six years. The rabbit-adapted (lapinised) virus is less virulent and is used throughout Africa and Asia; the immunity given lasts about two years. The egg-cultivated virus has not been extensively used. Calves born of immune dams lack rinderpest antibodies at birth but receive them in colostrum in the first few hours of life. The calf retains this immunity for several months and cannot be actively immunised satisfactorily until the age of eight months.

Laboratory Diagnosis.—A rapid post-mortem diagnosis of rinderpest can be made by placing a small fragment of infected tissue (*e.g.* lymph gland) and specific antiserum in adjacent cells in an agar-gel diffusion plate side by side with known positive and negative controls. Lines of precipitation form within a few hours at room temperature and the specific antigen of the rinderpest virus can be identified with certainty. The virus is isolated by the inoculation of tissue cultures or susceptible cattle with suspensions of infected tissue. It can be identified in complement-fixation and agar gel diffusion tests and in neutralisation tests in which immune rabbits or cattle are challenged with the freshly isolated strain.

ADENOVIRUSES

Adenoviruses derive their name from the fact that they were first isolated from fragments of adenoid tissue removed surgically and grown in tissue culture. They are able to live in both tonsillar and adenoid tissue in a latent or masked form without any apparent harm to the individual. In other situations, however, adenoviruses cause a wide variety of clinical syndromes including coryza, pharyngitis, sporadic or endemic acute respiratory tract infections, pneumonia, acute conjunctivitis, and epidemic kerato-conjunctivitis. The adenovirus group consists of 31 human, 11 simian, and 2 bovine serotypes as well as the canine hepatitis virus, a murine adenovirus, and an avian adenovirus GAL (Pereira *et al.*, 1963).

Properties of the viruses.—The elementary bodies are roughly spherical and approximately 100 mμ in diameter. When seen in electron microscopical preparations stained by uranyl acetate they have a hexagonal outline and a central electron dense mass. The external structure of the virus particle has been studied by a negative staining technique in which the virus is treated with phosphotungstic acid and sprayed on to electron microscope grids (Horne & Wildy, 1963). By this method the capsids are seen to have cubical symmetry and are revealed as regular icosahedra each with 252 spherical surface subunits 7 mμ in diameter (Fig. 24). There is no pericapsidal membrane. Within the capsid there is a DNA core.

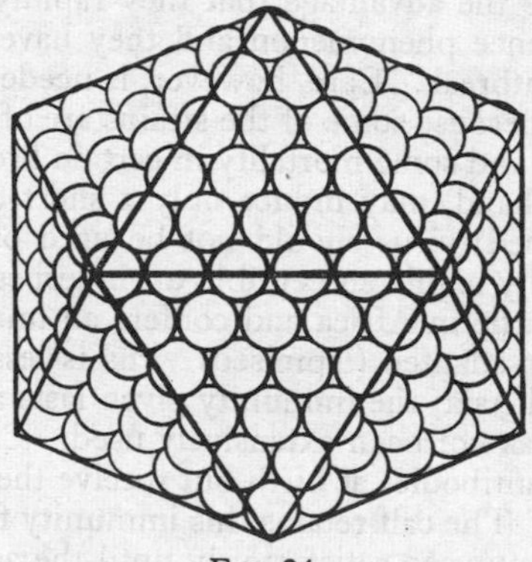

FIG. 24
Diagram to show the icosohedral structure of an adenovirus and the surface capsomeres. (Horne, R. W., 1963). Reprinted with permission. Copyright © 1963 by *Scientific American*, Inc. all rights reserved.

Cultivation.—All the adenoviruses can be cultivated with a cytopathic effect in tissue cultures. Human strains grow most abundantly in continuous lines of human malignant cells such as HEp2, HeLa or KB, or in primary cultures of human amnion, while simian strains grow best in monkey kidney cells. Strains of either origin can be adapted to grow in heterologous cells in tissue culture; although on primary isolation the cytopathic effect may be quite obvious, repeated passages with large inocula may be required to establish a human strain in monkey kidney cells or vice versa. Most strains can also be adapted to grow in rabbit or pig kidney cells or in bovine embryonic tissues.

The range of susceptible tissue culture host cells varies for different types of adenoviruses and although types 1 to 9 are readily propagated in HeLa cells, types 10, 12, 13, 15 and 17 require several serial passages with large inocula before they can be obtained in reasonable quantity. Inhibitors of the growth of adenoviruses are sometimes present in the calf, ox or horse serum commonly used as an ingredient of the tissue culture medium. For work with adenoviruses, 20–40 per cent. human serum in Earle's balanced salt solution is recommended as the growth medium for the host cells. Before inoculation, this medium should be removed and the monolayers should be washed three times with balanced salt solution to remove antibodies. The cells may then be maintained with medium 199 containing up to 7·5 per cent. chicken serum.

Adenoviruses produce both early and late cytopathic effects. The early effect is visible within a few hours of inoculation and is due to a soluble protein (the β component of antigen B) which has a toxic action on the cells and is separable from the viruses themselves. This is not a progressive change and it can be neutralised by immune sera.

Late cytopathic effects are of two types. The first is given by serotypes 1, 2, 5 and 6 and is the clumping of the cells into grape-like clusters. The changes develop over a period of several days and are progressive and irreversible. The infected cells are refractile, rounded off and granular in appearance; bridges of more normal cells link the infected nuclei. The infected cells can usually be stained with neutral red and are therefore still viable. Acidophilic inclusions are seen, and later nuclear enlargement with the formation of large irregular intranuclear inclusions develops. The second effect is given by Types 3, 4 and 7 viruses which are more constantly associated with disease than the first group. These viruses have a shorter growth cycle and often within 48 hours produce a marked cytopathic effect with the formation of large basophilic intranuclear inclusions 3–7 μ in diameter which are Feulgen positive and are rosette shaped with a honeycombed appearance. Treatment with deoxyribonuclease destroys the Feulgen positive characteristic and indicates the DNA content of the adenoviruses. These inclusions are crystalline in nature and under the electron microscope are seen to be composed of virions arranged in a cubic body-centred lattice.

Growth Cycle.—The virus is absorbed slowly by the cell before it begins to multiply in the nucleus. Thus with type 5 there is a latent period of 12 hours during which the virus goes into an eclipse phase. This is followed by a period of rapid increase which lasts some eight hours and thereafter multiplication proceeds at a slower rate for over thirty hours. Liberation of the virus from the host cell is slow and incomplete; only about 6 per cent. of the virus is released spontaneously. The rate of viral multiplication varies for the different types of adenoviruses; types 3, 4 and 7 have a shorter growth cycle than types 1, 2, 5 and 6.

Viability.—Adenoviruses are more stable than the myxoviruses.

They remain viable after 7 days at 36° C., 14 days at room temperature (22°–23° C.), and 70 days at 4° C. They are totally inactivated by two and a half to five min. at 56° C. They are not inactivated by ether and are stable within the pH range from 6 to 9·5, though at pH 3 and pH 10 or above partial but not always complete loss of infectivity results.

Antigenic Characters.—The 31 established human serotypes and the types affecting animals are distinguished by neutralisation tests performed with rabbit antisera. Sero-types 16 and 25 cross-react markedly and types 3, 7 and 14 are also related antigenically. Cross reacting types can be distinguished by haemagglutination inhibition tests (*vide infra*) although this technique reveals a relationship between types 10 and 19. Type 7 strains have been divided into 7 and 7a.

All strains possess a common soluble antigen which fixes complement. The antigenic composition of the adenoviruses can be studied with agar gel diffusion and chromatography methods and Pereira (1960) has shown that three antigens, A, B and C, can be separated. Antigen A is the group specific component α plus DNA; antigen C is the type specific component γ plus DNA; and antigen B is a complex of a trypsin sensitive β component with γ (*vide supra*).

Haemagglutination.—Nearly all adenoviruses agglutinate the red blood cells of one or other of a number of animals. Rat, mouse, and rhesus monkey erythrocytes are most commonly clumped. Four groups of adenoviruses can be distinguished by their power to agglutinate rhesus and rat cells; Group I contains types 3, 7, 11, 14, 16, 20, 21, 25 and 28 and agglutinates rhesus but not rat erythrocytes; Group 2 contains types 8, 9, 10, 13, 15, 17, 19, 22, 23, 24, 26 and 27 and agglutinates rat cells and rhesus cells only to a low titre; Group 3 contains types 1, 2, 4, 5 and 6 and agglutinates rat cells partially; and Group 4 which contains types 12 and 18 does not agglutinate either type of cell.

Pathogenesis.—Adenoviruses do not as a rule produce clinical disease in laboratory animals. It should however be noted that types 7, 12, 18 and 31 produce malignant tumours in baby hamsters. In man, infection with adenoviruses results in catarrhal inflammation of the mucous membranes of the eye and the respiratory tract, sometimes with enlargement of the regional lymph nodes. Adenoviruses have been recovered from enlarged mesenteric lymph glands removed at operation from cases of suspected appendicitis, from infants with intussusception and also from glands pressing on bronchi in bronchiectasis in children.

Types 1, 2, 5 and 6 are for the most part associated with mild, sporadic illnesses and are the common types found latent in human tonsils and adenoids. Types 3, 4, 7, 14 and 21 are more frequently found in association with small epidemics of acute respiratory disease in closed communities.

Acute pharyngitis is probably the most frequent manifestation of adenovirus infection. About half the cases are febrile, and coryzal symptoms and cough are frequent. Young children of pre-school age are commonly infected, often on repeated occasions. Most children have antibodies to types 1, 2, 3 and 5 by the time they begin school life.

Pharyngoconjunctival fever.—The triad of fever, pharyngitis and conjunctivitis lasting for about one week is a characteristic of infections with types 3, 7a and 14. This syndrome is encountered more frequently in the summer months, when it may spread rapidly amongst the members of a family and be associated with outbreaks in schools, day-nurseries or holiday camps.

Acute Respiratory Disease (ARD) is a feverish coryza which, unlike virus influenza, has a gradual onset. Headache, sore throat and cough are common but not severe. This illness seldom has clear-cut characters in civilian practice, and the diagnosis is usually only made when epidemics occur in such communities as large military camps.

Pneumonia.—The illness resembles primary atypical pneumonia. In children, type 7a is a frequent cause of the condition and in adults it occurs as a complication of ARD due to types 4 and 7.

Acute follicular conjunctivitis occurs principally in adults. The disease begins with a unilateral non-purulent inflammation of the conjunctiva with enlargement of the submucous lymphoid follicles and swelling of the pre-auricular lymph node. Fever and systemic effects are usually absent. After a few days the other eye shows a similar involvement and the condition usually clears up within a week. Types 3 and 7a have been isolated from these cases.

Epidemic kerato-conjunctivitis.—This condition is due to infection with the single adenovirus type 8. Factory workers are principally involved, especially those whose trade exposes them to the risk of small corneal abrasions from dust or metal particles such as are disseminated in arc welding and riveting. The acute phase of the infection may last for several weeks and healing is slow. Type 8 virus can easily be spread by contaminated towels to other members of a patient's family. Epidemics have been recorded where the virus was spread amongst patients in an ophthalmic clinic by means of contaminated eye solutions and instruments.

Epidemiology.—Adenoviruses are widespread in the continents of Europe and North America. In respiratory disease the viruses are spread by the inhalation of infected particles and possibly through contamination of the conjunctiva by infected fingers or droplet-spray. The seasonal incidence is maximal in the winter. Pharyngoconjunctival fever has a maximal incidence in the summer months, and types 3 and 7a viruses have been thought to be spread in swimming-bath water. In addition to being present in the exudates of the oropharynx and the eye, adenoviruses have been recovered from faeces and from the mesenteric lymph nodes. Adenoviruses types from 9 to 28, excluding types 14 and 21, have been recovered almost exclusively from the intestinal tract. The significance of the presence of adenoviruses in the intestine is still in doubt.

Clinical Syndromes due to Adenoviruses

Disease	Associated Adenovirus Type
Acute respiratory disease	**4**, **7**, 3, 14.
Acute febrile pharyngitis . . .	**1**, **2**, **3**, **5**.
Pharyngoconjunctival fever . . .	**3**, **7a**, 1, 2, 5, 6, 14.
Virus pneumonia:	
(*a*) in infants	**7a**, 1, 3.
(*b*) in adults	**4**, **7**, 3.
Acute follicular conjunctivitis . . .	**3**, **7a**, 1, 2, 5, 6, 14.
Epidemic kerato-conjunctivitis . . .	**8**, 3, 7a, 9.

The most common types are given in heavy figures.

Laboratory Diagnosis

Virus isolation is carried out by the inoculation of monolayer tissue cultures of human cells, preferably HeLa, HEp2 or primary cultures of human amnion, in which adenoviruses produce a characteristic cytopathic effect. They can be identified as members of the adenovirus group by their capacity to fix complement with a known positive human or rabbit antiserum. The type is determined in neutralisation tests with type-specific rabbit antisera.

Serological Tests.—Infection with any one type of adenovirus stimulates a rising titre of complement-fixing antibodies to the group soluble antigen. This provides a simple and practical test for the detection of infections with the adenovirus group although it does not identify the type of the infecting strain. Complement-fixing antibodies often rise from very low levels to titres of 1 in 128. The technique of the complement-fixation test is that described in Chapter 54. The antigen used is prepared from a heavy culture of HeLa cells infected with a large inoculum of an undiluted seed stock of any adenovirus type and incubated for about five days (for at least two days after the completion of the cytopathic effect). After thorough homogenisation in a blender and clarification by centrifugation at 2500 r.p.m. for twenty minutes the antigen is titrated against a positive serum and is then ready for use.

Rises of type-specific antibodies to the adenoviruses can be measured in neutralisation tests against serotypes in HeLa cell tissue cultures.

Prophylaxis.—The use of adenovirus vaccines of formol-inactivated cultures has been discontinued because of the possibility of tumour production.

Canine Hepatitis.—Infectious canine hepatitis or Rubarth's disease is widespread in Britain and in the continents of Europe and North America. The disease at one time was confused with canine distemper, but is a distinct entity caused by a different virus. Young dogs and puppies soon after weaning are most susceptible; infection also occurs in foxes, in which it takes the form of an acute encephalitis. After an incubation period of six to nine days, dogs suffer from high fever, vomiting, diarrhoea and abdominal pain. Petechiae of the gums and inflammation and engorgement of the tonsils are common. Icterus is unusual. The disease has a rapid course and 25 per cent. of the animals infected die within a few days of the onset. At autopsy the predominant features are subcutaneous oedema and a haemorrhagic peritoneal exudate. The liver is pale and swollen; histologically the endothelial cells of the sinusoids and the Küpffer cells show marked degeneration and the presence of acidophilic intranuclear inclusion bodies. The gall-bladder mucosa is markedly oedematous and the wall thickened.

The virus is excreted in the urine for many weeks after full recovery and it is from this source that the dissemination of the virus is maintained. The virus may also be spread on the hands of animal handlers contaminated by infected saliva.

Properties of the Virus.—The virion is 65 mμ in diameter and in negatively stained preparations has the electron microscopical appearances of the adenovirus. Antigenically the virus shares the group complement-fixing antigen with the human adenoviruses but it is distinct from them in neutralisation tests. The virus can be grown in cultures of dog, ferret, or pig kidney or testis. In monolayers it produces clearly defined plaques.

Vaccines.—Several vaccines which contain living attenuated strains of the canine hepatitis virus are available. One is combined in a single prophylactic dose with an attenuated strain of the canine distemper virus. Another reinforces the antigenic stimulus of the attenuated hepatitis virus with two doses of inactivated virus.

Virus Pneumonia

This condition is in effect a syndrome of variable symptoms and signs which usually arc lcss prominent than would be expected from the appearances of the soft patchy areas of consolidation that are seen at the bases of the lungs on radiological examination. There is no response to antibiotic therapy (but see Q fever, psittacosis, and primary atypical pneumonia).

Aetiology.—Although there is evidence to associate a wide variety of infective agents with the syndrome, it is true to say that the cause of many of these cases is yet to be determined. Pneumonia of this type is found in Q fever, due to infection with *Cox. burnetii*, and a similar illness is caused by the psittacosis and Eaton's agents. The influenza viruses and the respiratory syncytial virus, the Sendai virus, together with certain members of the group of adenoviruses (especially types 4, 7 and 7a) are able to cause pneumonia of this type. The measles virus occasionally causes an interstitial pneumonia (Hecht's disease) which is characterised by the formation of giant-cells with intranuclear and cytoplasmic inclusions.

Although virus pneumonias resemble the syndrome known as *Primary Atypical Pneumonia* (see p. 501) they may be differentiated from it by certain clinical and radiological features and by the absence of the cold agglutinins and agglutinins to *Streptococcus M.G.* which may occur in the latter condition. The cause of a high proportion of cases of primary atypical pneumonia is Eaton's agent (Cook *et al.*, 1960, Liu, 1957) which is *Mycoplasma pneumoniae*, a pleuropneumonia-like organism. Because *M. pneumoniae* is cultivatable on serum agar it is not a virus and it is described with the other mycoplasmas.

Laboratory Diagnosis.—Paired samples of serum should be tested for cold agglutinins and *Streptococcus MG* agglutinins. Antibodies to influenza and para-influenza viruses can be detected by haemagglutination or haemadsorption inhibition techniques. Antibodies to *M. pneumoniae*, *Cox. burnetii*, psittacosis, the influenza A, B and C and para-influenza viruses, the respiratory syncytical virus and the group of adenoviruses are detected by complement-fixation. The sputum should be examined bacteriologically, and virologically as in psittacosis. Blood cultures and animal inoculations may be required if Q fever is suspected.

RHINOVIRUSES

The viruses of this group are responsible for the most frequent of all human infections, the "common cold". Most people suffer from two to four colds every year and, although the condition is not a severe one, secondary bacterial infection often follows with temporary incapacity. These viruses are the cause of the loss of many millions of man-hours of work.

Properties of the viruses.—The virions are spheres about 30 mμ in diameter. Since growth is inhibited by 5-fluoro-uracil they probably contain RNA. They can be distinguished from most ECHO and Coxsackie viruses by the fact that their growth is not inhibited by benzimidazole. There are no reports that the rhinoviruses can cause haemagglutination. Rhinoviruses, together with other very small viruses, are classified as picornaviruses.

Cultivation.—The viruses are divided into two groups according to the tissues of optimal growth. "M" strains grow and produce a cytopathic effect in monkey kidney monolayers and also in continuous lines of malignant human cells such as HeLa and HEp2. "H" strains are most easily isolated in human embryonic kidney cultures but can, with rather more difficulty, also be grown in diploid cells from human embryonic lung (Hayflick & Moorehead, 1961, HeLa and KB cells; Taylor Robinson, Hucker & Tyrell, 1962).

Both M and H strains require for their growth a temperature of 33° C., a pH lower than that commonly used, and the use of revolving drums to maintain the oxygen tension of the cell cultures by rotation. Infected cultures are maintained in a medium containing 0·03 per cent. sodium bicarbonate, 0·25 per cent. lactalbumin hydrolysate and 2·0 per cent. calf serum in Hanks' saline with antibiotics.

Viability.—Rhinoviruses can be preserved at −76° C. and survive freeze drying rather better than most picornaviruses. Drying in air at atmospheric temperature quickly inactivates the viruses. They are stable to heat treatment at 50° C. for 30 min. but are sensitive to pH fluctuations and are quickly inactivated at pH 5·3. They survive overnight exposure to 20 per cent. ether.

Pathogenesis.—When rhinoviruses are instilled into the nose of human volunteers a mild sore throat and cough are the premonitory signs which precede the profuse nasal discharge of a typical common cold. The incubation period is 48–96 hr. Chimpanzees are the only other creatures known to be susceptible to these viruses. The viruses can be recovered from the secretion of the nose and throat but only rarely from the faeces.

Epidemiology.—The incidence of colds is greatest in the winter months when outside temperatures are falling but the reasons for the seasonal variation has never been satisfactorily explained. Deliberate exposure of volunteers to wet and chilling does not increase their susceptibility to colds. Common colds are probably transmitted by the same mechanisms as those in influenza and other respiratory infections. About 10 per cent. of colds compel their victims to absent themselves from work. Colds in the home are often introduced by pre-school and school children who contract the infection from their playmates. In general, adults under the age of thirty are more susceptible than those over forty (Lidwell & Williams, 1961).

Laboratory Diagnosis.—This rests on the isolation of the causative virus in tissue culture and the neutralisation of its cytopathic effect by antisera. Antibodies in sera can be titrated according to their ability to reduce the number of microplaques which a fixed dose of virus will produce in a monolayer of susceptible cells.

Prophylaxis.—An experimental vaccine containing a single inactivated virus strain injected intramuscularly is effective in stimulating the production of protective antibodies against that strain (Doggett, Bynoe & Tyrrell, 1963). The multiplicity of serotypes to be found in the community, however, makes it likely that for any vaccine to be effective it would require to contain a large number of different virus strains.

Miscellaneous Viruses Associated with Colds.—A number of these agents mostly picornaviruses are closely associated with cold-like illnesses. COE virus has been isolated in Great Britain and in the United States of America from patients suffering from febrile colds and sore throats. This virus has been identified as Coxsackie virus A21. A serological survey in Great Britain has shown that the incidence of infection with the COE virus is low in children under the age of ten years and rises steadily with age. By the age of fifty years, 50 per cent. of individuals have antibodies to the virus and there is a significantly higher proportion of infection in males (Pereira and Pereira, 1959).

ECHO 28 includes the J.H. and 2060 viruses which were isolated from feverish colds. These viruses are intermediate in their properties between the ECHO and Rhinoviruses.

REO viruses (respiratory enteric orphan viruses), see p. 441, which at one time were classified as ECHO 10 have occasionally been recovered from mild fevers in children but have been more constantly associated with diarrhoea than with respiratory symptoms.

Para-influenza viruses, the respiratory syncytial virus, the adenoviruses, and Eaton's agent have all been found in association with cold-like illness.

REFERENCES

Burnet, F. M. (1960). *Principles of Animal Virology*. p. 359. New York: Academic Press.

Chanock, R. M., Parrot, R. H., Cook, K., Andrews, B. E., Bell, J. A., Reichelderfer, T., Kapikan, A. Z., Mastrota, F. M. & Huebner, R. J. (1958). Newly recognised myxoviruses from children with respiratory disease. *New Engl. J. Med.*, **258**, 207.

Cook, M. K., Andrews, B. E., Fox, H. H., Turner, H. C., James, W. D. & Chanock, R. M. (1959). Antigenic relationships among the "newer" myxoviruses (parainfluenza). *Amer. J. Hyg.*, **69**, 250.

Cook, M. K., Chanock, R. M., Fox, H. H., Huebner, R. J., Buescher, E. L. & Johnson, R. T. (1960). Role of Eaton's agent in disease of lower respiratory tract. *Brit. med. J.*, **1**, 905.

Doggett, J. E., Bynoe, M. L. & Tyrell, D. A. J. (1963). Some attempts to produce an experimental vaccine with rhinoviruses. *Brit. med. J.*, **1**, 34.

Ghosh Ray, B. & Swain, R. H. A. (1953). Serum antibodies in mumps. *Brit. J. exp. Path.*, **34**, 501.

Ghosh Ray, B. & Swain, R. H. A. (1954). An investigation of the mumps virus by electron microscopy. *J. Path. Bact.*, **67**, 247.

Hayflick, L. & Moorhead, P. S. (1961). The serial cultivation of human diploid cell strains. *Exp. Cell. Res.*, **25**, 585.

Hambling, M. H. (1964). A survey of antibodies to respiratory syncytial virus in the population. *Brit. med. J.*, **1**, 1223.

Holzel, A., Parker, L., Paterson, W. H., White, L. L. R., Thompson, K. M. & Tobin, J. O'H. (1963). The isolation of respiratory syncytical virus from children with acute respiratory disease. *Lancet*, **1**, 295.

Horne, R. W. (1963). The structure of viruses. *Sci. Amer.*, **208**, 48.

Horne, R. W. & Wildy, P. (1963). Virus structure revealed by negative staining. *Advanc. Virus Res.*, **10**, 101.

Lidwell, O. M. & Williams, R. E. O. (1961). The epidemiology of the common cold. *J. Hyg.* (*Camb.*), **59**, 309, 331.

Lief, F. S. & Henle, W. (1956). Studies on the soluble antigen of the influenza virus. *Virology*, **2**, 753.

Liu, C. (1957). Studies on primary atypical pneumonia. *J. exp. Med.*, **106**, 455.

Medical Research Council Report (1958). Trials of an asian influenza vaccine. *Brit. med. J.*, **1**, 415.

Miller, D. L. (1964). Frequency of complications in measles 1963. *Brit. med. J.*, **2**, 75.

Pereira, H. G. (1960). Antigenic structure of non-infectious adenovirus particles. *Nature* (*Lond.*), **186**, 571.

Pereira, H. G., Huebner, R. J., Ginsberg, H. S. & Van der Veen, J. (1963). A short description of the adenovirus group. *Virology*, **20**, 613.

Pereira, M. S. (1958). Typing of Q-phase influenza-A virus. *Lancet*, **2**, 668.

Pereira, M. S. & Pereira, H. G. (1959). COE virus, properties and prevalence in Great Britain. *Lancet*, **2**, 539.

Pereira, H. G., Pereira, M. S. & Law, V. G. (1964). Antigenic variants of influenza A2 virus. *Bull World Hlth. Org.*, **31**, 129.

Pickles, W. N., Burnet, F. M. & McArthur, N. (1947). Epidemic respiratory infection in rural population. *J. Hyg.* (*Camb.*), **45**, 469.

Taylor-Robinson, D., Hucker, D. & Tyrell, D. A. J. (1962). Studies on the pathogenicity for tissue cultures of some viruses isolated from common colds. *Brit. J. exp. Path.*, **43**, 189.

Vogel, J. & Shelokov, A. (1957). Absorption-haemagglutination test for influenza virus in monkey tissue culture. *Science*, **126**, 358.

Waterson, A. P. (1962). Two kinds of myxovirus. *Nature* (*Lond.*), **193**, 1163.

CHAPTER 34

ENTEROVIRUSES; REOVIRUSES

THOSE viruses which multiply predominantly within the cells of the intestinal tract of man are grouped together and are known as the Enteroviruses. In this category are three smaller groups; the poliovirus subgroup consisting of the three poliomyelitis viruses; at least 30 ECHO viruses; and 30 Coxsackie viruses. Most are within the size range 25–33 mμ, ether resistant, and are antigenically distinct from each other. They can be isolated from human faeces in tissue culture, and in the case of Coxsackie viruses also by the inoculation of infant mice. As well as causing poliomyelitis these viruses give rise to a wide variety of acute feverish illnesses in man.

The enteroviruses are included in a larger group, the *Picornaviruses*, that also includes similar viruses such as the *Rhinoviruses* which cause common colds, the virus causing foot and mouth disease in farm animals, and a variety of other viruses many of which are pathogenic for different animals.

POLIOMYELITIS

Usually infection with the poliovirus is quite inapparent and the individual, although at the time excreting the virus, is unaware of any ill effects. Occasionally he may have a minor illness with, at most, symptoms of fever, headache and vomiting. In a smaller proportion of infections there are signs of a meningeal reaction of some severity and these may subside or proceed to involvement of the central nervous system with localisation of the virus either in the anterior horn cells of the spinal cord or in the region of the respiratory and vasomotor centres in the medulla. The clinical diagnosis of poliomyelitis based on the signs of paralysis is made in less than one in a thousand infections.

The Properties of Poliovirus hominis.—The poliovirus is a spherical particle 27 mμ in diameter; it is the smallest known human pathogen. The virion is in the form of an icosohedron with, perhaps, 32 protein capsomeres enclosing a RNA core which constitutes 25–30 per cent. of the particle.

Two outstanding characteristics of the virus are its affinity for nervous tissue and its narrow animal host range. The only animals readily susceptible are the primates, though it has been possible to adapt some strains to grow in small rodents and chick embryos. Cynomolgus and rhesus monkeys can be infected by the oral route and develop paralysis; in chimpanzees, however, the infection is often asymptomatic. Under the influence of cortisone, monkeys become more susceptible to small parenteral doses of the virus. The animals develop a viraemia which is suppressed when antibodies appear, and later they excrete the virus in their faeces. Poliomyelitis viruses are most easily isolated and cultivated in *in vitro* tissue cultures of monkey kidney or in HeLa cells where their cytopathic effect becomes rapidly apparent. They can also be grown in a wide variety of human cells in tissue culture explants, *e.g.* embryonic skin, muscle, kidney, tonsil, prepuce, testis and uterus; monkey testis or lung can also be used.

Viability.—The poliovirus is one of the most stable known. In aqueous suspensions of human faeces at 4° C. it survives for many months, and in pieces of spinal cord in 50 per cent. glycerol in normal saline it remains viable for periods of eight years or more. It can be preserved for many months or years at −20° C. or −70° C. Unlike most other viruses its infectivity is not well preserved by freeze drying. In human stools the virus may survive at room temperature for as short a time as one day or for as long as several weeks, depending on the amount of virus present, the pH, the amount of faecal moisture and other environmental conditions. The virus is readily killed by moist heat at 50°–55° C. but milk, cream and ice-cream exert a protective effect so that the virus in these foodstuffs may survive exposure to heat at 60° C. It is destroyed by the process of pasteurisation of milk at 62° C., but the safety margin is not sufficient for certain inactivation and the flash method at 72° C. is to be preferred.

In infected human spinal cord the virus is rapidly inactivated at pH values below 2 or over 11; it survives for ten days at 4° C. in 1 per cent. phenol, 18 hr. at 4° C. in ether, and 0·1 per cent. sodium desoxycholate. Inactivation of poliovirus in tissue culture fluids is complete after seven days exposure to 0·025 per cent. formaldehyde at 37° C., but its antigenicity is retained so that it can be used as an immunising agent. The most active disinfectants are oxidising agents such as potassium permanganate and hypochlorites. In the absence of organic matter free chlorine in a strength of 0·05 parts per million will inactivate the virus, but higher concentrations than this are needed to disinfect swimming-bath water or materials contaminated by faeces.

Antigenic Characters.—Three immunological types of the virus have been identified by neutralisation tests carried out in the monkey or in tissue cultures. The prototype strains of type 1 are the Brunhilde and Mahoney strains; type 2, which includes the rodent adapted strains, the Lansing and MEF1 strains; and type 3, the Leon and Saukett strains. The three types are immunologically distinct, but overlapping in neutralisation tests is not infrequent. Type 1 is the common epidemic type, type 2 is usually associated with endemic infections, and type 3 occasionally causes epidemics. The size, chemical and physical properties, and the resistance of the three types are all identical.

In partially purified preparations of polioviruses there are four antigens which differ in size, density, chemical composition, infectivity and antigenic characters. These particles can be separated by sedimentation in a sucrose density gradient, and two of them, the D and C particles, can be distinguished according to their predominant antigenic reactions. D particles have the characteristics of infective virus, are well defined and type specific; they are of uniform appearance in electron micrographs and contain 25–30 per cent. RNA and about 70 per cent. protein. The C antigen configuration is associated with particles which are less electron dense and which are structurally impaired so that they have a ring or "doughnut" appearance; they are devoid of RNA and have the power to react with antibodies which appear very early in the serum of acute cases of poliomyelitis. If D particles are exposed to heat or to ultra-violet light, C antigen is produced. D particles in concentrated preparations give type-specific reactions in complement-fixation tests and in precipitin reactions carried out by the agar gel diffusion method. C particle preparations also react specifically but are liable to react heterotypically with antibodies to all the three virus types. The preparation of purified suspensions of D particles for use in diagnostic serological work, although highly desirable, is still a matter of considerable technical difficulty.

Pathogenesis.—The only natural source of the virus is man; the virus is spread from person to person, and no intermediate host is known. The human reservoir of infection consists of persons who excrete the virus in their faeces and perhaps less commonly in their oropharyngeal secretions. The great majority of these people have no paralytic manifestations of the infection and suffer no illness; the virus they excrete enters the new host by ingestion or inhalation.

In paralytic poliomyelitis, the virus can be found in the faeces for a few days preceding the onset of acute symptoms and is present in over 80 per cent. of cases in the stool during the first 14 days. After three weeks some 50 per cent. of patients still excrete the virus and at five to six weeks 25 per cent. Only a few cases continue to excrete the virus after the twelfth week. No permanent carriers are known. The virus can be isolated from the oropharynx of many cases for a few days before and after the onset of the illness.

There is still some doubt as to the route by which the virus is disseminated throughout the body. One suggestion is that there is a primary focus of viral multiplication and that from this site the virus is disseminated in the blood stream. It is probable that on entering the body the virus first invades the lymphoid tissues in the upper respiratory tract or the Peyer's patches of the small intestine and the associated mesenteric lymph glands; during the next seven days large amounts of virus are produced locally in these extraneural sites until there is a spill over into the lymphatics and carriage into the blood stream. In those cases which die of an overwhelming infection within a short time from the onset, the Peyer's patches and the mesenteric lymph nodes are found to be greatly swollen and inflamed and to contain large amounts of virus (see Fig. 25).

The viraemic phase marks the end of the incubation period and is manifest in the patient by the fever and generalised toxic symptoms; it is followed by a period of about 48 hours of relative well-being (the disease is biphasic) while the virus is invading nerve tissue, and then, in serious cases, the signs of paralysis appear. Viraemia has been proved to occur after experimental infection of monkeys and has been demonstrated on several occasions in man. It is probable that the process can be arrested at various stages so that the virus may multiply in the intestine without ever reaching the blood stream, or once in the blood stream the virus may be overcome by the patient's natural defence mechanisms before it can reach nerve cells. Even if the virus destroys nerve cells, it is only when certain critical areas are involved that paralysis results. In this way it is possible to explain abortive and non-paralytic forms of poliomyelitis. It must be stated, however, that it is not yet known whether viraemia is a constant feature of the disease and that no adequate explanation has yet been offered of the manner whereby the virus enters the nerve cells in paralytic poliomyelitis.

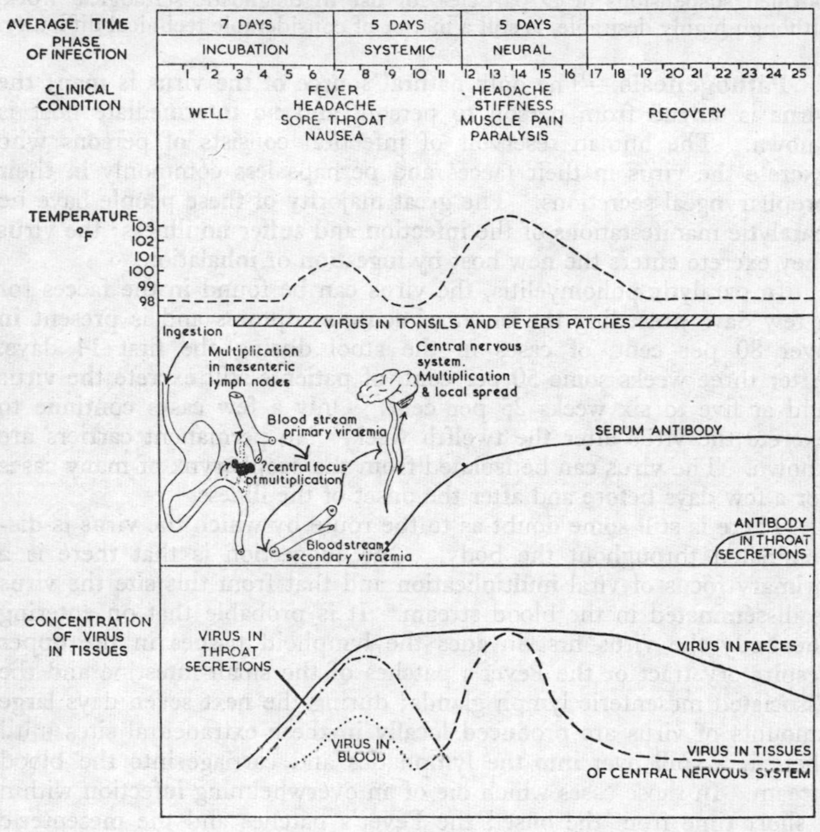

FIG. 25

A diagram to show the correlation between the clinical and pathological events occurring in a paralytic case of poliomyelitis.

An alternative explanation of the pathogenesis of poliomyelitis is that the virus is first deposited on the mucous membranes of the mouth or intestine where it enters the peripheral nerve endings. The virus then ascends along the axons to reach the peripheral ganglia and then the central nervous system. Virus multiplication follows with the production of lesions which may be small and heal quickly or which may progress to involve vital areas and cause paralysis. The evidence to support this view depends on the findings of lesions in the regional ganglia. It is, however, possible that such changes are caused not by the ascending spread of the virus but by its effect as it spreads outwards from the central nervous system. In general, it may be stated that there is considerable doubt as to whether the poliomyelitis virus can enter through intact nerve endings. In the experimental monkey, however, it is known that the virus can enter a nerve which has been deliberately cut and that it can travel along the proximal fibres to reach the central nervous system; such a sequence of events may occasionally occur in man and is thought to happen after tonsillectomy.

Factors Predisposing to Infection.—There are a number of factors which are known to shorten the incubation period, enhance the severity of the infection, and promote the localisation of the virus in the central nervous system, thus predisposing to paralysis. Muscular activity during the pre-paralytic phase of the illness leads to paralysis of the limbs used. Pregnant women are more susceptible than non-pregnant women. Poliomyelitis occurring near full term is apt to be severe and may assume the bulbar form. Tonsillectomy carries an increased risk of bulbar poliomyelitis, and this risk persists for several months or even years after the operation.

Paralytic poliomyelitis may also occur in children who have received immunising injections of alum-containing diphtheria toxoid, particularly when combined with pertussis antigens. It is probable that the irritant properties of the alum or other adjuvants used in these vaccines is more important than the nature of the vaccine. A similar effect has followed the use of penicillin, arsenicals and heavy metals in mass campaigns against yaws. Paralysis occurs in the limb which receives the inoculation, and its incidence is approximately 1 in 37,000 injections. There is much doubt about the manner in which the paralysis is precipitated; the irritant inoculum in the muscles may render the anterior horn cells of the corresponding segment of the cord more susceptible to virus invasion or perhaps it may provide a site for the local proliferation of the virus circulating in the blood.

In paralytic poliomyelitis it sometimes happens that the patient has a double infection and that both the poliomyelitis virus and a Coxsackie virus (see p. 438) can be recovered from the faeces. Viruses of Coxsackie group A occur with significantly greater frequency than those of group B in paralytic poliomyelitis. The constancy of the association of the poliomyelitis and Coxsackie group A viruses has been sufficient to suggest that infection with the latter predisposes to paralysis. Coxsackie B viruses are not associated with paralytic poliomyelitis and it is of interest to note that, in contrast to group A viruses, they have an interfering action which spares the mouse from the effects of experimental poliomyelitis.

Epidemiology

Poliomyelitis occurs throughout the world, but in temperate climates assumes an epidemiological pattern quite different from that found in the tropics. In Europe, North America and Australia the disease is endemic with periodic epidemic increases, usually in the late summer; in the tropics it occurs uniformly throughout the whole year without any tendency to seasonal variation. As hygiene improves, however, the epidemic pattern changes.

At the beginning of the century, paralytic poliomyelitis was known as "Infantile Paralysis" because it most frequently attacked children under 5 years old. Since the Second World War, however, the position has changed and only one-third of the patients are under 5 years of age, one-third are in the age-group 5–15 years and the remaining third are over 15. No age is exempt, and poliomyelitis has been recorded at the age of 70 years. In places where overcrowding and poor sanitation permit rapid dissemination of the virus, poliomyelitis remains a disease of infancy, and by the age of 4 years practically all the children have acquired immunity to all the three virus types. It is established that infants are less likely to develop paralysis than older children, but the peak incidence is still in the 1–3 year-olds: in recent epidemics over 60 per cent. of fatal cases have been in patients over 15 years old in whom the infection tends to be more severe.

The higher standard of hygiene in some countries impedes spread of the virus over wide areas and individuals or whole communities may escape infection for many years. In this way it may happen that a large part of a population lacks immunity to the polioviruses and that when infection is introduced it spreads so rapidly among susceptible persons that an epidemic results. The introduction of more virulent strains may also be a factor in epidemic spread. It is difficult to know which of these factors was more important when in this country in 1947 the incidence of poliomyelitis rose from the usual figure of 4 per 100,000 to 18 per 100,000 of the population. A preponderance of the clinical infections has been caused by type 1 virus.

Poliomyelitis is often contracted during a period of quite close proximity to an infected person; the virus may be inhaled in infected particles or ingested. It is thought that the virus is frequently transferred by the hands of persons who are excreting the virus or by those who have touched contaminated fomites.

Faeces provide a rich and persistent source of the virus; it has been calculated that one gram of stool may contain several million infective doses of the virus. Sewage in urban populations contains the virus throughout the summer and early winter months, while poliomyelitis is prevalent. Water supplies may occasionally be contaminated by sewage, and in rural areas this may be a means by which infection is spread. There is little evidence, however, that the virus can survive the purification processes used for a piped water supply, and urban water-borne epidemics have not been described. Faecal pollution of swimming-baths has often been thought to spread the infection, but there is little direct evidence on this point and with adequate chlorination the risk is small. Flies may carry the virus to food on their feet or by regurgitating after feeding on exposed faeces or sewage.

Immunity is permanent to the virus type causing the infection. Although the three virus types are antigenically distinct there is some evidence to suggest that prior infection with type 2 virus may confer a measure of resistance to the paralytic disease caused by type 1.

Virus neutralising antibodies are formed early during the disease (often before the seventh day) and persist for several decades. Complement-fixing antibodies are of much shorter duration.

Laboratory Diagnosis

Virus Isolation.—The virus may be recovered from faeces or throat swabs taken early during the disease. Two such specimens should be collected on successive days as early as possible in the course of the disease. A 10 per cent. faecal suspension is made in Hanks' balanced salt solution containing 100 units of penicillin and 100 μg. of streptomycin per ml. and is then centrifuged to remove coarse particles. Throat swabs are treated in a similar fashion. The material is then used to inoculate four monolayer tissue cultures of monkey kidney, human amnion, HeLa, HEp2 or other cells. If the virus is growing, a cytopathic effect is usually seen in the cells within 48 hours. Identification of the virus type is carried out by a neutralisation test in which a measured dose of virus (approx. 100 TCD 50) is exposed to the action of standard type-specific antisera. It is convenient to dilute the virus isolate 1 in 100 and 1 in 100,000 and to mix these two dilutions with a suitable amount of the standard antisera. In fatal cases specimens obtained at autopsy should include the cervical and lumbar enlargements of the spinal cord, the medulla, mesenteric lymph nodes and portions of small intestine and colon with their contents. After being homogenised, these tissues are treated in the same way as faeces. All types of infected material can be preserved in the refrigerator at 4° C. but better results are obtained when storage is at $-30°$ C. Tissues should be placed in 50 per cent. glycerol saline before storage.

It must be remembered that any poliovirus isolated from a patient may be either a "wild" virulent virus or an attenuated vaccine strain. The only certain way to distinguish between these two possibilities is to carry out virulence tests in the monkey, but with attenuated strains of polioviruses types 1 and 2 there are certain genetic, in-vitro, "marker" characteristics which are sufficiently stable to be helpful.

One marker that has been much used is the *intratypic* antigenic structure of the virus which is characteristic for each strain. The rate of inactivation of a poliovirus by its own homologous antiserum (calculated as the K value) is faster than that achieved by antisera to other strains of the same type. Thus, when antisera to attenuated strains are set up against the vaccine viruses the K value is higher than if wild viruses had been used (McBride, 1959; Gard, 1960). A second marker, the A (aluminium) marker, rests on the fact that attenuated strains are not inactivated by heat for 15 min. at 50° C. in the presence of 10mM $AlCl_3$, whereas wild strains treated in this way are inactivated and lose 3–4 log. 10 units of their infectivity (Melnick, 1962). Other markers which may be used include (1) the T or ret/40 marker (Lwoff and Lwoff, 1960) which employs the fact that neurovirulent polioviruses are more thermo-resistant than attenuated strains, (2) the *d* (bicarbonate) marker which uses the observation that strains with reduced virulence have a low plating efficiency in an acid medium with a low bicarbonate content in the overlay, whereas virulent viruses grow well under these conditions (Dulbecco and Vogt, 1958), and (3) the M marker which rests on the fact that virulent polioviruses grow well with the production of large plaques on a stable line of monkey kidney cells while attenuated strains grow less well with small plaques.

The use of these markers is confined to polioviruses types 1 and 2; poliovirus type 3 is genetically so unstable that only virulence tests in the monkey serve to differentiate the wild from the attenuated viruses.

Serological Tests.—Paired samples of serum are required; the first must be taken as soon as possible after the onset of the disease and the second after an interval of three to four weeks. Neutralisation tests are usually employed with all the three virus types. If the first sample has been taken sufficiently early it is often possible to show a significant rise of antibodies to the infecting virus type, but in practice this may not always be achieved because of the insidious nature of the onset. Antibody tends to rise rapidly, and titres of 1000 or higher are usual by the end of the third week of the disease. In type 1 infection some type 2 antibody may develop as well. Complement-fixation and flocculation tests are not yet in general use for routine diagnostic work.

Prophylaxis and Control

Since it has proved impractical to prevent the widespread dissemination of the virus and because it is impossible to recognise the trivial infections that the poliomyelitis viruses cause, it has become obvious that the disease can only be controlled by raising the immunity of the population to a high level.

Active immunisation with a formol-inactivated vaccine has been advocated by Salk for this purpose. The vaccine contains strains of the three types of virus inactivated by exposure to formaldehyde. In the vaccine used in America, type 1 is represented by the Mahoney strain, type 2 by MEF1, and type 3 by Saukett. A second vaccine of this type was developed in Britain and for greater safety less virulent strains were employed; the type 1 virus used was Brunenders, an attenuated variant of Brunhilde, type 2 was a strain of MEF1 adapted to suckling mice and the type 3 virus was again Saukett. Both vaccines have been used extensively and many millions of people have received them without ill effect; they cause no local or general reactions and each has been proved to lower significantly the incidence of paralytic poliomyelitis. Initially two doses of 1·0 ml. of the vaccine are given intramuscularly at an interval of three weeks. Two booster doses are required, one six to nine months after the second dose and the last a year or two later.

Until 1960 the antigenic efficiency of different batches of the inactivated vaccine was sometimes variable. The type 2 virus component was satisfactory and in most cases so was the type 3, but the antigenicity of the type 1 component was such that up to about 15 per cent. of those inoculated failed to produce antibody after two doses of the vaccine. New vaccines overcome this difficulty and contain a ten-fold increase in the concentration of the type 1 virus. Two injections of these vaccines evoke a good antibody response in 95 per cent. of susceptible children between the ages of 4 months and 14–15 years; a third injection given 7–12 months later results in a satisfactory antibody titre in almost 100 per cent. of the recipients. Antibodies first appear 7–10 days after the second inoculation, reach a maximum after about three weeks, and then gradually decline, so that after two years their level is about 20 per cent. of the peak titre. Thereafter the level decreases at a slower rate. In individuals who have received three doses of a good vaccine a satisfactory antibody titre is maintained for some five years.

The inactivated poliovirus vaccine may be used simultaneously with the triple vaccine against diphtheria, pertussis and tetanus or it may be combined with it in a quadruple vaccine (Butler *et al.*, 1962). The latter has not been recommended for general use in Britain.

Live attenuated poliovirus vaccines are now used extensively in many countries including Britain. The virus strains used in these vaccines are attenuated and lack all power to produce paralysis even when injected directly into the brain or spinal cord of monkeys. They were obtained by cultivating wild, but relatively avirulent, polioviruses in monolayer cultures of monkey kidney cells in which plaques were produced. By selection of a single plaque, pure clones of viruses were obtained and passaged until neurovirulence was lost. The strains most commonly used were developed by Sabin (1959a) and are designated as follows: Type 1 strain (LSc 2 ab), Type 2 strain (P712, Ch 2 ab) and Type 3 strain (Leon, 12 ab).

Live attenuated vaccines have the great advantage that they are given orally and are therefore much easier to administer; large numbers of persons can be immunised by feeding the vaccine during a very short space of time. In addition this vaccine is much more economical in use than the inactivated vaccine because it is much simpler to prepare and the virus dose required ($10^5 - 10^{5 \cdot 5}$ TCD 50) is approximately one ten thousandth part of the virus content of a single inoculation of the inactivated vaccine.

The immunity which follows feeding the attenuated viruses is effective in over 90 per cent. of the subjects and the antibody response is as good as that induced by inactivated vaccines. The duration of the immunity follows the same general pattern as that produced by the use of inactivated vaccines but there is as yet no evidence on which to assess whether or not it will last any longer. In addition to evoking the production of humoral antibodies the growth of the vaccine strains in the gut creates a state of cellular resistance whereby the subsequent establishment of polioviruses in the intestine is prevented.

Administration of the attenuated strains in Great Britain is carried out by feeding a trivalent oral vaccine on three separate occasions spaced at four to eight week intervals. Older children and adults receive the vaccine on a lump of sugar or in syrup (BP); in the case of infant) it can be given directly from a dropper. The dose is 0·15 ml. (3 drops and contains all three of the Sabin strains; Type 1 $10^{5\cdot7}$ TCD 50, Type 2 $10^{5\cdot0}$ TCD 50, and Type 3 $10^{5\cdot5}$ TCD 50. An alternative schedule recommended by Sabin employs monovalent vaccines which are given in similar doses in the order of types 1, 3 and 2 at intervals of at least four and preferably six weeks.

Attenuated vaccines have the advantage that they can be administered very easily and quickly in mass vaccination campaigns. When used in this way in the face of a commencing epidemic they have been successful in halting the spread of infection. Whole communities can be protected in this way and many hope that by these methods wild polioviruses may be eliminated and the disease of poliomyelitis will be eradicated.

There has been much controversy over the relative merits of the inactivated and the attenuated vaccines. In summary it may be said that both are highly effective immunising agents and both give very similar immunological responses. The inactivated vaccine can be accepted as safe without question but doubts exist about the possibility that the attenuated polioviruses will, as they are repeatedly transferred naturally from man to man, revert to a more neurotropic form and eventually resume their power to cause paralysis.

There is now little doubt that a small number of cases of paralytic poliomyelitis, that occurred in the U.S.A., were very closely associated with the use of the living vaccine. The risk to children under 15 years of age, however, is very small, and has been calculated for Type 1 as 1 in 6,000,000, for Type 2 as 1 in 50,000,000, and is greatest with Type 3 at 1 in 2,500,000 vaccine doses. In adults the risk is greater and the position may be serious because a significant proportion of the total number of paralytic cases are associated with the use of the vaccine; e.g. 24 out of 56 in 1963 and 10 out of 14 in 1964 (Henderson *et al.*, 1964). For an account of the inoculation schedules at present used see Chapter 43.

Passive immunity can be conferred by injecting gamma globulin. The doses recommended are as follows: for persons over the age of 7 years 1·5 g., for the age-group 1–6 years 1·0 g., and for infants under 1 year old 500 mg. To afford protection gamma globulin must be used as soon as possible after exposure or when possible, before the risk is taken. As it is in short supply and of rather doubtful value, gamma globulin is reserved for special occasions; it is used for pregnant women after exposure, for children after tonsillectomy at epidemic periods, and for laboratory workers accidentally contaminated by the virus. It should *not* be used for family contacts of a recognised case.

ECHO VIRUSES

When tissue cultures began to be used for the isolation of poliomyelitis viruses from stools it was soon found that many other viruses also could be recovered from the intestinal tract. These viruses can only be isolated in tissue cultures, optimally in those from monkey kidneys. Originally they were called "Orphan" viruses because they seemed unrelated to known diseases, and since they were present in faeces they were named "Enteric, Cytopathogenic, Human, Orphan *i.e.* ECHO viruses".

Properties of the Viruses.—By definition ECHO viruses are (1) cytopathogenic for monkey and human cells in tissue culture; (2) non-pathogenic for suckling mice and other laboratory animals; (3) unrelated to other known cytopathogenic viruses, *e.g.* poliomyelitis, Coxsackie B, herpes simplex, influenza, mumps, measles, varicella, and the adenoviruses; (4) neutralised by human gamma globulin; (5) ether resistant; (6) possessed of complement-fixing antigens; (7) characterised by plaques (see p. 79) different from those of the poliomyelitis viruses; (8) in the size range 23–35 mμ. ECHO type 10 is now regarded as the prototype of a new group, the reoviruses (see p. 441).

The ECHO viruses are in general similar to the poliomyelitis viruses in size, stability and resistance. They contain at least 25–30 per cent. RNA. They survive long periods at 4° C., are not inactivated at 37° C., and are stable from pH3 to pH11. In general, they are killed by heat for 30 min. at 65° C., survive well at −70° C., but lose much of their activity on freeze-drying. Continuous cell lines, *e.g.* HeLa, are not suitable for attempts at ECHO virus isolation, as the cytopathic effect may be absent or very slow to appear.

Cultivation.—Most strains grow well in epithelial cells from the kidneys of rhesus or cynomolgus monkeys and also in human amnion, human embryo kidney, lung or skin muscle. Growth is good in continuous lines such as HeLa or HEp2 but the cytopathic effect may be slow to appear or absent.

When ECHO viruses are seeded in dilute inocula on to the surface of a sheet of tissue culture cells, each single infective particle sets up an area of cell lysis or a plaque (see p. 79) which is easily recognised. Types 7, 8 and 12 produce large circular plaques with clearly defined edges and a diameter after a week's growth of 1 cm. Types 1, 3, 4, 6, 9, 11, 13, 14 and 16 produce irregularly shaped plaques which develop slowly and seldom reach 0·5 cm. in diameter (Hsiung, 1962).

ECHO viruses are pathogenic for rhesus and cynomolgus monkeys; types 2, 3, 4, 7, 9, 13, 14, 16 and 18 induce a febrile illness with viraemia and an antigenic response (Wenner, 1962). ECHO 9, especially after repeated passage in tissue culture, produces a fatal paralysis in mice resembling that caused by the Coxsackie viruses.

Haemagglutination of human group O erythrocytes is caused by types 3, 6, 7, 10, 11, 12, 13 and 19. These strains react with a receptor on human group O cells which is distinct from that of the myxoviruses. The haemagglutinin is not separable from the virus particle.

Antigenic Characters.—Twenty-eight distinct antigenic types have so far been distinguished by neutralisation tests in tissue cultures. Cross reactions occur between types 1, 8, 12, and 13 in neutralisation tests. Antigenic variation is known to occur in types 6, 9 and 10, and may be a common occurrence under natural conditions. The specificity of strains may be altered by cultivation in the presence of a heterologous antiserum.

Pathogenesis.—As knowledge of them has increased the ECHO viruses have lost their "orphan" status and now only two remain, types 15 and 17, that have never been clearly associated with disease.

ECHO virus infections are preceded by a short incubation period, usually of three to five days, and may take the form of simple fever, aseptic meningitis, diarrhoeal diseases or respiratory illnesses. A rubelliform rash may complicate these disease patterns or may occur as the sole manifestation of infection.

The sources of infection are human cases or carriers excreting ECHO viruses in their faeces or oropharyngeal secretions. When the viruses enter the body they multiply in epithelial cells in either the intestine or the respiratory tract. Some types, *e.g.* 6, 9, 11, 16 and 18, are able to penetrate the epithelial barrier of the gut to reach the bloodstream and multiply in secondary target organs. The viraemic phase may begin five days before the beginning of the illness and continue until 24 hours after the onset. Altogether, eleven types, 2, 3, 4, 7, 9, 11, 14, 15, 16, 18 and 19, have been recovered from the cerebrospinal fluid in cases of aseptic meningitis. ECHO 9 appears to be able to invade nervous tissue and infection with it is sometimes accompanied by mild transient paralysis. Recovery from ECHO virus infections is almost invariably rapid and complete; the number of human fatalities which can be ascribed with certainty to these viruses is exceedingly small.

ECHO viruses are not infrequently found in the stools of healthy young children, but the significance of this finding is not yet clear. There is little evidence to suggest that they are intestinal commensals and it is more probable that they are carried for undefined periods after mild or inapparent infections.

Epidemiology.—ECHO viruses occur in all parts of the world. They are found more frequently in children than in adults and are more prevalent in the summer and autumn months in temperate climates. The method of spread of the viruses is the same as that of the polioviruses and they are widely and rapidly disseminated when hygiene and sanitation are poor. In closed communities of children and in schools the viruses are transmitted easily so that almost inevitably a very high proportion of individuals are infected and excrete the virus.

All the ECHO types, with the exception of types 15 and 17, have been associated with sporadic cases of aseptic meningitis or one of the other disease patterns already mentioned. In the erruptive fevers caused by types 9 and 16 the aetiological relationship between the rash and the infective agent is well established. A number of the types, notably 4, 6, 9, 16, 20 and 28, have considerable epidemic potentialities (Sabin, 1960).

ECHO 9 epidemics have been common in Europe and North America and have taken the form of large outbreaks of a disease typically characterised by a biphasic fever, a sore throat, an exanthem in the form of macular or maculopapular rash on the face, neck and chest, and in 56 per cent., on the trunk and extremities. A minority of patients showed clinical signs of meningitis but many without distinct clinical signs showed a pleocytosis of the cerebrospinal fluid. On one occasion ECHO 9 was recovered from the medulla of an infant who died in coma.

ECHO 16 epidemics have been called "Boston Fever" after the city where the illness was first reported. Clinically the infection starts with a sharp fever, abdominal pains and a mild sore throat. Commonly in children there appears, 24–48 hours after defervescence, a pink, discrete macular or maculopapular rash mostly on the face, chest and back. Aseptic meningitis is uncommon.

ECHO 4 and 6 epidemics have been associated with considerable outbreaks of aseptic meningitis in children and adults.

ECHO 18 has been recovered from the faeces of many infants in an outbreak of diarrhoea. The children had no rash and no involvement of the central nervous system or meningeal reaction.

ECHO 20 was recovered from the throats of children suffering from cold-like illnesses and respiratory tract infections.

ECHO 28 or the J.H. or 2060 virus is the cause of a common cold illness and has been the cause of epidemics amongst army recruits in the U.S.A.

Laboratory Diagnosis.—ECHO viruses are readily isolated from throat swabs, stools or cerebrospinal fluid; they are present in 80 per cent. of cases in the faeces for two weeks after the onset. The procedure is that described for poliomyelitis and involves the inoculation of monolayers of monkey kidney tissue cultures. Human amnion cells may be used, but HeLa and other continuous lines of human cells are unsuitable. Strains are identified by testing first against pools of known antisera and then by neutralisation by a single type specific antiserum (Hambling, Davis and Macrae, 1963). Infections with more than one ECHO type can sometimes be revealed by the different types of plaques produced in monolayer cultures. Serological tests are burdensome, and unless there is some indication of the prevailing type it is often impractical to set up the many neutralisation tests required.

Other Enteroviruses.—ECHO-like viruses have been frequently isolated from animals. Monkeys appear to carry them asymptomatically and their presence is frequently detected by a cytopathic effect observed in uninoculated monkey kidney tissue culture cells. Often the cells show marked vacuolation and the viruses responsible have been known as "foamy agents". There are at least 25 enteric cytopathogenic monkey orphan (ECMO viruses). Similar agents have been recovered from bovines (ECBO viruses) and from swine (ECSO viruses). Further investigation is required into the relationship of these animal viruses to human enteric viruses and the possibility of their transfer from one host to another.

COXSACKIE VIRUSES

The third group of the enterovirus family contains the thirty Coxsackie viruses which cause such diverse illnesses as aseptic meningitis, epidemic myalgia or pleurodynia, herpangina and neonatal myocarditis.

Properties of the Viruses.—The virus particles are 25–35 mμ in diameter. One strain (group A type 10) has been obtained in a highly purified state from the carcases of infected mice by a combination of the processes of salting out and ultra-centrifugation; its elementary bodies when stored at 4° C. formed dodecahedral crystals about 100 mμ in diameter. The crystals have a high infectivity titre and contain a mixture of infective and non-infective units. About 4 per cent. of the virus particle is made up of RNA. In their reactions to chemical and physical agents Coxsackie viruses do not differ materially from other enteroviruses.

The most outstanding characteristic of the Coxsackie viruses is their pathogenicity for newborn mice and hamsters. It is during the first 48 hr. of life that these animals are fully susceptible to infection; thereafter they acquire a natural resistance and after the age of five days they can no longer be infected. By definition Coxsackie viruses are unable to infect adult mice. Two broad groups of the viruses have been made according to the histological nature and the situation of the lesions they produce in mice.

Group A viruses, of which there are 24, cause a single lesion, a widespread severe myositis involving skeletal muscle throughout the whole body. The principal muscles to be involved are those of the hind limbs, and in life the mice appear to have a flaccid paralysis. Usually the signs of infection appear four or five days after inoculation and progress until the animal dies four or five days later.

Group B viruses, of which there are six, cause widespread lesions in many organs. The myositis produced is characterised by focal lesions and gives rise to tremors, incoordination and a paralysis resembling the spastic type. The viruses also cause areas of necrosis in the brown fat lobules, especially those in the interscapular and cervical pads of brown fat. They also cause meningoencephalitis and pancreatitis. The incubation period of group B infections in mice is prolonged and symptoms may not be obvious until the tenth day after inoculation. Inoculated mice must be kept under observation for three weeks.

Haemagglutination.—Types A 27 and B 3 agglutinate human group O cells and type A 7 will agglutinate fowl cells which are sensitive to the vaccinia haemagglutinin.

Cultivation.—Tissue cultures are of limited value in isolating the viruses. Types A 9 and B 1, 2, 3, 4 and 5 grow well in monkey kidney monolayers and produce a cytopathic effect resembling that of the poliomyelitis viruses. These strains do not produce a cytopathic effect in human amnion or diploid cells. Types A 11, 13, 15 and 18 will grow in HeLa but not in monkey kidney cells. In general, however, the cytopathic effect in HeLa cells is variable and slow to develop. Explants of human uterus in plasma clot cultures are susceptible to those strains which grow in monkey kidney cells. Types A 1, 2, 4, 5, 6, 19 and 22 do not produce a cytopathic effect in tissue culture and to isolate them it is necessary to inoculate infant mice (Wenner and Lenahan, 1962).

In monkeys Coxsackie viruses do not produce clinical diseases, but after inoculation a viraemia is developed and later the virus is excreted for several weeks in the faeces. Types A 7 and A 14, however, possess the power to cause a mild paralysis in monkeys with lesions in the central nervous system resembling those of poliomyelitis. Type A 7, which has caused paralytic disease in man, is identical with the Russian AB IV strain which was at first thought to constitute a fourth type of the poliomyelitis virus.

Antigenic Characteristics.—Thirty antigenic types have been defined by cross-neutralisation tests in mice or tissue culture, and cross-complement-fixation reactions. Twenty-four have the pathogenicity of group A and six the characters of group B. Each of the six group B types are subject to antigenic variation and sera from convalescent cases may show heterotypic responses. Coxsackie A 9 is intermediate in some of its properties between the ECHO and Coxsackie groups and has some antigenic relationship with A 23 and ECHO 9.

Pathogenesis.—Coxsackie viruses are widespread in alimentary tracts of children and young adults and are disseminated in the summer and autumn months to a considerable proportion of children, especially those living under unhygienic conditions. The viruses are present in the gut for short periods, sometimes as little as a week; they are excreted in the faeces and have been recovered from sewage and flies. Their association with human infection is seen in the table on p. 440.

Clinically aseptic meningitis has the same manifestations whether it is caused by the Coxsackie, ECHO or poliomyelitis viruses. It is discussed further on p. 442. Epidemic myalgia or Bornholm disease, so-called because it was first described on the Danish island of Bornholm, is characterised by fever and the sudden onset of agonising stitch-like pains in the muscles of the chest, epigastrium or hypochondrium. Although the disease is most frequently recognised in its epidemic form, many sporadic cases also occur. Epidemic myalgia may be complicated by pleurisy and pericarditis. Herpangina is a sudden feverish illness of young children; the lesions in the mouth are highly characteristic and consist of papules on the anterior pillars of the fauces which soon become vesicles and finally shallow ulcers with a greyish base and a punched-out edge. In newborn infants severe and often fatal myocarditis has been reported and the causative virus has been found in high concentrations in the myocardium at autopsy. It may be that the newborn baby acquires the virus from its mother, and that, like the infant mouse, it is highly susceptible to infection.

Coxsackie B viruses are able also to produce myocarditis in adults of all age groups but this occurrence is much rarer than in infants.

In the respiratory tract Coxsackie A 21 (COE) has caused epidemics of colds in camps of military recruits and B strains have been associated with acute infections, bronchitis, and pneumonia in young children.

"Hand, foot, and mouth" disease presents as painful stomatitis with a vesicular erruption on the hands and feet. Typically it lasts for about a week (sometimes less); the majority of cases are seen in the summer in children aged 1–10 years.

Clinical Syndrome	Poliovirus Types	Coxsackie Viruses Types		ECHO Viruses Types
		A	B	
Neuronal damage				
Paralysis, sustained	1, 2, 3	4, 7, 9, 23.		2, 4, 9, 11, 13, 16.
Paralysis, transient	1, 2, 3	2, 9.	3, 4, 5.	1, 9, 16.
Encephalitis	1, 2, 3	—	3*.	9, 19.
Aseptic meningitis	1, 2, 3	2, 4, 7, 9, 23*.	1, 2, 3, 4, 5*, 6.	1, 2, 3, **4***, 5, **6***, 7, **9***, 11, 12, 13, 14, 15, 16, 18, 19, 20, 21, 22, 25.
Enteritis	—	—		**6***, 8, 11, 14, 18, 19, 20, 22, 23, 24, 28.
Herpangina	—	2, 3, 4, 5, 6, 8, 10.	—	—
Epidemic pleurodynia (Bornholm disease)	—	—	1, 2*, 3*, 4*, 5*.	—
Colds and respiratory illnesses	—	21* (COE).	1, 3.	6, 8, 11, 20*, 22, 25, 28*.
Myocarditis	1, 2, 3	—	2, 3, 4, 5.	—
Pericarditis	—	—	2, 3, 4, 5.	—
Rashes, maculopapular or vesicular		2, 4, 9, 16*, 23.	1, 3, 5. —	2, 4, 6, **9***, 14, **16***, 18.
"Hand, foot and mouth disease"	—	5, 16.	—	

The relationship between enteroviruses serotypes and clinical syndromes. Figures in heavy type indicate the commoner serotypes.

An asterisk indicates strains known to have been associated with epidemics.

Epidemiology.—Aseptic meningitis, epidemic myalgia and herpangina all occur characteristically as epidemics. The peak incidence is usually in the summer months and large epidemics may occur. In the summer of 1951 a widespread epidemic of Bornholm disease occurred in Great Britain and in 1959 a high incidence of aseptic meningitis due to Coxsackie viruses was reported in Scotland. Usually half the persons involved in epidemics are under the age of ten years and three-quarters under twenty. Herpangina is seen in very young children under five years of age in day nurseries and kindergarten schools, where it spreads rapidly. Sporadic cases of all the clinical forms of infection occur and often the patients are young adults who have acquired the infection presumably from family contacts. For a review of the Coxsackie viruses see Plager (1962).

Laboratory Diagnosis

Virus Isolation.—The virus can readily be isolated from throat swabs or faeces during the first two weeks of the infection and can also be recovered from the cerebrospinal fluid from cases of aseptic meningitis. Stools and throat swabs are treated with antibiotics and clarified by slow centrifugation in the manner used in isolation of the poliomyelitis viruses. The first step is to inoculate monkey kidney tissue cultures and HeLa cells. Human amnion cells may also be used but the viruses do not grow readily in them on primary isolation. Cytopathogenic agents growing in these cultures will include all the group B types and group A type 9. If this procedure yields no virus the specimens should be inoculated into mice no older than 48 hours by the combined intracerebral and intraperitoneal routes. The optimum age of mice for inoculation is 24 hours for group B and 48 hours for Group A viruses. Subsequently viruses will be placed in their appropriate groups according to the histological appearances of the lesions they produce. The causal relationship of a newly isolated virus to the illness should be confirmed by demonstrating a rising titre of homologous antibodies in the patient's serum. The final identification of the numerical serotype is carried out by neutralisation tests in tissue cultures or, if this is not possible, in infant mice. The procedures are burdensome, for there are thirty possible type-specific antisera to set against the unknown virus and, unless some information is available as to the prevalent infecting type, it may require much time to complete the task.

Serological Tests.—Neutralisation and complement-fixation reactions may be of value provided that the first serum has been taken within three days of the onset of the disease. Again the large number of viruses in the group often makes these tests impractical unless there is some clue as to the nature of the prevailing virus.

REOVIRUSES

Viruses of this group were at first classified as ECHO 10 but subsequently it was found that their larger size and other properties excluded them from the ECHO group. They were first called "Respiratory Enteric Orphan" viruses by Sabin (1959b) and the initial letters of this phrase gives the name REO. Despite the name, however, the pathogenicity of reovirus for man has not been clearly established. Although they have been isolated frequently from body secretions and excretions their pathological effects are questionable. They have been recovered from cases of diarrhoea in children and less frequently from mild febrile upper respiratory tract infections (Macrae, 1962).

Properties of the viruses.—The virus particle is 70 mμ in diameter and icosohedral in shape. The RNA core is enclosed in a capsid composed of 92 spherical capsomeres. All the reoviruses agglutinate human Group O erythrocytes. There are three serological types distinguished by haemagglutination inhibition tests; all three share a common complement-fixing antigen.

Cultivation.—The viruses grow well in monkey kidney tissue cultures in which they produce characteristic RNA-containing intracytoplastic inclusions. Strains isolated in tissue culture can be adapted to growth in suckling mice. The type 3 prototype strain sets up a fatal infection characterised before death by jaundice, a typical oily appearance of the fur, ataxia and peritonitis.

Aseptic Meningitis

Physicians are familiar with an acute feverish illness in which all the classical signs of meningeal irritation are present and yet the cerebrospinal fluid is bacteriologically sterile. The condition has been known as "abacterial", "serous", "virus", "lymphocytic" and "benign", but no one term is precisely accurate and the name "aseptic" is retained on the ground of common usage. The cell count in the cerebrospinal fluid is raised and figures between 50 and 2000 per cu. mm. have been recorded. The cells are predominantly lymphocytes and no bacteria can be seen in stained smears or obtained in culture. The protein content is always raised, usually to 80 or 100 mg. per 100 ml.; the figure may, however, be as low as 50 mg. per 100 ml. and the increase may not be apparent until several days after the onset of infection.

It must be remembered that this clinical syndrome may be associated with bacterial as well as viral infections. Tuberculous meningitis, middle ear disease, subdural abscesses, leptospiral meningitis, and even pyogenic meningitis under antibiotic therapy can all be associated with such a clinical picture.

Primary virus infections giving rise to aseptic meningitis are caused by poliomyelitis viruses (non-paralytic poliomyelitis); Coxsackie viruses especially group B; ECHO viruses; lymphocytic choriomeningitis virus; herpes simplex virus; certain arboviruses, *e.g.* louping ill, western equine encephalitis and Russian spring-summer encephalitis. In addition aseptic meningitis occurs as a complication of the following: mumps, chickenpox, measles, herpes zoster, infective hepatitis, sandfly fever and Jennerian vaccination.

Teschen Disease

Teschen Disease is an acute encephalomyelitis in pigs. The animals suffer from flaccid paralysis and develop lesions in the central nervous system which closely resemble those of human poliomyelitis. The causative virus is 25–30 mμ in diameter and has many of the general properties of the poliomyelitis viruses. It is, however, completely distinct antigenically and represents a unique type. The virus is excreted in the faeces and infection follows ingestion of contaminated food. Teschen disease is widespread on the continent of Europe, especially in Poland and Czechoslovakia, but has not been reported elsewhere. Sporadic cases of a similar though milder disease due to the related Talfan virus have been reported in Great Britain. The virus can be cultivated in pig or monkey kidney cells in which it produces a cytopathic effect like that of the polioviruses.

REFERENCES

BUTLER, N. R., BENSON, P. F., WILSON, B. D. R., PERKINS, F. T., UNGAR, J. & BEALE A. J. (1962). Poliomyelitis and triple antigen efficiency given separately and together. *Lancet*, **1**, 834.

DULBECCO, R. & VOGT, M. (1958). Study of the mutability of *d* lines of polioviruses. *Virology*, **5**, 220.

GARD, S. (1960). Immunological specificity within Type I poliovirus. *Bull. Wld. Hlth. Org.*, **22**, 235.

HAMBLING, M. H., DAVIS, P. M. & MACRAE, A. D. (1963). The typing of enteroviruses in tissue culture by neutralisation with composite antiserum pools. *J. Hyg. (Lond.)*, **61**, 479.

HENDERSON, D. A., WITTE, J. J., MORRIS, L. & LANGMUIR, A. D. (1964). Paralytic disease associated with oral polio vaccines. *J. Amer. med. Ass.*, **190**, 41.

HSIUNG, G. D. (1962). Further studies on characterisation and grouping of ECHO viruses. *Ann. N.Y. Acad. Sci.*, **101**, 413.

LWOFF, A. & LWOFF, W. (1960). Sur les facteurs du dévelopment viral et leur rôle dans l'évolution de l'infection. *Ann. Inst. Pasteur*, **98**, 173.

MACRAE, A. D. (1962). Reoviruses of man. *Ann. N.Y. Acad. Sci.*, **101**, 455.

MCBRIDE, W. D. (1959). Antigenic analysis of polioviruses by kinetic studies of serum neutralisation. *Virology*, **7**, 45.

MELNICK, J. L. (1962). Population genetics applied to live poliovirus vaccine. *Amer. J. publ. Hlth.*, **52**, 472.

PLAGER, H. (1962). The Coxsackie viruses. *Ann. N.Y. Acad. Sci.*, **101**, 390.

SABIN, A. B. (1959a). Present position of immunisation against poliomyelitis with live virus vaccines. *Brit. med. J.*, **1**, 663.

SABIN, A. B. (1959b). Reoviruses. *Science*, **130**, 1387.

SABIN, A. B. (1960). *Role of ECHO viruses in Human Disease.* Chapter 5 on Viral Infections of Infancy and Childhood, p. 55. New York: Hoeber-Harper.

WENNER, H. A. (1962). The ECHO viruses. *Ann. N.Y. Acad. Sci.*, **101**, 398.

WENNER, H. A. & LENAHAN, M. F. (1962). Propagation of Group A. Coxsackie viruses in tissue cultures. *Yale J. Biol. Med.*, **34**, 421.

CHAPTER 35

VIRAL HEPATITIS: INFECTIOUS MONONUCLEOSIS

VIRAL hepatitis includes two human diseases whose relationship to each other is still in doubt. Infectious hepatitis and serum hepatitis (homologous serum jaundice) are both characterised by the same clinical features of fever, nausea, malaise and jaundice. In both diseases severe degenerative changes occur in the parenchymal cells of the liver and marked impairment of hepatic function results. Usually, healing is remarkably complete and normal function is restored, but in a small proportion of patients relapses occur and occasionally the end-result may be multilobular cirrhosis of the liver.

Infectious hepatitis, or to use its older name "catarrhal jaundice", is a disease of children and young adults. It occurs endemically and more characteristically in epidemics in institutions, schools and in military camps. The virus is excreted in faeces and infection follows the ingestion of contaminated food; under conditions of communal living spread is facilitated and epidemics may occur.

Serum hepatitis is contracted when the virus is *injected* into a susceptible person; it occurs only after the injection of human serum or blood. Virus A is the name given to the agent associated with infectious hepatitis and virus B is associated with serum jaundice.

Properties of the viruses.—Different workers have claimed to have cultivated the viruses but their results have not so far been consistently reproducible in other laboratories. Amongst these claims, which all await confirmation, is that of Rightsel *et al.* (1961), who observed a cytopathic effect when a line of human cancer cells (Detroit 6) was inoculated with icterogenic serum or plasma. These workers who claimed the isolation of three serotypes of the virus, stated that it was 12–18 mμ in diameter, and reported that it survived after 30 min. at 60° C. The oral administration of one of the isolates failed to reproduce the disease but parenteral inoculation of human volunteers was followed by hepatitis. Davis (1961) found, in the sera of 14 of 22 children with infectious hepatitis, agents which produced a cytopathic effect on the cells of a line of human embryonic lung and showed that they were not known enteroviruses. Hillis (1962) recovered from the serum of 2 of 12 cases of acute hepatitis an agent which had a destructive effect on growing chimpanzee kidney cells.

Because the only known susceptible host has been man, much of the knowledge that we have of these viruses has been obtained from studies on human volunteers.

Virus A. Infectious Hepatitis.—The size of the virus particle is not known although it has been proved to be able to pass through a Seitz EK filter. The virus can be preserved for long periods in the frozen state—*e.g.* 18 months at −20° C. It survives heat at 56° C. for 30 min. and withstands chlorine at a concentration of one part per million for 30 min. and 10 per cent. ether at 4° C. for 24 hr. When given orally or parenterally to human volunteers the disease develops in 17–30 days and the virus is present in the blood and faeces in the pre-icteric and early icteric phases of the illness.

Virus B. Serum Hepatitis.—The virus, according to filtration experiments, is 26 mμ or less in diameter. It survives storage at room temperature for six months and can be kept at −20° C. for over four years; it is also well preserved by freeze drying. It has survived heat at 60° C. for four hours. Ultra-violet light has failed to inactivate the virus in plasma. The virus is not affected by 0·25 per cent. phenol, 0·05 per cent. merthiolate, nitrogen mustard in a concentration of 50 mg. per litre, or 10 per cent. ether. It is inactivated by sulphur mustard in a 0·005 M concentration.

Pathogenesis.—The only source of *infectious hepatitis* is man; the virus is present in his blood and intestine during the incubation period as well as in the pre-icteric and icteric phases of the acute illness. It is probable that most patients excrete the virus in the faeces for about one month after the onset but some, especially infants, may be faecal carriers for several months. The virus is also present in the blood stream, where it is known to have persisted for as long as eight months.

The only known source of *serum hepatitis* is human blood or serum or their products, and transmission occurs solely after the injection of these substances. When the donor of the blood or serum is traced it is seldom possible to elicit a history of previous jaundice. Sometimes the donors suspected as being the original source of infection develop jaundice many months later.

Minute amounts of blood or serum, as little as 0·01 ml., have often been known to have transmitted serum hepatitis. The disease develops after a remarkably long incubation period, which on average is about 80 days but may be as short as 40 days or as long as 160 days after the injection. The duration of infectivity following the jaundice is not known. In many cases the virus is in the blood for many months after recovery and long after the liver function tests have again given normal results. The longest recorded period for a person to have carried the virus in the blood is five and a half years. Patients with serum hepatitis do not seem to excrete the virus and their immediate contacts are not liable to contract the infection.

Epidemiology

Infectious Hepatitis exists throughout the world. It is essentially a disease of children and 65 per cent. of cases occur between the ages of 5 and 15. In young children, the disease may occur as an inapparent infection (*e.g.* in nurseries) or may manifest itself as an attack of diarrhoea. There is a seasonal trend with increased prevalence in the autumn and winter. Outbreaks in institutions, schools, mental hospitals and orphanages are common; often there is a characteristic interval of three to four weeks between the appearances of small crops of cases and this sequence may continue for months or even years, involving new members as they join the community. A similar sequence of infections is a familiar occurrence in large families. The disease has a special tendency to widespread epidemics amongst troops under wartime conditions. In the Mediterranean theatre in the Second World War, many thousands of young soldiers suffered from a severe form of infectious hepatitis. Communal living, poor sanitation and transfer by flies were all factors which aided the spread of infection. There are many examples of explosive waterborne epidemics, and many others have followed the contamination of foodstuffs by carriers. Shellfish, e.g. oysters and mussels, have been responsible for large-scale epidemics. It must also be remembered that, like serum hepatitis, the infection can be transmitted by the use of syringes and needles contaminated with blood. The subject of infectious hepatitis is studied in detail by MacCallum *et al.* (1951).

Serum Hepatitis.—On repeated occasions serum hepatitis has occurred in hospitals and clinics where syringes and needles were used without sterilisation between each inoculation. Since the introduction of proper cleaning and sterilising methods such outbreaks are rare and occur only when faulty technique prevents the destruction of the virus. In venereal clinics so-called "arsenical jaundice" in patients receiving courses of intravenous injections for syphilis used to be a common complication; for many years it was thought to be a true manifestation of the arsenical treatment, but when regular routine daily sterilisation of all syringes was introduced the condition virtually disappeared. Serum hepatitis has followed blood transfusions and more often the use of plasma and pooled serum but very rarely after the use of human gamma-globulin. Human serum has sometimes been used as a constituent of suspending or preservative solutions for yellow fever virus vaccines and on at least two occasions big epidemics of hepatitis occurred in service personnel receiving the vaccine.

A Comparison of Infectious and Serum Hepatitis.—The very considerable differences between these two diseases are shown on page 447, and they are sufficient to suggest that the causative viruses A and B are separate entities. The fact that a patient who has recovered from infectious hepatitis can still contract serum hepatitis and *vice versa* would support this view; but whether this represents two distinct viruses or antigenically dissimilar variants of the same virus is quite unknown.

Infectious hepatitis is an example of the familiar pattern of the natural history of many infectious diseases of man. Serum hepatitis, however, is quite different, for it is obviously an artificially induced condition; it cannot be produced by the ingestion of icterogenic serum and follows only after needle puncture. The condition is not contagious and the virus is not found in the stools. If serum hepatitis is a distinct entity there should be some means whereby it is spread naturally but this so far has eluded observation. Burnet (1960) has suggested that the virus may be transmitted from parent to offspring transplacentally and that as a consequence the new host has an immune-tolerance to the virus but remains a persistent carrier.

A Comparison of Infectious Hepatitis and Serum Hepatitis

Disease	Infective Hepatitis	Serum Hepatitis
Virus . . .	A	B
Infectiousness . .	Contagious.	Not contagious.
Incubation period .	15–40 days.	40–160 days.
Onset . . .	Acute.	Insidious.
Fever . . .	Over 38° C. (100° F.)	Low-grade.
Age	Children and young adults.	Any age.
Virus in blood . .	Three days before onset and in acute and convalescent phases.	In incubation period and acute phase.
Virus in faeces . .	In incubation period and acute phase.	Not present.
Longest known duration of carrier state:		
(*a*) Blood . .	8 months.	5 years.
(*b*) Faeces . .	16 months.	Not present.
Route of successful experimental transmission . . .	Oral and parenteral.	Parenteral only.
Seasonal incidence .	Autumn and winter.	All the year round.
Prophylactic value of gamma globulin .	Good.	Ineffective.
Immunity:		
(*a*) Homotypic .	Present.	Uncertain.
(*b*) Heterotypic .	None.	None.

Both types of hepatitis have indistinguishable clinical manifestations which may vary from the severe to mild and silent forms. In both the virus has been shown to be present in the blood in the presymptomatic period. Virus B, for instance, was demonstrated in the blood of one patient no less than 87 days before he developed the first symptoms of illness. It is therefore apparent that blood from supposedly normal donors who have never had hepatitis, may yet contain Virus A or Virus B, or both.

Prophylaxis and Control

Infectious Hepatitis.—An outbreak of the disease in schools and institutions is often largely due to poor personal hygiene and inadequate sanitary arrangements. All the hygienic measures which are required to control the spread of pathogenic intestinal bacteria should be enforced. It is of importance to make every effort to ensure that virus carriers do not act as food handlers. All needles, syringes, blood-counting pipettes and lancets that may have been in contact with patients with infectious hepatitis should be autoclaved. Passive protection against clinical infection may be conferred up to six days before the onset of symptoms by the use of gamma globulin (Moseley, Speers & Chin, 1963). The dose recommended for persons of the age of seven and over is 0·5 g. and for children below this age 0·25 g.

Serum Hepatitis.—People who have had jaundice should not be used as blood donors. Persons without a history of hepatitis, however, may have the virus in their blood and the problem of making blood and blood products safe for transfusion has not yet been completely solved. Exposure to ultra-violet light and treatment with nitrogen mustard have been recommended but are not always effective in killing the virus. The addition of sulphur-mustard (2,500 mg. per litre) and storage for 6 months at 70° F. has given more encouraging results. When pools of plasma are made and stored for use later, the risk of contaminating large volumes should be reduced by taking into each pool the plasma of not more than five donors. All transfusion apparatus, syringes, needles, blood-counting pipettes, lancets, etc., must be autoclaved before use. Such sterile precautions are required not only in transfusion work but in haematological, diabetic and venereal disease clinics, and indeed should be employed whenever the skin of the patient is punctured. Gamma globulin has been found to give no protection against serum hepatitis.

Laboratory Diagnosis

There are no specific laboratory tests that can be used to detect the virus or its antibody. Some help may however be obtained from biochemical tests of liver function and estimation of serum transaminase has proved valuable in this respect. Many unusual serological manifestations are found in infectious hepatitis and serum jaundice. Amongst these false positive Kahn and Wassermann reactions are frequent. About 70 per cent. of serum samples from cases of acute infectious hepatitis are able to agglutinate the erythrocytes of one-day-old chick embryos to a titre of 80 or above, and erythrocytes of rhesus monkeys at titres of 128 to 2048. These haemagglutination tests are of some limited diagnostic value because positive findings seldom occur in obstructive or toxic jaundice (McCollum *et al.*, 1959; Havens, 1960; Schmidt and Lenette, 1961). These reactions are not directly associated with action of the infectious hepatitis virus, and it is probable that the altered processes of protein production, occasioned by severe liver damage, result in the production of abnormal globulins which react with a wide variety of different bacterial and viral antigens.

INFECTIOUS MONONUCLEOSIS

Infectious mononucleosis or glandular fever is an acute feverish illness characterised by malaise, sore throat, enlargement of the lymph glands, a mononuclear blood picture, and heterophile antibodies in the blood. Liver function tests indicate that liver damage is constantly present. In about 40 per cent. of cases the spleen is palpable, and in about 10–20 per cent. a rubelliform rash is seen; jaundice and meningeal symptoms are rare complications but evidence of hepatitis can be elicited by liver function tests in the vast majority of cases. Three clinical forms, anginose, glandular and febrile, have been distinguished according to the predominant clinical features. The infection occurs most commonly among school children and young adults. The disease is often mild and probably ambulant undetected forms are frequent; it is rarely fatal. It is not highly infectious, although epidemics have occasionally been reported. There is some evidence to suggest that direct contact, *e.g.* kissing, may be a factor in the spread of the infection.

Aetiology.—The nature of the infective agent is unknown, but has been thought to be a virus on account of the infectious nature of the disease. In general, no laboratory animals can be infected and attempts to transmit the disease to man have usually failed. On one occasion when 250 ml. blood was transfused from a clinical case to a human volunteer the typical clinical picture of severe mononucleosis resulted. The cultivation of *Listeria monocytogenes* from the blood of a few cases has suggested that this organism may cause the infection in man, but a constant association with this or any other bacterium has never been demonstrated.

Laboratory Diagnosis.—Some 50–80 per cent. of patients develop heterophile antibodies which can be demonstrated by the Paul-Bunnell reaction (see Chapter 54). The characteristic blood picture also helps to establish the diagnosis; a relative or more usually an absolute increase in the number of lymphocytes, together with the presence of abnormal monocytes, is diagnostic. A proportion of cases whose clinical illness and blood picture conform to those of infective mononucleosis do not have a positive Paul-Bunnell reaction and are referred to as "sero-negative infectious mononucleosis".

Mouse Hepatitis

Weaned mice doubly infected with the mouse hepatitis virus and *Eperythrozoon coccoides* (a micro-organism related to *Haemobartonella*) develop a fatal hepatitis (Gledhill, Dick and Niven, 1955). Neither agent by itself can cause evident illness. In the presence of *E. coccoides* the virus multiplies more abundantly, but the nature of this synergism is not understood. A proportion of normal mice carry *E. coccoides* and are thereby rendered susceptible to virus infection.

The virus is 80–120 mμ in diameter, inactivated in 30 min. at 56° C. and is ether sensitive.

Hepatitis of Ducklings

This is an acute epizootic disease of young ducklings. It is a scheduled disease in Great Britain and is a rapidly fatal infection. Only young ducklings two to three weeks of age are affected; adult ducks, fowls and turkeys are resistant. Infected ducklings often die within a few hours of the onset of the disease; at autopsy the liver is enlarged with fatty change and shows subcapsular petechiae and larger haemorrhages. No inclusions have been described in the infected tissues. The virus can be isolated from the liver and other tissues by egg cultivation. It is 20–40 mμ in diameter and contains DNA. The chick embryo is not killed by the virus, but five days after inoculation a greenish discoloration of the liver and a viscid condition of the yolk sac is characteristic of the action of the virus. The virus does not agglutinate erythrocytes and is not related to the Newcastle virus. Ducks recovered from the disease are resistant to re-infection and their serum possesses neutralising antibodies. Active immunisation with vaccines of egg fluids or embryo livers has not proved satisfactory.

REFERENCES

Burnet, F. M. (1960). *Principles of Animal Virology*, p. 254. New York: Academic Press.

Davis, E. V. (1961). Isolation of viruses from children with infectious hepatitis. *Science*, **133**, 2059.

Gledhill, A. W., Dick, G. W. A. & Niven, J. S. F. (1955). Mouse hepatitis virus and its pathogenic action. *J. Path. Bact.*, **69**, 299.

Havens, W. P. (1960). Haemagglutination in hepatic disease. *Arch. intern. Med.*, **106**, 327.

Hillis, W. D. (1962). Destruction of chimpanzee kidney cells by sera from patients with acute infectious hepatitis. *Proc. Soc. exp. Biol. (N.Y.)*, **108**, 813.

MacCallum, F. O., McFarlan, A. M., Miles, J. A. R., Pollock, M. R. & Wilson, C. (1951). Infective Hepatitis. *Med. Res. Counc. Spec. Rep. Serv.*, No. 273. H.M.S.O., London.

McCollum, R. W., Bech, V., Isaacson, P. & Riordan, T. (1959). A survey for haemagglutinins in viral hepatitis. *Amer. J. Med.*, **27**, 703.

Moseley, W. H., Speers, J. F. & Chin, T. D. Y. (1963). Epidemiologic studies of a large urban outbreak of infectious hepatitis. *Amer. J. publ. Hlth.*, **53**, 1603.

Rightsel, W. A., Keltsch, R. A., Taylor, A. R. & Boggs, J. D. (1961). Status report on tissue-culture of cultivated hepatitis virus. *J. Amer. med. Ass.*, **177**, 671.

Schmidt, N. J. & Lennette, E. H. (1961). Recent advances in the serodiagnosis of virus infections. *Prog. med. Virol.*, **3**, 32.

CHAPTER 36

ARTHROPOD-BORNE (ARBO) VIRUSES

THE term *arbor-viruses* was a convenient abbreviation which was used as the name of a large group of viruses transmitted by arthropods. The name ARBOVIRUSES has recently been proposed for these viruses because it has no suggestion that these agents are of *arboreal* origin. Members of the group infect man and many other mammals and birds. Arthropods take in the virus when they feed on the blood of an infected animal and transmit it to a new host when they take their next meal. The viruses multiply within the body of the arthropod without damaging its tissues or producing disease. Those viruses which, like the rabbit myxomatosis virus, are merely conveyed mechanically on the soiled mouth parts or legs of the arthropods are by definition excluded from the arbor virus group.

Arboviruses are most prevalent in those parts of the world where tropical heat and rain encourage the abundant breeding of arthropods near to susceptible animals. Many of these viruses have complex infection cycles involving several vertebrate and invertebrate hosts.

The arboviruses, of which over 160 distinct prototypes exist, have been divided into groups on immunological grounds (WHO 1961). At present group A contains 17 types, group B 35, and group C 7; in addition there are 14 in the Bunyamwera group and 15 other groups each of which contain 2–6 members. There are 42 ungrouped viruses.

Properties of the Viruses.—The viruses are within the size range 20–50 mμ in diameter. They contain RNA and some of them appear to be spherical and enclosed by a covering membrane.

Host Range and Cultivation.—The viruses infect many animals both domestic such as horses, cattle, sheep, goats, pigs and poultry and wild animals including monkeys, many species of rodents, and birds. The suckling mouse is the most susceptible of all laboratory animals; adult mice may be resistant to infection with some strains by all routes of inoculation except the intracerebral. The viruses multiply in the chick embryo after inoculation into the yolk-sac or on to the chorio-allantoic membrane. They grow readily in tissue cultures of chicken and mouse embryo, or in pure cell lines often with marked cytopathic effects (Buckley, 1959). It is a characteristic of arbor viruses that in addition to growing in the tissues of vertebrate hosts they also multiply in the arthropod vector.

Haemagglutination.—Most members of the group agglutinate the erythrocytes of newly-hatched chicks or geese. Optimal conditions for haemagglutination vary for each of the virus groups.

Viability.—In aqueous suspensions arboviruses are unstable at room temperature; at $-20°$ C. they survive better but there is a slow progressive loss of infectivity over several months until it is lost at the end of about 9 to 12 months. In solid CO_2 at $-79°$ C. the viruses survive for several years provided that they have been placed in containers sealed so that the CO_2 does not gain access to them. Suspended in fluids containing serum or bovine albumen these viruses can be well preserved by freeze drying.

Formaldehyde even in very low concentrations, and 20 per cent. ether, inactivate the viruses; heat at 60° C. for ten minutes or ultraviolet light for ten to thirty minutes kills them. Sodium desoxycholate in a 0·1 per cent. concentration inactivates arboviruses but fails to affect enteroviruses. This is considered to be an excluding property in that no arbovirus has yet been shown to resist this chemical.

The effect of the pH of the suspending fluid is of the greatest importance in maintaining the infective titre of the virus. The majority of these viruses should be kept within the pH range 7–8, and for haemagglutination work the optimum pH for each must be determined.

Antigenic Structure.—There is a considerable degree of antigenic sharing amongst the arboviruses, and they have been classified into groups A, B and C and 16 other groups according to cross-reactions in haemagglutination-inhibition and complement-fixation reactions (see page 453). Antigens for serological reactions are usually obtained from the infected brain tissue of newborn mice, but occasionally infected liver or serum may be used. The details of the techniques of haemagglutination and haemagglutination-inhibition are described by Clarke and Casals (1958).

Pathogenesis.—In a considerable proportion of infections the arboviruses give rise to subclinical or minor illness but in those patients who develop encephalitis the effects are often severe. After an incubation period which may vary from 4–21 days there is a sudden onset of fever with signs resembling those seen in aseptic meningitis. Marked drowsiness or stupor is characteristic and the mortality, which varies with different viruses, is between 5 and 25 per cent. In elderly people the fatality rate is much higher, reaching 50–80 per cent.

The pathogenesis of these infections in man has not been well studied, but it is thought that the virus multiplies first in an extraneural situation and that a viraemic phase follows some two to three days before the onset of the clinical illness. In fatal cases there is a severe inflammatory reaction most pronounced in the cerebral cortex but involving all parts of the central nervous system.

Epidemiology.—To understand the epidemiology of the arbovirus infections a knowledge is necessary not only of the organisms themselves but also of the ecology of the arthropod vectors and non-human hosts of the viruses. Human infection is usually only an unimportant incident in the perpetuation of the virus in nature. Transmission of the virus from one vertebrate to the next may depend on more than one arthropod species, and several species of animals may be infected by the vector's bite. The chain of infection may simply be:

Vector→Vertebrate host→Vector→Vertebrate host

Group A	Group B	Group C	Other Groups
Mosquito-borne Eastern equine encephalomyelitis Western equine encephalomyelitis Venezuelan equine encephalomyelitis Chikungunya O'nyong-nyong Sindbis and 11 other viruses	*Mosquito-borne* Yellow fever Dengue types 1–4 St. Louis Japanese B West Nile Murray Valley Ilhéus Wesselbron and 16 other viruses *Tick-borne* Far Eastern Russian encephalitis Central European encephalitis Louping ill Omsk haemorrhagic fever Kyasanur forest disease Powassan and 2 other viruses	*Mosquito-borne* 7 viruses from Belém, Brazil	*Mosquito-borne* Bunyamera—14 viruses from Africa, North and South America, India, Slovakia, etc. California—5 viruses Bwamba —2 viruses Simbu —6 viruses Guamá —5 viruses *Phlebotomus-borne* Sandfly fever and 12 other groups of small numbers (2–8) of viruses

Classification of the arthropod-borne animal viruses. A selection including the more important viruses known to be associated with disease in man. There are, in addition, about 80 other arboviruses, some of which are associated with disease of animals and others not yet classified.

or it may be more complex:

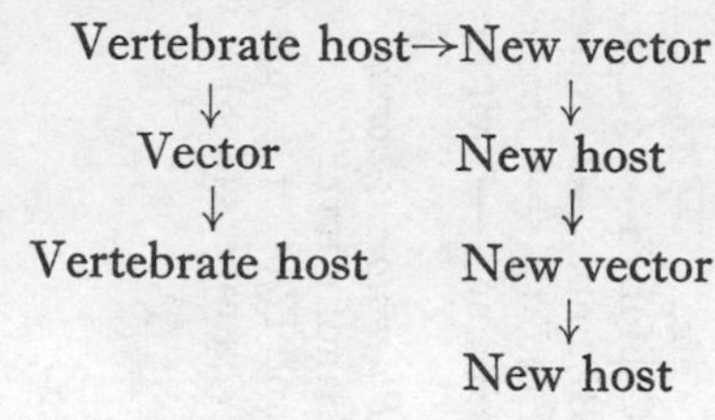

or again:

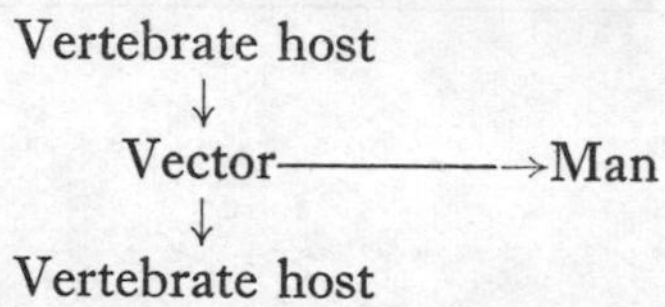

When the tick is the vector, the virus may be carried transovarially through several life cycles before the infection is again transmitted.

For further details on this subject the reader is referred to larger works, *e.g.* Smith (1959), Horsfall and Tamm (1959), Reeves (1961), McLean (1962).

Laboratory Diagnosis.—The virus may be isolated from the blood in the early stages of infection; it is often difficult to recover it from the cerebrospinal fluid. The virus may also be found in infected brain tissue of fatal cases. Suckling mice should be inoculated intracerebrally and intraperitoneally and eggs by the chorio-allantoic method. Tissue cultures of chick embryo fibroblasts or HeLa cells may also be used for certain strains. Chick embryos can be infected but usually only after adaptation. When the virus is recovered from the inoculated mice or embryos it is identified in suitable neutralisation, complement-fixation or haemagglutination-inhibition reactions. Adult goose erythrocytes are useful in haemadsorption tests in tissue cultures.

Serological tests for antibodies can be carried out using the haemagglutination-inhibition technique but the results are usually only group specific because of the common antigens shared by these viruses. For general diagnostic use the complement-fixation test using infected chick embryo antigens is satisfactory (Lenette *et al.*, 1956). Complement-fixation antibodies develop more slowly than neutralising or haemagglutination-inhibiting antibodies and thus they offer a better chance to demonstrate a significant rise of titre.

YELLOW FEVER

Yellow fever is primarily a disease of monkeys and possibly of some other forest animals. In nature the infection is transmitted from monkey to monkey by forest mosquitoes of the genera *Aedes* and *Haemagogus*; man is only involved incidentally when he is bitten by an infected mosquito. The human disease may vary from an almost symptomless infection to a severe jaundice with haemorrhage and death. Yellow fever is now a truly tropical disease and is endemic in large areas of equatorial South America and Africa.

Properties of the Virus.—From measurements by filtration the diameter of the virus is 17–28 mμ.

Host Range.—The yellow fever virus is pathogenic to all the species of South American monkeys but in many species of African monkeys it produces only viraemia and mild fever. Most African strains of the virus are highly pathogenic and kill the monkey by causing acute necrosis of the liver. Other strains have predominant neurotropic qualities but some may cause only a mild feverish illness. Adult mice can be infected by the intracerebral route, but not intraperitoneal inoculation. Infant mice are highly susceptible and can be infected by any route of inoculation. Guinea-pigs are susceptible after intracerebral inoculation, but different strains of the animals vary in their response to intraperitoneal inoculation. The rat and the rabbit are completely insusceptible. The virus can be readily cultivated in the chick embryo and in tissue cultures of chick or mouse embryos. Serial transfer of the virus in mice and other hosts readily modifies its pathogenicity for monkeys.

There is conclusive evidence that the yellow fever virus multiplies in the mosquito. *Aedes aegypti* becomes infected when it bites a host during the first three days of the disease and then after an interval of twelve days it is able to transmit the infection. The insect remains infective for life, but the virus is not transmitted through the egg to the next generation. Mosquitoes are the only blood-sucking arthropods known to play a part in the spread of yellow fever.

Viability.—The virus is extremely labile and is readily inactivated by heat and antiseptics. It is also rapidly inactivated if it is diluted in normal saline and to prevent this 10 per cent. normal serum or 0·75 per cent. bovine albumen should be added to the diluent. It survives in 50 per cent. glycerol saline at 0° C. for three months but is best preserved by freeze drying. It is well preserved at $-76°$ C. but care must be taken to avoid exposure to CO_2.

Antigenic Characters.—After infection with the yellow fever virus, neutralising, complement-fixing and haemagglutination-inhibiting antibodies appear. The first two of these antibodies are not identical and neutralisation appears some days before complement-fixation. In mild infections and after vaccination complement-fixing antibodies may be absent although the serum has definite neutralising qualities. The antigen used in the complement-fixation test is prepared from infected mouse brain or monkey liver and there is some evidence to suggest that it is not the virus itself which reacts but some product derived from the infected tissues. From cross-reactions in complement-fixation and haemagglutination-inhibition tests the virus has been placed in group B of the arbor viruses. It is related immunologically to dengue, Uganda S, and Zika viruses.

Pathogenesis.—After the virus has been injected through the skin by the mosquito it spreads to the local lymph glands, where it multiplies. After an incubation period of three to four days it invades the blood stream and is carried to the liver, spleen, bone marrow and kidneys, where it sets up necrotic processes. In fatal cases the pathological changes seen at autopsy are those of jaundice with haemorrhage into the gastric mucosa near the pylorus, and fatty change of the liver and kidneys. Histologically there is a characteristic coagulative hyaline necrosis (the "Councilman lesion") scattered diffusely throughout the liver. The necrotic changes are often most marked in the mid-zone of the lobules and are preceded or accompanied by cloudy swelling and fatty degeneration.

Yellow fever virus infection is sometimes accompanied by the formation of acidophilic intranuclear inclusion bodies (*Torres bodies*); they do not contain nucleic acid and probably do not consist of virus particles. These inclusions partially surround the nucleoli, are variable in size, granular in appearance and irregular in outline. *Torres bodies* are frequently found in the liver of the infected monkey but are uncommon in human tissues.

Epidemiology.—At one time yellow fever was prevalent in urban communities and the virus was transmitted from person to person by *Aedes aegypti.* This mosquito is essentially of a domestic type and breeds close to human dwellings; antimosquito measures have now eliminated the insect in most towns and "urban" yellow fever has been virtually eradicated.

Yellow fever, however, still occurs in people who live in remote rural parts in the tropics. It is referred to as "Jungle" or "Sylvatic" yellow fever and is perpetuated amongst the monkey population by different species of mosquitoes.

Tree-dwelling mosquitoes of the genus *Haemagogus* are responsible for the persistence of the disease in Central and South America and *Aedes africanus* in equatorial Africa.

Laboratory Diagnosis

The virus may be recovered from the blood during the first five days of the illness. The serum is injected intracerebrally in mice (preferably infant mice) and when the signs of encephalitis appear the animals are killed and an emulsion from their brains is prepared. Identification of the virus is carried out by neutralisation tests with a specific antiserum.

Serologically the diagnosis can be confirmed with neutralisation tests in adult mice on sera taken early in the disease and again during convalescence. A standard dose of a mouse-adapted strain of yellow fever virus (the French Neurotropic strain) is required in these tests. Neutralising antibodies develop early in the infection and are present on the fifth day. The antibody response in yellow fever is of two types, depending on whether the condition is primary or whether it occurs in an individual who has previously been infected with another agent belonging to group B of the arboviruses. In primary infections the antibodies produced are specific and enable the diagnosis to be made with certainty. In superimposed infections antibodies with wide cross-reactions with other arboviruses appear, and a specific diagnosis is virtually impossible. Complement-fixing antibodies appear later than the neutralising antibodies and persist for only a few months; in mild infections and after vaccination with the 17D egg-cultivated virus they are not developed. The complement-fixation test, however, provides satisfactory evidence that infection is due to yellow fever virus infection, especially when used on convalescent sera from known cases of primary infection (Theiler, 1959). In fatal cases the diagnosis of yellow fever may be made from the characteristic histological lesions seen in the liver (*vide supra*). When, for any reason, autopsy is impracticable, small specimens of liver tissue for histology can be obtained by the use of a *viscerotome*, which is inserted through the skin of the abdominal wall over the liver.

Prophylaxis

Vigorous mosquito control measures have virtually eliminated urban yellow fever. For protection against jungle yellow fever or for prevention of spread from endemic areas prophylactic vaccination is effective. The vaccine in general use contains a living attenuated strain of the virus (17D) and affords excellent protection; it is prepared from chick embryos inoculated with 17D and incubated at 37° C. for four days. The infected embryos are ground-up and freeze-dried in ampoules under dry nitrogen gas. The vaccine should be stored in the coldest part of a refrigerator (the ice chamber) and is reconstituted immediately before use with ice-cold physiological saline. Once made up, the virus must be used within thirty minutes and an ice-cold syringe should be used for the injections. As the virus is alive only one inoculation is required; the minimum dose of immunisation has been set at 500 LD50 and this is contained in a volume of 0·5 ml. It is most unusual for any local reaction to follow yellow fever immunisation; but general reaction with symptoms of encephalitis have occasionally been reported in infants, all of whom have recovered without sequelae. It is usually advised that children under the age of one year should not be vaccinated unless there is a great risk of yellow fever. Immunity is effective by the ninth day after inoculation. Full protection is maintained for at least eight years and in 70 per cent. of persons for nine years.

It is recommended that the vaccine should be given at least four days before smallpox vaccination or not until three weeks after a successful vaccination for fear of encephalitis. In West Africa, however, French workers have combined dried yellow fever vaccine, the Dakar vaccine (mouse neurotropic strain) with dried vaccinia virus in a suspending solution of gum arabic and have applied it to the scarified skin. Satisfactory levels of immunity against both diseases are achieved simultaneously, but the incidence of reaction was about 15 per cent.

DENGUE FEVER

Dengue is a mosquito-borne virus disease widespread in the tropics. The disease is benign but extremely prostrating with high fever, intense headache and very severe pain in the muscles, joints, bones, and behind the eyes. The fever may continue or may have a remission after the third day with a secondary rise three or four days later giving rise to the characteristic "saddleback" temperature chart. A maculo-papular or scarlatiniform rash appears on the third or fourth day and persists for about three days.

Properties of the Virus.—The dengue viruses have the general properties of the family of arboviruses. They are members of group B and are immunologically related to the yellow fever virus and to the Uganda S and Zika viruses. They do not infect the guinea-pig, rabbit, or cotton rat, and only cause inapparent infections in monkeys. Some strains have been adapted to adult or suckling mice and produce a flaccid paralysis in the animals. Other strains have been cultivated in the chick embryo, monkey kidney and hamster kidney tissue culture. There are at least four distinct immunological types.

Pathogenesis.—Dengue follows the introduction of the virus by the bite of the mosquito *Aedes aegypti* or of other *Aedes* species. At the site of the bite, a red papule 1–4 cm. in diameter is always present; the lesion is characteristic and is the site of local viral multiplication. Within 24 hours of the onset of the first fever the virus is in the blood stream and the disease begins. In the Philippines, Thailand and recently India, infection with types 3 and 4 has been found accompanied by a more severe form of the illness characterised by a petechial rash, epistaxis and gastrointestinal haemorrhage.

Dengue occurs in the eastern Mediterranean, Africa, India, the Far East and on many islands in the Pacific Ocean. The infection is transmitted by *Aedes aegyptae* and certain other species of mosquitoes and is perpetuated in a cycle of infection which includes monkeys or man. The mosquito becomes infective some seven to ten days after biting a dengue patient and remains so for the rest of its life. The virus is not, however, transmitted transovarially to the progeny of the insect. It is probable that there is a reservoir of infection in monkeys, or in other wild mammals. When cold weather renders the mosquito inactive, outbreaks of dengue cease, and it is only in those parts of the world where warm humid conditions persist throughout the year that dengue is constantly maintained.

Laboratory Diagnosis.—The virus may be isolated by the intracerebral inoculation of suckling mice with blood taken during the first three days of the illness. When the mice die the virus is identified by neutralisation tests with type-specific antisera. If the mice survive, the presence or absence of the virus can be determined by challenging the animals when they are four to six weeks old with an intracerebral inoculation of 100 LD50 of a mouse-adapted strain. If the mice are unaffected by the challenge they are presumed to have acquired a specific resistance from dengue virus in the original inoculum.

Neutralising antibodies appear within seven days of the onset of fever and complement-fixing antibodies about two weeks later. The haemagglutination-inhibition test is, however, the most useful because when the convalescent phase serum obtained within two days of defervescence is compared with the acute phase serum, a clear-cut rise of antibody titre can usually be demonstrated. Antigens of both type 1 and type 2 dengue viruses must be employed in these tests. Great care is required in the interpretation of serological findings because of the possibility of heterotypic responses following infection by other group B arboviruses.

Prophylaxis.—Control depends upon the eradication of the mosquito vector. The yellow fever (17D) vaccine gives no protection against dengue. There is no dengue virus vaccine available for use at present.

THE TICK-BORNE ENCEPHALITIS COMPLEX

The majority of arboviruses in Group B are mosquito-borne but six (perhaps more) are tick-borne, and constitute a family which includes the Louping Ill, Central European Tick-borne Fever (Russian spring-summer encephalitis), Far Eastern Russian Encephalitis, Omsk Haemorrhagic Fever, Kyasanur Forest Fever, and Powassan viruses.

The tick-borne viruses have the same general properties as other Group B arboviruses but with the following special features:—they can be cultivated in fertile eggs where they grow in the yolk sac and in the embryo, as well as producing pocks on the chorio-allantoic membrane. Growth occurs in HeLa cells, monkey kidney, human amnion, human embryo, chick and mouse embryo cells. Antigenically the family are closely related to each other in haemagglutination-inhibition tests and there is a lesser degree of crossing with other group B viruses.

The tick not only transmits infection through its bite but usually also constitutes a long-sustained reservoir of infection because it remains infected for long periods of time and transfers the virus transovarially to successive generations. It is rare for mammals and birds to act as natural reservoirs of infection but when domestic animals such as cattle and goats are infected they may excrete the viruses in their milk which may convey the infection to man.

Louping Ill.—This is primarily a disease of sheep characterised by an encephalomyelitis giving rise to cerebellar ataxia and disorder of nervous functions. It occurs in Scotland and the North of England and owes its name to the peculiar ataxic leaping (louping) movements of the animal. The vector is the tick *Ixodes ricinus*. Cattle, pigs and monkeys can also be infected. Man is, however, seldom infected and in Britain there are only some ten fully authenticated cases, mostly in shepherds or laboratory workers. The human disease takes the form of a mild meningitis from which recovery is complete. The diagnosis is made in the laboratory by isolating the virus from the cerebro-spinal fluid using young adult mice inoculated intracerebrally and by neutralisation tests for antibodies in the serum, also carried out in mice.

Central European Tick-borne Fever (Russian spring-summer encephalitis—Western form) is a biphasic illness with an influenza-like onset, followed by a period of apyrexia for 4–10 days and culminating in meningitis or meningo-encephalitis. Transient paralysis is not infrequent but complete recovery is the rule. Mild and inapparent infections also occur. Severe forms, with permanent paralysis and a fatal bulbo-spinal form, occur infrequently. The vector is *Ixodes ricinus*. About 60 per cent. of human cases have been attributed to the bite of the tick and 23 per cent. to drinking unboiled goat's milk.

Far East Russian Encephalitis (Russian spring-summer encephalitis—Eastern form) is due to infection with a closely related virus. The disease is serious and is commonly followed by flaccid paralysis resembling that of poliomyelitis, or by the signs of bulbar involvement. The vector is *Ixodes persulcatus*.

Omsk Haemorrhagic Fever is caused by an arbovirus transmitted by the ticks *Dermacentor pictus* and *D. marginatus*. The disease is the most serious for man of any caused by tick-borne viruses and takes the form of a diphasic illness with fever, lymphadenopathy, gastro-intestinal symptoms, and haemorrhages from the nose, stomach, colon and uterus.

Kyasanur Forest Fever is a disease found amongst forest workers in Mysore in Southern India. It begins about eight days after forest exposure with fever and a falling pulse rate; epistaxis, haemoptysis, bleeding from the gums, and other haemorrhagic incidents are common. There is a leucopenia and a thrombocytopenia. A biphasic form of the illness is reported in which, after an afebrile period of 9–21 days, there appear signs of involvement of the central nervous system including meningism, vertigo, tremors, and mental disturbance.

Kyasanur Forest Fever was unknown until 1955 when an epidemic of the disease amongst forest workers occurred simultaneously with an epizootic in the indigenous monkeys. The vector is he tick *Haemaphysalis spinigera* which disseminates the virus amongst monkeys, many of which have mild infections, and also amongst birds. Although monkeys form an important reservoir of infection, other animals, including small rodents and wild jungle birds, may also have this function. It is possible that the virus was conveyed to India in the years preceding 1955 by ticks transported there by migrating birds.

Powassan Virus is enzootic in Canada amongst squirrels and chipmunks. The vector is the tick *Dermacentor andersoni*.

Prophylaxis.—The destruction of the tick vectors of the viruses wherever this is possible is the logical control procedure. Otherwise, formalin inactivated vaccines containing egg or tissue culture propagated viruses have been used with some success to protect personnel obliged to enter tick-infested areas.

Sandfly Fever

Sandfly fever is also known as phlebotomous fever because the virus which causes it is transmitted by the sandfly *Phlebotomus papatasii*. The disease has an abrupt onset with high fever, severe headache, muscular aching, and pain behind the eyes. Photophobia, stiffness of the back and neck, and leucopenia are characteristic signs. There is no encephalitis and the cerebrospinal fluid is normal. Recovery is complete within a few days and fatality is almost unknown. The disease occurs commonly in countries bordering the Mediterranean and is seen also in Kenya, Egypt, Russia, China and India.

The sandfly fever virus is introduced by the female phlebotomus and an itching papule appears at the site of the bite. After an incubation period of three or four days the virus is liberated into the blood stream, where it may be found a day before and a day after the onset of the clinical illness.

The Properties of the Virus.—The diameter of the elementary bodies is 17–25 mμ. The virus agglutinates chick erythrocytes at 37° C. at pH 5·5–6·5 provided an alcohol soluble inhibitor is removed. It can be propagated in the brains of suckling mice by intracerebral inoculation. It can be cultivated in tissue cultures of human, monkey, hamster or mouse kidneys. Laboratory animals including monkeys and the chick embryo are not susceptible to the infection. Two distinct antigenic types, the Naples and the Sicilian strains, have been distinguished by Sabin (1955) and are not related to other groups of the arboviruses.

The diagnosis of sandfly fever is usually made on clinical and epidemiological grounds. Specific proof of infection with the sandfly fever virus can be obtained by isolation of the strains in suckling mice inoculated with blood taken on the first day of the fever. Further confirmation may be obtained by the demonstration of rising antibody titres in neutralisation, complement-fixation and haemagglutination-inhibition tests.

Phlebotomus papatasii is only about 2 mm. long and is able to pass through the mesh of ordinary screens and mosquito nets. Control measures are directed against the vector and comprise the regular and systematic application of DDT to the breeding grounds of the phlebotomus. Insect repellents such as dimethyl phthalate used at night are useful in preventing the disease.

Rift Valley Fever

This disease, which is also known as enzootic hepatitis, was first described by Daubney and Hudson in 1931 in Kenya, where there was an extremely severe epizootic amongst lambs. Most of the lambs died, but many of the ewes recovered. Native shepherds and European investigators of the epizootic developed a dengue-like fever with severe back pains.

The Rift Valley fever virus is about 23–35 mμ in diameter. It can be grown in fertile eggs and in tissue cultures of the suspended cell type; sarcoma cells of rat and mouse origin and fibroblasts from human and murine sources are susceptible. The infection can be transmitted by blood, liver or spleen tissue from infected sheep to cattle, mice, field voles, dormice and squirrels. Rabbits, guinea-pigs, birds and reptiles are not susceptible. The virus has the property of haemagglutination and has been designated as an arbovirus but it does not fall into any group.

The disease in lambs is characterised by marked necrosis of the liver with haemorrhages into other organs. Inclusion bodies are numerous in the liver. In man the disease is mild and resembles dengue with a typical "saddleback" temperature chart.

Rift Valley fever is transmitted by the bite of mosquitoes; three species of *Aedes* and several species of *Eretmapodites* transmit the virus to sheep and bovine, murine and human hosts.

The diagnosis may be made by the inoculation of suckling mice with blood taken from a case during the first 24 hr. of infection. When the infected animals die, the virus is identified by the characteristic lesions it produces in the liver and by neutralisation with specific antisera. In convalescence the diagnosis can be made by demonstrating the development of neutralising, complement-fixing, and haemagglutination-inhibiting antibodies. The results of these tests are remarkably specific and there is very little tendency to overlap with other arboviruses. Antibodies to the virus appear as early as four days after the onset of the clinical illness and they persist for as long as twelve years after recovery.

Arbovirus Infections of Animals

There are arboviruses which do not appear to be pathogenic for man but which cause epizootics and serious economic loss in domestic animals. These diseases include African horse-sickness and Blue tongue in sheep, both of which are midge-borne (*Culicoides spp.*) and also Nairobi sheep disease which is transmitted by the tick *Rhipicephalus appendiculatus*.

REFERENCES

Buckley, S. M. (1959). Propagation, cytopathogenicity, and haemagglutination-haemadsorption of some arthropod-borne viruses in tissue cultures. *Ann. N.Y. Acad. Sci.*, **81**, 172.

Clarke, D. H. & Casals, J. (1958). Techniques for haemagglutination and haemagglutination-inhibition with arthropod-borne viruses. *Amer. J. trop. Med.*, **7**, 561.

Horsfall, F. L. & Tamm, I. (1965). *Viral and Rickettsial Infections of Man*. 4th Ed. London: Pitman.

Lennette, E. H., Wiener, A., Neff, B. J. & Hoffman, M. N. (1956). A chick embryo-derived complement-fixing antigen for Western equine encephalomyelitis. *Proc. Soc. exp. Biol. (N.Y.)*, **92**, 575.

McLean, D. M. (1962). *The Arborvirus Group*. Chapters 36-55 in *Textbook of Virology*. Ed. Rhodes, A. J. & Van Rooyen, C. E. Baltimore: Williams & Wilkins.

Reeves, W. C. (1961). Overwintering of arthropod-borne viruses. *Progr. med. Virol.*, **3**, 59.

Sabin, A. B. (1955). Recent advances in our knowledge of dengue and sandfly fever. *Amer. J. trop. Med. & Hyg.*, **4**, 198.

Smith, C. E. Gordon (1959). Arthropod-borne viruses. *Brit. med. Bull.*, **15**, 235.

Theiler, M. (1959). Yellow fever. Chapter 15 in *Viral and Rickettsial Infections of Man*. Ed. Rivers, T. M. & Horsfall, F. L., p. 351. London: Pitman.

World Health Organisation (1961). Arthropod-borne viruses. *Wld. Hlth. Org. techn. Rep Ser.* No. 219.

CHAPTER 37

MISCELLANEOUS VIRUS INFECTIONS OF MAN AND ANIMALS

MANY of the viruses to be described in this chapter do not fall easily into the virus classification described on page 83 either because there is not yet sufficient information about them or because they may belong to groups so far undefined. A number of viruses of veterinary importance have also been included for convenience.

RUBELLA

Rubella or "German Measles" is a common and mild infectious disease characterised by a macular rash and enlargement of the cervical lymph glands.

Properties of the virus.—The virions are 120–180 mμ in diameter; they have a core about 130 mμ in diameter covered by a smooth outer membrane. The virus is inactivated by heat for 1 hour at 56° C. and is stable at −65° C. It is sensitive to ether, chloroform and desoxycholate.

Cultivation.—In primary cultures of human thyroid tissue and in the cells of a transformed rabbit kidney cell, RK13, the virus regularly produces a definite cytopathic effect with focal changes and intracytoplasmic inclusions (McCarthy, Taylor-Robinson & Pillinger, 1963). In primary human amnion and in embryonic-skin-muscle cultures the cytopathic effect is less regular. In primary cultures of kidney cells from vervet and patas monkeys and in the HeLa and Chang liver cell lines the virus grows without cytopathic effect. The presence of the virus, in the absence of any cytopathic effect, can be detected by its *interference* (see p. 74) with growth of a challenge dose of a virus such as ECHO 2 or 9, Coxsackie A9, or Sindbis. There are no confirmed reports of the growth of the rubella virus in the chick embryo.

Antigenicity.—Estimations of the antibody response in rubella infections can be carried out by serum neutralisation tests performed against the virus grown in the RK13 line (Dudgeon, Butler & Plotkin, 1964).

Pathogenesis.—The reservoir of infection is formed by human cases or carriers from whom the virus is transmitted in naso-pharyngeal secretions borne in the air or dust. The virus is inhaled and multiplies in the mucosa of the upper respiratory tract. After an incubation period, usually 16–18 days, there is a viraemic phase with fever and the localisation of the virus in the skin lesions and cervical glands. Complications are very uncommon but the following occur occasionally: meningo-encephalitis, neuritis, arthritis, synovitis and thrombocytopenia.

Epidemiology.—Rubella is world wide in distribution and occurs usually in epidemic form. It affects principally children but the disease is more common in adults than is measles. Epidemics have often occurred in military recruit camps and in university communities. A case is infectious for not more than four days after the onset of the catarrhal symptoms. In one series a little over one-third of contacts aged less than ten years were attacked and thereafter the rate fell sharply with advancing years. One attack of the disease usually confers immunity for life.

Rubella in pregnancy

During the viraemic phase of the illness the virus is able to cross the placental barrier in a pregnant woman and multiply in the differentiating cells of the human embryo. This passage happens most frequently during the first trimester of pregnancy, less frequently in the second and seldom in the third. The effect on the embryo is the production of congenital abnormalities of which deafness is the most frequent, and then, in order of incidence, congenital heart disease (persistent ductus arteriosus and ventricular septal defects are common), chorio-retinitis, cataract, mental defects, microcephaly, etc. The rubella virus has been recovered on several occasions from the tissues of malformed foetuses removed at hysterotomy from mothers who had suffered from rubella early in their pregnancies. There is no agreement on the assessment of the chances of an abnormal child being born to a woman who contracts rubella during pregnancy. In Britain and in Sweden 14 per cent. of children born after rubella in the first trimester of pregnancy showed malformation of one or more kinds; about 30 per cent. of these infants had some hearing loss, 20 per cent. chorio-retinitis, and 18 per cent. congenital heart disorders (Manson, Logan & Loy, 1960; Lundström, 1962). The incidence of prematurity and still births were also increased in women who had contracted rubella during the first trimester of pregnancy. Hill *et al.* (1958) estimated that the incidence of birth defects was 50 per cent. if rubella was contracted during the first month of pregnancy, 25 per cent. in the second month, 17 per cent. in the third, 11 per cent. in the fourth, and 6 per cent. in the fifth, but thereafter the risk disappeared. The children of mothers exposed to but not contracting rubella in their pregnancies show no increased frequency of malformations.

Laboratory Diagnosis.—The virus may be isolated from the blood in the viraemic phase, from throat washings and nasopharyngeal swabs during the three days after the onset of fever or from the tissues of the abnormal foetus of a mother infected during pregnancy (*vide supra*). Antibodies in the serum are estimated by neutralisation tests. Characteristically there is a lymphocytosis in the blood with the presence of plasma cells and Turk cells.

Prophylaxis.—No measures need to be taken to prevent the spread of this harmless infection amongst children and, indeed, many advocate that every effort should be taken to expose girls so that they are infected and acquire an immunity before they reach the age of marriage. In pregnant women exposed to infection normal gamma-globulin is effective in preventing the clinical disease. A dose of 1500 mgm. reduces the attack rate, if given within 28 days of exposure, to 1·13 per cent. (McDonald, 1963).

Although the rubella virus is notorious for the frequency with which it can induce congenital abnormalities, other viruses, notably the pox viruses, measles, mumps, influenza, varicella, hepatitis and the Coxsackie group, may also in lesser degree possess this property. The position is reviewed by Blattner & Heys (1961).

LYMPHOCYTIC CHORIOMENINGITIS

Benign lymphocytic chorio-meningitis is primarily an enzootic disease of wild mice. The virus is excreted in the urine and faeces and is transmissible in contaminated dust to man in whom it causes an influenza-like fever or a meningitis.

The properties of the virus.—The virions are 40–60 mμ in diameter. They are well preserved by freeze-drying or storage at −70° C. In whole infected tissue stored in 50 per cent. glycerol at 4° C. the virus survives for several years. The virus is inactivated by 10 per cent. ether overnight, 0·5 per cent. formalin, and 0·01 per cent. merthiolate. At pH values below 7 it is unstable.

Cultivation.—The virus grows on the chorio-allantoic membrane of 11–12 day-old chick embryos without pock production or any obvious effect on the embryo. Tissue culture cells of the chick, mouse, calves, and monkey support the growth of the virus but a cytopathic effect may not be obvious until the virus has been adapted by several passages.

When inoculated into healthy mice intracerebrally a severe encephalitis results in which the animals show marked muscular spasms and convulsions. In the guinea-pig the disease takes the form of generalised systemic infection. Rabbits are not susceptible.

Pathogenesis.—In man the most obvious clinical picture is that of aseptic meningitis but the infection may be inapparent or show itself as a severe influenzal illness or as an "atypical pneumonia".

The lymphocytic chorio-meningitis virus is essentially an inhabitant of mice and in these animals exists in a latent form which is transmitted by the mother to her young *in utero*. The virus is excreted by the mice in urine, faeces and nasal secretions. Most human infections are contracted from material contaminated by mice, and the most likely route of infection is thought to be through the respiratory mucosa.

Laboratory Diagnosis.—The cerebrospinal fluid shows a marked cellular response; 200–1000 cells per c.mm. are present and 90 per cent. are lymphocytes. The protein is raised to 60–100 mg. per 100 ml., but normal values are found for the chloride and sugar estimations; these findings help to distinguish lymphocytic chorio-meningitis from tuberculous meningitis. The virus may be isolated from the cerebrospinal fluid by intracerebral inoculation of adult mice. Virus identification is carried out by neutralisation tests or complement-fixation reactions with specific antisera.

Serological tests may give a retrospective diagnosis if virus isolation tests have not been carried out. Complement-fixing antibodies appear by the fourteenth day, but are slow to reach a peak. Three samples of serum are usually required to establish the existence of a rising titre of antibodies; the first should be taken as soon as possible after the onset of the illness, the second 14 days later and the third after an interval of four to five weeks.

There are no specific measures to control infection with this virus. Extermination of mice will usually eradicate the disease. Those whose work as laboratory assistants or rodent exterminators obliges them to come into contact with mice must take precautions to avoid inhaling infected material.

CYTOMEGALOVIRUSES

This group of viruses affects man, guinea-pigs, mice and other rodents, and pigs. Many of them have a marked predilection for growth in the salivary glands and all are highly species specific. The human infection is known as Cytomegalic Inclusion Disease and takes a number of clinical forms. These viruses are also sometimes known as *salivary gland* or *submaxillary viruses.*

Properties of the viruses.—Virus particles of two sizes have been described in ultra-thin sections of infected fibroblasts examined under the electron-microscope. Smaller particles, 80–100 mμ, are seen in the nucleus at an early stage of infection and larger particles, 150–500 mμ, are found in the cytoplasm. In the electron-microscope negatively stained particles are seen to have a structure like that of the herpes viruses with perhaps 162 capsomeres.

Host Range and Cultivation.—The disease occurs naturally in man and there are more than a hundred recorded fatal cases in children mostly under the age of two years. Monkeys, guinea-pigs and mice are also affected. The virus can be cultivated in roller-tube tissue cultures of fibroblasts from explanted fragments of adult human uterus, prepuce or embryonic skin-muscle. Strains of the virus are species specific, even in tissue culture, although the similarity of the cellular changes they produce suggests that they are biologically closely related.

Viability.—At 4° C. the virus loses its infectivity within a week but can be preserved in 50 per cent. glycerol for long periods at this temperature. It is destroyed by heat at 56° C. in 30 min., and is inactivated by exposure to 20 per cent. ether for two hours, and by storage at pH values below 5.

Pathogenesis.—In man infection may take one of the following five forms: (1) an inapparent infection involving only the salivary glands: (2) an overwhelming neonatal infection in a child born to a woman who presumably suffered from a symptomless viraemia during pregnancy. The disease begins shortly before or soon after birth, often in a premature infant. The infection is generalised and usually fatal; almost all the organs are involved but jaundice, haemorrhages, hepato- and splenomegaly are the dominant features, accompanied also by anuria, calcification of the brain, and bronchopneumonia: (3) in children of 3–6 months the disease may be associated with enteritis, upper respiratory tract infections and pertussis: (4) in older children aged 6 months to 2 years the disease may be associated with tumours or leukaemia and may be responsible for the later developments of microcephaly, intracerebral calcification, and hydrocephalus: (5) localised granulomata occur rarely.

Histologically large basophilic inclusion bodies in both the cytoplasm and the nucleus greatly distend the host cells and may measure as much as 40 μ in diameter. They are found in the epithelial cells of the liver and bile ducts, renal tubules, bronchi and lining cells of the alveoli, and in many other organs.

Epidemiology.—The disease is probably world wide and chiefly affects children up to the age of two years. Adults are rarely affected. Infection is probably transferred *in utero* in many cases but in general the manner of transmission is not clear as a considerable number of cases are contracted post-natally. The virus is, however, present in any tissue bearing inclusions and may be excreted in the saliva, faeces and urine, and in theory could be transmitted from these sources. A high incidence of complement-fixing antibodies in adults (Rowe *et al.*, 1956 & Rowe 1960) suggests that the infection is more common than had been thought, especially where socio-economic conditions are poor.

Laboratory Diagnosis.—The typical inclusions can be detected in cells in urinary sediments or in biopsy tissues. The virus can be isolated from throat swabs, gastric or bronchial washings, urine or tissue fragments by the inoculation of tissue cultures of human explanted tissues (*vide supra*). A complement-fixing test using as an antigen infected tissue culture fluids is valuable for diagnostic purposes and for serological surveys. Neutralisation tests arc used to identify the virus after isolation and to detect antibodies.

RABIES

This is a disease of all warm-blooded animals and especially of dogs. The virus is excreted in the saliva of the animals and is transmitted by biting.

Properties of the Virus.—The diameter of the virus particle measured by filtration is 100–150 mμ. In negatively stained preparations the virus is seen under the electron microscope to have a fine structure similar to that of the myxoviruses with an inner, continuous, flattened, ribbon-like, helix. It is probable that the nucleic acid is RNA.

Host Range and Cultivation.—There is a wide range of susceptible animals, including man and almost all mammals; the outcome of infection is nearly always fatal, with the exception that vampire bats are known to be able to transmit the virus for several months without showing any signs of the disease themselves. The virus invades the blood and the central nervous system of the host and is excreted in the saliva, milk and urine. These materials can be used to transmit the infection to laboratory animals, including rabbits, mice and guinea-pigs. Freshly isolated strains of the virus are known as "street virus" and will kill laboratory animals with a severe encephalitis after an incubation period which varies from one to twelve weeks according to the species inoculated. Multiple eosinophilic inclusions known as Negri bodies are found in the nerve cells especially in the hippocampus, and measure 0·5 μ to 20 μ in diameter. Negri bodies are specific in rabies infection and their detection in nerve tissue enables a diagnosis of rabies to be made.

Serial brain-to-brain passages of the virus in rabbits yields an attenuated or "fixed" strain of the virus which is no longer able to multiply in extraneural situations. Negri bodies are scanty in the brains of animals inoculated with the fixed virus. The virus grows in the tissues of 7-day-old chick embryos inoculated by any of the usual routes; the maximum yield of virus is obtained nine days after inoculation. The virus has been grown in monolayer cultures of the following cells, chick or mouse embryo, suckling hamster kidney and embryo rabbit brain. Most strains appear to grow poorly and do not produce any marked cytopathic effect.

Viability.—The infectivity of the virus in tissues kept at room temperatures is gradually lost in 7–14 days. At 4° C. the virus survives several weeks and in 50 per cent. glycerol saline at 4° C. for many months. The best diluent for the preservation of the virus is 2·5 per cent. normal guinea-pig serum in saline.

At 37° C., the virus survives five days, at 50° C. one hour, at 60° C. five min., and at 100° C. two to three min. Rabies virus is more resistant than vegetative bacteria to disinfectants; 0·5 per cent. formaldehyde fails to kill it in two months at 4° C., but 1·0 per cent. formaldehyde, 3 per cent. cresol and 0·1 per cent. mercuric chloride inactivate in 15 min.

Antigenic Characters.—All strains of the virus are antigenically similar. Antibodies in the serum after vaccination can be demonstrated by neutralisation and complement-fixation methods.

Pathogenesis.—The portal of entry is the bite and the rabies virus in the infected saliva is introduced into the depths of the wound. Occasionally the virus may gain access through a pre-existing scratch or abrasion if this has been contaminated by saliva. The virus multiplies locally in the tissues, invades damaged nerve fibres, and spreads centrally to reach the brain and spinal cord. It is not yet decided whether the virus travels along the axons of nerves or along perineural lymphatics. There is no evidence that the virus is spread through the blood stream or lymphatic channels, and it has only rarely been isolated from the cerebrospinal fluid.

The incubation period varies from ten days to two years after the bite of a rabid animal; its duration may depend on the distance the virus has to move from the point of entry to reach the brain. Average figures are: for bites on the leg 60 days, on the arm 40 days and on the head 30 days. The incubation period is shorter in children than in adults.

The first symptoms of the disease are headache, fever, a profound sense of apprehension, and a feeling of irritation at the site of the bite. The patients complain of a dry throat and thirst, but they will not drink. High fever, difficulty in swallowing and a fear of water (hydrophobia) become the dominant symptoms, and the patient passes into delirium with generalised convulsions. The outcome is invariably fatal and at autopsy there is a severe encephalitis, characterised by generalised hyperaemia and a pronounced cell destruction throughout the brain especially marked in the medulla. Demyelinisation is widespread and the cells of the posterior horn are severely damaged.

Epidemiology

The epidemiology of rabies is determined by the animal sources of infection. Dog and cat rabies constitute the most important source because 95 per cent. of human infections are derived from these animals. In the dog the incubation period is as a rule two to eight weeks, but it may be as long as eight months. The disease is characterised by two clinical forms. In "furious" rabies the animals become aggressive, vicious and excited; they snap and bite at the approach of any other creatures. In "dumb" rabies paralysis of the muscles of the head and neck occurs and the dog cannot chew its food; its owner, believing it has some object in its throat, may attempt to remove the obstruction and contaminate his hands with infected saliva. About 50 per cent. of rabid dogs excrete the virus in their saliva. They are infectious for only about ten days before their death.

Many species of wild animals suffer from rabies. One of the most important carriers is the fox, which may transmit the infection to farm animals. In Canada many cases of cattle rabies have been attributed to this means of spread. In Europe, Iran and the Middle East wolves, and jackals have transmitted the infection, and in India the mongoose. Other species which are able to transmit rabies are rats, badgers, opossums, musk-rats, racoons, skunks, chipmunks and squirrels.

Rabies may infect all the usual domestic animals, including the horse, cow, sheep, goat or pig. Often the animals are infected by the bite of rabid foxes, or other wild animals.

In Trinidad and South America rabies is transmitted by the vampire bat *Desmodus rotundus murinus*. The bat is the only species so far recognised as being latently infected with rabies virus. Fruit- and insect-eating bats are also known to harbour the virus, and when rabid are able to transmit the infection to other bats, animals and man.

Control.—It is only by complete eradication of the animal reservoir that rabies can be eliminated. This has been possible in Great Britain, where the strict enforcement of a six month period of quarantine has prevented the entry of infected animals for many years. The result has been that there is no longer any source of the virus to infect animals and there has been no case of rabies in the country since 1921.

In other countries it has not been possible to eliminate the animal reservoir so completely, and rabies still presents a major problem to many public health authorities. When the dog is the principal reservoir the disease can be brought under effective control by the active immunisation of pet dogs and by the destruction of all strays and wild dogs. An effective vaccine in general use contains the living avirulent egg-adapted Flury strain of the rabies virus. It is given in a dose of 3·0 ml. intramuscularly into the hind limb of the animal and an effective protection lasting three years is developed.

Laboratory Diagnosis

In man the clinical findings are so characteristic that laboratory confirmation is not usually necessary. The virus, however, is present in the saliva and may also be isolated from specimens of the nervous tissue and salivary glands obtained at autopsy. The material is first treated with antibiotics and then inoculated intracerebrally in mice; the animals develop a flaccid paralysis of the limbs and die within six to eight days.

In the dog the diagnosis depends on the demonstration of Negri bodies in the brain tissue and the isolation of the virus; there is no satisfactory serological test that can be used in life. If there is the slightest reason to suspect a dog of rabies, the animal should be kept in strict isolation and observed for a period of ten days; if it survives for this period, rabies may safely be excluded. If unmistakable symptoms of rabies are observed, the animal is killed (preferably with chloroform) and the diagnosis is confirmed by laboratory examination. If the laboratory is at some distance, the head is removed, wrapped in a cloth soaked in 50 per cent. glycerol saline, and forwarded in cracked ice. In the laboratory the scalp is reflected, the skull is opened by means of sterile bone forceps and the brain removed with aseptic precautions. The hippocampus, which is situated in the floor of the lateral ventricle, is dissected out, smears are made by squeezing a portion of the tissue between two slides, and pieces are also fixed for histological examination. In addition, a suspension is prepared for animal inoculation. The method of choice both for accuracy and speed is that of immune fluorescence. Conjugated antiserum is applied to thin sections or smears of brain or salivary gland which are then examined for fluorescence. By this technique a specific diagnosis can be made within a few hours (Goldwasser *et al.*, 1959, McQueen, Lewis, and Schneider, 1960). Smears may be fixed in methyl alcohol for five minutes, and stained by Giemsa's method or by Mann's method (see Chapter 45). For section, the tissue is fixed in Zenker's fluid and stained as above. The animal's salivary glands should also be removed and homogenised for mouse inoculation. The diagnosis depends on the finding of the characteristic Negri bodies in the cytoplasm of the nerve cells. These bodies are best seen when the animal has reached the paretic stage of the disease. Intracerebral inoculation of mice with brain emulsion is also carried out, and if the virus is present, paresis and death occur as described above.

Prophylaxis

When a person is bitten by a dog suffering from or suspected of rabies, the first step is the thorough cleaning of the bite wound with soap and water. The puncture wounds should then be thoroughly dried and cauterised with concentrated nitric acid applied with a capillary pipette; after a few moments a solution of sodium bicarbonate should be applied to neutralise the acid.

If the risk of rabies is great, as happens when there is a high probability that the animal concerned is rabid, and there are multiple bites on the head, face, neck or arms, immediate action is necessary and passive protection should be given at once by injecting hyper-immune horse serum or the gamma globulin obtained from it. The dose of the serum is 0·5 ml. per kg. body weight and that of the gamma globulin is at least 40 International Units (1 I.U. = 1 mg.) per kg. body weight. This injection must be followed by a minimum of 10, and preferably 14, injections of vaccine to stimulate active immunity; this is necessary because passively injected antibodies have a suppressive effect in the early stages of the development of antibodies by the patient himself.

Various vaccines are used to confer active immunity. One type in general use in many countries is the Semple vaccine which contains a 4 per cent. suspension of the brain of rabbits infected with the "fixed" rabies virus inactivated by 0·5 per cent. phenol. A number of similar vaccines prepared from infected rabbit or sheep brain are also used and inactivation is achieved by ultra-violet light, formalin or other agents. Vaccines of this type suffer from the serious disadvantage that the nervous tissue they contain may sensitise a small proportion (1 in 4,000 to 1 in 10,000) of persons being immunised who later may develop an encephalitis. In order to avoid such "neuro-paralytic accidents" other types of vaccines containing no nervous tissue have been developed. One such vaccine now on trial is the "Duck" vaccine which is prepared from cultures of the "fixed" virus in duck embryos inactivated with beta-propiolactone.

Attenuated strains of the living virus have also been developed and have been used in extensive trials. Of these the Flury low egg passage (LEP) strain, which has been carried through 40–60 egg passages, is now the virus used in the standard vaccine for the immunisation of dogs. A high passage strain (HEP) has been carried through more than 180 egg passages and is further attenuated to a degree where it can be used safely in man with a good antibody response (Fox, 1958).

In 1960 the W.H.O. Expert Committee made the following recommendations for protection against rabies:—

(1) For severe exposure in a non-immunised person—hyperimmune serum or gamma globulin followed by at least 10 injections of a vaccine. (The dose of the Semple vaccine is 2·0 ml.)

(2) When the exposure is not severe, or when the patient is seen for the first time seven days or more after the incident and no serum has been given—a course of 14 doses of vaccine.

(3) If the patient has received vaccine within the previous 15 years —two doses of vaccine spaced 7 days apart. If the interval is longer than 15 years a full course of 14 injections is needed.

(4) For prophylactic inoculation of those likely to be exposed in the future—five doses at monthly intervals of a vaccine, preferably not containing nervous tissue, are advised with booster doses spaced one to two years apart.

In Great Britain these immunising procedures are only required for returning travellers who have been exposed to the risk of rabies while abroad or for workers in quarantine establishments. Their use is *contra-indicated* for patients who could not have been exposed to any real risk of rabies.

INFECTIOUS WARTS

Warts occur so frequently that they constitute one of the most familiar of the virus infections of man. Although they vary considerably in shape, size, location, and age preference, the majority fall into two types. The first type comprises the common wart, *Verruca vulgaris* which usually takes the form of multiple, sessile, discrete, rounded papillomata on the hands, around the nail folds of the fingers, or on the wrists. The second type, the plantar wart or *Myrmecia* (ant hill) occurs on the soles of the feet and the palms of the hands, where its appearance is modified by pressure, so that it is flattened, and situated deep in the cutis, with a domed surface (Lyell & Miles, 1951). It is not yet decided whether these two types are spread by the same or different viruses. Another group is formed by genital warts, *Condylomata acuminata*, which are small, rough, fungating outgrowths, often pedunculated, situated on the prepuce and the coronal sulcus of the penis or on the labia and around the vulva. A small proportion of genital warts undergoes malignant change. Laryngeal warts may be small and flat or pedunculated.

Properties of the virus.—The virions are 55 mμ in diameter and have an icosohedral symmetry with 42 capsomeres on the surface. The nucleic acid is DNA. The virus resists ether and heat for 30 min. at 50° C. It is now placed in the PAPOVA group together with the related polyoma virus of mice, the vacuolating agents of monkeys (*e.g.* SV 40), and the rabbit papilloma virus.

Cultivation.—There have been a number of reports that the virus produces a cytopathic effect in primate cells in tissue culture but there has been no confirmation that virus reproduces under these conditions. The infection is not readily transmissible to animals but lesions have been produced with suspensions of wart tissue inoculated into the vagina of bitches. Bacteria free filtrates of wart tissue inoculated into the skin of human volunteers produce warts after an incubation period of six weeks to eight months.

Pathogenesis.—The source of infection is the infected blood or tissue shed from a damaged wart. Spread may occur directly by self-inoculation as in scratching or in the case of genital warts during sexual contact. Indirect spread is frequent and the virus enters through abrasions of the skin from contaminated fomites such as the instruments of barbers or chiropodists, the floors or towels of bathrooms, swimming baths, and communal washing places. Histologically, the essential feature of any human wart is the proliferation of the Malpighian layer of the skin. The appearances are extremely variable but in the case of verruca vulgaris they are those of the epithelium covered papillae arising from the deeper layers of the epidermis and protruding to form the bulk of the wart. Inclusion bodies are present in only a small number, about 4 per cent., of these lesions. In myrmecia the epithelial proliferation is accompanied by considerable hyper-keratosis. Intranuclear eosinophilic inclusions of Cowdry type B are present in 43 per cent. of warts of this type. Electron microscopical studies of thin sections of these warts have shown virus particles arranged in a crystalline lattice in the nuclei of the rete cells.

A great many warts, perhaps 50 per cent. or even more, disappear spontaneously and thus it is extremely difficult to assess the value of the many remedies advocated. If warts occur in inconvenient situations they may be removed surgically or destroyed by measures such as cautery, the application of liquid nitrogen, solid carbon dioxide, or deep X-rays.

FOOT-AND-MOUTH DISEASE

Foot-and-mouth disease is a highly contagious condition of cattle, pigs, sheep, goats and deer. It is characterised by vesicles on the feet and in the mouth along with constitutional symptoms of infection. The disease may also occur naturally in the hedgehog. The infection spreads rapidly among farm animals, and large epizootics are the cause of much economic loss in many parts of the world.

The Properties of the Virus.—The diameter is 20–25 mμ and the shape is roughly spherical or hexagonal. The nucleic acid is RNA. It is classified as a picorna virus (see p. 71).

Host Range and Cultivation.—The virus grows in cultures of bovine, pig, and sheep kidney cells, in embryonic guinea-pig tissues and in suspended cultures of bovine tongue epithelium. Strains have been adapted to growth in chick embryos by intravenous inoculation. Cattle, guinea-pigs, suckling mice, hamsters and new born rabbits are all highly susceptible. Human infections are rare and only a very small number of cases are recorded in which adequate virological proof of the nature of the infection was established.

Viability.—The virus is one of the most stable known, and its ability to survive drying for several weeks or even months on hay or other materials is responsible for the great facility of its spread in the field. The virus is resistant to ether, alcohol, chloroform, bile salts and heat for 30 min. at 56° C. It is readily destroyed at pH values below 6 and above 10. Immersion of infected tissue fragments, *e.g.* bovine tongue epithelium, in neutral glycerol saline at 4° C. preserves its infectivity indefinitely.

Antigenic Characters.—There are seven recognised antigenic types of the virus which have been differentiated by neutralisation tests in animals or tissue cultures and by complement-fixation. Three types are primarily European and are designed O (Oise), A (Allemagne), and C. Three South African types are called SAT 1, 2 and 3 and the seventh is known as Asia 1. A large number of variants of these strains has been recognised.

Pathogenesis.—Foot-and-mouth disease is spread from animal to animal by means of saliva which contains large amounts of the virus. The disease is highly contagious, and saliva and faeces contaminate the environment so that it spreads with great rapidity within a herd. After an incubation period of 24–48 hours a viraemic phase follows. The disease declares itself with fever, drooling of saliva, and the appearance of vesicles on the mucous membranes of the mouth, muzzle and feet. Foot-and-mouth disease is notifiable in Great Britain, and its importance is not on account of its ability to kill but by virtue of the loss of flesh, reduction of milk yield and loss of export value. Pigs, sheep, goats, deer, antelope and other ruminants are all subject to infection.

Epizootiology.—The foot-and-mouth disease virus is often introduced to a herd from far-distant parts. The viability of the virus makes it possible for it to be carried alive long distances in infected meat or on contaminated fomites. Migrating birds (especially starlings) have been thought to carry the virus, and there is some evidence to suggest that from time to time they have brought the infection to Great Britain from Belgium and the Low Countries. Pigs have frequently contracted the infection from eating swill containing infected fragments of meat imported from South America.

Laboratory Diagnosis.—Infected tissues (preferably bovine epithelium) from cases, especially when new types or subtypes of the virus are suspected, should be sent immersed in glycerol saline to the World Reference Laboratory, Animal Diseases Research Institute, Pirbright, Surrey, England.

Control.—In countries where the disease is not endemic, as in Great Britain, quarantine, slaughter of infected animals and their contacts, and disinfection of contaminated premises have proved both efficient and economic. In endemic areas vaccination is widely practised. A formol inactivated virus adsorbed to alum forms the most generally used vaccine but more recently living virus attenuated by cultivation in eggs, or mice, has given encouraging results.

For further information on the virus of foot-and-mouth disease the reader should consult a review by Brooksby (1958).

VESICULAR STOMATITIS

The disease occurs naturally among cattle, horse and swine. The disease is not a serious one, but because of the vesicles that occur in the mouth and on the tongue is easily mistaken for foot-and-mouth disease. The virus is antigenically distinct from the foot-and-mouth disease virus and is larger, being rod-shaped (170×70 mμ) with an internal core composed of a hollow helix. The nucleic acid is probably RNA. It can be cultivated without difficulty in the chick embryo and in monolayer cultures of chick, ox and pig tissues, where it has a cytopathic effect. The vesicular stomatitis virus gives plaques in monolayer culture of ox embryo kidney. There are two immunologically distinct strains. The virus has the same degree of resistance to physical and chemical agents as the foot-and-mouth disease virus. The disease is mild, and drastic control measures are not required.

VESICULAR EXANTHEMA

This disease occurs naturally only in pigs and, like foot-and-mouth disease, is characterised by vesicles on the mouth and feet. Cattle are resistant to the infection and the virus is only mildly pathogenic to horses. No lesions are produced in the foot-pad of the guinea-pig, a finding which differentiates the vesicular exanthema virus from those of vesicular stomatitis and foot-and-mouth disease. The virus is classified as a picorna virus and resembles the foot-and-mouth disease virus (q.v.) in its physical and chemical properties. It can be cultivated in tissue cultures of the skin, kidney or embryo of swine, dog, horse and cat with plaque production. Antigenically there are probably at least seven immunological types.

The Susceptibility of Animals to the Vesicular Viruses

Susceptible Animal	Foot-and-Mouth Disease	Vesicular Exanthema	Vesicular Stomatitis
Pig . . .	+	+	+
Horse	–	±	+
Cow	+	–	+
Guinea-pig . . .	+	–	+
Adult Mouse . .	±	–	–
Suckling mouse . .	+	–	+

SWINE FEVER

Swine fever is a highly contagious disease of pigs and is responsible for considerable and world-wide economic loss. The animals show fever, apathy, vomiting, eye-discharge, diarrhoea, and cutaneous haemorrhages with a high mortality.

The virus is a small one, probably 25–50 mμ in diameter. It is very stable and survives moderate heat and freezing well, persisting for long periods in cured ham, pickled pork, or garbage. The virus grows well in tissue cultures of swine kidney, testis or bone marrow, and in leucocytes of the "buffy coat" of pig blood. The cytopathic effect is however minimal. Some strains have been adapted to growth in duck and chick embryos. Antigenically only one type has been reported but variant strains occur from time to time.

Pathogenesis.—The natural mode of infection is by ingestion and very minute quantities of the virus will produce the disease in susceptible swine. Eye and nasal secretions, urine, faeces, and blood from an infected animal all contain the virus. The outstanding pathological changes are petechial haemorrhages on serous surfaces, haemorrhages into the bladder, kidney and epicardium, haemorrhagic lymphadenitis and leucopenia. Cases with secondary bacterial infection may show severe enteritis. Pigs that have recovered may remain infective several months; wild pigs are an important source of the virus. Transmission is often by way of infected swill containing scraps of contaminated pork. The virus may resist pickling, smoking and salting for up to six months though it is rapidly destroyed by putrefaction.

Laboratory diagnosis depends on the demonstration of the presence of the virus using known susceptible pigs. An agar gel diffusion test is also useful as an aid to the diagnosis of swine fever; pancreatic tissue from infected pigs contains a soluble antigen which will precipitate with serum from hyperimmunised pigs. Swine fever virus shares a common precipitating antigen and common antibodies with mucosal disease viruses of cattle. Some strains of the mucosal disease complex will protect pigs against swine fever and hyperimmune sera from pigs contain antibodies that neutralise both viruses.

Matumoto *et al.* (1961) described an *in vitro* method for the detection and measurement of swine fever virus, and also of antibody, and the uses of the test for diagnosis in outbreaks. It depends upon the absence of CPE of the swine fever virus when sown on swine kidney cell tissue culture in monolayer, even though it is actively multiplying. In the same tissue culture, Newcastle disease virus hardly grows and is not cytopathic as long as it is sown within the first five days of the growth of the pig kidney cells. However, in such a tissue culture, previously sown with the virus of swine fever, Newcastle disease virus multiplies and is cytopathic, even when sown on the third day of tissue culture growth. The test is spoken of as "exultation" of Newcastle disease virus and is named the END test.

Prophylaxis.—Passive immunisation using hyperimmune serum is valuable when the disease appears in a herd. For active immunisation several vaccines are in use. Virus inactivated with gentian violet is extensively and successfully used in one vaccine. Living viruses attenuated by passage in rabbits, goats, or in tissue culture of swine kidney give much promise but there is doubt as to whether their use is followed by abortions or malformations in the litters.

REFERENCES

Blattner, R. J. & Heys, F. M. (1961). Role of the viruses in the aetiology of congenital malformations. *Progr. med. Virol.*, **3**, 311.

Brooksby, J. B. (1958). The virus of foot-and-mouth disease. *Advanc. virus Res.*, **5**, 1.

Dudgeon, J. A., Butler, N. R. & Plotkin, S. A. (1964). Further serological studies on the rubella syndrome. *Brit. med. J.*, **2**, 155.

Fox, J. P. (1958). Prophylaxis against rabies in man. *Ann. N.Y. Acad. Sci.*, **70**, 480.

Goldwasser, R. A., Kissling, R. E., Carski, T. R. & Hosty, T. S. (1959). Fluorescent antibody staining of rabies virus antigens in the salivary glands of rabid animals. *Bull. Wld. Hlth. Org.*, **20**, 579.

Hill, A. B., Doll, R., Galloway, T. McL. & Hughes, J. P. W. (1958). Virus diseases in pregnancy and congenital defects. *Brit. J. prev. soc. Med.*, **12**, 1.

Lündstrom, R., (1962). Rubella during pregnancy. *Acta. paediat.* (*Uppsala*), suppl. 133.

Lyell, A. & Miles, J. A. R. (1951). The Myrmecia. A study of inclusion bodies in warts. *Brit. med. J. i*, 912-915.

Manson, M. M., Logan, W. P. D. & Loy, R. M. (1960). Rubella and other Virus Infections during Pregnancy. *Rep. publ. Hlth. med. Subj., London*, 1. London: H.M.S.O.

Matumoto, M., Kumgai, T., Shimizu, T. & Ikeda, S. (1961). A new *in vitro* method (END) for the detection and measurement of the hog cholera virus and its antibody. *J. Immunol.*, **87**, 257.

McCarthy, K., Taylor-Robinson, C. H. & Pillinger, S. E. (1963). Isolation of rubella virus from cases in Britain. *Lancet*, **2**, 593.

McDonald, J. C., (1963). Gamma globulin for prevention of rubella in pregnancy. *Brit. med. J.*, **2**, 416.

McQueen, J. L., Lewis, A. L. & Schneider, N. J. (1960). Rabies diagnosis by fluorescent antibody. *Amer. J. publ. Hlth.*, **50**, 1743.

Rowe, W. P. (1960). Salivary gland virus infections in children, p. 209 in *Viral Infections in Infancy & Childhood.* Ed. Rose. *Symposium No.* 10, *New York Academy of Science.* New York: Hoeber-Harper.

Rowe, W. P., Hartley, J. W., Waterman, S., Turner, H. C. & Huebner, R. J. (1956). Cytopathic agent resembling human salivary gland virus recovered from tissue cultures of human adenoids. *Proc. Soc. exp. Biol.* (*N.Y.*), **92**, 418.

World Health Organisation (1960). Expert committee on rabies. *Wld. Hlth. Org. tech. Rep. Ser. No.* 201.

CHAPTER 38

THE PSITTACOSIS, LYMPHOGRANULOMA, TRACHOMA GROUP OF "VIRUSES"

THE properties of these agents are so different from those of true viruses that there is considerable dispute as to their taxonomic position; many authors prefer to classify them with rickettsiae even though they have no arthropod vectors. The organisms have been shown by Perkins and Allison (1963) to possess cell walls which resemble those of bacteria and rickettsiae in that they owe their rigidity to a mucopeptide which contains the amino sugar *muramic acid* as a key constituent. The characteristic sensitivity of the group to penicillin, other antibiotics and lysozyme is due to the ability of these substances to inhibit the synthesis of cell wall mucopeptides. All the members of the group take Castaneda and Macchiavello stains in the same way as rickettsiae. The inclusion bodies produced are intracytoplasmic and basophilic; they consist of deoxyribonucleic acid-containing particles set in a matrix which is composed of glycogen and ribonucleic acid. They have a complex cycle of reproduction which terminates in binary fission of the particles and all share a common heat stable antigen. Certain members of the group cause the haemagglutination of red blood cells. In the case of the psittacosis virus mouse and hamster erythrocytes are agglutinated but not those of man or fowls. The haemagglutinin is smaller than the virus itself and is composed of lecithin and nucleoprotein; it does not react with the receptor areas for the myxoviruses.

PSITTACOSIS

Psittacosis is an epizootic disease of birds which may affect man. Psittacine birds such as parrots, parakeets, cockatoos and budgerigars are natural hosts of the infection, and pet birds of this type have often been the source of human infections. Ducks, pigeons, turkeys, fulmars and certain species of gulls are also affected, and in these hosts the disease is known as *ornithosis*.

In birds the disease is characterised by diarrhoea, emaciation and a purulent nasal discharge. Man is infected by inhaling dust which is heavily contaminated by exudates from affected birds. The resultant illness is pneumonic in type and in untreated cases may be severe with a 20 per cent. mortality. Often, however, the illness is mild and resembles an attack of influenza. There may be a mild feverish illness or, more severely, a patchy bronchopneumonia which usually involves the bases of the lungs. The carrier state may persist in the birds for many months and human cases have not infrequently been traced to apparently healthy birds which were later proved to have harboured the virus.

Properties of the Virus.—The mature elementary body is a sphere about 250 mμ in diameter; it stains blue with Castaneda's stain. Under the electron microscope the particle is seen to be covered with a membrane like a cell wall, and to have an irregular surface; the appearance has been likened to that of a wrinkled pea. During reproduction the virus passes through a regular sequence of morphological changes. On entering the cell cytoplasm it gives rise, after a few hours, to a vaguely defined mass seen only in ultra-thin sections under the electron microscope. After eight or nine hours a basophilic inclusion appears and increases in size as time passes. Within the inclusion a few large particles about 1·0 μ in diameter appear and these divide and subdivide by binary fission to give rise to large numbers of mature elementary bodies. The final effect is that the parasitised cell disintegrates and the virus is liberated into the intercellular spaces.

The psittacosis virus is inactivated in 10 min. by heat at 60° C. and 0·1 per cent. formalin and 0·5 per cent. phenol kill it in 24 hr. Yolk sac suspensions of the virus are inactivated in 30 min. by 10 per cent. ether. Stored in M/50 phosphate buffered saline at pH 7·6 at 4° C. the virus remains viable for two to three weeks. It is best preserved at $-70°$ C. when it retains its activity for several years. Potency is lost rapidly if glycerol is used as a preserving solution. Penicillin and the tetracyclines interfere with the growth cycle and cause the production of abnormal developmental forms within the cell. The virus is not sensitive to streptomycin and only a few strains are influenced by sulphonamides.

Culture.—The virus grows most readily in the cells of the yolk sac of six- to eight-day-old chick embryos and in the peritoneal cavity and spleen of mice. Inoculated on to the chorio-allantoic membrane it produces a slight generalised thickening with oedema. Chick embryos die within four days of inoculation and mice in four to six days. Intranasal instillation of the virus in mice causes pneumonia, and intracerebral inoculation a fatal encephalitis.

The virus of ornithosis resembles that of psittacosis very closely and it is distinguished mainly by its pathogenicity for certain laboratory animals in which it is nearer to the lymphogranuloma virus. There is evidence to suggest that the ornithosis virus possesses a type-specific antigen.

The lethal effect of these viruses may be due in part to an endotoxin, for large doses may kill the host before there has been time for the virus to multiply. Latent infection in psittacosis and ornithosis may be common; it is known that the virus may fail to reproduce within the cells of tissue cultures grown in nutritionally poor medium. Multiplication resumes when a satisfactory medium is provided.

These viruses have been adapted to grow in tissue cultures and have been propagated in the "L" strain of mouse fibroblasts, HeLa and HEp2 cell lines, as well as in human and mouse liver cells and chick embryo cells.

Antigenic Structure.—A heat-labile antigen is thought to be specific for the psittacosis virus itself; it is readily destroyed by heat at 60° C. and by phenol, acids, and papain. A second antigen is remarkably resistant to heat and resists boiling or even autoclaving at 135° C.; since it also resists proteolytic enzymes but is destroyed by periodate it is probably a carbohydrate. This antigen is shared by all the members of the virus group and is employed in the diagnostic complement-fixation reactions in general use. The antibody to this common antigen is not protective.

Laboratory Diagnosis

Human Infections.—The sputum, which contains the virus during the first few days of the infection, is emulsified in Hanks' solution containing no antibiotics. Treatment of the specimen with sulphonamides or penicillin is contra-indicated. The suspension is spun in the centrifuge at 1000 r.p.m. to deposit cells and debris. Inoculate four to six mice intraperitoneally with 0·5 ml. of the supernatant. If the psittacosis virus is present, some or all of the mice will die seven to ten days later and will show a glairy peritoneal exudate, and enlargement of the spleen and liver. Films of the peritoneal exudate and impression smears of the spleen when stained with Giemsa's or Castaneda's stains show typical virus inclusions and clusters of elementary bodies. To confirm the diagnosis a 10 per cent. suspension of the infected mouse spleens in Hanks' solution should be passed to further mice and an attempt should be made to protect some of these with an immune serum.

If the mice inoculated with human material survive for 10 days, they should be killed and the spleens examined microscopically for virus. If no virus is found, an emulsion of the spleens is injected intraperitoneally in four to six mice. If the animals of this second passage show no sign of disease the case is presumed negative; if they die, they are examined as above.

Eggs may be used as well as mice to isolate the virus, but often the sputum and the contained bacteria are so toxic that the embryo dies before the virus has time to multiply. Streptomycin added to the sputum suspension in concentrations up to 2000 μg. per ml. may be used to overcome this difficulty.

The sputum suspension in a dose of 0·1 ml. is inoculated into the yolk sac of six- to eight-day-old embryos. If the virus is present, the embryos will die three to four days later. Impression smears of the stalks of the infected yolk sacs should be stained by Castaneda's or Macchiavello's stains and examined microscopically for clusters of virus elementary bodies. Care is required to distinguish the virus from yolk sac granules which, however, are irregular in shape and size and are usually larger than the virus.

Serological confirmation of the diagnosis is obtained by the complement fixation test using the heat stable antigen. Serum samples are taken early in the disease and 10–14 days later. A four-fold or greater increase in titre provides firm evidence of infection. The single observation on a convalescent case of a serum titre of 32 or higher is highly suggestive of recent infection.

Avian Infections.—Great care must be taken by laboratory workers in handling dead birds and in performing the post-mortem examination, for the material is highly infective. The procedure is to remove the spleen and to prepare an emulsion from it. Mice and eggs are inoculated in the same way as for sputum from the human case.

If the birds have recovered, blood may be taken from the wing vein and a complement fixation test carried out. Positive reactions should, however, be interpreted with caution because psittacine birds and pigeons frequently have low levels of antibodies.

LYMPHOGRANULOMA VENEREUM

(*Lymphogranuloma inguinale or Climatic bubo*)

This disease is transmitted by venereal contact. After an incubation period of three to twenty-one days a small primary sore appears taking the form of a papule which becomes vesicular and then breaks to leave a shallow ulcer; in the male it may be situated on the glans penis or in the urethra, causing urethritis; in the female the vaginal wall or the cervix uteri are the common sites. The virus spreads from the primary site to involve the regional lymph nodes, where an inflammatory reaction and suppuration begin to develop about two weeks after the appearance of the primary sore. In the male, suppuration of the inguinal glands gives rise to a bubo, from which it is possible to aspirate pus. In the female, the lymphatic drainage carries the virus to lymph glands within the pelvis and inguinal buboes do not occur. As a late result of chronic inflammatory processes in the perianal tissues, rectal stricture, granulomatous involvement of the vulva, and elephantiasis of the genitalia may result.

Properties of the Virus.—The virus is a typical member of the psittacosis group. In morphology, viability and susceptibility to chemotherapeutic agents it resembles very closely the psittacosis virus.

Culture.—After adaptation, the virus grows abundantly in the yolk sac of developing chick embryos. Usually the embryos do not die until seven to nine days after inoculation. It will multiply in the mouse only after intracerebral inoculation and does grow in the peritoneal cavity. It does not infect birds.

Laboratory Diagnosis

Isolation of the virus may be achieved by the inoculation of pus from the bubo into the yolk sac of six- to eight-day-old chick embryos and by the inoculation of mice by the intracerebral route. If the pus is contaminated with bacteria it may be treated with streptomycin at a concentration of up to 2000 μg. per ml.; penicillin, tetracyclines and sulphonamides should *not* be used for the purpose as they may kill the virus.

Complement Fixation Tests are carried out using a heated antigen prepared from infected yolk sacs in the same way as for psittacosis. The test becomes positive two to four weeks after the onset of the infection. A titre of 32 or higher in a clinically acceptable case suggests active infection, but better evidence is obtained if a significant rise in titre can be demonstrated during the course of the disease. False positive reactions may be given by syphilitic sera.

Frei Test.—Patients with lymphogranuloma venereum react allergically when inactivated virus is inoculated intradermally. The antigen is prepared by phenolising a purified virus suspension from infected yolk sacs.[1] Originally pus from the bubo suitably diluted and inactivated at 60° C. was used for the purpose. The test is carried out by injecting 0·1 ml. of the antigen intracutaneously into one arm and a similar amount of control material from normal eggs into the other arm. A positive reaction takes four days to reach its maximum and consists of an area of erythema with a central indurated papule at least 7 mm. in diameter. Minor reactions, especially if accompanied by any change in the control inoculation, should be disregarded.

The Frei test remains positive many years after the active infection has subsided. Like the tuberculin reaction it is an indication that infection has, at some time, taken place. The test is positive when infection has been due to other members of the group and depends on hypersensitivity to the heat-stable antigen. The Frei test, therefore, is not specific for lymphogranuloma venereum. Barwell (1952) has shown, however, that if an acid extract of the virus is injected intradermally a reaction occurs which is specific for the lymphogranuloma virus.

Tetracyclines and, to a lesser degree, sulphonamides are effective as therapeutic agents.

TRACHOMA

Trachoma is a severe form of kerato-conjunctivitis which frequently damages the eye permanently, and causes blindness. It is highly prevalent in the East, the Middle East, Africa and parts of South America and occurs also in Eastern Europe. The infection is due to a virus of the psittacosis group and is spread from eye to eye directly by fingers and also by flies. The incubation period in human experimental infections is 4–7 days but under natural conditions it is probably longer. Secondary bacterial infection is present at all stages of the infection and plays an important accessary part in tissue damage.

Trachoma usually begins insidiously with some swelling and granularity of the upper eyelids, a variable amount of muco-purulent discharge and a preauricular adenitis. Follicles are soon formed in the conjunctivae and within a few weeks the condition passes to a chronic stage of kerato-conjunctivitis, when the cornea is invaded by inflammatory tissue which later becomes vascularised. The cicatricial tissue

[1] Available commercially as "Lygranum" (Squibb).

formed may impair vision and distort the eyelids. The recent developments in the study of the trachoma virus are described by Bernkopf (1962).

Properties of the Virus.—The elementary bodies are 0·2–0·6 μ in diameter, and electron microscopically have the "wrinkled pea" appearance of the psittacosis-lymphogranuloma group. Larger forms up to 1·5 μ in diameter are also seen. They are stained blue by Castaneda's stain and red by Macchiavello's stain.

The virus multiplies within the cytoplasm of the epithelial cells of the conjunctiva and passes through a cycle of morphological changes closely similar to that of the psittacosis virus (Armstrong, Valentine & Fildes, 1963). The first sign of infection is the appearance of an "initial body", a basophilic inclusion 0·3–0·8 μ in diameter. This body divides by fission and as the particles increase in number they become smaller and more acidophilic. The mature inclusion consists of a mass of elementary bodies which are stained purplish by Giemsa's stain; they are set in a matrix composed of glycogen. In the final stage of development the inclusion bodies often entirely replace the cytoplasm. Many different shapes and sizes of inclusions may be seen; they are usually known as *Halberstaedter-Prowazek* bodies and on their detection depends the confirmation of the clinical diagnosis. They are found most frequently in scrapings of the conjunctiva of the upper lids taken in the earlier phases of the disease.

The infection has been transmitted to human volunteers and to baboons. The virus can be cultivated if infected corneal scrapings are treated with streptomycin at a concentration of 20,000 μg/ml. (Sowa & Collier, 1960) to destroy bacterial contaminants and inoculated into the yolk sac of five- to seven-day-old chick embryos. Death of the embryo occurs irregularly during the first passages but later occurs five to seven days after inoculation. Virus cultured in this way has the typical morphology of the group and is infective when introduced into the cornea of human volunteers. Some strains (*e.g.* the T'ang strain) of the trachoma virus have been adapted to grow in the FL line of human amnion cells and in HeLa cells.

Laboratory Diagnosis

Films of the conjunctival exudate are unsatisfactory and it is essential to make smears of scrapings of the conjunctival epithelium on glass slides. For preliminary screening a dry unfixed film is stained for two min. with 5 per cent. (w/v) iodine in 10 per cent. potassium iodide. On examination with the $\frac{1}{6}$ in. objective inclusion bodies are seen as deep orange-brown masses against a clear background of cytoplasm. The nature of the inclusions can be confirmed by decolourising the film with absolute methyl alcohol which acts as a fixative before staining with Giemsa (Gilkes, Smith & Sowa, 1958). Fresh films may also be fixed for ten minutes in methyl alcohol and stained overnight with a 1 in 10 solution of Giemsa's stain. A search is then made for the basophilic

Halberstaedter-Prowazek inclusions. Immune-fluorescent staining by the indirect method using a serum with a high titre of antibodies against the group antigen of the psittacosis group of viruses can be used to give a rapid and specific diagnosis.

In the complement-fixation reaction an unheated, purified antigen is more effective than the group antigen in measuring antibody levels (Woolridge & Grayston, 1962). A neutralisation test using the virus grown in HeLa cells may also be used to estimate antibody levels in sera (Reeve & Graham, 1962).

Sulphonamides and tetracyclines are very valuable in the treatment of trachoma.

INCLUSION CONJUNCTIVITIS

A virus closely related to the trachoma virus causes inclusion blenorrhoea of the newborn or in adults; the inflammatory reaction is unlike that of trachoma in that it is more intense in the lower eyelids. The virus also causes urethritis and cervicitis in adults.

It is yet to be decided whether the virus of inclusion conjunctivitis, is a separate entity or whether it is a trachoma virus of low virulence. These two agents are sometimes referred to as the "TRIC" viruses.

The properties of the virus are those of the psittacosis-lymphogranuloma group; the inclusions formed in the epithelial cells are basophilic with a glycogen matrix and are indistinguishable morphologically from those of trachoma. When transmitted to human volunteers a severe conjunctivitis results, but there is no subsequent scarring or pannus (Jones & Collier, 1962); when inoculated into apes, a severe mucopurulent conjunctivitis is produced. The virus can be isolated from infected epithelium by the inoculation of the yolk sac of chick embryos and has been cultured in this way in series and in quantity.

Laboratory diagnosis is made by the examination of smears of corneal scrapings in the same way as for trachoma.

Epidemiology.—The reservoir of the infection is the human genital tract and the virus is spread by venereal contact. The virus may be present in cells without apparently causing any symptoms, for it has been detected in smears of the transitional epithelial cells just within the *os uteri* of apparently healthy women. In the male it has been found to be associated with a mild purulent urethritis. A proportion of cases of non-gonococcal ("non-specific") urethritis are due to infection with this virus. The disease has been known in the past as "swimming bath conjunctivitis" from the fact that many cases have occurred in bathers. It is probable that the water may have been infected by the discharges from the genital tracts of infected persons.

The virus may be transmitted from the cervix uteri to the baby's eye at birth, giving rise to a severe, acute, mucopurulent conjunctivitis ("inclusion blenorrhoea"). There is, however, no corneal ulceration and the lesions slowly heal without scarring. Therapy with tetracyclines or sulphonamides is effective.

For a valuable survey of the "TRIC" viruses see Jawetz (1964).

Cat Scratch Disease

Cat scratch disease is characterised by fever, malaise and adenitis. The primary lesion is usually a cat scratch or bite often developing into a cutaneous pustular lesion and followed by a marked adenitis and bubo formation. Mere contact with a cat, however, has sometimes been thought to cause the infection and has been followed by marked adenitis. Clinically the disease resembles many other infections of lymph glands especially lymphogranuloma venereum.

The disease is thought to be due to a virus and elementary bodies of the psittacosis type are said to have been found in stained preparations of pus. Monkeys have been infected by the inoculation of the pus and develop nodules at the site of injection and a lymphadenopathy.

In man the diagnosis depends on the use of an intradermal test with antigen prepared from pus from a lymph gland of an undoubted clinical case. A positive reaction consists of a firm papule 0·5–1·0 cm. in diameter within forty-eight hours of inoculation. Although the results of such tests appear to indicate that the antigen is specific, positive reactions should be interpreted with caution, since they may occur in normal people presumably as the result of previous undiagnosed infection. It is not yet clear whether cat scratch fever is a feline disease transmitted to man (e.g. feline pneumonitis) or is an infection of which the cat is merely a vector.

ENZOOTIC ABORTION IN EWES

Abortion and premature lambing is frequent in flocks on tick-free pastures in south-east Scotland and has been reported in New Zealand and Australia. The causative organism is a virus of the psittacosis-lymphogranuloma group (Stamp *et al.* 1950).

Properties of the Virus.—In size, morphology and staining reactions the ewe abortion virus is indistinguishable from other members of the group. It can be cultivated readily in the yolk sac of the developing chick embryo or on the chorio-allantoic membrane where it produces a marked generalised thickening. When injected intravenously into pregnant ewes abortion results, and when instilled intranasally in mice a pneumonia is produced. Cattle may be infected experimentally and abort, but the disease does not appear to occur naturally in bovines. The virus possesses the same heat-stable complement-fixing antigen that is found in all the other members of the group.

Laboratory Diagnosis.—The gross appearances of the aborted placenta and membranes are similar to those seen in the bovine as a result of infection with *Brucella abortus.* Films should be made from the diseased cotyledons, from the chorion, and from purulent discharges. On staining with Macchiavello's or Castaneda's stain, many clusters of virus elementary bodies can be seen within the cytoplasm of cells. The virus may be isolated by the egg cultivation methods used for psittacosis; usually seven to eight days pass after inoculation into the yolk sac before the embryos die.

Epidemiology.—Abortion and premature lambing are the only striking features of the infection and usually take place late in pregnancy, often in the last two or three weeks of the gestation period. The infected membranes and discharges contain huge amounts of the virus and are able to contaminate the pastures and lambing pens very heavily. Probably infected pastures are the common source of infection. However, lambs born of infected ewes may survive and carry the virus in their tissues until maturity. When such animals are themselves fertilised they are frequently liable to abort and in one experiment 27 per cent. lambed with infected foetal membranes (McEwen, Littlejohn & Foggie 1951). It is possible that the ewe abortion virus occasionally infects man; there is one case recorded of a laboratory worker who contracted the infection.

Control.—A vaccine prepared from formolised yolk sac cultures of the virus (McEwen, Dow & Anderson, 1955) precipitated with alum and suspended in mineral oil, has been shown to stimulate the production of virus-neutralising antibodies. The use of this vaccine by subcutaneous inoculation before service has proved highly effective in reducing the incidence of ewe abortion.

Feline Pneumonitis

The aetiological agents responsible for the common forms of respiratory infections in the domesticated cat are ill understood. "Cat flu" is a very common and highly contagious illness, and much remains to be done in the study of this condition. From some types of cases American workers have isolated a virus which has all the morphological and cultural characteristics of the psittacosis-lymphogranuloma group. The feline pneumonitis virus has a similar host range to the other members of the group and after infection neutralising and complement-fixing antibodies appear. The significance and the incidence of infections with this virus in cats in Great Britain has yet to be determined.

Murine Pneumonitis

Several viruses associated with pneumonitis in mice have been described. Nigg's mouse pneumonitis was isolated from a healthy colony and has all the morphological and general characters of the psittacosis, lymphogranuloma group. Horsfall and Hahn's pneumonia virus of mice (PVM) has been isolated from healthy mice as well as from patients with pneumonia. This virus agglutinates mouse and hamster red blood cells. The natural occurrence of mouse pneumonitis viruses must be borne in mind when human material is inoculated. The instillation of sputum suspensions into the nares of mice under ether anaesthesia may well activate a latent pneumonitis virus being carried by the animal. Furthermore, it is probable that mouse pneumonitis viruses occasionally cause disease in man.

REFERENCES

Psittacosis.

Perkins, H. R. & Allison, A. C. (1963). Cell wall constituents of rickettsiae and psittacosis-lymphogranuloma organisms. *J. gen. Microbiol.*, **30**, 469.

Lymphogranuloma venereum.

Barwell, C. F. (1952). Some observations of the antigenic structure of psittacosis and lymphogranuloma venereum viruses. Treatment of virus suspension by various agents and the specific activity of acid extracts. *Brit. J. exp. Path.*, **33**, 268.

Trachoma.

Armstrong, J. A., Valentine, R. C. & Fildes, C. (1963). Structure and replication of the trachoma agent in cell cultures, as shown by electron microscopy. *J. gen. Microbiol.*, **30**, 59.

Bernkopf, H. (1962). Trachoma virus—recent developments. *Progr. med. Virol.*, **4**, 119.

GILKES, M. J., SMITH, C. H. & SOWA, J. (1958). Staining of the inclusion bodies of trachoma and inclusion conjunctivitis. *Brit. J. Ophthal.*, **42**, 473.

JAWETZ, E. (1964). Agents of trachoma and inclusion conjunctivitis *Ann. Rev. Microbiol.* **18**. 301.

REEVE, P. & GRAHAM, D. M. (1962). A neutralisation test for trachoma and inclusion blenorrhoea viruses grown in HeLa cell cultures. *J. gen. Microbiol.*, **27**, 177.

SOWA, J. & COLLIER, L. H. (1960). Isolation of trachoma virus from patients in West Africa. *J. Hyg.* (*Lond.*), **58**, 99.

WOOLRIDGE, R. L. & GRAYSTON, J. T. (1962). Further studies with a complement fixation test for trachoma. *Ann. N.Y. Acad. Sci.*, **98**, 314.

Inclusion Conjunctivitis.

JONES, B. R. & COLLIER, L. H. (1962). Inoculation of man with inclusion blenorrhoea virus. *Ann. N.Y. Acad. Sci.*, **98**, 212.

Enzootic Abortion of Ewes.

MCEWEN, A. D., DOW, J. B. & ANDERSON, R. D. (1955). Enzootic abortion in ewes. An adjuvant vaccine prepared from eggs. *Vet Rec.*, **67**, 393.

MCEWEN, A. D., LITTLEJOHN, A. L. & FOGGIE, A. (1951). Enzootic abortion in ewes. Some aspects of infection and resistance. *Vet. Rec.*, **63**, 489.

STAMP, J. T., MCEWEN, A. D., WATT, T. A. & NISBETT, D. L. (1950). Enzootic abortion in ewes. Transmission of the disease. *Vet. Rec.*, **62**, 251.

CHAPTER 39

RICKETTSIAE; COXIELLA; PLEUROPNEUMONIA ORGANISMS; BARTONELLA

THE *Rickettsiae* occupy a biological position which is intermediate between that of the smaller bacteria and the larger viruses. They resemble the former in that they are visible with the light microscope, are known to divide by binary fission, have cell walls which contain the amino sugar muramic acid, and are susceptible to the action of antibiotics. It is, however, undisputed that, like the viruses, they are obligate intracellular parasites. A further distinctive property of rickettsiae is that they occur under natural conditions in the alimentary tract of such blood-sucking arthropods as lice, fleas, mites, and ticks. Some have no relationship to human disease, but others when transmitted to unnatural hosts, such as man, cause severe diseases. The typhus fevers are due to infection by rickettsiae of various species and it is convenient to arrange these diseases according to the arthropod vectors which transmit them.

1. *Louse-borne typhus*	
(*a*) Epidemic typhus	*Rickettsia prowazekii*
(*b*) Recrudescent typhus (Brill's Disease)	*R. prowazekii*
(*c*) Trench fever	*R. quintana*
2. *Flea-borne typhus*	
Murine endemic typhus Tabardillo	*R. mooseri* (*R. typhi*)
3. *Tick-borne typhus*	
(*a*) Rocky Mountain spotted fever	*R. rickettsii*
(*b*) South African tick bite fever	*R. rickettsii* var. *pijperi*
(*c*) Mediterranean fever (fièvre boutonneuse)	*R. conorii*
4. *Mite-borne typhus*	
(*a*) Scrub typhus (Tsutsugamushi fever)	*R. tsutsugamushi*
(*b*) Rickettsialpox	*R. akari*

Morphology and Staining.—Cocco-bacilli measuring approximately 0·35 μ in length and 0·25 μ in width. They are usually described as Gram-negative though they are only faintly stained by watery solutions of aniline dyes. They are, however, readily stained blue with Castaneda or Giemsa's stains; with Macchiavello's stain they appear red against a blue background. Pleomorphism is frequent and the organisms may occur singly, in pairs or short chains or as filaments. *R. prowazekii* has a tendency to show slender filamentous forms whereas *R. mooseri* shows shorter and broader rod-forms. Bipolarity with a suggestion of the presence of metachromatic granules is often evident in *R. tsutsugamushi*. In smears or sections of infected tissues, clumps and masses of rickettsiae are often seen lying within the cytoplasm of endothelial and serosal cells (*e.g.* in the cells lining the tunica vaginalis in experimentally infected guinea-pigs). Under the electron microscope they appear to have a mucoid envelope, a cell wall, and an electron-dense mass resembling a nucleus.

Viability.—In general, rickettsiae are easily destroyed by heat, drying and chemical disinfectants. They die within a few hours at room temperature but may be preserved well in glycerol saline at 0° C. or by freeze-drying emulsions of infected tissue suspended in sterile skimmed milk.

Under certain circumstances they may survive drying for long periods and it is known that the dried faeces of lice and fleas may remain infective for months.

Rickettsial growth is inhibited by chloramphenicol and tetracyclines which are effective therapeutic agents. Sulphonamides accelerate the growth of the organisms, but para-amino-benzoic acid exerts a marked inhibitory effect and has been used with some success in treatment.

Laboratory Diagnosis

Cultivation.—The most satisfactory method for primary isolation is the inoculation of adult male guinea-pigs or mice. Whole blood or ground-up blood clot taken during the height of the patient's fever is injected by the intraperitoneal route. The first signs of infection in the guinea-pig are seen after nine or ten days, when the animal's temperature rises to 41° C. to 42° C.; it remains above normal for four to eight days. If the animals are killed at the height of their fever rickettsiae can be demonstrated in Giemsa stained films of the peritoneal exudate and in impression smears from the spleen. Usually the animals recover, but *R. tsutsugamushi* is highly pathogenic and often kills both mice and guinea-pigs within a few days. Some members of the group may produce transient and very mild infections. In the case of *R. mooseri* however, well-marked swelling and oedema of the scrotum occurs with inflammation of the tunica vaginalis. Stained smears from the tunica show intracytoplasmic rickettsiae in the serosal and endothelial cells. Those members of the group causing epidemic and endemic typhus fevers are seen in clusters in the cell cytoplasm and those causing spotted fever are also seen within the nucleus. In human tissues the cells most frequently infected are the endothelial cells and the smooth muscle fibres around small blood vessels. It seems that rickettsiae grow best in cells whose metabolic activity is depressed by measures which reduce the oxidative processes of the cell (*e.g.* a lowering of the temperature or a reduction of the oxygen tension).

All strains of rickettsiae can be cultivated in the yolk sac of the chick embryo. Using this method and incubating the eggs at 32° C. big yields of the organisms can be obtained for vaccine production or for the preparation of serological antigens. The method is only of limited value in primary isolation. Tissue cultures of mouse lymphosarcoma cells (Bozeman *et al.*, 1956) and rat fibroblasts (Schaechter, Bozeman & Smadel, 1957) can also serve as hosts for these organisms.

Antigenic Structure.—Each species of rickettsia possesses its own specific antigens which provoke the production of homologous antibodies. These antibodies can be measured by agglutination and neutralisation tests, but are more conveniently demonstrated by the method of complement fixation. In washed and carefully purified rickettsial suspensions only the type-specific antigens remain, and by demonstration of these it is possible to differentiate epidemic from murine typhus, and both of these from the spotted fevers. Fluorescent antibody staining offers a highly specific method which can be applied either to the estimation and identification of antibodies in sera (Goldwasser & Shepard, 1959) or to the identification of the rickettsiae themselves in the tissues of ticks or animals (Shepard & Goldwasser, 1960). Strains of *R. tsutsugamushi* are antigenically so heterogeneous that the complement fixation reaction is of doubtful value in the diagnosis of scrub typhus. There is also a soluble antigen which is group specific and is probably derived from the mucoid envelope of the organisms. It reacts with antibodies in the sera of cases of both epidemic and murine typhus though not with those from spotted fever. It must be emphasised that the antigens required for the specific complement fixation reactions are both difficult and expensive to prepare and that these tests are of necessity only carried out in a small number of reference laboratories.

The Weil-Felix Reaction.—The rickettsiae of epidemic, endemic and mite-borne typhus and those of the spotted fevers contain in varying amounts an alkali-stable carbohydrate hapten which is shared by a non-flagellate strain of *Proteus* and some of its variants. This hapten is a somatic constituent of these bacilli, which are readily agglutinated by the sera of convalescent cases of typhus.

The reaction, first described by Weil and Felix, is very simple to carry out and of great practical importance in the diagnosis of rickettsial infections. By the end of the first week of the illness in epidemic typhus the titre of agglutinins for Proteus OX 19 has usually reached a figure of 200 and a peak of 1000–5000 is reached at the end of the second week. The agglutinins tend to disappear a few months after recovery and thus a positive Weil-Felix reaction is a useful indication of recent infection. Complement fixing antibodies persist for much longer periods and by providing evidence of past infection, their presence enables a retrospective diagnosis to be made.

The Weil-Felix reaction is performed in the same manner as the Widal test except that an O-agglutinable suspension of Proteus X 19 is used as the agglutinins are of the O type. As this organism may revert to the H form it should be grown on dry agar, and subcultures made from non-spreading separate colonies.[1] The tubes are incubated at 50° C. for four hours and then overnight at 37° C., after which final readings are made. The results of the Weil-Felix test should be interpreted strictly in relation to the clinical findings, for a positive reaction is occasionally observed in other diseases such as undulant fever, malaria, infectious mononucleosis and tuberculosis. The agglutination reactions with this and other *Proteus* suspensions in rickettsial infections are shown in the table below.

		Proteus OX 19	OX 2	OX K
Epidemic	Louse-borne	+++	±	−
Brill's disease	Louse-borne	Usually	negative	−
Murine typhus	Flea-borne	+++	+	−
Tsutsugamushi fever	Mite borne	−	−	+++
Rocky Mountain spotted fever	Tick-borne	+++	++	−
Fièvre boutonneuse	Tick-borne	++	++	−
South African tick-bite fever	Tick-borne	++	++	−

Epidemiology

Epidemic typhus fever, known also as Classical or European typhus fever, is caused by *R. prowazekii*. It is spread from man to man by the bite of the human body louse (*Pediculus corporis*) or more doubtfully by the head louse (*P. capitis*). Although potentially world wide, the location of the disease is now limited to the Balkans and the Middle East, North Africa, Asia, Mexico and the Andes. Lice become infected when they bite either patients suffering from typhus fever or carriers in whom the infection has persisted in latent form for many years. When the infected blood reaches the intestine of the louse, the rickettsiae invade the epithelial cells and multiply until the host cells distend and rupture. As a result, the faeces become heavily laden with the organisms and when they are discharged on the skin, the rickettsiae are readily introduced into the human host through the abrasions caused by scratching or through fresh biting wounds. When standards of personal hygiene are low and when a considerable proportion of the population are infested with lice, typhus fever may assume epidemic proportions. Such conditions may arise in time of war, and if a reservoir of the rickettsiae in the form of a carrier of the latent infection is introduced into the community, typhus breaks out. The epidemic in Naples during the Second World War began in this way, but was quickly controlled by measures which were taken against the lice that were transmitting the infection. It was possible to delouse the persons of the affected community as well as their clothes, bedding and dwelling-places by the use of a residual insecticide DDT (dichloro-diphenyl-

[1] A standard suspension can be obtained from the Central Public Health Laboratory, Colindale, London.

trichloro-ethane) which was readily applied by being blown forcibly through an insufflator. The result of prompt and thorough use of DDT was that the epidemic was cut short before it could spread throughout the whole city.

Rickettsiae may persist alive in the tissues of recovered patients for as long as twenty years without manifest symptoms. Occasionally, however, they become active once more and cause a recurrence of typhus fever often in an atypical clinical form. Recrudescent typhus fever is known as *Brill's disease.*

Murine typhus is caused by *R. mooseri* (*R. typhi*) and is primarily a disease of rats, amongst which it is spread by the rat flea (*Xenopsylla cheopis*) and the rat louse (*Polypax spinulosus*). Occasionally the rat fleas carry the infection to man, and sporadic *endemic* typhus fever occurs. This disease is world wide and is most frequent in areas where rat infestation is high. In Mexico it is known as Tabardillo, from the cloak-like distribution of the rash. The disease has sometimes spread in epidemic form in man, but the vector responsible is not certainly known.

Spotted Fever. Rocky Mountain spotted fever was first recognised by Ricketts in western Montana in America. The causative organism is *R. rickettsii.* Spotted fever also occurs in North Africa along the shores of the Mediterranean, where it is named "fièvre boutonneuse" and is caused by *R. conorii.* In Kenya and South Africa similar infections are due to *R. rickettsii* var. *pijperi* and other rickettsiae. Spotted fever also exists in Mexico, Brazil and Colombia. The organisms are transmitted by ticks usually of the Ixodidae family, e.g. *Dermacentor andersoni*, a vector of Rocky Mountain spotted fever. Rickettsiae enter the human host either by the bite of the tick or through minute abrasions such as may occur when an engorged tick is crushed in the fingers. Fresh tick faeces are infectious, but dried faeces, in contrast to those of lice in epidemic typhus fever, are non-infective. Normally *R. rickettsii* inhabits healthy ticks and is passed transovarially throughout the life cycle. Vertebrate hosts such as horses and dogs are occasionally bitten by ticks and become for a time reservoirs of infection. After feeding on such animals, engorged ticks are a common source of infection for man.

Scrub typhus is caused by *R. tsutsugamushi* and is transmitted by the bite of the larvae of mites (*Trombicula akamushi* or *T. deliensis*). The larvae become infected after biting an infected host and the rickettsiae are then carried to the adult mite and thence throughout the life cycle to the egg and to the larvae once more. The infection is transmitted by the young larvae which bite only once and which usually feed on wild rats and other rodents. The larvae are found on low-lying humid vegetation and on moist ground, whence they can readily attack man. Scrub typhus is very difficult to control because the mites and their larvae can be eradicated only by clearing away large areas of vegetation and drying the ground where camps or houses are to be sited. Miticidal chemicals such as dimethyl phthalate are used as an ointment to act as a repellent, and chemoprophylaxis with chloramphenicol is of considerable value.

Rickettsialpox is a mild disease which occurs in the U.S.A., West and South Africa and the U.S.S.R. It is caused by *R. akari* which antigenically is closely related to members of the tick borne group especially *R. rickettsii* and *R. conorii*. The reservoir of infection is the house mouse and the infection is spread to man by the bite of the common mouse mite *Allodermanyssus sanguineus*. No Weil-Felix antibodies are produced in man and complement fixation and neutralisation tests are used for diagnostic serology. *R. akari* causes a marked scrotal reaction in mice and guinea pigs five days after intraperitoneal inoculation.

Prophylaxis.—Active immunisation against typhus is usually carried out with a formolised vaccine of the Cox type for which the rickettsiae have been cultivated in the yolk sacs of developing chick embryos. A vaccine of this type containing *R. prowazekii* is used against epidemic typhus and one containing *R. mooseri* against endemic typhus. A similar vaccine containing *R. rickettsii* is employed against Rocky Mountain spotted fever. The latter is given early in the summer months before the ticks are active.

Cox-type vaccines are administered in three 1·0 ml. doses at intervals of seven to fourteen days. Booster doses of 1·0 ml. are needed at yearly intervals or more frequently if the risk is great. Antibodies may persist for some years after inoculation. The booster dose results in a prompt rise of circulating antibodies reaching a peak in about ten days. A second type of vaccine prepared from "strain E", a living attenuated strain of *R. prowazekii*, is at present under trial and shows considerable promise. Although reactions have followed the use of this vaccine it has caused no harm and has given a firm immunity against epidemic typhus for as long as five years (Fox, 1956).

In scrub typhus formolised vaccines of *R. tsutsugamushi* have proved to be ineffective. A vaccine of a living strain is under trial and the infection it establishes is controlled after some ten days by chloramphenicol therapy. The procedure is, however, not without risk, and on account of the antigenic heterogeneity of the *R. tsutsugamushi* its effectiveness is in some doubt.

Chemotherapy.—Tetracyclines, chloramphenicol and para-aminobenzoic acid all exhibit a rickettsiostatic effect. The tetracyclines and chloramphenicol are more or less equally effective against louse-borne, flea-borne, tick-borne and mite-borne typhus fevers.

Trench Fever, a form of louse-borne typhus fever, is caused by *Rickettsia quintana*. The disease occurred in both world wars and was shown to be transmitted from man to man by the human louse. *R. quintana* has been propagated in the intestinal epithelial cells of lice, but not in egg or tissue cultures. There are no specific laboratory tests for Trench fever.

Heartwater Disease of cattle, sheep and goats is caused by *Cowdria ruminantium*. It occurs in Central, East and West Africa and the infection is spread by the bite of the "bont" tick (*Amblyomma hebraeum*). Affected animals develop high fever, gastroenteritis, and oedematous swellings, the most characteristic of which is the hydropericardium, which gives the disease its name. Rickettsiae are found in large numbers in the endothelial cells of capillaries of many internal organs, especially those of the brain and renal glomeruli. It is thought that the serum from recovered animals can transmit a mild infection to young calves and it has been used in attempts to procure active immunisation.

TICK-BORNE FEVER of sheep in Great Britain has been regarded as a rickettsial infection and inclusion bodies are observed within the cytoplasm of granular leucocytes and monocytes. The organism is also found in cattle and goats.

Q FEVER

Q fever is an acute systemic infection usually characterised by an interstitial pneumonia; unlike other rickettsial infections it has no rash. The name of the disease is derived not from Queensland in Australia, where it was first recognised, but from the letter Q in "Query", because for some time its aetiology was uncertain. The signs and symptoms are usually referable to the respiratory system but are very inconstant. Often the first indications of the diagnosis are the characteristic multiple, patchy areas of infiltration or the segmental consolidation seen on radiological examination differing somewhat from the more circumscribed lesions of a "primary atypical pneumonia". Very rarely the disease may declare itself with the prolonged fever and embolic signs of subacute bacterial endocarditis.

Coxiella burnetii is the causative organism. It is an obligate intracellular parasite, pleomorphic in appearance, and measuring 0·25 μ by 0·5 μ to 1·5 μ in length. It is frequently seen as a diplobacillus and closely resembles the *Rickettsiae* in its morphology. The infective property of *Cox. burnetii* has been passed through a collodion membrane of an average diameter of 400 mμ. The organism infects guinea-pigs, hamsters, mice and the cells of the yolk sac of the developing chick embryo. It appears as clumps or masses within the cytoplasm of endothelial and serosal cells such as those lining the peritoneal cavity. *Cox. burnetii* is remarkably resistant to desiccation and may survive for long periods in the tissues or faeces of infected ticks. It remains viable for several days in water or milk. It can withstand heat at 60° C. for one hour, survives 1·0 per cent. phenol for one hour, and 1 in 1000 merthiolate for a week.

Cox. burnetii thus possesses properties which are distinct from those of all the other members of the family *Rickettsiaceae*. It is filterable, highly resistant to heat and disinfectants, does not produce a rash in infected persons and does not elicit the agglutinin to the *Proteus* X strains which characterises the typhus fevers. For these reasons the organism is no longer regarded as a true *Rickettsia* and has been designated the prototype of a new genus—*Coxiella*.

Epidemiology.—*Cox. burnetii* is the cause of enzootic infections in domesticated animals such as cattle, sheep and goats. The disease is found throughout the world and has been reported in fifty different countries, including the United Kingdom. Apparently healthy animals may excrete coxiellae in their milk and also during parturition, when huge numbers of the organism are present in the placenta and the birth fluids. Man may be infected by drinking contaminated milk or, more commonly, by inhaling the infected dust from the straw and bedding soiled by the animals. There are many instances on record of the infection of workers by the inhalation of infected material in the laboratory. The infection is prevalent in many wild rodents, particularly in the bandicoot in Australia and in pigeons and other birds. *Cox. burnetii* is conveyed from animal to animal by the bite of ticks. More than twenty species of ticks mostly of the Ixodidae and Argasidae families are known vectors. It is uncommon for the organism to be carried throughout all stages of the life cycle of the tick and for most the part these arthropods are infected from the animal reservoir (Stoker & Marmion, 1955). Ticks seldom if ever transmit the disease to man. The risk of person-to-person transmission of Q fever is small, and strict isolation precautions are not needed, but infection has occurred from the necropsy of a fatal case.

Laboratory Diagnosis

This depends on the recovery of *Cox. burnetii* from the blood in the early febrile stages of the illness and on the results of serological tests for specific antibodies. The Weil-Felix reaction is negative.

Isolation of the Causative Organism.—Heparinised blood should be inoculated into as many susceptible hosts as possible, *e.g.* intraperitoneally into guinea-pigs, and hamsters and into the yolk sacs of five- to six-day-old chick embryos. Guinea-pigs and hamsters do not die from the infection and seldom show any obvious sign of disease. The animals must be carefully observed for signs of illness and the rectal temperature should be recorded twice daily. When any definite fever or illness is detected, the animals should be killed and blood and tissue extracts from them should be injected into fresh animals. Smears from the spleen, liver and from the yolk sacs of chick embryos of sluggish movement should be stained by Castaneda's and Macchiavello's stains and examined for the presence of rickettsia-like organisms. Animals which do not sicken should be bled by cardiac puncture after two weeks and the serum examined for antibodies to *Cox. burnetii.*

For *Complement-fixation tests* killed antigens of egg adapted strains of *Cox. burnetii* are used. The Henzerling strain (Italian) and the Nine Mile strain (American) obtained from infected yolk sacs are in general use. Freshly isolated strains do not react well with sera in early convalescence and it is only after adaption to the egg that fully reactive antigens can be prepared (Stoker, Page & Marmion, 1955). The methods used to make the antigen and to carry out the test are similar to those used in psittacosis. Antibody titres rise from an initial low level to figures ranging from 64 to over 1000 in convalescence. Three samples of serum should be tested, the first taken at the onset of the illness, and the second and third at ten-day intervals thereafter.

Control measures for Q fever must include the adequate pasteurisation of milk. Coxiellae may not all be killed at 62° C. for 30 min., but are killed at 63° C. for 30 min. The "flash" method of pasteurisation (72° C. for 15 sec.) is adequate to eliminate viable *Cox. burnetii* from raw milk (Enright, Sadler & Thomas, 1957). In the laboratory great care must be taken with infected animals and eggs and they should always be handled within special inoculation cabinets, where the risk of contamination of the air is eliminated. All carcases and eggs should be immersed in disinfectant solution and then incinerated. The use of a vaccine of the Cox type if available is indicated for laboratory personnel and for persons whose work brings them into contact with live or dead animals.

Both chloramphenicol and the tetracyclines are effective therapeutically in Q fever.

PLEUROPNEUMONIA-LIKE ORGANISMS

Mycoplasmas

The pleuropneumonia-like organisms (PPLO) are very small parasitic or saprophytic microorganisms characterised by their lack of a rigid cell wall, great variability of cell morphology and characteristic "fried-egg" colony morphology on agar culture medium. They are almost ubiquitous in nature. The best known members of the group have been recognised for many years as the cause of great epizootics of severe respiratory disease of cattle, sheep and goats; others cause chronic respiratory disease in poultry and many different animals. Recently it has been established that Eaton's agent, which has been proved to be a cause of primary atypical pneumonia in man, is not a virus but is capable of growth on inanimate culture media, and is for this and other reasons a true mycoplasma (Chanock, Hayflick & Barile, 1962). It has been given the name of *Mycoplasma pneumoniae*. A considerable number of pleuropneumonia-like organisms are found as commensals in the oral cavity and in the genital tract in man, and in cattle, dogs and other animals. Mycoplasmas have been isolated from various pathological conditions of the female genito-urinary tract and from non-gonococcal urethritis in man, but the aetiological role of these organisms has not been proved. One species, *M. laidlawii*, is a saprophyte that can be recovered from sewage, manure, soil, etc.

The organisms are classified as the genus *Mycoplasma* (in the order *Mycoplasmatales*) which at present contains sixteen distinct species. They are small but variable in size, the smaller viable forms measuring 0·125–0·3 μ in diameter and being capable of passing through bacteria-stopping filters. They differ from other bacteria in that they lack a rigid cell wall, a deficiency that results in extreme variations in their morphology being produced by changes in their environmental circumstances. They are Gram-negative, non-motile and non-sporing. They can be cultivated in the absence of living cells in nutrient media heavily enriched with serum and most species have been found to require cholesterol or related steroids as an essential metabolite (Rodwell, 1963). It is a characteristic of the genus that their growth is inhibited by organic gold salts *in vivo*. For reviews of the properties of mycoplasmas see Edward (1954), Adler & Shifrine (1960) and Klieneberger-Nobel (1962).

Morphology.—The appearances of mycoplasmas are best seen in agar block preparations (Ørskov's method) or in impression smears made from young colonies grown on solid media. Dark ground microscopy of wet films offers the best results. In fluid cultures, stained films are often unsatisfactory. The organisms are highly pleomorphic and show granules of various sizes, disc-like and amoeboid structures, as well as rings, clubs, filaments (up to 100 μ long) and vibrionic and starlike forms. The smallest viable granules, or coccoid forms, which are filter-passing, are often called *elementary corpuscles*.

These many diverse forms are due in part to the fragility of the organism and its lack of a cell wall and in part to its reproductive process which is not confined to simple binary fission. Environmental influences, osmotic pressure (Leach, 1962), and trauma to the organism when films are being made all influence its morphology.

Klieneberger-Nobel (1962) has described successive phases of growth beginning with a granule (elementary corpuscle) 0·125–0·3 μ in diameter which is the minimal reproductive unit. This granule flattens on the surface or in the agar to give an irregularly shaped mass (0·4–0·9 μ in diameter) and as growth proceeds dense concentrations of material appear within the cytoplasm and are often placed at the periphery of the cell. The large body undergoes multiple fission, the cytoplasmic concentrations being separated to give newly formed granules which then give rise to a new generation of the larger elements. A similar process is observed in fluid cultures; there is a tendency for the granules and larger cells to form filaments which later become transformed into chains of small bodies which divide up, to liberate these as granules. Granules may remain attached to the parent cell or may be cast loose so that many differing configurations may arise.

Staining.—The organisms are Gram-negative but stain poorly with the usual aniline dyes. They stain satisfactorily with Giemsa by the prolonged method. On agar the organisms may be stained by Dienes' stain; colonies of mycoplasma retain the blue stain for two days while those of nearly all other bacterial colonies lose the colour in half an hour. *M. gallinarum*, however, is an exception. Dienes' stain contains azure II 0·25 g., methylene blue 0·5 g., maltose 2·0 g., Na_2CO_3 0·05 g., benzoic acid 0·04 g. and distilled water 20·0 ml. Mycoplasmae in tissues can be stained by an intensified Giemsa method (Goodburn & Marmion, 1962) in which the section is pre-treated for 2 minutes with a freshly made 1·0 per cent. w/v solution of potassium permanganate before overnight staining with 1 in 25 Giemsa's stain. Final differentiation is with 0·5 per cent. w/v acetic acid.

Cultural characters.—Cultures of most strains can be obtained aerobically on serum enriched media although some (e.g. *M. salivarium*) require 10 per cent. CO_2 for growth. For primary isolation from material contaminated with other bacteria the following selective medium can be used. PPLO agar (Difco) is enriched with 20 per cent. *unheated* horse serum, 10 per cent. of an extract of fresh yeast (see Chapter 47) but never heated over 75° C., and deoxyribonucleic acid (sodium salt of nucleic acid from thymus gland, BDH) 20 μg per ml. Penicillin 50 units per ml. and thallium acetate 0·25 mg. per ml. are added to control Gram-negative and Gram-positive bacterial contaminants. The final pH of the medium should be brought to pH 7·8–8·0 (Edward, 1947) by adding 2·8 ml. of M/1 K_2HPO_4 for each 100 ml. medium. Subcultures are made by excising a block of agar bearing one or more colonies and transferring it to a fresh semi-solid agar plate (enriched as above and with or without the selective agents). The agar base can be made conveniently by adding 10 ml. PPLO agar to 90 ml. PPLO broth (Difco). Growth visible microscopically occurs in 2–12 days under aerobic conditions; it is not readily discernible by the naked eye. In fluid medium it is seen as a very faint general cloudiness or granularity. On inoculation on solid agar the small granules seep into the agar medium and are caught in the fibrillary meshwork of the agar gel. They grow upwards to reach the surface where a thin layer of growth spreads outwards from the centre of the colony in the film of water on the agar surface. The colonies are seen to have an irregular but entire edge, the centre is heaped up, often granular, and is surrounded by a thin transparent peripheral rim. Most species give this typical "fried egg" appearance but some, e.g. *Mycoplasma pneumoniae,* may not. In cross section the colony has the outline of a drawing pin. The central portion of the colony is adherent to the agar. At three to four days, depending on the medium and the strain, the colonies measure 20–600 μ in diameter and can be seen only with the plate microscope; by about 7–12 days they may reach approximately 2–3 mm. in diameter and will then be visible to the naked eye. The morphology of the colony varies with the species; it can be studied in unstained agar block preparations using phase contrast microscopy or after staining by Dienes' method (*vide supra*). A rapid identification of the colony may be made by staining with specific fluorescein labelled antisera (Marmion & Hers, 1963). Sheep or guinea-pig blood cells are lysed by some strains including *M. pneumoniae.* For this purpose one part of 50 per cent. cells in Alsever's solution is added to three parts of 1 per cent. Bacto agar in normal saline and is layered over a 2–5 day old culture. Haemolysis of the α or β type appears after reincubation for 24 hr. and is seen as zones 2–5 mm. in diameter around the colonies. When 0·5 per cent. benzidine is incorporated in the blood agar, hydrogen peroxide is formed causing a blackening of the colonies which makes them more easily counted. *M. pneumoniae* can be cultivated by the amniotic inoculation of 13-day-old chick embryos; the organism is recovered from the lungs of the embryos after 6–7 days' incubation at 35° C. This organism can also be cultivated in primary monkey kidney and in continuous lines of human amnion and human embryonic lung cells where a cytopathic effect is detectable by Giemsa or minimal fluorescent stains (Eaton *et al.*, 1962).

Biochemical Reactions.—*M. pneumoniae* ferments glucose, maltose, mannose, dextrin, starch and xylose without gas formation and can thereby be distinguished from two human commensal mycoplasmas, *M. salivarium* and *M. hominis*, which do not attack carbohydrates. Another human commensal, *M. fermentans*, attacks most of these carbohydrates but fails to ferment mannose or xylose. *M. mycoides* ferments glucose, maltose, mannose, dextrin, starch, fructose and glycogen. *M. agalactiae* and *M. gallinarum* do not attack carbohydrates.

It should be noted that horse serum is not suitable as an enrichment for the sugar containing media because it contains maltases and diastases which may engender false positive reactions. Human or rabbit serum may however be used.

Viability.—Cultures on solid media remain viable at 4° C. for periods of up to 2 weeks but fluid cultures at this temperature die out more rapidly. Cultures on semi-solid agar stay alive without subculture for 6–12 months if preserved at −20° C. or lower. Mycoplasmas are readily destroyed by heat. Depending on the type of culture medium used *M. pneumoniae* will survive 4 hr. at 20° C. and 15 min. at 56° C. This organism is inactivated by ether and its growth like that of mycoplasmas generally is inhibited *in vivo* by sodium aurothiomalate.

Antigenic characters.—Each species of mycoplasma appears to be antigenically distinct and little or no sharing of antigens has been reported. There are two antigenic varieties of *M. hominis* and three of *M. laidlawii*, the saprophyte from sewage.

Animal pathogenicity.—When *M. pneumoniae* is introduced intranasally into hamsters or cotton rats it causes a patchy bronchopneumonia which can be seen at necropsy in animals killed about 12 days after inoculation.

M. mycoides is pathogenic for cattle, sheep and goats but not for rabbits, guinea-pigs or rats. After simple inoculation in cattle the natural disease does not follow although an extensive local inflammatory reaction is developed. It is difficult to reproduce typical bovine contagious pleuropneumonia by any form of inoculation but in some breeds of cattle it can be achieved by obliging them to inhale a fine spray of virulent culture. For further details of the pathogenicity of animal mycoplasmas see Turner (1959).

Epidemiology

The only pleuropneumonia organism known definitely to be pathogenic for man is *M. pneumoniae* (Eaton's agent). It causes that form of atypical pneumonia in which the patients develop serum agglutinins against *Streptococcus MG* and against human erythrocytes in the cold

(Chanock *et al.*, 1961; Goodburn, Marmion & Kendall, 1963). The organism has been proved to have caused outbreaks of acute respiratory disease and pneumonia in closed communities such as boarding schools and military barracks. It is probable that surveys at present in progress will show that Eaton's agent is distributed widely and somewhat irregularly in the general population and that it is responsible for a variable proportion of cases of respiratory infections at all ages.

M. hominis is of doubtful pathogenicity; it has been found in the genital tract (particularly in the urethra and the vagina) in about 2 per cent. of healthy blood donors and children, and in 56 per cent. of women and 24 per cent. of men attending venereal disease clinics (Card, 1959). The role of the organism in "non-specific" or non-gonococcal urethritis is uncertain. The mycoplasmas can become established in the vagina when the pH is raised above 4·0; bacterial infections that raise the pH enhance the growth of mycoplasmas. The normal male urethra, because of its high pH, is a good site for growth. The major mode of spread in man is by sexual contact.

M. mycoides has been known for many years as the cause of contagious bovine pleuropneumonia, epizootics of which have been responsible for enormous economic losses in cattle and sheep. The disease still exists in many parts of the world but has been eradicated in Western Europe and North America. The clinical disease takes the form of a chronic interstitial pneumonia with sero-fibrinous pleurisy and oedema of the interlobular septae of the lungs; it may be acute in onset and rapidly fatal but frequently it is subacute or chronic with organisation of the exudate. In many of the latter cases areas of segmented necrosis occur in the lung tissue and subsequently become encapsulated. The organisms may persist in the lesions for many months and such animals form a reservoir of infection which is responsible for the perpetuation of the disease. The disease is spread by droplet infection during close proximity between infected and susceptible animals. Epidemiological control is difficult because about 20 per cent. of infected animals suffer only from inapparent or subclinical forms of the illness and 10 per cent. become chronic carriers; these animals form a reservoir of infection that can be detected only by serological means.

M. agalactiae causes a generalised infection in sheep and goats with lesions localising in the joints, eyes and mammary glands. Infection is by ingestion of foodstuffs contaminated with purulent discharges.

M. gallisepticum is a primary cause of chronic respiratory disease in fowls, turkeys and other birds; a disease of considerable economic importance. Other species of mycoplasma have been found as commensals or as pathogens in pigs, dogs, rats and mice.

Chemotherapy.—Mycoplasmas are insensitive to sulphonamides and penicillin but sensitive to chloramphenicol, tetracycline, neomycin and kanamycin and tylosin tartrate. Species vary in their sensitivity to streptomycin and erythromycin. In general, human infections with these organisms respond to treatment with tetracyclines.

Prophylaxis.—Of the many types of vaccines that have been used against bovine pleuropneumonia the living chick embryo vaccine of

Sheriff and Piercy (1952) is perhaps the most effective, but in some breeds of cattle carries a grave risk of severe reactions and the loss of small numbers of animals.

Relationship to "L-forms" of bacteria.—The lack of a rigid cell wall and the similarity in morphology and colonial characters between mycoplasmas and L-forms of bacteria has suggested to some that it may be possible for transformation to occur and that bacteria may give rise to mycoplasmas or the reverse. The L-forms of bacteria are variants lacking a rigid cell wall and their origin is practically always the result of artificial procedures which are carried out in the laboratory; they have not been found to occur as pathogens in nature. The distinctness of the antigenic characters of the various species of mycoplasmas, their widespread distribution in nature, and their cholesterol requirement would tilt the balance of evidence in favour of the view that they are separate entities devoid of a bacterial origin (Klieneberger-Nobel, 1962).

Primary Atypical Pneumonia

There is now sufficient justification for regarding primary atypical pneumonia (PAP) as a separate entity that differs clinically and aetiologically from the primary and secondary virus pneumonias. The disease is characterised by moderately severe respiratory involvement with bronchitis and pulmonary consolidation. The lung changes are usually unilateral with patchy opacities often seen on radiological examination to extend fan-wise towards the lower lobe. Less severe febrile respiratory manifestations may occur, especially in children. Characteristically the patients develop serum agglutinins for *Streptococcus MG*, and for human erythrocytes tested in the cold. The cause of the condition is Eaton's agent which was for many years thought to be a virus but is now known to be a pleuropneumonia-like organism and is named *M. pneumoniae*. Antibodies to this agent are developed during the infection and can be demonstrated by neutralisation, complement fixation, and immune fluorescence. In one series of patients developing antibodies to *M. pneumoniae*, 47 per cent. also developed cold agglutinins with or without antibodies to *Streptococcus MG* (Mufson *et al.*, 1962). However, 92 per cent. of the sera containing cold agglutinins contain antibodies to *M. pneumoniae*. The nature of these reactions has not yet been elucidated.

Laboratory diagnosis.—This usually depends on the demonstration of rising titres of cold agglutinins and of antibodies for *Streptococcus MG*, combined when possible, with estimations of antibodies to *M. pneumoniae* by complement fixation (Chanock *et al.*, 1962), or immune fluorescent methods (Goodburn & Marmion, 1962).

The causative organism may be isolated by the direct cultivation of sputum or swabs on a selective culture medium. Proof that the suspected colonies are those of mycoplasmas is obtained by showing (*a*) that the colony stains positively with Dienes' stain, (*b*) that its central area is adherent to the agar, (*c*) subcultures from it will not grow in serum free media. The fermentation reactions are then checked but the final identification of the colonies is always made by the fluorescent antibody technique using a known positive serum.

BARTONELLA BACILLIFORMIS

This organism is the cause of two quite distinct clinical conditions: Oroya fever, characterised by intermittent pyrexia, anaemia and high mortality, and Verruga peruana, a benign, nodular skin eruption. The organism under natural conditions grows on or in the erythrocytes of man or in the cytoplasm of his tissue cells. These infections are found only in mountainous districts in South America (Peru, Ecuador and Colombia). The disease is transmitted by the bite of sandflies, *Phlebotomus verrucarum* in Peru and *P. colombianum* in Colombia.

The infective agent is seen in red blood cells as minute rod-shaped forms 0·3–2·5 μ in length; it is extremely pleomorphic and coccal forms are frequently found. The organism is actively motile, with 1–10 flagella attached at one pole of the bacillus. Flagella are not seen in blood films but are regularly present in cultures. The organism is Gram-negative, non-sporing, non-encapsulated and an obligate aerobe. It can be grown on semi-solid agar enriched with 10 per cent. rabbit blood at 28° C. or on a tryptone-serum medium (Gieman, 1941). It can survive many weeks in blood or blood cultures. Inoculated intracutaneously in monkeys, *Bartonella bacilliformis* produces Verruga regularly, but Oroya fever is manifest only occasionally unless the animals have previously been splenectomised. *Haemobartonella muris* is found in wild rodents and in many strains of laboratory rats. A considerable proportion of the animals show no sign of disease and react only mildly if inoculated with the organism. It has been observed that after splenectomy in rats, organisms which closely resemble *Bartonella moniliformis* frequently appear in the red cells; the infection is associated with marked anaemia and often has a fatal result. Presumably latent infection is prevalent in rats associated with a certain degree of natural immunity which is broken down by removal of the spleen. The infection is louse-borne.

Other species of *Haemobartonella* have been described in mice, guinea-pigs, squirrels, bovines and dogs.

It should be noted that these organisms are unusual in that they can be cultivated artificially and show a marked tendency in nature to multiply within the host's cells. *Bartonella* and *Haemobartonella* constitute two genera of the family *Bartonellaceae* and have been brought together with the *Rickettsiaceae* in the order *Rickettsiales*. For a review of the Bartonellaceae see Peters and Wigand (1955).

REFERENCES

Rickettsiae.

Bozeman, F. M., Hopps, W. E., Danauskas, J. X., Jackson, E. B. & Smadel, J. E. (1956). Study on the growth of rickettsiae. *J. Immunol.*, **76**, 475

ENRIGHT, J. B., SADLER, W. W. & THOMAS, R. C. (1957). Pasteurisation of Milk Containing the Organism of Q Fever. *Amer. J. publ. Hlth*, **47**, 695.

FOX, J. P. (1956). Immunisation against epidemic typhus. *Amer. J. trop. Med. Hyg.*, **5**, 464.

GOLDWASSER, R. A. & SHEPARD, C. C. (1959). Fluorescent antibody methods in the differentiation of murine and epidemic typhus sera; specificity changes resulting from previous immunisation. *J. Immunol.*, **82**, 375.

SCHAECHTER, M., BOZEMAN, F. M. & SMADEL, J. E. (1957). Study on the growth of rickettsiae. *Virology*, **3**, 160.

SHEPARD, C. C. & GOLDWASSER, R. A. (1960). Fluorescent antibody staining as a means of detecting Rocky Mountain spotted fever infection in individual ticks. *Amer. J. Hyg.*, **72**, 120.

STOKER, M. G. P. & MARMION, B. P. (1955). The spread of Q fever from animals to man: the natural history of a rickettsial disease. *Bull. Wld. Hlth Org.*, **13**, 781.

STOKER, M. G. P., PAGE, Z. & MARMION, B. P. (1955). Problems in the diagnosis of Q fever by complement fixation tests. *Bull. Wld. Hlth Org.*, **13**, 807.

Pleuropneumonia organisms.

ADLER, H. E. & SHIFRINE, M. (1960). Nutrition, metabolism, and pathogenicity of mycoplasmas. *Ann. Rev. Microbiol.*, **14**, 141.

CARD, D. W. (1959). PPLO of human genital origin. Serological classification of strains and antibody distribution in man. *Brit. J. vener. Dis.*, **35**, 27.

CHANOCK, R. M., HAYFLICK, L. & BARILE, M. F. (1962). Growth on artificial medium of an agent associated with atypical pneumonia and its identification as a PPLO *Proc. nat. Acad. Sci. (Wash.)*, **48**, 41.

CHANOCK, R. M., MUFSON, M. A., BLOOM, H. H., JAMES, W. D., FOX, H. H. & KINGSTON, J. R. (1961). Eaton agent pneumonia. *J. Amer. med. Ass.*, **175**, 213.

CHANOCK, R. M., JAMES, W. D., FOX, H. H., TURNER, M. A., MUFSON, M. A. & HAYFLICK, L. (1962). Growth of Eaton PPLO in broth and preparation of complement-fixing antigen. *Proc. Soc. exp. Biol. (N.Y.)*, **110**, 884.

EATON, M. D., FARNHAM, E., LEVINTHAL, J. D. & SCALA, A. R. (1962). Cytopathic effect of atypical pneumonia organism in cultures of human tissue. *J. Bact.*, **84**, 1330.

EDWARD, D. G. FF. (1947). A selective medium for pleuropneumonia-like organisms. *J. gen. Microbiol.*, **1**, 238.

EDWARD, D. G. FF. (1954). The pleuropneumonia group of organisms; a review, together with some new observations. *J. gen. Microbiol.*, **10**, 27.

GOODBURN, G. M. & MARMION, B. P. (1962). A study of the properties of Eaton's primary atypical pneumonia organism. *J. gen. Microbiol.*, **29**, 271.

GOODBURN, G. M., MARMION, B. P. & KENDALL, E. J. C. (1963). Infection with Eaton's primary atypical pneumonia agent in England. *Brit. med. J.*, **i**, 1266.

KLIENEBERGER-NOBEL, E. (1962). *Pleuropneumonia-like Organisms (PPLO). Mycoplasmataceae*. London: Academic Press.

LEACH, R. H. (1962). The osmotic requirements for growth of Mycoplasma. *J. gen. Microbiol.*, **27**, 345.

MARMION, B. P. & HERS, J. F. Ph. (1963). Observations on Eaton primary atypical pneumonia agent and analogous problems in animals (1962). Proceedings Conference on Newer Respiratory Viruses. *Amer. Rev. resp. Dis.*, **88**, 198.

MUFSON, M. A., BLOOM, H. H., MANKO, M. A., KINGSTON, J. R. & CHANOCK, R. H. (1962). *Eaton agent: a review*. *Amer. J. publ. Hlth*, **52**, 925.

RODWELL, A. W. (1963). The steroid growth-requirement of Mycoplasma mycoides. *J, gen. Microbiol.*, **32**, 91.

SHERIFF, D. & PIERCY, S. E. (1952). Experiments with an avianised strain of the organism of contagious bovine pleuropneumonia. *Vet. Rec.*, **64**, 615.

TURNER, A. W. (1959). Pleuro-pneumonia group of diseases. Chapter 14 in vol. 2, *Infectious Diseases of Animals. Diseases due to Bacteria*. Ed. Stableforth, A. W. & Galloway, I. A. London: Butterworths.

Bartonella.

GIEMAN, Q. M. (1941). New Media for the growth of *Bartonella bacilliformis*. *Proc. Soc. exp. Biol. (N.Y.)*, **47**, 329.

PETERS, D. & WIGAND, R. (1955). Bartonellaceae. *Bact. Rev.*, **19**, 150.

CHAPTER 40

PATHOGENIC FUNGI

INFECTIONS produced by the true fungi, or *Eumycetes* (p. 7), are usually designated "mycoses". These infections are of less importance in medicine than bacterial and viral infections. Some fungal infections are very common, e.g. ringworm infections of skin, hair and nails, and candida infections of the skin and mucous membranes, but these infections are superficial and rarely a danger to life. Deep and systemic fungal infections, which may often be fatal, are relatively uncommon in Britain. The pathogenic fungi are insusceptible to the antibiotics that are used successfully in the treatment of bacterial infections and there is a lack of useful and effective antifungal drugs that can be administered systemically. Because of their drug-resistance, the fungal infections, particularly infections with *Candida albicans*, have become more prominent since the advent of the antibiotics. Thus, effective treatment of a bacterial infection with antibiotics may lead to an intractable secondary infection with fungi.

The *Eumycetes* can be divided into four morphological groups, each of which includes some pathogenic varieties. (1) The *moulds* (filamentous or mycelial fungi) grow as long filaments (hyphae) which branch and interlace to form a meshwork (mycelium), and reproduce by the formation of various kinds of spores. The major part of the mycelium, the *vegetative mycelium*, grows on and penetrates into the substrate, absorbing nutrients for growth; sometimes it forms asexual thallospores. Other hyphae constitute the *aerial mycelium* and protrude from the vegetative mycelium into the air; they form and disseminate into the air various kinds of spores. When grown to a large size on artificial medium, the mycelium is seen as a filamentous mould colony; this may become powdery on its surface due to the abundant formation of spores. The filamentous fungi usually are only locally invasive in the body and spread to fresh hosts by their spores, *e.g.* the ringworm fungi.

(2) The *yeasts* are unicellular fungi which occur mainly as single spherical or ellipsoidal cells and reproduce by budding. On artificial media they form compact colonies with a creamy, mucoid or pasty consistence (*e.g.* like those of staphylococcus). They grow diffusely through fluid media and may spread readily through the animal body, e.g. *Cryptococcus neoformans*.

(3) The *yeast-like fungi* grow partly as yeasts and partly as long filamentous cells joined end to end, forming a "pseudomycelium", e.g. *Candida albicans*.

(4) The *dimorphic fungi* grow either as filaments or as yeasts, according to the cultural conditions. Growth usually takes place in the mycelial form (the saprophytic phase) on culture media at 22° C. and in the soil, but in the yeast form (the parasitic phase) on media at 37° C. and in the animal body; e.g. *Blastomyces dermatitidis*.

Fungi are aerobic and all cultures are incubated aerobically. Culture tubes and bottles are best stoppered with cotton-wool, and if screw-capped bottles are used, the caps should be left loose.

Systematic Classification

The systematic classification of the fungi is made on different lines from the simple morphological classification given above. Four classes are distinguished, mainly according to the nature of their sexual spores. (1) The *Phycomycetes* form non-septate hyphae, asexual "sporangiospores" contained within a swollen spore case, or "sporangium", borne at the ends of aerial hyphae, and sexual spores of the "oospore" or "zygospore" varieties. (2) The *Ascomycetes* form septate hyphae, various kinds of asexual spores including "conidia" which are abstricted successively from the ends of specialised (often aerial) hyphae called "conidiophores", and sexual "ascospores" formed, usually eight together, within a sac or "ascus". (3) The *Basidiomycetes* form septate hyphae and sexual "basidiospores", usually four in number, from the ends of club-shaped structures called "basidia". (4) The *Fungi imperfecti* include the fungi that do not have a sexual stage and thus cannot be placed with certainty in one of the other three classes. Many imperfect fungi form septate hyphae and asexual conidia resembling those of *Ascomycetes*, and their closest affinities lie with this class. A majority of the pathogenic moulds, yeasts, yeast-like fungi and dimorphic fungi belong to the group *Fungi imperfecti*.

Common Saprophytic Moulds

Many species of non-pathogenic moulds occur in the soil and on decomposing organic matter. Aerial dissemination of their spores is widespread and they are commonly found contaminating exposed bacteriological culture media, human foodstuffs and specimens taken from the surfaces of the body. They also occur as secondary invaders, *e.g.* in the external ear or lung. *Their presence in diagnostic cultures must not be taken as denoting an aetiological relationship.* Varieties commonly encountered include *Rhizopus*, *Mucor* (e.g. *M. mucedo*), *Aspergillus* (e.g. *A. niger*) and *Penicillium* (e.g. *P. expansum*). *Rhizopus* and *Mucor* are phycomycetes with non-septate hyphae, asexual sporangiospores, and sexual zygospores which are formed by conjugation of two hyphae at their tips. *Aspergillus* and *Penicillium* species are either ascomycetes or fungi imperfecti, having septate hyphae, asexual conidia and in some cases sexual ascospores. Their colonies are commonly pigmented yellow, green or black. The conidial chains of *Aspergillus* arise from finger-like "sterigmata" which radiate without branching from the expanded bulbous tip of the conidiophore. Those of *Penicillium* arise brush-like from sterigmata borne on the tips of several terminal branches of the conidiophore (Fig. 26). The important antibiotic substance, penicillin, is derived from *Penicillium notatum* and *P. chrysogenum*.

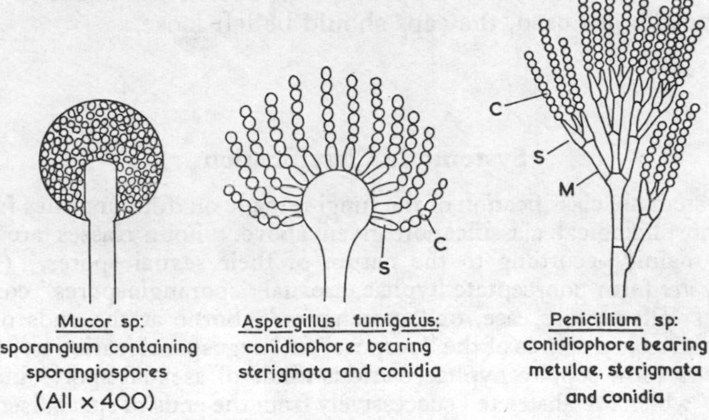

Fig. 26

THE DERMATOPHYTES OR RINGWORM FUNGI

Tinea, or ringworm, is caused by three related genera of filamentous *Fungi imperfecti*, namely *Microsporum*, *Trichophyton* and *Epidermophyton*. These are dermatophytic fungi, having the unusual ability of digesting and utilising keratin, and being specialised for parasitising the keratinous structures of the body, *i.e.* the horny outer layer of the skin, the hairs and the nails. They do not invade the underlying living tissues that form the keratin, or the deeper tissues and organs of the body. The skin lesions are varied and may include inflammation, scaling, hyperkeratosis, vesiculation, pustulation, maceration or ulceration; secondary suppurative infection with pyogenic bacteria may ensue. In ringworm of the body, the spreading edge of the lesion is commonly seen as a red inflammatory ring (*e.g.* 5-50 mm. diam.) studded with vesicles and pustules, whilst the recovering central region is scaly and less reddened. Infected hairs become weakened and readily broken off, so that bald patches are produced; in some cases they show a characteristic green fluorescence under ultra-violet irradiation. Infected nails become deformed, discoloured, brittle and broken.

In their host the fungi occur in only two forms: (1) as a *vegetative mycelium* which grows through the keratinous structures, and (2) as chains of *arthrospores* formed by the septation of hyphae into short cylindrical or rounded segments which become widened and thick-walled. The arthrospores are capable of infecting intact skin on which they are deposited, but they more readily infect skin subjected to minor injury by rubbing, scratching or prolonged moistening. They germinate and give rise to hyphae which spread as a mycelium through the whole depth of the horny layer and extend radially into adjoining areas of skin. The mechanism whereby this superficial fungal growth causes inflammation of the skin is uncertain; the liberation of toxic products from the digested keratin or an allergic response to fungal antigens may be responsible. In hair-infecting species, the hyphae grow down the walls of the hair follicles that they encounter as they spread through the skin; they pass over into the shaft of the hair and grow in the newly keratinised zone just above the root bulb. After two to three weeks' growth has carried the first infected part of the hair above the skin surface, this part has become so weakened that it breaks off leaving a short (2 mm.) stump. (This happens in most types of infection, but in infections with *Trichophyton violaceum* and *T. sulphureum* (*T. tonsurans*) the hairs break off at the mouth of the follicle, to give a "black dot" appearance.)

Hyphae in skin, nail or hair eventually give rise to arthrospores. In hair, the arthrospore formation may be "endothrix", *i.e.* from hyphae within the hair shaft, or "ectothrix", *i.e.* from hyphae that have grown out over the surface of the hair. In the latter case, the affected part of the hair comes to bear a thick white coat of spores several layers deep. Some species form small arthrospores, of 2-3 μ diameter, and others form large spores of 4-6 μ (Fig. 27).

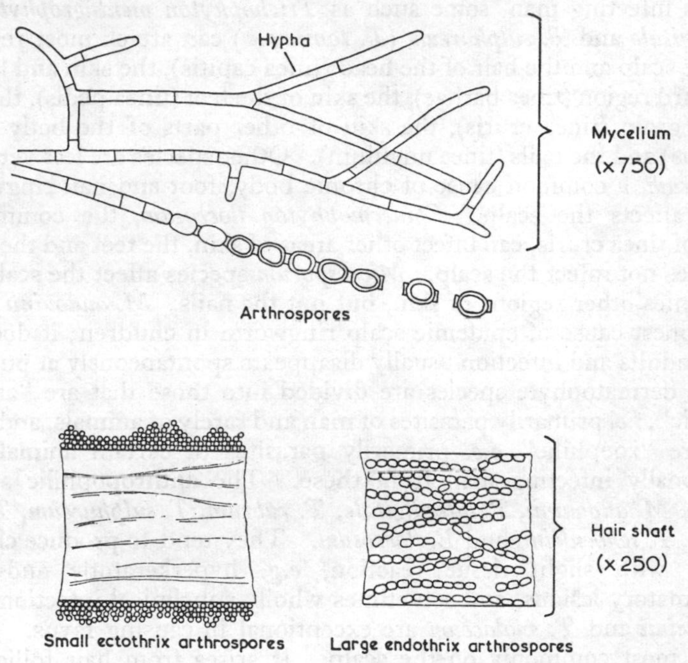

FIG. 27

Forms of ringworm fungi seen *in vivo* in skin, nail or hair.

Immunological and Hypersensitive Reactions.—The blood of patients with superficial dermatomycoses cannot be shown to contain agglutinins, precipitins or complement-fixing antibodies. Nevertheless, patient's serum and normal human serum may contain fungistatic substances. Moreover, some kind of immunity mechanism appears to be operative in producing the eventual spontaneous healing of the affected parts. Many patients, especially those with trichophyton infections, develop a widespread cutaneous hypersensitiveness to the antigenic products of the fungus. In the course of the infection, secondary generalised skin eruptions of an allergic nature may occur, *i.e.* "dermatophytids" or "trichophytids", which are apparently due to blood-borne spread of fungal fragments or antigens. The commonest manifestation is a series of vesicles (pomphlox) on the fingers and hands, though other parts of the skin are sometimes also affected. No fungus is found in these allergic lesions. Evidence of hypersensitiveness may be elicited by injecting extracts of the organism, *e.g.* trichophyton; this usually evokes an inflammatory reaction after 24-48 hr., like the tuberculin reaction. The reactions are not species specific.

Species; Sources and Modes of Infection

The various dermatophyte species differ in their adaptation to different regions of the body and to different animal hosts. Among species infecting man, some such as *Trichophyton mentagrophytes*, *T. interdigitale* and *T. sulphureum* (*T. tonsurans*) can attack most regions: *e.g.* the scalp and the hair of the head (tinea capitis), the skin and hair of the beard region (tinea barbae), the skin of the feet (tinea pedis), the skin of the groin (tinea cruris), the skin of other parts of the body (tinea corporis) and the nails (tinea unguium). Other species are less versatile. *T. rubrum*, a common cause of chronic body, foot and nail ringworm. rarely affects the scalp. *Epidermophyton floccosum*, the commonest cause of tinea cruris, can infect other areas of skin, the feet and the nails, but does not infect the scalp. *Microsporum* species affect the scalp and sometimes other regions of skin, but not the nails. *M. audouinii* is the commonest cause of epidemic scalp ringworm in children; it does not attack adults and infection usually disappears spontaneously at puberty.

The dermatophyte species are divided into those that are "anthropophilic", *i.e.* primarily parasites of man and rarely of animals, and those that are "zoophilic", *i.e.* primarily parasites of certain animals and occasionally infecting man from these. The anthropophilic species include *M. audouinii*, *T. interdigitale*, *T. rubrum*, *T. sulphureum*, *T. violaceum*, *T. schoenleinii* and *E. floccosum*. They tend to produce chronic lesions with slight tissue reaction, *e.g.* hyperkeratotic and non-inflammatory lesions, and sometimes wholly subclinical infections. *T. schoenleinii* and *T. violaceum* are exceptional in causing favus. Favus occurs most commonly on the scalp. It arises from hair follicles as minute yellow-red papules; these grow to form cup-shaped yellow "scutula", or crusts of mycelium, and ultimately destroy the involved hairs. The zoophilic species include *M. canis* (cat and dog), *M. gypseum* (horse and soil), *T. mentagrophytes* (cat, dog, mouse, ox, horse, soil). *T. verrucosum* (ox and horse), *T. quinckeanum* (mouse favus) and *M. equinum* and *T. equinum* (horse). When these fungi infect man (as do the first four), they tend to cause an acute inflammatory lesion (kerion) with vesiculation and perhaps suppuration, easy to cure and often healing spontaneously.

Ringworm due to an anthropophilic species is contracted by man from another infected man, as in the epidemic spread of tinea capitis due to *M. audouinii* and tinea pedis ("athlete's foot") due to *T. interdigitale* or *T. rubrum*. Infections by zoophilic species are contracted from infected pets, farm animals or vermin, and rarely from infected humans. It is thus important to identify the species causing an infection if an indication is required as to whether the source should be sought among human or animal contacts. Infected cats and dogs should be destroyed if it is considered necessary to eliminate them as a source of infection in a household, since they cannot be effectively treated.

The fungus is spread by contact and through the air in the form of arthrospores. These spores are shed from the affected parts, often in scales of skin, in fragments of hair or nail, and in finer debris. They are highly resistant to environmental conditions and may remain alive for years in infected premises and survive on clothing through many successive launderings. They can be killed by brief boiling. Formalin may be used for disinfecting shoes, socks and other articles. The relative importance of the different mechanisms and vehicles of spread is unknown.

M. gypseum has been found in soil and it is believed that it is capable of growing saprophytically in soil as well as of growing parasitically in the human or animal body. If this belief is correct, the soil may occasionally act as a source of infections for man and animals.

Ringworm in Animals

Ringworm in dogs and cats is usually caused by *M. canis*, but other fungi, e.g. *M. gypseum*, *M. audouinii*, *T. mentagrophytes* and *T. quinckeanum*, are sometimes responsible. Although cats frequently fail to show clinical symptoms, bare patches with broken hairs may be seen on the head, face and paws. In dogs the lesions are more obvious, circular bare areas appearing on any part of the body. Ringworm in cattle is especially prevalent in young animals, the commonest pathogen being *T. verrucosum*. The lesions vary from small circumscribed hairless areas to extensive white or yellowish-brown crusts on the head, neck or other parts of the body. Ringworm in the horse may be caused by species of *Microsporum* and *Trichophyton*, the commonest being *M. equinum*, *M. gypseum*, *T. mentagrophytes* and *T. equinum*. Typical lesions are circumscribed bare patches or plaques covered by a soft crust which is easily removed. Ringworm in sheep and goats is rare, but pigs are susceptible to infection with *T. mentagrophytes*. In favus of poultry, the lesions are mostly confined to the comb and wattles as dirty white crusts of fungus tissue. In more generalised infections the base of the feathers and the skin may be involved. The causal fungus *T. gallinae* (*Achorion gallinae*) is transmissible to man.

Laboratory Diagnosis of Ringworm

The presence of fungus is demonstrated by direct microscopic examination of a specimen of the infected skin, hair or nail. Identification of the genus and species requires isolation of the organism in artificial culture.

Collection of Specimens.—The specimen must be taken with care.

A preliminary cleansing of the lesion with 70 per cent. alcohol reduces bacterial contamination. Scales of skin (*e.g.* 2-3 mm. diameter) are scraped with a blunt scalpel from the active periphery of the inflamed area, avoiding white macerated material in flexures. The domes of vesicles are snipped off for examination. The scales may be stored in small packages or envelopes made of clean folded paper, and bacterial contaminants are partly eliminated after a few weeks of such storage; fungus spores remain viable. In the case of infected nails, the affected parts are clipped off for examination and scrapings are also taken from the deeper parts with a blunt scalpel.

Infected hairs must be chosen carefully. It is useless to take *healthy* hairs from the infected regions of skin. The stumps of broken hairs should be plucked with fine forceps, or else lustreless hairs may be taken. Intrafollicular fragments of hairs broken at the follicle mouths may be extracted with a cutting needle. If the infecting fungus is *M. audouinii*, *M. canis* or *T. schoenleinii*, the infected hairs may be recognised by their fluorescence under ultra-violet irradiation. The head is viewed in a darkened room under filtered ultra-violet radiation from a Wood's lamp. (A suitable lamp is a 125 watts ultra-violet black glass lamp, Type MBW/V, General Electric Co., with a choke for A.C. 230 volts, Type Z 1832H, and a 10 mfd condenser Type Z 1850. By filtration through sodium-barium-silicate glass containing nickel oxide it yields only rays outside the visible spectrum with fungi not causing fluorescence.) Specimens for dispatch to the laboratory are best sent in packages of clean folded paper.

Microscopic Examination of Skin, Nail and Hair.—The specimen must be "cleared", *i.e.* rendered transparent, to allow observation of the fungi within it. This is done by hydrolysing and partly dissolving the keratin with alkali. The fragments of skin, hair or nail are placed in a drop of 10–30 per cent. potassium or sodium hydroxide solution on a glass slide, and a coverslip is applied. The preparation is left for a while at room temperature, or is warmed very gently to hasten digestion. Thin scales of skin may be cleared within several minutes at room temperature, whilst a piece of nail may require up to three hours at 37° C., the solution being replenished as necessary. Thick pieces of nail may be incubated with the alkali in a small tube. Excessive digestion must be avoided. When ready, the coverslip is squeezed down gently under blotting-paper to give a thin film without disruption of the specimen. The specimen is then examined microscopically in the unstained condition using a 4 mm. objective. It is convenient first to examine the specimen widely with a low power (16 mm.) objective and then to search suspicious areas with the high power (4 mm.) one. Mycelium, chains of arthrospores and free arthrospores may be seen and their recognition permits a diagnosis of fungus infection. Artefacts may be mistaken for fungal elements by inexperienced observers; *e.g.* oil or fat droplets, air bubbles and spaces between epithelial cells. Thus, cholesterol crystals having the appearance of chains of spores, so-called "mosaic fungus", are often seen between the epithelial cells of skin specimens. These artefacts can be recognised by their failure to stain with lactophenol blue.

Staining is usually unnecessary in routine diagnostic work, but it should be carried out if there is doubt as to the nature of any fungus-like elements in the specimen. The alkali is replaced by lactophenol blue stain; a drop of stain is placed at one edge of the coverslip and the alkali is withdrawn at the other side by application of blotting-paper, the process being continued until the lactophenol blue has entirely replaced the colourless alkali. The slide is warmed gently and excess stain is removed by pressing lightly under blotting-paper.

With specimens of hair, the size and arrangement of the arthrospores affords some indication of the variety of fungus. Thus, *Microsporum* species and *T. mentagrophytes* give small-spored ectothrix infections, *T. verrucosum* large-spored ectothrix infections, and *T. sulphureum* and *T. violaceum* large-spored endothrix infections. In favus due to *T. schoenleinii* the infection is endothrix and it is further distinguished by the presence of air bubbles in the hair.

Culture.—In artificial culture the dermatophyte fungi produce a variety of spore-forms additional to the arthrospores found *in vivo*. These include small unicellular "microconidia" and large multicellular "macroconidia" (Fig. 28). The genera are distinguished according to the morphology of their macroconidia, and the species according to other microscopic features and the naked-eye morphology of their colonies.

Primary culture. Skin, hair and nail specimens are likely to bear contaminating bacteria; these may be reduced by storage in paper envelopes for one or more weeks, or by immersion in 70 per cent. ethyl alcohol for 2–3 min. Since the dermatophytes are aerobic, surface cultures are grown on agar slopes in tubes or vials stoppered with cotton-wool. Fungal growth is favoured by a high sugar concentration and is relatively tolerant of acidity. Sugar-containing media of low pH are therefore selective for fungi and restrain the growth of most bacterial contaminants. Sabouraud's glucose peptone agar at pH 5·4 or malt extract agar at pH 5·4 are recommended. The malt agar may be made more selective for fungi by addition of 0·036 per cent. potassium tellurite, and Sabouraud's medium may be supplemented with 10 mg. thiamine per l. to promote spore formation in *T. verrucosum*, *T. violaceum* and *T. schoenleinii*.

The fragments of skin, hair or nail are planted with a firm straight-pointed wire. Nickel-chrome wire SWG 18 is suitable for this and other manipulations of fungi. After sterilisation by flaming, the wire must be given sufficient time to cool, or be cooled by pressing into the sterile medium, before being used to transfer fungal material. At intervals of about 1 cm., three or four fragments are pressed into the surface of the agar so as to be partly submerged. The cultures should be incubated at 28° C. and they can usually be identified within 2 weeks, but none should be discarded as negative until it has been incubated for at least 3 weeks. Incubation at room temperature (20° C.) is adequate, but less satisfactory than incubation at 28° C. The cultures should be examined every three or four days for the appearance of growth around the edges of the implanted specimen. The fungal colony spreads outwards over the medium and usually extends beyond any contaminating bacterial growth. Material should be taken from near the edge of the colony and transplanted to a fresh slope in order to obtain a pure culture; a single speck of material is planted in the middle of the slope to yield a giant colony suitable for observation of naked-eye morphology. Material from the primary culture may also be subcultivated by Riddell's slide culture method to facilitate observation of its microscopic morphology.

Naked-eye examination of morphology of colonies.—The texture and colour of the colony are observed on both its upper and lower sides, and note should be taken of any diffusible pigment entering the medium. Most species form large, spreading filamentous colonies and the rhizoid hyphal outgrowth may give the appearance of radial striation (*e.g.* in *M. canis*). The filamentous structure of the vegetative mycelium is usually soon obscured by a velvety, cottony or powdery covering of aerial mycelium and spores. *T. verrucosum*, *T. violaceum* and *T. schoenleinii* are exceptionally slow growing and form compact bacteria-like colonies which are at first smooth and waxy, and later become corrugated and covered with a sparse velvety growth of aerial mycelium. In most species the colonies ultimately develop some degree of pigmentation, commonly cream-pink, buff or yellow-green, though non-pigmented variant strains may be encountered. *T. rubrum* is distinguished by its formation of a red pigment (brown to rose-purple) which colours the underside of the colony and sometimes the aerial mycelium, and rarely diffuses into the medium. *T. violaceum* forms a deep violet pigment mainly confined to the colony. The colony of *T. sulphureum* changes from white to sulphur yellow as the spores are formed, and its centre eventually becomes folded and crateriform. White variants of this species have been termed *T. tonsurans*. The colony of *T. mentagrophytes* becomes covered with buff-coloured spores and forms a brown-red pigment which diffuses for a short distance into the agar. *Microsporum* colonies become covered with buff-coloured spores, whilst the underlying medium is tinted yellow-orange by *M. canis* and salmon-pink by *M. audouinii*. The colony of *E. floccosum* is green-brown and radially furrowed.

Microscopical Examination of Culture.—A "needle-mount" is made as soon as spore formation is sufficiently advanced at the centre of the colony. Some sporing mycelium is removed on the point of an inoculating wire and transferred into a drop of lactophenol blue stain on a microscope slide. There it is teased out using two wires or dissecting needles. A coverslip is applied and excess stain removed after some minutes by pressing down gently under blotting-paper. The needle-mount is then examined microscopically, first with the low-power objective and then with the 4 mm. dry objective.

An alternative method of preparing a needle-mount avoids the trapping of bubbles of air in the specimen. The fragment of colonial material is transferred to, and teased out in a drop of 95 per cent. ethyl alcohol on a slide and, just before the alcohol has evaporated completely, a drop of lactophenol blue is added and a coverslip applied.

A search is first made for the presence of *macroconidia*. These are large, elongated bodies which are formed at the tips of certain hyphae and, when mature, are divided by visible transverse septa into several (*e.g.* 2–10) segments or cells. Those of *Microsporum* are largest, 40–150$\mu \times$ 8–15μ, and fusiform with pointed ends. Those of *Trichophyton* are smallest, 10–50$\mu \times$ 4–6μ, and generally cylindrical, though sometimes curved, with a rounded free end. Those of *Epidermophyton* are 30–40$\mu \times$ 10μ, and pear-shaped with the narrow end attached to the conidiophore (Fig. 28). Unfortunately, macroconidia are rare or absent in Sabouraud agar cultures of certain species, e.g. *M. audouinii* and most *Trichophyton* species.

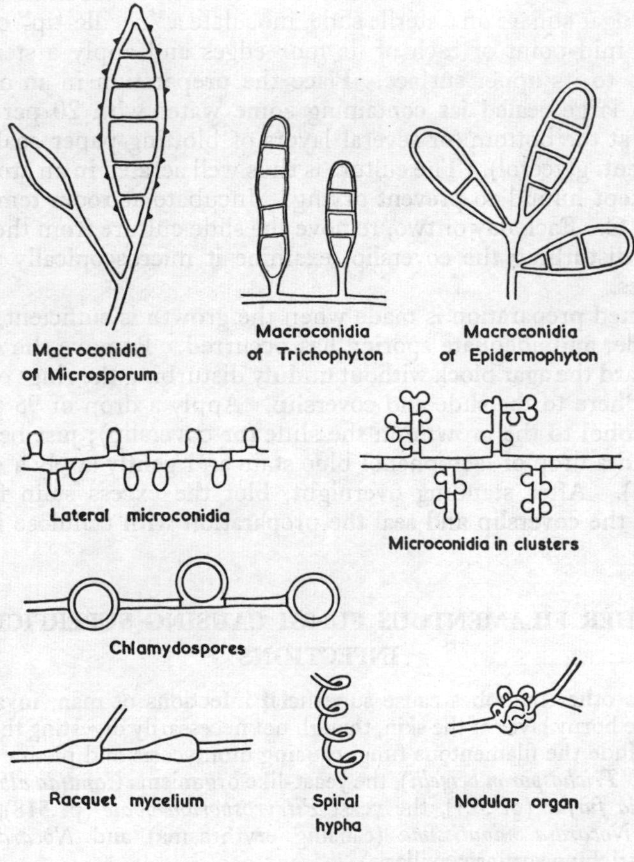

FIG. 28

Types of spores and abnormal mycelial forms found in artificial cultures of ringworm fungi. (×600.)

The smaller *microconidia* are usually numerous, though they are rare or absent in *T. verrucosum*, *T. violaceum*, *T. schoenleinii* and *E. floccosum*. Microconidia are single cells of 2–6μ diam., spherical, pear-shaped or elongated, and borne singly from the sides of the hyphae or in grape-like clusters on short stalks. Several species usually show a number of *chlamydospores* (e.g. *T. sulphureum*, *T. verrucosum*, *T. violaceum*, *T. schoenleinii* and *E. floccosum*); these are large, roughly spherical cells with very thick walls and are borne singly in the length of the vegetative hypha, bulging to one side, or at its end.

Slide Culture by Riddell's Method.—The fungus may be subcultivated on an agar block held between a slide and coverslip. This enables the arrangement of mycelium and spores to be observed undisturbed at various stages during the course of growth. Fill a Petri dish to the depth of about 2 mm. with Sabouraud's medium (10 ml. agar per 9 cm. dish). When set, cut the agar into square blocks, 1 cm. × 1 cm., with a sterile blade. The dishful of blocks may be stored at 4° C. until required. Place an agar square on a sterile slide, inoculate a "needle-tip" of culture into the mid-point of each of its four edges and apply a sterile $\frac{7}{8}$ in. coverslip to its upper surface. Place the preparation in an open rack within a large sealed jar containing some water with 20 per cent. of glycerol at the bottom (or several layers of blotting-paper soaked with 20 per cent. glycerol). The culture is thus well aerated in an atmosphere that is kept humid to prevent drying. Incubate at room temperature or at 28° C. Each day or two, remove the slide culture from the jar and, without disturbing the coverslip, examine it microscopically with dry objectives.

A stained preparation is made when the growth is sufficient, *e.g.* 1–3 mm. wide, and adequate sporing has occurred. Remove the coverslip and discard the agar block without unduly disturbing the rings of growth which adhere to the slide and coverslip. Apply a drop of 95 per cent. ethyl alcohol to the growth on the slide (or coverslip); just before this dries, add a drop of lactophenol blue stain and gently apply a coverslip (or slide). After standing overnight, blot the excess stain from the edges of the coverslip and seal the preparation with cellulose lacquer.

OTHER FILAMENTOUS FUNGI CAUSING SUPERFICIAL INFECTIONS

Various other microbes cause superficial infections of man, invading the hair or the horny layer of the skin, though not necessarily digesting the keratin. They include the filamentous fungi causing otomycosis and piedra (*Piedraia hortai* and *Trichosporon beigelii*), the yeast-like organisms *Candida albicans* and *Malassezia furfur* (p. 524), the yeast *Pitryrosporum ovale* (p. 518), and the bacteria *Nocardia minutissima* (causing erythrasma) and *Nocardia tenuis* (causing trichinocardiosis axillaris).

Aspergillus Species Causing Otomycosis

Fungal otomycosis is a subacute or chronic infection of the skin of the external auditory meatus and is commonly associated with bacterial infection. *Aspergillus niger* and *A. flavus* are the fungi most frequently present, but species of *Penicillium*, *Mucor* and *Rhizopus* occur in some cases. For diagnosis, the mycelium or conidiophore heads must be demonstrated in films of exudate mounted in 10–20 per cent. sodium hydroxide. The species may be identified by culture on Sabouraud's medium.

FILAMENTOUS FUNGI CAUSING DEEP INFECTIONS

Broncho-pulmonary infections

Various normally saprophytic species of *Aspergillus*, *Penicillium*, *Mucor* and *Rhizopus* are found in infections of the bronchi and lungs in man and animals. *Aspergillus fumigatus* is the most important of these. Birds, *e.g.* penguins, are especially susceptible to a primary and frequently fatal pulmonary aspergillosis. The infection may be acute, as in the commonly fatal Brooder pneumonia of chicks, or chronic, with the formation of yellow caseous nodules in the lungs.

In man, the fungal infection appears usually to supervene on a pre-existing pulmonary disease such as bronchiectasis, tuberculosis or pneumonia. It occurs most frequently in agricultural workers and other persons who commonly inhale dusts of organic materials heavily contaminated with fungus spores. The fungus may grow in the damaged bronchus or lung tissue so that it forms a compact mass of mycelium called a mycetoma. In some cases broncho-pulmonary infection with *A. fumigatus* causes an asthmatic disease with plugging of bronchi by exudate containing mucus, fibrin and eosinophils. Rarely, *A. fumigatus* produces a severe pulmonary infection that is apparently primary.

Laboratory diagnosis.—Diagnosis depends on microscopical and cultural demonstration of the presence of abundant fungal elements in repeated specimens of sputum. The fungi are common contaminants in the home, hospital and laboratory, so that the occasional finding of a few fungal elements in sputum is of no diagnostic value. Since contaminating spores may germinate and the fungi overgrow other organisms, the examination of postal specimens or specimens stored at room temperature is usually worthless. Storage, if unavoidable, should be at *c.* 4° C.

The sputum should be examined microscopically not only in Gram-stained smears but also in unstained wet films. If no fungi are seen in these the sputum should be liquefied either by heating at 100° C. for 5 min. after the addition of two volumes of 4 per cent. sodium hydroxide or by digestion with pancreatin; it should then be centrifuged and a wet film of the deposit should be examined.

Cultures of sputum should be made on two plates of Sabouraud's glucose agar and two plates of blood agar containing 30 units of penicillin and 30 μg of streptomycin per ml. One plate of each kind should be incubated at 37° C., the other at room temperature or 28° C. Tubes of Sabouraud's broth should also be inoculated if material on dry swabs has to be examined; after 3 or 4 days the broth cultures are subcultured on plates.

A. fumigatus generally forms smoky-green colonies, but cultures from sputum or resected mycetoma sometimes yield white, very poorly sporing colonies. For detailed information enabling the identification of *A. fumigatus* and other *Aspergillus* species the reader should consult Thom and Raper (1945).

Precipitating antibodies to an antigenic extract of *A. fumigatus* may be demonstrated in the serum of patients by an agar-gel double diffusion test. A positive result confirms the significance of the finding of the fungus in the patient's sputum.

Farmer's lung. This disease is the result of a hypersensitivity reaction in the lungs to antigens in dust from mouldy hay. It occurs in persons who are exposed to inhalation of such dust and who, on repeated exposure, develop increasing hypersensitivity. Ultimately a very limited exposure may cause severe pulmonary symptoms.

The hay that is liable to cause farmer's lung is hay that has become heated spontaneously to at least 50° C. during maturation and contains more thermophilic moulds and actinomycetes, and their spores, than good hay. Pepys *et al.* (1963) have shown that pure cultures of the thermophilic actinomycetes *Thermopolyspora polyspora* and *Micromonospora vulgaris* grown in sterilised hay produce antigens that react in agar-gel diffusion tests and immunoelectrophoresis tests with the majority (90 per cent.) of sera from patients with farmer's lung. Cultures of other actinomycetes, of fungi such as *A. fumigatus* and *Mucor pusillus*, and of bacteria found in hay did not produce these farmer's lung hay antigens. When patients with a history of farmer's lung inhaled an aerosol containing an extract of *T. polyspora* culture they developed within 5–7 hr. systemic and pulmonary symptoms resembling those of attacks of farmer's lung.

It has been proposed that farmer's lung may be diagnosed by agar-gel precipitation tests made with the patient's serum and an antigenic extract of *T. polyspora*, but a minority of false-positive and false-negative results may be given by these tests.

Maduromycosis

Mycetoma or Madura foot in man can be produced not only by actinomycetes such as *Nocardia madurae*, *Noc. pelletieri* and *Streptomyces somaliensis*, but also by a variety of fungi including *Madurella mycetomi*, *M. grisei*, *Allescheria boydii* (*Monosporium apiospermum*), *Phialophora jeanselmei* and *Cephalosporium falciforme*. These fungi are thought to occur as saprophytes in the soil and on vegetable matter, and to enter the tissues of the foot through thorn pricks and other minor injuries. For diagnosis, some pus is obtained from a sinus or aspirated from an unopened abscess. It is spread thinly in a sterile Petri dish and searched for the presence of granules about 0·5–2·0 mm. in diameter. Granules are mounted on a slide in a drop of 10 per cent. sodium hydroxide, gently crushed under a coverslip and examined without staining. In addition, granules are crushed between two slides and the slide preparations fixed by flaming and stained, one by Gram's method and the other by the modified Ziehl-Neelsen method, as in the diagnosis of actinomycosis. The fungal granules consist of a mass of hyphae 2–5 μ wide and thus are readily distinguishable from the 1 μ hyphae of actinomycetes. Chlamydospores may be present and the peripheral hyphae may bear "clubs" similar to those in actinomycotic granules. Cultures are grown on Sabouraud's glucose agar for at least three weeks at room temperature or at 22° C.; granules washed in sterile saline are inoculated on a number of slopes. *Monosporium apiospermum* grows rapidly as a white cottony colony in which ovoid conidia, about 6×9 μ, are borne singly at the ends of conidiophores. *Madurella* colonies grow slowly and are dark grey or black in colour.

Chromoblastomycosis in man is a chronic verrucous and granulomatous infection of the skin and subcutaneous tissue which extends slowly along the lymphatics. It occurs in North and South America, Russia, South Africa and Japan, and is caused by the filamentous fungi *Hormodendrum pedrosoi*, *H. compactum* and *Phialophora verrucosa.* These live saprophytically on wood and vegetation and are commonly introduced through the skin of the legs by an injury with wood. Pus or crusts from the warty lesions are examined in a wet film with 10 per cent. sodium hydroxide. The fungi appear as spherical, dark brown thick-walled cells, about 5–10 μ in diameter, occurring in small clusters and characteristically dividing by septation. Cultures are grown on Sabouraud's glucose agar for at least three weeks at 22° C. Brown-black or green-black mycelial colonies slowly develop. They contain hyphae 2–3 μ wide and characteristic conidiophores on aerial hyphae. The conidia are oval single cells, 1·5–3 $\mu \times$ 3–6 μ, but more nearly spherical in *H. compactum. P. verrucosa* forms the conidia at the cup-like ends of flask-shaped conidiophores. *Hormodendrum* species produce these and also two other kinds of conidiophores, one forming the conidia in branching chains from its end and the other bearing the conidia around its sides.

Mucormycosis.—Disease of animals, and rarely man, may be caused by certain species of *Mucor*, *Absidia* and *Rhizopus*, the lesions being either granulomatous or ulcerative.

PATHOGENIC YEASTS

Cryptococcus neoformans (Torula histolytica)

C. neoformans is a true yeast which reproduces by budding and does not give rise to a mycelium or pseudomycelium. It occurs as spherical cells, 5–20 μ in diameter, Gram-positive and surrounded by a very wide, gelatinous capsule, which is visible in India ink preparations. It produces sporadic, commonly fatal infections (cryptococcosis or torulosis) in man, dog, cat, horse, ox and pig. The infections are subacute or chronic, and most commonly affect the meninges and brain, though sometimes the lungs or skin. In cattle, outbreaks of cryptococcal mastitis and metritis occur.

Infection is not transmitted from man to man. Its source is unknown, but the infection may be endogenous, from animals and birds, or from the soil. *C. neoformans* is commonly present in the droppings of birds. Cryptococcus strains have also been found on the skin and in the gut of healthy persons; these were culturally identical with *C. neoformans* but much less pathogenic for experimental animals (mice). The yeast withstands drying in soil and dust, and it is thought usually to enter the body by inhalation, but maybe sometimes through the skin or intestine.

Laboratory Diagnosis.—The specimens taken for examination may include cerebrospinal fluid (or its centrifuged deposit), sputum, or pus from acneform skin lesions. These are observed microscopically, with condenser defocused, in an unstained wet film under a coverslip and in a second wet film mixed with an equal volume of India ink. The presence of budding, thick-walled, nearly spherical cells with capsules is diagnostic. The yeasts and their capsules stain strongly in tissue sections treated by the periodic acid Schiff method.

Cultures are made on Sabouraud's glucose agar at 37° C. and at 22° C., and on blood agar at 37° C., incubating for at least two weeks. Sputum and exudate contaminated with bacteria should be cultivated on the tellurite malt agar that is selective for the yeasts. Cultures are cream to light brown in colour, and become mucoid rapidly at 37° C. and slowly at 22° C. Before becoming mucoid, the colonies may be similar to those of *Staph. albus*. Films of the cultures show the capsulated yeast cells and no mycelium.

The pathogenicity of a strain can be demonstrated by injecting mice intraperitoneally with 0·5 ml. of a saline suspension of an infected exudate or a 1 per cent. (v/v) suspension of a pure culture. The mouse dies within three to four weeks with gelatinous masses of yeast in the abdomen and brain.

Pityrosporum ovale

P. ovale, or the "bottle bacillus", is a small Gram-positive yeast. It is a common commensal of normal skin and occurs on dandruff scales, being regarded by some authors as causative of dandruff and seborrhoeic dermatitis, though there is little evidence to support this belief. It is ovoid or flask-shaped, 1–2$\mu \times$2–4μ, and reproduces by a process intermediate between budding and fission; the bud is separated from the parent cell by a septum formed across its relatively large base. The organism can be grown on nutrient agar smeared with butter fat which supplies oleic acid.

PATHOGENIC YEAST-LIKE FUNGI

Candida albicans (Monilia albicans, M. psilosis)

Candida organisms grow partly as spherical or oval yeast cells (blastospores) 2·5–4·0 μ in diameter, which reproduce by budding, and partly as a pseudomycelium of non-branching filamentous cells which divide by constriction and give rise to yeast cells by budding from these division sites (Fig. 29). Both forms are thin walled, Gram-positive and non-capsulate. Some of the yeast cells enlarge, form thick walls and become resting chlamydospores 7–17 μ in diameter. Ascospores are never formed. An abundance of easily assimilable nutrients and sufficient aeration encourages growth in the yeast form, whereas nutritionally poor media (e.g. corn meal agar) and poorly aerated conditions in cultures below the surface of agar or liquid media favour mycelial growth and chlamydospore formation. Conditions in the body generally give both yeast and mycelial growth.

Occurrence and pathogenicity.—*C. albicans* is the only important pathogenic species in the genus *Candida*. It is a common cause of acute and subacute infections (candidiasis, or moniliasis) in man, animals and birds. Other species of *Candida* include *C. tropicalis* (*Monilia candida*), *C. pseudotropicalis* (*M. mortifera*), *C. krusei*, *C. parakrusei* (*M. parapsilosis*), *C. stellatoidea* and *C. guilliermondii*; these, like *C. albicans*, occur as commensals in the human and animal body, but they only rarely cause disease. *C. tropicalis*, however, has been found, apparently as the causal pathogen, in oral and vaginal thrush and, more rarely, in broncho-pulmonary infections, osteomyelitis, pyelonephritis and septicaemia.

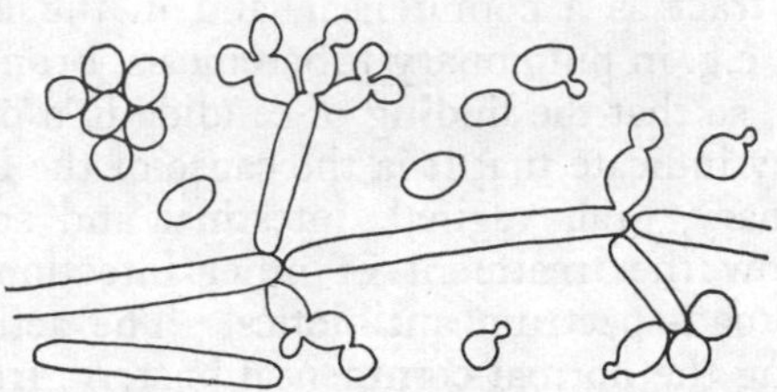

Candida albicans: hyphae forming a pseudomycelium and giving rise to budding yeast-like cells (blastospores) (×1000)

FIG. 29

C. albicans is pathogenic when injected intravenously in rabbits, guinea-pigs and mice. The other species of *Candida* are generally entirely non-pathogenic in laboratory animals. *C. tropicalis*, however, when injected in fairly large doses, is pathogenic in mice, though not in rabbits.

In man, *C. albicans* produces superficial infections of the skin (cutaneous candidiasis) and mucous membranes (oral and vaginal thrush); it also causes broncho-pulmonary infections, secondary intestinal infections and, though much less frequently, septicaemia and deep, blood-borne infections, e.g. meningitis, endocarditis and pyelonephritis. Infection is generally dependent on a weakening of the body defence mechanisms, e.g. by diabetes, leukaemia, iron-deficiency anaemia, neonatal debility, senility, alcoholism, drug addiction, antibiotic therapy and cortisone therapy. Infection of the *skin* is promoted by prolonged exposure to moisture and the lesions, characterised by erythema, exudation and desquamation, are generally localised in damp folds (intertriginous candidiasis), e.g. in the axillae, groin, infra-mammary areas, interdigital clefts, umbilicus and gluteal folds, and, in infants, in the napkin area; cutaneous candidiasis is also frequent in persons whose occupations involve frequent immersion in water. Infection may involve the *nails* and lead to chronic paronychia and oonychia.

Oral thrush is especially common in infants; creamy white patches of exudate form on a red, raw, inflamed mucous membrane in the mouth and throat, and on the tongue. In adults, denture sore mouth and angular cheilitis may be caused by infection with candida.

Vaginal thrush (candida vulvovaginitis) occurs commonly in pregnancy, remitting after parturition, and in diabetes. Vaginal discharges due to infection with candida generally contain little or no pus, and are relatively acid (pH 4·3–5·2), whereas discharges that are purulent and less acid (pH 5·2–6·4) are usually due to infection with *Trichomonas vaginalis* or pyogenic bacteria, e.g. gonococcus, *Strept. pyogenes*, *Staph. aureus* and coliform bacilli (Boycott, 1961).

Bronchial and pulmonary candidiasis may occur, with the production of mucoid, gelatinous sputum containing numerous candida organisms. It must be noted, however, that *C. albicans* is commonly present in the upper respiratory tract as a commensal, and in the lower tract as a secondary invader, e.g. in pulmonary tuberculosis, bronchial carcinoma and bronchiectasis, so that the finding of candida in a patient's sputum does not necessarily indicate that it is the cause of the illness.

Broncho-pulmonary, oral, vaginal, intestinal and septicaemic candidiasis often follow the treatment of other infections (e.g. chronic bronchitis) with broad-spectrum antibiotics. The action of the antibiotic in eliminating the normal commensal bacteria from the mucous membrane is probably responsible, at least in part, for the facilitation of infection with candida.

Avian moniliasis is an infection of the upper alimentary canal of chickens, turkeys and pigeons, the lesions being mostly confined to the crop and proventriculus. Although usually of sporadic occurrence, epidemics of "thrush" with an average mortality of over 60 per cent. have occurred, the species responsible being *Candida albicans* and *C. krusei*. Moniliasis has occurred in pigs, probably as a result of feeding antibiotic-supplemented food, whilst in cattle thrush-like lesions have been observed in the rumen and intestinal mucosa.

Source of Infection.—*C. albicans* is a common commensal of man and animals, occurring in the mouth, nose, throat, intestine, vagina and skin; it occurs in the mouth and in the faeces of 20–30 per cent. of healthy persons. Infection is thus usually endogenous, but occasionally it is exogenous and contagious. Infants, for instance, may be infected from their mothers or from other infants during an epidemic in a maternity hospital. Artificially fed babies are more often affected than breast fed babies. Unless aseptic precautions are taken, infection may be spread among pregnant women by the obstetrician's gloved hand. *C. albicans* is found on the bedding of patients and in the air, and it may be spread by contact or by air-borne infected dust.

C. tropicalis, *C. pseudotropicalis*, *C. krusei*, *C. parakrusei*, *C. stellatoidea* and *C. guilliermondii* have all been isolated from the human nose, throat, alimentary tract, vagina and skin, where they appear to be commensal. *C. stellatoidea* occurs frequently in the vagina and urethra. These species probably also occur in many non-human sources, e.g. in vegetation.

Laboratory Diagnosis

Since *C. albicans* commonly occurs as a commensal in the same situations as it causes infection, the mere demonstration of its presence is not proof of infection. This diagnosis requires demonstration that the organism is *abundantly present* on several occasions, and also the exclusion of other possible causative agents. Specimens must be examined with minimum delay to avoid multiplication of originally scanty, contaminating yeasts.

Sputum and exudate, e.g. mucous patches from mouth or vagina, should be examined microscopically in Gram-stained smears and in unstained wet films. Skin and nail scrapings are examined in a wet film with 10–20 per cent. sodium hydroxide. Budding yeast cells mixed with long filaments are indicative of a yeast-like fungus. The cells and filaments stain Gram-positively and they are clearly much larger (e.g. 2–4 fold in diameter) than the commensal bacteria that are generally also present in the specimens.

For culture, exudate may be collected on dry swabs or, preferably, swabs soaked in Sabouraud broth. The cultures are grown on plates of blood agar at 37° C. and on Sabouraud's glucose agar at 37° C. and at 22° C. Specimens of faeces or sputum should be cultivated on the selective tellurite malt agar or penicillin-streptomycin blood agar to control the growth of bacterial contaminants. In two to three days, large creamy bacteria-like colonies develop on the Sabouraud's medium and smaller grey colonies on blood agar. The culture, which has a characteristic odour, is examined in an unstained wet film, or a Gram film, for budding yeast forms. A pure culture is isolated by picking a colony from one of the primary plates or, if necessary to ensure purity, from a secondary plating, and grown on a slope of Sabouraud's glucose agar for 48 hr. at 37° C. The pure culture is then identified by the following examinations, which distinguish *C. albicans* from the other candida species (see table). For further information on the identification of *Candida* spp., see Benham (1957).

Examination of pure culture for identification of species.—(1) The naked-eye appearances of the 48-hr. Sabouraud slope culture are noted. Growths of *C. albicans* and most other candida organisms are raised, white, moist and creamy; that of *C. krusei* is flat and dry.

(2) A portion of the culture is examined in a wet film with India ink to confirm the yeast-like morphology and absence of capsules that are characteristic of *Candida* spp. The culture should consist mainly of round or oval budding cells (blastospores) with an occasional, usually short filament. The blastospores of *C. krusei* are longer and narrower than those of the other species.

(3) A subculture is grown in a tube of 10 ml. of Sabouraud's glucose broth (pH 5·4) for 48 hr. at 37° C. The culture is examined for the presence of a pellicle on its surface. Cultures of *C. tropicalis* and *C. krusei* form pellicles, but those of *C. albicans* and other species do not.

(4) The pure culture or, preferably, its subculture in Sabouraud

Differential characters of *Candida* species
(modified from Martin *et al.*, 1937, who give illustrations)

Species	Growth on Sabouraud's agar (pH 5·4) for 48 hr at 37°C	Surface film of growth on Sabouraud's broth after 48 hr at 37°C	Colonies on blood agar (pH 7·4) after 10 days at 37°C	Growth in corn meal agar for 2-4 days at 18-22°C	Production of acid (A) and gas (G) after 48 hr at 37°C in broth with 2 per cent. of			
					Glucose	Maltose	Sucrose	Lactose
C. albicans	Creamy	None	Medium sized (*c.* 1·5 mm.), circular, smooth, grey	Branched "tree-like" mycelium *with chlamydospores* at tips of most branches	AG	AG	A	—
C. tropicalis	Variable	Narrow film with bubbles	Large, grey, mycelial fringe	Branched mycelium; many scattered blastospores; no chlamydospores	AG	AG	AG	—
C. pseudotropicalis	Variable	None	Small (*c.* 0·5 mm.)	Poor, branched mycelium; no chlamydospores	AG	—	AG	AG
C. krusei	Flat, dry	Thick film	Small, round or irregular, flat or heaped (0·2-1·0 mm.)	"Crossed sticks" mycelium; no chlamydospores	AG	—	—	—
C. parakrusei	Creamy	None	Small, very white	Branched mycelium; no chlamydospores	AG or A	—	—	—
C. stellatoidea	Creamy	None	Star-shaped, large	Mycelium; large, dense, ball-like clusters of blastospores; usually no chlamydospores	AG	AG	—	—
C. guilliermondii	Creamy	None	Medium sized, dull grey	Good mycelium; no chlamydospores	—	—	—	—

broth is plated out on a blood agar plate (pH 7·4) and the plate incubated for 10 days at 37° C. The appearance of the colonies is noted; it is characteristic of the species (see p. 522), but experience is necessary if reliance is to be placed on this criterion.

(5) The pure culture is subcultured twice or thrice on ordinary nutrient agar (no added glucose, pH 7·4) and material from the last of these glucose-free cultures is used to inoculate chlamydospore medium and sugar fermentation test media.

(6) A test for the formation of *chlamydospores* and *mycelium* is made by growing a deep-streak culture of the organism for 2 days, or more, at 18-22° C. in a plate of corn meal agar (Benham, 1931) or, preferably, zein agar (Reid, Jones and Carter, 1953), rice extract agar (Taschdjian, (1953) or rice starch and Tween agar (Taschdjian, 1957; Rosenthal and Furnari, 1959). Chlamydospores are produced more rapidly (within 24 hr.) and profusely on zein agar and rice agars than on corn meal agar. A stiff wire bearing the inoculum is cut in strokes through the substance of the shallow layer of agar. As the culture grows it is observed *in situ* under the low power (16 mm.) and high power (4 mm.) objectives of the microscope, the whole plate being placed on the microscope stage. A filamentous pseudomycelium is formed by all species of *Candida*, but is absent in cultures of *Cryptococcus*, *Saccharomyces* and other yeasts. *C. albicans* produces a well developed branching "tree-like" pseudomycelium which consists of hyphal cells, 2–3 μ wide, separated by transverse septa and which develops large spherical thick-walled chlamydospores, 6–9 microns in diameter, at the tips of most branches, and clusters of smaller, oval, thin-walled blastospores (*c.* $2{\cdot}5 \times 4\ \mu$) at the junctions of the filamentous cells. Other species of *Candida* (except, occasionally, *C. stellatoidea*) do not form chlamydospores; the appearances of their pseudomycelia are given on p. 522. Candida organisms do not produce ascospores. Chlamydospore formation is considered to be the most important distinguishing feature of *C. albicans*.

(7) Fermentation tests are made in tubes of 10 ml. of nutrient broth (pH 7·2) to which a separately sterilised (20 per cent.) solution of sugar is added to give a final sugar concentration of 3 per cent. Bromothymol blue is used as indicator and Durham tubes are used to show the production of gas. The standard peptone water medium containing 1 per cent. of sugar is almost as satisfactory. The tubes are inoculated heavily from a culture on glucose-free nutrient agar and are incubated at 37° C. for 10 days. Fermentation is usually apparent in 48 hr.

C. albicans ferments glucose and maltose to give acid and gas, sucrose to acid only and fails to ferment lactose. Other species give different reactions, as shown on page 522.

Widra (1957) has described a method in which the yeast is grown as a stab culture in phenol red agar base (Difco) containing 3 per cent. of sugar. After inoculation, the medium is covered to a depth of 1–1½ cm. with melted Vaspar (one part of yellow petroleum jelly mixed with one part of paraffin wax) and the tubes are incubated at 37° C. for 5 days. Production of acid is shown by change of the indicator from orange to yellow along the line of the stab and the production of gas is shown by the collection of bubbles under the Vaspar. Readings are made at 1, 3 and 5 days since the rate of fermentation is significant in some cases. Thus *C. tropicalis* ferments sucrose within 24 hr., but maltose only in 3–5 days.

(8) Pathogenicity is demonstrated by injecting a rabbit intravenously with 1 ml. of a 1 per cent. suspension of packed yeast cells in saline; the animal dies in four to five days and small abscesses are seen throughout the cortex of its kidneys. Only *C. albicans*, of all the species of *Candida*, is pathogenic in the rabbit.

Immunology.—Agglutinating antibodies are found in the blood of many patients. However, they are found also in normal persons, so that their demonstration is of little diagnostic value. The various species of *Candida* are closely related antigenically. By means of slide agglutination tests with monospecific and absorbed antisera Tsuchiya *et al.* (1961) have demonstrated the presence of several different kinds of thermolabile and thermostable antigens in different species of *Candida*, some of which antigens are shared by most of the species.

Chemotherapy. Candida organisms are highly resistant to the antibiotics used for the treatment of bacterial infections and they are liable to proliferate excessively during therapy with a broad spectrum antibiotic that eliminates the commensal bacterial flora. They are, however, susceptible to the antibiotic, nystatin, produced by *Streptomyces noursei*. This is the drug of choice for the treatment of candidiasis. Administration is usually topical: tablets are taken by mouth for oral and intestinal infections, and ointment and powder is applied to skin lesions. Nystatin is poorly absorbed from the intestine, but there have been reports of systemic, urinary and pulmonary infections responding to oral treatment.

For further information on *Candida albicans* the reader should consult the book by Winner and Hurley (1964).

Malassezia furfur.—This is a yeast-like fungus which causes the superficial skin infection known as pityriasis versicolor, a chronic asymptomatic infection producing irregular brownish and desquamating macules. Diagnosis is confirmed by microscopic examination of skin scales mounted in 10–20 per cent. sodium hydroxide; the fungus is seen as clusters of round, budding thick-walled cells, 3–8 μ in diameter, together with short fragments of mycelium.

DIMORPHIC FUNGI CAUSING DEEP INFECTIONS

Sporotrichum schenckii

This fungus is the cause of sporotrichosis in man, horses, cats, dogs, rats and other animals. The infection is chronic, giving firm nodules in the subcutaneous tissue with subsequent inflammation and ulceration of the overlying skin, and spread along the draining lymphatics. Blood-borne dissemination is rare, but when it occurs is often fatal.

Source of Infection.—The fungus is primarily a saprophyte, that grows on dead plant material and wood. It can also infect living plants, *e.g.* being commonly present on the thorny plant, berberis, and is found in the soil and in dust on the coats of animals. Man and animals are infected from such contaminated materials through an injury to the skin, *e.g.* by an infected thorn or splinter of wood. Infection is most frequent in farm workers, gardeners and manual labourers. Men are sometimes infected by contact with infected animals, and occasionally by an animal bite or sting, but natural spread from man to man has not been recorded. The infection is remarkably susceptible to treatment with potassium iodide.

Laboratory Diagnosis.—The fungus occurs in the yeast form (parasitic phase) when in animal tissues. However, *it can rarely be seen in exudates and tissue sections from human lesions*, so that direct microscopic examination of these is of no positive diagnostic value.

In artificial culture, the fungus grows in the yeast form at 37° C. and in the mycelial form (saprophytic phase) at 22° C. Pus swabbed from an ulcer or, preferably, aspirated from an unruptured abscess, is heavily inoculated on to blood agar and Sabouraud's glucose agar. After 2–3 days at 37° C. on blood agar, the colonies are moist, wrinkled and cream-coloured, and consist of Gram-positive budding yeast cells which are fusiform, cigar-like or oval in shape, and about 3–5 μ in length. After 3–5 days at 22° C. on Sabouraud's medium, the colonies are small, white and waxy; later, they become wrinkled, membranous and pigmented cream, brown or black, but never develop a cottony aerial mycelium. These colonies are composed of a mycelium (2–3 μ diameter) bearing pear-shaped conidia (3–6 μ long) which radiate from the tips of hyphae as a cluster or project from their sides as a sheath.

Animal inoculation may be attempted. A suspension of pus or culture is injected intraperitoneally into mice. The animals develop peritonitis and the fusiform and oval yeast cells may be demonstrated both extracellularly and intracellularly in macrophages.

Blastomyces dermatitidis

This dimorphic fungus is the cause of North American blastomycosis, a chronic suppurative and granulomatous infection of man. *Cutaneous blastomycosis* is usually a primary infection of the skin; there is papule and pustule formation followed by ulceration and a slow peripheral spread in the skin, but no systemic dissemination. *Systemic blastomycosis* usually results from a primary infection of the lungs with subsequent blood-borne dissemination to the skin, subcutaneous tissues, bones, kidneys, brain and other organs. Natural infections also occur in dogs and horses.

Source of Infection.—This is unknown. The fungus has not been found as a saprophyte in the soil or elsewhere, and apparently does not spread from man to man or from animal to man. It presumably enters the body by inoculation through the skin or by inhalation into the lungs.

Laboratory Diagnosis.—Pus or tissue scrapings are examined microscopically in an unstained wet film; this may be mounted with 10 per cent. sodium hydroxide if the specimen requires to be rendered more transparent. When in tissues, the fungus occurs in the yeast form (parasitic phase) and is seen as thick-walled spherical cells which are 8–15 μ in diameter, occur either free or within phagocytes, and on budding *bear only single buds*.

In artificial culture the fungus grows in the yeast form at 37° C. and in the mycelial form (saprophytic phase) at 22° C. Growth is slow, taking one to three weeks at either temperature. On blood agar at 37° C. it forms wrinkled, creamy or waxy colonies consisting of budding yeast cells as seen in tissues. On Sabouraud's glucose agar at 22° C. the colonies are initially like those of the yeast form, but eventually become covered with a white cottony aerial mycelium which later turns brown. The 22° C. colony comprises a mycelium of broad, thick-walled and closely septate hyphae, later developing many round or oval conidia, 3–5 μ in diameter, and eventually many smooth and thick-walled chlamydospores, 7–18 μ in diameter.

If pus or culture is inoculated intraperitoneally in mice, the budding yeast forms are later seen in the peritoneal exudate.

Paracoccidioides brasiliensis

This dimorphic fungus causes South American blastomycosis, a chronic granulomatous infection of the skin, mucosae, lymph nodes and internal organs. The source of infection is unknown. It occurs chiefly in manual workers in rural areas and does not spread from man to man.

Pus or tissue examined in a wet film with sodium hydroxide shows thick-walled yeast cells, 10–60 μ in diameter; some of these bear single buds, as in *B. dermatitidis*, but others bear ***multiple buds radiating from their surface***. After several days on blood agar at 37° C. the fungus forms moist wrinkled creamy colonies of yeast cells. In two to three weeks on Sabouraud's agar at 22° C. it forms white wrinkled cottony colonies which later turn brown; these consist of a septate mycelium bearing a few round or oval conidia. Pus and yeast-form cultures are pathogenic when inoculated intraperitoneally in mice; in five to six weeks, nodules containing budding yeast cells are found in the mesentery.

Histoplasma capsulatum

This dimorphic fungus is the cause of histoplasmosis, a granulomatous disease which occurs in man either as a primary benign, usually asymptomatic infection of the lungs, or, rarely, as a progressive, usually fatal systemic infection involving the reticulo-endothelial tissues; in the latter case the primary infection is often extra-pulmonary, *e.g.* in the skin, upper respiratory tract, mouth or intestine. The disease is endemic in the Mississippi valley, but sporadic cases occur throughout the world. Natural infections also occur in cows, horses, dogs, cats, rodents and other animals.

Source of Infection.—The fungus is found in the soil of endemic areas, but whether it grows in the soil as a saprophyte or enters the soil from small infected animals, is uncertain. It has been frequently found in the droppings of bats. Infection seems mainly to occur by inhalation of infected soil dust. It does not spread from man to man.

Laboratory Diagnosis.—The fungus occurs as the yeast form when in the tissues. Characteristically it is an *intracellular parasite of reticulo-endothelial macrophages.* Smears of sputum, blood, sternal bone marrow, lymph-node pulp and mucosal lesion scrapings are stained with Giemsa's stain. Numerous capsulate oval yeast cells, 1–5 μ in diameter, are seen within the macrophages and a very few extracellularly (Fig. 30, left).

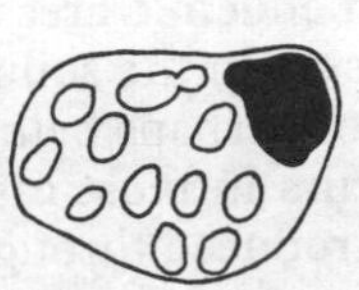
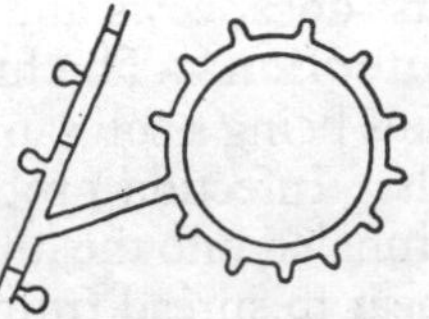

Histoplasma capsulatum: left, yeast-like cells in macrophage; right, mycelium from culture bearing microconidia and a tuberculate chlamydospore. (x1000)

FIG. 30

Sputum, gastric washings and other clinical specimens are cultivated on blood agar at 37° C. (or glucose blood agar containing penicillin and streptomycin to control bacterial contaminants, p. 771) and Sabouraud's glucose agar at 22° C. On blood agar at 37° C., the colonies are moist, wrinkled and creamy, and consist of budding yeast cells. On Sabouraud's medium at 22° C., they are slow growing, cottony in appearance due to development of an aerial mycelium, white at first and later turning brownish; they consist of septate mycelium bearing small lateral conidia (2–3 μ in diameter) and eventually form large round "tuberculate" chlamydospores, 7–15 μ in diameter; the latter are characterised by a covering of small rounded tubercles projecting from the outer surface of the thick spore wall and they are diagnostic of *H. capsulatum* (Fig. 30, right).

The fungus is pathogenic to laboratory animals. Mice injected intraperitoneally with infected material or culture die after varying periods of time.

Immune and Hypersensitive Reactions.—Within a few weeks of first becoming infected, the patients develop complement-fixing antibodies in their blood and become hypersensitive to *H. capsulatum* antigens. Hypersensitivity is demonstrated by injecting intradermally 0·1 ml. of a 1 in 100 dilution of a standardised preparation "histoplasmin"; this gives rise in 24–48 hr. to an area of induration more than 0·5 cm. in diameter. The significance of a positive histoplasmin reaction is analogous to that of a positive tuberculin reaction, indicating present *or* past infection. Partial cross-reactions may be given with blastomyces and coccidioides antigens, which should therefore be tested simultaneously for quantitative comparison. Surveys have shown that histoplasmosis is not endemic in Britain.

Coccidioides immitis

This is another dimorphic fungus and is the cause of coccidioidomycosis, a granulomatous disease affecting man either as a primary benign, often asymptomatic infection of the lungs or, occasionally, as a progressive and fatal infection that disseminates to lungs, skin, bones, meninges and other organs. Coccidioidomycosis is endemic in the arid south-west of the United States of America, and also occurs endemically or sporadically in various other parts of the world. Natural infections occur in rodents, dogs, cows and sheep in endemic areas.

Source of Infection.—The fungus occurs in the soil in the endemic localities, perhaps being a soil saprophyte or perhaps being derived from infected animals. Infection probably occurs in most cases by infected soil dust being inhaled into the lungs or introduced through injured skin. It does not appear to spread from man to man or from animals to man. *The arthrospores formed in artificial cultures readily become airborne and are highly infective, so that infection is liable to occur in laboratory workers unless special precautions are taken.*

Laboratory Diagnosis.—The fungus occurs in the tissues as non-budding, spherical thick-walled sporangia. These are 20–70 μ in diameter and contain numerous small spherical endospores (2–5 μ diam.). The spores are liberated by rupture of the sporangium and subsequently themselves develop into sporangia (Fig. 31, left). Sputum and

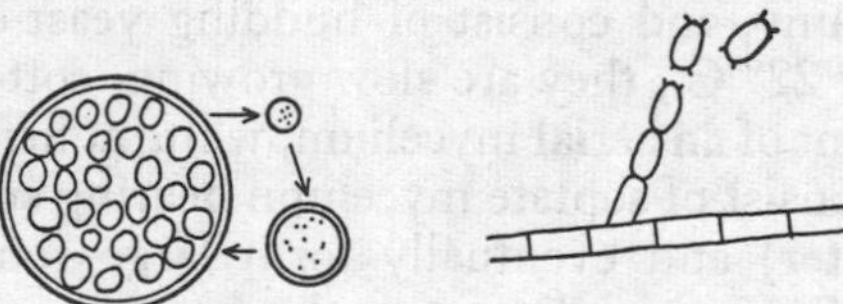

Coccidioides immitis: left, mature spherule containing endospores and immature spherules as found in tissues; right, mycelium segmenting to form arthrospores in culture. (×500)

Fig. 31

other infective materials from patients are examined in wet films with 10 per cent. sodium hydroxide in order to demonstrate these forms.

When infected materials are cultivated on blood agar at 37° C. and on Sabouraud's glucose agar at 22° C., the growth is mycelial in both cases. The colonies are whitish, at first moist and membranous, but later becoming cottony with the development of an abundant aerial mycelium. The hyphae segment into arthrospores (about 3 × 4 μ) which become very thick-walled and are highly infective (Fig. 31, right).

Cultures and infected exudates are pathogenic for mice and cause demonstrable infection one to two weeks after intraperitoneal injection.

Immune and Hypersensitive Reactions.—Precipitins and complement-fixing antibodies appear in the patient's blood in severe primary infections. Hypersensitivity to *C. immitis* antigens appears during the first or second week of severe or mild illness. Intradermal injection of 0·1 ml. of a 1 in 100 dilution of standardised "coccidioidin" gives rise to an area of erythema and induration of at least 0·5 cm. in diameter. Patients with disseminated coccidioidomycosis usually fail to give a reaction. A positive coccidioidin reaction has a significance analogous to that of a positive tuberculin reaction.

Rhinosporidium seeberi

Rhinosporidiosis is a chronic polyp-forming infection of the submucous tissue of the nose, eyes, ears and larynx, and occasionally of the genitalia and skin. It is commonest in India and occurs sporadically in man, horses and cows. The source of infection is unknown, though persons swimming in rivers and stagnant water are frequently infected. The causative organism, *Rhinosporidium seeberi*, has not been cultured, but its appearance in tissues suggests that it is a fungus. For microscopic diagnosis, material is taken from a polyp and squeezed in water between a slide and coverslip. Free thick-walled spherical spores about 5–7 μ in diameter are seen and various stages of their growth into spherical sporangia of 200–300 μ diameter. The sporangia contain thousands of spores and eventually release these by bursting at a pore.

REFERENCES

Benham, R. W. (1931). Certain monilias parasitic on man. Their identification by morphology and by agglutination. *J. infect. Dis.*, **49**, 183.

Benham, R. W. (1957). Species of candida most frequently isolated from man: methods and criteria for their identification. *J. chron. Dis.*, **5**, 460.

Boycott, J. A. (1961). The nature of vaginal discharge. *Lancet*, **1**, 1071.

Conant, N. F., Smith, D. T., Baker, R. D., Callaway, J. L. & Martin, D. S. (1954). *Manual of Clinical Mycology*, 2nd ed. Philadelphia: Saunders.

Martin, D. S., Jones, C. P., Yao, K. F. & Lee, L. E. Jr. (1937). A practical classification of the monilias. *J. Bact.*, **34**, 99.

Pepys, J., Jenkins, P. A., Festenstein, G. N., Gregory, P. H., Lacey, M. E. & Skinner, F. A. (1963). Farmer's lung, thermophilic actinomycetes as a source of "Farmer's lung hay" antigen. *Lancet*, **2**, 607.

Reid, J. D., Jones, M. M. & Carter, E. B. (1953). A simple, clear medium for demonstration of chlamydospores of *Candida albicans*. *Amer. J. clin. Path.*, **23**, 938.

Riddell, R. W. (1951). Laboratory diagnosis of common fungus infections. In *Recent Advances in Clinical Pathology*, 2nd ed., S. C. Dyke, p. 77. London: Churchill.

Rosenthal, S. A. & Furnari, D. (1959). Chlamydospore production by *Candida albicans*. Comparison of dehydrated rice extract agar with other media. *J. invest. Derm.*, **32**, 115.

Taschdjian, C. L. (1953). A simply prepared identification medium for *Caudida albicans*. *Mycologia*, **45**, 474.

Taschdjian, C. L. (1957). Routine identification of *Candida albicans*: current methods and a new medium. *Mycologia*, **49**, 332.

Thom, C. & Raper, K. B. (1945). *A manual of the aspergilli*. Baltimore: Williams & Wilkins Co.

Tsuchiya, T., Fukazawa, Y. & Kawakita, S. (1961). Serological classification of the genus *Candida*. In *Studies on Candidiasis in Japan*. Pp. 34–46. Research Committee of Candidiasis, Education Ministry of Japan. Tokyo.

Widra, A. (1957). An improved fermentation method for rapid identification of candida species. *J. infect. Dis.*, **100**, 70.

Winner, H. I. & Hurley, R. (1964). *Candida albicans*. London: J. A. Churchill.

CHAPTER 41

PROTOZOA

MALARIA PLASMODIA; BABESIAE; TRYPANOSOMES; LEISHMANIAE; INTESTINAL PROTOZOA

PROTOZOA are the lowest and simplest of animals; they are unicellular but may display a considerable measure of differentiation and possess such specialised structures as undulating membranes, cilia, and flagella. A number of protozoa are parasites of man and domestic animals and of these the malarial parasite, trypanosomes, amoebae, leishmaniae, toxoplasmae, and trichomonas are the most important. The immunology of protozoan infections is not yet well understood but during recent years new serological techniques have been applied to the study of these diseases and for further information and a full bibliography on this subject the reader is referred to Fulton (1963).

THE MALARIA PLASMODIA

Malaria is a protozoal disease of man in which the causative organism, *Plasmodium*, invades certain tissue cells and red cells of the blood. Analogous diseases occur in other animals but as far as is known their plasmodia are non-infectious to man. An exception may be those infecting certain chimpanzees which appear to be closely related to *Pl. malariae* of man.

Malaria is an illness with intermittent pyrexia, splenic enlargement and response to alkaloids of the cinchona group and other drugs. It occurs widely thoughout the world in areas where there is a mean annual isotherm of more than 16° C. (60° F.) suitable for the breeding of a large number of *anopheline* mosquitoes and a dense population of susceptible human hosts, as an endemic disease with periodic exacerbations. The great advances in the practical control of malaria which have taken place have altered the natural history of the disease in many areas but left it unaffected in others. Where there is little or no control the disease is characterised by a high morbidity and relatively low mortality directly attributable to malaria. It has, however, far-reaching effects because of the lowered resistance of those affected to other diseases.

Infants are infected at an early age and throughout their lives may be repeatedly reinfected; many die during early age either directly or from intercurrent disease. Those who survive have a variable degree of immunity together with proliferation of the reticulo-endothelial system and splenic enlargement. Thus the frequency of enlarged spleen is a useful indication of the degree of infection in a community.

There are four well-defined species of malaria plasmodium infecting man. *Plasmodium vivax* is responsible for benign tertian malaria and is the most widespread, *Plasmodium falciparum* is the cause of malignant tertian malaria, *Plasmodium malariae* of quartan malaria and *Plasmodium ovale*, the least frequently found, is a cause of some infections in Africa.

Plasmodium knowlesii, a natural cause of chimpanzee malaria, may be capable of transmission to man and may be a reservoir of human infection.

These plasmodia belong to the order *Haemosporidia* of the class Sporozoa. They have a sexual cycle with sporogony in the mosquito, and an asexual cycle with schizogony in man. A number of different phases occur, three in man. The complete life-cycle requires alternation between the two hosts.

Some features of the malaria parasites can be observed in unstained preparations but the features of importance in the diagnosis of malaria are best seen in preparations with one of the Romanowsky stains, *e.g.* Leishman's.

Outline of the Life History of the Malaria Plasmodium.—It is introduced into the body by the bite of the mosquito (*vide infra*) as a minute spindle-shaped motile cell, or sporozoite, containing nuclear material in the form of a chromatin granule. The sporozoite rapidly leaves the general circulation and invades tissue cells, particularly those of the liver, to commence the *pre-erythrocytic* phase of the asexual cycle. In these cells the sporozoites develop into large schizonts which divide to form merozoites and these are liberated when the host cell bursts. Some merozoites initiate the exo-erythrocytic phase by parasitising other tissue cells; others invade red cells to start the *erythrocytic* phase and enter the circulation (Fig. 32). In the red cells the merozoites grow at the expense of the cells to form a trophozoite and altered blood pigment accumulates as brownish granules. It may display amoeboid movement and protrude pseudopodia. More than one trophozoite may attack a single corpuscle. The corpuscle may show considerable alteration in size as the trophozoite develops. The trophozoite tends to assume a characteristic ring-form due to the formation of a vacuole-like structure, with the chromatin granule at one side, so that the whole organism resembles a signet-ring. When fully grown it is more or less rounded, and may appear to occupy the greater part of the corpuscle. These mature trophozoites usually contain a considerable amount of blood pigment.

When fully developed, the trophozoite becomes a schizont, and schizogony takes place. The pigment accumulates towards the centre, the chromatin breaks up into smaller particles, the protoplasm subdivides and forms a number of small round or oval merozoites (about 2 μ in diameter) each containing a fragment of the original chromatin. The residual protoplasm and pigment remain in the centre of the group of merozoites. The number of merozoites resulting from schizogony varies with the different species. Finally the individual merozoites are liberated as free structures in the blood. The merozoite attacks another red cell and thus the asexual cycle is repeated.

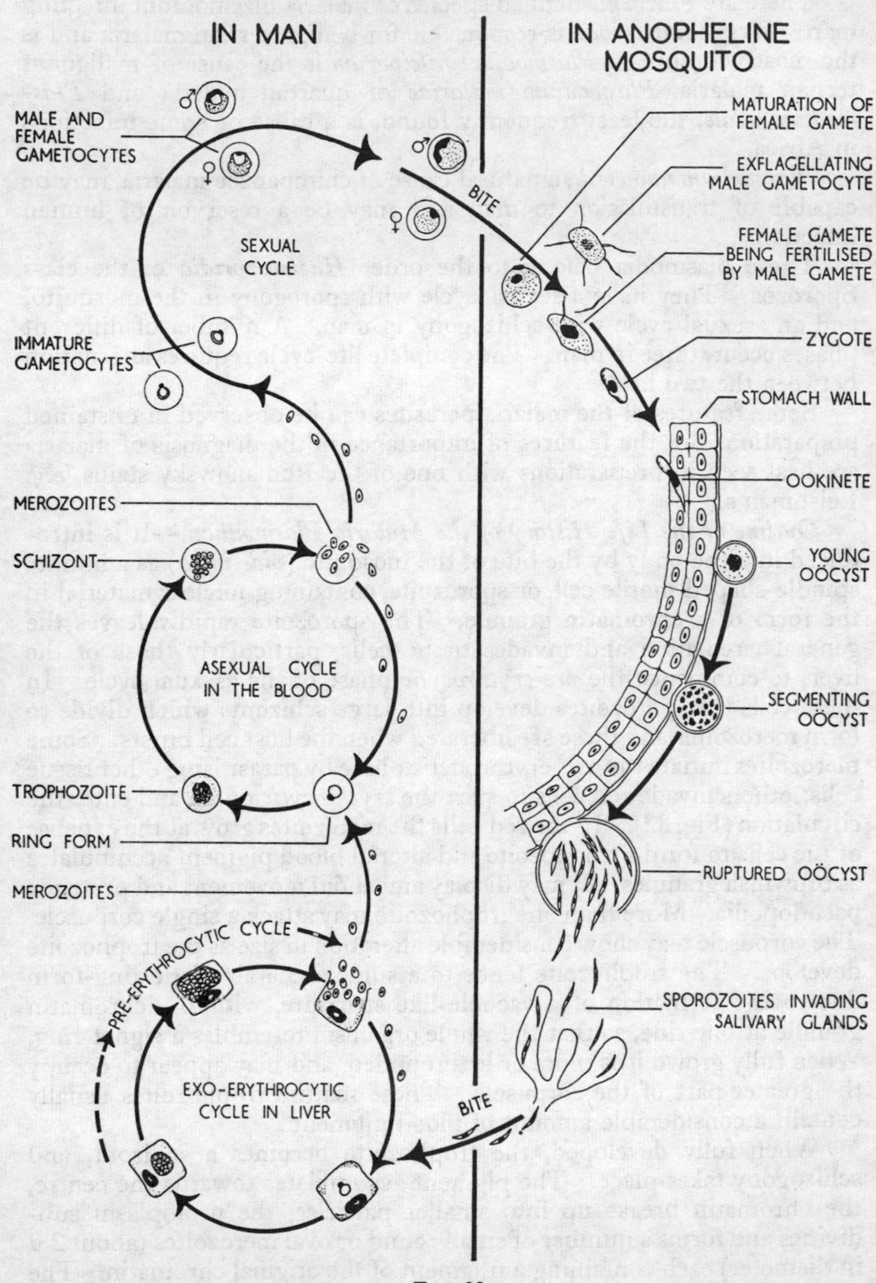

FIG. 32

Reproductive cycles of the malarial parasite *Plasmodium vivax*.[1]

[1] Modified from Blacklock and Southwell *A Guide to Human Parasitology*, 6th Edition (1958). London: Lewis.

In *Plasmodium vivax* and *Plasmodium malariae* infections exo-erythrocytic schizogony carries on in parallel with erythrocytic development and frequently persists for long periods after the parasite has left the peripheral blood. This leads to long latent periods and relapses as erythrocytic invasion is always liable to occur. In *Plasmodium falciparum* infections exo-erythrocytic schizogony does not persist along with erythrocytic development so that once the erythrocytic parasite has been eradicated relapse does not occur.

The length of time the organism takes to complete the asexual cycle varies with the species:

Plasmodium vivax	Two days.
Plasmodium malariae	Three days.
Plasmodium falciparum	One or two days.

If the majority of the parasites in the body mature at the same time schizogony will be synchronous and fever, possibly rigor, will occur; thus in *Pl. vivax* infection the febrile paroxysm occurs every second day (tertian malaria) and in *Pl. malariae* infection every third day (quartan malaria).[1] This clinical picture is now relatively rare however, especially as a result of extensive drug treatment and prophylaxis, and maturation is asynchronous and fever irregular. Multiple infection with the same species may take place and more rarely more than one species may infect the same individual.

In malignant malaria the parasite leaves the peripheral blood before it becomes a mature trophozoite, and schizogony occurs, as a rule, only in the blood of internal organs.

Differentiation of the Malaria Plasmodia

While some of the organisms develop into schizonts, others become gametocytes. In the case of *Plasmodium vivax* and *Plasmodium malariae*, these are rounded and about the same size as a mature trophozoite. The gametocytes of *Plasmodium falciparum* are sausage-shaped or crescentic, with the envelope of the corpuscle stretched across the poles of the crescent. Male and female gametocytes are distinguished, and designated respectively micro- and macro-gametocytes, the former generally smaller than the latter. The female form of *Plasmodium falciparum* is narrower than the male. The micro-gametocyte, as compared with the macro-gametocyte, contains a nuclear structure that is relatively large, diffuse and often disposed across the body in the form of a spindle. The protoplasm stains faintly and the pigment is diffuse. In the macro-gametocyte the protoplasm stains dark blue, the nucleus is small, compact and often peripheral in situation; but in the female gametocyte of *Plamodium falciparum* the nucleus is situated centrally with the pigment accumulated round it.

[1] The terms "tertian" and "quartan" are derived from the occurrence of the successive attacks on the third and fourth days respectively, counting the day of the previous attack as the first.

	P. vivax (*Benign tertian*)	P. malariae (*Quartan*)	P. falciparum (*Malignant*)
Asexual life-cycle	48 hours	72 hours	24 to 48 hours
Trophozoites in fresh unstained preparations of blood . .	Not refractile, hyaline, not easily observed; usually one organism only in red cell; active movement	Refractile, "frosted-glass" appearance; more easily observed; less amoeboid and active	Small, about $\frac{1}{5}$ or $\frac{1}{6}$ of diameter of red cell; often more than one organism in cell; active at first
Pigment in trophozoites .	Fine, yellowish-brown, and evenly distributed	Coarse, brownish-black	Scanty, fine
Ring forms (stained preparations) .	Large, irregular, not well defined, about $\frac{1}{3}$ diameter of red cell; usually single chromatin granule	Thick round rings, about $\frac{1}{3}$ diameter of red cell; often in the form of equatorial bands	Small, multiple, thin; often 2 chromatin granules; often situated at the edge of red cell; about $\frac{1}{5}$ or $\frac{1}{6}$ diameter of red cell
Red cells (stained preparations) .	Swollen, pale, showing deeply stained rose to purple points, "Schüffner's dots"	Not altered	Shrivelled, deeper colour, but may be swollen and pale; may have a few cleft-like irregular purple dots, "Maurer's dots"
Schizonts (stained preparations) .	Large, mulberry-like; about same size as red cell; 12-25 oval merozoites	Small, "daisy-head"-like; smaller than red cell; 6-16 round merozoites	Small; segmentation irregular; 8-32 (usually 12) very small merozoites; *rarely seen in peripheral blood*
Gametocytes .	Rounded; macro-gametocyte about one and a half times the size of red cell	Rounded; about the same size as red cell or smaller	Elongated, crescentic or sausage-shaped

These gametocytes remain unchanged in the blood until it is withdrawn from the body, *e.g.* by the mosquito or when a drop is exposed to air and transferred to a warm stage for microscopic observation. In the stomach of the mosquito the following changes occur. The gametocytes of the crescent type become rounded. The female gametocytes undergo "maturation" by the formation of one or two "polar bodies" which contain part of the original nuclear chromatin, and are protruded and detached. The mature macro-gametocyte constitutes the macro-gamete. From the male cell, four to eight flagella-like structures are quickly protruded ("exflagellation"); these are long, slender processes with somewhat enlarged free ends, each containing a chromatin granule derived from the parent nucleus, and are the micro-gametes; they are ultimately detached, and move with a kind of lashing motility. A micro- and a macro-gamete unite to form the zygote which develops movement (oökinete), elongates slightly and penetrates the stomach wall, embedding itself under the outer layer or between muscle fibres; it becomes spheroidal, forms an encysting membrane (oöcyst) and increases in size until it projects into the body cavity; division into rounded sporoblasts (or sporoblastoids) occurs, and these divide again into the spindle-shaped sporozoites, thousands of which are formed from the original oöcyst. The cyst ultimately ruptures and the sporozoites are set free in the body cavity and settle in the salivary gland, from which they are injected with the salivary secretion when the insect bites. This phase in the life history is that of sporogony (as contrasted with asexual schizogony in the human subject) and takes seven to ten days under favourable temperature conditions.

Plasmodium ovale resembles *Plasmodium malariae*, but the erythrocytes are often markedly enlarged, oval in shape, show an irregular outline, and exhibit to a marked degree stippling (Schüffner's dots) as seen in the benign tertian form of malaria. The schizont comprises six to twelve merozoites. The illness is tertian in periodicity. The infection has been transmitted experimentally by the bite of *Anopheles maculipennis*.

Certain other supposed sub-species of *Plasmodium* have also been described.

Laboratory diagnosis

It cannot be too strongly stressed that in the early stages of a primary attack of malaria, particularly malignant tertian infection, the clinical picture is quite unlike that classically associated with malaria; it may simulate any other febrile disease. Meticulous care in the preparation and staining of blood smears is important if scanty or delicate trophozoites are not to be missed with serious consequences to the patient.

Thin Blood Films.—Two or three films are made on microscope slides or ¾-in. square No. 1 coverslips, which have been carefully cleansed and polished with a smooth cloth. Slides are generally preferred for the purpose as they are more easily handled than coverslips, though with skill better blood films can be made on coverslips.

Films on Slides.—The blood is obtained by puncturing the lobe of the ear, or the finger close to the base of the nail. The needle is sterilised by flaming or by some other efficient process and the area to be punctured is cleansed with 70 per cent. alcohol or 90 per cent. isopropyl alcohol. Touch the exuding drop of blood with the surface of a slide close to one end; place the narrow edge of a second slide, kept at an angle of 45°, on the drop of blood and allow the blood to spread out across the slide in this angle before drawing out the film; now spread the blood uniformly on the slide in the form of a thin film (see Fig. 33).

Films on Coverslips.—Touch the drop of blood (obtained as above) with the surface of a coverslip held by the edges between the thumb and first finger of one hand, and place a second coverslip over the first so that the drop spreads out between them. Then, at once, take the second slip by the edges between the thumb and forefinger of the other hand, and slide the two apart without exerting pressure.

The films are allowed to dry, and are then fixed and stained with Leishman's stain. They are mounted and examined, first with a dry $\frac{1}{6}$-in. lens, and later with the oil-immersion objective. In searching for crescents it is advisable to use the former. The $\frac{1}{7}$-in. oil-immersion lens is particularly useful for this purpose.

It is essential that the film should be well stained; otherwise it is useless searching for the parasite. A valuable guide is the staining of the leucocytes in the film; if this is satisfactory, malaria parasites should be detectable.

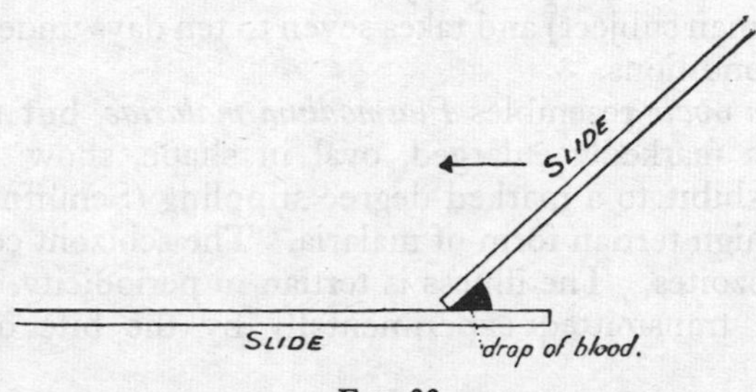

FIG. 33

Thick Blood Films.—As a routine measure, and especially when the organisms are likely to be scanty, thick films should be prepared and examined. A large drop of blood is deposited on a slide, and spread with the head of a pin in the form of a thick film about $\frac{3}{4}$ in. in diameter, the density being such that the hands of a watch can just be seen through the film; it is thoroughly dried, *e.g.* in the incubator. The unfixed film can be stained by Field's stain (p. 669) or for thirty minutes in Leishman's stain diluted one part in twenty with distilled water buffered at pH 7·2. Dilute Giemsa's stain may also be used. Alternatively the haemoglobin is removed by treating with acid-alcohol (alcohol 50 ml., hydrochloric acid 10 drops) or a mixture of 4 parts of 2·5 per cent. glacial acetic acid in distilled water and 1 part of 2 per cent. crystalline tartaric acid in distilled water, and then washing in water. The film can now be stained by Leishman's or Giemsa's stains.

Fresh Preparations of Blood.—A drop of blood is deposited on a slide, covered with a coverslip, and the edges of the glass are smeared with vaseline to prevent drying of the film. A warm-stage apparatus should be used during the microscopic examination.

Only stained films are examined as a rule in routine work. They should, if possible, be taken during the pyrexia and no anti-malarial drugs should have been administered beforehand. The organisms can be recognised by their various characteristic appearances, and it is possible to determine the species or type present (see p. 534). It must be remembered, however, that the young trophozoites of the three types may be almost indistinguishable from one another, and if only young forms are present in the film, it may be difficult to determine the species. To inexperienced workers, artificial appearances may sometimes simulate malaria parasites, and a blood platelet overlying a red corpuscle may be mistaken for a young form of the plasmodium. In some cases prolonged search may be required. It is advisable, in searching thin films for scanty malaria organisms, to examine particularly the edges of the film; parasites may be more numerous there than in the centre. The thick-film method greatly facilitates the detection of the parasite. The absence of parasites during an apyrexial interval by no means excludes malaria and repeated examination of films may be required before the diagnosis can be established.

Malaria organisms can sometimes be detected in *films from bone marrow aspirated by sternal puncture*, and in some cases this method may be used for diagnostic purposes.

For further reading see Shute & Maryon (1960).

BABESIAE (or PIROPLASMS)

These protozoal organisms (classified with the Sporozoa) produce disease in various domestic animals, but are not known to infect the human subject.

They invade red blood corpuscles like the malaria plasmodia, and multiple infection of these cells is characteristic. The individual organisms are generally pyriform bodies about 2 μ to 4 μ in length, containing a well-defined chromatin structure. The central part of the organism often stains less deeply than the periphery, and ring-forms like those of the malaria parasite may be observed. Some species show small rod-shaped forms. Multiplication occurs by binary fission, and pairs of individuals partially attached to one another may be seen inside the red cells. For microscopic demonstration, blood films are stained by a Romanowsky stain, *e.g.* Leishman's or Giemsa's. These organisms are usually transmitted by ticks, of which the eggs may become infected. For detailed information regarding the biology and life-cycle of these organisms, one of the works on protozoology should be consulted.

Babesia bigemina causes Red Water fever of cattle, *Babesia canis* Biliary fever in dogs and *Babesia* (or *Theileria*) *parva* East African Coast fever in cattle.

TRYPANOSOMES

Protozoa of the class Mastigophora. Infection with these organisms is designated by the general term Trypanosomiasis.

Three species which are pathogenic to man have been described: *Trypanosoma gambiense* and *Trypanosoma rhodesiense* of African Sleeping Sickness, and *Trypanosoma cruzi* of Brazilian trypanosomiasis (Chagas' disease). It is doubtful whether the first two are separate species. The last-named is sometimes classified in a separate genus, *Schizotrypanum.*

The organisms of African trypanosomiasis are transmitted by the tsetse fly (*Glossina spp.*), and the disease is limited to areas where the vector occurs, between about 15° N. and 25° S. During development of the disease the patient has febrile periods before becoming apathetic and sleepy by day (sleeping sickness). Without treatment paralysis develops later and the patient dies. There are clinical differences between typical cases of East African trypanosomiasis (*T. rhodesiense*) and those of West African disease (*T. gambiense*) but frequently the demarcation is not clear cut.

The flies bite mainly during the daylight hours: after inoculation of the parasites there is local multiplication and sometimes irritation but this often passes unnoticed and the trypanosomes invade the blood. They may be seen by microscopic examination of the blood at this stage in infections due to *T. rhodesiense* but very rarely when *T. gambiense* is responsible; in the latter infection adenitis is more common and examination of gland juice obtained by needle puncture will reveal the trypanosomes. In both forms of sleeping sickness the central nervous system is involved, within a few weeks in *T. rhodesiense* infections and after 6 months or more in *T. gambiense* infections. Changes in the cerebrospinal fluid occur and demonstration of the trypanosomes may be possible. Diagnosis may be obscured by insufficient treatment or chemoprophylaxis.

The trypanosome has a definite cycle of development in both human and insect hosts. The cycle in the tsetse fly follows ingestion of the trypanosomal (blood) form from a human host and leads to the development of the *metacyclic* form in the salivary glands rendering the saliva infective for new hosts by inoculation into the wound when the insect bites. There is a definite barrier to development in the fly and the percentage in which the trypanosome succeeds in establishing itself is low. Prevention is possible by the local destruction of the tsetse fly in areas where it is known to occur.

Infection with *Trypanosoma cruzi* occurs in parts of Central and South America. This organism develops in the hind-gut of the insect vector (winged bugs) and is transmitted by their droppings being deposited on mucous membranes—*e.g.* the conjunctivae. Young children are most frequently infected and the disease is seen in the acute form with fever, adenitis, progressive anaemia and a characteristic oedema of one eye. In the chronic form cardiac symptoms predominate because of a parasitic myocarditis. The trypanosome is readily found in the blood in the early stages, but disappears as the disease becomes chronic and penetrates tissue cells where it assumes a leishmanial form ($1{\cdot}5 \times 4\ \mu$) and forms cyst-like agglomerations.

Trypanosoma gambiense

Biological Characters.—This organism is an elongated, sinuous, fusiform structure, 12–40 μ long by 1·5–3 μ broad, with a longitudinal undulating membrane, and a flagellum projecting from one end. It is motile and, in moving, the flagellum is anterior. In stained preparations two nuclear structures are noted, the larger or trophonucleus situated about the middle of the organism, and the smaller micro- or kinetonucleus (or kinetoplast) at the posterior end. The latter stains deeply and is surrounded by an unstained halo. Two constituent structures have been distinguished in the kinetoplast: a granule (blepharoplast) from which the axoneme arises (*vide infra*) and the "parabasal" body. Chromatin-like granules are seen in the protoplasm independently of the nuclei. From the blepharoplast arises a filament, the axoneme, which forms the free edge of the undulating membrane and is continued into the flagellum, forming its central core. This structure stains like chromatin. Morphological variation (polymorphism) is noted among individual organisms, some being relatively long and slender with long "free" flagella, other shorter and broader and with a short flagellum or lacking a free flagellum (Fig. 34). Intermediate forms are also observed.

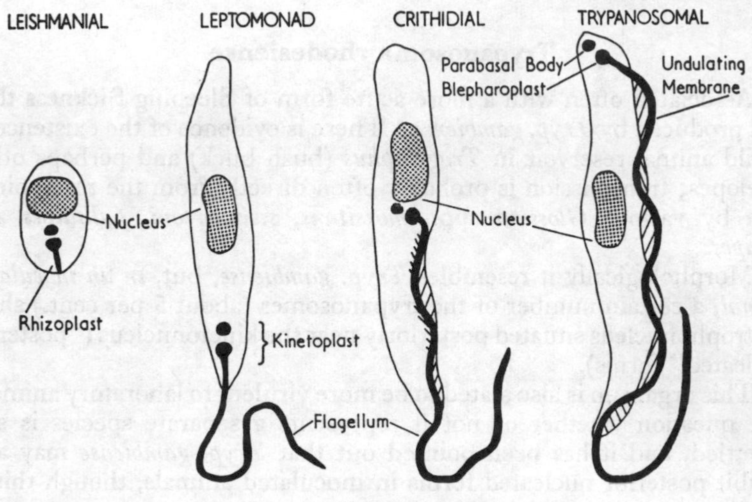

FIG. 34
Forms of Trypanosomidae.

Multiplication is by longitudinal fission.

Cultivation of trypanosomes. See Chapter 47.

Pathogenesis.—The infection is transmitted mainly by *Glossina palpalis* and by *G. tachinoides*; possibly wild animals are reservoirs of infection but transmission is largely from man to man. Shortly after blood from an infected person is ingested by the insect, transmission is possible in a mechanical fashion. A later stage of infectivity occurs after about 20 days; the trypanosomes have multiplied in the intestine and passed to the proventriculus, the salivary gland and proboscis. Multiplying in the insect, the organism may show considerable change of form. Crithidial forms, in which the kinetoplast is anterior to the nucleus, occur. From these crithidia in the salivary gland the so-called "metacyclic" forms develop, *i.e.* resembling the short and broad trypanosomes seen in the blood (*vide supra*). The fly does not become infective until the metacyclic forms are present in the salivary gland.

In man fever may develop within a few weeks of infection or may be long delayed; trypanosomes may be so scanty in the blood as to be very difficult to find. The superficial lymph glands, *e.g.* posterior cervical, become enlarged, and trypanosomes can be demonstrated by puncture and aspiration with a syringe. In the advanced stages of the disease, when the characteristic lethargy has developed, the parasites can be detected in the cerebrospinal fluid.

Monkeys injected with infective material develop a disease which is more or less similar to human trypanosomiasis.

Guinea-pigs can be infected, and trypanosomes appear in considerable numbers in the blood, but the infection is either unassociated with any obvious pathological condition, or the resulting disease is very chronic in its course.

Trypanosoma rhodesiense

Associated often with a more acute form of Sleeping Sickness than that produced by *Tryp. gambiense.* There is evidence of the existence of a wild animal reservoir in *Tragelaphus* (bush buck) and perhaps other antelopes; transmission is probably often directly from the reservoir to man by various *Glossina* spp., *morsitans*, *swinnertoni*, *pallidipes* and *fuscipes*.

Morphologically it resembles *Tryp. gambiense*, but, *in an inoculated animal*, a certain number of the trypanosomes (about 5 per cent.) show the trophonucleus situated posteriorly near the kinetonucleus ("posterior nucleated" forms).

This organism is also stated to be more virulent to laboratory animals. The question whether or not it represents a separate species is still unsettled, and it has been pointed out that *Tryp. gambiense* may also exhibit posterior nucleated forms in inoculated animals, though this is infrequent.

It has been supposed that this organism may be identical with *Tryp. brucei*, the organism of Nagana, but it has been shown by inoculation of man that *Tryp. brucei* is not pathogenic to the human subject.

Trypanosoma (or Schizotrypanum) cruzi

The cause of human trypanosomiasis in Brazil (Chagas' disease).

Its first development after infection occurs in the endothelial and tissue cells of internal organs, in the muscles and in the heart wall. It is non-flagellate at first, and resembles *Leishmania* (*vide infra*). It may, however, appear in the blood as a typical flagellate trypanosome with a very prominent kinetonucleus.

Certain other vertebrate hosts harbour the organism, *e.g.* the armadillo and opossum.

It is transmitted by Reduviid bugs, e.g. *Panstrongylus megistus* (syn. *Conorhinus megistus*). These bugs are readily infected experimentally, unlike *Glossina* flies with African trypanosomes, and may be used in laboratory diagnosis of *Tryp. cruzi* infections by allowing them to feed on suspect cases, and recovering the trypanosome from their droppings (xenodiagnosis).

Various laboratory animals are susceptible to experimental inoculation, *e.g.* guinea-pigs, white rats, monkeys.

Laboratory Diagnosis

Examination of the Primary Lesion.—This is of no great practical value as the lesion is not often noticed, but if it is, fluid from it may be examined for trypanosomes as detailed below.

Microscopic Examination of the Peripheral Blood.—As trypanosomes are scanty in the early stages and especially in *Tryp. gambiense* infections "thick films" are prepared and stained by Leishman's stain as in malaria diagnosis (*q.v.*). Unstained ("wet") preparations of the blood may be examined with advantage.

A method of concentrating trypanosomes in the blood has been applied as follows: 5–10 ml. of blood are withdrawn from a vein into 20 ml. of 1 per cent. sodium citrate solution, and the mixture is centrifuged for about ten minutes; the plasma and the leucocyte layer on the surface of the blood sediment are withdrawn and re-centrifuged; this is repeated two or three times; the deposit is examined, in the form of fresh preparations and stained films, after each centrifuging.

Examination of Gland Juice.—If superficial lymph glands are enlarged, puncture and aspiration with a syringe may be carried out, and the "juice" examined microscopically. The syringe should be perfectly dry if this procedure is to be successful.

Examination of the CSF—In the lethargic state, 10 ml. of cerebrospinal fluid are withdrawn, and centrifuged for 15–20 min.; the deposit is then examined either in the form of a fresh preparation under a coverslip ringed with nail varnish, or in stained films.

Animal Inoculation.—Blood, gland "juice" or an emulsion of an excised gland injected into a guinea-pig may yield a positive diagnosis where other methods fail. The blood of the animal is examined, in fresh preparations of stained films, at daily intervals after the inoculation.

Culture.—Material obtained as for animal inoculation may be cultured in suitable media such as NNN medium.

Trypanosomiasis of Animals

Trypanosome infections occur in a variety of animals. Different species of trypanosomes are recognised. These have the general characters of the genus as described in the case of *Tryp. gambiense*, but show variations in certain of their characters.

Tryp. brucei is the organism of Nagana or Tsetse Fly Disease occurring in horses, other equidae, dogs and cattle in Africa; it is transmitted by *Glossina morsitans* and certain other species of *Glossina.* It is sluggish in movement and corresponds in its morphology with *Tryp. rhodesiense* (*vide supra*), showing posterior nucleated forms.

Tryp. vivax, so called in virtue of its active movement, and *Tryp. congolense* produce infections in domesticated animals in Africa and are transmitted by tsetse flies. *Tryp. vivax* possesses a "free" flagellum. *Tryp. congolense* is a smaller organism (9–18 μ long) and has no free flagellum.

Tryp. equinum is the organism of Mal de Caderas, a South American disease of horses. A feature of the organism is the inconspicuous kinetonucleus which stains feebly.

Tryp. evansi is the organism of Surra affecting domesticated animals (including camels) in various parts of the world. It is actively motile, with a free flagellum and a blunt posterior end. It is conveyed mechanically by *Stomoxys* and Tabanid flies.

Tryp. equiperdum occurs in horses, producing the disease known as Dourine; the infection is transmitted by coitus. The organism shows a free flagellum and is very similar to *Tryp. evansi.*

Tryp. lewisi is an exceedingly common blood parasite of rats, and is world-wide in distribution. It is an actively motile, narrow trypanosome, with a pointed posterior end and anteriorly a free flagellum. The kinetonucleus is rod-shaped and stains deeply. It produces little disturbance in the health of the host. Infection is transmitted by rat fleas.

Tryp. theileri occurs in cattle in South Africa. It is unusually large (25–70 μ in length). The flagellum is free. It is possibly transmitted by a Tabanid fly. The pathogenicity of this organism is doubtful.

For further details of the pathogenic trypanosomes see Wenyon (1926) and Faust & Russell (1964).

LEISHMANIAE

These are pathogenic protozoa with certain biological relationships to the trypanosomes. They are parasitic in man, dogs and a number of wild animals. Sandflies are intermediate hosts and vectors. There are complex relationships between host, parasite, vector and environment producing a varied epidemiological picture. In man leishmaniasis is either (*a*) *Visceral* (*Kala Azar*), due to *Leishmania donovani* occurring predominantly in children in North Africa, and in both children and adults in parts of East Africa, the Indian sub-continent and the Far East, or (*b*) *Cutaneous* (*Oriental sore* or *Tropical sore*), due to *Leishmania tropica* which predominates in the Near and Middle East, and *Muco-cutaneous* (*Espundia* or *Uta*) due to *Leishmania brasiliensis* in South America.

Leishmania donovani

Visceral leishmaniasis (*Kala Azar*) is a disease with a lengthy incubation period, insidious onset and a chronic course with much involvement of the reticulo-endothelial system as shown by leucopenia, anaemia and enlargement of the spleen and liver. The mortality of the fully developed disease is high but the use of residual insecticides in recent years has much reduced the incidence. Transmission of the disease is by the sand-fly (*Phlebotomus* spp.). Hot and moist conditions, such as are found along great rivers in south Asia favour the vector and a crowded population ensures spread of the disease which in the past periodically assumed epidemic proportions.

When the insect ingests infected blood the organisms become transformed to leptomonads in the gut of the vector and undergo multiplication, ultimately migrating to the buccal cavity from which they are inoculated when the insect bites another person.

Leishmania donovani is typically intracellular in the tissues, situated in the endothelial cells of the spleen, liver, bone marrow and lymphatic glands. It may also be found, though infrequently, in large mononuclear cells in the peripheral blood. One endothelial cell may contain a considerable number of organisms.

In morphology it is a round or oval organism about 2–5 μ in its longest diameter. Sometimes in films from the blood in the spleen and bone marrow, torpedo-shaped forms are seen.

Stained with a Romanowsky stain, two nuclear structures are observed, one large and rounded (macronucleus), and the other small, deeply staining, and rod-shaped (kinetoplast). As in the trypanosomes, this latter structure consists of a parabasal body and a prolongation corresponding to the axoneme (rhizoplast). The protoplasm may be vacuolated (*vide supra*). The organism multiplies by binary fission.

Cultures can be obtained from the spleen on NNN medium incubated at 20°–24° C. In culture the organisms increase in size and elongate; the kinetoplast becomes situated at one end, and from it a flagellum arises. No undulating membrane develops. Thus, *Leishmania* in culture assumes the biological characters of a leptomonad.

Monkeys and dogs can be infected experimentally. The Chinese hamster (*Cricetulus griseus*) is susceptible to inoculation and has been used for experimental studies.

In certain parts of the world human leishmaniasis is associated with the same infection among dogs which may act as reservoirs of the disease.

Laboratory Diagnosis

Gland Puncture.—Gland "juice" is aspirated from the inguinal or femoral lymphatic glands; films are made and stained with Leishman's stain as in malaria diagnosis. This method gives excellent results in a large proportion of cases and is without risk to the patient.

Bone-marrow Aspiration (from the sternum or tibia).—Films are prepared from the marrow and stained as above.

Spleen Puncture.—Fluid is aspirated from the enlarged spleen with a fine hypodermic needle attached to a dry syringe and films are prepared as above. The procedure is not without risk in inexperienced hands and liver puncture is preferred.

Culture.—Aspirated spleen, bone marrow, or gland "juice" is cultured on NNN medium.

Blood Films (*Thick*).—These are prepared as in malaria diagnosis. This method is sometimes successful, especially in India, but is too unreliable for routine diagnosis.

Any one of the above methods may be negative while others are positive and, for tests of cure, as well as diagnosis, it is therefore advisable to use more than one method.

Experimental inoculation—in monkeys or hamsters—with the material obtained by spleen, gland, liver or bone-marrow puncture, though of value for experimental work cannot be regarded as a practical method for routine purposes.

Leucopenia is invariable in uncomplicated kala-azar and there is a relative lymphocytosis.

The *aldehyde reaction* has also been used in the diagnosis of the disease. For this purpose about 5 ml. of blood are withdrawn and allowed to clot. The serum is separated and to 1 ml. are added 2 drops of commercial formalin. A positive reaction is indicated by an immediate opacity, followed within thirty minutes by the development of a firm white gelatinous coagulum (like boiled egg albumin); mere jellification is not accepted as a positive result. This method is commonly used in India, but it has been found unreliable in the diagnosis of kala-azar in other countries.

The *complement-fixation test* is sometimes of definite value; the antigen can be prepared from cultures of the organism.

Leishmania tropica

In cutaneous leishmaniasis there are single or multiple indolent ulcers on exposed surfaces of the body; there is no systemic involvement and the infection spontaneously disappears in a few years leaving disfiguring scars.

The parasite is found in a wide variety of mammals which act as reservoirs of human infection which is more common among children.

This organism is similar to *Leishmania donovani* and shows the same intracellular distribution. Besides the characteristic oval forms, elongated organisms may be noted. In culture on NNN medium leptomonas forms develop as in the case of *Leishmania donovani*. Monkeys and dogs can be infected experimentally. Transmission is probably by *Phlebotomus papatasii* and *Phlebotomus sergenti*.

Diagnosis.—Films are made from the scrapings from the sore (preferably at the margin) after carefully cleansing the surface and removing the surface discharge. They are stained with Leishman's stain.

Leishmania brasiliensis

South American muco-cutaneous leishmaniasis (Uta, Espundia or Forest yaws) is a chronic ulceration of exposed parts of the body and secondary ulceration may occur in mucosae of the mouth and upper respiratory tract. The disease is mainly contracted in low-lying forest regions by adult males since they are more frequently exposed.

The organism is morphologically indistinguishable from *L. donovani* but is antigenically distinct. It is found in the edges of the early cutaneous ulcers but is later scanty, and also in the regional lymph nodes draining the ulcer. The mucosal lesions are secondary to blood spread and the parasite can usually be seen in preparations made by scratching the intact mucosa around the lesion.

Montenegro's test is a skin test in which 0·1 ml. of a suspension of a culture of *L. brasiliensis* is injected intradermally. Infected cases give a reaction in 48–72 hours. Alternatively a polysaccharide antigen isolated from the organism may be used.

THE INTESTINAL PROTOZOA

Entamoeba histolytica

Of half a dozen species of amoebae found in the human alimentary tract only one is pathogenic, namely *Entamoeba histolytica*, the causative organism of amoebiasis. This disease varies from a mild colic to acute dysentery with necrosis and ulceration of the large bowel, the passage of blood and mucus in the stool and occasionally perforation. Metastatic complications after lymphatic and blood stream invasion may follow with the formation of amoebic abscesses in the liver, brain and lungs. In contrast to bacillary dysentery the incubation period is measurable in weeks rather than days; the onset of symptoms is usually more gradual and the character of the stools differs from those of bacillary dysentery.

Biological Characters.—The two "types" or races of amoeba are the small (average size 9–15 μ) and the large (average size 18–30 μ). The vegetative forms are rounded, elongated or irregular amoebae. The cytoplasm consists of a clear hyaline ectoplasm, and a granular, often vacuolated endoplasm, but this differentiation is not always readily observed. In their most active condition the amoebae show flowing movements of their protoplasm and rapidly protrude and retract pseudopodia, which may be composed at first mostly of ectoplasm. These movements lead to changes in shape and also to active progression, often likened to the motion of a snail. The nucleus is round or oval, and in the unstained condition is not easily distinguished. It is situated in the endoplasm, usually excentric in position. It is poor in chromatin, and the nuclear membrane is thin. The chromatin granules are small, and are collected in a ring just inside the nuclear membrane. The nucleus shows a small central karyosome. The amoebae ingest red corpuscles, leucocytes and tissue cells, which are observed in the endoplasm, but ingested bacteria are less frequently found. The ingested erythrocytes appear smaller than normal. The vegetative forms after leaving the body tend to become rounded and immobile, and soon die and disintegrate. Multiplication is by mitotic binary fission.

Under certain conditions encystment occurs. Cysts are spherical, with a thin, hyaline, refractile cyst wall, which gives them a distinct double contour. The contents are finely granular. The average diameter is 6–11 μ for the small race and 11–18 μ for the large. The cysts usually contain multiple nuclei, *not more than four*, a glycogen mass, and also thick rod-shaped or oval structures which stain deeply with haematoxylin and are called "chromatoid bodies" or "chromidial bars" (see Fig. 35).

The cysts are developed by division of the vegetative form into smaller and rounded "precystic" forms.

The newly formed cyst has only one nucleus, which later divides into two, with further division to four. The glycogen mass is best seen in young cysts, staining brown with iodine, but is apparently used up as the cyst matures. In unstained preparations the chromatoid bodies appear as refractile structures.

Methods of microscopic demonstration and staining are referred to under dysentery diagnosis.

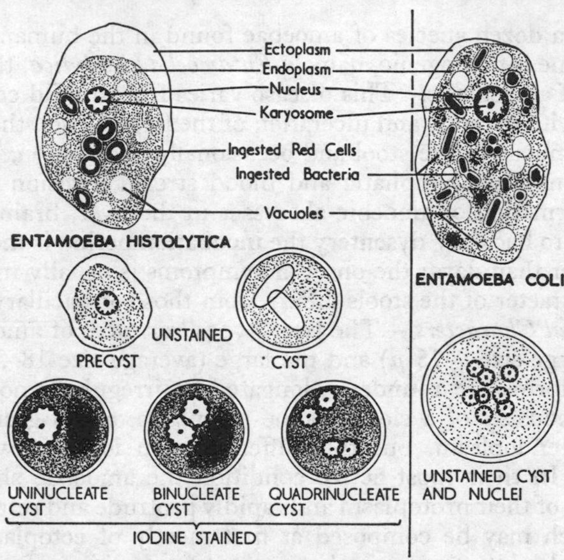

FIG. 35

Stages in the development of *Entamoeba histolytica* and *Entamoeba coli*.

Pathogenesis.—In the early stage of amoebic dysentery the vegetative forms are present in considerable numbers in the large intestine and in the stools. They penetrate the mucosa of the large bowel and disintegrate the tissue by their pseudopodia and possibly also by means of a liquefying ferment. The submucosa is invaded, and, occasionally, small veins are penetrated from which the amoebae may be carried to the liver. In the bowel, oval or irregular ulcers are developed with undermined edges, which may sometimes lead to perforation of the bowel wall with resulting peritonitis. Other complications are stricture, intussusception and fistulae. Unless secondary infection occurs there is little inflammatory reaction (cf. bacillary dysentery). Invasion of the liver occurs through the portal circulation and results in lobular necrosis of the liver with abscess formation ("tropical abscess"), which may extend into the peritoneal or pleural cavities or into lung. The abscess contains a slimy chocolate coloured pus consisting of necrotic tissue and altered blood with relatively few leucocytes or pus cells. The amoebae are found mainly in the wall of the abscess and may not be seen in the pus when it is first evacuated; no cysts are found in these tissues.

Cysts may be detected in the stools, often in large numbers, either in chronic cases or asymptomatic carriers. After apparent recovery a patient may remain a carrier. The cyst represents a resting phase with increased powers of resistance to survive outside of the body and is the form in which the organism is transmitted from person to person, although it is possible in rare instances that immediate ingestion of food or drink contaminated with fresh amoebae could cause infection.

Epidemiology.—*Entamoeba histolytica* is found in the intestine of man and a number of other mammals, the most important of which are the monkey (many species) and the rat (*Rattus norvegicus*). The life-cycle is relatively simple alternating between trophozoites and cystic forms, only the latter being of importance in the spread of infection as the trophozoite is highly sensitive to environmental influences outside of the host, especially oxidation and drying. The cysts are discharged with the stools but only those in the quadrinucleate state are infective when swallowed by new hosts. Those that pass the hazard of the gastric juices hatch in the small and large intestine to form trophozoites. In the majority of individuals so affected the trophozoites remain free-living in the lumen of the intestine and it is from these that cysts are formed in the largest numbers, up to 50,000,000 a day. Such large numbers may however alternate with small numbers so that they may be difficult to demonstrate. The cysts are viable outside the body, provided they are kept moist, for several weeks in faeces at room temperature and for several months in water and sewage at low temperatures. Most modern sewage schemes will kill cysts but cesspools will not.

The most important sources of the cyst are chronic cases or asymptomatic carriers of the protozoa since in the acute tissue invasive stage cysts are not formed. Such persons are found widely distributed in tropical, sub-tropical and temperate regions though their numbers vary with the sanitary conditions of the community. Thus in underdeveloped areas 50 per cent. or more of persons may harbour the organism whilst in the United Kingdom the figure is less than 5 per cent. Amoebiasis however is confined to tropical and sub-tropical regions so that factors promoting invasiveness of the parasites must be peculiar to these areas. Thus the state of nutrition of the host and his resistance may be of importance though there is little clear evidence of any relationship between these and the prevalence of the disease. Foreigners, especially Europeans, entering an endemic area of dysentery are highly susceptible to infection. The qualitative nature of the diet may be important since communities having a high starch diet may have high carrier rates but a low incidence of clinical disease.

Thus it is becoming increasingly clear that *Ent. histolytica* exists in both commensal and pathogenic forms. This difference may be correlated with size so that small amoebae are believed to be non-pathogenic and some, though not all, of the large ones pathogenic. Whether non-pathogenic commensal forms become pathogenic or are entirely different strains is unknown (Hoare & Neal, 1955). The amoebae from cases of amoebic dysentery are invasive whilst those from healthy carriers are not. These "carrier" strains cannot be enhanced in virulence although attenuated virulent strains may be restored in virulence by passage. It has been maintained that the associated bacterial flora of the gut plays a part in invasion of the tissues by amoebae otherwise not invasive and this is substantiated by the beneficial effects of antibacterial antibiotics in the treatment of intestinal amoebiasis, and the necessity of the presence of bacteria in cultivating amoebae under laboratory conditions.

Prophylaxis.—This involves the enforcement of good general sanitation and personal hygiene in the community. Water supplies must be efficiently filtered and faeces disposed of so that water and food cannot be contaminated. The preparation of food must be carefully supervised so that wherever possible it is cooked, and special attention paid to vegetables and salads which may have been cultivated on contaminated soil. Food-handlers must be regularly examined for intestinal infection and hand-washing after defaecation strictly enforced.

Cases of dysentery may be isolated but as they are not highly infective in the acute phase it is more important to ensure that they are thoroughly treated to prevent chronic disease and the development of the carrier state. Carriers when diagnosed may be treated with antibiotic drugs, *e.g.* tetracyclines.

Laboratory Diagnosis of Amoebic Dysentery

Collection of Specimens of Stools.—The stool should be examined as soon as possible after being passed and while still warm. This is most successfully done by looking at the freshly passed stool in a bed-pan and selecting for examination a portion that looks suspicious such as blood-stained mucus which is characteristic of the acute stage of the infection. Alternatively the specimen, unmixed with urine, may be collected in a faeces specimen tube provided with a cork carrying a metal spoon or scoop which fits into the tube, and by means of which faecal matter may be collected. A satisfactory alternative is the Universal container.

Swabs taken directly from the ulcers in the colon or fragments of tissue from the edge of the ulcer taken during sigmoidoscopy offer the best chance of finding the amoebae in chronic cases.

Microscopic Examination.—This requires care and considerable experience for reliable results. A microscope slide is gently warmed over the Bunsen flame, and on the middle of one half of the slide a large drop of normal saline solution is placed and, on the other, a drop of Lugol's iodine. A loopful of the mucous discharge or the stool is emulsified in the saline drop and another loopful in the iodine solution. (A preparation in 1 per cent. watery eosin also assists in the detection of protozoa.) If specks of blood-stained mucus are observed in the specimen, these should be examined. The preparations are covered with No. 1 cover-slips, and examined first with the low-power objective and then with the $\frac{2}{3}$-in. and, if necessary, the oil-immersion lens. It is advantageous to use a "warm stage" attached to the microscope in examining fresh preparations for amoebae (Chapter 44). Phase-contrast microscopy is specially applicable for demonstrating cytological features of the protozoa.

Vegetative amoebae can usually be recognised without difficulty. In the saline preparations *Entamoeba histolytica* may often be identified by its active characteristic, amoeboid movement and the inclusion in the cytoplasm of numerous red corpuscles. On the other hand, immobile vegetative amoebae without ingested corpuscles present considerable difficulty in their identification. Large phagocytic cells (macrophages) may be found in dysenteric stools, and may be mistaken for immobile amoebae by inexperienced workers. They often show vacuolation, and may even contain red corpuscles. They are practically immobile, and the nucleus, unless degenerate, occupying one-fourth or one-fifth of the whole cell, is definitely larger than that of an amoeba, and is not of the ring-like or "vesicular" type. This distinction is seen in the iodine preparation. In a heat-fixed film these macrophage cells and their nuclei can be stained with methylene blue, while amoebae cannot thus be demonstrated.

The differences in the morphology of protozoal cysts as seen in iodine-stained preparations makes it possible to diagnose amoebic dysentery in the absence of motile amoebae. It must, however, be emphasised that considerable experience is necessary before the laboratory worker can distinguish pathogenic from non-pathogenic cysts, and that it is often a difficult matter to make this diagnosis with certainty.

Where pathogenic amoebae cannot be detected, the microscopic examination of a wet film of the faeces often yields information of diagnostic importance. In a case of bacillary infection there is usually an abundant and characteristic cellular exudate. The cells present are mostly polymorph leucocytes with a varying number of red cells, and in the early stages, numerous epithelial cells. In addition to these, macrophages are frequently a characteristic feature of the exudate. The leucocytes, as a rule, show marked degeneration.

In amoebic dysentery there are few leucocytes unless the case is complicated by bacterial infection. Other characters of the amoebic exudate are pyknotic bodies, sloughed mucosal cells, altered erythrocytes, eosinophils, goblet cells and Charcot-Leyden crystals.

This microscopic examination is therefore an important step in diagnosis: the finding of the characteristic *Ent. histolytica* establishes a diagnosis of amoebic dysentery, while an abundant cell exudate and the absence of amoebae would indicate bacillary dysentery.

This provisional diagnosis enables a report to be made at once as to the nature of the dysentery, so that treatment can be initiated without delay.

Where no amoebae can be found, and if a diagnosis of bacillary dysentery cannot be established, it is essential that further microscopic examinations be carried out before amoebic infection is excluded.

Demonstration of Amoebic Cysts by the Flotation Method (Faust *et al.*, 1939).—A dense, but finely divided, watery suspension of faeces is prepared in a mortar and then strained through previously wetted wire gauze. The suspension is centrifuged for five minutes at 2000 to 3000 r.p.m. in a conical tube. The contents of the tube except the lowest inch of deposit are discarded and to the residue, zinc sulphate solution of sp. gr. 1·25 is added in fractions, thorough mixing being effected by stirring with a glass rod. The mixture is finally centrifuged for three minutes. At this stage the cysts float to the surface and are concentrated there. A loopful of the surface scum is removed and mixed on a slide with a loopful of Lugol's iodine, a cover-slip is superimposed and the preparation is examined microscopically.

Stained preparations are of assistance in the identification of intestinal amoebae. Films are made on cover-slips from the stool and are fixed "wet" by floating the cover-slips (film downwards) in a fixing solution consisting of 2 parts saturated perchloride of mercury in saline, with 1 part absolute alcohol. They are then stained with iron-haematoxylin.

An alternative method is that of Dobell, in which the preparation is mordanted with ammonium molybdate and then stained with an aqueous solution of haematoxylin.

Serological Diagnosis.—Complement-fixation tests can occasionally be of value in the diagnosis of extra-intestinal amoebiasis but the sera of many patients tends to be anti-complementary and the test is difficult to perform and interpret. The antigen, from *Ent. histolytica* must be satisfactorily prepared and the possibility of there being strains of differing antigenic structure indicates the desirability of a polyvalent antigen-preparation.

Cultivation.—*Ent. histolytica* can be cultured artificially by the method of Dobell and Laidlaw or a modification of their method (p. 775).

Non-pathogenic amoebae

Entamoeba coli.—A non-pathogenic intestinal amoeba which, in diagnosis, must be carefully differentiated from *Ent. histolytica.*

The vegetative forms closely resemble those of *Ent. histolytica,* but the cytoplasm is not so distinctly differentiated into endo- and ecto-plasm. The pseudopodia are small and blunt and not so refractile as those of *Ent. histolytica.* The nucleus is usually central in position, easily distinguishable, rich in chromatin which is sometimes arranged in quadrant form, and has a thick, refractile, nuclear membrane. The karyosome is well marked. *Amoeboid movement is negligible or sluggish.* It has been generally agreed that no ingested red cells are seen in the cytoplasm (when this organism is noted in a case of dysentery). It has been pointed out, however, that *in vitro* this organism can ingest red cells as readily as *Ent. histolytica.* Bacteria are ingested often in large numbers. The cysts are larger (15-30 μ) than those of *Ent. histolytica,* the cyst wall is thick, and there may be more than four nuclei, *e.g.* frequently eight. No bar-shaped chromatoid bodies are observed in the fully developed cysts which occur in the faeces.

Endolimax nana.—A frequent non-pathogenic intestinal amoeba. The vegetative form is 10 μ in diameter or less. In unstained preparations the nucleus is not distinct, but when stained by haematoxylin it is easily demonstrated, and shows a large, irregular, excentric karyosome.

The cysts are oval, and about the same size as the vegetative form. They contain one, two or four small nuclei, but no chromatoid bodies.

Iodamoeba bütschlii and Dientamoeba fragilis are also included among the intestinal amoebae of man, but need not be described here. Their characters may be ascertained by reference to works on protozoology (Hoare, 1949).

Entamoeba hartmanii (*Ent. dispar*) resembles the small form of *Ent. histolytica* but is now recognised as a separate non-pathogenic species. Thus amoebae less than 10 μ in size may be either *Ent. hartmanii* or *Ent. histolytica* and this presents considerable diagnostic difficulty to the microscopist. The trophozoites are small 3–10 μ with nuclei a little smaller than those of *Ent. histolytica* but the peripheral chromatin is in discrete masses like that of *Ent. coli*.

Entamoeba gingivalis.—This organism occurs in considerable numbers in pathological conditions of the mouth, *e.g.* pyorrhoea, gingivitis, dental caries, but has no definite aetiological relationship to these conditions. It is about 10–20 μ in diameter and resembles *Ent. histolytica* in many respects, showing active amoeboid movement and differentiation of the cytoplasm into ecto- and endo-plasm; the nucleus is indistinct in unstained preparations; the organism possesses the property of ingesting free cells, *e.g.* leucocytes.

Balantidium coli

Balantidium coli is a ciliated protozoon and is the only member of the class *Ciliophora* pathogenic to man. It can cause ulceration of the intestinal wall with symptoms of colitis, diarrhoea or dysentery (balantidial dysentery). The vegetative form is larger than other human intestinal protozoa measuring 60 by 40 μ. The body is uniformly covered with short cilia and at the anterior end is a groove leading to a mouth opening. There is a nucleus and the cytoplasm contains vacuoles. Encystation occurs with the formation of a thick-walled cyst and the cysts may remain alive for weeks in moist faeces. When swallowed the cyst germinates in the intestine, setting free vegetative ciliates.

Balantidiosis is common among pigs which are the natural host and probably form the source of infection for man. The disease may occur in temperate climes, particularly among persons who come into contact with pigs.

Intestinal Flagellates

These organisms are often associated with dysentery and diarrhoea particularly in the tropics, but their pathogenicity is doubtful, and they may occur as commensals.

Trichomonas hominis.—Is pear-shaped, 9–15 μ long, and shows a nucleus and cytostome. It possesses three to five flagella projecting from the broad end, and also another flagellum forming the border of an undulating membrane and with the free part projecting from the pointed posterior end.

An organism which is biologically similar to *Trich. hominis* may occur in the vagina, and has been named *Trich. vaginalis*. It may be found in cases of vaginitis, and there is a considerable body of evidence in support of its pathogenicity. For recognition of *Trich. vaginalis* and its characteristic jerky movements, "wet" preparations of vaginal secretion should be examined first with low magnification and then with the $\frac{1}{6}$-in. lens of a phase-contrast or dark ground microscope. Dried films stained by Leishman's stain may also be used for diagnostic examination. Its morphological features are similar to those of *Trich. hominis*.

Chilomastix mesnili.—Resembles *Trich. hominis*, but has no undulating membrane and only three flagella. It has an elongated slit-like cytostome. Cysts can easily be recognised; they are oval, about 8 μ in their long diameter, and contain one nucleus.

Giardia (or *Lamblia*) *intestinalis*.—Inhabits the duodenum and jejunum.

Main characters:—somewhat flattened in shape; flat surface pear-shaped; bilaterally symmetrical; 10–18 μ in its long diameter; a large sucking disk, on one surface; two nuclei with karyosomes; two long median parallel axostyles which represent skeletal structures, with blepharoplasts at each end; eight flagella in pairs—two arising from the anterior blepharoplasts (the broad end is spoken of as anterior), two arising near the anterior blepharoplasts but following the axostyles to the posterior edge of the sucker before diverging, two arising at the posterior edge of the sucker and rooted in the axostyles, and two arising from the posterior blepharoplasts.

The cysts are characteristic: oval in shape, about 10–15 μ long, with two or four nuclei (the cyst containing two organisms formed by subdivision); the parallel axostyles are observable.

Giardia intestinalis has been found in the faeces of young children suffering from subacute diarrhoea with bulky offensive stools. Infection occurs particularly in day and residential nurseries and there may be many symptomless carriers. The giardia can be eliminated from the bowels of cases and carriers by treatment with mepacrine (0·1–0·3 g. daily for six days).

For further reading on intestinal protozoa see Wenyon (1926) and Faust & Russell (1964).

Toxoplasma

Human toxoplasmosis is due to infection with *Toxoplasma gondii* a protozoon parasite of many mammals and birds. Human clinical disease is rare. In human congenital toxoplasmosis acute involvement of every organ can occur and may lead to foetal death or malformation at birth, and subsequent encephalitis associated with chorio-retinitis. Post-natal active disease may show with fever and jaundice resembling haemolytic disease of the newborn. Infection acquired after birth is usually mild and, as indicated by antibody studies, is often sub-clinical. If more severe there may be fever, lymphadenopathy and lymphocytosis resembling glandular fever, or exanthematous blood infection with pneumonitis in adults.

The infection in the new-born appears to be derived from the mother *in utero*, the maternal infection being inapparent. In other cases transmission may occur by droplet infection or contact with excreta or infected tissue.

The organism occurs in the form of oval or crescentic bodies, about 6–7 $\mu \times$ 2–4 μ, which are found in endothelial and large mononuclear cells, but also in the free state. With a Romanowsky stain, *e.g.* Giemsa, it shows a reddish nuclear structure and blue cytoplasm. It can be transmitted experimentally to various animals, *e.g.* guinea-pigs, mice and other laboratory rodents. The origin of human infection has not been defined but similar organisms cause natural infections in many animals throughout the world. Strains isolated from human infections display immunological homogeneity.

For diagnosis during life, body fluids may be inoculated into laboratory rodents. The inoculation of material into young mice by the intracerebral *and* intraperitoneal routes at the same time is recommended. A *complement-fixation* test using a toxoplasma-containing material as antigen is available for diagnosis. A *neutralisation* test (Macdonald, 1949) using the chorio-allantoic membrane of the chick embryo has also been found satisfactory. Another laboratory test which has been used in diagnosis is the *cytoplasm-modifying antibody reaction* of Sabin and Feldman. It is based on the fact that the organism when acted on *in vitro* by a specific antibody fails to take up, and stain with, methylene blue. The organisms used in the test are obtained from peritoneal exudate of experimentally inoculated mice. For details of the method and interpretation of the results reference should be made to Sabin & Feldman (1948, 1949), and Beverley & Beattie (1952, 1958).

More recently introduced serological tests include a fluorescence inhibition test (Goldman, 1957), a quantitative direct agglutination test (Fulton & Turk, 1959) using preserved dead parasites, and a simple slide test depending on the flocculation of polymethylmethacrylate particles coated with toxoplasma antigen by serum antibodies (Sim & Lind, 1960). These tests still require to be fully evaluated.

REFERENCES

Beverley, J. K. A. & Beattie, C. P. (1952). Standardisation of dye test for toxoplasmosis. *J. clin. Path.*, **5**, 350.

Beverley, J. K. A. & Beattie, C. P. (1958). Glandular toxoplasmosis. *Lancet*, **2**, 379.

Faust, E. C., & Russell, P. F. (1964). *Craig & Faust's Clinical Parasitology* (7th ed.). London: Kimpton.

Faust, E. C., Sawitz, W., Tobie, J., Odom, V., Peres, C. & Lencicome, D. P. (1939). Comparative efficiency of various techniques for the diagnosis of protozoa and helminths in faeces. *J. Parasit.*, **25**, 241.

Fulton, J. D. (1963). Acquired immunity: Protozoal infections. Chapter 7 in *Modern Trends in Immunology*. Ed. Cruickshank. London: Butterworth.

Fulton, J. D. & Turk, J. L. (1959). Direct agglutination test for toxoplasmosis. *Lancet*, **2**, 1068.

GOLDMAN, M. (1957). Staining *Toxoplasma gondii* with fluorescein-labelled antibody. *J. exp. Med.*, **105**, 549, 557.

HOARE, C. A. (1949). *Handbook of Medical Protozoology*. London: Baillière, Tindall & Cox.

HOARE, C. A. & NEAL, R. A. (1955). *Mechanisms of Microbial Pathogenicity*, p. 230. Cambridge University Press.

MACDONALD, A. (1949). Serological diagnosis of human toxoplasmosis. *Lancet*, **1**, 950.

SABIN, A. B. & FELDMAN, H. A. (1948). Dyes as microchemical indicators of a new immunity phenomenon affecting a protozoon parasite (toxoplasma). *Science*, **108**, 660.

SABIN, A. B. & FELDMAN, H. A. (1949). Antibodies in congenital toxoplasmosis. *Paediatrics*, **4**, 660.

SHUTE, P. G. & MARYON, M. (1960). *Techniques for the Study of Malaria*. London: Churchill.

SIM, J. C. & LIND, K. (1960). A toxoplasma flocculation test. *Acta. path. microbiol. scand.*, **50**, 445.

WENYON, C. M. (1926). *Protozoology*. London: Baillière, Tindall & Cox.

PART IV

APPLIED MICROBIOLOGY

CHAPTER 42

THE LABORATORY DIAGNOSIS OF COMMON INFECTIVE SYNDROMES

THE practice of good clinical medicine requires the intelligent use of laboratory services. The aid of the bacteriology department is necessary for the accurate diagnosis of many common infections and selection of a suitable antimicrobial agent for the treatment of the patient may be impossible without knowledge of the *in vitro* sensitivity of the causal microorganism. The bacteriological results, however, should always be interpreted in relation to clinical findings and the results of other investigations.

Sterile containers and swabs of various types are provided by the laboratory, but unless the clinician accepts responsibility for the careful collection and prompt submission of suitable specimens, laboratory examinations may be useless. Prolonged transport can result in the death of some delicate bacteria and viruses whereas other clinically insignificant bacteria may be able to multiply in the material sent for examination. The effect of delay in transit can sometimes be overcome by the use of special transport media. Specimens *must be* clearly labelled and accompanied by a completed laboratory request form giving relevant clinical details. This information is often essential in deciding how a particular specimen will be treated in the laboratory. The laboratory diagnosis of an infection can be accomplished in two different ways: either the microorganism responsible for the infection can be isolated and identified, or serological evidence of the host's reaction to the pathogen can be detected.

I. Isolation of the Causal Microorganism

Bacteria

Isolation of the causal bacterium is the most satisfactory method of laboratory diagnosis. This may be relatively easy to do, but sometimes it is difficult or even impossible. The evaluation of cultures inoculated with samples taken from sites which have a normal bacterial flora requires experience. Here potentially pathogenic bacteria have to be distinguished from commensal organisms and isolation of a potential pathogen is not necessarily significant.

The way in which a specimen is treated in the laboratory largely depends on its source and nature although the routine method may be modified if there are special circumstances noted in the patient's history.

The laboratory examination of bacteriological specimens, however, follows a standard pattern.

1. Direct Films.—Films made from the material submitted are usually examined after they have been stained, but some direct films, *e.g.* those made from faeces and urine, may yield additional information if they are examined unstained ("wet films"). Gram's method is the staining technique universally used and, if tuberculous infection is suspected, Ziehl-Neelsen-stained films are also prepared. In addition films stained by Leishman's method or another Romanowsky stain may be necessary to study the nature of the cells in an exudate.

2. Culture.—The specimen is inoculated on to solid and into fluid culture media.

(a) *Solid Media.*—Blood agar is the most widely used medium in diagnostic bacteriology and plates of this medium, seeded with the material sent for examination, are often incubated in a variety of different atmospheric conditions. These range from the presence of air (aerobic conditions) through varying degrees of reduced oxygen tension to completely anaerobic conditions; the addition of carbon dioxide may be necessary for the growth of certain bacteria. On blood agar, colonies of many of the common pathogens can be recognised after overnight incubation. Other types of media in routine use include *specially enriched media* which promote the growth of exacting pathogens, *e.g.* heated blood agar for isolation of the gonococcus, and *selective media* which inhibit some organisms but allow others to grow. Many selective media have been devised to facilitate the isolation of a particular pathogen from a mixture of commensal organisms, *e.g.* desoxycholate-citrate agar for the isolation of intestinal pathogens.

(b) *Fluid Media.*—Bacteria may not grow on solid media if only a few viable organisms are present in the specimen, or if the material submitted contains substances that inhibit bacterial growth (*e.g.* antibiotics). Inoculation of a suitable fluid medium, however, not only ensures the rapid multiplication of small numbers of organisms but also dilutes the concentration of inhibitory substances and this may allow growth to take place. Note, however, that such cultures yield no information about the number of organisms actually present in the original specimen. Growth in fluid media is investigated by making films from the broth and subculturing on to solid media. The most important fluid medium for general use is Robertson's cooked-meat broth which grows both aerobic and anaerobic organisms.

3. Antibiotic Sensitivity Tests.—By determining the sensitivity of pathogenic bacteria to the various antibiotics the laboratory can aid the practitioner in the treatment of bacterial diseases. In general there is good agreement between the in-vitro sensitivity of the infecting organism to a given antibiotic and the clinical response observed when that drug is given to the patient.

The simplest way to carry out these tests is by the disk diffusion method. Here a number of paper disks or tablets containing different antibiotics are placed on the surface of an agar plate that has been uniformly spread with the test organism. After overnight incubation the plate is examined for zones of inhibition of growth around the various disks. The size of these zones indicates the degree of sensitivity to the antibiotic contained in the disk: growth right up to the disk margin indicates great resistance. To speed laboratory reporting it is sometimes possible to use the specimen submitted, *e.g.* pus, urine, as the inoculum instead of the isolated pathogen. This is called primary sensitivity testing.

Viruses

The isolation of viruses is time-consuming, expensive and requires special laboratory resources. Attempts to isolate viruses are often futile unless the specimens are collected in the very early stages of the illness; the specimens must be promptly preserved, and sent to the laboratory by a very rapid method.

Swabs on wooden applicator sticks are the most suitable for taking materials from the throat, mouth, skin lesions, rectum, vagina, etc. Immediately after use the stick is broken to a short length and the swab is inserted into a screw cap container to which has been added about 2 ml. of a suitable transport medium (*e.g.* medium 199 or 1 per cent. skim milk) containing 50 units penicillin and 50 μg. streptomycin per ml. Samples of faeces should also be placed in a transport medium.

Specimens for virus isolation should be placed at temperatures below 4° C. without delay after collection, and they must be kept at these temperatures until the tests are carried out. It is often convenient in hospital practice to store the specimen in the ice trays of a domestic refrigerator. For transport to the laboratory the specimens in their containers may be surrounded with ice, or preferably an ice-salt mixture, in a suitable jar or tin. *Do not send such specimens by post.* The best way of transmitting frozen specimens to a laboratory at some distance is to pack them in a special insulated box or thermos flask surrounded by "dry ice" (*i.e.* solid carbon dioxide). Such containers are sometimes available on demand at the laboratory.

II. Serological Diagnosis

Serological tests to detect antibodies against the infecting microorganism provide a useful means of indirect diagnosis. These tests are of especial value in virology where isolation of the virus responsible for the infection may be difficult or impossible. In diagnosing bacterial infections, however, serological methods are less often used but there are two particular instances where such tests are routine, *viz.* the examination of the patient's serum for agglutinating antibodies against the salmonellae responsible for enteric fever (Widal Reaction) and *Brucella abortus* when investigating the cause of an unknown fever, and the examination of the patient's serum for complement-fixing or flocculating antibodies in the diagnosis of syphilis.

Serological Diagnosis of Virus Infections.—Serological tests for complement-fixing, neutralising and haemagglutination inhibiting antibodies, often give valuable diagnostic information; they form the usual routine means of laboratory investigation in some virus infections. Since small traces of antibody may persist long after recovery and are frequently demonstrable in normal healthy individuals the examination of a single sample of serum seldom yields information of any value. Exceptions are seen in cases of infections with the psittacosis and lymphogranuloma venereum viruses where the single observation of a high antibody titre may be significant. In most other infections the results of serological tests are of diagnostic significance only if it has been shown that there has been at least a fourfold rise of antibody titre during the period between the onset of the illness and convalescence.

It is therefore essential to send at least two samples of serum to the laboratory; the first taken as soon as possible after the onset of the disease, and the second after about three weeks. Details of the optimum times for the collection of sera are given in Appendix IV at the end of this chapter.

For the tests, 1–2 ml. of clear serum showing no trace of haemolysis is required The serum should be removed from the clot within 24 hr. of collection and then kept at 4° C. or lower. When both acute and convalescent samples have been collected they may be sent to the laboratory by post. Whole blood is unsuitable for transmission by post and should not be sent.

RESPIRATORY TRACT INFECTIONS

Infections of the Upper Respiratory Tract

The upper respiratory tract is frequently involved in general and localised infections involving the mouth, oropharynx, nose, nasopharynx, larynx and trachea. The primary infection is often viral in origin and secondary bacterial infection is most often due to the potential pathogens resident in the upper respiratory tract, *e.g.* pneumococci, streptococci, *H. influenzae* and staphylococci. The area affected is usually obvious and examination will be directed to the site affected. The most useful procedure is to take a swab direct from the surface; if exudate, membrane or pus is present some of this should be sampled. Films may be prepared from the swabs after cultures have been inoculated, or smears may be prepared directly from the membranes, exudate or surface by means of a swab or loop and stained by suitable stains.

Acute mouth infections, such as *stomatitis*, are commoner in young babies, children and older persons, especially when the patient is debilitated as the result of intercurrent disease, or when the mouth has not been given proper hygiene. The more common organisms involved are aerobic and anaerobic streptococci, Vincent's organisms, and Candida species; viruses involved may be those of herpes simplex, Coxsackie group A, measles, smallpox, etc. More rarely *Treponema pallidum* and *Treponema pertenue* are responsible.

Sore Throat.—This syndrome, characterised by acute inflammation of the tonsillar and faucial areas (acute tonsillitis, acute pharyngitis) with or without exudate, which may be loose or adherent, is most commonly due to *Strept. pyogenes.* But many cases of acute sore throat, and especially the milder cases, are virus infections (mostly adenoviruses), and it is important to distinguish between streptococcal and non-streptococcal infections since the former respond to penicillin therapy which is also effective in preventing septic and non-septic complications, including acute rheumatic fever. Virus infections, on the other hand, do not respond to antibiotics and should not be treated with these drugs unless there is evidence of a secondary bacterial infection. Other causes of sore throat with exudate are diphtheria and Vincent's angina; exudate is also frequently present in certain forms of mononucleosis (glandular fever), in agranulocytosis and in the leukaemias. An important contributing factor in the last three of these diseases is the diminution or inefficiency of the granular white cells which normally act as scavengers in keeping the mucous membranes clean.

Acute adenitis, sinusitis, otitis media, rhinitis, laryngitis, tracheitis, may accompany or follow the acute throat infection. Chronic diseases may be due to leprosy, syphilis and tuberculosis. Actinomycosis with involvement of deeper tissues and the formation of abscesses is a rare cause of infection in the cervico-facial region.

Diagnostic procedures.—A throat swab specimen is taken. The patient holds his mouth open and breathes deeply. A good light should be placed to illuminate the throat. A clean wooden tongue depressor or the handle of a clean spoon should be used to press down the tongue. The throat swab is then quickly placed in the throat and rubbed gently but firmly over the tonsils, the posterior pharyngeal wall and, particularly, on any areas of purulent exudate.

Direct Film.—A direct film may on occasion be helpful if the causative organism has a characteristic morphology. A clinical diagnosis of Vincent's infection may be confirmed by demonstrating the characteristic morphology of *Borrelia vincentii* and the accompanying fusiform bacilli; these organisms are in any case virtually impossible to cultivate. The observation of many "yeasts" in the direct film confirms the diagnosis of thrush, and films may be of limited assistance in the presumptive diagnosis of diphtheria, especially if membrane is present. However, direct films are valueless in the differentiation of most other acute infections because the normal commensal flora are similar in morphology to the specific pathogens.

Suitable material should be examined by dark-ground microscopy to exclude treponemal infection such as syphilis and yaws if this is suspected, and scrapings from suspicious lesions may be stained by the Ziehl-Neelsen technique for mycobacteria.

Throat washings may be taken for the isolation of viruses and for direct examination to detect antigen by the fluorescent antibody technique (Chapter 54).

Culture.—The specimen is plated on to blood-agar plates which are incubated aerobically, anaerobically and in the presence of carbon dioxide. Penicillin disks are useful for the differentiation of streptococci, yeasts and *Haemophilus* species. Heated blood agar is used for *Haemophilus inflenzae* and neisseriae: Sabouraud's medium is used for cultivating Candida and other fungi, and a tellurite medium and Loeffler's serum are inoculated if infection with *Corynebacterium diphtheriae* is suspected.

The interpretation of results of culture of material from the respiratory tract requires a knowledge of the commensal flora of the upper respiratory tract, which is as follows:

anterior nares: staphylococcus, including *Staph. albus* and *Staph. aureus* (30–50 per cent.), diphtheroids.

nasopharynx: alpha-haemolytic streptococci, neisseriae, staphylococcus and more rarely pneumococcus.

mouth: alpha-haemolytic streptococci predominate.

oropharynx: alpha-haemolytic streptococci, pneumococci (30–40 per cent.), *Haemophilus species* (40–60 per cent.), neisseriae and diphtheroids. More rarely *Strept. pyogenes* and *Neisseria meningitidis* (see Report, 1939).

Salivary and other upper respiratory tract secretions contain vast numbers of these commensals and sputum will be contaminated with them. Some of these commensal organisms, *e.g.* pneumococci, *Haemophilus* species are potential pathogens causing secondary bacterial infections; the rôle of others is doubtful.

In health it is practically impossible to recover organisms from levels of the respiratory tract below the middle of the larynx.

Infections of the Lower Respiratory Tract

The lower respiratory tract (bronchi, bronchioles and lung tissue) is usually infected by pathogenic microorganisms from the upper respiratory tract and by spread through the blood and lymph channels; more rarely there is direct extension of infection from other affected tissues, such as the liver. The mucous membrane of this part of the respiratory tract is probably sterile in health, but direct examination involves bronchoscopy or lung biopsy, neither of which is indicated in the normal course of the diagnosis of infection.

Sputum from patients with acute bronchitis, acute exacerbations of chronic bronchitis, bronchiolitis and pneumonia, should be examined bacteriologically. In most cases the sputum will consist of a mixture of exudate from the affected mucous membrane or lung tissue and saliva. The more purulent material is likely to contain specific pathogens and therefore examination should be directed to this part by spreading the sputum in a dish so that the purulent material may be picked directly with a loop. Alternatively, the sputum may be homogenised either by adding saponin and incubating for half an hour, or by shaking the sputum with glass beads; in this way random sampling of the sputum specimen will include any pathogens present.

Direct Film.—Films should be made from the sputum and stained by Gram's method. They are of limited value and give no indication of the number of viable organisms present: further the presence of commensal organisms in saliva may confuse the picture. Direct films are of more value in the diagnosis of specific infections of the lung, such as pneumococcal and staphylococcal infections. If tuberculosis is suspected, a direct film stained by Ziehl-Neelsen's method is examined for acid- and alcohol-fast bacilli.

CULTURE.—Sputum is plated on blood agar for aerobic, anaerobic and carbon dioxide incubation and heated blood agar incubated in carbon dioxide with diagnostic antimicrobial disks. An optochin disk may be placed on the plates for the differentiation of pneumococci from *Strept. viridans*. In specific infections the significant organisms such as pneumococci, *Haemophilus influenzae* and *Staphylococcus aureus* are usually isolated in large numbers. If tuberculosis is suspected the sputum is concentrated prior to culture and sometimes guinea-pig inoculation is also performed. The methods are detailed in Chapter 14.

ACUTE INTESTINAL INFECTIONS

Acute diarrhoea with or without vomiting is a very common complaint that may be due to a variety of causes. Infection with known or unknown bacteria, viruses or protozoa is a major contributor but specific bacterial pathogens can be recovered from not more than around 20 per cent. of the "infective diarrhoeas." The most common identifiable intestinal pathogen in Britain is *Shigella sonnei*; the salmonella species, enteropathogenic *Esch. coli*, and the food poisoning enterotoxic strains of *Staph. aureus* and *Cl. welchii* are less commonly incriminated. The aid of the laboratory is essential in arriving at a diagnosis and specimens of faeces should be sent for bacteriological examination. A specific infection must never be excluded on the basis of one negative report and a series of specimens may have to be submitted for investigation.

Specimen Collection

A sample of faeces is a much better specimen than a rectal swab. However, if a large number of contacts of a patient with an infective diarrhoea have to be investigated it is often more convenient to take rectal swabs. When this is done it is necessary to ensure that these swabs sample the contents of the *rectum* and that they are not merely placed in the anal orifice. Faeces should be passed into a clean pot which does not contain any antiseptic and the specimen should be collected free from urine. A sample of the specimen is transferred with the spoon provided to a sterile glass universal container and this should be sent to the laboratory as soon as possible. Alternatively, a sample of the faeces in the pot may be sent on a swab. If delay is inevitable, it is an advantage to transport the specimen in glycerol saline because this prevents the intestinal commensal organisms overgrowing any enteric pathogens that may be present (see Appendix I). If amoebic dysentery is suspected the specimen must be available for examination *within a few minutes* of being passed if the motile vegetative form of *Entamoeba histolytica* is to be recognised. The record of the history sent with the specimen should include information about recent foreign travel as patients who have been abroad are more likely to be infested with intestinal protozoa and worms.

Laboratory Examination

Appearance.—The specimen is examined naked-eye for mucus, fresh blood, altered blood (melaena) and for the presence of whole worms or tapeworm segments.

Wet Films.—These films, made by suspending the faeces in saline, are *not* prepared as a routine in all laboratories. They are examined for red blood cells and pus cells, the vegetative forms of protozoa such as *Entamoeba histolytica*, the cysts of intestinal protozoa and the ova of intestinal worms. If the presence of cysts or ova is suspected, films should be made after the concentration of the faeces, *e.g.* by the zinc sulphate flotation method (Chapter 41).

Stained Films.—Gram-stained films are of limited value in the bacteriological examination of faeces. In staphylococcal enterocolitis, however, the stool is watery and Gram-stained films show many clusters of Gram-positive cocci with few, if any, other organisms.

Culture.—If the faeces are formed, a little of the specimen should be emulsified in saline or peptone water and this suspension is used to inoculate solid media; in the case of fluid faeces, an effort should be made to select flakes of mucus for culture. The solid media routinely used in Britain are MacConkey's medium, desoxycholate-citrate-agar (DCA) and Wilson and Blair's medium. Fluid enrichment media such as selenite F and tetrathionate broths, which allow the multiplication of enteric pathogens but inhibit the growth of intestinal commensal organisms, are also inoculated with the sample: after 24 hr. incubation the broths are subcultured on one or more of the selective solid media named above. The resulting growths on the solid media are dealt with as follows.

On MacConkey's medium and DCA the Gram-negative intestinal bacilli produce pink colonies if the organism ferments the lactose in the medium and pale colonies if it fails to do so. Pink colonies are usually abundant on the MacConkey plate but they tend to be scanty on the more inhibitory DCA medium; most of these lactose-fermenting organisms belong to the genus Escherichia and the rest of them are other intestinal commensals such as Klebsiella species. Therefore, when a search for intestinal pathogens is being made, pink colonies can be disregarded as a rule. There are, however, two important exceptions to this: *Shigella sonnei* is a late-lactose fermenter and may produce *slightly pink* colonies after overnight culture, and the enteropathogenic strains of *Escherichia coli*, which can cause severe diarrhoea in infancy, produce colonies morphologically indistinguishable from other strains of *Esch. coli*. Thus when faeces from young children are being examined, several pink colonies, preferably about ten, should be picked from the MacConkey plate and serologically tested on a slide against a polyvalent enteropathogenic *Esch. coli* antiserum. If agglutination takes place, further tests are made with individual type-specific sera to allow provisional identification of the type. This must be confirmed by setting up a tube agglutination test and showing that a boiled suspension of the organism is agglutinated by dilutions of the monospecific antiserum up to the stated titre.

The organisms that produce pale colonies may be salmonellae or shigellae but they may also be Proteus species, non-lactose-fermenting strains of *Esch. coli* or some other gut commensal organism. Therefore all pale (and slightly pink) colonies are subjected to biochemical investigation. Their activity is tested by picking a single pale colony and inoculating a tube of peptone water (to test for motility and indole production), a series of peptone waters containing different carbohydrates (subsequently examined for the formation of acid and/or gas), a urea slope (to test for urease activity) and an agar slope (the growth on this to be used for agglutination tests if necessary). It is wise also to "plate out" the pale colony on MacConkey's medium and to examine the resulting growth to make sure that it is pure. Alternatively, biochemical activity can be tested by the use of composite media such as those described by Gillies (Chapter 47). If the results of the biochemical tests are consistent with the organism being a salmonella or a shigella, slide agglutination tests are carried out with polyvalent antisera; if these are positive, provisional identification is made by further slide agglutination tests with monospecific antisera. In every case, final identification must depend on the result of tube agglutination tests. Most laboratories have only a limited range of antisera and although these are sufficient for the recognition of the common salmonella and shigella types, unusual species may have to be sent to a reference laboratory for identification.

On Wilson and Blair's medium jet black or dark green colonies with a metallic lustre are selected for further examination. Such colonies are typically produced by some of the salmonellae, *Salmonella typhi*, and *Salmonella paratyphi* in particular, and they are investigated in the same way as pale colonies on MacConkey's medium or DCA.

In addition to the routine methods of culture described above, faeces from patients suspected of having food poisoning are sometimes examined for *Staphylococcus aureus* and "heat-resistant" strains of *Clostridium welchii*. If present in fairly large numbers, *Staph. aureus* can be isolated by inoculating the faeces directly on to blood agar, although there is always the risk that the culture will be overgrown by *Proteus* species. For this reason direct plating on a selective medium such as salt-milk agar is to be preferred. It may be possible to isolate *Staph. aureus* from faeces that contain only small numbers of this organism by inoculating a salt cooked-meat broth with the faeces and incubating this overnight before subculturing the broth on solid media. The isolation of a few *Staph. aureus* from a specimen of faeces, however, is of doubtful significance for some 20 per cent. of normal people carry *Staph. aureus* in their faeces. It should also be remembered that staphylococcal enterotoxin is more resistant to heat than *Staph. aureus* and it is therefore possible for a patient to suffer from staphylococcal food poisoning even when *Staph. aureus* is not isolated from either the faeces or the suspect food.

The spores of the food-poisoning strains of *Cl. welchii* withstand boiling for 1 hr. and this property is employed in isolating these strains from faeces (see Chapter 27 for a detailed description of the method). Again the significance of these organisms in faeces requires critical evaluation because they can be found in the faeces of 5–30 per cent. of apparently healthy people.

URINARY TRACT INFECTIONS

The diagnosis of urinary tract infection cannot be made without bacteriological examination of the urine. Patients with classic symptoms of urinary infection may have a sterile urine and asymptomatic patients may have significant bacteriuria. The chemotherapy of proven infection may be controlled by in-vitro sensitivity tests and the outcome assessed by examination of the urine at the conclusion of treatment. Follow-up of patients who have had a urinary infection is essential because relapse may be clinically silent.

Specimen Collection

Specimens are usually collected in universal containers, but for the collection of mid-stream specimens from females it is an advantage to provide a wide-mouthed container such as a 12-oz. honey-pot. Alternatively, disposable plastic pots with tight-fitting lids can be used for urine specimens.

From male patients a mid-stream specimen of urine (MSU) should be submitted: the prepuce is retracted, the glans penis cleansed with soap and water and the middle of the urinary flow collected. Formerly, for bacteriological examination, a catheter specimen of urine (CSU) was always collected from female patients so that contamination of the specimen with organisms from the ano-genital region was avoided. This practice, however, is no longer regarded as justifiable because catheterisation may introduce infection—a risk, under ideal conditions, estimated at between 2 and 6 per cent. As a result voided specimens are now submitted from women and, if carefully taken, these compare satisfactorily with catheter specimens. To collect a voided specimen, the ano-genital region should be thoroughly cleansed and antiseptic, *e.g.* chlorhexidine or cetrimide, may be applied to the labia. The patient then passes urine with the labia separated and the middle of the stream is collected for examination. Note, however, that a perfunctory wash of the vulva, and this is often all that can be carried out where toilet facilities are limited, is of no value.

Once collected, the specimen must be transported to the laboratory without delay because urine is an excellent culture medium supporting the rapid growth of many bacteria. If delay of more than 1–2 hr. is unavoidable the multiplication of bacteria in the urine should be prevented by storage in a refrigerator, or the specimen may be transported in some form of special container that maintains a low temperature. A simple container which utilises a standard one pint vacuum flask has been devised for this purpose (Elliott and Sleigh 1963).

Laboratory Examination

"Routine" examination of the urine, *vide infra*, is still carried out in most bacteriological laboratories. In recent years, however, the trend has been to apply various quantitative methods: the enumeration of the number of bacteria in each ml. of freshly voided urine has allowed the development of the concept of significant bacteriuria, and the introduction of a simplified method has revived interest in measuring the urinary white cell excretion rate.

ROUTINE EXAMINATION.—The urine is centrifuged, and wet and Gram-stained films are made from the deposit which is also inoculated on to blood agar and MacConkey agar plates. The supernatant may be kept for chemical examination. The wet film is examined at this stage for pus cells, red blood cells and organisms; if many bacteria are seen, a primary sensitivity test is set up. The following day the stained film and the cultures are examined. If the primary sensitivity test plate has been omitted or if it cannot be interpreted with certainty, another sensitivity test is carried out when the organism has been cultured. This time the isolated organism and not the urine deposit is used as inoculum for the sensitivity test plate.

Interpretation.—Pyuria is variable in degree in urinary infections. It is almost always present and is often gross in acute infections but in chronic infections it may be absent. Squamous epithelial cells and lactobacilli seen in urinary deposits from women indicate vulval contamination. Culture may yield no growth of bacteria, a growth indicating contamination, or a growth signifying infection. A scanty growth of several different organisms usually indicates non-pathogenic contaminants, e.g. *Staph. albus*, micrococci, diphtheroid organisms. A heavier growth of one or two bacterial species indicates infection and the types of organism isolated may vary with the patient's history. In acute uncomplicated and untreated infections the growth is usually of a single organism which in some 80 per cent. of cases is *Escherichia coli.* In chronic infections, where there is often established disease of the urinary tract, the cultures are more likely to contain more than one organism and *Klebsiella*, *Proteus* and *Pseudomonas* species and *Strept. faecalis* are common.

Quantitative Examination

WHITE CELL EXCRETION RATE.—Although gross pyuria is easy to detect there is no general agreement about the significance of an occasional pus cell seen in a urine deposit. The original quantitative method, that of Addis, had a number of disadvantages and the technique of Houghton and Pears (1957) is generally used nowadays although, for reasons already discussed, mid-stream rather than catheter specimens should be examined. In order to determine the excretion rate of white cells the total volume of urine voided must be measured and the time during which it has collected in the bladder must be known. Ten ml. of this urine are centrifuged, nine ml. of the supernatant discarded and the deposit is re-suspended in the remaining one ml. This concentrates the cellular elements, and the leucocytes and non-squamous epithelial cells present are then counted in a Fuchs-Rosenthal chamber. The number of these cells excreted in each hour can then be calculated.

White cell excretion rates greater than 200,000 cells per hour are probably abnormal; rates between 100,000 and 200,000 cells per hour are considered of doubtful significance, and rates less than 100,000 cells per hour are taken as normal. Raised cell excretion rates are found in acute and chronic pyelonephritis, acute and chronic glomerulonephritis, and hypertension; they are noted occasionally in other systemic diseases and sometimes have no detectable cause. In chronic pyelonephritis the cell excretion rate may be raised at a time when pathogenic organisms are absent from the urine and such a finding points to the silent progression of the disease.

Bacterial Counts.—The results of culture are not always clear-cut, and in recent years studies of the actual number of bacteria present in otherwise normal but contaminated and infected urines have been made. Viable counts may be performed either by a pour-plate method or by inoculating the surface of media with known volumes of urine. Colony counts are made after incubation for 24–48 hr.

When properly taken urine specimens are examined, contamination never produces more than 10^4 organisms per ml. and usually accounts for less than 10^3 organisms per ml. These counts, inconstant and varying from specimen to specimen taken from the same patient, represent bacteria from the urethra and external genitalia which have entered the urine during collection of the specimen. Infected urines contain more than 10^4 organisms per ml., usually more than 10^5 organisms per ml. and often up to 10^8 organisms per ml. These high counts, fairly constant in serial specimens taken from the same patient, are the result of bacterial multiplication in the urine within the urinary tract.

Significant bacteriuria (counts greater than 10^5 organisms per ml.) may sometimes be found, in the absence of symptoms or pyuria, in patients who subsequently develop clinical symptoms of urinary infection. Evidence is accumulating of an association between asymptomatic bacteriuria and pyelonephritis.

Semi-quantitative Culture of Urine

Although quantitative urine culture yields extra information it is time-consuming and also requires considerable amounts of laboratory materials. Consequently, a number of semi-quantitative methods have been introduced and the results of these simplified techniques compare well with quantitative examinations carried out on the same specimen. In the semi-quantitative methods a loop of standard diameter is charged with the uncentrifuged urine and plated-out on solid media in a standard way (see McGeachie and Kennedy, 1963). After overnight incubation the plate is read and the results evaluated in accordance with a pre-arranged scheme. There is no reason why a simple method such as this should not be used routinely in diagnostic laboratories.

MENINGITIS

The clinical signs of meningeal irritation always suggest infection of the meninges but they may occur in association with certain other acute infections not involving the meninges (meningismus) and they may also be seen in patients with non-infective conditions such as subarachnoid haemorrhage. Infants, however, may have meningitis without the usual localising signs. Patients suspected of having meningitis should always have a specimen of cerebrospinal fluid (CSF) examined in the laboratory. Prompt identification of the causal organism is important because until an exact bacteriological diagnosis has been made the proper antimicrobial therapy cannot be prescribed.

Infection with the meningococcus is the most common type of acute purulent meningitis in Britain, followed by infections with *Haemophilus influenzae* (confined to pre-school children, mostly under 3 years of age) and the pneumococcus. Infection with enterobacteria (salmonellae, coliform organisms) occurs in early infancy.

Specimen Collection

When cerebrospinal fluid is obtained by lumbar puncture it is essential to take rigorous precautions to prevent the introduction of infection. (It is safe to remove 5-10 ml. of CSF *as long as intracranial pressure is not increased.*) The sample is best collected in one or two sterile screw-capped containers. Test-tubes with cotton-wool plugs should not be used because if they are shaken or fall over the CSF may be absorbed by the plug. The specimen must be dispatched to the laboratory at once; delay may result in the death of delicate pathogens such as meningococci, the disintegration of leucocytes and the reduction in the concentration of sugar in the CSF.

Laboratory Examination

APPEARANCE.—Normal CSF is clear and colourless. Increase in the number of cells, or the presence of many bacteria, makes the fluid opalescent or turbid; fibrinous clots may be seen if the protein content is increased. Fresh blood in the CSF is usually the result of local bleeding at the site of the lumbar puncture and if a series of samples is collected in several containers it may be seen that most of the blood is mixed with the fluid which has escaped first. When the CSF is centrifuged, the supernatant fluid will be clear if the bleeding has been recent; if the supernatant fluid is yellow this indicates that the bleeding into the CSF has taken place at least 12 hours ago and this finding is usually associated with subarachnoid haemorrhage.

CYTOLOGICAL EXAMINATION.—The number of leucocytes in the CSF is enumerated using a white-blood-cell-count pipette and a special counting chamber. Cerebrospinal fluid normally contains 3 or less leucocytes per cu. mm. If the number of cells is increased a film of the centrifuged deposit, stained by Leishman's method, should be examined so that a differential cell count can be carried out.

In acute bacterial meningitis there is a great increase in the number of leucocytes in the CSF. Up to several thousand cells per cu. mm. is a common finding and early in the disease almost all of them are polymorphs. In tuberculous meningitis there are fewer cells in the CSF (200–500 per cu. mm.) and lymphocytes predominate, but some polymorphs are usually present. Virus infections of the meninges result in an "aseptic" type of meningitis; between 50 and 1000 cells per cu. mm. are found and they are virtually all lymphocytes.

BIOCHEMICAL EXAMINATION.—Part of the specimen should be submitted for quantitative biochemical estimation of the protein, sugar (glucose) and chloride content of the fluid (see p. 569). The Lange colloidal gold test depends on the relationship between gamma-globulins and other protein fractions in the CSF. Three abnormal types of curve are recognised, the paretic, the luetic and the meningitic.

EXAMINATION FOR MICROORGANISMS

BACTERIA.—The three bacterial species most often responsible for an acute purulent meningitis are the meningococcus, the pneumococcus and *Haemophilus influenzae*. These organisms usually reach the meninges by way of the blood stream and it is sometimes possible to isolate them simultaneously from blood cultures. Meningitis, however, can result from the direct spread of bacteria to the meninges from infections in neighbouring structures such as the middle ear and paranasal or frontal sinuses. Bacteria may also gain access to the meninges after careless lumbar puncture or from infected neurosurgical wounds. Thus a wide variety of organisms including *Staphylococcus aureus*, *Streptococcus pyogenes*, *Pseudomonas pyocyanea*, *Escherichia coli* and anaerobic organisms such as *Bacteroides* species and anaerobic streptococci can cause meningitis. Leptospires e.g. *L. canicola* and *Listeria monocytogenes* occasionally cause meningeal infection. *Mycobacterium tuberculosis* produces a less acute form of meningitis.

The CSF is centrifuged and films are made from the deposit. If clots are present additional films are prepared by spreading out the coagulum on a glass slide. Films are stained by Gram's method and, should a tuberculous infection be suspected, by the Ziehl-Neelsen method as well. It is often possible at this stage to make a provisional diagnosis by examination of the stained films alone, especially if the patient has not received any antibiotics, and this allows the appropriate treatment to be given without delay. In tuberculous meningitis a prolonged and thorough search of several thick films is often necessary before acid- and alcohol-fast bacilli are discovered.

The centrifuged deposit is inoculated on blood and heated blood agar plates that are then incubated, aerobically, anaerobically and in an atmosphere containing 5–10 per cent. carbon dioxide. If bacteria have been seen in the stained films a primary sensitivity test should also be set up. The plates are examined after overnight incubation, and in many cases a good growth of the pathogen will have taken place. However, it may be necessary to reincubate the plates for another 24 hr. before satisfactory growth is obtained. The organisms isolated on culture are identified in the usual way. If the cultures are sterile and if tuberculous meningitis is suspected the deposit should be inoculated, without prior concentration, on to slopes of Lowenstein-Jensen medium and also injected into guinea-pigs which are examined after the usual interval of 4 to 8 weeks.

When patients are thought to have either meningovascular or neurosyphilis the standard serological tests for syphilis should be performed on the CSF.

VIRUSES.—The viruses that are most often responsible for aseptic meningitis are the enteroviruses (ECHO, Coxsackie and less frequently poliomyelitis), the virus of lymphocytic choriomeningitis and herpes simplex virus. Aseptic meningitis may also occur as a complication of other virus diseases such as mumps (sometimes unassociated with parotitis), chickenpox, measles, infective hepatitis and herpes zoster. ECHO and Coxsackie viruses can usually be isolated directly from the CSF. They may also be present in the faeces. A sample of CSF should be sent as early as possible and faeces may also be submitted. Second samples of both specimens should be sent two or three days later. If faeces are not available, a rectal swab is a reasonably satisfactory alternative. These viruses may also be recovered from throat swabs or oropharyngeal washings but, in the case of the polioviruses, with considerably less frequency. Cerebrospinal fluid from cases of aseptic meningitis seldom, if ever, contains polioviruses. These materials may be held for up to 24 hr. at 0°–4° C., in a domestic refrigerator, but for longer periods they should be preserved frozen at −30° C. or in 50 per cent. glycerol saline.

FINDINGS IN THE CEREBROSPINAL FLUID IN DIFFERENT TYPES OF MENINGITIS

Test	Normal	Acute Bacterial Meningitis	Tuberculous Meningitis	Aseptic Meningitis
Appearance	clear and colourless	turbid	clear or opalescent	usually clear
Total protein	15–40 mg/100 ml.	greatly increased	moderately increased	slightly increased
Sugar	50–70 mg/100 ml.	greatly reduced	reduced	normal
Chloride	700–740 mg/100 ml.	reduced	reduced	normal
Cell count	0–3 lymphocytes per cu. mm.	greatly increased—all polymorphs	increased—mainly lymphocytes, some polymorphs	increased—lymphocytes predominate
Culture on artificial media	sterile	causal bacterium isolated	*M. tuberculosis* isolated	sterile

WOUND INFECTIONS

Wound infections may be *endogenous* or *exogenous*. Endogenous infections (*auto-infection*) are caused by organisms that were leading a commensal existence elsewhere in the host's body; for example abdominal surgical wounds may become infected with organisms from the large bowel after an operation that has involved incision of the colon. In exogenous infections the source of the infecting organism is outwith the host who becomes infected; *cross-infection* is a particular example of exogenous infection where the causal organism is spread from person to person. Infection may occur after accidental or intentional trauma of the skin or other tissues; the latter type is often called "post-operative sepsis".

Specimen Collection

Pus or exudate from infected wounds is usually sampled by means of a swab which must be well soaked in the exudate (Appendix 3). A specimen of the pus itself is always preferable and may often be obtained by using a syringe or pipette to transfer the material to a sterile tube or screw-capped bottle. If only a small amount of exudate is available it should be allowed to run into a capillary tube; after sealing both ends the tube can be sent to the laboratory. Pieces of tissue removed at operation, or curettings from infected sinuses and other tissues are sometimes sent for bacteriological examination: these specimens are homogenised in a tissue grinder with a little broth and subsequently treated in the same way as exudates. Delay in the transit of specimens to the laboratory must be avoided, especially in the case of swabs where the exudate may dry into the cotton-wool.

Laboratory Examination

The pus should, if possible, be examined for any unusual features such as granules which are characteristic of some forms of actinomycotic infection. If granules are present they can easily be separated by shaking up the pus with water in a test-tube, allowing them to sediment and collecting them in a capillary pipette. The granules are then crushed to make films and inoculated on to culture media.

Direct Films.—Films made from pus may be of value. They are stained by Gram's method and, if indicated, by the Ziehl-Neelsen method. It is difficult, however, to make good films from swabs, and quite impossible if the swab is dry. To avoid contamination, either the swab must be rubbed on to the surface of a sterile slide or the smear made after all the culture media have been inoculated; the latter procedure is usually followed and a poor film, not representative of the actual exudate, is often the result. The examination of material on swabs for mycobacteria is almost always unsatisfactory.

In good films made from the exudate, polymorphs in various stages of disintegration will be seen with bacteria of one or more types. Gram-positive branching filaments suggest actinomycosis, and the demonstration of acid- and alcohol-fast bacilli indicates a tuberculous infection.

CULTURE.—A large variety of aerobic and anaerobic bacteria, occurring either singly or in combination, are involved in wound infections. The commonest pyogens are *Staphylococcus aureus*, *Streptococcus pyogenes* and anaerobic streptococci, coliform bacilli such as *Esch. coli* and *Proteus* spp. and *Pseudomonas pyocyanea*. Among other species more rarely encountered are *Pasteurella septica* (from animal bites), *Corynebacterium diphtheriae* (in wound diphtheria) and *Bacillus anthracis* (malignant pustule). In long-standing infections that are slow to heal, and in pus showing no other microorganisms the possibility of infection due to *Mycobacterium tuberculosis* and *Actinomyces israelii* must be considered. Anaerobic organisms, in particular clostridia (notably *Cl. welchii*), *Bacteroides* spp. and anaerobic streptococci may be very important in wound infections, especially in abdominal wounds, traumatic wounds and wherever devitalised tissues provide suitably anaerobic conditions. Infection with aerobic bacteria may encourage the growth of clostridial pathogens, leading to tetanus and gas gangrene.

The swab or the exudate is inoculated on to two blood agar plates, one for aerobic, the other for anaerobic incubation, and also into a tube of Robertson's cooked meat broth. In addition some bacteriologists inoculate special media such as MacConkey's medium (to facilitate the differentiation of coliform organisms), double strength (4 per cent.) agar (to inhibit the swarming of *Proteus* spp. and so make possible the more rapid isolation of other pathogens present), crystal violet blood agar (to assist the separation of *Strept. pyogenes* in mixed infections), and neomycin egg-yolk agar (for the rapid identification of *Cl. welchii*).

Primary sensitivity tests are usually carried out on the diagnostic plates and the disks used have the added advantage of providing areas on the plates that are locally selective for certain species, thus facilitating their isolation and identification. Neomycin disks, each containing 100 μg., are particularly useful in this respect for the isolation of clostridia on anaerobic media.

The culture plates are examined after overnight incubation. Should there be growth in the cooked meat broth but no growth on the solid media the broth must be subcultured aerobically and anaerobically.

Pure or mixed growths of pathogens are reported along with the results of the *in vitro* sensitivity tests; if the primary sensitivity plate cannot be read with certainty a secondary sensitivity test is set up using the isolated organism in pure culture as inoculum. Scanty growths of skin commensal organisms such as *Staphylococcus albus* and diphtheroids are usually disregarded, as are growths likely to be due to extraneous contaminants, *e.g.* a *few* colonies of *Esch. coli* isolated from a perineal wound. Sometimes the significance of the growth is difficult to assess but the problem can often be resolved by examining a further carefully taken specimen from the lesion.

If there is no growth after 24 hr., the culture plates and the cooked-meat broth are reincubated for another 24 hr.; if the cultures are still sterile they may be discarded, unless there is an indication for a further period of incubation before finally concluding that no growth will take place, *e.g.* in isolating slow-growing pathogens such as *Actinomyces israelii.*

If tuberculous infection is suspected and if the pus has not yielded any growth on ordinary culture media, it may be possible to use the pus as inoculum for Löwenstein-Jensen or similar medium and for injecting into guinea-pigs. If the pus is viscid, or if ordinary culture has shown it to contain other organisms, it must be treated before these further investigations can be undertaken.

GENITAL TRACT INFECTIONS

Infection of the upper part of the female genital tract (salpingitis and oophoritis) may be part of a generalised infection or it may be localised, but in either case bacteriological diagnosis by examination of specimens obtained from the accessible lower tract is rarely possible.

Acute infections in the female are fairly common after delivery, *e.g.* puerperal sepsis or septic abortion. Acute cervicitis also occurs in non-pregnant women and some cases are venereal in origin. Where possible, cervical swabs should be taken with the aid of a speculum under direct vision but more frequently only a high vaginal swab is taken and this makes bacteriological diagnosis more difficult because of the presence of a complicated vaginal commensal flora which is variable and poorly classified.

Acute and chronic vaginitis and vulvo-vaginitis may be due to a variety of causes and many organisms may be responsible. Acute vaginitis due to *Trichomonas vaginalis* and vaginal thrush (particularly in pregnant women) are the most important infections. Exudate can be readily obtained by swabbing and direct smears made on slides for microscopic examination: or exudate may be collected by pipette or spoon for wet films.

In the male, acute urethritis and prostatitis are fairly common; many cases have a venereal origin.

Direct Films.—The discharge from female patients with leucorrhoea should be examined by direct microscopy ("wet film") for the presence of *Trichomonas vaginalis* as soon as possible after it has been obtained from the patient. Gram-stained smears of the discharge show the presence of inflammatory cells and in vaginal candidiasis "yeasts" are seen, but the morphology of the other flora present is not sufficiently characteristic to allow further differentiation from the commensal flora.

The microscopic diagnosis of acute gonhorroeal infection requires investigation of smears made from the cervix, urethral exudate and Bartholin's glands.

In the male, urethral discharge is less likely to be contaminated with organisms from the perineum than in the female although it should be remembered that the distal urethra does possess a commensal flora of diphtheroid bacilli, streptococci and *Staph. albus* and the presence of these bacteria is unlikely to be related to infection. Infection of the prostate gland is frequently difficult to diagnose; if there is no urethral discharge prostatic massage may provide exudate for examination.

The examination of a chancre requires careful collection of exudate and preparation for dark-field microscopy (Chapter 29).

CULTURE.—Vaginal, cervical, urethral and gland exudates must be cultured on as wide a range of media as is practicable. For the gonococcus, blood and heated blood agar may be inoculated and incubated in 5 per cent. carbon dioxide; this may be obviated if a medium containing mucin is used. Ristocetin or Vancomycin added to the medium makes it more selective for the gonococcus. If there is a delay in transit to the laboratory, transport media should be used.

The presence of well defined pathogens not normally found in the genital tract, e.g. *Strept. pyogenes*, even in small numbers, is probably significant of infection; others such as *Staph. aureus*, anaerobic streptococci and *Esch. coli* if present in considerable numbers are likely to be significant but the presence of other organisms closely resembling the normal flora of the female tract is difficult to assess in most cases.

CONJUNCTIVAL INFECTIONS

A variety of bacteria may produce acute conjunctivitis. The gonococcus produces severe ophthalmia neonatorum and *Staph. aureus* is a common cause of "sticky eye" in newborn babies in maternity hospitals. Pneumococcus, *Haemophilus influenzae* (Koch-Weeks bacillus) and *Moraxella lacunata* are other common infecting species. Certain adenoviruses and other viruses produce conjunctivitis together with an upper respiratory infection, and the TRIC. agents (p. 484) cause acute and chronic infections, *e.g.* inclusion blennorrhoea and trachoma. Severe infections with *Ps. pyocyanea* have followed the use of contaminated "eye-drops".

Purulent exudate from an inflamed conjunctiva should be treated as pus. Direct microscopy frequently shows microorganisms and a presumptive diagnosis can then be made: this is particularly important in the early detection of gonococcal ophthalmia. Small numbers of Gram-positive cocci, small Gram-negative bacilli or Gram-positive bacilli may indicate no more than the normal commensal flora but the pneumococcus, gonococcus, *Haemophilus* spp., moraxella, *Staph. aureus* and coliform bacilli may be seen in numbers sufficient to suggest a diagnosis. The cultures must always be incubated in the presence of carbon dioxide.

In many cases there is a minimum of exudate and diagnosis is facilitated by the inoculation of media and the preparation of smears for direct microscopy at the bedside. For this purpose a platinum loop (diameter 1 mm.) and slopes of heated blood agar in 1-oz. screw-capped bottles are useful.

Many cases of conjunctival inflammation are not bacterial in origin and attention must be directed towards the demonstration of viruses in such instances. Material taken with a platinum loop from the conjunctiva is spread on slides, stained with Giemsa's stain and examined for inclusion bodies.

PYREXIA OF UNCERTAIN ORIGIN

Patients who have a significant and persistent fever (greater than 100° F.), the cause of which cannot be readily diagnosed on clinical examination, are classified as having a "pyrexia of uncertain origin" (PUO). Many such cases are due to infection and their diagnosis will depend upon the employment of any methods to demonstrate the presence of a specific pathogen in the tissues; thus while every effort must be made to recover the causative organism, recourse to indirect methods of diagnosis must also be made, particularly serological methods to demonstrate the presence of specific antibody. Further, it is frequently necessary to repeat examinations a number of times since negative results do not always exclude the possibility of infection.

The procedure to be followed is usually along the following lines:

(1) Examination of the Blood

(*a*) Blood Films.—Direct films of the patient's blood should be prepared and examined to exclude the presence of circulating parasites such as plasmodia; this examination will also indicate the white cell picture of the peripheral blood and this information may be a help in diagnosis.

(*b*) Blood Culture.—This should be carried out on several occasions each day or on successive days. In cases of bacteraemia such as subacute bacterial endocarditis the number of organisms in the blood may be very small; to increase the chance of their recovery a series of cultures over a period of several hours should be taken. The presence of antibacterial agents increases the difficulty of recovering the causative organism and, with the exceptions of benzylpenicillin and sulphonamides, their inhibitory effects can best be countered by dilution of the blood.

(*c*) Animal Inoculation.—In some infections, *e.g.* leptospirosis, brucellosis and rickettsial diseases, animal inoculation carried out with freshly drawn blood may be more successful than attempts at culture in artificial media.

(*d*) Examination of the Serum.—Part of the blood drawn for blood culture may be set aside and allowed to clot and the serum used for antibody studies. Serological studies should be done at intervals of 5–10 days during the acute phase of the disease and later during the convalescent stages. This allows demonstration of any rise or fall in the amount of antibody; the unequivocal interpretation of a single result is often impossible. Examinations should always be made for antibodies to the enteric group of salmonellae (Widal test) and the brucella species.

It may be necessary to carry out as many tests as the laboratory is able to perform, in which case fairly large quantities of serum will be required (up to 10 ml.). If possible, indication of the most likely causes of the infection is helpful as this will direct attention to a more limited number of tests.

(2) **Examination of the Urine**

Routine examination should be carried out to exclude infection of the urinary tract and it should be remembered that urinary tract pathogens such as *Esch. coli* may be present only on intermittent occasions in chronic pyelonephritis. Occasionally *Salmonella* spp. can be isolated from the urine. Repeated examinations may be necessary.

If genito-urinary tuberculosis is suspected a 24 hr specimen of urine or three entire early morning specimens should be submitted; pyuria is usually present and *Myco. tuberculosis* may be seen after centrifugation and staining of the urine deposit; in leptospirosis, leptospires may be demonstrated by dark field examinations of the fresh urine.

(3) **Examination of Faeces**

This should be carried out particularly for organisms of the enteric and dysentery groups and for other causes of intestinal disease, including protozoa and the ova of helminths. In suspected virus infections it is advisable to match isolation of a virus with rises in the homologous antibody titre of the serum.

(4) **Examination of Tissues**

Biopsy of tissue such as a lymph gland may be carried out. The tissue is best cultured, *e.g.* for *M. tuberculosis*, after grinding it in a homogeniser or tissue blender. It is essential to avoid contamination, especially when fluid cultures are used for the cultivation of the pathogens.

(5) **Examination of Other Body Fluids**

Other body fluids should be examined microscopically and by culture if clinical signs or symptoms indicate this. Aspiration of secretions such as bile may be advisable to confirm suspected infection of the gall-bladder, liver or biliary passages, cerebrospinal fluid in meningitis and bone marrow in enteric fever.

(6) **Skin Tests**

In a number of subacute and chronic infections, hypersensitivity to the constituents of the causative organism develops. The inoculation of small quantities of suitable preparations of these bacterial products, ***e.g.*** tuberculin, brucellin, the Frei antigen, results in a localised delayed-type hypersensitivity reaction at the site of inoculation in patients with present or past infection. The results of such tests may be helpful in making a diagnosis.

POXVIRUS INFECTIONS

Variola: Vaccinia: Cowpox: Varicella.—The tests used for these infections are both rapid and sensitive, so that within 48 hr. of collection of the material the laboratory can make at least a provisional diagnosis of variola. It is of the utmost importance to employ these tests when there is even the slightest possibility of smallpox and they may give valuable information in many atypical or unusually severe cases of chickenpox. They may also be used in the investigation of vaccinial lesions and in Kaposi's varicelliform dermatitis.

An essential precaution for the worker who collects or handles material from suspect cases of smallpox is that he should have been satisfactorily vaccinated during the preceding twelve months. Specimens must be taken from the patient at as early a stage of the disease as possible and for this purpose the following apparatus is required: six well-cleaned, grease-free slides, a scalpel or needle, forceps, three to four capillary tubes, throat swabs, a screw-capped vial, ether, a spirit lamp, and suitable wooden boxes in which to transmit the specimens by post. The variola-vaccinia group of viruses are stable at atmospheric temperatures especially in dried material protected from sunlight, and are thus an exception to the rule that precludes the despatch of such material by post. The following specimens are required:

1. Pre-eruptive or viraemic stage. A sample of 5–8 ml. of whole blood should be taken at the first indication of illness in all persons known to have been in contact with a case of smallpox.

2. Maculo-papular stage. Clean the site of the lesion with ether especially if any ointment has been applied. Scrape six or more of lesions and transfer the material to the slides making a minimum of six reasonably thick films. Dry the films in air; *do not heat them.*

3. Vesicular stage. Collect vesicle fluid from several intact vesicles into capillary tubes and seal the ends of the tubes in a flame. If this is not possible take up material from the lesions on throat swabs and also make smears on slides from scrapings from the bases of the lesions.

4. Pustular or crusted stage. Remove 4–6 crusts with forceps and place them in the screw-capped bottle.

Send all the specimens together with the needle or scalpel blade used without delay to the laboratory.

The tests used will differentiate variola from vaccinia and cowpox, and all three from varicella and herpes simplex. The distinction between variola and vaccinia is, however, a matter of some difficulty and depends largely on the appearance of the lesions produced by the two viruses on the chorio-allantoic membrane.

Serological tests for antibodies seldom give information in time to be of use in the early diagnosis of smallpox; their main value is in establishing the nature of the infection in retrospect. When, however, the hypersensitive state has been established by vaccination in the past, infection with the variola virus occasions an accelerated outpouring of antibodies. The demonstration of a rapid increase in the amount of antibody in these circumstances may give valuable diagnostic information, in cases of suspected smallpox where a small number of lesions has escaped observation and no material has been taken for virus identification, or in cases of *variola sine eruptione*. If the patient has been recently vaccinated it will, however, not be possible to demonstrate a significant rise in antibody titre. Paired samples of sera are required together with full information of the vaccination history of the patient.

INFLUENZAL INFECTIONS

During the first 2–3 days of the acute phase of an "influenzal" illness the patient is instructed to cough vigorously and then to gargle immediately with five ml. of normal saline. The contents of the mouth are expectorated into a 1 oz. wide-necked screw-capped vial containing 2 ml. of medium 199 with added antibiotics. In the case of young children who cannot gargle a well-taken throat swab is satisfactory. The specimen is placed at once in the freezing coils of a refrigerator. For transport to the laboratory it can be placed in a jar surrounded by an ice and salt mixture or preferably in a special insulated box in which it is covered with fragments of solid CO_2 (−70° C.). An important exception to this procedure is needed when infection with the respiratory syncytial virus is suspected because this virus is inactivated by temperatures around 0° C. In this case the specimen should be sent very rapidly to the laboratory unfrozen. It is improbable that virus will be isolated from the patient after the third day of the illness.

It is convenient to take the first sample of blood (5–10 ml.) at the same time as the throat washings. A second sample of blood is required 10–16 days later. *On no account must either sample of blood be frozen.*

In fatal cases the autopsy should be performed with minimal delay and specimens of lung tissue involved in areas of consolidation or congestion should be frozen and sent without delay to the laboratory.

The influenza viruses A, B & C, the four para-influenza viruses, the adenoviruses, the respiratory syncytial virus, and the rhinoviruses can be isolated by the inoculation of tissue cultures. In addition influenza viruses A, B and C can be isolated by the inoculation of the amniotic cavity of the developing chick embryo. The best conditions for the growth of the virus, e.g. the most suitable tissue culture cells and the optimum temperature are given in the chapters referring to each of the individual viruses. Chapter 57 gives details of the techniques required.

Paired sera are examined by complement-fixation or haemagglutination inhibition with the following antigens: influenza A, B & C, para-influenza 1, 2 & 3, adenovirus, respiratory syncytial virus, psittacosis, etc. (see Chapter 54). A four-fold or greater rise in antibody titre between the acute and convalescent sera is accepted as indicating recent infection.

APPENDIX 1

CONTAINERS AND SWABS FOR THE COLLECTION OF SPECIMENS

Specimens for bacteriological investigation should be forwarded as soon as possible to the laboratory in robust, leak-proof, sterile containers. It is essential that each container should bear the name of the patient from whom the specimen is submitted and the accompanying form should be accurately completed. Relevant clinical data must indicate the probable clinical diagnosis, information regarding recent or current chemotherapy and, especially if a serological investigation is required, relevant details of previous immunisation should be given.

Glass Tubes and Universal Containers.—These are suitable for submission of specimens of exudate, pus, blood, cerebrospinal fluid, urine and faeces. Strong glass test-tubes, $4 \times \frac{5}{8}$ in., with rubber bungs or bark corks, may be used. They should be sterilised in the autoclave with the bungs or corks loosely fitted and thereafter pressed in. Tubes with bark corks may be sterilised in the hot-air oven.

The screw-capped bottle known as a universal container is recommended; it consists of a strong moulded glass bottle, $3\frac{1}{4}$ in. high $\times$ $1\frac{1}{8}$ in. diameter, capacity 1 oz. (28 ml.), with a flat base and wide mouth. These bottles are supplied already cleaned and capped in 1-gross boxes. They are sterilised by autoclaving with the caps loosely screwed on; after sterilisation the caps are tightened. They cannot be sterilised in the hot-air oven, as the rubber washers will not withstand the temperature.

The screw-capped universal container has many advantages over the glass tube. It is stronger, and the screw cap keeps the mouth of the container sterile whereas dust collects at the rim of a stoppered tube. The contents of a universal container cannot leak or become contaminated and, as it is quite stable on its base, it is particularly convenient when specimens are taken at the bedside.

For the collection of serous fluids, *e.g.* pleural fluid, the universal container is suitable. The addition of 0·3 ml. of a 20 per cent. solution of sodium citrate to the container prior to autoclaving (with the cap fitted) is recommended for the collection of fluids that may coagulate on standing. This avoids difficulty in performing cell counts or centrifuging procedures with such fluids.

Blood may be submitted in a universal container but a small quantity for serological investigation is more conveniently sent in a sterile glass tube fitted with a rubber bung. The blood clot may be cultured in selective medium, *e.g.* for enteric organisms. Blood intended primarily for blood culture should be submitted in a special blood culture bottle.

For the collection of *faeces*, a small squat bottle of about 2 oz. capacity, or a glass specimen tube 2 in. × 1 in., fitted with a bark cork in which a small metal spoon is fixed, is sometimes used. Such containers have the disadvantage that any fermentation of the faeces tends to blow out the cork and cause leakage of the contents. The corks have to be discarded after use. The shoulder on the bottle makes cleaning difficult.

For small quantities of faeces the universal container is recommended. A small spoon made of tin plate $3\frac{3}{8} \times \frac{3}{8}$ in. may be included in the container prior to sterilisation. A portion of faeces is taken up in the spoon and the whole dropped into the container and the cap screwed on. Alternatively, a wide-mouth 2-oz. screw-capped jar, known as a "pomade pot", is used and the faeces taken up in small cardboard spoons (such as are used for ice-cream cartons). These containers may be transmitted to the laboratory by post, the package labelled "Pathological Specimen".

When there is likely to be a delay of some hours before laboratory cultivation can be carried out, neutral glycerol-saline should be added to the faeces.

For small quantities of *urine*, *e.g.* for the diagnosis of most cases of urinary tract infection, the universal container is used (but see p. 564). For larger quantities, *e.g.* complete early morning specimens, 20-oz. screw-capped bottles are convenient.

WAXED CARDBOARD CARTONS.—For the collection of *sputum* and *faeces* when the specimen is not to be sent by post, screw-capped waxed cardboard cartons of 2 oz. capacity (such as are used for cream and ice-cream) are suitable. After the specimen has been examined in the laboratory the carton and contents are burned. Because of postal regulations the waxed carton cannot be sent through the post. Disposable aluminium containers (2 in. in diameter by 1 in. deep) are now available; they cost about 3d. each, can be dispatched by post, and are suitable for the collection of specimens of faeces or sputum. They should be destroyed in a furnace after use.

SWABS.—A swab usually consists of a piece of aluminium or tinned iron wire, 15 gauge and 6 in. long. One end is made rough for about $\frac{1}{2}$ in. by squeezing it in a small metal vice or cutting edge of pliers. Around this end a thin pledget of absorbent cotton-wool is tightly wrapped for about $\frac{3}{4}$ in. The wire is placed in a narrow thick-walled test-tube, 5 in. $\times$ $\frac{1}{2}$ in., and the top of the tube is plugged with cotton-wool. Alternatively, and where swabs have to be sent by post, the wire should be $4\frac{1}{2}$ in. long and the top inserted into a bark cork which stoppers the tube. The tube with swab should be sterilised in the autoclave and not in the hot-air oven, as in the latter the wool may char and give rise to tar-like products which may be inimical to bacteria on the swab. It is important to autoclave cork-stoppered tubes with the cork loose and to press in the cork after sterilisation. Tubes plugged with cotton wool should be dried after autoclaving.

Instead of wire, swabs may be prepared from thin wooden sticks $6\frac{1}{2}$ in. long that are specially made for the purpose, and are known as "Peerless" wooden applicators. A cotton-wool pledget is wrapped round one end as above, and the tube is plugged with cotton-wool. They cannot be used conveniently with a bark cork, but have the advantage that the stick can be broken off short when the swab has to be placed in transport medium in a screw-capped container.

When taking specimens from babies and young children it is often necessary to employ a very fine swab so that small orifices, such as the aural meatus, may be negotiated without gross contamination from the external surfaces. These are made in the same way as the swabs described above but with fine rigid wire such as that supplied as ENT probes by George Stone and Son, 35 High Park Street, Liverpool 8. To avoid damage to the tissues, the end of the wire should be fused in a Bunsen flame before fixing a tiny pledget of cotton wool to it.

Swabs are very useful for taking specimens from:

(*a*) Throat: in cases of suspected diphtheria, tonsillitis, etc.

(*b*) Wounds, discharging ears, or surgical conditions, *e.g.* fistula, sinus, etc.: Some of the purulent material is taken up on the cotton wool.

(*c*) Post-nasal or naso-pharyngeal space: for this purpose the terminal $\frac{3}{4}$ in. is bent through an angle of 45 degrees, and in use is inserted behind the soft palate. This procedure is useful for obtaining specimens from suspected meningococcal carriers and for the early diagnosis of whooping-cough.

For the diagnosis of whooping-cough a "pernasal" swab may be conveniently used: this is made from 7 in. of flexible copper wire or nichrome SWG 25 (0·51 mm. diameter), the terminal $\frac{1}{4}$ in. being bent back to take the pledget of cotton-wool, a very thin layer of which is wound firmly round it. The swab is contained in a $6 \times \frac{1}{2}$ in. test-tube plugged with cotton-wool. The swab is passed gently back from one nostril, along the floor of the nasal cavity until it reaches the posterior wall of the nasopharynx, rotated gently and it is then withdrawn.

(*d*) Rectum: rectal swabs are very useful in bacillary dysentery cases or contacts, especially in young children.

(*e*) Cervix uteri: in gonorrhoea and puerperal infections. A longer wire, 9 in., is preferable for these specimens.

Where some time may elapse before the swab is examined and especially where delicate pathogens are concerned, *e.g.* meningococcus or *Bord. pertussis*, it is advantageous to place the swab in transport medium. A bark cork is used as a stopper and the wire pushed through the cork so that the cotton-wool is clear of the agar. After the specimen has been taken, the swab is inserted into the tube and the wire pushed down until the cotton-wool pledget is in contact with the transport medium.

A special method for preserving the viability of the gonococcus in swabs is described in Chapter 47. The problem of bacterial survival is not confined to the *Neisseria*, since slow-drying is known to be lethal to most bacterial species. Transport media for various species are described in Chapter 47. Rubbo and Benjamin (1951), as a result of their comparative findings with many different pathogens, recommend the use of a serum-coated cotton-wool swab to prolong viability. The swabs are prepared by dipping the cotton-wool on a wooden applicator into undiluted ox serum for 10–30 sec., spreading them out on sheets of blotting-paper, drying in an incubator at 37° C. for about half an hour, and finally sterilising in the autoclave at 121° C. for 20 min. The finished product is a compact honey-coloured pledget, 3–5 mm. in diameter, in which the cotton-wool fibres are firmly bound to each other and to the applicator. Clinicians may need to be warned about the unusual appearance of these swabs so that they will not think they have already been used. For a more detailed account of swabs and swabbing methods see Cruickshank (1953).

APPENDIX 2

POSTAL REGULATIONS

The Postmaster-General has laid down the following instructions for sending pathological material through the post and these should be rigorously observed:

"ARTICLES SENT FOR MEDICAL EXAMINATION OR ANALYSIS.—Deleterious liquids or substances, though otherwise prohibited from transmission by post, may be sent for medical examination or analysis to a recognised Medical Laboratory or Institute, whether or not belonging to a Public Health Authority or to a qualified Medical Practitioner or Veterinary Surgeon within the United Kingdom, by *letter post, and on no account by parcel post*, under the following condition:

"Any such liquid or substance must be enclosed in a receptacle, hermetically sealed or otherwise securely closed, which receptacle must itself be placed in a strong wooden, leather or metal case in such a way that it cannot shift about, and with a sufficient quantity of some absorbent material (such as sawdust or cotton-wool) so packed about the receptacle as absolutely to prevent any possible leakage from the package in the event of damage to the receptacle. The packet so made up must be conspicuously marked 'Fragile with care' and bear the words 'Pathological Specimen'.

"Any packet of the kind found in the parcel post, or found in the letter post not packed and marked as directed, will be at once stopped and destroyed with all its wrappings and enclosures. Further, any person who sends by post a deleterious liquid or substance for medical examination or analysis otherwise than as provided by these regulations is liable to prosecution.

"If receptacles are supplied by a Laboratory or Institute, they should be submitted to the Secretary, General Post Office, in order to ascertain whether they are regarded as complying with the regulations."

The following receptacles have been approved by the Postmaster-General:

For universal containers, media bottles and 2-oz. pots, a leatherboard box, internal size $4\frac{3}{8}$ in. × $2\frac{1}{8}$ in. × $1\frac{7}{8}$ in. deep with metal-bound edges and full-depth lid, is used. The glass container is wrapped in a piece of cellulose tissue, 19 in. × $4\frac{1}{2}$ in., and then fits securely in the box which is placed in a shaped gummed envelope having a tag for the postage stamps.

Swabs or cultures in tubes are wrapped in cellulose tissue and placed in hinged metal boxes having rounded corners, size $6\frac{1}{4}$ in. long, $2\frac{1}{2}$ in. wide and 1 in. deep. Leatherboard boxes with metal-bound edges of the same size are also permitted. These are placed in stout manilla envelopes which have a tag at the end for the postage stamps.

For the 8-oz. pots and the 1-lb. jars, a larger piece of cellulose tissue is required, while the leatherboard box is similar in construction to the one mentioned above and large enough to take these receptacles.

Gummed labels printed with the name and address of the laboratory and the information required by the Post Office Regulations are often issued by laboratories when sending out the postal materials.

APPENDIX 3

THE LABORATORY DIAGNOSIS OF VIRUS INFECTIONS OF MAN

Disease	Detection of Virus			Detection of Serum Antibodies	
	Material Required	Transport to Laboratory	Tests Used	Dates for Collection of Sera	Tests Used
Variola; (See p 576). Vaccinia; Cowpox.	1. Serum in pre-eruptive phase. 2. 6 films on slides made from scrapings of macules and papules. 3. Vesicle fluid in capillary tubes. 4. Crusts in screw capped bottles.	By hand or by post. ,, ,, ,,	Virus cultivation Microscopy for elementary bodies. Cultures on allantoic membrane. Complement fixation, agar gel precipitation, for viral antigen.	Before 5th and after 15th day.	Comp. fixation; Neutralisation.
Varicella; Herpes zoster.	Vesicle fluid.	By hand or by post.	Microscopy for elementary bodies and giant cells. Complement fixation for viral antigen. Tissue culture.	Before 5th and after 15th day.	Comp. fixation.
Herpes simplex.	1. Vesicle fluid. 2. Crusts or scrapings from bases of lesions on slides. 3. Skin or brain from autopsy.	Frozen. Frozen. In glycerol saline and frozen.	Egg, animal, or tissue culture inoculation.	Before 5th and after 15th day.	Comp. fixation; Neutralisation.

Influenza (See p. 577)	1. Throat washings in first 48 hours.	Frozen.	Egg, ferret or tissue culture inoculation.	Before 3rd and after 15th day.	Comp. fixation; Haemagglutination-inhibition.
	2. Throat swab (children).	Frozen.			
	3. Lung tissue at autopsy.	Frozen.			
Acute Respiratory Disease due to: (*a*) Para-influenza viruses, etc.	Throat washings or throat swabs.	Frozen.	Tissue culture inoculation.	Before 3rd and after 15th day.	Neutralisation; Comp. fixation.
(*b*) Adenoviruses.	1. Throat washings or throat swab. 2. Conjunctival swab. 3. Sputum.	By hand or by post.	Tissue culture inoculation.	Before 3rd day and after 15th day.	Comp. fixation (group); Neutralisation (type).
Measles.	Throat and oral swab.	Immediate.	Tissue culture inoculation.	Before 3rd day and after 15th day.	Neutralisation; Comp. fixation.
Mumps.	1. Saliva during first 3 days.	Frozen.	Egg inoculation.	During first 6 days and after 21st day.	Comp. fixation; Haemagglutination-inhibition.
	2. Cerebrospinal fluid in first 3 days of encephalitis.	Frozen.	Egg inoculation.		
Psittacosis.	1. Sputum } 2. Citrated blood. } in acute phase.	Frozen.	Egg or animal inoculation.	After 21st day, and if possible before 6th day.	Comp. fixation.
	3. Lung and spleen from autopsy.	Frozen.	Egg or animal inoculation.		
Lymphogranuloma venereum.	1. Pus from bubo.	Frozen.	Animal or egg inoculation.	After 21st day, and if possible before 10th day.	Comp. fixation.
	2. Biopsy material.	One portion of biopsy material to be frozen another fixed in Zenker's fluid.	Histological picture. Frei's test positive after 2 weeks.		

THE LABORATORY DIAGNOSIS OF VIRUS INFECTIONS OF MAN—*continued.*

Diseases	Detection of Virus			Detection of Serum Antibodies	
	Material Required	Transport to Laboratory	Tests Used	Dates for Collection of Sera	Tests Used
Primary atypical pneumonia.	Sputum in first four days.	Frozen.	Animal, egg or tissue culture inoculation. Special medium for PPLO.	Before 7th and after 14th day.	Comp. fixation for Q. fever, psittacosis, influenza; Mycoplasma Strep. M.G. agglut.; Cold. agglutinins.
Trachoma; Inclusion conjunctivitis.	Smears of scrapings from tarsal conjunctiva.	By hand or post.	Microscopy for elementary bodies and inclusions. Egg or tissue culture inoculation.		Comp. fixation.
Rickettsial infections.	Whole blood.	Immediate.	Animal or egg inoculation.	Before 6th day. After 21st day.	Weil-Felix, agglutination and Comp. fixation.
Rabies.	1. Saliva.	Frozen.	Animal inoculation.		
	2. Animal brain. One half in glycerol saline. One half in Zenker's solution.	By hand or post.	Animal inoculation. Examination for Negri bodies.		Neutralisation.
Encephalitis (Herpes; Louping ill, and Arthropod borne virus infections).	1. CSF in first four days.	Frozen.	Animal inoculation.	Before 5th and after 14th day.	Haemagglutination inhibition; Neutralisation; Comp. fixation.
	2. Brain from autopsy in glycerol saline.	Frozen.			
Lymphocytic choriomeningitis.	1. CSF. 2. Citrated blood. } in first 4 days.	Frozen.	Animal inoculation.	Before 10th day, after 21st day and again after 50 days.	Comp. fixation.

Poliomyelitis (See p. 431).	1. Whole blood during prodromal period.	By hand or frozen.	Inoculation of animal or tissue cultures.	Before 3rd and after 14th day.	Neutralisation; Comp. fixation.
	2. Pharyngeal swab during first week.	By hand or frozen.			
	3. Faeces.	By hand or post.			
	4. Brain or spinal cord from autopsy.	In glycerol saline by hand or post.	Inoculation of animal or tissue cultures.		
ECHO Virus infections; Coxsackie Virus Infections; Bornholm Disease; Herpangina; Aseptic Meningitis.	1. Faeces or rectal swabs } during first 3 days. 2. Swabs from oral lesions } during first 3 days. 3. CSF.	By hand or frozen.	Suckling mouse inoculation. Tissue culture inoculation.	Before 5th and after 21st day.	Neutralisation; Comp. fixation.

Note.—At present there are no diagnostic tests available in infective hepatitis or homologous serum jaundice.

Routine tests for all the virus infections listed may not be available. In special emergencies the laboratory should always be consulted.

This table has been modified from that in *Virus and Rickettsial Diseases*. Edward Arnold and Company, London (1961).

APPENDIX 4

THE LABORATORY DIAGNOSIS OF BACTERIAL INFECTIONS OF MAN

Nature of Infection	Specimens to be submitted for examination	Media for primary inoculation	Atmosphere for incubation	Techniques and selective agents for separation	Further steps for identification of the causal organism	Indirect methods of diagnosis	Antibiograms. Fixed: Sensitive	Antibiograms. Fixed: Resistant	Antibiograms. Variable
Actinomycosis and related infections.	Exudate. Tissue.	Blood agar. Shake culture in glucose agar.	Aerobic. Micro-aerophilic. Anaerobic.	Prolonged culture. Washing of granules.			P.S.C.T.		
Anthrax.	Exudate. Blood culture. (Sputum, Faeces.)	Nutrient agar. Blood agar.	Aerobic.		Animal pathogenicity.		P.C.T.		
Brucellosis.	Blood culture. Serum.	Liver infusion agar and broth. Blood agar.	Aerobic. Air + CO_2.		Dye sensitivity tests. Animal pathogenicity. Specific antisera.	Agglutination tests. Brucellin skin test.	S.C.T.E.		
Cholera.	Faeces.	Alkaline selective medium.	Aerobic.	Surface growth on alkaline peptone water.	Haemolysis. Biochemical tests. Specific antisera.				
Clostridial.	Exudate. Tissue. Blood culture.	Blood agar. Cooked-meat broth.	Anaerobic.	Neomycin. Differential heating.	Biochemical tests. Toxin neutralisation tests. Animal pathogenicity.		C.T.	N.	Su.P.S.
Diphtheria.	Exudate (membrane). Throat swab.	Blood agar. Loeffler's medium. Blood tellurite media.	Aerobic.		Biochemical tests. Toxin neutralisation tests. Animal pathogenicity.		P.E.		
Gonococcal.	Exudate from urethra, cervix, conjunctiva. Serum.	Blood agar. Heated blood agar.	Air + CO_2 (high humidity).		Oxidase test. Biochemical tests.	Complement fixation test.	C.T.K.		Su.P.

Haemophilus.	Sputum. Exudate from eye. CSF. Blood culture.	Blood agar. Heated blood agar.	Aerobic. Air + CO_2.	Penicillin.	Growth requirement. Specific antisera.*		S.C.T.	P.	
L eptospiral.	Blood culture. Serum. Urine.	Serum broth.	Aerobic. Micro-aerophilic.	Animal inoculation.	Dark ground microscopy. Specif c antisera.	Agglutination tests.	P.S.T.		
Meningococcal.	CSF. Blood culture. Post nasal swabs (carriers).	Blood agar. Heated blood agar.	Air + CO_2 (high humidity). Anaerobic.		Oxidase test. Biochemical tests. Specific antisera.*		Su.P.C.		
Pasteurella.	Exudate. Aspirate (bubo). Blood culture. Sputum. Serum.	Blood agar. Nutrient agar.	Aerobic.		Biochemical tests. Animal pathogenicity.	Agglutination tests.*	S.C.T.		T.
Pneumococcal.	Sputum. CSF. Blood culture. Exudate. Throat swab.	Blood agar.	Air + CO_2. Anaerobic.	Optochin.	Biochemical tests. Specific antisera.* Animal pathogenicity.		P.C.E.	S.	Su.
Proteus.	Urine. Exudate.	MacConkey's medium. 4% agar.	Aerobic.	Inhibition of swarming.	Biochemical tests.		K.	T.	Su.S.C.A.G.
Pseudomonas.	Urine. Exudate. CSF.	Blood agar Nutrient agar.	Aerobic.	Chloroxylenol or Cetrimide.	Pigment production. Oxidase test. Phage typing.* Pyocine typing.*		Colo. Poly.		Su.C.T.K.G.
Salmonella — Enteric Fever.	Blood culture. Faeces. Urine. Serum.	MacConkey's medium. DCA Wilson & Blair's medium.	Aerobic.	Enrichment broth media.	Biochemical tests. Specific antisera. Phage typing.*	Agglutination tests. (Widal reaction.)	C.A.		T.
Salmonella — Food poisoning.	Faeces. Vomit. Food. Blood culture.	MacConkey's medium. DCA Wilson & Blair's medium.	Aerobic.	Enrichment broth media.	Biochemical tests. Specific antisera. Phage typing.*		C.A.		T.
Shigella.	Faeces.	MacConkey's medium. DCA	Aerobic.	Enrichment broth media.	Biochemical tests. Specific antisera. Colicine typing.*				Su.S.C.T.N. Colo.

Nature of Infection	Specimens to be submitted for examination	Media for primary inoculation	Atmosphere for incubation	Techniques and selective agents for separation	Further steps for identification of the causal organism	Indirect methods of diagnosis	Antibiograms. Fixed: Sensitive	Antibiograms. Fixed: Resistant	Antibiograms. Variable
Staphylococcal.	Exudates. Anterior nares, Flexures } Carriers. Tissue. Blood culture. Serum.	Blood agar.	Aerobic.	7–10% NaCl. Polymyxin agar.	Coagulase test. Phage typing.*	Anti α-staphylolysin.*	Ox.		P.S.C.T.E.A.
Streptococcal caused by *Strept. pyogenes.*	Exudates. Throat swab. High vaginal swab. Blood culture. Serum.	Blood agar.	Aerobic. Anaerobic.	Crystal violet.	Bacitracin sensitivity—Lancefield Group A. Griffith typing.*	Antistreptolysin O.*	P.C.E.	S.	T.
Streptococcal caused by other streptococci.	Exudate. Blood culture.	Blood agar.	Aerobic. Anaerobic.	Crystal violet.	Bacitracin resistance—other Lancefield Groups.		E.	S.	P.C.T.
Treponemal.	Exudate. Serum.				Dark ground microscopy.	Complement fixation tests. Flocculation tests. Immobilisation and fluorescent antibody tests.*	P.C.T.		
Tuberculosis.	Sputum. Exudate. Urine. CSF	Egg media e.g. Löwenstein-Jensen.	Aerobic.	Concentration and preparation of specimen.	Differentiation from atypical forms by various tests.	Tuberculin skin test.			S.I.Pas.T.
Whooping Cough.	Pharyngeal/laryngeal swab. Cough plate. Throat washings.	Special blood media e.g. Bordet-Gengou.	Aerobic.	Penicillin.	Specific antisera.		C.T.		

Antibiograms
Fixed, (sensitive/resistant) = invariable results of *in vitro* tests.
Variable = strains vary significantly in their sensitivity to the antibiotics listed.

A = Ampicillin.	G = Gentamicin.	P = Penicillin.
C = Chloramphenicol.	K = Kanamycin.	Poly = Polymyxin B.
Colo = Colomycin (polymyxin E).	N = Neomycin.	S = Streptomycin.
E = Erythromycin.	Ox = Cloxacillin.	Su = Sulphonamides.
I = Isonicotinic acid hydrazide.	Pas = Para-amino-salicylic acid.	T = Tetracyclines.

* Tests requiring special laboratory facilities.

APPENDIX 5

DOCUMENTATION OF SPECIMENS IN THE LABORATORY

Specimens should be dealt with as expeditiously as possible after arrival at the laboratory, and efforts to deliver the material rapidly from the patient must not be vitiated by unnecessary delays consequent upon specimens lying about unattended. Great care must be taken to identify specimens and request forms on arrival at the laboratory so that when their future separation occurs no mistake will arise: this is best carried out by having a responsible person label all specimens and corresponding forms with a duplicate serial number. For this purpose serial numbers printed on gummed paper, in duplicate, triplicate, etc., may be purchased; these are also useful for identifying tubes and culture plates that are used for the examination of the specimen. Different colours and prefixes may be usefully employed to distinguish different types of specimen or series of examinations and this facilitates record keeping and identification, *e.g.* T for tuberculosis, U for urine examination. These serial numbers can be used for chronological clerking of specimens which serves as a cross reference system to an alphabetical filing system.

In most cases it is valuable to examine and report on each specimen in the light of previous knowledge of the patient. The information given by practitioners on bacteriological request forms is not usually sufficient for this and it is preferable to have the results of previous bacteriological examination available in each case. This can be done by filing the results of all examinations on a card for each patient; it is more informative and less time consuming if all laboratory findings are recorded on the reverse side of each request form and to file this in a small envelope or folder for each patient along with a copy of the report issued. This occupies less filing space. The colour of the folders may be changed at six month intervals and one year's work is kept readily available. At the end of each six month period files more than one year old are removed for storage and later destroyed.

As each specimen arrives at the laboratory, the file for the patient is withdrawn and it accompanies the specimen throughout its examination; in this way the bacteriologist may direct his examination and interpret his findings in the light of all the previous reports.

REFERENCES

CRUICKSHANK, R. (1953). Clinical pathology in general practice—taking swabs. *Brit. med. J.*, **2**, 1095.

ELLIOT, W. A., & SLEIGH, J. D. (1963). Container for transport of urine specimens at low temperature. *Brit. med. J.*, **1**, 1142.

HOUGHTON, B. J. & PEARS, M.A. (1957). Cell excretion in normal urine. *Brit. med. J.*, **1**, 622.

McGEACHIE, J. & KENNEDY, A. C. (1963). Simplified quantitative methods for bacteriuria and pyuria. *J. clin. Path.*, **16**, 32.

REPORT (1939). A study of the Nasopharyngeal Bacterial Flora of Different Groups of Persons observed in London and South-East England during the years 1930 to 1937. STRAKER, EDITH, HILL, A. B. & LOVELL, R. *H.M.S.O.*

RUBBO, S. D. & BENJAMIN, M. (1951). Some observations on survival of pathogenic bacteria on cotton-wool swabs. Development of a new type of swab. *Brit. med. J.*, **1**, 983.

GENERAL READING

BEDSON, S. P., DOWNIE, A. W., MACCALLUM, F. O. & STEWART-HARRIS, C. H. (1961). *Virus and Rickettsial Diseases of Man*, 3rd ed. London: Arnold.

STOKES, E. JOAN (1960). *Clinical Bacteriology*, 2nd ed. London: Arnold.

THOMSON, W. A. R. (ed.) (1966). *Calling the Laboratory*, 2nd ed. Edinburgh: Livingstone.

CHAPTER 43

PROPHYLACTIC IMMUNISATION

In recent years there has developed an increasing interest in the role of immunisation in the control of communicable diseases. This fresh interest in immunisation probably derives from a number of contributory factors, *e.g.* the dramatic success of national programmes for the control of diphtheria by immunisation; the publicity given to large-scale campaigns for the control of diphtheria, tuberculosis and poliomyelitis by prophylactic vaccines; the wider knowledge made available through international bodies like WHO of the prevalence and economic importance of communicable diseases in developing countries; the need for protection against the introduction of quarantinable diseases like smallpox and yellow fever; and the growing realisation that treatment with antimicrobial drugs has definite limitations and disadvantages.

The Rationale of Immunisation

The objective of immunisation is to produce, without harm to the recipient, a degree of resistance as great as, or greater than, that which follows a clinical attack of the natural infection. With this objective in mind, those communicable or infectious diseases amenable to control by vaccination may be considered in four main groups; toxic, acute bacterial, chronic bacterial, viral and rickettsial infections. In the first group, *e.g.* diphtheria and tetanus, the brunt of the infection is due to a specific poison or toxin which can be purified artificially, rendered harmless by treatment with formaldehyde (=toxoid) and used as an effective antigen or prophylactic, particularly if it is adsorbed on to a mineral carrier, *e.g.* aluminium hydroxide or aluminium phosphate. (These alum salts are tissue irritants and therefore should be used in the lowest concentration required for an adjuvant action.) The potency of toxoid antigens can be measured and standardised with great accuracy, and the amount of antitoxin that is produced in the inoculated person gives a reliable indication of the degree of resistance to infection in that individual.

Among the acute bacterial infections there are two categories as far as immunisation procedures are concerned: (*a*) pyogenic infections (staphylococcal, streptococcal and pneumococcal) against which vaccines are largely ineffective, since there are many different antigenic types within the species, *e.g.* pneumococcus type 1, 2, 3, etc., so that an infection (or immunisation) with one type does not protect against infection with other types; (*b*) infections like whooping-cough, cholera, plague and anthrax, where there is one antigenic type of organism, so that a vaccine prepared with the infecting organism might be expected to give a reasonable degree of protection. However, these organisms contain many different antigenic components, of which probably only one or two are particularly concerned with the virulence of the organism. It is important to try to identify and certainly to preserve these so-called "protective antigens" in vaccine preparations.

Another difficulty is that in bacterial infections like whooping-cough and cholera, the infection affects predominantly the epithelial surfaces so that antibodies produced as a result of vaccination may not gain easy access to the site where the pathogen is producing the infection. For this and other reasons it was essential to test vaccines against whooping-cough and cholera in properly controlled field trials, so that objective assessment of their value could be obtained.

So far, the assumption has been implicit that the production of a specific protecting antibody is the main requirement for effective immunisation, although it should be noted that immunity may persist long after such antibodies cease to be demonstrable, as in whooping-cough. When the chronic bacterial infections are considered (*e.g.* typhoid, brucellosis, tuberculosis), it must be concluded from knowledge of the natural behaviour of these infections that the specific humoral antibodies which can at present be identified play little part in overcoming the infection. Thus, antibodies to the specific antigens of the typhoid and brucella bacteria are demonstrable in the blood of the patient within a week of onset of the clinical illness, but the fever may go on for many weeks before clinical recovery. In addition, relapses in these *continued fevers* are not uncommon despite the presence of high concentrations of specific antibodies. In contrast to the acute bacterial infections, the infecting organisms in chronic infections are for the most part intracellular parasites, and it seems likely that what is called *cellular immunity* may be more important in overcoming the infection than the presence of humoral antibodies. It may be noted that in tuberculosis and brucellosis a living attenuated vaccine is needed to produce immunity. The development of tissue hypersensitivity probably plays a part in raising resistance to infection or re-infection in these and some other infections.

In the viral infections it is known that humoral antibodies may be protective, but, again, cellular immunity seems to be important in some diseases. Thus, children with hypo-gammaglobulinaemia can recover from infections like measles, chickenpox and mumps with an apparently good immunity without detectable humoral antibody, whereas they rapidly succumb to acute bacterial or toxic infections. Such children can also be successfully vaccinated with smallpox vaccine (and with BCG). But again, repeated attacks of herpes simplex occur in the presence of humoral antibodies. These findings indicate that specific humoral antibodies do not play a major role in recovery from some virus diseases. On the other hand, immunity to certain infections seems to be equated with the presence of antibody; human gammaglobulin can be used effectively to protect against measles and killed viral vaccines, which probably act mainly in virtue of the production of humoral antibody, can protect against diseases like poliomyelitis and influenza.

Immune Response and Duration of Immunity

The newborn baby may contain in its blood antibodies to the agents of certain toxic, bacterial and viral infections according as the corresponding antibodies are present in the mother's blood. This passive immunity gives protection to the infant at a time when it is poorly equipped to produce specific antibodies, but it interferes to a varying extent with the infant's capacity to respond to the stimulus of toxoids or vaccines in the early months of life. For example, killed poliomyelitis vaccines elicit little or no antibody response in most children under 6 months of age because of the presence of maternal antibody. The capacity of the infant's tissues to produce specific antibody to injected antigens is, in any case, poorly developed in the first few months of life although some response is obtained to powerful antigens such as alum-adsorbed toxoids. It should be noted that the newborn infant will respond to living vaccines, *e.g.* BCG and smallpox vaccines.

When a good specific antibody response is being sought to a toxoid or killed antigen, the usual procedure is to give two or three doses of the antigen at intervals of several weeks. The first dose of antigen evokes a poor antibody response after a latent period of approximately two weeks, but after the second dose the amount of antibody produced is multiplied tenfold and after a third dose may be increased a hundredfold. The first or "priming" dose of toxoid will be more effective the larger it is; or if it is released slowly as from a mineral carrier; or if it is mixed with certain bacterial vaccines, *e.g.* tetanus toxoid plus typhoid vaccine, diphtheria toxoid plus pertussis vaccine. The second and subsequent doses are effectivc in much smaller amounts than the first, and without the help of adjuvants. With toxoids the response is much better if the two doses are spaced out at an interval of four to eight weeks, and, provided the priming dose is adequate, the response to the second dose will still be maximal even if given six to twelve months after the first. It is not known whether this delayed secondary response is applicable also to killed bacterial or viral vaccines: certainly with Salk-type polio vaccines, it is considered advisable to give the second dose not later than four weeks after the first dose. Where there is reason to believe that a community has acquired a basic immunity from the widespread occurrence of clinical or inapparent infection, as in influenza, one dose of antigen will act as the secondary stimulus.

As regards the duration of immunity after the basic course, this can be measured precisely in the case of toxic infections according to the level of specific antitoxin in the blood, or, less precisely, in diphtheria by the Schick test. Recent studies have shown that an adequate concentration of diphtheria antitoxin may persist in the blood of children for several years after primary immunisation in early infancy. After a primary course of three doses of tetanus toxoid, a satisfactory antitoxin titre may be present for as long as ten years.

The duration of immunity after injections of killed bacterial vaccines cannot be equated with the presence of demonstrable antibody; for example, after a course of three doses of pertussis vaccine given to children (average age one year) there was no change in the degree of protection in successive six months during a follow-up period of two-and-a-half years, although antibodies were no longer demonstrable in a considerable proportion of the children within a year after immunisation. Again, in the chronic bacterial infections, there is no correlation between antibody titres and clinical protection, as was shown by the controlled studies of typhoid vaccines in Yugoslavia. In the viral infections, although antibody titres are accepted as a measure of the degree of protection, there are certain anomalous findings: for example, high titres of neutralising antibody have been found in the early stages of fatal infections in smallpox.

For these bacterial and viral infections, therefore, the only reliable measure of the duration of immunity after vaccination is a careful assessment of the attack rate over a period of time, preferably in comparable groups of vaccinated and non-vaccinated children.

Controlled Field and Laboratory Studies of Prophylactic Vaccines

Evaluation of prophylactic vaccines and toxoids by means of carefully designed field trials has in the past two decades resulted in a revolutionary change in the accuracy with which the degree of protection afforded to the inoculated can be assessed. Public health programmes for the use of vaccines so tested can now be planned with the assurance that a known degree of effectiveness will be obtained. Vaccines submitted to controlled field trials so far include those against whooping-cough, tuberculosis, typhoid fever, influenza and poliomyelitis. It will be noted that although BCG and typhoid vaccines had been available and in use for many years prior to the time the new methods of field testing were generally applied, they had ultimately to be submitted to controlled trials before a true assessment of their value could be made. It is only by statistically acceptable studies which give unbiased information that controversy is settled and confident use can be made of the vaccines on a large scale.

Well-planned studies, though costly, save money, time and misplaced effort in the long run and can give information not otherwise obtainable on dosage, combined antigens, duration of immunity and the like. Combined field and laboratory studies of vaccines aim at providing confidence in the efficacy of future vaccination programmes. Sufficient confidence can only rarely be attained if the studies do not observe two basic principles, which may be called (1) the principle of comparability and (2) the principle of reproducibility.

(1) *The Principle of Comparability* ensures confidence that an observed degree of protection apparently conferred upon a population group by vaccination was due to the vaccination and not to other chance influences. It requires comparison of the incidence of the disease in two or more groups, and precautions to ensure that these groups can be regarded as identical in all respects except for the factor of vaccination.

The most convincing evidence will be obtained if one of the groups in a field trial ("the control group") remains unvaccinated, or is vaccinated with an unrelated vaccine. If it is not feasible to have a control group, comparisons may be made between groups inoculated with vaccines that are prepared in different ways, or sometimes between groups treated with the same vaccine but using a different dosage schedule.

(2) *The Principle of Reproducibility* ensures confidence in obtaining, in future vaccination programmes, the same degree of protection as was observed in the initial field trial. It requires precautions to ensure that the vaccine which was proved to be of value in the field trial can be prepared again and can, if possible, be validly tested in a laboratory assay.

A field trial can only show whether or not the actual preparation of vaccine used in the trial was successful. What is then needed is confidence in the ability to reproduce this particular preparation or of pre paring an equally or more efficient preparation. The preparation method must therefore be meticulously described and the laboratory studies must include assays of different vaccine preparations in experimental animals, in order to develop a laboratory method yielding results that parallel those obtained in the field; this procedure permits the assessment of the protective value of future vaccine preparations by laboratory assay alone.

If the essential protective antigen of a microorganism could be isolated, identified and quantitatively assessed with chemical exactitude and if the mechanism of the production of immunity by the host were understood, there would clearly be no need to do more than to measure the amount of protective antigen in the first successful vaccines tested. It could then be ensured that all subsequent vaccines contained similar or greater amounts of the essential constituent.

Such measurement can be made with some approach to accuracy with toxoids such as the diphtheria or tetanus prophylactics, but with most bacterial and virus vaccines, killed or living, this is not possible, and the principle of reproducibility must therefore be carefully observed. It is then necessary to compare a series of vaccines in field studies and at the same time to submit them to as many laboratory studies as possible in the hope that variations of protective power in the field will occur and will be reflected in one or more laboratory tests. The laboratory test which gives results most closely corresponding to the protective value may then be adopted as the test for future batches of vaccine.

Examples of Controlled Trials of Prophylactic Vaccines.— Some examples are given of well-conducted field trials that have given valuable information on the usefulness of prophylactic vaccination against certain infectious diseases in defined communities.

(*a*) *Whooping-cough.*—In whooping-cough, following the earlier studies of Kendrick and Eldering in Grand Rapids, Michigan, a continuing series of controlled field and laboratory trials of pertussis vaccines have been carried out in the United Kingdom. Altogether some 50,000 children in the age range 6 months to 2 years were inoculated and 25 different vaccines were tested. The following is an extract from the last of three reports (Report, 1959a):

> "The results of the trials clearly showed that it was possible by vaccination to produce a high degree of protection against the disease, as shown by the substantial reduction in the attack rate amongst home contacts, and, in those cases where vaccination failed to give complete protection, to reduce the severity and duration of the disease. The results also showed that the different vaccines employed varied a great deal in their protective action; the poorest gave an attack rate in home contacts of 87 per cent., and the most effective an attack rate of 4 per cent." (see Fig. 36).

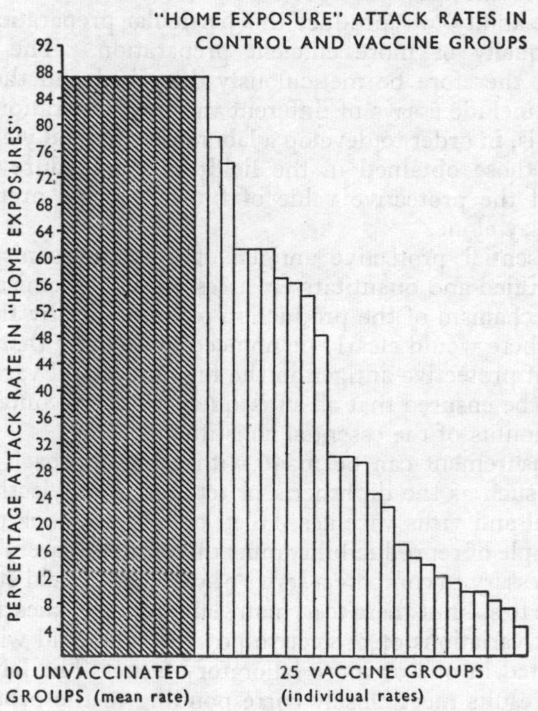

FIG. 36

(*A Symposium on Immunization in Childhood.* Edinburgh: Livingstone, 1960.)

In regard to laboratory assays of potency, three methods of evaluation were used: agglutinin response in the inoculated children, agglutinin response in mice, and the mouse-brain protection test. The first two of these tests correlated well with attack rates in inoculated children with most of the vaccines tested, but there was a lack of corrrelation with a purified antigenic fraction of *B. pertussis* (the Pillemer fraction) which gave good protection clinically but a poor agglutinin response in mice. It was therefore considered that the mouse-brain protection test was the most satisfactory in assessing prophylactic potency. The correlation between field trials and laboratory tests is shown in Fig. 37.

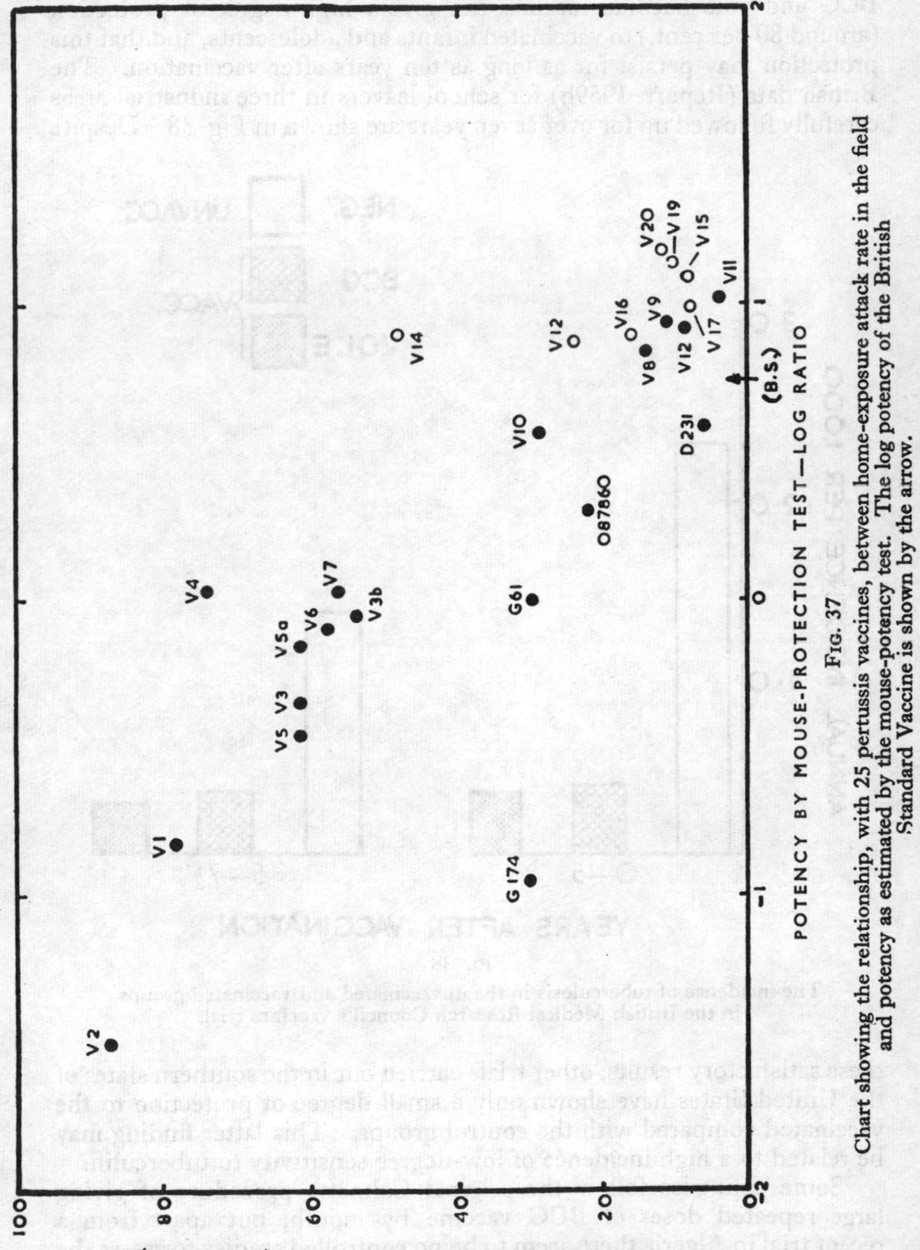

Fig. 37

Chart showing the relationship, with 25 pertussis vaccines, between home-exposure attack rate in the field and potency as estimated by the mouse-potency test. The log potency of the British Standard Vaccine is shown by the arrow.

(*b*) *Tuberculosis.*—Despite epidemiological evidence, particularly from Scandinavian countries, of the protective effect of BCG vaccination, there were until recently very few well-controlled trials from which a critical assessment of the vaccine could be made. Now, controlled field trials in different age-groups and communities have shown that BCG and vole bacillus vaccines can give a high degree of protection (around 80 per cent.) to vaccinated infants and adolescents, and that this protection may persist for as long as ten years after vaccination. The British data (Report, 1959b) for school leavers in three industrial areas carefully followed up for over seven years are shown in Fig. 38. Despite

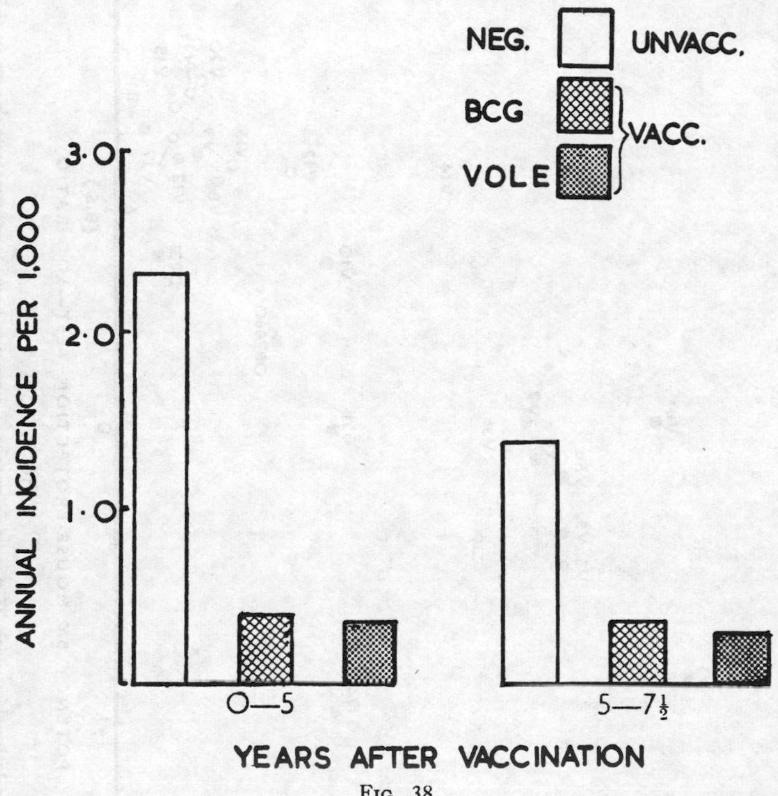

Fig. 38

The incidence of tuberculosis in the unvaccinated and vaccinated groups in the British Medical Research Council's vaccines trial.

these satisfactory results, other trials carried out in the southern states of the United States have shown only a small degree of protection to the vaccinated compared with the control groups. This latter finding may be related to a high incidence of low-degree sensitivity to tuberculin.

Some countries follow the original Calmette procedure of giving large repeated doses of BCG vaccine by mouth, but apart from a recent trial in Algeria there seem to be no controlled studies to assess the protective value of the oral route of vaccination.

(*c*) *Poliomyelitis.*—The relatively low incidence of paralytic poliomyelitis, even in well-developed countries, has meant that a critical evaluation of polio vaccine would require very large numbers of children. Such a study was carried out in the United States of America where over half a million school-children aged 6–8 years were involved in a strictly controlled trial in 1954. The overall attack rate of paralytic poliomyelitis in the vaccinated and placebo groups was in the ratio of 1 : 3·5. This ratio was much greater for the grave bulbo-spinal (1 : 18) than for spinal poliomyelitis (1 : 2·5) and was progressively greater in the 6, 7 and 8 year old children (see table p. 598). Subsequent trials carried out in the United Kingdom and Sweden have supported the American conclusion that killed poliovirus vaccine can give a high degree of protection.

Paralytic Poliomyelitis Cases by Age and Vaccination Status

Age (1 May 1954)	Vaccinated	Placebo	Per cent. Effectiveness	SL
6 years:				
Number	16	21		NS
Rate per 100,000	37	49	24	
7 years:				
Number	12	48		0·001
Rate per 100,000	16	64	75	
8 years:				
Number	4	29		0·001
Rate per 100,000	7	53	87	
9 years:				
Number	1	9		0·01
Rate per 100,000	4	37	89	
All ages (6–10 and over):				
Number	33	110		0·001
Rate per 100,000	16	55	71	

SL = level of statistical significance.
NS = not significant at level of 0·05.

Presently a live, attenuated polio vaccine, often called 'Sabin vaccine,' which can be given orally has become widely used. It may be taken in syrup, candy or on a lump of sugar either as monovalent vaccine, usually in the order type 1, type 3 and type 2 polio vaccines, at 4–8 weekly intervals or as 3 doses of a trivalent vaccine at 4–8 weekly intervals. The advantages of the living oral vaccine are ease of administration, cheapness and the establishment of a local gut immunity which interferes with parasitisation by the virulent wild strains. There may be some increase in neurovirulence for the monkey in vaccine strains that have become established in the intestine but, despite some reported cases of poliomyelitis, mostly in adults, with the type 3 vaccine strain in U.S.A. and Canada, it may be accepted that oral vaccination is safe and effective.

(*d*) *Typhoid.*—Although it has been assumed for many years that anti-typhoid vaccination has made a major contribution to the control of typhoid, particularly for the armed forces in times of war, certain anomalous findings among vaccinated troops during and after the second world war raised doubts and called for a fresh critical assessment of typhoid vaccination. A controlled trial of two vaccines (heat-killed phenol-preserved, and alcohol-killed alcohol-preserved) with a control group given a Flexner dysentery vaccine, was carried out in an endemic typhoid area in Yugoslavia, involving over 35,000 inoculated persons in the age range 5–40 years. The results, over a two-year follow-up period (1954–55), showed a significant degree of protection in those receiving the phenolised vaccine, whereas there was insignificant protection with the alcoholised vaccine (Report, 1957). It is interesting that in the following three years provisional data showed that those who received two doses of phenolised vaccine in 1954 and a booster in 1955 still showed a significantly lower attack rate than the control group (see table below).

Typhoid Cases in Vaccinated Groups

Vaccine	1954		1955		1956	1957	1958	Total cases
	No. of vacc.	No. of cases	No. of vacc.	No. of cases	No. of cases	No. of cases	No. of cases	
Alcohol	12,017	17	8,913	6	1	0	6	30
Phenol	11,503	7	8,595	2	1	1	2	13
Control	11,988	23	9,002	8	4	6	9	50
Total	35,508	47	26,510	16	6	7	17	93

Further controlled field trials of typhoid vaccines have since been carried out in British Guiana, Yugoslavia, Poland and U.S.S.R. In the British Guiana trial (Ashcroft *et al.*, 1964) about 72,000 school children aged 5–15 years were randomly allocated to one of three vaccine groups receiving two 0·5 ml. injections, at about 5 weeks' interval, of, respectively, acetone-killed typhoid vaccine, heat-killed phenolised typhoid vaccine and tetanus toxoid (as control). The average annual attack rates per 10,000 in the three groups in a 26 months follow-up period were, in the same order, 1·0, 3·6 and 14·2, thus confirming the protective value of the phenolised vaccine but also demonstrating a much higher prophylactic effectiveness of the acetone-killed vaccine. These findings were corroborated in the second Yugoslav trial although the degree of protection was not so high.

Hazards of Immunisation

It is axiomatic that prophylactic agents, before they are issued for use, should have been shown to be safe as well as effective, and the Therapeutics Substances Act regulations require certain tests for sterility and toxicity to be carried out on these prophylactics. Nonetheless, there are certain incidental hazards associated with the injection of immunising agents, and the first of these relates to the syringe and needle to be used for the injection. The best way to ensure that a syringe and needle are sterile is to heat the assembled outfit in a hot air oven at a temperature of 160° C. for one hour. The next best is the use of high pressure steam in an autoclave or pressure cooker, which, with the syringe dismantled, can again ensure absolute sterility, *i.e.* the destruction of both sporing and non-sporing micro-organisms. Although boiling does not kill the more resistant sporing organisms, this procedure is accepted as reasonably safe for the re-sterilisation of syringes that have already been properly sterilised in a hot air oven or autoclave. In other words, where many injections are being given, as at a baby clinic, repeated boiling of the syringe and needle for ten minutes is accepted as adequate protection against the risk of transference of infection. A sterile syringe and needle must be used for each injection to avoid the risk of transferring the agent of homologous serum hepatitis, for a syringe, if used for repeated injections with a fresh sterile needle each time, may carry over minimal amounts of tissue fluid. The skin should, of course, be cleansed and preferably treated with a quick acting antiseptic such as 2 per cent. iodine in 70 per cent. alcohol immediately before the injection. For smallpox vaccination, the skin should simply be cleansed with soap or methylated ether and then allowed to dry. It is unwise to give an injection to a child who is obviously suffering from skin sepsis; and smallpox vaccination should be avoided in a child with eczema, because of the risk of generalised vaccinial skin lesions (p. 378).

In regard to reactions, there is as a rule little or no local or systemic reaction following the injection of plain toxoids, but when alum is added to the toxoid there is usually some local reaction because of the irritant effect of the alum. For this reason the injection should be given deep subcutaneously or intramuscularly, so that any fibrous nodule at the site of injection is not easily felt. With killed vaccines, the amount of local or systemic reaction is usually greater than with toxoids and with both TAB and pertussis vaccines there may be local swelling associated with some febrile reaction within the first 24–72 hr. after inoculation. After injections of pertussis vaccine, cases of encephalopathy, manifested by convulsions and coma and followed sometimes by mental deterioration, have been reported. It is impossible to estimate the risk of this hazard, but it occurs in probably less than one in 1 million injections and has been noted particularly in the U.S.A. In view of this rare hazard, it is advisable to avoid giving pertussis vaccine to children with a history of repeated convulsions and to children who are convalescent from some other illness.

There is very little risk of reaction following the use of poliomyelitis virus vaccines. A few instances of allergic reactions in patients who were already hypersensitive to penicillin have been recorded, but as manufacturers are giving up the use of penicillin in the production of poliovirus vaccine, this hazard is not likely to occur in future. Both local and systemic reactions to influenza virus vaccine may occur in a low percentage of persons; here and also in the use of yellow fever vaccine, enquiry should be made about the patient's sensitivity to egg since these vaccines are prepared from chick embryo tissue.

With smallpox vaccine there is the recognised, if small, risk of post-vaccinal encephalitis when primary vaccination is carried out on a school child or adult. It is perhaps not so widely known that the risk of post-vaccinal encephalitis seems to be rather greater in children under 1 year of age (15·8 per million) than in children between 1 and 4 years of age (2·1 per million). Again, generalised vaccinia is more likely to occur in infants (51 per million) than in 1 to 4 year olds (23 per million). But these hazards are admittedly very small and should not necessarily influence the doctor in deciding on the most convenient time for giving particular inoculations.

A complication that has attracted considerable attention in recent years is the so-called "provocation" poliomyelitis, which may occur as a paralysis in the inoculated limb in children within a month of receiving some prophylactic inoculation. In an MRC investigation (Report, 1956), the overall incidence of provocation poliomyelitis was 1 per 37,000 inoculations. The risk, however, was greatest with a mixed diphtheria-pertussis vaccine containing alum, where the rate was 1 in 15,000 injections. Significant, but smaller risks, were observed with the diphtheria prophylactics APT and PTAP, and with the mixed diphtheria-pertussis vaccine without alum. No significant risk was found after plain pertussis vaccine, TAF or formol toxoid, or smallpox vaccine. Because of the hazard associated with an alum-containing combined prophylactic the Ministry of Health have advised against the use of such prophylactic agents. Studies both in this country and in Canada indicate that the hazard associated with combined diphtheria-pertussis or with the triple diphtheria-tetanus-pertussis vaccine is so small as to warrant the continued use of combined prophylactics because of their administrative and other advantages. Purified diphtheria toxoid is *per se* a poor antigen.

IMMUNISATION SCHEDULES

The aim of immunisation programmes is the control of infection in the community rather than individual protection. A lower level of immunity than is necessary for solid individual protection can effectively reduce the incidence of communicable diseases if a high proportion of the susceptible community is immunised. Thus, in diphtheria, there is a rapid reduction in both morbidity and mortality when 60–70 per cent. of the pre-school and school children are effectively immunised. It is stated that smallpox may be controlled when approximately 80 per cent. of the whole community has been successfully vaccinated. Tetanus is an exception to this general rule in that protection of a proportion of the population does not reduce the risk to the non-immunised individual.

For countries with well-developed systems for the collection of morbidity and mortality data relating to communicable diseases plus good medical services, it should be relatively easy to decide what vaccinations should be carried out and how best the programme can be effected. Nonetheless, delays and lack of co-ordination in the application of knowledge frequently occur even when a good organisation is available. There is also the risk that the incidence and importance of a disease may be under-estimated or miscalculated if notification is poor, or mortality rates are falling, *e.g.* in tuberculosis and whooping-cough, or deaths are attributed to secondary causes, *e.g.* bronchopneumonia following measles or whooping-cough. In countries with limited medical services it is essential that strenuous efforts be made to provide satisfactory vital statistics and, by sample surveys or other means, to obtain a reasonably accurate assessment of the main causes of morbidity and mortality.

In the United Kingdom most of the immunisation work is done either at child welfare clinics or by the family doctor or paediatrician. While there are obvious advantages in having the immunisations carried out by the family doctor (and the available evidence indicates that the proportion of immunisations done by practitioners is steadily increasing) it is essential that there should be a well-organised system for ensuring that the child receives its injections at the appropriate age and time intervals and that there is an efficient system of recording the immunisations.

An immunisation campaign carried out without provision for its continuation as a routine procedure will not give satisfactory results—except where complete eradication is achieved. Therefore, in planning immunisation schedules, provision must be made to ensure receptivity by the public and, particularly, to secure the co-operation of parents who have to bring their children to the doctor or clinic for repeated inoculations. These measures are essential for the successful execution of the programme.

Knowledge about the duration of immunity following the primary course of immunisation and after booster (or recall) injections is not yet sufficiently precise in a number of communicable diseases. The number and timetable of booster doses must, therefore, be left rather elastic. The need to use efficient prophylactics and, wherever possible, vaccines that can be standardised, cannot be over-emphasised since the continuance of immunisation programmes with the co-operation and confidence of the public depends on the successful results of these procedures.

The two schedules set out below are suggested models (*a*) for areas with well-developed medical services, and (*b*) for developing areas with inadequate medical services.

It is envisaged that schedule (*b*) will be used in countries with a low incidence of clinical poliomyelitis. In such areas poliomyelitis vaccine should not be employed routinely, but should be available to those at special risk of clinical disease.

(a) *Suggested Schedule of Immunisation in Areas with Adequate Public Health Medical Services*

Age	Visit	Vaccine	Injection	Interval
1 to 6 months	1	Diphtheria, Tetanus, Pertussis	1	
				4–6 weeks
	2	Diphtheria, Tetanus, Pertussis	2	
				4–6 weeks
	3	Diphtheria, Tetanus, Pertussis	3	
7 to 11 months	4	Poliomyelitis (oral)*	–	
				4–8 weeks
	5	Poliomyelitis (oral)	–	
				4–8 weeks
	6	Poliomyelitis (oral)	–	
18 to 21 months	7	Diphtheria, Tetanus, Pertussis	4	
Smallpox vaccination during the first 2 years, preferably in the second year				
School entry		Diphtheria and Tetanus		
8 to 12 years		Diphtheria and Tetanus Smallpox revaccination		
Over 12 years		BCG		

* *Poliomyelitis.*—If a child has had two doses only of Salk vaccine he should receive two further doses of oral vaccine to complete the primary course. The second dose could be at a convenient time such as school entry.

Children who have already started a course of immunisation with killed vaccine may, at the doctor's discretion, either complete the course or be given oral vaccine, as follows:—

(i) If a child has had only *one* injection of Salk vaccine, a full course of three doses of oral vaccine should be administered.

(ii) If a child, aged 5–12 years, has had *three* injections of Salk vaccine, the fourth injection may be replaced by one dose of oral vaccine.

Tuberculosis.—BCG vaccination. High prevalence areas: first vaccination within first four weeks of life or, where the modified vaccination schedule is used, BCG vaccine may be given at the same time as the second dose of triple vaccine at 4 to 8 months of age. Pre-vaccination tuberculin testing may have to be done at this age, depending upon the infection risk during the first year of life. Re-vaccination at school entry and at school leaving age, after tuberculin test.

(b) *Suggested Schedule of Immunisation in Areas with Inadequate Medical Services*

Age	Prophylactic Vaccine	Visit
0–4 weeks	(1) BCG vaccination.	1st
3–9 months	(2) Smallpox vaccination. (3) Diphtheria-pertussis-tetanus (triple vaccine with alum): 2 doses at an interval of one month. The first injection could be given at the time of smallpox vaccination. Smallpox vaccination is verified at the second visit. Failures of smallpox vaccination are re-vaccinated.	2nd and 3rd
School entry or soon thereafter.	(4) Diphtheria/tetanus booster (plain or with alum). (5) TAB vaccination: 2 doses at an interval of one month. (6) Smallpox re-vaccination: at the time of second TAB injection.	4th and 5th
10–14 years	(7) BCG re-vaccination (in tuberculin negative reactors). (8) Smallpox re-vaccination. (9) TAB booster.	6th and 7th

Low prevalence areas: first vaccination—in school or before leaving school after tuberculin test. Re-vaccination may be performed on military recruits, students, and on the occasion of routine examination of other occupational groups.

REFERENCES

Ashcroft, M. T., Ritchie, J. M. & Nicholson, C. C. (1964). Controlled field trial in British Guiana school children of heat-killed phenolized and acetone-killed lyophilized typhoid vaccines. *Amer. J. Hyg.*, 79, 196.

Report (1956). Poliomyelitis and prophylactic inoculation against diphtheria, whooping-cough, and smallpox. *Lancet*, **2**, 1223.

Report (1957). Field and laboratory studies with typhoid vaccines. *Bull. Wld. Hlth. Org.*, **16**, 897.

Report (1959a). Vaccination against whooping-cough. *Brit. med. J.*, **1**, 994.

Report (1959b). BCG and vole bacillus vaccines in the prevention of tuberculosis in adolescents. *Brit. med. J.*, **2**, 379.

GENERAL REFERENCES

A Symposium on Immunization in Childhood. Edinburgh: E. & S. Livingstone, 1959.

The Role of Immunization in Communicable Disease Control. Public Health Papers No. 8. Geneva: World Health Organization, 1961.

Control of Communicable Diseases in Man. 10th Ed., 1965. New York: American Public Health Association.

PART V

TECHNICAL METHODS

CHAPTER 44

MICROSCOPY

THE study of the morphology of very small organisms is of such importance that the microbiologist must of necessity be a competent microscopist. It is of paramount importance for him to obtain the best possible performance from his instrument and for this a sound knowledge of the basic optical principles involved and an understanding of the construction of the microscope are essential.

Microscopes designed by different manufacturers differ enormously in their outward appearance, but essentially most consist of three parts—the stand, the body and the train of optical lenses. A typical monocular microscope suitable for microbiology is seen in Fig. 39.

The stand comprises a heavy foot, often horse-shoe shaped (1), to give stability and the limb (5) which bears the optical system. The limb is attached to the foot by a hinged joint so that the microscope can be set at a comfortable angle for the observer. The optical system is mounted in the tube which is usually in two parts, (*a*) an external tube (9) which bears at its lower end a revolving nose-piece (15) in which interchangeable objective lenses of various magnifications are fitted (16 & 17), and (*b*) an inner draw-tube (13) which carries the eye-piece (12) at its upper end. This whole assembly is held in position by the body (8) which houses two mechanisms, the coarse (7) and fine adjustments (6) whereby the height of the tube can be adjusted in such a way that the objective can be positioned at its optimal working distance (its focal length) from the object (19) to be examined. These focusing mechanisms are operated by milled heads situated on the two sides of the body. The milled head of the fine adjustment is usually graduated in $\frac{1}{50}$ths and one division corresponds to a movement of 0·002 mm. of the tube. The stage (18) is a platform which accommodates a glass microscope slide on which the object to be examined (19) is mounted; it is attached to the limb immediately below the level of the objective lens and has an aperture in its centre to permit light to reach the object. The stage may be of the fixed type fitted with two spring clips or of the mechanical type that can be moved in two planes by rack and pinion mechanisms (3). A mechanical stage is of great advantage because it controls small movements of the object accurately and it is really necessary when a large area of the microscopic preparation has to be searched, as in the examination of films of sputum for tubercle bacilli or of blood for malaria parasites. It is possible to obtain attachable mechanical stages for almost all microscopes but the type that is built into the instrument is much more stable and greatly to be preferred.

In some modern microscopes the objective is held in a fixed position and the distance between it and the object is adjusted by the *downward movement of the stage* which is controlled by coarse and fine adjustment screws similar to those used in other models to move the tube. For those accustomed to the standard microscope great care is at first required to avoid the risk of damage to both object and objective.

Beneath the stage is the substage (24) which carries a condenser (20) whose lenses focus light from the illuminating source on the plane of the object. The height of the condenser, and therefore the focus of the light, can be varied at will by a rack and pinion mechanism (2). The horizontal position of the condenser can be adjusted in two planes by centring screws (21). Immediately

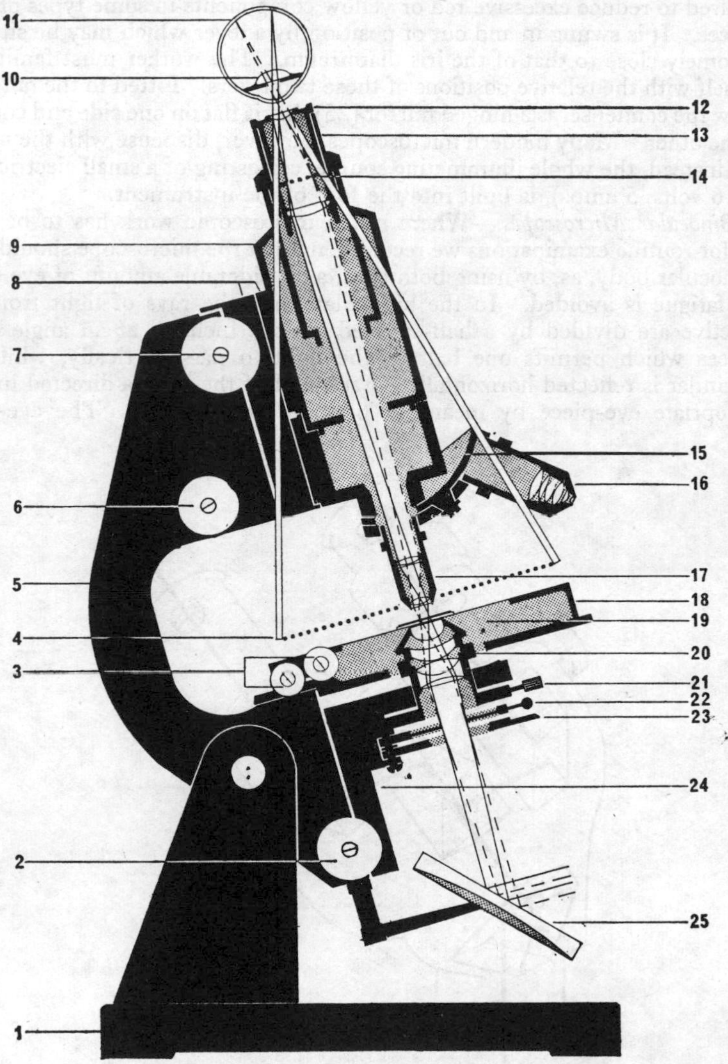

FIG. 39

A diagram illustrating the component parts of a monocular microscope and the paths of the optical rays. (1) Foot; (2) Adjusting screw for height of condenser; (3) Controls for mechanical stage; (4) Enlarged virtual image; (5) Limb; (6) Fine adjustment; (7) Coarse adjustment; (8) Body; (9) External tube; (10) Lens of observer's eye; (11) Retina; (12) Eye-piece; (13) Inner draw-tube; (14) Primary image, real and enlarged by objective; (15) Revolving nose-piece; (16) High-power objective; (17) Low-power objective; (18) Stage; (19) Object; (20) Condenser; (21) Centring screw for condenser; (22) Iris diaphragm; (23) Ring filter holder; (24) Substage; (25) Mirror.

below the condenser and incorporated in the same mount is the substage iris diaphragm operated by a small lever which protrudes to one side (22). Opening or closing this iris diaphragm controls the amount of light reaching the object. Just below the iris diaphragm is a ring-shaped filter holder (23) designed to carry circular coloured glass filters (*e.g.* a blue "daylight" filter) required to reduce excessive red or yellow components in some types of light sources. It is swung in and out of position by a lever which may be situated tiresomely close to that of the iris diaphragm. The worker must familiarise himself with the relative positions of these two levers. Fitted to the tail piece below the condenser is a hinged mirror (25) that is flat on one side and concave on the other. Many modern microscopes, however, dispense with the mirror and, instead, the whole illuminating source, consisting of a small electric bulb (*e.g.* 6 volts, 5 amps), is built into the foot of the instrument.

Binocular Microscopes.—Where much microscopic work has to be done and for routine examinations we recommend that the microscope should have a binocular body, as, by using both eyes, a considerable amount of eye strain and fatigue is avoided. In the binocular body the rays of light from the objective are divided by a half-silvered surface inclined at an angle of 45 degrees which permits one half of the light to pass vertically, while the remainder is reflected horizontally. Each half of the rays is directed into its appropriate eye-piece by means of prisms (see Fig. 40). The eye-piece

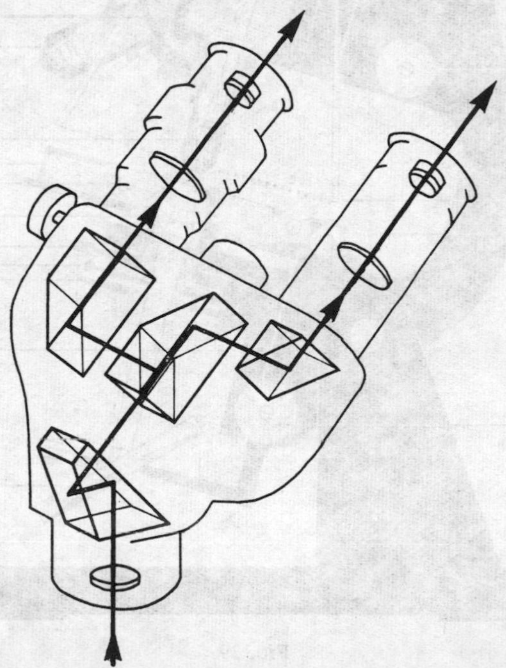

Fig. 40
A diagram to illustrate the optical path in the binocular head of a microscope.

sockets can be adjusted to the interpupillary distance of the observer, while one of the ocular tubes is adjustable to correct individual differences between the two eyes.

Inclined binocular microscopes are very suitable for routine use, as the eye-pieces are inclined towards the observer and it is not necessary to tilt the stand as with the straight binocular or monocular bodies. Consequently the stage is kept horizontal and this is of particular advantage when dealing with wet films or using dark-ground illumination. (Similarly an inclined eye-piece fitting for a monocular tube may be obtained.)

It should be noted that the inclined binocular body may increase the actual magnification by 1½ times. This factor shown as 1·5 × is engraved on the body. Lower-power eye-pieces only should be used; 6 × is the most convenient, and 8 × is the highest practicable for routine use.

Binocular microscopes have interchangeable monocular and binocular bodies, which are removable without disturbing the objectives, so that a monocular body can readily be used for photography, micrometry, etc.

MAGNIFICATION

The purpose of the microscope is to produce an enlarged image of objects too small to be observed with the naked eye; the degree of enlargement is the *magnification* of the instrument. It is perfectly possible to design an optical system which will give enormous magnifications, *e.g.* hundreds of thousands of times, but after a certain point detail and sharpness begin to be lost. A common example of this is seen when a magnifying glass is used to examine a newspaper photograph; the effect is not to reveal more detail, instead the picture is broken down to a series of black and white dots. Magnification of this type which does not increase the detail observed is known as "*empty magnification*" and is of no value to the microbiologist. As will be seen later there is a fundamental limit to the amount of detail or "*useful magnification*" of any optical system and this is imposed by the wavelength of the light rays used.

The Formation of the Image.—It is the lenses composing the objective which initiate the magnifying processes. An objective operates at a distance from the object that is roughly equivalent to its focal length, and admits rays that are transmitted to form a real, inverted, enlarged image (the primary image) in the upper part of the tube. At this point there is interposed another lens—the field lens—whose function is to collect the diverging rays of the primary image (Fig. 39 (14)) so that they pass through the eye lens of the eye-piece which magnifies the image still further. The field lens is accommodated in the lower plane of the eye-piece. Rays as they leave the eye-piece to reach the lens of the observer's eye (10) are once more divergent and thus the image seen by the retina (11) is virtual, appearing to be some 10 in. in front of the eyes (see Fig. 39 (4)).

The magnification of a microscope is the product of the separate magnifications of the objective and the eye-piece and depends on the following factors:

(1) The optical tube length.
(2) The focal length of the objective.
(3) The magnifying power of the eye-piece.

1. The *optical tube length* is the distance between the posterior principal plane of the lens system of the objective and the plane of the image in the upper part of the draw-tube. This distance is difficult to determine but, for practical purposes, may be taken as equal to the *mechanical tube length* which is the distance between the point where the objective fits into the lower end of the body or the nose-piece and the eye lens of the eye-piece, a measurement easily made with a ruler (see Fig. 41). Most modern microscopes have a mechanical tube length of 160 mm., but a few manufacturers employ 170 mm.

Objectives are designed to work at a definite tube length and any variation from this distance may seriously impair the quality of the image. This must be borne in mind when buying new objectives, particularly when high-power apochromatic or achromatic lenses are needed.

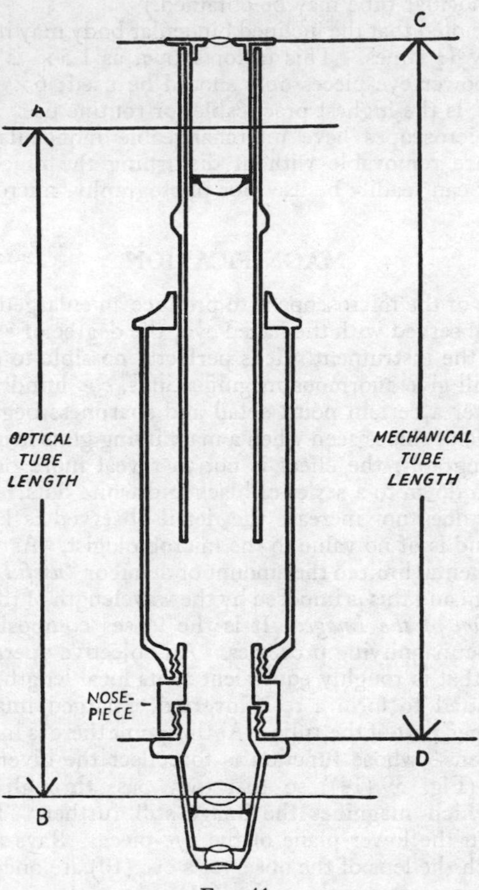

FIG. 41

A diagram to illustrate the optical tube of a monocular microscope.

Many microscopes have an extensile draw-tube that can be used to vary the optical tube length but its use is only required in correcting for coverslip thickness or possibly in calibrating an eye-piece micrometer. The tube length should *not* be used to obtain greater magnification because a serious distortion of the final image results.

2. The *magnification of an objective* is obtained as follows:

$$\text{Magnification of objective} = \frac{\text{size of image}}{\text{size of object}}$$

$$= \frac{\text{distance of image from objective}}{\text{distance of object from objective}}$$

$$= \frac{\text{mechanical tube length}}{\text{focal length of objective}}.$$

Examples

(*a*) 16 mm. ($\frac{2}{3}$ in.) objective $=\frac{160}{16}=10$.
(*b*) 4 mm. ($\frac{1}{6}$ in.) objective $=\frac{160}{4}=40$.
(*c*) 2 mm. ($\frac{1}{12}$ in.) objective $=\frac{160}{2}=80$.

The 2 mm. objective has, in reality, a shorter focal length than that by which it is designated, and gives a magnification of 95–100 diameters according to the make. Makers now engrave the initial magnification on the objective mount and refer to the objective by its magnification as well as by the numerical aperture (*vide infra*) thus, the 16 mm. ($\frac{2}{3}$ in.) objective is designated 10/0·28, the 4 mm. ($\frac{1}{6}$ in.) is 40/0·65, and the 2 mm. ($\frac{1}{12}$ in.) is 95–100/1·28 (or 1·3).

3. The *magnification of the eye-piece* is clearly engraved on the mount by the makers.

4. The *total magnification of the microscope* is:

$$\frac{\text{Tube length}}{\text{Focal length of objective}} \times \text{eye-piece magnification}$$

or

$$\text{Objective magnification} \times \text{eye-piece magnification.}$$

NUMERICAL APERTURE

Objectives are rated not only by their focal length but also by their angles of aperture which determine their light gathering powers. A method of expressing the fraction of a wave front admitted to a lens is the use of the measurement of the *Numerical Aperture* (NA). The numerical aperture may be defined simply as the ratio of the diameter of the lens to its focal length.[1] It is expressed mathematically as follows:

$$\text{NA} = n \text{ Sin U}$$

where n is the refractive index of the medium between object and objective (air, 1·0; cedar-wood immersion oil, approximately 1·5), and 2U the *angle of aperture—i.e.* the angle formed by the two extreme rays of light, which, starting from the centre point of the object, reach the eye of the observer (see Fig. 42).

$$\text{That is, DAC} = 2\text{U}$$
$$\text{BAC} = \text{U}$$
$$\text{Sin U} = \frac{\text{EF}}{\text{EA}}$$

It is thus seen that the numerical aperture, other things being equal, depends on EF, which is half the diameter of the lens. Objectives, therefore, may have equal focal lengths, but different numerical apertures depending on the diameter of the front lens.

The theoretical limit of the angle DAC is 180°—*i.e.* when the objective is actually on the object—and therefore the theoretical limit of U is 90°. The greatest possible NA of a dry lens cannot exceed 1, since the refractive index of air (n) = 1, and Sin 90° = 1. Actually the highest practical NA of a dry lens is 0·95. On the other hand, the introduction of cedar-oil between the

[1] The numerical aperture has been expressed in this manner to simplify description, but this is true only for objectives of long focal length, where EA is approximately equal to FA (see Fig.42). With short-focus lenses of high numerical aperture this definition is not correct. The length EA is then much greater than the distance of the objective from the slide (FA).

objective and object gives *n* a value of 1·5. The highest theoretical value, therefore, of *n* Sin U for an oil-immersion objective is 1·5 × Sin 90°—*i.e.* 1·5. In practice, however, the highest NA of an oil-immersion objective (attained in an apochromat) is 1·4. The ordinary $\frac{1}{12}$-in. objective for bacteriological purpose has a NA of 1·28 or 1·3.

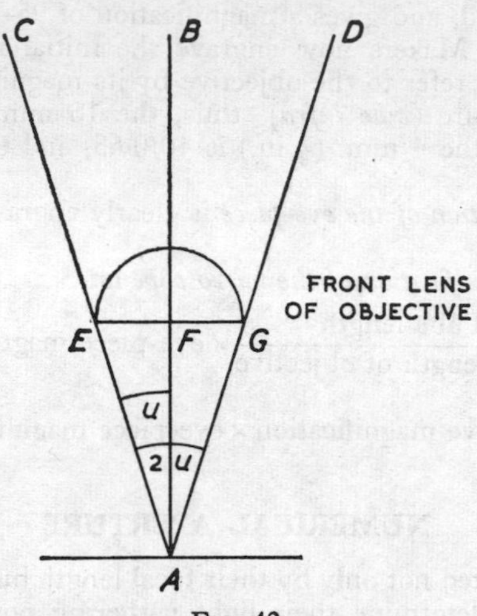

FIG. 42

Diagram to illustrate numerical aperture.

RESOLUTION

The limit of useful magnification is set by the resolving power of the microscope, *i.e.* its ability to reveal closely adjacent structural details as separate and distinct; expressed quantitatively it is its *capacity* to distinguish two neighbouring points as separate entities. It is this power which determines the amount of structural detail that can be observed microscopically. The minimum resolvable distance between two luminous points (r) is given by the formula

$$r = \frac{0{\cdot}61 \times \lambda}{\text{NA}}$$

where λ is the wavelength of the light used. In practice, with axial illumination, two points any closer together than about half the wavelength of the light cannot be resolved. Thus, if green light of wavelength $0{\cdot}55 \times 10^{-4}$ cm. and an objective of N.A. 1·4 are used

$$r = \frac{0{\cdot}61 \times 0{\cdot}55 \times 10^{-4} \text{ cm.}}{1{\cdot}4}$$
$$= 0{\cdot}24 \times 10^{-4} \text{ cm.} = 240 \text{ m}\mu.$$

Under working conditions the limit of resolution is reached at about 0·00025 mm. (250 mμ.). Thus, using ordinary microscopic methods with an apochromatic objective of NA 1·4, and a high-power compensating eye-piece used at the optimal tube length, the whole optical system and illuminant being carefully centred, stained particles of 250 mμ. can be seen. It should be realised that when the bodies observed have been coated with a mordant, as in Paschen's stain for the vaccinia virus, the stained virus particles may have been rendered larger than the natural ones and are thereby brought within the limits of resolution.

If ultraviolet light is used as the illuminating source greater resolution may be obtained because the wavelength is shorter (about half that of visible light) and thus an effective NA of approximately 2·5 can be obtained. The method, however, requires an optical system composed of quartz lenses because ordinary glass offers too much resistance to the path of the rays; this, with the necessity for photographic recording, makes the apparatus expensive and complicated to use.

In the electron microscope the illumination is provided by a beam of electrons that has an equivalent wavelength as small as 1/100,000th that of ordinary light. The efficiency of the lens systems of the electron microscope, however, does not match that of optical lenses and the resolution of this instrument is therefore only about 250 times better than that of the best light microscope.

DEFINITION

Definition, not to be confused with resolution, is the capacity of an objective to render the outline of the image of the object clear and distinct. It depends on the elimination of optical aberrations inherent in the glass of the lenses.

Spherical aberration is due to the fact that rays passing, for example, through the edge of a lens will seldom be brought to precisely the same focus as those passing nearer the centre (see Fig. 43); the result may be serious distortion of the image.

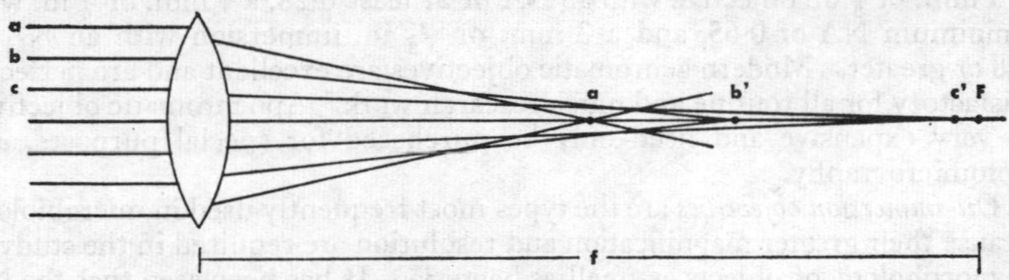

FIG. 43

Diagram to illustrate spherical aberration. Light entering a convex lens is brought to a focus at point F, the focal length of the lens being *f*. Rays *a*, *b* and *c* are refracted to different degrees to reach focus points *a'*, *b'* and *c'*, which are situated at points apart from each other. The result in an uncorrected lens system would be multiple superimposed images and great blurring.

Chromatic aberration occurs because white light as it traverses a lens is diffracted as it would be in a prism to its various component colours, each with its own wavelength (see Fig. 44). The rays of different wavelengths are

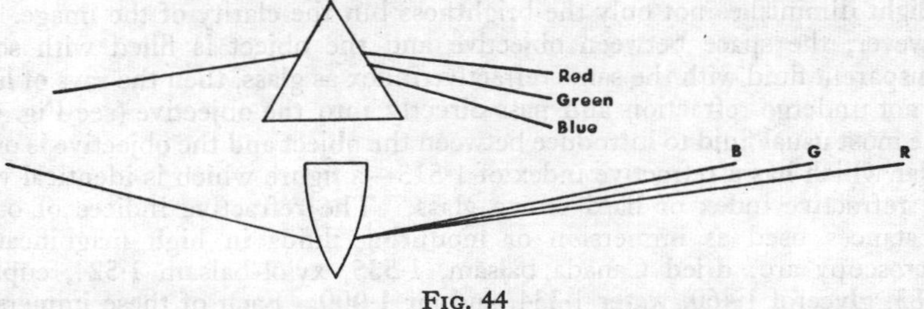

FIG. 44

A diagram to illustrate chromatic aberration.

refracted by the lens to varying extents and may not always be recombined in the same focus. Blue rays, for example, are refracted more and come to a focus nearer to the lens than red rays; the result may be a hazy image fringed with the colours of the spectrum (see Fig. 44).

Aberrations are *corrected* by the makers of better quality lenses by combining lenses of different dispersive qualities. Crown glass has a low dispersive power and is used for convex lenses, while flint glass, which has a high dispersive power, is used for concave lenses. In this manner the colours of the spectrum are recombined to form white light and lenses of this type are known as *achromatic lenses*. The best performance from lenses of this type is obtained when monochromatic green light is used.

THE LENSES OF THE MICROSCOPE

OBJECTIVES

Microscope objectives are constructed from an intricate assembly of lenses; even the lower powers contain up to four lenses and higher powers eight or more. Essentially the qualities of any objective depend on (1) brightness of image, which, other things being equal, varies as the *square* of the NA; and (2) the resolution and definition which vary directly as the NA. The depth of focus, while not entirely dependent on the NA, varies in inverse proportion to it. In general, it may be said that in the case of two objectives of equal focal length, the one with the higher NA is to be preferred as the better lens.

In microbiology three objectives are generally adequate for most purposes; a 16 mm. or $\frac{2}{3}$ in. objective with an NA of at least 0·28, a 4 mm. or $\frac{1}{6}$ in. with a minimum NA of 0·65, and a 2 mm. or $\frac{1}{12}$ in. immersion with an NA of 1·28 or greater. Modern achromatic objectives are excellent and are perfectly satisfactory for all routine and much research work. Apochromatic objectives are very expensive and need only be purchased for special purposes, *e.g.* photomicrography.

Oil-immersion objectives are the types most frequently used in microbiology because their greater magnification and resolution are required in the study of the morphology of objects as small as bacteria. It has been seen that the NA of an objective depends on the angle of the cone of rays that it can admit from the object and that any factor which reduces the rays accepted impairs the quality of the image. In the case of the 2 mm. ($\frac{1}{12}$ in.) objective such a factor is the air between the front lens of the objective and the coverslip. The 2 mm. objective works very close to the object and rays passing from a dense medium (glass of the coverslip) to a less dense medium (air) are refracted obliquely outwards so that many may miss the front lens of the objective altogether. As the brightness of the image depends upon the amount of light entering the objective, and the resolution depends on the effective aperture, this refraction of light diminishes not only the brightness but the clarity of the image. If, however, the space between objective and the object is filled with some transparent fluid with the same refractive index as glass, then the rays of light do not undergo refraction and pass directly into the objective (see Fig. 45). The most usual fluid to introduce between the object and the objective is oil of cedar which has a refractive index of 1·515—a figure which is identical with the refractive index of hard crown glass. The refractive indices of other substances used as immersion or mounting fluids in high magnification microscopy are: dried Canada balsam, 1·535, xylol-balsam 1·524, euparal 1·483, glycerol 1·460, water 1·334, and air 1·000. Each of these immersion fluids has its own place in microscopy according to the type of lens being used.

The newer designs of objectives are so constructed that the optical train is accommodated in a spring-loaded mount which effectively eliminates the risk to the unwary worker of racking down the objective and damaging the cover-slip and slide.

Some objectives are fitted with an adjustable collar that may be turned to move the two back combinations of lenses in order to correct any spherical aberration introduced by the thickness of the coverslip.

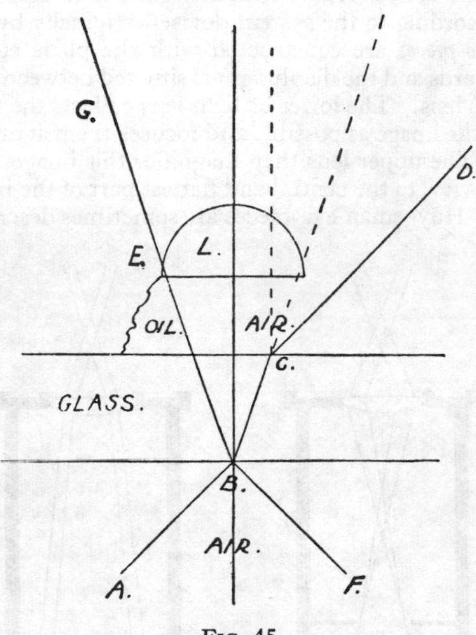

FIG. 45

Diagram showing the paths of rays through (1) a dry lens (on right), and (2) an oil-immersion lens (on left) (*after* Spitta).

Note the refraction of the oblique ray ABCD in passing from the glass slide to air, as compared with the ray FBEG. L is the front lens of the objective.

Apochromatic objectives represent the highest degree of optical perfection and in consequence are very costly; it is only in critical research work that it is possible to justify the expense of these lenses. In the apochromatic objective, light of at least three different wavelengths (colours) may be united, the aberrations are less, and the NA is usually higher, *e.g.* a good oil immersion apochromat may have an NA of approximately 1·4. Apochromats owe this property of almost complete colour correction to the use of the mineral fluorite which endows the objectives with a brilliance and crispness of image not attainable with ordinary lenses, and enables the maximum resolving power to be obtained. Fluorite is so valuable optically because it possesses a high degree of transparency; a low refractive index; and extremely small dispersion. A series of objectives containing a certain amount of fluorite, which are intermediate between apochromatic and achromatic objectives are known as "semi-apochromatic" or "fluorite" lenses; some of them have a performance which approximates to that of apochromatic objectives.

Apochromatic objectives must always be used with "compensating" eye-pieces (*vide infra*) and a properly centred condenser (*q.v.*).

EYE PIECES

The functions of the eye-piece are (1) the magnification of the real image, (2) the formation of a virtual image of the real image produced by the objective, and (3) to carry measuring scales, markers, cross-hairs, etc. There are many different types of eye-pieces but the most generally useful are simple and comprise two plano-convex lenses with a circular field diaphragm interposed between them according to the system devised originally by Huygens.

Huygenian eye-pieces are constructed with the plane surface of the two lenses facing upwards and the diaphragm is situated between them at the focus of the upper (eye) lens. The lower or field lens collects the rays from as wide a field of view of the image as possible and focuses them at or near the plane of the diaphragm. The upper lens then magnifies this image. The diaphragm limits the field of view to the central and flattest part of the image and reduces glare (Fig. 46A). Huygenian eye-pieces are sometimes described as ' negative

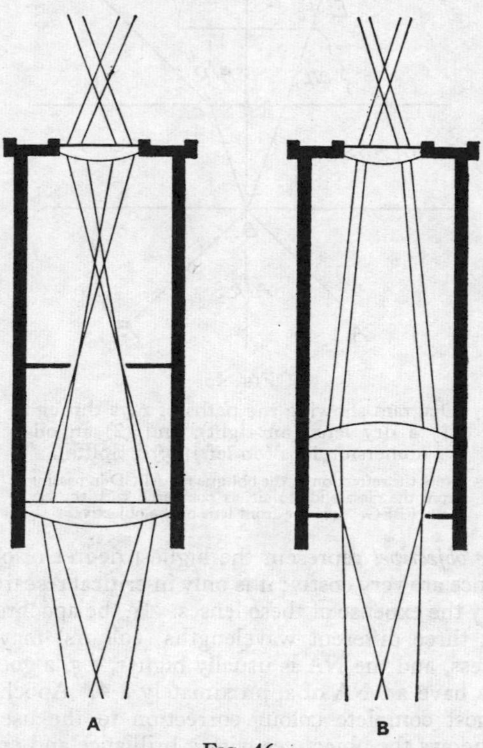

FIG. 46
Diagram to illustrate the optical paths in A–an Huygenian eye-piece and B–a Ramsden eye-piece.

oculars" because the focus occurs within the eye-piece. In microbiology a 10 × Huygenian eye-piece with a monocular tube is most generally useful but a 5 × ocular is also useful for locating the object without altering the objective. It is not practical to use this type of eye-piece at a magnification above 12 × and even this magnification gives some haziness of outline and distortion. With binocular microscopes, 6 × or 8 × eye-pieces are perfectly sufficient as, owing to the division of the rays, less light enters each eye-piece. With 10× oculars definition is lost and the field is apt to be too dark when ordinary illuminants are used.

Ramsden or positive eye-pieces are constructed with the convex surface of both lenses facing inwards, the two together forming a single lens unit. In this type of ocular the diaphragm is placed externally *below* the lower lens and in this way has the advantage that any aberration or distortion of the lenses affects equally the image itself and the view of any scale placed on the external diaphragm (Fig. 46B). They are therefore admirable for micrometry and give more accurate results than Huygenian eye-pieces.

Compensating eye-pieces are of the positive type and usually contain a triplet system as the lower lens component. Aberrations are carefully corrected by the makers and they are designed specifically for use with particular objectives. They have an important function in correcting the chromatic difference of magnification inherent in apochromatic lenses. Although designed specifically for use with apochromatic objectives, they can with advantage be used with high power achromats; their use, however, with lower power achromats is to be avoided.

CONDENSERS

The function of the condenser is to focus light on the object; it is mounted in the substage with a rack and pinion mechanism for adjusting the focus and should be fitted with centring screws for critical work with highly corrected lenses.

Abbé condensers are the simplest form of "chromatic" condensers and are often fitted to student microscopes. They are composed of two lenses neither of which is corrected for spherical or chromatic aberration. They are, however, cheap and easily fitted and may be satisfactory for low power work. They should seldom be used in microbiology because they give a poor image at higher magnifications. The light rays are not brought to an accurate focus and only a poor image of the light source can be obtained. Thus, there is flooding of the image with stray light and considerable glare results. In designing apochromatic and semi-apochromatic objectives it is assumed that the light reaching the lenses is corrected and it is essential that a condenser of similar optical quality is used with them.

Aplanatic condensers contain a third or middle lens which corrects for spherical aberration but not for colour. Such condensers give reasonable results especially when used with monochromatic light.

Achromatic condensers, which approach objectives in their complexity, give the best results because they place most of the light where it is needed, *i.e.* in the plane of the object, and very little escapes to produce glare.

The NA of a condenser should ideally be equal to that of the objective. A good achromatic condenser has an NA of 1·37 and supplies a solid cone of light to the limit of its aperture. This is adequate to fill the aperture of the highest power objective and is sufficient to meet the needs of all the commonly used objectives. The NA of such a condenser can be adjusted to that of lower power objectives by the use of the iris diaphragm mounted below the lowest lens component. It must be remembered that the highest NA of any dry lens is 1·0 and that for critical high-power work it is necessary to introduce immersion oil (refractive index = 1·50) between the top lens of the condenser and the lower surface of the microscopic slide.

Centration of the Condenser

If the condenser mount of the microscope possesses centring screws, the centration of the condenser with respect to the objectives must be checked from time to time as follows. After the microscope and the illuminant have been set up as described (see p. 625), close the condenser iris diaphragm to its limit. Rack down the condenser until the image of the condenser iris appears in the field. If it is not concentric, adjust the centring screws until it is so. It will be of advantage to open up the condenser iris until its aperture is almost that of the field for the final centration. Then open the iris diaphragm fully and rack up the condenser to its normal position.

For more detailed accounts of the microscope and its uses see Barer (1959) and Wredden (1947).

Brief Specification of a Microscope suitable for Routine Bacteriological Work

Microscope, with coarse and fine adjustments, fitted with a removable inclined binocular body. Built-in mechanical stage with verniers, quadruple nose-piece, rackwork substage with centring screws.

Objectives

Achromatic 10× (16-mm.).
,, 40× (4-mm.).
Fluorite 45× (3·5-mm.) oil-imm. (magnification and focal length may vary slightly according to make).
Achromatic 95× (2-mm. or $\frac{1}{12}$-in.) oil-imm.

Paired Eye-pieces

6× and 8×.

Condenser

Aplanatic or achromatic.

Note.—(*a*) Some makers supply a 10× objective specially computed to work with compensating eye-pieces. As it is an advantage to use this type of eye-piece with the other three objectives, it is recommended that this objective and compensating eye-pieces should be specified when ordering.

(*b*) If micrometry or photographic work is to be done, an interchangeable monocular tube is required.

(*c*) For dark-ground illumination, a special concentric condenser is necessary, and also a funnel stop for the $\frac{1}{12}$-in. objective.

(*d*) When more than one condenser is used it is advisable to have a substage in which the condensers can easily be changed.

MICROSCOPE LAMPS

The clarity and sharpness of the microscope image depend not only on the excellence of the optical system but also on the illuminant employed. For a monocular instrument with an Abbé condenser, and particularly for lower powers, a 40- or 60-watt opal bulb in a simple lamp housing is sufficient, but for a modern instrument with an inclined binocular body, well corrected oil-immersion objectives and an aplanatic or achromatic condenser, this type of illuminant is far from satisfactory. Unless the bulb is much over-run there is not sufficient light to see small details, and the advantages of modern optical systems can be nullified by poor illumination. If the opal bulb lamp is used it is of advantage to over-run the bulb, *e.g.* a 200-volt bulb on a 240-volt mains supply. The life of the bulb is shortened, but that is not a serious matter compared with the illumination obtained. The opal bulb should be in a well ventilated housing with a hood over the aperture to prevent direct light from reaching the eyes and should preferably be fitted with an iris diaphragm. The latter is very useful for centring the light in the microscope field and helps to diminish glare. The amount of light required for a good visual image depends on many factors: the intensity of the bulb, the magnification used (for example less light is required for a 16-mm. objective than a 2-mm.), the amount of light in the room (less light is required if the microscope is at the back of the room than on the bench at the window), and the time of day (much more illumination is required if there is sunshine than on a dull day or in the evening). With microscopical work, therefore, the amount of illumination required is always changing and a sliding variable resistance of 250 ohms to carry 0·75 or 1 amp. fitted with a switch is strongly recommended. This is most desirable if an over-run bulb is used, and an absolute necessity if a high-intensity projection type of bulb is employed. The resistance is placed in series with the opal bulb and in series with the primary winding of the transformer if a low-voltage projection bulb is used.

The full resistance should always be used when the lamp is switched on so that the bulb warms up comparatively slowly, and then the slide of the resistance is moved until optimum illumination is reached. With a change of objective the slide is easily adjusted to suit the intensity of light required, and this method of control is of great value when much microscopic work is done and where the objectives are changed frequently as in histological work.

High-intensity Lamps

With binocular microscopes the amount of light reaching each tube is only about one-third of that of a monocular instrument as light is absorbed by the glass prisms. In consequence a more intense source of light must be used. In order that the whole of the field shall be evenly illuminated, a corrected lamp condenser lens is necessary and this must be capable of being focussed. An iris diaphragm in front of this condenser is essential, and provision for a filter holder, preferably of the sliding type, should be made.

High-intensity lamps of this type are produced by several makers and a model specially suitable for high-power microscopy has been described (McCartney, 1951). This lamp uses a large "solid source" filament bulb of 12 volt 250 watts capacity, but it is actually run at 6 volts and the intensity is controlled by a sliding resistance in the primary of the transformer. The lamp is not only suitable for ordinary microscopy but is useful for dark-ground illumination and phase-contrast microscopy. Its high intensity ensures ample illumination even with dense filters. It is particularly useful for photomicrography.

It may be desirable sometimes to have a more intense beam of light than is possible with a 6-volt transformer, as when filters are required, with dark-ground illumination, or when high-power photomicrography is undertaken. In these cases a 9-volt transformer to take 18 amps. and tapped at 6 volts should be used. The 6-volt tapping is employed for ordinary work and the higher voltage output only for special purposes.

Other sources of light may be used for special types of work, such as a mercury vapour lamp for fluorescence microscopy, or even a high-intensity DC arc-lamp as in cinephotomicrography.

Light Filters

A blue daylight filter such as is supplied by most manufacturers should be fitted in the substage ring underneath the microscope condenser when artificial light is used. Filters, however, are not specially required in bacteriological work except for the methods used in fluorescent microscopy p. 632. Where much microscopic work has to be carried out, particularly with unstained objects as in dark-ground illumination or phase-contrast microscopy, the use of a pale-green filter, Wratten No. 66 (supplied by Kodak Ltd.) can be recommended. This filter cuts out glare, sharpens detail and is very restful to the eyes. After a short time in use, the green colour is not noticed. It can also be recommended when searching for malaria parasites or tubercle bacilli. In the latter case the organisms appear darker and are more easily recognised when only scanty bacilli are present.

ILLUMINATION OF THE OBJECT

It is common practice in microbiology to use a high-intensity lamp with a binocular microscope and it is important for the worker to obtain the full advantage of this apparatus. It must be remembered that high-intensity lamps have their own optical axis which must be aligned with the optical axis of the microscope. It is recommended that the *Köhler method* of illumination is used because it has the great advantage of providing a variable, uniformly illuminated field of view even with an irregular light source. The essential features of Köhler illumination are (1) the condenser lens of the lamp focuses an enlarged image of the light source (the filament) on the iris diaphragm of the substage condenser; (2) the image of the iris diaphragm in front of the lamp condenser is focused on the object plane by means of the substage condenser.

Method of using a high-intensity lamp:

(1) Rack up fully the substage condenser of the microscope.

(2) Check that lamp filament has been centred correctly with respect to the lamp condenser lens.

(3) Place the lamp so that its distance from the mirror is 8–10 in.

(4) Switch on the lamp, open its iris fully and decrease the resistance so that there is a bright beam of light shining on the plane side of the mirror. Adjust the lamp by altering its vertical tilt and by moving the base so that the beam of light is in the centre of the mirror.

It is important to ensure that (*a*) before switching on the lamp the full resistance is in and then for the illumination to be increased or decreased as desired, and (*b*) before switching off the lamp the bulb is dimmed to the full amount. If these precautions are taken, the life of the bulb will be much prolonged.

(5) Close the substage iris diaphragm and focus the lamp condenser so that a sharp image of the filament is obtained on the closed diaphragm. A small hand mirror, placed in a suitable place on the bench, facilitates this manoeuvre.

(6) Open the substage iris diaphragm and move the lamp backwards or forwards until the size of the image of the filament is large enough to fill the lowest lens of the microscope condenser.

(7) Pull back the resistance until the light is much dimmed, place a stained specimen with good contrast on the stage and focus it with the objective to be used.

(8) Close the lamp iris and adjust the mirror so that the image of this iris is in the centre of the field.

(9) Open the lamp iris until its image just fills the field.

(10) Remove the eye piece and inspect the back lens of the objective. An image of the filament should be seen to be symmetrically placed and large enough to fill the back lens of the objective.

To obtain the maximum definition, the lamp iris should be closed and focussed in the field for each objective. These adjustments, with practice, should only take a few seconds; they are possible with the 16 mm., 4 mm. and 3·5 mm. oil immersion objectives but not with the 2 mm. oil immersion objective.

DARK-GROUND ILLUMINATION

This method renders visible delicate organisms, such as the spirochaete of syphilis, which cannot be seen in unstained preparations with an ordinary microscope.

By means of a special condenser the specimen is illuminated by oblique light only. The rays do not enter the tube of the microscope, and, in consequence, do not reach the eye of the observer unless they are "scattered" by objects (*e.g.* bacteria) of different refractive index from the medium in which they are suspended. As a result, the organisms appear brightly illuminated on a dark background.

Three requisites are necessary for adapting a microscope for dark-ground illumination:

(1) A "dark-ground" condenser.

(2) A suitable illuminant of sufficient intensity.

(3) A stop which reduces the numerical aperture of the objective to less than 1·0, *if the ordinary oil-immersion lens is used.*

The Condenser.—A special condenser must be employed and may be of the paraboloid or of the concentric spherical reflecting type. The latter is recommended. The function of the special condenser is to focus the light on the object, the paths of the rays being such that no direct light passes into the front of the lens. Figure 47 shows the paths of rays through the concentric reflecting condenser. The condenser should be furnished with a centring device, and it must be emphasised here that success with dark-ground illumination depends on the accurate centring of the condenser. There must be immersion oil between the slide and condenser.

The Illuminant.—A lamp of sufficiently powerful intensity should be employed.

If direct current only is available, the small arc lamp or the "pointolite" lamp (a proprietary name applied to a lamp consisting of two tungsten electrodes in a vacuum across which an arc is struck) should be used. The "pointolite" is more convenient to use than the arc lamp.

Alternating current is now almost universal, and high-intensity low-voltage lamps worked through a transformer and having a condensing lens are satisfactory for this purpose (p. 619). Complete lamps are obtainable from several makers.

The Funnel Stop.—When the objectives employed for dark-ground illumination have a numerical aperture of more than 1·0 (as in the case of ordinary oil-immersion lenses), a special stop to reduce the NA to less than 1·0 must be employed. This consists of a small funnel-shaped piece of metal or vulcanite which fits into the objective behind the back lens. It is advisable to procure the stop from the maker of the lens employed. The stop is easily inserted and removed, and the objective can at once be converted for ordinary use.

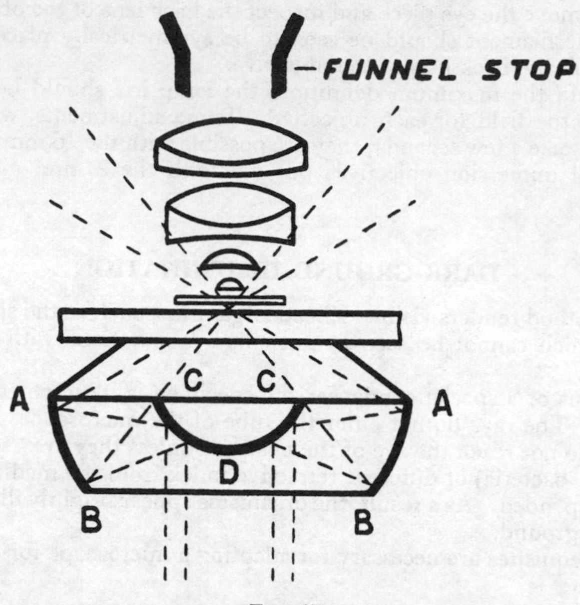

FIG. 47

Diagram showing the paths of rays through the condenser and a $\frac{1}{12}$-in. oil-immersion lens fitted with a funnel stop. AB and CDC are reflecting surfaces. The surface at CC is opaque. (*After* E. Leitz.)

Alternatively an *objective adaptor*, with a small iris diaphragm, may be used. The front part of the oil-immersion objective is removed and screwed to the adaptor, which then takes the place of the objective on the nose-piece. The numerical aperture of the objective may be reduced as desired by manipulating the iris diaphragm in the adaptor. Some makers incorporate an iris diaphragm in the mount of the objective itself so that it can be used for bright or dark-ground illumination without further alteration.

Certain manufacturers have introduced for dark-ground illumination with bicentric condensers, special oil-immersion fluorite objectives, which are used without a funnel stop. These are 2 mm. NA 1·15, and 3.5 mm. NA 0·95. The latter lens (referred to on p. 618) can be recommended for routine dark-ground observation at low magnification.

The Preparation.—The preparation should be as thin as possible in order to secure a satisfactory dark background, and so that the moving objects shall, as far as possible, be in one plane. A preparation which is too thick greatly diminishes the contrast in the dark field, and in order to obtain satisfactory contrast the objective has to be stopped down considerably, thus diminishing its resolving power. The preparation should not be too dense, otherwise there is an excessive number of particles which "scatter" the light. This causes lack of contrast even to a greater degree than a thick preparation. Some manufacturers supply special cells for dark-ground work so that when the coverslip is placed over the cell the preparation has a definite and uniform thickness.

The thickness of the slide employed is important. The slides should be 1·0–1·1 mm. thick, and when a suitable supply has been obtained they should be used only for dark-ground work. They should be thoroughly clean and free from grease. The object to be examined must be at the focus of the condenser, the focal length of which is about 1·2 mm. If, therefore, too thick a slide is used, the focus of the condenser will be below the specimen and poor illumination will result; if the slide is too thin, the distance between the condenser and slide is such that a large amount of oil must be employed to make contact.

Method of using Dark-Ground Illumination with the Oil-Immersion Objective

The microscope with special condenser, and with the NA of the objective reduced by a funnel stop or iris diaphragm adaptor, is placed in front of the illuminant. It is advisable to have the microscope in the upright position and not inclined, to avoid running of the oil. The condensing lens of the lamp is adjusted so that a slightly converging beam of light is obtained. With the plane side of the mirror, direct the light into the dark-ground condenser. Using the low-power ($\frac{2}{3}$-in. or 16 mm.) objective, focus the surface of the condenser so that the engraved concentric rings on the surface come into view. These rings show the centre of the condenser, and if the condenser is out of centre adjust the centring screws so that the rings become concentric with the edge of the field.

Should the condenser have no engraved rings the centring may be accomplished as follows.

A slide preparation is placed on the stage, and oil contact between it and the condenser established. The preparation is focussed with the $\frac{2}{3}$-in. objective, and, if the mirror is properly adjusted, a bright ring of light is noticed in the field. Focus the condenser cautiously up or down so that the ring of light contracts to the smallest bright spot obtainable. If this spot of light is not in the centre of the field, alter the centring screws of the condenser accordingly.

The accurate centring of the condenser is of the utmost importance and the time spent in this manipulation will be amply rewarded by the brilliant illumination obtained. The preparation to be examined must be covered with a No. 1 coverslip, and it is advisable to ring round the coverslip with petroleum jelly to prevent evaporation. Place a large drop of immersion oil upon the under surface of the slide and also on the upper lens of the condenser, and a similar drop on the coverslip. Place the slide on the microscope stage, taking care that the upper surface of the condenser is well below the slide. Rack up the condenser until oil-contact is made between the whole surface of the upper lens of the condenser and the slide; then bring the oil-immersion lens into position so that it touches the oil on the coverslip. Now carefully focus the specimen. A slight adjustment of the condenser, up or down, may be necessary, and some manipulation of the mirror may also be required. After a little practice an evenly illuminated field with an intensely dark background and brilliantly lit objects may be obtained with a minimum of trouble.

Where much dark-ground work has to be done, it is recommended that a microscope be reserved solely for this work and kept ready with the illuminant in position, so that it is always available for immediate use. It is convenient to have the lamp and microscope fixed to a board for this purpose. The microscope, when not in use, should be covered to exclude dust.

After use, the condenser and objective should be carefully wiped free from oil.

Dark-Ground Illumination with Low- and Medium-Power Lenses

Dark-ground illumination is easily obtained with a low-power lens whose NA does not exceed 0·3, *e.g.* the ⅔-in. objective, by placing a central patch or stop below the condenser. Most manufacturers supply a set of stops which fit into the ring below the iris diaphragm. Alternatively, a circle of glass with a central patch of black gummed-paper about 10–12 mm. in diameter may be used. The ordinary source of illumination is quite sufficient. Such dark-ground illumination may be used for observing slide-agglutination and for cells, casts, etc., in urinary deposits. With the higher power dry lenses, however, it is not so easy to secure satisfactory dark-ground illumination unless special condensers are used. Some microscope manufacturers make dry dark-ground condensers to work with ⅙-in. objectives up to numerical apertures of 0·65, but these are expensive and usually require a high-intensity lamp to work satisfactorily. The results, however, are very beautiful.

Where the NA of the objective does not exceed 0·65, dark-ground illumination can be secured with an "achromatic" or "aplanatic" condenser (not Abbé condenser), an expanding iris or suitably large central stop being used. As such condensers are suitable for ordinary microscopy it is possible to change over from direct transmitted light to dark-ground illumination, without removing the condenser, by merely inserting the stop. A high-intensity illuminant is, however, necessary, and immersion oil is placed between the condenser and slide (*vide supra*). An intermediate objective adaptor with iris diaphragm is often of value in reducing the NA of the ⅙-in. objective sufficiently to obtain a uniform dark field.

PRACTICAL INSTRUCTIONS FOR THE USE OF A MICROSCOPE

When an observer has to examine a specimen for a long time, as when scanning a film for tubercle bacilli or malaria parasites, he must adopt a comfortable position with the height of his chair adjusted so that the oculars of the microscope are level with his eyes. Many workers who wear spectacles are able to dispense with them when using a microscope. If, however, the visual defect is that of astigmatism spectacles will often need to be worn, and if this is so workers must take care to avoid contact between the eye-piece and the spectacle lenses or they may scratch each other. If a monocular microscope is used the worker should keep both eyes open if possible, in order to reduce strain. It is wise to ease the burden on the eye by changing from one eye to the other from time to time. Both forearms should rest on the table, and if there is no mechanical stage the slide is moved with the left hand while the right hand controls the fine adjustment. Before beginning to examine a specimen the microscope is checked to ensure that:

(1) the objectives are clean and free from immersion oil;
(2) the eye pieces are free from dust;
(3) the plane side of the mirror is in position;
(4) the substage condenser is racked up until its top surface is 1–2 mm. below the object slide.

For microbiological work it is recommended that artificial light should always be used. A 60-watt opal bulb or a high-intensity lamp (see p. 619) is employed according to the type of microscope used. It is not advisable to place the microscope at a window because daylight, and especially bright sunlight, entering the eyes renders vision less acute. A suitable arrangement is to use the microscope on a table at one side of a room so that the observer's back is to the window.

When examining an object, using a simple 40- or 60-watt opal bulb lamp, the manipulations of the microscope should be carried out in the following order:

(1) Set up the microscope, place the object on the stage, and adjust the plane side of the mirror to the illuminant so that the light is reflected into the condenser.

(2) Focus the specimen with the low-power objective, using the coarse adjustment.

(3) Manipulate the mirror until the image of the illuminant is seen in the centre of the field; if the lamp has an iris diaphragm this should be closed and the mirror adjusted until the aperture of the iris is concentric with the edge of the field. Rack the condenser up or down until the edge of the iris is sharply focussed.

It is essential, particularly when examining tissues, to use the low power first, in order to locate organisms and observe the tissue changes. A suitable field having been obtained, the slide must be kept in place by means of the right-hand clip if a mechanical stage is not used.

(4) Rack up the objective a short distance and place a drop of cedar-wood immersion oil on the portion of the specimen immediately below the objective.

(5) Raise the condenser so that its upper surface is practically level with the stage. (This is not necessary if the lamp iris has been focussed as in (3).)

(6) Make sure that the iris diaphragm of the substage condenser is widely open.

(7) Rotate the nose-piece until the oil-immersion lens is in position.

(8) With the eye at the level of the stage and using the coarse adjustment lower the objective until it makes contact with the oil; at this moment the drop of oil "lights up". Next, the objective is gently lowered a little further towards the slide but great care must be exercised not to carry this movement too far or too harshly. The working distance of oil-immersion lenses is extremely short and there is a great risk that with pressure, the tiny front lens of the objective may be displaced and its performance ruined. Some modern objectives, but not all, have a special guarding device to prevent this, or are set in a spring-loaded mount.

(9) Apply the eye to the microscope and observe if the field is well illuminated; if not, adjust the mirror until maximum illumination is secured.

(10) Next, slowly and carefully *focus up* with the coarse adjustment until the object is brought into view and then use the fine adjustment to secure a sharp focus.

In using a binocular microscope the same directions should be observed, but, in addition, the eye-pieces should be adjusted to the correct interpupillary distance of the observer when the specimen is focussed with the low-power objective (*vide* direction No. 2).

CARE OF THE MICROSCOPE

The microscope is an instrument of precision, and care must be taken to preserve its accuracy. The instrument should be kept at a uniform temperature and not exposed to sunlight or any source of heat. When not in use it must be protected from dust under a transparent plastic cover or in its box. Failing these, it should be covered with a clean cloth. The microscope should be cleaned at intervals, and its working surfaces very lightly smeared with soft paraffin. With binocular microscopes dust may collect on the surfaces of the prisms. This may be removed by passing a soft-camel-hair brush down the eye-piece tubes after removing the eye-pieces. On no account must the prism case be opened and the prisms removed, as this will completely alter the optical alignment and necessitate the return of the instrument to the maker before it can be used again.

If the microscope has to be moved, it should be lifted by the upright limb and not held by the body-tube.

The oil-immersion objective must be cleaned each day after use by wiping the front lens with a well-washed silk or cotton handkerchief. Alternatively, a fine tissue paper known as "lens paper" may be used (books of which are supplied by most manufacturers), and this is very suitable for the purpose. Oil remaining on the lens-front dries and becomes sticky; later it hardens and is then difficult to remove. Canada balsam accidentally present on the lens from a mounted microscopic specimen may also dry hard in the same way. When cleaning the objective *do not use alcohol*, as the cement that unites the component lenses may be soluble in alcohol, and, in consequence, the lens systems may become disorganised and the objective spoiled. Benzol or xylol must be used to remove dried oil, and if the oil is hard, repeated applications on a soft cloth are necessary.

Dry objectives—e.g. $\frac{2}{3}$-in. and $\frac{1}{6}$-in.—are cleaned with a piece of well-washed silk or fine cotton, or lens paper. If any oil or Canada balsam is accidentally present on the front lens it must be removed with a soft cloth moistened in benzol or xylol and the lens quickly dried with a soft cloth. On no account must the component parts of an objective be unscrewed.

Eye-pieces from time to time may be contaminated with dust and fuzzy specks are seen in the field of view. The trouble is easily located because the specks move when the eye-piece is rotated in its mount. If the dust is situated on the upper lens the specks will move if the eye-piece is raised a little with one hand while the upper lens is unscrewed with the other. If the dirt is on the bottom lens the specks will move when the lower component is rotated. When the position of the dirt has been located, remove it by blowing a jet of dry air on it with bellows or a large rubber teat. Alternatively, use a soft camel-hair brush. If the brush is held for a few seconds against a hot electric bulb it acquires an electric charge and will then attract dust particles easily. If these methods fail then use a silk cloth or lens paper moistened with *distilled* water. Never rub the surface of a lens with a dry cloth because any hard particles on its surface may scratch the glass.

COMMON DIFFICULTIES IN MICROSCOPY

A number of troubles may be encountered by those beginning microscopy and the following hints are given to help overcome them:

1. *Inability to obtain a sharp image with the oil immersion objective*:

(*a*) Check that there is no dirt or dried oil adherent to the front lens of the objective. If there is clean it off (*vide supra*).

(*b*) Check that the microscope slide carrying the object has not been put in upside down.

(*c*) Check that the immersion oil being used is not so viscous that the slide adheres firmly to the objective and travels upwards with movements of the coarse adjustment.

(*d*) Check whether the specimen slide and coverslip has a film of dried immersion oil and dirt left on it by a previous viewer.

(*e*) Some high-power objectives have so short a working distance that a thick coverslip or a thick layer of Canada balsam beneath the coverslip may prevent the objective approaching near enough to bring the object within its focal length.

If none of these steps improves matters, exchange the objective with one from another microscope; if a sharp image is obtained with the new objective the faulty one should be returned to the makers.

2. *A dark shadow passes into the field* with loss of definition of the image. This is usually caused by the movement of an air bubble in the immersion oil. The trouble may be cured by raising the objective so that the contact between the oil and the objective is broken and then refocussing. If this fails, clean objective and coverslip with a little xylol and begin again.

3. *Poor illumination or the field of view in semi-darkness*:

(*a*) Check that the flat and NOT the concave surface of the mirror is being used and adjust the mirror so that the light beam fills the field of view.

(*b*) Check that the condenser has been racked up to its full height. Occasionally it slips downwards in its mounting ring and must be pressed up as far as possible before it can be racked up close to the microscope slide.

(*c*) Check that the substage iris diaphragm is fully open.

EXAMINATION OF LIVING UNSTAINED ORGANISMS

In the case of bacteria, "hanging-drop" preparations are frequently used for this purpose, and a glass slide having a circular concavity in the centre is employed.

There should be no difficulty in observing a satisfactory specimen if the following procedure is adopted:

(1) By means of a match dipped in petroleum jelly, a ring or square (according to the shape and size of the coverslip) is outlined round the concavity.

(2) With a wire loop place a drop of fluid containing the organisms on a coverslip laid on the bench.

For this purpose a fluid culture is used or the condensation fluid of a slope culture. A further alternative is to emulsify a small amount of culture from the surface of a solid medium in a drop of broth or normal saline, taking care that the emulsion is not too dense.

(3) Invert the slide over the coverslip, allowing the glass to adhere to the jelly, and quickly turn round the slide so that the coverslip is uppermost. The drop should then be "hanging" from the coverslip in the centre of the concavity.

(4) Place the slide on the microscope, rack down the condenser slightly and partially close the iris diaphragm. (Excessive illumination renders the organisms invisible.)

(5) With the low power objective, focus the edge of the drop so that it appears across the centre of the field.

(6) Turn the high-power ($\frac{1}{6}$-in. or 4-mm.) lens into position and focus the

edge of the drop. Obtain the best illumination by lowering or raising the condenser, and secure sharp definition by reducing the aperture of the iris diaphragm.

Instead of employing a hanging-drop preparation, a film of the fluid between an ordinary slide and coverslip may be used, but in this case the edge of the coverslip should be sealed with vaseline or nail varnish to prevent evaporation of the fluid.

Motility of organisms can be detected in this way, and their shape, approximate size and general structure can be observed. *It is advisable to use the high-power dry lens* and not the oil-immersion objective. Owing to the viscosity of the oil, the coverslip is apt to move during focussing, and currents are thus caused in the fluid, which produce an appearance of motility in the organisms.

It is essential to distinguish between true motility, where the organism changes its position in the field, and Brownian movement, which is an oscillatory movement possessed by all small bodies (whether living or not) suspended in fluid.

A warm stage is very convenient when examining fresh unstained preparations for amoebae and other protozoa. There are several types of warm stage available, some of which consist of a thin, flat metal box filled with hot water, or through which warm water can circulate, and having an aperture in the centre by which the light passes to the preparation. Improved forms are electrically heated and have an automatic temperature control. The warm stage keeps the preparation at body temperature, and enables the movements of organisms to be studied, as these movements may cease if the material is kept for any length of time at room temperature.

A simple warm stage may easily be improvised from a sheet of thin copper (18-gauge) shaped like the letter T, with the long arm 5–6 in. in length. The top of the T is the size of a microscope slide (3 in. × 1 in.) and in the centre is an aperture $\frac{1}{2}$ in. in diameter. The copper T is placed on the microscope stage with the long arm projecting forward, and the aperture over the condenser. The preparation is placed on the copper strip and secured by the stage clips. The projecting part of the T is warmed by means of a small Bunsen flame or spirit lamp. Care must be taken that the preparation is not overheated.

MICROMETRY

In bacteriological work the unit of measurement is 0·001 mm., designated a *micron* or μ. The measurement of microscopic objects is accomplished by means of the stage micrometer in conjunction with a micrometer eye-piece. The stage micrometer consists of a 3 × 1 in. slide on which is a millimetre scale graduated in hundredths of a millimetre. This scale may be engraved, but is usually made by a photographic process. The micrometer eye-piece consists of a special eye-piece in which a graduated scale, mounted on the diaphragm of a positive type eye-piece, can be focussed by means of the movable eye-lens.

When measurements are to be made, the micrometer eye-piece is inserted into the draw-tube, the tube length is accurately noted, and the rulings on the stage micrometer focussed by the appropriate objective according to the size of the object to be measured. The number of divisions on the eye-piece scale corresponding to a definite number of divisions of the millimetre stage scale is determined. The stage micrometer is removed, and the object to be measured is next focussed. The number of divisions of the eye-piece scale which just cover the object are noted.

The millimetre value of each division of the eye-piece scale depends on the objective used and the tube length employed, and is usually determined each time a measurement is taken. Sometimes it is advisable to increase or diminish the draw-tube length or to move the adjustable collar of the objective so that the stage and eye-piece scales coincide or bear a geometric relation to each other—*e.g.* 1 division of the former to 10 of the latter.

Example: Using a $\frac{1}{12}$-in. objective and a 6× micrometer eye-piece at 165 mm. tube length, it was found that 100 divisions on the eye-piece scale exactly covered 11 divisions of the stage micrometer. Each division of the stage micrometer is $\frac{1}{100}$ mm.

100 eye-piece divisions = 11 stage divisions = 0·11 mm.
1 eye-piece division = 0·0011 mm.
1 eye-piece division, therefore, with the given objective, eye-piece and tube length = 1·1 μ.

The stage micrometer was removed and a stained slide of blood showing malaria crescents was substituted. The diameter of a red blood corpuscle covered 7 divisions of the eye-piece scale—*i.e.* 7·7 μ. A polymorph leucocyte covered 11 divisions, while the length of a malaria crescent was equal to 10 divisions, showing the sizes of these objects to be 12·1 μ and 11 μ respectively.

If the draw-tube is so adjusted that 1 division of the stage micrometer equals 10 of the eye-piece scale, then each division of the latter corresponds to 1 μ.

The Screw Micrometer Eye-piece employs a vertical fine hair line which is made to traverse a fixed scale situated on the eye-piece diaphragm. The eye-piece is of the Ramsden, or compensating, type and is fitted with an accurate screw contained in a drum which is divided into a hundred parts, each of which represents a displacement of 0·01 mm. of the hair line. The fixed scale is not intended for direct measurement but is constructed so that with each complete revolution of the drum the hair line traverses one division. Calibration is made by comparison with a stage micrometer (Needham, 1958) in the way described for the eye-piece micrometer (*vide supra*). The screw micrometer eye-piece is more precise and accurate than the eye-piece micrometer and measurements to one-hundredths of the fixed scale divisions are possible.

Photographic Method of Micrometry.—An accurate method is to photograph a film of the organisms or cells under a high magnification. Without disturbing the microscope or camera, the slide is removed from the microscope stage and the stage micrometer substituted. A photograph of the stage micrometer is then taken at exactly the same magnification. By means of a pair of fine dividers the length of the organism on the print is taken, and its exact measurement found by applying this distance to the micrometer print.

Electron-microscopical Method of Micrometry.—Optical methods of micrometry have, to a large extent, been replaced by electron-microscopical techniques. A suitable suspension of the organism to be measured is made and to it is added a suspension of latex particles of known diameter (*e.g.* 250 or 80 mμ). Measurements of the organism and the reference particles on the electron micrograph give a highly accurate estimate of size. It must, however, be remembered that during examination in the electron microscope an organism may be distorted by drying or heat. Most of these difficulties, however, can be overcome by careful fixation (see pp. 639-640).

PHASE CONTRAST MICROSCOPY

One of the difficulties of examining microscopically living, unstained biological specimens is that they are immersed in a fluid of almost the same refractive index as themselves. In order to see them distinctly it is necessary either (*a*) to close considerably the iris diaphragm, thereby reducing the numerical aperture, or (*b*) to use dark-ground illumination. The latter procedure is satisfactory with very small or slender objects such as spirochaetes, but its use in bacteriology is limited.

By means of phase contrast microscopy, it is possible to examine living cells with the full aperture of the objective. In consequence internal details are effectively brought out.

Phase contrast microscopy can be used with any type of microscope, either monocular or binocular.

It is necessary to have:

(1) A special condenser which usually incorporates a rotating metal disk carrying a series of annular diaphragms. These are disks of glass rendered opaque but with a narrow ring of clear glass. Each objective requires a different size of annulus according to its numerical aperture; thus, for the 16-mm. objective the ring is narrow and about 4½ mm. in diameter, whereas for the 2-mm. objective it is wider and about 18 mm. in diameter. The size of the annulus is such that the condenser forms an image of it in the back focal plane of the objective.

(2) Special phase objectives. These are ordinary objectives at the back of which, *i.e.* in its back focal plane, is inserted a phase plate consisting of a disk of glass having a circular trough etched in it and of such a depth that the light after passing through it has a phase difference of a quarter of a wave-length compared with the rest of the plate (see Fig. 48).

The objective is focussed on the specimen. The appropriate annulus for the objective is rotated into position under the condenser. The condenser is then focussed so that the image of the annulus is superimposed on the phase plate at the back of the objective. A special telescope (supplied with the outfit) is inserted in place of the eye-piece and through it the back focal plane of the objective is observed. The annulus and phase ring should coincide. If they are not exactly coincident the centring screws under the condenser are adjusted to achieve this. The eye-piece is now re-inserted and the specimen examined.

All powers of the microscope can be used, provided that each objective has its own phase plate fitted, and there is an appropriate annulus for it below the condenser.

The *optical principal* briefly is as follows. If a diffraction grating is examined under the microscope, diffraction spectra are formed in the back focal plane of the objective. The detail observed in the image is due to interference between the direct and diffracted beams. Unstained objects such as bacteria or cells may be considered as similar to a diffraction grating; that is, the detail consists of alternate strips of material with slightly different refractive indices, through which light acquires small phase differences, and these form the image. With ordinary illumination, however, such slight differences are almost completely obscured by the intensity of the direct light beam, and hardly any detail can be observed at all.

As will be seen from Fig. 48, the direct light from the annular diaphragm passes only through the trough in the phase plate. The diffracted beam having a slightly different path goes through the thicker glass of the phase plate outside the trough and in consequence is retarded one-quarter of a

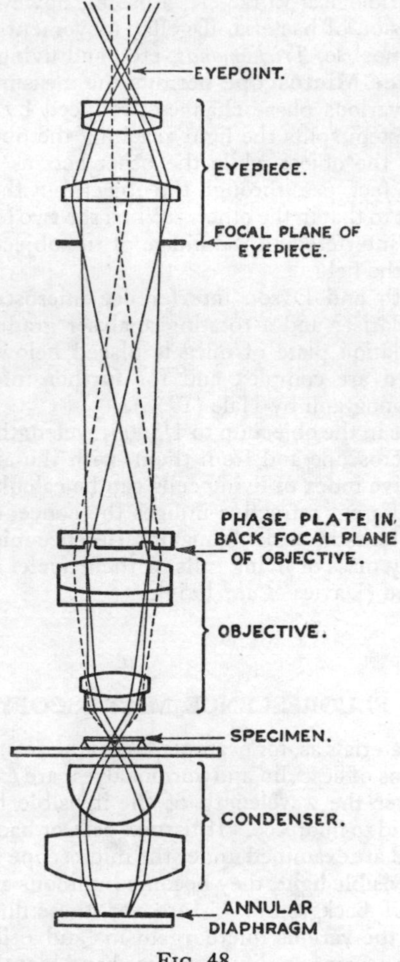

FIG. 48

Diagram illustrating the paths of light rays in phase contrast microscopy.
Reproduced by permission of American Optical Company.

wavelength with respect to the direct beam. When these two beams (direct and diffracted) unite they are not in phase, and these phase differences are apparent as appreciable changes in intensity. The details of the object stand out sharply and distinctly on a grey background, and being observed at full aperture, there is maximum resolution.

As there is a great difference in intensity between the direct beam and the diffracted beam, the trough of the phase plate through which the direct beam passes is covered with a light-absorbing material, usually a thin deposit of silver or other metal, so that the intensity of the direct beam is much reduced and approaches that of the diffracted beam. In consequence of this, and as the illumination is much restricted by the narrow annular diaphragm, a high-intensity lamp must be used.

Phase contrast microscopy is most valuable in general biology, but has less application in bacteriological work. It is useful, however, in examining the growth and subdivision of bacteria, flagellar movement, intestinal and other protozoa, such as amoebae, *Trichomonas*, etc., and living blood cells.

The Interference Microscope permits the measurement as well as the observation of the various phase changes produced by transparent objects. The illumination system splits the light reaching the object into two beams; one passes through the object while the other acts as a comparison beam. Both beams may, in fact, pass through the object, but the image in one is out of focus with respect to that in the other. When the two beams are recombined they are allowed to interfere and the image of the object is defined by interference contrast in the field.

The Baker-Smith and Dyson interference microscopes both employ a built-in rotating polariser and a rotating analyser graduated in degrees. A quarter wave retardation plate of mica is placed below the analyser. The optical systems used are complex and for further information the reader should consult a monograph by Hale (1958).

Phase differences in the object up to 1/300 wavelength can be measured by the interference microscope and from them, with the aid of a mathematical formula, the refractive index of living cells can be calculated. By immersing cells in media of different refractive indices the concentration of dried substances in them can be estimated. Thus, interference microscopy can be used to determine the dry mass of living cells or their nuclei and as a quantitative cytochemical method (Davies *et al.*, 1954).

FLUORESCENCE MICROSCOPY

When certain materials as, for example, uranium ores, uranium glass, oil or fat droplets, solutions of aesculin and various dyes, are exposed to ultra-violet (UV) light, they alter the wavelength of the invisible light and so become luminous and are said to fluoresce. If tissues, cells or bacteria are stained with a fluorescent dye and are examined under the microscope with ultra-violet light instead of ordinary visible light, they become luminous and are seen as bright objects against a dark background. Moreover, these fluorescent dyes have a selective action for the various microorganisms and cells and for their constituents which thus become readily recognised and identified. Dyes specially suited for fluorescent staining are auramine O, acridine orange R, berberine sulphate, primulin, thioflavin S, trypaflavine, thiazo-yellow G, and morin.

Immunofluorescence

Certain other fluorescent dyes can be used to label serum antibodies. They are coupled to gamma globulins (or to any chosen protein) by chemically reactive groups and render the resulting conjugates fluorescent. Two dyes are used, fluorescein isothiocyanate which has a brilliant apple-green colour, and lissamine rhodamine B (RB200) which has an orange colour. Labelled antisera have an important application in immunological work and the techniques of immunofluorescence are described in Chapter 54 and by Nairn (1964).

Many manufacturers supply complete units for fluorescent microscopy but it is possible to adapt the ordinary microscope for this work.

The most satisfactory light source is a high pressure mercury vapour lamp and is preferred to the tungsten or carbon arc lamps formerly used because it emits a very powerful beam of ultra-violet light at a steady intensity. The wavelength range required is 290–325 mμ for fluorescein and 310–350 mμ for rhodamine; these two dyes have emission peaks at 525 mμ and 595 mμ respectively. The HB200 (Osram[1]) lamp is recommended for this purpose and has a wavelength range of 280–600 mμ with peaks at 365 and 435 mμ. The lamp requires a special starter unit to provide a high tension initial impulse to start the mercury arc, followed by a continuous flow of low tension current to maintain the lamp. The average life of an HB200 lamp is 200 hr. and it is wise to keep a record of the burning time. The lamp should be enclosed in a protective housing because there is a small risk of explosion that increases when the lamp is used beyond its stated life. Within the housing an aluminium-coated reflecting mirror is needed and adequate centring devices are required.

The collector lens of the lamp should be made of ultra-violet transmitting crown glass or, better still, of "fused quartz" (quartz glass) because it is more heat-resistant than ordinary glass. Quartz condensers, and lenses in the optical path are, however, quite unnecessary and in any case they are extremely expensive. Thus, the absence of quartz condensers and lenses should on no account discourage the worker from undertaking fluorescence microscopy; the one essential is a satisfactory light source.

Condensers.—Two types of substage condenser may be used. For fluorochrome stained preparations a bright ground, three lens, aplanatic condenser is satisfactory, but for immune fluorescence a dark ground condenser gives better results, especially with the higher powered dry or oil immersion objectives.

Objectives.—Achromats are preferred to apochromats because the glass of their lenses has less tendency to fluoresce.

Filter systems.—(a) Primary filters. Light of wavelength 480 mμ is required and satisfactory filters, which must be sited close to the lamp, are available from Kodak Wratten 18B, Chance Pilkington OX7, in Great Britain, U.G.1 of Schott & Genossen in West Germany, and Corning 5840 in the U.S.A. (b) Secondary filters are situated in the eye-pieces and have the dual purpose of cutting off any UV rays which might damage the cornea of the observer's eye while at the same time giving a satisfactory colour contrast. A Kodak Wratten 2B filter is satisfactory, but a variety of green-yellow filters may be used.

Immersion oil.—Special non-fluorescent immersion oil is essential and that supplied by E. Leitz & Co. is recommended.

Staining with Fluorochrome Dyes

AURAMINE O.—This dye can be substituted for carbol fuchsin in the Ziehl-Neelsen method with the effect that the tubercle bacilli fluoresce and become much easier to detect.

[1] Manufactured by the German "Osram" Company and marketed in the U.K. under the name of "Neron".

Method

The following are required:

Staining solution

Auramine "O"	0·3 g.
Phenol	3·0 g.
Distilled Water	97·0 ml.

Dissolve the phenol in water with gentle heat. Add the auramine gradually and shake vigorously until dissolved. Filter and store in a dark stoppered bottle.

Decolourising solution. 75 per cent. industrial alcohol containing 0·5 per cent. NaCl and 0·5 per cent. HCl.

Potassium Permanganate Solution. 1 in 1000.

Stain a thin smear of sputum with auramine solution for 15 min. Rinse under the tap and decolourise for 5 min., with the acid-alcohol. Wash well in tap water, apply permanganate solution for 30 sec., wash well in tap water and allow to dry. (Do not use blotting paper to dry.)

The film is examined dry with a $\frac{1}{6}$-in. (4 mm.) objective, or preferably with an 8-mm. objective and a high-power eye-piece. The tubercle bacilli are seen as yellow luminous organisms in a dark field. A darkened room is an advantage. When fluorescent bacilli have been detected with the low power objective their morphology is checked by observation under the oil immersion objective.

This method has the advantage that large areas of a film of sputum can be scanned in a short space of time.

Acridine Orange R.—This dye has a marked affinity for the nucleic acids found in host cell-parasite relationships. When cells stained with this dye are viewed with UV light the RNA components fluoresce with shades of orange and red while the DNA components take on shades of green. The method is of great value in studying the growth of animal viruses and bacteriophages in their respective host cells (Anderson, Armstrong, and Niven, 1959).

Method

Coverslip preparations of living cells, tissue cultures or exudates are used. The following are required:

1. 3 per cent. HCl in 95 per cent. alcohol.
2. Citrate-phosphate buffer pH 3·8 (see Chapter 50).
3. Stock Acridine Orange R 0·1 per cent. in distilled water.

Solutions 2 and 3 are prepared freshly each week and stored at 4° C.

Proceed as follows:

1. Dilute the stock acridine orange solution 1 in 10 with the buffer on the day of use.
2. Place the coverslip without delay in acid-alcohol for 5 min.
3. Rinse for 2 min. in two changes of buffer.
4. Stain in the 0·01 per cent. acridine orange for 4–10 min.
5. Wash in two changes of buffer for 2 min.
6. Mount in buffer.
7. Ring the coverslip with nail varnish.

ELECTRON MICROSCOPY

With improvement in design and the evolution of new preparatory techniques, the modern electron microscope has become indispensable in microbiological research. The greatly increased resolving power of the instrument enables details of the fine structure and of the nature of the component parts of bacteria, viruses, cells and tissues to be visualised in a way that is impossible with the light microscope.

Although the electron microscope is complex, costly and technically difficult to maintain, the principles of its construction are closely paralleled by those of the optical microscope and easily understood. The resolution of the light microscope depends on the wavelength of the light used and the numerical aperture of the lens (see p. 611). When electrons move they behave somewhat like light waves and have properties of refraction, diffraction and interference. The wavelength of electrons is inversely proportional to their velocity and the particular wavelength used in an electron microscope is $\frac{1}{20}$ of an Ångström unit, *i.e.* about 100,000 times shorter than that of ordinary light, and thus high resolution and great magnifications are possible. Theoretically, if conditions were identical in the optical and electron microscopes, resolution down to $\frac{1}{40}$ Å would be possible. However, the NA of an electron microscope lens is very small (the diameter of the aperture is only a few microns) and does not approach the width of that of an optical microscope objective. In practice, the best resolution that can be obtained is 3–5 Å, i.e. 0·3–0·5 mμ. Thus the resolution of the electron microscope is approximately a hundred times better than that of the light microscope.

The electron microscope (see Fig. 49) consists of a column or "stack" (4) at the top of which is mounted the source of illumination, the "electron gun" (6) which emits electrons from a hot tungsten-wire filament (7). Beneath this filament a cathode shield (8) is placed. A high voltage (5) which can be varied from 50 to 100 kV. is applied to the anode. The life of the tungsten wire filament is limited and it usually requires to be replaced after some 15 hr. viewing. A pencil beam of electrons (9) moving at high velocity is projected through the hole in the anode and onwards down the stack. The high accelerating voltage used must be stabilised with an accuracy better than 1 in 100,000 in order to ensure uniform velocity of the electrons. Because the electron beam would be scattered by any atoms with which it might collide, the air in the stack is completely evacuated and a vacuum of the order of 10^{-6} mm. Hg. is maintained (3).

As in the light microscope, focussing and magnification are achieved by a series of "lenses" which, in fact, are accurately controlled electromagnetic fields. There is a condenser lens system (10 and 11) which bends the rays of electrons so that a parallel beam is directed onto the object (12) placed below it. The electrons are scattered to a degree that is proportional to the thickness and density of the various parts of the specimen. An objective lens (14) gathers the scattered electrons through a very small aperture (13) and brings them to a focus where a real primary image (2) is formed and is magnified about a hundred times. Two "projector" lenses (16), which have the function of the eye-piece of the light microscope, magnify a part of the primary image a further 300–500 times. The focal length of electromagnetic lenses can be changed by varying the current flowing through the lens and thus a continuously variable magnification is obtained and controlled at the turn of a dial.

The final image (18) is observed on a fluorescent screen (19) situated at the

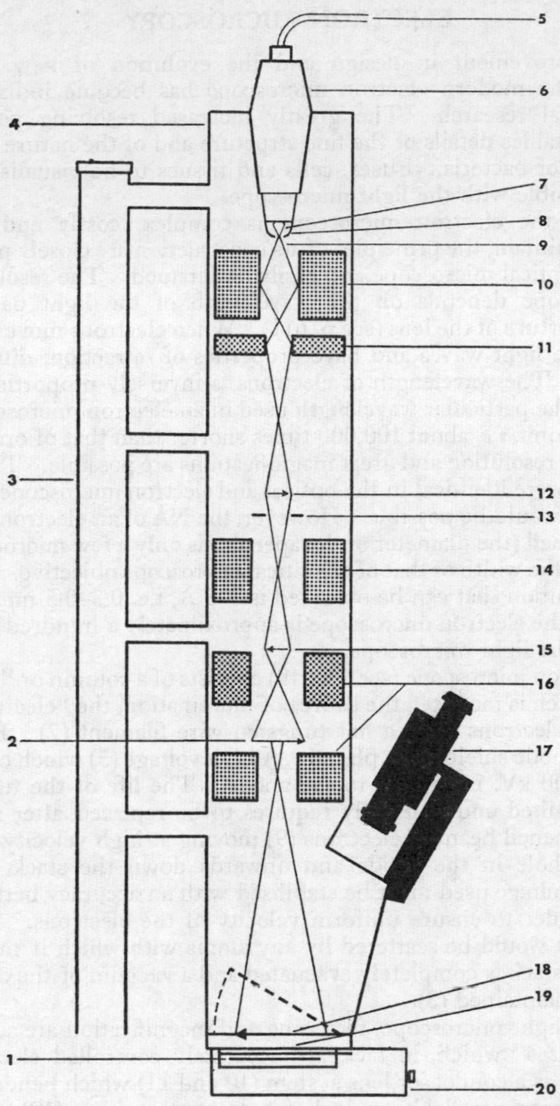

FIG. 49

A diagram to show the optical system and component parts of an electron microscope. (1) Photographic plate; (2) Primary image; (3) Connections from stack to vacuum pumps; (4) Stack; (5) 100,000-volt supply; (6) Electron gun; (7) Hot tungsten-wire filament; (8) Cathode shield; (9) Electron beam; (10) First condenser lens; (11) Second condenser lens; (12) Object; (13) Objective aperture; (14) Objective lens; (15) Intermediate image; (16) First and second projector lenses; (17) Focussing binoculars; (18) Final image; (19) Fluorescent screen; (20) Camera.

lower end of the stack and is viewed through a glass window. The screen can be withdrawn by a lever to allow the electrons to impinge on a photographic plate (1) or film held in a camera (20) placed immediately below. Owing to the high resolving powers of the electron microscope it is possible to take negatives at any magnification from 2000 to 100,000 and these may be enlarged photographically up to ten times. Thus, a useful magnification of up to 1,000,000 diameters can be obtained.

The specimen to be examined is placed in a special holder and then introduced into the stack between the condenser and objective lenses through an air lock. Finally, when the vacuum has been restored, it is lowered into position by a lever and its examination can be made. A 10 × binocular microscope (17) is used to facilitate accurate focussing before taking photographs.

The controls of the electron microscope are accommodated in panels on its desk. They include dials for variation of the magnification, a mechanical stage to move the specimen, switches and meters to control and check the voltage used, vacuum gauges, and controls for electron optical alignment. The electronic circuits for stabilising and controlling the high voltage and lens currents form a separate unit, as also do the rotary and diffusion pumps.

THE PREPARATION OF MATERIALS FOR ELECTRON MICROSCOPY

The electron beam, with an accelerating voltage of 50–100 kV., has a very poor penetrating power and for this reason only small objects or very thin sections of tissues can be examined in the electron microscope. The specimens must be mounted on films no thicker than 20 mμ and of high transparency to electrons. Such films are naturally very fragile and have to be mounted on small copper supporting discs that are perforated with many apertures regularly arranged to form a 40,000 per sq. in. mesh. Suitable grids for the AEI and other electron microscopes can be obtained from Smethurst Highlight Ltd., Bolton, Lancs.

They are made with a shiny surface on one side and a matt surface on the other for maximum adhesion of the film. Handling grids of this type requires very fine pointed forceps and is easier if the grids are bent very slightly. Traces of fluid may adhere to the points of the forceps as the grids are being manipulated through various solutions rendering the grids adherent, with the risk of damage to or loss of the specimen. This difficulty can be avoided if it is made a rule always to take a strip of filter paper and blot away traces of fluid from between the points of the forceps before transferring the grid to any dry surface.

Preparation of Support Films

Collodion Cast on Water.—The following are required:

(*a*) A 2 per cent. solution of nitrocellulose in amyl acetate ("Collodion").

(*b*) A brass ring $\frac{1}{4}$ in. deep and about 3 in. in diameter which is covered on one side by a disk of fine copper gauze (200 in. mesh).

(*c*) A 4-in. Petri dish or a shallow glass bowl of similar diameter standing on the lid of a 6-in. Petri dish.

PROCEDURE

1. Place the ring, gauze side uppermost, in the small Petri dish and pour in clean distilled water until it is covered and the water just reaches the brim of the dish.

2. Pick up electron microscope grids with fine forceps, moisten them carefully and place them in even rows, shiny surface down, on to the copper gauze.

3. The surface of the water is now cleaned by allowing two drops of the collodion to fall on it from a dropping pipette. A solid film is formed within a few seconds entrapping any dust particles on the surface and is then swept away with a glass rod.

4. A second film is now formed in the same way.

5. With minimum disturbance pipette the water out of the Petri dish into the surrounding trough. The collodion membrane sinks gently on to the grids on the copper gauze.

6. The gauze on its ring is now lifted from the dish and set to dry over calcium chloride in a desiccator.

7. When the grids are required for use they are freed by cutting the membrane at their edges with a fine needle, and then transferred to a holding clip.

Formvar Cast on Glass.—The following are required:

(*a*) A 0·125 per cent. solution of polyvinyl formal (Formvar) in chloroform.

(*b*) Microscope slides and short length of glass rod cleaned with a detergent and polished with a clean cloth.

(*c*) The materials required for collodion films.

PROCEDURE

1. Place a drop of the Formvar solution on a microscope slide and spread it to cover the whole surface with the glass rod. Allow a few seconds for the chloroform to evaporate. Ideally the film should have a pale straw colour.

2. Breathe heavily on the film.

3. Float off the Formvar membrane by lowering the slide at a shallow angle into the water in a Petri dish in which grids have been placed on copper gauze (*vide supra*).

4. Proceed as in making collodion films.

Formvar films are much stronger than collodion films and resist the heat of the electron beam much better. They suffer, however, from the disadvantage that they may have a coarser grained surface than collodion and thus are not desirable if the specimen to be viewed is comprised of small particles or macro-molecules.

Evaporated Carbon Films are prepared by the method of Bradley (1961). They can be obtained by evaporating carbon on to the surface of a glass slide and floated off as for Formvar. They have a thickness of only 50 Å. They have the finest grain of any film so far described. They are, however, fragile and some workers prefer to evaporate a layer of carbon 20–50 Å thick on to a grid previously covered with a collodion membrane.

Preparation of Suspensions of Microorganisms for Electron Microscopy

Suitable cultures containing large numbers of bacteria or virus particles must be obtained. In the case of viruses an infectivity or haemagglutinating titre of 10^7 or greater is desirable. The original cultures are centrifuged to deposit the microorganisms into a pellet which is then resuspended in a small volume of sterile culture medium. Extracts of virus infected cells or tissues may require several cycles of differential centrifugation.

Fixation

Bacteria and the larger viruses require some form of fixation though this may be omitted with some of the smaller viruses. Usually the suspension or the centrifuged pellet is added directly to the fixing solution. If sections are to be cut the pellet may be embedded in 2·0 per cent. molten agar (Difco, Noble agar, *vide infra*).

The following three fixatives are of general usefulness:

Kellenberger's Method for the Fixation of Microorganisms (Kellenberger, Ryter & Séchaud, 1958).

Prepare the following:

(1) Michaelis veronal-acetate buffer:

Sodium barbitone	2·94 g.
Sodium acetate (hydrated)	1·94 g.
Sodium chloride	3·40 g.
Distilled water to make	100 ml.

(2) Kellenberger buffer:

Veronal-acetate buffer	5·0 ml.
Distilled water	13·0 ml.
0·1 *N* HCl	7·0 ml.
$M/1$ $CaCl_2$	0·25 ml.

Adjust to pH=6·0 with the 0·1*N* HCl or buffer.
Prepare freshly on the day of use.

(3) Kellenberger fixative:

Osmium tetroxide	0·1 g.
Kellenberger buffer	10·0 ml.

The pH does not change.

(4) Tryptone medium:

Bacto-Tryptone (Difco)	1·0 g.
Sodium chloride	0·5 g.
Distilled water to make	100 ml.

(5) Sterile agar solution:

Agar (Noble)	2·0 g.
Distilled water to make	100 ml.

Sterilise in the autoclave in 5 or 10 ml. amounts.

(6) Kellenberger washing solution:

Uranyl acetate	0·5 g.
Kellenberger buffer to make	100 ml.

This solution keeps for several weeks at 4° C.

Procedure

(1) Mix 30 ml. of a suitable suspension of microorganisms with 3·0 ml. of Kellenberger fixative. Centrifuge 5 min. at 1800 G.
(2) Decant the supernatant and resuspend the deposit in 1·0 ml. of Kellenberger fixative to which has been added 0·1 ml. of tryptone medium.
(3) Stand overnight (about 16 hr.) at room temperature.
(4) Add 8·0 ml. Kellenberger buffer and centrifuge 5 min. at 1800 G.
(5) Decant the supernatant and resuspend the pellet in distilled water for direct electron microscopy.

(6) If ultra-thin sections are to be cut proceed as follows:
(*a*) add about 0·03 ml. of molten agar at 45° C. to the suspension and mix carefully;
(*b*) pour a drop of the molten agar suspension on to a clean microscope slide and allow it to set firm;
(*c*) cut the solid drop of agar into 1-mm. cubes with a razor blade;
(*d*) place the cubes into the uranyl acetate washing solution for 2 hr. at room temperature.

The cubes are now ready for dehydration and embedding.

For the techniques of embedding and the preparation and staining of ultra-thin sections, the reader is referred to Glauert (1961) and to Pease (1960).

Palade's Fixative (Palade 1952)

(1) Osmium tetroxide . . . . 1·0 g.
Distilled water . . . . . . 50 ml.
Store in a clean dark glass bottle away from the light. It keeps for several months at 4° C.

(2) Sodium barbitone . . . . 2·89 g.
Sodium acetate (hydrated) . . . . . 1·9 g.
Distilled water . . . . 100 ml.

(3) Prepare the fixative as follows:
Mix together—
2 per cent. osmium tetroxide . . . . . 12·5 ml.
Veronal-acetate buffer . . . . . . 5·0 ml.
0·1 *N* HCl . . . . approx. 5·0 ml.
Distilled water . . . . 2·5 ml.
Adjust to pH 7·3–7·4 using 0·1 *N* HCl. The fixative can be stored for a few days at 4° C. It is used mainly for fixing protozoa, cells and tissues.

Glutaraldehyde Fixation

(1) Stock solution 25 per cent. of glutaraldehyde (L. Light, Colnbrook).
(2) Phosphate buffer pH 7·4 (p. 854)

Fixative
Glutaraldehyde . . . . 5 ml.
0·1 M phosphate buffer . . . . . . 20 ml.

If sections are to be stained with lead salts, substitute 0·067 *M* sodium cacodylate for the phosphate buffered saline in order to avoid the precipitation of lead.
Adjust to pH 7·4.

Glutaraldehyde is an excellent fixative and much superior to formaldehyde.

Mounting.—The fixed bacteria are spun down in the centrifuge and resuspended into a suitable volume in distilled water. A light or phase contrast microscope is used to ensure that the suspension is neither too dense nor too dilute. A drop of the suspension is now placed on the surface of a supporting film on a grid. This can be done with a *very finely drawn* Pasteur pipette or a platinum loop. Experience is required to judge the size of drop used but it must not be so large that fluid spills and flows off the grid to adhere to its under side. After 2–3 min. the organisms have settled on to the film and the fluid is removed by touching the drop with a fine strip of filter paper. The grid is now dried for a few hours over calcium chloride in a desiccator and is ready for examination.

Contrast Enhancement

Microorganisms fixed in this manner are seen in outline under the electron microscope but if their components and the minute details of their structure is to be seen some form of contrast enhancement is required (Valentine, 1961). This is usually achieved by the use of "shadow casting" or by negative or positive staining techniques.

Shadow casting or metal shadowing consists of a technique whereby an atomic vapour of electron dense material is directed at an angle and deposited over the specimen. Heavy metals such as gold, platinum, palladium or their alloys are evaporated under a high vacuum in a special plant designed for the purpose (Bradley, 1961). The effect is that the side of the object farthest from the source of the heavy metal vapour is protected from the impinging atoms; these areas are more electron transparent than the overlaid areas and in electron micrographs look like shadows. The method is of particular value in the examination of bacteria bearing flagella, fimbriae and also in visualising the filaments of spirochaetes.

Negative Staining.—When virus particles or other small objects are added to a neutral solution of potassium phosphotungstate and the mixture is transferred to electron microscope grids the particles appear under the electron microscope as surrounded by an electron-dense background. Furthermore, any surface contours and depressions attract the tungstate so that details of the external characters of the object are revealed (Horne & Wildy, 1963). The method has been particularly successful in the study of the fine structure of animal viruses and bacteriophages but has many applications in microbiology.

Phosphotungstate Staining.—The method is that of Brenner & Horne (1959). Specimens for examination are suspended in a volatile buffer such as 1 per cent. ammonium acetate and then are added to an equal volume of 2·0 per cent. phosphotungstic acid adjusted to pH 7·0 by the use of *N*/1 KOH. The mixture is placed on electron microscope grids in the way described or sprayed on them with a "Vaponefrin" spray (Horne & Naginton, 1959). Sometimes the phosphotungstate fails to spread and forms dense masses in which the particles are completely buried. This may be corrected by the addition of a trace of serum albumin to reduce the surface tension or by reducing the concentration of phosphotungstate. If, on the other hand, the phosphotungstate spreads too widely and forms only a thin film the trouble can sometimes be overcome by increasing the tungstate concentration and/or diluting the virus preparation a little.

Uranyl acetate in a 1 per cent. solution can be used in a similar way. It does not produce so great a contrast as phosphotungstate but is valuable for the very smallest particles and macromolecules. The deposited uranyl acetate has an even texture and is less "grainy" than phosphotungstate.

Positive staining has its main application in microbiology in the enhancement of the contrast in ultra-thin sections of bacteria, protozoa and other cells. Solutions of heavy metal compounds such as phosphotungstic acid, phosphomolybic acid, uranyl acetate, barium hydroxide, lead acetate and lead tartrate are all used.

Much information is obtained from the study of ultra-thin sections and the techniques involved include embedding in epoxy resins, the use of the ultra microtome and special staining methods. For the details of these techniques the reader is referred to Glauert & Phillips (1961) and Pease (1960).

REFERENCES

Anderson, E. A., Armstrong, J. A. & Niven, J. S. F. (1959). Fluorescence microscopy; observations of virus growth with aminoacridines. *Symposium Society General Microbiology* No. IX, p. 224. Cambridge Univ. Press.

Barer, R. (1959). *Lecture Notes on the Use of the Microscope.* 2nd ed. Oxford: Blackwell.

Bradley, D. E. (1961). The preparation of specimen support films. Chap. 3 in *Techniques for Electron Microscopy.* Ed. Kay, D. Oxford: Blackwell.

Brenner, S. & Horne, R. W. (1959). A negative staining method for high resolution electron microscopy of viruses. *Biochim biophys. Acta (Amst.)*, **34**, 103.

Davies, H. G., Wilkins, M. F. H., Chayen, J. & La Cour, L. F. (1954). The use of the interference microscope to determine dry mass in living cells and as a quantitative cytochemical method. *Quart. J. micr. Sci.*, **95**, 271.

Glauert, A. M. (1961). The fixation, embedding, and staining of biological specimens. Chap. 8 in *Techniques for Electron Microscopy.* Ed. Kay, D. Oxford: Blackwell.

Glauert, A. M. & Phillips, R. (1961). The preparation of thin sections. *Ibid.*, Chap. 9.

Hale, A. J. (1958). *The Interference Microscope.* Edinburgh: Livingstone.

Horne, R. W. & Naginton, J. (1959). Electron microscope studies of the development of and structure of poliomyelitis virus. *J. molec. Biol.*, **1**, 333.

Horne, R. W. & Wildy, P. (1963). Virus structure revealed by negative staining. *Advanc. Virus Res.*, **10**, 101.

Kellenberger, E., Ryter, A. & Séchaud, J. (1958). Electron microscope study of DNA containing plasms. *J. biophys. biochem. Cytol.*, **4**, 671.

McCartney, J. E. (1951). An improved microscope lamp. *J. clin. Path.*, **4**, 234.

Nairn, R. C. (1964). 2nd ed. *Fluorescent Protein Tracing.* Edinburgh: Livingstone.

Needham, G. H. (1958). *The Practical Use of the Microscope.* Springfield: Thomas.

Palade, G. E. (1952). A study of fixation for electron microscopy. *J. exp. Med.*, **95**, 285.

Pease, D. C. (1960). *Histological Techniques for Electron Microscopy.* New York & London: Academic Press.

Valentine, R. C. (1961). Contrast enhancement in the electron microscopy of viruses. *Advanc. Virus Res.*, **8**, 287.

Wredden, J. H. (1947). *The Microscope.* London: Churchill.

CHAPTER 45

STAINING METHODS

As bacteria consist of clear protoplasmic matter, differing but slightly in refractive index from the medium in which they are growing, it is difficult with the ordinary microscope, except when special methods of illumination are used, to see them in the unstained condition. Staining, therefore, is of primary importance for the recognition of bacteria.

The use and general principles of bacterial staining have been discussed in Chapter 2.

METHODS OF MAKING FILM OR SMEAR PREPARATIONS

Before describing the various staining processes, details of the methods employed in making films must be considered.

Film preparations are made either on coverslips or on the ordinary 3 × 1 in. glass slides, usually the latter. It is essential that the coverslips or slides should be perfectly clean and free from grease, otherwise uneven films will result.

Coverslips.—These should be ¾ or ⅞ in. square, and of No. 1 thickness, *i.e.* 0·1 mm. thick. (Thicker coverslips—No. 2—may prevent the oil-immersion objective from coming near enough for the specimen to be focussed.) They are cleaned by placing them in a mixture of nitric acid, 6 parts; potassium bichromate, 6 parts; water, 100 parts. They should be dropped one by one into the fluid. The solution is contained in an evaporating dish and boiled. Alternatively, they may be cleaned in the dichromate-sulphuric acid solution (p. 661) by the method described for slides on p. 862. The coverslips are then well washed, first in tap water and later in distilled water, and stored in a stoppered jar in 50 per cent. alcohol. Before use they are dried with a soft clean cloth, such as an old handkerchief. For routine use, the coverslips may be sufficiently clean as supplied by the maker and require only to be wiped free from grit and dust with a clean dry cloth.

Slides.—These may be treated in a manner similar to coverslips. A quicker and quite satisfactory method for ordinary routine use is to wipe the slide with a clean dry cotton cloth and then, holding its end with forceps, roast it free from grease by passing it 6–12 times through a blue Bunsen flame. The heating should be as strong as is possible without cracking the slide. Cracking is rendered less likely by allowing the slide to cool somewhat before laying down, or by laying it on a warmed metal rack. Another method of cleaning is to moisten the finger with water, rub it on the surface of some fine sand soap, and then smear the surface of the slide. After removing the soapy film with a clean cloth the surface is clean and free from grease. For special purposes, such as the staining of flagella, slides are cleaned with hot dichromate-sulphuric acid solution followed by flaming, as described on p. 661. If the slide is perfectly clean a drop of water can be spread over its surface in a thin even film; otherwise the water collects into small drops and a film cannot be made.

After the films have been made and examined the slides should be discarded. ***They should not be cleaned and used again, since it is difficult to ensure that all organisms are removed.***

In the case of fluid material, *e.g.* broth cultures, urine, sputum, pus, etc., one loopful (or more) is taken up with the inoculating wire (p. 791) and spread thinly on the slide. A little experience will soon determine the amount required, and in spreading the films it will be found that there are both thick and thin portions, which is not disadvantageous. The slide is then held in the palm of the hand high over a Bunsen flame and dried. The film is fixed by passing the *dried* slide, film downwards, three times slowly through the flame, or by heating through the glass slide. In the latter method the slide is held, film upwards, in the top of the Bunsen flame for a few seconds so that the slide becomes hot. Care must be taken not to char the film, and when the slide is just too hot to be borne on the back of the hand, fixation is complete.

In making films on coverslips and staining them, Cornet's forceps are used to hold the slip in a horizontal position, the forceps resting on the bench.

With solid material, such as cultures on agar, etc., it is necessary to place a loopful of clean water on the slide. The loop is then sterilised and a minute quantity of material, obtained by just touching the growth, is transferred to the drop, thoroughly emulsified, and the mixture is spread evenly on the slide. The resulting film is fixed and dried as above. *Beginners are apt to take more material than necessary from the culture and thus make too thick a film.*

STAINING OF FILMS

The stains are poured directly or filtered on to the slide. When staining is completed, the dye is washed off with water, and the slide is allowed to dry in the vertical position or is placed between two sheets of white fluffless blotting paper or filter paper. The drying of the film is completed over the Bunsen flame. Such stained films may be mounted in Canada balsam under a coverslip, or may be examined unmounted with the oil-immersion lens, a small drop of cedar-wood oil being placed directly on the film. If it is desired to mount the preparation later, the oil can be removed with xylol or benzol (*i.e.* benzene).

STAINING OF TISSUE SECTIONS

The sections being embedded in paraffin (p. 678), it is necessary to remove the paraffin so that a watery stain may penetrate. The paraffin is first removed with xylol (xylene) or benzol (benzene), the xylol or benzol is then removed with alcohol (95 per cent. ethanol), and the alcohol is replaced with water. The staining is then done. After staining, the section must be dehydrated with absolute alcohol, cleared in xylol and mounted in Canada balsam under a coverslip. The Canada balsam (which is a resin) is dissolved in xylol in order to render it suitable in consistency.

Alcohol (*Ethanol*) *Solutions.*—The reagents most commonly employed in preparation of sections are "absolute alcohol", which is 100 per cent. ethanol, and "95 per cent. alcohol", which is a 95 per cent. solution of ethanol in water by volume (*i.e.* 95 ml. absolute alcohol plus water to give 100 ml. solution).

Industrial methylated spirit (not mineralised) may be used for making up stains, decolourising stained preparations, dehydrating tissues and treating sections. The type known as "Toilet spirit, acetone free (66 O.P.)" is quite satisfactory for use instead of 95 per cent. alcohol. Similarly, industrial methylated spirit, absolute (74 O.P.), can be used instead of absolute alcohol. Not only are these industrial spirits much cheaper than rectified spirit (90 per cent. alcohol) and absolute alcohol, but permits for obtaining them duty-free are more readily granted by the Customs Authorities.

Technique.—The slide bearing the paraffin section is placed in a jar of xylol for some minutes to remove the paraffin. The section is then treated with a few drops of absolute alcohol (ethanol), when it immediately becomes opaque. A few drops of 50 per cent. alcohol are poured on, and the slide is finally washed gently in water. If the tissue has been fixed in any mercuric chloride preparation, such as Zenker's fluid, the section should be treated with Gram's iodine solution for a few minutes (p. 650), then with 95 per cent. alcohol and finally with water. The sections are now ready to be stained by the appropriate method. After staining and washing with water, the slide is wiped all round the section with a clean cloth to remove excess of water. The bulk of the water in the section may be removed by pressing between fluffless blotting paper. The section is treated *immediately* with a few drops of 95 per cent. alcohol and then with absolute alcohol. The slide is again wiped all round the section, a few more drops of absolute alcohol are poured on and the slide is then immersed in xylol. When cleared, the slide is removed, and excess of xylol round the section is wiped away, a drop of Canada balsam is applied and the section mounted under a No. 1 coverslip. It is essential that the section should not be allowed to dry at any period of the process, and that dehydration with absolute alcohol should be complete in order that the section may be thoroughly cleared.

When the bacteria are readily decolourised with alcohol, aniline-xylol (aniline, 2 parts; xylol, 1 part) should be used for dehydration. After washing, when the slide has been wiped round the section, the preparation is blotted and then treated with the aniline-xylol mixture, which clears as well as dehydrates. The aniline-xylol is then replaced with xylol. This can be done conveniently by holding the slide almost vertically and dropping xylol from a drop bottle on to the slide just above the section. The xylol flows over the section and quickly removes the aniline. The preparation is mounted immediately in Canada balsam.

DPX Mounting Medium

A mounting medium that replaces Canada balsam has been devised by Kirkpatrick and Lendrum (1939, 1941). It consists of polystyrene (a synthetic resin) dissolved in xylol, with a plasticiser—dibutyl phthalate—to ensure flexibility. There is, however, much shrinkage and the mounting fluid should be applied generously. The mountant termed DPX is made up as follows:

Mix dibutyl phthalate (B.D.H.)	5 ml.
with pure xylol	35 ml.
and dissolve "Distrene 80"[1]	10 g.

DPX medium is water-clear, inert and does not become acid or cause fading of stained preparations. It is used in the same way as Canada balsam.

If polystyrene of a low molecular weight (about 3000) is used, much less xylol is required and no plasticiser need be added. Moreover, there is practically no shrinkage, which is a great advantage over DPX.

SIMPLE STAINS

These show not only the presence of organisms but also the nature of the cellular content in exudates.

[1] Normally obtainable from Messrs. Honeywill & Stein, Ltd., 21 St. James's Square, London, S.W.1.

METHYLENE BLUE

Of the many preparations of this dye, Löffler's methylene blue is generally the most useful:

Saturated solution of methylene blue in alcohol	300 ml.
KOH, 0·01 per cent. in water	1000 ml.

Films.—Stain for 3 min., then wash with water. This preparation does not readily over-stain.

Sections.—Stain for 5 min. or longer. The application of the alcohol during dehydration is sufficient for differentiation. Aniline-xylol can also be used for dehydration and clearing.

Polychrome Methylene Blue

This is made by allowing Löffler's methylene blue to "ripen" slowly. The stain is kept in bottles, which are half filled and shaken at intervals to aerate thoroughly the contents. The slow oxidation of the methylene blue forms a violet compound that gives the stain its polychrome properties. The ripening takes 12 months or more to complete. The preparation is used in a manner similar to Löffler's methylene blue; it is employed in McFadyean's reaction (p. 295).

Borax Methylene Blue (Masson)

This gives similar staining results to polychrome methylene blue.

Methylene blue	20 g.
Borax	50 g.
Water	1000 ml.

Warm the water to 60° C., stir in the solids, and allow to cool slowly. This staining solution improves with age.

DILUTE CARBOL FUCHSIN

Made by diluting Ziehl-Neelsen's stain (p. 654) with 10–15 times its volume of water. Stain for 10–25 sec. and wash well with water. Over-staining must be avoided, as this is an intense stain, and prolonged application colours the cell protoplasm in addition to nuclei and bacteria.

NEGATIVE STAINING

"Negative Staining" is exemplified by Burri's India ink method, which was formerly used for the spirochaete of syphilis. A small quantity of India ink is mixed on a slide with the culture or other material containing bacteria, and then by means of another slide or loop a thin film is made; this is allowed to dry before being examined. The bacteria or spirochaetes are seen as clear transparent objects on a dark-brown background. (See also India ink methods for capsules, p. 659.)

FLEMING'S NIGROSIN METHOD

A 10 per cent. solution of nigrosin (G. T. Gurr) is made in warm distilled water (solution is effected in about an hour) and filtered. Formalin 0·5 per cent. (*i.e.* formaldehyde 0·19 per cent.) is added as a preservative. A small drop of the dye is placed on a slide, bacteria are mixed with it and a smear is made with a loop or another slide. A number of preparations can be made on the same slide. Dry and examine.

Nigrosin gives an absolutely homogeneous background, and this is the simplest method of making a preliminary examination of a culture to show shape, size and arrangement of bacteria. Most bacteria stand out as clear objects on a dark field, but some bacilli, such as those of the coliform and haemophilic groups, show in their central portion a slightly dark patch somewhat resembling a nucleus. This is attributed to the fact that in drying they develop a shallow depression in which some of the nigrosin lies. In the spore-bearing anaerobes the spores are larger than the bacilli, so that when the nigrosin film is slightly thicker than usual the spores stand out as bright clear spaces while the bacillary bodies are slightly overlaid with the nigrosin.

GRAM'S STAINING METHOD

This is the most important staining method in bacteriology, and must be employed for the diagnostic identification of various organisms. The principle of the method has been dealt with in Chapter 2.

Certain bacteria when treated with one of the basic para-rosaniline dyes such as methyl violet, crystal violet or gentian violet (which is a mixture of the two preceding dyes), and then with iodine, "fix" the stain so that subsequent treatment with a decolourising agent—*e.g.* alcohol or acetone—does not remove the colour. Other organisms, however, are decolourised by this process. If a mixture of various organisms are thus stained and subjected to the decolourising agent, it is found that some species retain the dye, and these are termed "Gram-positive", whereas others are completely decolourised and are termed "Gram-negative". In order to render the decolourised organisms visible, and to distinguish them from those retaining the colour, a contrast or counterstain is then applied. This counterstain is usually red, in order that the Gram-negative organisms may easily be differentiated from the Gram-positive organisms, which retain the original violet stain.

If Gram's method is properly carried out, Gram-positive organisms and fibrin are stained dark violet in colour. Gram-negative organisms, the nuclei and protoplasm of pus cells and tissue cells are stained pink with the counterstain. To obviate errors from overdecolourising, a control film of a known Gram-positive organism (*e.g.* a pure culture of *Staphylococcus aureus*) may be made at one side of the film to be examined. For the recognition of Gram-negative organisms such as gonococci or meningococci in pus, this control must retain the violet stain while the nuclei of the pus cells are stained only with the counterstain.

In the original method of Gram (1884), the smear was stained with aniline-gentian violet, treated with Lugol's iodine (iodine 1 g., KI 2 g., water 300 ml.), decolourised with absolute alcohol, and counterstained with Bismarck brown. Later modifications, however, have given better results.

KOPELOFF AND BEERMAN'S (1922) MODIFICATION

(Decolourisation with acetone)

This method, which is a modification of Burke's (1922) method, is recommended for general use.

Solutions required

(1) Methyl violet stain.

Solution A:

Methyl violet 6B	10 g.
Distilled water	1000 ml.

Solution B:

Sodium bicarbonate ($NaHCO_3$)	50 g.
Distilled water	1000 ml.

Shortly before use, mix 30 volumes of solution A with 8 volumes of solution B. (The mixture is apt to precipitate within a few days and so cannot be kept. Methyl violet solution *without* the addition of bicarbonate acts almost as well in Gram staining and has the advantage of keeping indefinitely. For critical work, however, a freshly made mixture of stain with bicarbonate is to be preferred.)

(2) Iodine solution.

Iodine	20 g.
Normal solution of sodium hydroxide (*i.e.* 1*N* NaOH, or 4 per cent. NaOH)	100 ml.
Distilled water	900 ml.

Dissolve the iodine in the NaOH solution and, when it is dissolved, add the distilled water.

(3) Basic fuchsin stain.

Basic fuchsin	0·5 or 1·0 g.
Distilled water	1000 ml.

Procedure for staining films

(1) Make a smear on a slide according to the instructions given on p. 643. Dry thoroughly in cool air or in warm air *far above* a Bunsen flame. Then, fix by flaming in the usual way (p. 644).

(2) Cover the whole slide with methyl violet stain and allow this to remain on the slide for about 5 min.

(3) Tip off the methyl violet stain, hold the slide at a steep slope and wash off the residual stain with an *excess* of iodine solution; begin by pouring the iodine on the upper end of the slide and rapidly work downwards. (It is important to use enough iodine solution to wash away all the crystalline deposit that forms when the stain and the iodine mix.)

(4) Cover the whole slide with fresh iodine solution and leave it thus for about 2 min.

(5) Decolourise with acetone (100 per cent.). First tip off the iodine and hold the slide at a steep slope. Then pour acetone over the slide from its upper end, soas to cover its whole surface. Decolourisation is very rapid, and is usually complete in 2–3 sec. After this period of contact the acetone must *at once* be removed by washing thoroughly with water under a running tap. To avoid delay, the tap should be running before the acetone is applied to the slide.

(Kopeloff and Beerman recommended that the acetone should be added to the slide drop by drop until no colour is seen in the washings; they noted that decolourisation generally requires less than 10 sec. and that the time should be reduced to a minimum. We have found that, with thin smears, successful results are obtained more consistently if the acetone is flooded over the slide and then washed off with water after only 2 seconds' contact.)

(6) Cover the whole slide with basic fuchsin stain and allow this to remain for about 30 sec.

(7) Wash thoroughly (for *c.* 5 sec.) in water from the tap, blot and dry in air.

Normally a Gram-stained film is examined under oil-immersion without mounting under a coverslip. The oil can be removed with xylol or benzol if it is desired to preserve the film.

Procedure for staining sections

(1) Remove paraffin with xylol or benzol.

(2) Treat the section with absolute alcohol (ethanol) and wash in tap water.

(3) Cover the slide with methyl violet stain and allow to act for 5 min.

(4) Wash off stain with an excess of iodine solution, cover with more iodine and allow to act for 2 min.

(5) Decolourise with acetone (*vide supra*). The visible violet staining should be removed from the section and this may take one or two seconds longer than is necessary in the decolourisation of films.

(6) Wash slide in water from tap.

(7) Counterstain with basic fuchsin for 30 sec.

(8) Wipe carefully around the section to remove as much water as possible. dehydrate quickly in absolute alcohol, clear in xylol or benzol and mount in Canada balsam or DPX.

Use of acetone-alcohol as decolouriser

Kopeloff and Beerman's method is sometimes modified by the substitution of acetone-alcohol in the place of pure acetone as decolouriser. Acetone-alcohol is a mixture of 1 volume of acetone with 1 volume of 95 per cent. ethyl alcohol (ethanol). It acts rather more slowly than pure acetone and decolourisation may be prolonged to 10 sec. or more, and can be more carefully adjusted in duration. It is not, however, considered to be quite as satisfactory as pure acetone in producing specific differential decolourisation.

BURKE'S (1922) MODIFICATION OF GRAM'S METHOD

(Decolourisation with acetone)

(1) Make smear, dry in air, and fix by flaming.

(2) Cover the slide with 1 per cent. aqueous methyl violet (or crystal violet). Then add 5 drops of a 5 per cent. solution of sodium bicarbonate to the dye on the slide, mix, and allow to act for 3 min.

(3) Tip off the stain and flush the slide freely with iodine solution (iodine 10 g., potassium iodide 20 g., and distilled water 1000 ml.). Cover slide with fresh iodine solution and allow to act for 1–2 min.

(4) Wash in water from tap, blot off all free water, but do not allow smear to dry. (Alternatively, blot the iodine from the slide.)

(5) Decolourise with acetone (100 per cent.) or acetone-ether (1 volume of ether and 2 volumes of acetone). Cover the slide with the decolouriser, stand for a few seconds, drain off, cover with fresh decolouriser for 1–2 sec. and drain off. Decolourisation usually requires a total duration of contact of less than 10 sec.

(6) At once blot slide and allow to dry in air.

(7) Counterstain for 10 sec. or longer with a 2 per cent. aqueous solution of safranine (or neutral red).

(8) Wash off counterstain by flushing with water for a few seconds, blot and allow to dry in air.

JENSEN'S MODIFICATION OF GRAM'S METHOD

(Decolourisation with alcohol)

This modification can be recommended for routine bacteriological work. It has been used especially in examination of exudates for gonococci and meningococci.

Solutions required

(1) Methyl violet stain:

Methyl violet 6B (or crystal violet)	5 g.
Distilled water	1000 ml.

The solution should be made up in bulk and filtered. It keeps indefinitely, and does not precipitate, but should be filtered again before use.

(2) Iodine solution[1]:

Iodine	10 g.
Potassium iodide	20 g.
Distilled water	1000 ml.

Dissolve 20 g. potassium iodide in 250 ml. water, and then add 10 g. iodine; when dissolved, make up to 1000 ml. with water.

(3) Counterstain—Neutral red solution:

Neutral red	1 g.
1 per cent. acetic acid	2 ml.
Distilled water	1000 ml.

Procedure for films

These are made, dried and fixed in the usual way.

(1) Cover the slide with methyl violet solution and allow to act for about 30 sec.

(2) Pour off stain and, holding the slide at an angle downwards, pour on the iodine solution so that it washes away the methyl violet. Cover the slide with fresh iodine and allow to act for about 30 sec.

[1] Iodine solution does not keep well and it is convenient, especially where stains are distributed from a central source, to have potassium iodide and iodine mixed ready for solution when required. Potassium iodide tends to be hygroscopic and must be dried, otherwise the mixture becomes sticky and lumpy. Place the potassium iodide in a thin layer in a Petri dish overnight in a desiccator over calcium chloride. Mix two parts of potassium iodide by weight with one part of iodine in a mortar. Weigh out at once amounts of 7·5 grams and place them in 1-oz. screw-capped bottles (p. 725) and screw down the caps. This is sufficient for 250 ml. of solution. The mixture keeps indefinitely and easily "pours" from the bottle. For use, place the contents of one bottle into an empty 10-oz. screw-capped bottle. Add about 50 ml. distilled water and agitate until the iodine is dissolved. Make up to 250 ml. with distilled water.

(3) Wash off the iodine with absolute alcohol (ethanol) and treat with fresh alcohol, tilting the slide from side to side until colour ceases to come out of the preparation. This is easily seen by holding the slide against a white background.

(4) Wash with water.

(5) Apply the counterstain for 1–2 min.

(6) Wash with water and dry between blotting paper.

This method is very simple and gives excellent results with freedom from deposit. Safranine, 0·5 per cent. in distilled water, may be substituted for neutral red as counterstain. Basic fuchsin, 0·05 per cent., may be used for up to 30 sec., but dilute carbol fuchsin should not be used because it tends to stain Gram-negative bacteria so intensely that they may appear Gram-positive.

For the gonococcus and meningococcus in films, *Sandiford's counterstain* is useful, particularly when the organisms are scanty.

Malachite green	0·05 g.
Pyronine	0·15 g.
Distilled water	to 100 ml.

(The stain keeps for about a month only.) Apply the counterstain for 2 min., flood off with water (but do not wash) and blot. Cells and nuclei stain bluish green. Gram-positive organisms are purple-black and gonococci red. It should be noted that not all samples of pyronine are satisfactory for this stain, so that with each new purchase of pyronine the made-up stain should be tested on a film known to contain gonococci or meningococci.

WEIGERT'S MODIFICATION OF GRAM'S METHOD

(Decolourisation with aniline-xylol)

Solutions required

(1) Carbol gentian violet.

Saturated alcoholic solution of gentian violet	1 part
5 per cent. solution of phenol in distilled water	10 parts

(This mixture should be made up each day, as it tends to precipitate.)

(2) Gram's (Lugol's) iodine.

Iodine	1 g.
Potassium iodide	2 g.
Distilled water	300 ml.

(3) Aniline-xylol.

Aniline	2 parts
Xylol	1 part

(4) Dilute carbol fuchsin.

Ziehl-Neelsen's carbol fuchsin (p. 654)	1 part
Distilled water	9 parts

(5) Carmalum solution.

Carminic acid	1 g.
Potassium alum	10 g.
Distilled water	200 ml.

Dissolve with gentle heat; filter and add 1 ml. formalin as preservative.

Procedure for films

These are made, dried and fixed in the usual manner.

(1) Stain with carbol gentian violet for 2–3 min.

(2) Pour off stain, replace with Gram's iodine solution and allow to act for 1 min.

(3) Dry thoroughly by blotting.

(4) Decolourise with aniline-xylol, using several changes until the stain ceases to be removed.

Now examine at this stage under the low power of the microscope; the nuclei of the pus cells should be of a pale-violet colour; if the nuclei are deeply stained, then decolourisation is incomplete.

(5) Wash with several changes of xylol and dry.

(6) Counterstain with dilute carbol fuchsin for 10–25 sec. Wash with water and dry.

Procedure for sections

Weigert's modification is specially recommended for the staining of sections.

After removing the paraffin with xylol or benzol, treating with alcohol and washing with water, counterstain first with carmalum for 10 min. and then proceed as above. After (5) the sections will be cleared and can at once be mounted in Canada balsam or DPX.

CLAUDIUS'S (1897) MODIFICATION OF GRAM'S METHOD

(Counterstaining with picric acid)

This method, which gives very pale, "transparent" counterstaining, is recommended for the demonstration of fungi in tissue sections.

(1) Stain with 1 per cent. aqueous methyl violet for 1–2 min.

(2) Wash in water.

(3) Flood slide with a half-saturated watery solution of picric acid (*i.e.* 0·6 per cent.). Cover slide with fresh picric acid and allow to act for 1–2 min.

(4) Remove excess picric acid solution with blotting paper.

(5) Decolourise with chloroform (or, preferably, aniline containing 0·1 per cent. picric acid) until no more violet comes away in the decolouriser.

(6) Rinse with xylol and mount in Canada balsam.

PRESTON AND MORRELL'S (1962) MODIFICATION OF GRAM'S METHOD

(Decolourisation with iodine-acetone)

This method is recommended as giving reliable results without the need for taking great care in adjusting the duration of decolourisation.

Solutions required

(1) Ammonium oxalate-crystal violet.

Crystal violet	20 g.
Methylated spirit (64 O.P.)	200 ml.
Ammonium oxalate, 1 per cent. in water . . .	800 ml.

(2) Iodine solution

Iodine	10 g.
Potassium iodide	20 g.
Distilled water	1000 ml.

(3) Liquor iodi fortis (BP)

Iodine	10 g.
Potassium iodide	6 g.
Methylated spirit (74 O.P.)	90 ml.
Distilled water	10 ml.

(4) Iodine-acetone.

Liquor iodi fortis	35 ml.
Acetone	965 ml.

(5) Dilute carbol fuchsin.

Ziehl-Neelsen's (strong) carbol fuchsin (p. 654) .	50 ml.
Distilled water	950 ml.

Procedure for films

(1) Cover slide with ammonium oxalate-crystal violet and allow to act for about 30 sec.

(2) Pour off and wash freely with iodine solution. Cover with fresh iodine solution and allow to act for about 30 sec.

(3) Pour off iodine solution and wash freely with iodine-acetone. Cover with fresh iodine-acetone and allow to act for about 30 sec.

(4) Wash thoroughly with water.

(5) Counterstain with dilute carbol fuchsin for about 30 sec.

(6) Wash with water, blot and dry.

It is essential that the whole slide is flooded with each reagent in turn, and that the previous reagent is thoroughly removed at each step.

STAINING OF TUBERCLE AND OTHER ACID-FAST BACILLI

ZIEHL-NEELSEN METHOD

This method is a modification of Ehrlich's (1882) original method for the differential staining of acid-fast bacilli with aniline-gentian violet followed by strong nitric acid. It incorporates improvements suggested, successively, by Ziehl and Neelsen, and is described in a footnote in a paper by Johne (1885).

The ordinary aniline dye solutions do not readily penetrate the substance of the tubercle bacillus and are therefore unsuitable for staining it. However, by the use of a powerful staining solution that contains phenol, and the application of heat, the dye can be made to penetrate the bacillus. Once stained, the tubercle bacillus will withstand the action of powerful decolourising agents for a considerable time and thus still retains the stain when everything else in the microscopic preparation has been decolourised.

The stain used consists of basic fuchsin, with phenol added. The dye is basic and its combination with a mineral acid produces a compound that is yellowish brown in colour and is readily dissolved out of all structures except acid-fast bacteria. Any strong acid can be used as a decolourising agent, but

20 per cent. sulphuric acid (by volume) is usually employed. Acid-alcohol (p. 655) may also be used.

In order to show structures and cells, including non-acid-fast bacteria, that have been decolourised, and to form a contrast with the red-stained bacilli, the preparation is counterstained with methylene blue or malachite green.

Solutions required

(1) Ziehl-Neelsen's (strong) carbol fuchsin.

Basic fuchsin	10 g.
Absolute alcohol (ethanol)	100 ml.
Solution of phenol (5 per cent. in water) . .	1000 ml.

Dissolve the dye in the alcohol and add to the phenol solution.

An alternative and quicker preparation is as follows:

Basic fuchsin (powder)	5 g.
Phenol (crystalline)	25 g.
Alcohol (95 per cent. or absolute)	50 ml.
Distilled water	500 ml.

Dissolve the fuchsin in the phenol by placing them in a one-litre flask over a boiling waterbath for about 5 min., shaking the contents from time to time. When there is complete solution add the alcohol and mix thoroughly. Then add the distilled water. Filter the mixture before use.

(2) Sulphuric acid, 20 per cent. solution.

Place 800 ml. water in a large flask. Add 200 ml. concentrated sulphuric acid (about 98 per cent.; about 1·835 g. per ml.). The acid should be poured slowly down the side of the flask into the water. The mixture will become hot. Finally, mix gently.

Note.—The acid must be added to the water. It is *dangerous* to add the water to the acid. Great care must be taken to avoid spilling the acid on skin or clothing, or elsewhere. Especial care must be taken to avoid splashing or spurting into the eye. In event of such an accident occurring the eye should at once be washed with an excess of clean water.

(3) Alcohol 95 per cent.

Ethanol 95 ml. plus water to 100 ml.

(4) Counterstain.

Löffler's methylene blue (p. 646).

Procedure for films.

These are made, dried and fixed by flaming in the usual manner.

(1) Cover the slide with filtered carbol fuchsin and heat until steam rises. Allow the preparation to stain for 5 min., heat being applied at intervals to keep the stain hot. The stain must not be allowed to evaporate and dry on the slide; if necessary, pour on more carbol fuchsin to keep the whole slide covered with liquid.

(*Note.*—The slide may be heated with a torch prepared by twisting a *small* piece of cotton wool on to the tip of an inoculating wire and soaking it in methylated spirit before lighting. When steam rises from the slide, remove and extinguish the torch. After about 1 min. re-charge the torch with spirit, re-light it, and again heat the slide until the steam rises. Continue in this way for 5 min.)

(2) Wash with water.

(3) Cover the slide with 20 per cent. sulphuric acid. The red colour of the preparation is changed to yellowish brown. After about a minute in the acid, wash the slide with water, and pour on more acid. Repeat this process several times. The object of the washing is to remove the compound of acid with stain and allow fresh acid to gain access to the preparation. The decolourisation is finished when, after washing, the film is only very faintly pink.

Decolourisation generally requires contact with sulphuric acid for a total time of at least 10 min.

(4) Wash the slide well in water.

(5) Treat with 95 per cent. alcohol for 2 min. This step is optional, and may be omitted; see below.

(6) Wash with water.

(7) Counterstain with Löffler's methylene blue or dilute malachite green for 15–20 sec.

(8) Wash, blot, dry and mount.

Acid-fast bacilli stain bright red, while the tissue cells and other organisms are stained blue or green according to the counterstain used. If tissue cells appear red, the preparation has not been adequately decolourised with sulphuric acid.

Note.—The practice of using staining jars in the Ziehl-Neelsen method is to be condemned, as with a positive sputum, stained tubercle bacilli may become detached and float about in the staining fluid or decolourising agent. After a number of strongly positive films have been passed through the staining jars the number of free stained tubercle bacilli may be considerable. Negative material may, during the staining process, pick up these bacilli and so appear positive when examined microscopically. These false positives can give rise to serious errors of diagnosis. Each slide, therefore, should be stained individually by pouring on the stain from a bottle, the washing done with a stream of tap water and the subsequent decolourising and staining fluids added to the film from bottles. When drying with blotting paper, a fresh clean piece of paper is used for each slide and then discarded. The practice of using a number of large sheets for drying a succession of slides is also condemned as tubercle bacilli from a positive film may adhere to the blotting paper and subsequently be transferred to a negative film.

Use of alcohol for secondary decolourisation.—After primary decolourisation with sulphuric acid, the film may be treated with 95 per cent. alcohol as a secondary decolouriser (step 5, above). The basis of this practice is the fact that tubercle bacilli are alcohol-fast as well as acid-fast. One advantage of using alcohol is that decolourisation is completed more quickly and the margins and underside of the slide are more completely cleaned and freed from deposits of stain.

Another advantage of using alcohol when the staining is being done for identification of tubercle bacilli, is that certain other acid-fast bacilli, which may be encountered in pathological specimens and may otherwise be confused with tubercle bacilli, are decolourised by alcohol. Thus, specimens of urine often contain the smegma bacillus, an acid-fast bacillus that is a harmless commensal inhabitant in the region of the urethral orifice. Some, though not all strains of smegma bacillus are decolourised with alcohol and the use of alcohol thus lessens, though it does not entirely remove the likelihood of confusion arising in the diagnosis of urinary tract tuberculosis.

Acid-alcohol as decolouriser.—Instead of employing 20 per cent. sulphuric acid as a decolourising agent, 3 per cent. hydrochloric acid in 95 per cent. alcohol (industrial methylated spirit) may be used (*i.e.* concentrated HCl, 3 ml., and 95 per cent. alcohol, 97 ml.). The necessity for subsequent treatment with alcohol, as in the original method, is obviated. Acid-alcohol is a more expensive reagent than sulphuric acid, but it is much less corrosive and more convenient to make up and employ, while its use definitely excludes organisms that are acid-fast but not alcohol-fast.

Malachite green as counterstain.—Malachite green is also recommended as a counterstain in the Ziehl-Neelsen method. A stock solution of 1 per cent. in distilled water is made, and for use a small quantity is diluted with distilled water in a drop-bottle so that 15–20 seconds' application of the weak stain gives the background a pale green tint. Deep counterstaining must be avoided. The pale green background is pleasant for the eyes, and is required for the method in which a deep blue-green filter is used for the easy recognition of tubercle bacilli.

Procedure for sections

Sections are treated with xylol to remove paraffin, then with alcohol, and finally are washed in water.

(1) Stain with Ziehl-Neelsen's stain as described for films, but heat gently, otherwise the section may become detached from the slide.

(2) Wash with water.

(3) Decolourise with 20 per cent. sulphuric acid or acid-alcohol as for films. The process takes longer owing to the thickness of the section, and care must be exercised in washing to retain the section on the slide.

(4) Wash well with water.

(5) Counterstain with methylene blue or malachite green for ½–1 min.

(6) Wash with water.

(7) Wipe the slide dry all round the section, blot with filter paper or fluffless blotting paper, and treat with a few drops of absolute alcohol. Pour on more absolute alcohol, wipe the slide again and clear in xylol.

(8) Mount in Canada balsam or DPX.

Modification of Ziehl-Neelsen method for staining of leprosy bacilli

Leprosy bacilli are also acid-fast, but usually to a lesser degree than the tubercle bacillus. They are stained in films or sections in the same way as the tubercle bacillus, except that 5 per cent. sulphuric acid is used for decolourisation.

STAINING OF DIPHTHERIA BACILLUS AND VOLUTIN-CONTAINING ORGANISMS

The diphtheria bacillus gives its characteristic volutin-staining reactions best in a young culture (18–24 hr.) on a blood or serum medium.

ALBERT'S METHOD

Laybourn's (1924) modification, in which malachite green is substituted for methyl green, is given here instead of the original method. It is recommended for routine use.

Albert's stain

Toluidine blue	1·5 g.
Malachite green	2·0 g.
Glacial acetic acid	10 ml.
Alcohol (95 per cent. ethanol)	20 ml.
Distilled water	1000 ml.

Dissolve the dyes in the alcohol and add to the water and acetic acid. Allow to stand for one day and then filter.

Albert's iodine

Iodine	6 g.
Potassium iodide	9 g.
Distilled water	900 ml.

Note.—The iodine solution used in Jensen's modification of Gram's method (p. 650) works equally well.

Procedure

(1) Make film, dry in air, and fix by heat.
(2) Cover slide with Albert's stain and allow to act for 3–5 min.
(3) Wash in water and blot dry.
(4) Cover slide with Albert's iodine and allow to act for 1 min.
(5) Wash and blot dry.

By this method the granules stain bluish black, the protoplasm green and other organisms mostly light green.

NEISSER'S METHOD (Modified)

The following modification of Neisser's method gives better results than the original:

Neisser's methylene blue stain.

Methylene blue	1 g.
Ethyl alcohol (95 per cent.)	50 ml.
Glacial acetic acid	50 ml.
Distilled water	1000 ml.

Procedure

(1) Stain with Neisser's methylene blue for 3 min.

(2) Wash off with dilute iodine solution (iodine solution of Kopeloff and Beerman's modification of Gram's method, p. 648, diluted 1 in 10 with water) and leave some of this solution on the slide for 1 min.

(3) Wash in water.

(4) Counterstain with neutral red solution for 3 min., using the same solution as that employed in Jensen's modification of Gram's method (p. 650).

(5) Wash in water and dry.

By this method the bacilli exhibit deep blue granules and the remainder of the organism assumes a pink colour.

STAINING OF SPORES

If spore-bearing organisms are stained with ordinary dyes, or by Gram's stain, the body of the bacillus is deeply coloured, whereas the spore is unstained and appears as a clear area in the organism. This is the way in which spores are most commonly observed. If desired, however, it is possible by vigorous staining procedures to introduce dye into the substance of the spore. When thus stained, the spore tends to retain the dye after treatment with decolourising agents, and in this respect behaves similarly to the tubercle bacillus (q.v.).

ACID-FAST STAIN FOR SPORES

Films, which must be thin, are made, dried and fixed in the usual manner with the minimum amount of heating.

(1) Stain with Ziehl-Neelsen's carbol fuchsin (p. 654) for 3–5 min., heating the preparation until steam rises.

(2) Wash in water.

(3) Treat with $\frac{1}{4}$ or $\frac{1}{2}$ per cent. sulphuric acid for one to several minutes, the period being determined by trial for each culture. *Alternatively*, excellent results are obtained by decolourising in a 2 per cent. solution of nitric acid in absolute ethyl alcohol; the slide is dipped once rapidly in the solution and immediately washed in water.

(4) Wash with water.

(5) Counterstain with 1 per cent. aqueous methylene blue for 3 min.

(6) Wash in water, blot and dry.

The spores are stained bright red and the protoplasm of the bacilli blue.

It should be noted that the spores of some bacteria are decolourised more readily than those of others and that lipid inclusion granules may stain dark red, appearing like small spherical spores.

Nigrosin method (see also p. 646).—As an alternative to counterstaining with methylene blue in the acid-fast staining method for spores, a drop of 10 per cent. nigrosin solution may be spread thinly over the dried, decolourised film with the edge of another slide. This provides a dark background which outlines the unstained bacillary bodies.

MALACHITE GREEN STAIN FOR SPORES

(Method of Schaeffer and Fulton, modified by Ashby (1938))

Films are dried and fixed with minimal flaming.

(1) Place the slide over a beaker of boiling water, resting it on the rim with the bacterial film uppermost.

(2) When, within several seconds, large droplets have condensed on the underside of the slide, flood it with a 5 per cent. aqueous solution of malachite green and leave to act for 1 min. while the water continues to boil.

(3) Wash in cold water.

(4) Treat with 0·5 per cent. safranine or 0·05 per cent. basic fuchsin for 30 sec.

(5) Wash and dry.

This method colours the spores green and the vegetative bacilli red. Lipid granules are unstained.

STAINING OF CAPSULES

Capsules.—The capsules of bacteria present in animal tissues, blood, serous fluids and pus are often clearly stained when these materials are treated by one of the common stains such as basic fuchsin, polychrome methylene blue, Leishman's stain (p. 665) and Gram's stain (which colours them with the red counterstain). Special capsule stains may be of little advantage in such cases. On the other hand, when artificial cultures of bacteria are being examined, the capsules normally are not coloured by ordinary staining methods and special methods must be employed for their demonstration, *e.g.* "negative" or "relief" staining.

The best method for staining capsules on bacteria from cultures in either liquid or solid media is the wet-film India ink method. Dry-film negative staining methods using India ink, nigrosin or eosin are somewhat less reliable since occasionally shrinkage spaces give the appearance of capsules around bacteria that are non-capsulate and occasionally, especially in thick films, capsules may be shrunken or obscured to the point that they are rendered invisible. Dry film methods in which *positive* staining of capsules is attempted are the least reliable and are not recommended. The advantages and disadvantages of all these different methods are discussed by Duguid (1951).

Loose slime.—Many capsulate and some non-capsulate bacteria secrete extracellularly a viscid material, generally polysaccharide in composition. This may be seen in preparations made by some of the methods used for staining of capsules. The wet-film India ink method and the dry-film eosin method (see below) are recommended for this purpose. The slime appears as irregular masses of amorphous material lying between the bacteria and outside the capsules of capsulate ones.

DEMONSTRATION OF CAPSULES IN WET INDIA INK FILMS

If a permanent preparation is required for demonstration of bacterial capsules, it is necessary that a dry-film method should be employed, as described below; otherwise capsules are best observed in very thin wet films of India ink. This is the simplest, most informative and most generally applicable method of demonstrating capsules. The capsules do not become shrunken, since they are not dried or fixed, and they are clearly apparent even when very narrow.

A microscope slide is carefully wiped free from grit particles. A loopful of India ink is placed on it. A small portion of solid bacterial culture is emulsified in the drop of ink, or else a loopful of a liquid culture is mixed with the ink. A clean coverslip is placed on the ink drop; it is pressed down firmly through a sheet of blotting paper so that the ink film becomes very thin and thus pale in colour. The film should be so thin that the bacterial cell with its capsule is "gripped" between the slide and coverslip, neither being overlaid by ink nor being capable of moving about.

Some practice is required in making satisfactory films. A *large* loopful of ink should be used and a *very small* speck of solid culture material. The latter is rubbed on the slide just beside the drop of ink before mixing it into the ink.

On microscopical examination with the oil-immersion objective the highly refractile outline of the bacterium is seen. Between this refractile surface-membrane and the dark background of ink particles there is a clear space which represents the bacterial capsule; the capsular zone may be from a fraction of a micron to several microns in width. Non-capsulated bacteria do not show this clear zone; the ink particles directly abut the refractile cell wall and, in consequence, these bacteria are not easily seen. When solid bacterial culture is newly mixed with the ink, any *loose slime* in it can be seen as irregular strands and masses, lighter than the ink, which gradually disperse from the bacteria and dissolve in the ink. Loose slime is generally invisible if the preparations are made from cultures in a liquid medium.

Note.—Sometimes a bottle of India ink becomes contaminated with a capsulated saprophytic bacterium. To avoid error from this cause, a film of the ink alone should be examined microscopically and proved to be free from capsulated bacteria.

Use of phase-contrast microscope.—It is recommended that wet India ink films should be examined with a phase-contrast microscope. Since the bodies of the bacteria are not stained in such films their outlines are only faintly visible under the ordinary microscope. With the phase-contrast microscope the bodies of the bacteria appear dark and are seen in clear contrast to the bright capsular zones surrounding them.

DEMONSTRATION OF CAPSULES IN DRY INDIA INK FILMS

(Method of Butt, Bonynge and Joyce (1936))

(1) Place a loopful of 6 per cent. glucose in water at one end of a slide. Add a small amount of bacterial culture to this and mix to form an even suspension. Add a loopful of India ink to the drop, and mix.

(2) Spread the mixture over the slide in a thin film with the edge of a second glass slide. Dry thoroughly by waving in the air.

(3) Fix the film by pouring over it some undiluted Leishman stain or methyl alcohol. Drain off excess at once and dry thoroughly by warming over a flame.

(4) Drop on methyl violet solution as used in Gram's stain, and stain for one or two minutes. Wash in water. Blot and dry over a flame.

(5) Examine directly with the oil-immersion objective.

DEMONSTRATION OF CAPSULES BY RELIEF STAINING WITH EOSIN

(Method of Howie and Kirkpatrick (1934))

Staining solution:

10 per cent. water-soluble eosin, "yellowish" or "bluish", or erythrosin in distilled water	4 parts
Serum (human, rabbit, sheep or ox, heated at 56° C. for thirty minutes)	1 part
Crystal of thymol.	

Allow the mixture to stand at room temperature for several days. Centrifuge and store the supernatant fluid at room temperature; it will keep for several months.

On a slide with a 1-mm. diameter wire loop, mix one drop of exudate (or fluid culture, or a suspension in *broth* from an agar slope culture) with one drop of Ziehl-Neelsen's carbol fuchsin stain diluted 1 : 5, and allow to stain for half a minute. Then add one drop of the eosin solution and leave for about 1 min. Spread a film with cigarette paper or with the edge of another slide as in making a blood film. Allow to dry (do not heat), and examine with the oil-immersion objective.

If intense colouration of the bacterium is not essential, the preliminary staining with dilute carbol fuchsin may be omitted. Films of capsulated organisms prepared by this method show a practically homogeneous red background with an unstained capsular area prominently shown, and the bodies of the organisms stained red of about the same intensity as the background or slightly darker. The capsules are thus seen by "relief staining". If free slime is present in the culture, it is often seen as a light granular or fibrous deposit distributed throughout the red background between the bacilli.

DEMONSTRATION OF FLAGELLA

Because of their extreme thinness, flagella are best demonstrated with the electron microscope; metal-shadowed films or films made with phosphotungstic acid (PTA) for "negative staining" are employed. Flagella can also be demonstrated by the light microscope, using special staining methods which require most careful attention to details of technique. To make possible their resolution, the flagella must be thickened at least ten-fold by a superficial deposition of stain. In spite of this, their characteristic arrangement and wave form are generally distinguishable.

STAINING OF FLAGELLA BY LEIFSON'S METHOD

(Modification used at Microbiology Department, Lister Institute of Preventive Medicine)

The stain, basic fuchsin with tannic acid, is deposited on the bacteria and flagella from an evaporating alcoholic solution. The degree of staining is controlled by an exact determination of the duration of exposure. Good results depend to a large extent on preliminary thorough cleaning and flaming of the glass slides.

(1) Clean the slides with absolute alcohol, rubbing with a fine cotton cloth. Then immerse them in concentrated sulphuric acid saturated with potassium dichromate (p. 864) for several days at room temperature or for an hour at 90° C. (In the latter case it is advisable to place the beaker of solution in a strong metal container with sand while heating.) *During all subsequent stages until staining is complete, take care not to finger the slides, even at their edges, and do not let them touch surfaces not properly cleaned and grease-free.* Using forceps, transfer the slides to cleaned Coplin jars in which they will be kept for rinsing, drying and storing; do not overcrowd. Rinse thoroughly with tap water and finally with distilled water. Allow to drain and dry in air with the jar inverted on clean blotting-paper. Store with the jar closed to prevent contamination by air-borne dust. Just before use, flame the slide for a few seconds, passing it with each face downwards about six times through a blue Bunsen flame. Place on a clean warmed metal rack and allow to cool. Mark or number the slide with a diamond while holding with forceps.

(2) Fix the broth culture, or saline suspension of an agar culture, by adding formalin to give a final formaldehyde concentration of 1–2 per cent. (w/v). Sediment the bacilli by centrifuging at 2000–3000 r.p.m., preferably in a horizontal centrifuge. Decant the supernatant liquid and gently resuspend the bacilli in distilled water by rotating the tube alternately in opposite directions, rolling it between the palms of the hand. Centrifuge again and gently resuspend in fresh distilled water so as to obtain a final suspension which is only slightly cloudy (*e.g.* equal to Brown's opacity standard no. 1, see p. 873). With a flamed platinum loop, place a large loopful of the suspension on the prepared slide and gently spread over an area 1–2 cm. in diameter. Allow to dry in air at room temperature or in an incubator at 37° C. Do not fix film.

(3) The stain is prepared as follows:

Tannic acid	10 g.
Sodium chloride	5 g.
Basic fuchsin	4 g.

Thoroughly mix the powdered ingredients in these proportions and store dry in a stoppered container. Prepare the solution by adding 1·9 g. of the powder mixture to 33 ml. of 95 per cent. ethyl alcohol and, when mostly dissolved (*e.g.* in ten minutes), adding distilled water to make a final volume of 100 ml. Adjust the pH to 5·0 (at least within 0·2) by addition of NaOH or HCl, using a pH meter (p. 850). Store the solution in a stoppered bottle in the refrigerator at 3°–5° C., where it may remain stable for several weeks.

Alternatively, prepare three stock solutions: (1) tannic acid, 3·0 per cent. (w/v) in water with 0·2 per cent. (w/v) phenol as preservative; (2) sodium chloride, 1·5 per cent. (w/v) in water; and (3) basic fuchsin, 1·2 per cent. (w/v) in 95 per cent. ethyl alcohol. (The basic fuchsin must have a pH of 5·0; it may be compounded thus by mixing one part of pararosaniline hydrochloride with three parts of pararosaniline acetate. Allow several hours for solution in the alcohol.) Mix the three solutions in exactly equal proportions to prepare the stain.

(4) Place the prepared slide horizontally on a carefully levelled staining rack. Pipette exactly 1 ml. stain on to the slide so that it covers the whole surface. Leave at room temperature for exactly the required time, using a stop watch. Several similar preparations should be stained for different times, *e.g.* for 6, 8, 10 and 12 min., so that the best may be chosen. The optimal duration of staining will vary with the batch of stain, the room temperature and other factors; the apparent thickness of the flagella increases with the duration of staining. Rinse off the stain gently by placing the slide under a slowly running water tap; do not pour off stain before rinsing. Counterstain with methylene blue, *e.g.* with borax methylene blue (p. 646) for 30 min. to colour the bacterial protoplast. Wash with water, rinse with distilled water, drain, dry in air and examine by oil-immersion.

STAINING OF INTRACELLULAR LIPID WITH SUDAN BLACK

BURDON'S (1946) METHOD

Sudan black stain:

Sudan black B powder	0·3 g.
70 per cent. ethyl alcohol	100 ml.

Shake thoroughly at intervals and stand overnight before use. Keep in a well-stoppered bottle.

Procedure

(1) Make a film, dry in air and fix by flaming.

(2) Cover the entire slide with Sudan black stain and leave at room temperature for 15 min.

(3) Drain off excess stain, blot, and dry in air.

(4) Rinse thoroughly with xylol and again blot dry.

(5) Counterstain lightly by covering with 0·5 per cent. aqueous safranine or dilute carbol fuchsin (p. 646) for 5–10 sec.; rinse with tap water, blot and dry.

Lipid inclusion granules are stained blue-black or blue-grey, while the bacterial cytoplasm is stained light pink.

STAINING OF CELL POLYSACCHARIDES BY THE PERIODIC ACID SCHIFF (PAS) METHOD

HOTCHKISS, 1948

The polysaccharide constituents of bacteria and fungi are oxidised by periodate to form polyaldehydes which yield red-coloured compounds with Schiff's fuchsin-sulphite; the proteins and nucleic acids remain uncoloured. The method may be used to reveal fungal elements in sections of infected animal tissue; the fungi stain red, while the tissue material, except glycogen and mucin, fails to take the stain.

Periodate Solution.—Dissolve 0·8 g. periodic acid in 20 ml. distilled water; add 10 ml. of 0·2 *M* sodium acetate and 70 ml. ethyl alcohol. The solution may be used for several days if protected from undue exposure to light.

Reducing Rinse.—Dissolve 10 g. potassium iodide and 10 g. sodium thiosulphate pentahydrate in 200 ml. distilled water. Add, with stirring, 300 ml. ethyl alcohol, and then 5 ml. of 2 *N* hydrochloric acid. The sulphur which slowly precipitates may be allowed to settle out.

Fuchsin-Sulphite Solution.—Dissolve 2 g. basic fuchsin in 400 ml. boiling water, cool to 50° C. and filter. To the filtrate add 10 ml. of 2 *N* hydrochloric acid and 4 g. potassium metabisulphite. Stopper and leave in a dark cool place overnight. Add 1 g. decolourising charcoal, mix and filter promptly. Add up to 10 ml. or more 2 *N* hydrochloric acid until the mixture when drying in a thin film on glass does not become pink. Preserved in the dark and well stoppered, the stain remains effective for several weeks.

Sulphite Wash.—Add 2 g. potassium metabisulphite and 5 ml. concentrated hydrochloric acid to 500 ml. distilled water. This should be freshly prepared.

Procedure

(1) Dry films in air and fix by flaming. For sections, fix tissue with usual fixatives; bring to 70 per cent. ethyl alcohol and wash thoroughly with this.

(2) Treat with periodate solution for 5 min. at room temperature. Rinse with 70 per cent. alcohol.

(3) Treat with reducing rinse for 5 min. Rinse with 70 per cent. alcohol.

(4) Stain with fuchsin-sulphite for 15–45 min.

(5) Wash twice or thrice with sulphite wash solution. Wash with water.

(6) Counterstain, if desired, with dilute aqueous malachite green (*e.g.* 0·002 g. per 100 ml.).

(7) Wash with water. Dehydrate and mount by the usual methods.

Control sections are prepared similarly, omitting step (2).

Unless easily soluble polysaccharides such as glycogen are to be demonstrated, the method may be simplified by substituting distilled water for the alcohol in the periodate solution and by substituting tap water for rinsing in steps (1)–(3), *e.g.* see below.

MODIFIED PAS STAIN FOR FUNGI IN TISSUE SECTIONS

(1) Bring sections to distilled water.

(2) Treat for 5 min. with a freshly prepared 1 per cent. solution of periodic acid in water.

(3) Wash in running tap water for 15 min. and rinse in distilled water.
(4) Stain with fuchsin-sulphite for 15 min.
(5) Wash twice with sulphite wash solution for 5 min.
(6) Wash in running tap water for 5 min. and rinse in distilled water.
(7) Counterstain with dilute aqueous malachite green or with 0·1 per cent. light green in 90 per cent. alcohol for 1 min.
(8) Dehydrate rapidly in absolute alcohol, clear in benzol and mount in Canada balsam.

IMPRESSION PREPARATIONS

KLIENEBERGER, 1934; BISSET, 1938

These have been used in the morphological study of the pleuropneumonia group of organisms and of "rough" and "smooth" colonies of various bacteria.

The essential part of the technique is to remove a small slab about 2 mm. thick of the solid medium (*e.g.* serum-agar) on which the organism is growing and place it colony downwards on a coverslip. The whole is immersed in fixative, so that the fixing fluid penetrates through the agar to reach the colony. When the bacteria are fixed, the agar is removed carefully from the coverslip which is well washed for two hours in distilled water, suitably stained and mounted. As fixative Bouin's fluid (p. 677) may be used, or Flemming's solution (p. 678). For staining, methylene blue or dilute carbol fuchsin may be employed, but Giemsa's stain, applied by the slow method (p. 668), is the most satisfactory for the pleuropneumonia organism. The agar slabs, after fixation, may also be embedded, and vertical sections of the colony cut with a microtome.

DEMONSTRATION OF NUCLEAR MATERIAL IN BACTERIA

ROBINOW'S (1944, 1949) METHOD

The nuclear bodies of bacteria can be differentiated from the cytoplasm if the cells are first treated with 1 *N* HCl at 60° C. and then stained with Giemsa's solution.

Method

Fixation

Cut a small square from an agar plate on which the organisms are growing in a thin layer and place it in a deep dish (well sealed with a greased glass plate) in which 5 ml. of 2 per cent. osmium tetroxide, wetting three layers of glass balls, produces a strong concentration of osmic vapour. Expose the agar for 2–3 min. in the vapour.

Place the square face downwards on a clean coverslip, remove the agar, dry the film of fixed bacteria deposited on the coverslip and fix in warm alcohol-mercuric-chloride (Schaudinn's fluid, p. 667) for 5 min. Wash in water and store in 70 per cent. alcohol.

(*Note.*—If osmium tetroxide is not available, a simpler method of fixation is to immerse the agar square, bacteria-carrying side uppermost, in a shallow layer of methyl alcohol for 5 min. The agar block is dried in air before pressing on a slide or coverslip for transfer of the bacteria. Secondary fixation in Schaudinn's fluid may be omitted.)

Staining

Transfer films from 70 per cent. alcohol to 1 *N* HCl at 60° C. for 10 min. to "hydrolyse". Rinse in tap water and twice in distilled water and float on a staining solution made with 2–3 drops of Giemsa stain (G. T. Gurr's R66 Giemsa stain) per ml. of phosphate buffer (p. 666). Stain for 30 min. at 37° C., rinse and mount in water, and examine at once. This method shows the chromatic structures quite clearly.

If sealed with wax, water mounted preparations will keep their colour contrast for a few days.

Feulgen staining of deoxyribonucleic acid in the nuclear bodies may be effected by staining with Schiff's fuchsin-sulphite (p. 663) for 1 hr. at 15–20° C. instead of staining with the Giemsa stain in the above method.

To demonstrate the *cell wall*, make impression preparations fixed in Bouin's fluid, as described on p. 663. Mordant for 20–30 min. with 5–10 per cent. tannic acid and stain with 0·02 per cent. crystal violet in water for about 1 min. Mount in water.

THE ROMANOWSKY STAINS

The original Romanowsky stain was made by dissolving in methyl alcohol the compound formed by the interaction of watery solutions of eosin and zinc-free methylene blue. The original stain has now been replaced by various modifications which are easier to use and give better results; these are: Leishman's, Wright's, Jenner's and Giemsa's stains. The peculiar property of the Romanowsky stains is that they impart a reddish-purple colour to the chromatin of malaria and other parasites. This colour is due to a substance which forms when methylene blue is "ripened", either by age, as in polychrome methylene blue, or by heating with sodium carbonate. The latter method is employed in the manufacture of Leishman's and Wright's stains. The ripened methylene blue is mixed with a solution of water-soluble eosin, when a precipitate, due to the combination of these dyes, is formed. The precipitate is washed with distilled water, dried and dissolved in pure methyl alcohol. (The methyl alcohol, i.e. methanol, must be "pure, for analysis", and have a pH of 6·5. If too acid, the reaction must be adjusted by the addition of 0·01 *N* NaOH.) Each modification of the Romanowsky stain varies according to the "ripening" and the relative proportions of methylene blue and eosin.

According to the nature of the microscopic preparation, different stains are employed. Thus, for the cytological examination of blood, Jenner's stain may be used, but Leishman's stain is now generally employed; for the malaria parasite and trypanosomes, Leishman's and Wright's modifications give the best results, while the pathogenic spirochaetes (particularly the *Treponema pallidum* of syphilis) and certain protozoa can be demonstrated best by Giemsa's stain. Wright's stain, which should be purchased ready for use, is applied in the same way as Leishman's.

The Romanowsky stains are usually diluted for staining purposes with distilled water, when a precipitate is formed which is removed by subsequent washing.

LEISHMAN'S STAIN

This stain may be purchased ready for use or made by dissolving 0·15 g. of Leishman's powder in 100 ml. pure methyl alcohol. The powder is ground in a mortar with a little methyl alcohol ("pure for analysis", pH 6·5), the residue of undissolved stain allowed to settle and the fluid decanted into a bottle. The residue in the mortar is treated with more methyl alcohol, and the process is repeated until all the stain goes into solution. The remainder of the methyl alcohol is now added. The stain can be used within an hour or two of making.

Films

Dry unfixed films are used. The stain is first used undiluted, and the methyl alcohol fixes the film. The stain is then diluted with distilled water, and the staining proper carried out.

(1) Pour the undiluted stain on the unfixed film and allow it to act for 1 min.

(2) By means of a pipette and rubber teat add double the volume of distilled water to the slide, mixing the fluids by alternately sucking them up in the pipette and expelling them. Allow the diluted stain to act for 12 min.

(3) Flood the slide gently with distilled water, allowing the preparation to differentiate in the distilled water until the film appears bright pink in colour —usually about 30 sec.

(4) Remove the excess of water with blotting paper and dry in the air.

It is important that the reaction of the distilled water be neither acid nor alkaline. Any slight variations from neutrality may alter considerably the colour of granules in white blood corpuscles, etc., and give rise to supposed "pathological" appearances in cells which are really normal. A simple method of ensuring a suitable reaction of the distilled water is to keep large bottles of it—*e.g.* aspirator bottles—specially for these stains. Add 2 or 3 drops of 1 per cent. aqueous neutral red solution. The usual reaction of distilled water is slightly acid, and a few drops of 1 per cent. sodium carbonate solution should be added until the solution shows the faintest possible suggestion of pink colour.

Much trouble will be eliminated if a buffer solution is used instead of distilled water for diluting the stain and washing the slide. It is made as follows:

Na_2HPO_4 (anhydrous)	5·447 g.
KH_2PO_4	4·752 g.

Mix together in a mortar and keep as such. The buffer mixture is quite stable.

Add 1 g. of buffer mixture to 2 litres of distilled water and this gives a pH of 7·0, which is suitable for most work.

Some samples of stain may require a slightly more acid solution, of pH 6·8. For this mix

Na_2HPO_4 (anhydrous)	4·539 g.
KH_2PO_4	5·940 g.

Add 1 g. of the mixture to 2 litres of distilled water.

Note.—When staining is excessively bluish, as in old films, good differentiation is obtained by brief washing with 1 per cent. NaH_2PO_4.

Shute (1950) maintains that fifteen seconds' fixation with the undiluted stain is sufficient and that only four drops of stain are necessary. The slide is rocked for 12–15 sec. and then eight to twelve drops of water are added and thoroughly mixed. Staining proceeds for 15 min. and the diluted stain is flooded off in 2–3 sec. only. If washed for longer, Schüffner's dots will not be seen. Shute advocates a pH of 7·2 for the diluting fluid.

For demonstrating Schüffner's dots in Benign Tertian Malaria the use of

Giemsa's stain following Leishman's stain has been recommended by Dinscombe (1945).

Fix thin blood film with Leishman's stain for 15–60 sec. Dilute with twice the volume of buffer solution at pH 7·0 and stain for 15 min.

Wash off with dilute Giemsa's stain (*e.g.* G. T. Gurr's R66)—1 drop of stain to 1 ml. buffer solution at pH 7·0—and stain with this for a further 30 min.

Wash with buffer solution.

Blot and dry.

Sections

(1) Treat the section with xylol to remove the paraffin, then with alcohol and finally distilled water.

(2) Drain off the excess of water and stain for 5–10 min. with a mixture of 1 part Leishman's stain and 2 parts of distilled water or buffer solution.

(3) Wash with distilled water.

(4) Differentiate with a weak solution of acetic acid (1 : 1500), controlling the differentiation under the low power of the microscope until the protoplasm of the cells is pink and only the nuclei are blue.

(5) Wash with distilled water or buffer solution.

(6) Blot, dehydrate with a few drops of absolute alcohol, clear in xylol and mount in Canada balsam or preferably DPX mounting medium (p. 645).

Note.—If the eosin tint is too pronounced, it can be lightened by the use of very dilute caustic soda solution (1 in 7000) which is washed off whenever the desired colour has been obtained.

GIEMSA'S STAIN

This consists of a number of compounds made by mixing different proportions of methylene blue and eosin. These have been designated Azur I, Azur II and Azur II-eosin. The preparation can be purchased made up, but batches may vary considerably.

We can recommend the following method of preparation devised by Lillie (1943), which gives consistent and reliable results. It is excellent for staining blood films for malaria parasites, and also mouse or rat blood for trypanosomes.

(1) *Azure B Eosinate.*—Dissolve 10 g. methylene blue in 600 ml. distilled water. Add 6·0 ml. concentrated sulphuric acid. Bring to the boil and add 2·5 g. potassium bichromate dissolved in 25 ml. distilled water. Boil for 20 min. Cool to 10° C. or lower (place in refrigerator overnight). When cold add 21 g. dry sodium bicarbonate slowly with frequent shaking. Then add a 5 per cent. solution of eosin (yellowish) and shake constantly until the margin of the fluid appears pale blue or bluish-pink. About 205 ml. will be required, and 150 ml. of this can be added at once. Filter immediately, preferably on a vacuum funnel with hard paper. When the fluid has been drawn through and the surface begins to crack, add 50 ml. distilled water. Allow to drain, and wash again with a second 50 ml. distilled water. Now wash with 40 ml. alcohol (95 per cent.) and repeat with a second 40 ml. alcohol. Dry the precipitate at room temperature or 37° C. (not higher). This constitutes Azure B eosinate.

(2) *Azure A Eosinate.*—Proceed exactly as above, but use 5·0 g. potassium bichromate (in place of 2·5 g.) and dissolve it in 50 ml. distilled water.

(3) *Methylene Blue Eosinate.*—Dissolve 10 g. methylene blue in 600 ml.

cold distilled water and precipitate as before with 5 per cent. eosin solution, filtering and drying as above.

To make the finished stain, grind the three eosinates separately into fine powder in separate clean mortars. Then weigh out 500 mg. azure B eosinate, 100 mg. azure A eosinate, 400 mg. methylene blue eosinate, and 200 mg. finely ground methylene blue. Decant the mixed powder on to the surface of 200 ml. solvent, allowing it to settle in gradually. Then shake frequently for two or three days, keeping the bottle between 50° and 60° C. between shakings. The solvent consists of equal volumes of methyl alcohol (A.R.) and glycerol (A.R.). The proportion of stains given above should yield a satisfactory staining picture. The diluting fluid is buffer solution pH 7·0 (p. 665).

This stain may be used in a manner somewhat similar to Leishman's preparation (the "rapid method"), or prolonged staining may be carried out, as, for example, in staining spirochaetes (the "slow method"). In both cases the preparation must be fixed prior to staining, either with methyl alcohol (methanol) for 3 min., or with absolute alcohol (ethanol) for 15 min.

Rapid Method

(1) Fix films in methyl alcohol for 3 min.

(2) Stain in a mixture of 1 part stain and 10 parts buffer solution pH 7·0 for 1 hr.

(3) Wash with buffer solution, allowing the preparation to differentiate for about 30 sec.

(4) Blot and allow to dry in the air.

This method of staining gives excellent results with thin blood films for malaria parasites, Shüffner's dots being well defined. Trypanosomes are also well demonstrated.

A rapid method with the application of heat is useful for demonstrating spirochaetes.

Fix preparations with absolute alcohol (15 min.) or by drawing three times through a flame. Prepare a fresh solution of 10 drops of Giemsa's solution with 10 ml. of buffer solution of pH 7·0 (p. 666), shake gently and cover the fixed film with the diluted stain. Warm till steam rises, allow to cool for 15 sec., then pour off and replace with fresh stain and heat again. Repeat the procedure four or five times, wash in distilled water, dry and mount.

Slow Method

This is a specially valuable method for demonstrating objects difficult to stain in the ordinary way, *e.g.* certain pathogenic spirochaetes. The principle is to allow the diluted stain to act for a considerable period. As the mixture of stain and water causes a fine precipitate, care has to be taken that this does not deposit on the film.

Slides.—The film is fixed in methyl alcohol for 3 min. A mixture is made in a Petri dish in the proportion of 1 ml. of stain to 20 ml. of buffer solution, pH 7·0. A piece of thin glass rod is placed in the Petri dish, and the slides, after fixing, are laid film downwards in the fluid with one end of the slide resting on the glass rod so that there is sufficient staining fluid between the film and the bottom of the dish. After staining for 16–24 hr., the slides are washed in a stream of buffer solution, allowed to dry in air and mounted. There should be no deposit of precipitated stain on the preparation.

Adachi's Modification.—This method has been utilised for staining the flagella of *Spirillum minus* (p. 270) and can also be applied in the staining of delicate spirochaetes. Fix the preparation for 30–60 sec. with osmic acid vapour over the following solution: osmic acid 1 g., distilled water 100 ml., 10 drops of 5 per cent. mercuric chloride; and then stain overnight in dilute Giemsa's solution (*vide supra*) to each 10 ml. of which 0·6 ml. of 1 per cent. potassium carbonate has been added.

FIELD'S (1941) RAPID METHOD OF STAINING THICK BLOOD FILMS FOR MALARIA PARASITES

This method can be recommended for routine use.

In preparing the blood films it is important to ensure that they are not too thick. Drying may be assisted by placing the film in the incubator. After the film is quite dry it may be passed very rapidly two or three times through a Bunsen or spirit flame, each passage occupying two to three seconds. When cool the film is ready for staining.

Field's Stain

(Obtainable also in tablet form)

Solution A (methylene blue):

Methylene blue	1·3 g.
Na_2HPO_4 (anhydrous)	5·0 g.
(If Na_2HPO_4, 12 H_2O, is used, 12·6 g.)	

Dissolve in 50 ml. distilled water, bring to the boil and evaporate almost to dryness in a waterbath, then add KH_2PO_4 (anhydrous) 6·25 g. Add 500 ml. of freshly boiled and still warm distilled water, stir until the stain is completely dissolved and set aside for 24 hr. Filter before use. If a scum forms during use, filter again.

Alternatively, if Azur I is available there is no need to carry out the polychroming of the methylene blue as outlined above, and *Solution A* can be made as follows:

Methylene blue	0·8 g.
Azur I	0·5 g.
Na_2HPO_4 (anhydrous)	5·0 g.
(Na_2HPO_4, 12 H_2O, 12·6 g.)	
KH_2PO_4 (anhydrous)	6·25 g.
(KH_2PO_4, 2 H_2O, 8·0 g.)	
Distilled water	500 ml.

The phosphate salts are first dissolved in freshly boiled and still warm distilled water and the stain is then added. Set aside for 24 hr. and filter before use.

Solution B (eosin):

Eosin	1·3 g.
Na_2HPO_4 (anhydrous)	5·0 g.
(Na_2HPO_4, 12 H_2O, 12·6 g.)	
KH_2PO_4 (anhydrous)	6·25 g.
(KH_2PO_4, 2 H_2O, 8·0 g.)	
Distilled water	500 ml.

The phosphate salts are first dissolved in freshly boiled and still warm distilled water, then the stain is added. Set aside for 24 hr. and filter before use.

The stains are kept in covered jars, the level being maintained by the addition of fresh stain as necessary. The same solution may be used continuously for many weeks without apparent deterioration, but the eosin solution should be renewed when it becomes greenish from the slight carry-over of methylene blue (*vide infra*). If solutions show a growth of bacteria or moulds they should be discarded and replaced from stock solutions which, if stored carefully, will remain satisfactory up to a year.

Method of Staining

(1) Dip the slide into the Solution A for 1–2 sec. only.

(2) Remove slide and immediately rinse *gently* in a jar of clean distilled or tap water until the stain ceases to flow from the film and the glass of the slide is free from stain.

(3) Dip the slide into Solution B for 1–2 sec. only.

(4) Rinse *gently* for 2–3 sec. in clean water.

(5) Place *vertically* against a rack to drain and dry.

The relative times may require slight adjustment to suit different batches of stain.

Films up to 3 wk. old may benefit from immersion in phosphate buffer solution (as used for dissolving the stains) until haemoglobin begins to diffuse out. The film is stained in the ordinary way. Unduly thick films should be similarly immersed before staining to remove the greater part of the haemoglobin. The phosphate buffer solution may be used in place of water for rinsing between Solutions A and B.

Another method of staining thick blood films for malaria parasites is that of Simeons (1942).

STAINING OF SPIROCHAETES

FONTANA'S METHOD FOR FILMS

Solutions required:

(*a*) *Fixative*:

Acetic acid	1 ml.
Formalin	2 ml.
Distilled water	100 ml.

(*b*) *Mordant*:

Phenol	1 g.
Tannic acid	5 g.
Distilled water	100 ml.

(*c*) *Ammoniated silver nitrate*:

Add 10 per cent. ammonia to 0·5 per cent. solution of silver nitrate in distilled water until the precipitate formed just dissolves. Now add more silver nitrate solution drop by drop until the precipitate returns and does not redissolve.

(1) Treat the film three times, 30 sec. each time, with the fixative.

(2) Wash off the fixative with absolute alcohol and allow the alcohol to act for 3 min.

(3) Drain off the excess of alcohol and carefully burn off the remainder until the film is dry.

(4) Pour on the mordant, heating till steam rises, and allow it to act for 30 sec.

(5) Wash well in distilled water and again dry the slide.

(6) Treat with ammoniated silver nitrate, heating till steam rises, for 30 sec., when the film becomes brown in colour.

(7) Wash well in distilled water, dry and mount in Canada balsam.

It is essential that the specimen be mounted in balsam under a coverslip before examination, as some immersion oils cause the film to fade at once.

The spirochaetes are stained brownish-black on a brownish-yellow background.

BECKER'S METHOD (MODIFIED)

The fixative and mordant are as in Fontana's method.

Staining solution:

Basic fuchsin (saturated alcoholic solution) . . .	45 ml.
Shunk's mordant B (95 or 100 per cent. ethanol 16 ml. and aniline oil 4 ml.)	18 ml.
Distilled water	100 ml.

Mix the Shunk's mordant with the alcoholic fuchsin and then add the distilled water. (The glassware should be dry.)

Procedure

(1) Filter stain and reagents into jars for use.
(2) Make film and dry in air.
(3) Place in fixative for 1–3 min.
(4) Wash in water for *c.* 30 sec.
(5) Treat with mordant for 3–5 min.
(6) Wash in water for *c.* 30 sec.
(7) Place in staining solution for 3–5 min.
(8) Wash well in water and drain dry.

LEVADITI'S METHOD OF STAINING SPIROCHAETES IN TISSUES

Pyridine Modification

This method is more rapid than the original technique.

(1) Fix the tissue, which must be in small pieces 1 mm. thick, in 10 per cent. formalin for 24 hr.

(2) Wash the tissue for 1 hr. in water and thereafter place it in 96–98 per cent. alcohol for 24 hr.

(3) Place the tissue in a 1 per cent. solution of silver nitrate (to which one-tenth of the volume of pure pyridine has been added) for 2 hr. at room temperature, and thereafter at about 50° C. for 4–6 hr. It is then rapidly washed in 10 per cent. pyridine solution.

(4) Transfer to the reducing fluid, which consists of:

Formalin 4 per cent.	100 parts

to which are added immediately before use:

Acetone (pure)	10 parts
Pyridine (pure)	15 parts

Keep the tissue in this fluid for two days at room temperature in the dark.

(5) After washing well with water, dehydrate the tissue with increasing strengths of alcohol and embed in paraffin (p. 678). Thin sections are cut and mounted in the usual way. After removing the paraffin with xylol the sections are immediately mounted in Canada balsam.

STAINING OF AMOEBAE AND OTHER INTESTINAL PROTOZOA IN FAECES

Iron haematoxylin stain

Fix wet smears in Schaudinn's fluid (p. 677) for 5 min. or longer.

Wash the films in 50 per cent. alcohol and apply Gram's iodine for 2 min. to remove the mercury salt, remove the iodine with alcohol and wash the films in water.

Stain with iron haematoxylin for 10–20 min.

Iron Haematoxylin:

(*a*) Haematoxylin	1 g.
Absolute alcohol	100 ml.
(*b*) Liquor ferri perchlor. 30 per cent.	4 ml.
Concentrated hydrochloric acid	1 ml.
Distilled water	100 ml.

Mix equal parts of (*a*) and (*b*) immediately before using.

After staining, wash films in water, pass through alcohol, clear with xylol and mount in balsam, as in the treatment of tissue sections.

Preparations may be counterstained with van Gieson's stain for 15–30 sec.

Saturated aqueous solution of acid fuchsin	1–3 parts
Saturated aqueous solution of picric acid	100 parts

Dehydrate rapidly with absolute alcohol, clear in xylol and mount in balsam. Fixed wet preparations must be treated in the same manner as sections and never be allowed to become dry.

Dobell's (1942) Method

Fix films as above, and after washing in distilled water, mordant for 10 min. in 2 per cent. watery solution of ammonium molybdate.

Wash in distilled water and stain for 10 min. with 0·2 per cent. haematoxylin solution in water (the haematoxylin should be fresh, not "ripened").

Wash in distilled water and transfer to tap water for about 30 min., *i.e.* until the film assumes a blue colour. Dehydrate with alcohol, clear with xylol and mount in balsam.

STAINING OF FUNGI IN WET MOUNTS WITH LACTOPHENOL BLUE

Staining solution:

Phenol crystals	20 g.
Lactic acid	20 ml.
Glycerol	40 ml.
Distilled water	20 ml.
Cotton blue (or methyl blue)	0·075 g.

Dissolve the phenol crystals in the liquids by gentle warming and then add the dye.

"Needle-mount" Method

(1) Place a drop of the stain on a slide and in this gently tease a fragment of the culture with needles.

(2) Apply a coverslip with little pressure, as far as possible eliminating bubbles. With blotting-paper remove the excess stain exuding at the edges of the coverslip.

(3) After several hours or a day, seal the edges with cellulose lacquer to make a permanent preparation. (*Note.*—Some staining occurs rapidly, but the preparation improves on standing for several hours.)

Staining of slide culture preparations. Slides or coverslips bearing fungus grown ***in situ*** by the slide culture method are mounted undisturbed with a drop of lactophenol blue.

It is an advantage to treat needle-mount and slide culture preparations with 95 per cent. alcohol before applying the lactophenol blue stain; the stain is added while the preparation is still moist with alcohol. This procedure helps to obviate the trapping of bubbles of air in the specimen.

STAINING OF VIRUS INCLUSION AND ELEMENTARY BODIES, AND RICKETTSIAE

INCLUSION BODIES

For intranuclear and cytoplasmic inclusions Giemsa's stain, p. 667, is satisfactory when such forms are of a basophilic nature as in psittacosis. For acidophilic inclusion bodies other stains give more satisfactory results.

Mann's Methyl-Blue Eosin Stain

1 per cent. aqueous solution of methyl blue	35 parts
1 per cent. aqueous solution of eosin	45 parts
Distilled water	100 parts

Fix tissues in Bouin's solution (p. 677) or Zenker's fluid (p. 676), and cut paraffin sections in the usual way. Stain for 12 hr. in the incubator at 37° C. Rinse the section in water, differentiate under the microscope in 70 per cent. alcohol to each ml. of which has been added one drop of saturated aqueous Orange G solution, dehydrate and mount in balsam.

In Ford's modification the sections are stained for 3 hr. at 37° C., treated with 40 per cent. formaldehyde (strong formalin) for 5 sec., washed in water, differentiated and mounted as above. This method is especially useful for staining the Negri bodies in rabies.

ELEMENTARY BODIES

Giemsa's Stain

This has already been described on p. 667, and whilst satisfactory for the elementary bodies of vaccinia and psittacosis, it has been replaced by other methods that are quicker, free from deposit and give more consistent results.

Gutstein's Method

This method is valuable for staining the elementary bodies of the variola-vaccinia group of viruses in smears made from scrapings of skin lesions and elsewhere.

Solution 1.	Methyl violet	1 g.
	Distilled water	100 ml.
Solution 2.	Sodium carbonate	2 g.
	Distilled water	100 ml.

Prepare films of infected material and if much protein is present rinse first in saline and then in distilled water. Fix in methyl alcohol for 20–30 min. Place the slide, film facing downwards, supported on two pieces of capillary tubing in a Petri dish.

Mix equal volumes of solutions 1 and 2, filter, and run the stain under the slide in the Petri dish.

Cover the Petri dish, and incubate at 37° C. for 20–30 min. Remove the slide, rinse in distilled water, and leave to dry in air.

Castaneda's Stain (Bedson's modification)

This method is useful for rickettsiae as well as for virus particles.

Reagents

(1) 1·0 *N* HCl.

(2) *Formaldehyde buffer*.—Add 40 ml. commercial formalin (previously neutralised with 1·0 *N* NaOH in the presence of phenol red) to 960 ml. Sørensen's (Geigy, 1962) *M*/15 phosphate buffer pH 7·2.

(3) *Stock Azur II*.—Dissolve 1 g. Azur II (Gurr) in 100 ml. distilled water. Filter.

(4) *Counterstain*.—Dissolve 0·25 g. safranine in 100 ml. distilled water. Filter.

Procedure

(1) Fix the film in 1·0 *N* HCl for 2 min.

(2) Wash thoroughly with distilled water to remove acid.

(3) Dilute the azure II stock solution 1 in 10 with formaldehyde buffer and use this to stain the smear for 20 min.

(4) Wash thoroughly with distilled water.

(5) Counterstain with 0·25 per cent. safranine for 6–8 sec. (not longer).

(6) Wash in running water, blot and dry.

The rickettsiae remain blue while the protoplasm and nuclei of the cells are red.

Nicholau's Stain

Stain

Isamine blue	1·0 g.
Phenol	3·0 g.
Ethanol	10·0 ml.
Distilled water	100 ml.

This stain keeps indefinitely, does not precipitate and, even in thick films containing much protein, shows clearly defined virus particles.

Procedure

Fix smears with gentle heat or methanol. Cover with stain and heat until the stain steams, but does *not* boil. After 5 min. rinse the smear and blot dry.

Macchiavello's Method for staining Rickettsiae

This method is very suitable for staining rickettsiae in films from tissues.

Make a film in the usual way and dry in air. Warm the slide gently and stain for 4 min. with 0·25 per cent. basic fuchsin (in distilled water) which has been adjusted to pH 7·2–7·4 with alkali and filtered through paper.

Then wash oft the stain rapidly with 0·5 per cent. citric acid and after this with tap water.

Finally, stain with 1 per cent. watery methylene blue for a few seconds.

The rickettsiae are coloured red, tissue cells blue.

FIXATION AND EMBEDDING OF TISSUES; SECTION CUTTING

As the ordinary routine bacteriological investigation of tissues is carried out almost exclusively with paraffin sections, this technique only will be described.

The fixed tissue is embedded in paraffin wax to support it during the cutting of the section, and the section is held together by the wax in the process of transferring it to the slide.

The paraffin wax must completely permeate the tissue, but before it can do so, all water must be removed from the material and replaced by a fluid with which melted paraffin will mix.

Water, therefore, is first removed with several changes of alcohol; the alcohol is replaced by some fluid—such as xylol, benzol, acetone, chloroform —which is a solvent of both alcohol and paraffin wax, and the tissue is finally embedded in melted paraffin.

Before removing the water from the tissue preparatory to embedding, the tissue must be suitably fixed and hardened.

The essentials for obtaining good sections are:

(1) The tissue must be fresh.

(2) It must be properly fixed by using small pieces and employing a large amount of fixing fluid.

(3) The appropriate fixing fluid must be employed for the particular investigation required.

(4) The tissue must not remain too long in the embedding bath.

FIXATIVES

FORMALIN

Formalin is a 38–40 per cent. (weight/volume) solution of formaldehyde (H.CHO) in water containing 10 per cent. methanol to inhibit polymerisation (*i.e.* 38–40 g. H.CHO per 100 ml. solution).

Ten per cent. commercial formalin in normal saline solution is a good fixative for general use. Its advantages are: it is easily prepared, has good penetrating qualities, does not shrink the tissues, and permits considerable latitude in the time during which specimens may be left in it. Moreover, the subsequent handling of the material is much easier in our experience than in the case of mercuric chloride fixatives, such as Zenker's fluid. Formalin fixation is not so good as other methods where fine detail has to be observed, as, for example, in material containing protozoa. For general routine use, however, it is the most convenient and useful of fixatives. Tissue should be cut into thin slices, about 4 mm. thick, and dropped into a large bulk of fixative. The fluid may be changed at the end of 24 hr., and fixation is usually complete in 48 hr. Specimens are then washed in running water for an hour and transferred to 50 per cent. alcohol. In the latter fluid they may be kept for a considerable time without deterioration.

Formalin tends to become acid owing to the formation of formic acid. The strong formalin should be kept neutral by the addition of excess of magnesium carbonate. The clear supernatant fluid is decanted off when formalin dilutions are required.

ZENKER'S FLUID

Mercuric chloride	50 g.
Potassium bichromate	25 g.
Sodium sulphate	10 g.
Water	1000 ml.

Immediately before use, add 5 ml. of glacial acetic acid per 100 ml. of fluid.

The fluid should be warmed to body temperature and only small pieces of tissue must be placed in it. Fixation is complete in 24 hr., and thereafter the pieces of tissue are washed in running water for 24 hr. to remove the potassium bichromate and mercuric chloride. The tissue is then transferred to 50 per cent. alcohol.

It is essential that all the mercuric chloride should be removed, otherwise a deposit will appear in the sections. The bulk of it is removed by washing. The remainder can be removed with iodine during the dehydration stage in alcohol. The material after washing is transferred to 50 per cent., and later to 70 per cent. alcohol to which sufficient iodine has been added to make the fluid dark brown in colour. (It is convenient to keep a saturated solution of iodine in 90 per cent. alcohol in a drop-bottle, and add a few drops as required.) If the alcohol becomes clear more iodine is added until the fluid remains brown. This indicates that all the mercury salt has been dissolved out by the iodine-alcohol.

Cut sections fixed on slides can also be treated with iodine—*e.g.* Gram's iodine—for 3–5 min., to remove mercuric chloride.

Animal tissues fixed in Zenker's fluid are more difficult to cut, and sections are apt to float off the slide, particularly if fixation has been unduly prolonged.

ZENKER-FORMOL FLUID

This is similar to Zenker's fluid except that the acetic acid is omitted and 5 ml. of formalin are added per 100 ml. immediately before use. It is a useful general fixative for animal tissues.

MERCURIC-CHLORIDE-FORMALIN SOLUTION

Mercuric chloride, saturated aqueous solution	90 ml.
Formalin, commercial	10 ml.

Small portions of tissue must be used and fixation is complete in 1–12 hr. Then transfer to alcohol and iodine as after Zenker's fluid (q.v.). This fluid fixes with the minimum amount of distortion and the finer cytological details of the cells are retained. It is useful when staining virus inclusion bodies.

"SUSA" FIXATIVE (M. Heidenhain)

Mercuric chloride	45 g.
Distilled water	800 ml.
Sodium chloride	5 g.
Trichloracetic acid	20 g.
Acetic acid (glacial)	40 ml.
Formalin (40 per cent. formaldehyde)	200 ml.

This is one of the best fixatives for both normal and pathological tissues. Pieces of tissue not thicker than 1 cm. should be fixed for 3–24 hr., depending on the thickness. The material should be transferred *direct* to 95 per cent. alcohol. Lower grades of alcohol, or water, may cause undue swelling of connective tissue. Add to the alcohol sufficient of a saturated solution of iodine in 95 per cent. alcohol to give a brown colour. If the latter fades, more iodine should be added.

The advantages of "Susa" fixative are rapid and even fixation with little shrinkage of connective tissue. The transference direct to 95 per cent. alcohol shortens the time of dehydration, while tissues thus fixed are easy to cut.

BOUIN'S FLUID

This fixative is useful for the investigation of virus inclusion bodies.

Saturated aqueous solution of picric acid	75 parts
Formalin	25 parts
Glacial acetic acid	5 parts

This solution keeps well. Use thin pieces of tissue not exceeding 10 mm. thick. Fix for 1–12 hr. according to thickness and density of tissue. Wash in 50 per cent. alcohol (not water), then 70 per cent. until the picric acid is removed.

SCHAUDINN'S FLUID

Absolute ethyl alcohol	100 ml.
Saturated aqueous solution of mercuric chloride	200 ml.

This is an important fixative for protozoa. It may be used cold or warmed to 60° C., when it is more quickly penetrating. It is also a suitable fixative for wet films.

FLEMMING'S FLUID

Osmic acid	0·1 g.
Chromic acid	0·2 g.
Glacial acetic acid	0·1 ml.
Water	100 ml.

The osmic and chromic acids, when mixed, will keep for only 3–4 wk. The acetic acid should be added immediately before use.

EMBEDDING AND SECTION CUTTING

After fixation by any of the above-mentioned methods and transference to 50 per cent. alcohol, *small pieces* of tissue are treated as follows:

(1) Place in 90 per cent. alcohol for 2–5 hr.

(2) Transfer to absolute alcohol for 2 hr.

(3) Complete the dehydration in fresh absolute alcohol for 2 hr.

(4) Transfer to a mixture of absolute alcohol and chloroform (equal parts) till tissue sinks, or overnight.

(5) Place in pure chloroform for 6 hr.

(6) Transfer the tissue for 1 hr. to a mixture of equal parts of chloroform and paraffin wax, which is kept melted in the paraffin oven.

(7) Place in pure melted paraffin in the oven at 55° C. for 2 hr., preferably in a vacuum embedding oven.

The tissue is embedded in blocks of paraffin. These are cut out, trimmed with a knife, and sections 5 μ thick are cut by means of a microtome. The sections are flattened on warm water, floated on to slides and allowed to dry. Albuminised slides are useful where the staining process involves heating, and where animal tissue is used, especially after fixation with Zenker's fluid. The slides are coated with albumin either by means of a small piece of chamois leather or by the finger tip. The albumin solution is made by adding three parts of distilled water to one part of egg-white and shaking thoroughly. The mixture is filtered through muslin into a bottle, and a crystal of thymol is added as a preservative. It is usual to coat a number of slides and, after drying, these are stored until required. The albuminised side may be identified by breathing gently on the slide; it is not dimmed by the breath, whereas the plain side is.

For additional details, reference must be made to works on histology.

REFERENCES

Ashby, G. K. (1938). Simplified Schaeffer spore stain. *Science*, **87**, 443.

Bisset, K. A. (1938). The structure of "rough" and "smooth" colonies. *J. Path. Bact.*, **47**, 223.

Burdon, K. L. (1946). Fatty material in bacteria and fungi revealed by staining dried, fixed slide preparations. *J. Bact.*, 52, 665.

Burke, V. (1922). Notes on the gram stain with description of a new method. *J. Bact.*, **7**, 159.

Butt, E. M., Bonynge, C. W. & Joyce, R. L. (1936). The demonstration of capsules about haemolytic streptococci with India ink or azo blue. *J. infect. Dis.*, **58**, 5.

Claudius, M. (1897). Méthode de coloration a la fois simple et contrastante des microbes. *Ann. Inst. Pasteur*, **77**, 332.

DINSCOMBE, G. (1945). The demonstration of Schüffner's dots in benign tertian malaria. *Brit. med. J.*, **1**, 298.

DOBELL, C. (1942). Some new methods for studying intestinal amoebae and other protozoa. *Parasitology*, **34**, 109.

DUGUID, J. P. (1951). The demonstration of bacterial capsules and slime. *J. Path. Bact.*, **63**, 673.

EHRLICH, P. (1882). Aus dem Verein für innere medizin zu Berlin. *Dtsch. med. Wsch.*, **8**, 269.

FIELD, J. W. (1941). Further notes on a method of staining malarial parasites in thick blood films. *Trans. roy. Soc. Trop. Med. Hyg.*, **35**, 35.

GEIGY (1962). *Documenta Geigy Scientific Tables*, 6th ed. p. 314. Ed. K. Diem. Manchester: Geigypharmaceuticals.

GRAM, C. (1884). Ueber die isolirte Färbung der Schizomyceten in Schnitt-und Trockenpräparaten. *Fortschritte der Medicin*, **2**, 185. See "The differential staining of Schizomycetes in tissue sections and in dried preparations" p. 215 in *Milestones in Microbiology* ed. T. D. Brock (1961). London: Prentice-Hall.

HOTCHKISS, R. D. (1948). A microchemical reaction resulting in the staining of polysaccharide structures in fixed tissue preparations. *Archiv. Biochem.*, **16**, 131.

HOWIE, J. W. & KIRKPATRICK, J. (1934). Observations on bacterial capsules as demonstrated by a simple method. *J. Path. Bact.*, **39**, 165.

JOHNE, A. (1885). Einzweiffelöser Fall von congenitaler Tuberkulose. *Fortschr. Med.*, **3**, 198 (footnote p. 200).

KIRKPATRICK, J. & LENDRUM, A. C. (1939). A mounting medium for microscopical preparations giving good preservation of colour. *J. Path. Bact.*, **49**, 592.

KIRKPATRICK, J. & LENDRUM, A. C. (1941). Further observations on the use of synthetic resin as a substitute for Canada balsam. Precipitation of paraffin wax in the medium and an improved plasticiser. *J. Path. Bact.*, **53**, 441.

KLIENEBERGER, E. (1934). The colonial development of the organisms of pleuropneumonia and agalactia on serum agar and variations in the morphology under different conditions of growth. *J. Path. Bact.*, **39**, 409.

KOPELOFF, N. & BEERMAN, P. (1922). Modified Gram stains. *J. Infect. Dis.*, **31**, 480.

LAYBOURN, R. L. (1924). A modification of Albert's stain for the diphtheria bacillus. *J. Amer. med. Assoc.*, **83**, 121.

LILLIE, R. D. (1943). Giemsa stain of quite constant composition and performance, made in the laboratory from eosin and methylene blue. *U.S. Publ. Health Rep.*, **58**, 449.

PRESTON, N. W. & MORRELL, A. (1962). Reproducible results with the Gram stain. *J. Path. Bact.*, **84**, 241.

ROBINOW, C. F. (1944). Cytological observations on *Bact. coli*, *Proteus vulgaris*, and various aerobic spore-forming bacteria with special reference to the nuclear structures. *J. Hyg.* (*Lond.*), **43**, 413.

ROBINOW, C. F. (1949). In *The Bacterial Cell*, by R. J. Dubos, Cambridge, Mass., Harvard Univ. Press, Addendum.

SHUTE, P. G. (1950). Thin and thick films showing malarial parasites on the same slide and in the same microscope field. *Trans. roy. Soc. trop. Med. Hyg.*, **43**, 364.

SIMEONS, A. T. W. (1942). Economy and simplification in staining blood slides. *Indian Med. Gaz.* **77**, 725.

CHAPTER 46

STERILISATION

STERILISATION is the freeing of an article from all living organisms, including bacteria and their spores. The sterilisation of culture media, containers and instruments is essential in bacteriological work for the isolation and maintenance of pure cultures. In surgery and medicine, the sterilisation of instruments, drugs and other supplies is important for the prevention of infection.

Sterilisation can be effected in a variety of ways which can be conveniently categorised as follows.

I. PHYSICAL METHODS.
- (a) *Heat.*
  - (1) Dry heat (including infra-red radiation).
  - (2) Moist heat.
- (b) *Radiation.*
  - (1) Ultra-violet radiation.
  - (2) Ionising radiation.
- (c) *Filtration.*

II. CHEMICAL METHODS.

Heat is most often employed, since it is generally the simplest and most reliable means of sterilisation. Bacteria-stopping filters are used to sterilise liquids that would be spoiled by heat, *e.g.* blood serum, antibiotic solutions, and in which contamination by filter-passing viruses is improbable or unimportant. Chemical agents are generally less reliable than heat; they are used mainly for disinfecting the skin, floors, furniture and other articles that cannot be heated effectively without damage.

Once articles have been rendered sterile they must be protected from contact with unsterile objects and from exposure to airborne dust or else they will become recontaminated. To ensure maintenance of sterility, articles are usually enclosed in a dust-proof container or wrapping before being sterilised. Subsequently they remain protected by it until required for use.

STERILISATION BY HEAT

Heat can be applied in two forms: (1) dry heat and (2) moist heat. Moist heat is more effective than dry heat, sterilising at lower temperatures in a given time and in shorter times at the same temperature. Moist heat kills microorganisms probably by coagulating and denaturing their enzymes and structural proteins, a process in which water participates. *Sterilisation,* i.e. *killing of the most resistant spores, generally requires moist heat at* 121° C. *for* 15–30 *minutes.* Culture media, since they contain water, must be sterilised by moist heat. Dry heat is believed to kill microorganisms by promoting a destructive oxidation of essential cell constituents. *Killing of the most resistant spores by dry heat requires a temperature of about* 160° *C. for* 60 *minutes.* This high temperature causes slight charring of paper, cotton and other organic materials. Dry heat is employed mainly for glassware, syringes, metal instruments and paper-wrapped goods which are not spoiled by the high temperature and are required dry. It is also used for anhydrous fats, oils and powders which are impermeable to moisture and thus are incapable of sterilisation by moist heat.

Factors Influencing Sterilisation by Heat

The factors to be considered are the temperature and time of exposure, the number of vegetative microorganisms and spores present, the species, strain and spore-forming ability of the microorganisms and the nature of the material that contains the microorganisms.

(1) The *temperature* and *time* required for killing are inversely related, shorter times sufficing at higher temperatures. Thus, the minimal moist-heat sterilising times for the most resistant kind of spores known (those of a thermophilic *Bacillus* species) were found in tests of corn juice at pH 6·0 containing 200,000 spores per ml. to be: 22 hr. at 100° C., 11½ hr. at 105° C., 3¾ hr. at 110° C., 84 min. at 115° C., 23 min. at 120° C., 8 min. at 125° C., 3½ min. at 130° C. and 1½ min. at 135° C. Published findings on resistant spores show many discrepancies, but their collation suggests that in practice the following may be taken as equivalent minimal sterilising exposures:

Moist Heat		Dry Heat	
Temperature	Sterilising Time	Temperature	Sterilising Time
100° C.	20 hours	120° C.	8 hours
110° C.	2½ hours	140° C.	2½ hours
115° C.	45 minutes	160° C.	1 hour
121° C.	15 minutes	170° C.	40 minutes
126° C.	6 minutes	180° C.	20 minutes
134° C.	2 minutes		
150° C.	instantaneous		

For surgical and bacteriological sterilisation, most authorities consider that a 10–12 minute exposure of the organisms to moist heat at 121° C. is generally sufficient. This ensures killing of all pathogenic sporing organisms and all saprophytes except for some strict thermophiles which cannot grow at less than 40° C., and so cause no trouble in media stored and used at lower temperatures (*e.g.* incubated at 37° C.).

The minimal sterilising times just recommended are the times for which the microbes themselves are held at the appropriate temperature, *and do not include heating-up time.* When an article is being sterilised by exposure in hot air, hot water or steam, the total duration of the exposure must include time for the article to become heated up to the sterilising temperature, in addition to the recommended minimal sterilising time at that temperature. The amount of time to be allowed for heating up (or *heat-penetration time*) will be discussed later for the individual methods.

(2) The *number of microorganisms and spores* affects the rapidity of sterilisation. The susceptibility and duration of survival on heating varies considerably among the individual cells, even in a pure culture. The number of survivors diminishes exponentially with the duration of heating, and the time for complete sterilisation increases with the number initially present. Thus, when an exposure of 23 min. at 120° C. was required to sterilise a suspension of 200,000 spores per ml. only 17 min. was required for one of 2000 spores per ml. In practice it is advantageous to minimise bacterial contamination by cleansing procedures before applying heat for the purpose of sterilisation.

(3) The *species*, *strain* and *spore-forming ability* of the microbe greatly affect its susceptibility to heat. The amount of heat required to kill a given variety is normally stated in terms of the temperature and time of exposure, either as the *thermal death point*, i.e. the lowest temperature to give complete killing in aqueous suspension within 10 min., or, preferably, as the *thermal death time*, i.e. the shortest time for complete killing at a stated temperature. The tests are made under strictly standardised conditions, *e.g.* with sealed 9 mm. diameter hard glass tubes containing 1–2 ml. of a suspension of 50,000,000 organisms per ml. in a phosphate buffer solution at pH 7·0.

Susceptibility to Moist Heat.—The vegetative forms of most bacteria, yeasts and fungi, and most animal viruses, are killed in 10 min. by a temperature between 50° C. (e.g. *N. gonorrhoeae*) and 65° C. (e.g. *Staph. aureus*). Extreme susceptibility is shown by *Tr. pallidum* which is killed in 10 min. at about 43° C., and extreme resistance by thermophilic saprophytic bacilli, e.g. *B. stearothermophilus*, whose vegetative forms can grow at temperatures of up to nearly 80° C. A few animal viruses are more resistant than the majority: that of poliomyelitis may require heating at 75° C. for 30 min. and that of homologous serum hepatitis, when in serum, at 60° C. for 10 hr. Many bacteriophages are more resistant than their host bacterium, and it is often possible to kill the latter by heating at 60° C. for 15–30 min. without affecting the phage; these phages are killed by temperatures in the range 65°–80° C.

The spore forms of actinomycetes, yeasts and fungi are more resistant than the vegetative forms, though not as highly resistant as bacterial spores. The more susceptible kinds are killed at 70° C. in 5 min. and the more resistant at 80°–90° C. in 30 min.

The spores of bacterial species are killed by moist heat in 10 min. at temperatures mainly in the range 100°–121° C. Their resistance may vary considerably between different strains of the same species. Thus, spores of most strains of *Cl. tetani* and *Cl. welchii* are killed by boiling at 100° C. for 10 min., but exceptional strains of either species may resist boiling for 1–3 hr. Such strains of *Cl. tetani* are the most resistant pathogens capable of infecting wounds and their degree of resistance thus determines the minimum standards for surgical sterilisation: *i.e.* 121° C. for 12 min. or 115° C. for 30 min., exclusive of heating-up time. *Cl. botulinum*, the cause of botulism food-poisoning, forms spores that at pH 7·0 may resist boiling at 100° C. for up to 8 hr. and autoclaving at 115° C. for 10–40 min.; these limits determine the standards of heat processing employed in the preservation of non-acid canned foods.

Susceptibility to Dry Heat.—For vegetative bacteria, dry heat at 100° C. for 60 min. is required to kill strains that would succumb to moist heat at 60° C. in 30 min. Fungal spores are killed in hot air at 115° C. within 60 min., and bacterial spores at temperatures in the range 120°–160° C.

(4) The ***nature of the material*** in which the organisms are heated may affect the rate of killing. A high content of organic substances generally tends to protect spores and vegetative organisms against the lethal action of heat. Proteins, gelatin, sugars, starch, nucleic acids, fats and oils all act in this way. The effect of fats and oils is greatest with moist heat since they prevent access of moisture to the microbes. The presence of an organic or inorganic disinfectant has the opposite effect and facilitates killing by heat. The pH is important; the heat resistance of spores is greatest in neutral media (pH 7·0) and is diminished with increasing acidity or alkalinity. Thus, spores of *Cl. tetani* whose killing required moist heat at 100° C. for 29 min. at pH 7·2, were killed in only 11 min. at pH 10·2 or pH 4·1. Acidity (*e.g.* pH 4) not only enhances the killing of the spores of *Cl. botulinum* but also inhibits growth and this explains the safety of acid fruits preserved by brief heating at 100° C. The effect of alkali may be put to practical use in the sterilisation of metal instruments; boiling in water containing 2 per cent. sodium carbonate gives as effective killing in 10 min. as boiling in plain water for several hours.

The conditions under which sporulating bacteria are grown may influence the heat resistance of the spores. Thus, spores formed by soil and intestinal bacteria in artificial cultures are sometimes less resistant than those formed in the organism's natural habitat.

METHODS OF STERILISATION BY DRY HEAT

(i) *Red Heat.*—Inoculating wires, points of forceps and searing spatulas are sterilised by holding them in the flame of a Bunsen burner until they are seen to be red hot.

(ii) *Flaming.*—This method is used for sterilising scalpels, needles, the mouths of culture tubes, cotton-wool stoppers, and glass slides and coverslips. It involves passing the article through the Bunsen flame without allowing it to become red hot. When a slide or other glass article is heated sufficiently for sterilisation, it is apt to crack if placed at once on a cold surface. Needles, scalpels and basins are sometimes treated by immersing them in methylated spirit and burning off the spirit, but this does not produce a sufficiently high temperature for sterilisation.

(iii) *Hot-Air Oven.*—This is the main means of sterilisation by dry heat. The oven is usually heated by electricity and has a thermostat that maintains the chamber air constantly at the chosen temperature. Preferably, it should have a fan or turbo-blower to assist the circulation of air and so ensure rapid, uniform heating of the load (Darmady & Brock, 1954). Exposure at a temperature of 160° C. for 1 hr. is generally employed.

This is the best method of sterilising dry glassware such as test-tubes, Petri dishes, flasks, pipettes and instruments such as forceps, scalpels, scissors, throat swabs and assembled *all-glass* syringes. Before sterilisation, test-tubes and flasks should be plugged with cotton-wool stoppers; other glassware, *e.g.* pipettes, may be wrapped in kraft paper. Certain brands of cotton-wool give off volatile substances during sterilisation, that condense on the glass and later may interfere with the growth of sensitive bacteria, *e.g.* pneumococcus. Slip-on metal caps may be substituted for cotton-wool. Although screw-capped bottles themselves will withstand the temperature of the hot-air oven, the ordinary rubber liners or washers in their caps will not, and bottles already capped should therefore be autoclaved unless the liners are made of silicone rubber.

The hot-air oven is also used for sterilising dry materials in sealed containers, and powders, fats, oils and greases (*e.g.* petroleum jelly) that are impermeable to moisture. These materials are penetrated very slowly by heat and must therefore be sterilised in small lots or shallow layers, *e.g.* in packets not exceeding 10 g. and in layers not exceeding 0·5 cm. depth in a Petri dish.

Glassware should be perfectly dry before being placed in the sterilising oven; wet glassware is liable to be cracked and should first be dried in a "drying oven" at about 100° C. The sterilising oven must not be overloaded and spaces must be left for circulation of air through the load. It may be cold or warm when loaded, and is then heated up to the sterilising temperature in the course of 1–2 hr. The *holding period* of 1 hr. at 160° C. is timed as beginning when the thermometer first shows that the oven air has reached 160° C. Finally, the oven is allowed to cool gradually during about 2 hr. before the door is opened, since glassware may be cracked by sudden or uneven cooling.

A holding period of 1 hr. at 160° C. is generally considered sufficient for loads of a kind that will heat up rapidly and reach 160° C. soon after the oven air does so; *e.g.* loosely packed loads of simple glassware and metal instruments, especially if the oven is equipped with a fan. An exposure of 2-2½ hr. at 160° C. is preferable for loads likely to require a longer heating-up time: *e.g.* heavy loads in an oven without a fan, assembled *all-glass* syringes packed in test-tubes and slowly heating materials such as powders, oils and greases. Two hours at 170° C. is sometimes used.

(iv) *Infra-red radiation.*—A recent method of dry heat sterilisation is the use of infra-red radiation. The source employed is an electrically heated element; the infra-red rays are directed on to the object to be sterilised and temperatures of 180° C. can be attained. The application of this method is considered in the section dealing with the sterilisation of syringes. Using a special chamber high temperature (200° C. or more) heating produced by infra-red rays *in vacuo* has been employed as a means of sterilising surgical instruments. Cooling is hastened and oxidation prevented during the cooling period by admitting filtered nitrogen to the chamber.

METHODS OF STERILISATION BY MOIST HEAT

Moist heat can be employed:

(i) at temperatures below 100° C.;
(ii) at a temperature of 100° C. (either in boiling water or in free steam); or
(iii) at temperatures above 100° C. (in saturated steam under increased pressure).

Only the third procedure fully ensures sterilisation and killing of the most highly resistant spores. Killing by moist heat requires contact of the hot water or steam with the microorganisms, and if these are protected from wetting, as by grease or by a sealed impervious container, they will be subject only to the weaker effect of dry heat at the same temperature.

Saturated steam is a more efficient sterilising agent than hot air, partly because it provides the greater lethal action of moist heat and partly because it is quicker in heating up the exposed articles and in penetrating porous materials such as cotton-wool stoppers, paper and cloth wrappers, bundles of surgical linen and the interstices of hollow apparatus. When the steam contacts the cooler surface of the article, it condenses into a small volume of water and liberates its large latent heat to that surface (*e.g.* 1600 ml. steam at 100° C. and atmospheric pressure condenses into 1 ml. water at 100° C. liberating 518 calories of heat). The contraction in volume causes immediate suction of more steam to the same site and the process thus continues rapidly until the article is heated to the temperature of the steam. The condensation water ensures the effective "moist" conditions for killing of the exposed microbes. Pure steam is used and the presence of air avoided, since air hinders penetration by the steam.

Steam sterilisation is especially suitable for culture media and aqueous solutions, since the atmosphere of steam prevents the loss of water by evaporation during heating. To avoid drenching of cotton-wool stoppers in a steamer or autoclave, the stoppers should be covered with kraft paper; thus a wire basket of test-tubes is covered by a single sheet of paper turned down at the edges.

(i) Moist Heat at Temperatures below 100° C.

The best known example of moist heat at a relatively low temperature being used as a "sterilising" agent is in the pasteurisation of milk. The temperature employed is either 63° C. for 30 min. (the "holder" method) or 72° C. for 20 sec. (the "flash" method) and these processes will destroy all the non-spore-forming pathogens such as *Myco. tuberculosis*, *Br. abortus* and various salmonellae that may be found in milk.

The sterilisation of serum or body fluids containing coagulable protein can sometimes be effected by heating for 1 hr. at 56° C. on several successive days. It may be necessary to repeat the heating eight times to ensure complete sterilisation. Care must be taken not to allow the temperature to rise above 59° C., as inspissation may occur. The exposure to 56° C. is best carried out in a waterbath, but a 56° C. oven may be used. This procedure is not always effective if certain resistant types of sporing organisms are present.

Vaccines prepared from cultures of non-sporing bacteria may be sterilised in a special waterbath ("vaccine bath") at a comparatively low temperature, 1 hr. at 60° C. being *usually* sufficient. Higher temperatures may diminish the immunising power of the vaccine.

(ii) Moist Heat at a Temperature of 100° C.

Boiling at 100° C.—A suitable form of boiling bath is the fish-kettle type made of enamel-ware or tinned copper. It should have a removable tray provided with a raised edge to prevent cylindrical instruments from falling off. Boiling at 100° C. for 5–10 min. is sufficient to kill all non-sporing and many, but not all, sporing organisms, *e.g.* not the spores of exceptional *Cl. tetani* strains that may survive boiling for 1–3 hr. The method thus does not ensure sterility, but it has been found satisfactory for certain purposes in bacteriology and medicine where absolute sterility is not essential or better methods are unavailable. It may be used for tubing, pipettes, measuring cylinders, rubber stoppers, instruments such as scalpels, forceps and scissors, and syringes of the metal and glass type that do not stand higher temperatures. If the water supply is "hard", distilled water should be used, otherwise the instruments on removal become covered with a film of calcium salts. Sterilisation may be promoted by the addition of 2 per cent. sodium carbonate to the water.

The instruments and other articles are removed from the boiling water with long-handled forceps which have been stored in 3 per cent. lysol (saponated cresol) solution to a level approaching the finger grips. Before taking into the hand, which should be dry, the newly boiled instrument is held by the forceps for a few moments while it dries by evaporation. If it were taken into the hand while still wet, its working end (*e.g.* scalpel blade or syringe needle) would be liable to contamination with skin bacteria floating down from the fingers in the film of water.

The interior of a test-tube may be sterilised quickly for ordinary purposes by boiling water in it.

Steaming at 100° C.—Pure steam in equilibrium with water boiling at normal atmospheric pressure (760 mm. Hg) has a temperature of 100° C.; at the lower pressures found at high altitudes the temperature is slightly less, *e.g.* 99° C. at 1000 feet, 97° C. at 3000 feet and 95° C. at 5000 feet. Because of its convenience, "steaming" at 100° C. is commonly used for the sterilisation of culture media such as broth and nutrient agar, although it is not as certainly effective as autoclaving. A Koch or Arnold steam steriliser ("steamer") heated by steam, gas or electricity is employed. In its simplest form this is a vertical metal cylinder with a removable conical lid (having a small opening for the escaping steam) and containing water which is boiled by a heater under the cylinder; but various modifications are available. A perforated tray situated above the water bears the articles to be sterilised. The apparatus is inexpensive and simple to operate. Bottles of medium may be introduced or removed while steaming is in progress, but unnecessary opening of the steamer, with the consequent introduction of cool air, should be avoided. Sterilisation may be effected in two ways:

(a) *By a single exposure at* 100° C. *for* 90 *min.*—The spores of some thermophilic and rare mesophilic bacteria can survive this treatment, but in practice it seldom fails to sterilise. The steaming period of 90 min. includes the time required for the tubes and bottles of media to be heated up from room temperature to 100° C. This may be about 15–20 min. for tubes or bottles containing up to 100 ml., 30 min. for bottles of 600 ml. and 45 min. for a flask of 5 litres. For the larger volumes it is advisable to increase the total steaming period by an appropriate amount.

(b) *By intermittent exposure at* 100° C., e.g. *for* 20–45 *min. on each of three successive days.*—The principle of this intermittent method of sterilisation, or "Tyndallisation", is that one exposure suffices to kill the vegetative organisms; between the heatings the spores, being in a favourable nutrient medium, become vegetative forms which are killed during the subsequent heating. The duration of each steaming should be sufficient to heat up the medium to 100° C., *i.e.* 20 min. for lots up to 100 ml. and longer for larger volumes (see (a) above). The method is used for media containing sugars that may be decomposed at higher temperatures, and for gelatin media which after prolonged heating fail to solidify on cooling. Thermophilic, anaerobic and other bacteria whose spores will not germinate in the particular medium and under the conditions of storage between the heatings, may escape being killed.

(iii) Moist Heat at Temperatures above 100° C.

Sterilisation in the Autoclave

Water boils when its vapour pressure equals the pressure of the surrounding atmosphere. This occurs at 100° C. for normal atmospheric pressure (*i.e.* 760 mm. Hg, 14·7 lb. per square inch absolute pressure or 0 lb. per sq. in. "gauge pressure"). Thus, when water is boiled within a closed vessel at increased pressure, the temperature at which it boils, and that of the steam it forms, will rise above 100° C.

This is the principle employed in the autoclave, which therefore provides a means of subjecting articles to moist heat at temperatures higher than 100° C. "Autoclaving" is the most reliable method and the method most widely used for sterilisation of culture media and surgical supplies.

In the autoclave all parts of the load to be sterilised must be permeated by steam. Ideally the steam should be *hot* and not only *saturated* (*i.e.* at the point of condensing to liquid water) but also *dry* (*i.e.* free from particles of liquid water). Only limited deviations from this ideal are allowable (M.R.C. Report 1964). Such dry, saturated steam effects sterilisation by virtue of its high temperature, its wealth of latent heat, the condensate (water) it produces and the contraction in volume that takes place when it condenses. Once the whole of the load has been heated-up to the temperature of the steam there is a minimum holding time at that temperature necessary for sterilisation. The minimum holding times are 2 min. at not less than 134° C. (30 lb. per sq. in. gauge pressure); 12 min. at not less than 121° C. (15 lb. per sq. in. gauge pressure) and 30 min. at not less than 115° C. (10 lb. per sq. in. gauge pressure). A 50 per cent. safety period is usually added to these minimum holding times and they become 3, 18 and 45 min. respectively.

The exact temperature attained depends not only upon the pressure employed but also on whether any air is present with the steam. The temperature of the steam at different pressures, when all, half or none of the original air content has been discharged from the autoclave chamber, is shown below:

Gauge Pressure *i.e.* pressure above atmospheric (lb./sq. in.)	Temperature in Degrees Centigrade		
	Complete air discharge	Half air discharge	No air discharge
0	100	—	—
5	109	94	72
10	115	105	90
15	121	112	100
20	126	118	109
25	130	124	115
30	134	128	121

The Importance of Air Discharge.—All the air must be removed from the autoclave chamber and articles of the load, so that the latter are exposed to pure steam during the period of sterilisation. There are three reasons for this: (1) the admixture of air with steam results in a lower temperature being achieved at the chosen pressure; (2) the air hinders penetration of the steam into the interstices of porous materials, surgical dressings especially, and the narrow openings of containers, syringes, etc.; and (3) the air, being denser than the steam, tends to form a separate and cooler layer in the lower part of the autoclave, and so prevents adequate heating of the articles there (*e.g.* in an autoclave with no air discharge, a temperature of only 70° C. was recorded at the bottom when that at the top was 115° C.).

There is one exception to the necessity for complete air discharge from the load. Hermetically sealed bottles and ampoules of aqueous solutions and culture media are satisfactorily sterilised in spite of the presence of some air within them. The contained water provides the conditions for moist-heat sterilisation, making unnecessary the entry of steam for this purpose, and the contents are heated to the same temperature as the chamber steam, though to a higher pressure, by conduction of heat through the container walls.

The Simple Non-jacketed Laboratory Autoclave

The simplest form of laboratory autoclave, the so-called "pressure-cooker" type (see figure), consists of a vertical or horizontal cylinder of gun-metal or stainless steel in a supporting frame or case. The size may be up to about 18 in. in diameter and 30 in. in length. The lid (or door) is fastened by screw clamps, and is rendered air-tight by means of an asbestos washer. The cylinder contains water up to a certain level (*e.g.* 3½ in. for a vertical autoclave of 19 in. internal height) and this is heated by a gas burner or electric heater below the cylinder. The bottles, tubes, etc., to be sterilised are placed on a perforated tray situated above the water level. The apparatus is furnished on its lid or upper side with a discharge tap for air and steam, a pressure gauge and a safety valve that can be set to blow off at any desired pressure.

Directions for Using the Simple Autoclave.—See that there is sufficient water in the cylinder. Insert material to be sterilised and turn on the heater. Place the lid in position, see that the discharge tap is *open* and then screw down the lid. Adjust the safety valve to the required pressure; in some varieties of autoclave this adjustment has to be determined previously by trial. As steam rises from the boiling water, it mixes with the air in the chamber and carries this out through the discharge tap. *Allow the steam and air mixture to escape freely until all the air has been eliminated from the autoclave.* A means of testing this is to lead a rubber tube from the discharge tap into a pail of cold water. The steam condenses within the water, while the air rises in bubbles to the surface. When the latter cease, the air discharge is seen to be as complete as is possible with this type of autoclave. After some trials it will be known what period of discharge to allow under normal operating conditions.

Now close the discharge tap. The steam pressure rises until it reaches the desired level, *e.g.* 15 lb. per sq. in. for 121° C., when the safety valve opens and allows the excess steam to escape. From exactly this point begin the *holding period*, continuing exposure at 15 lb. pressure for the appropriate time, *i.e.* usually 15 min. for aqueous media in lots up to 100 ml. and longer for the large volumes that heat up more slowly. Then turn off the heater and allow the autoclave to cool until the pressure gauge indicates that the inside is at atmospheric pressure (0 lb. per sq. in.). At once open the discharge tap slowly to allow the air to enter the autoclave. If the tap is opened while the chamber pressure is still high, and the pressure is reduced too rapidly, liquid media will tend to boil violently and spill from their containers. On the other hand, if the tap is not opened until the pressure has fallen much below atmospheric pressure, an excessive amount of water will be evaporated and lost from the media. (When spontaneous cooling is too slow, *e.g.* taking about 1 hr., the discharge tap may be opened very slightly so as to cause a gradual reduction to atmospheric pressure during 15–30 min.).

Deficiencies of the Simple Autoclave.—The simple form of laboratory autoclave is effective when carefully operated, but has several important disadvantages. The method of air discharge is inefficient, especially for a large and heavily loaded chamber, and it is difficult to decide when the discharge is complete. If, as a result, the discharge tap is closed and the holding period begun while there is still some air present in the chamber and load, the temperature produced at 15 lb. pressure will not be as high as 121° C. This failure to achieve the proper temperature is likely to pass undetected, since these simple autoclaves are not furnished with a thermometer showing the temperature in the lowest and coolest part of the chamber. The operation of the autoclave is controlled solely by the pressure gauge and it is very common for such gauges to become inaccurate.

The simple autoclave also lacks means for *drying* the load after sterilisation. This is desirable for apparatus wrapped in paper or cloth, and is essential for surgical linen and dressings. Although dry when put into the autoclave, these articles are moistened by the condensation of the steam. When damp, paper and cloth wrappings, even in several layers, are unable to prevent the entry of contaminating bacteria. ***It is therefore important to avoid placing the sterilised articles in contact with unsterile objects until their wrappings are dry.***

A wide variety of autoclaves are manufactured which incorporate various devices to overcome these and other difficulties, some being specialised for particular purposes. Many autoclaves at present in hospitals and laboratories have been badly designed or wrongly installed, and cannot ensure sterilisation. In recent years there has been a great increase in interest in these problems prompted particularly by the work of Bowie (1955) and Howie and Timbury (1956). In 1957 the Medical Research Council set up a working party to examine the whole question of sterilisation by steam under increased pressure and their report (M.R.C. Report 1964) is very comprehensive. The following description is given of an autoclave suitable for either laboratory or surgical purposes.

Steam-Jacketed Autoclave with Automatic Air and Condensate Discharge

Most are horizontal cylinders (*e.g.* 20 in. diam. by 30 in.) of rustless metal (*e.g.* Monel metal). There is a trend, however, to make the chamber rectangular as bottles and all surgical materials are more conveniently loaded into an autoclave of this shape. At the front is a swing door fastened by bolts and nuts, or preferably by a "capstan head" which operates radial bolts and automatically remains locked while the chamber pressure is raised. A pressure-locked safety door is a valuable guard against the possibility of a dangerous explosion through premature opening by the operator.

The autoclave (see figure) also possesses: (1) a supply of steam from an external source, *e.g.* an independent boiler beside the autoclave or, more usually, the main steam supply of the building; (2) a steam jacket which heats the side walls independently of the presence of steam in the

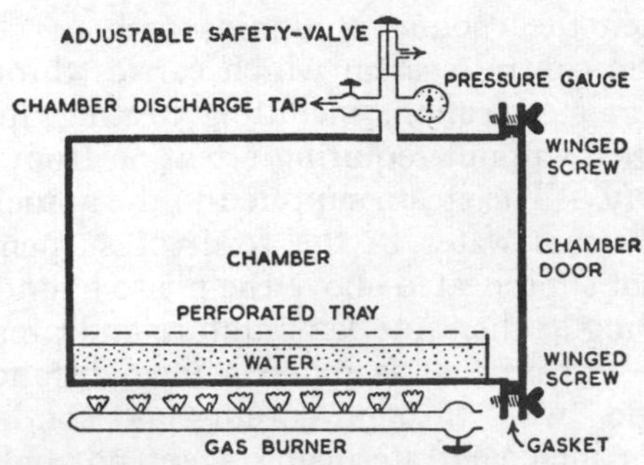

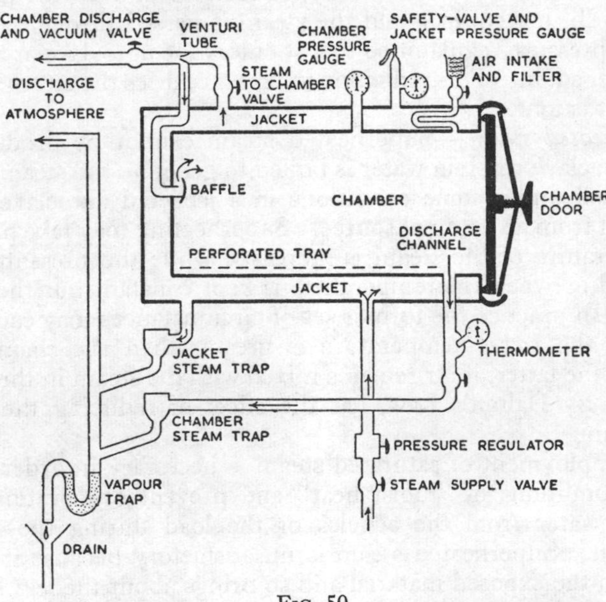

FIG. 50

AUTOCLAVES. *Above:* Simple non-jacketed autoclave. *Below:* Steam-jacketed autoclave with automatic gravity discharge of air and condensate, and system for drying by vacuum and intake of filtered air.

chamber and so facilitates drying of the load; (3) a channel for discharging air and condensate by gravity from the bottom of the chamber, with a "no-return" valve and a thermostatic valve ("steam trap") to control this discharge automatically; (4) a thermometer indicating the temperature in the discharge channel above the steam trap, *i.e.* approximately that of the lowest and coolest part of the chamber; (5) a vacuum system which may be used to assist drying of the load; and (6) an air-intake with a self-sterilising filter for introducing warm sterile air into the chamber. It appears that glass fibre woven into sheet form provides the most reliable filter and that the working life of such a filter is at least one year (M.R.C. Report 1964). It may also have (7) a cooling system to hasten the cooling of liquids without violent boiling, and (8) an automatic control system which carries through exactly a pre-selected cycle of sterilisation, including heating-up, holding, cooling and drying stages, without requiring attention from the operator.

Steam Supply.—The steam supplied to the autoclave should be *dry*, *i.e.* free from excess water in the form of suspended droplets, and *saturated*, *i.e.* not superheated above the phase boundary of equilibrium with water boiling at the same temperature and pressure.

Wet steam.—Steam that is piped a long distance from the boiler tends to become "wet" through cooling and condensation, and such wet steam is an inefficient sterilising agent not only because it soaks porous materials and so hinders further penetration but also because the particles of water possess no latent heat. However, the pressure of the main steam supply should be between 40 and 75 lb. per sq. in. (ideally 55 lb. per sq. in.), and the steam is passed through a reducing valve and pressure regulator so that it enters the autoclave at a pressure of 15 lb. per sq. in. This reduction in pressure dries the steam usually to a sufficient extent.

Superheated steam.—Superheated steam cannot be produced in a simple autoclave wherein water is boiled to generate the steam, but may be produced under some conditions in a jacketed autoclave supplied with steam from an external source. Superheating may take place when the temperature of the steam is increased while the pressure remains unchanged or when the temperature is kept constant but the pressure reduced. In practice the former set of circumstances may cause superheating if the jacket temperature is greater than the chamber temperature; the latter, if air remains mixed with the steam in the chamber since this, by Dalton's Law, has the effect of reducing the pressure of the steam.

The employment of saturated steam is necessary in order to maintain the conditions of "moist heat" and prevent evaporation of condensation water from the articles of the load during the period of sterilisation. Superheated steam is unsatisfactory because it abstracts water from the exposed material and so brings about the less lethal, yet more destructive, conditions of "dry heat".

Starting of Autoclave and Heating of Jacket.—The steam is first introduced into the jacket, a space between the double side-walls of the chamber. The jacket is kept filled with steam at 121° C. throughout the whole day, both during and between the successive steamings in the chamber. Some steam is continually condensing into water on the walls of the jacket and this condensate is drained away through a jacket discharge channel controlled by a thermostatic "jacket steam trap". Care must be taken to ensure that there is no obstruction to this discharge.

Loading of Chamber.—When the jacket is heated, the load is packed into the chamber. Articles requiring different treatment should not be included in the same load, *e.g.* aqueous media in unsealed containers together with wrapped goods requiring drying. The articles should be arranged loosely to allow free circulation of steam and displacement of air. For further details see the section dealing with sterilisation of individual articles.

Heating-up and Air-displacement Period.—The door is closed and steam allowed to enter the chamber through a baffle high up at the back. The steam for the chamber is drawn from the jacket, which thus acts as a reservoir between the chamber and the supply line; the same pressure and therefore temperature, must be maintained in the chamber as in the jacket. The steam tends to float as a layer above the cooler and denser air, and as more is introduced it displaces the air downwards through the articles of the load and out through the chamber discharge channel which leads from the bottom of the chamber near the front. The condensation water formed on the cool load and chamber door also drains through this channel. The channel's thermostatic steam trap remains open while steam mixed with air and condensate passes through it to the drain and atmospheric vent, but as soon as all free air has been eliminated and the arrival of pure steam raises the trap's temperature to 121° C., it automatically closes and prevents further escape. About 5 or 10 min. may be taken for this displacement of air by steam.

Holding Period of Sterilisation.—The holding period at 121° C. is timed as starting when the thermometer in the discharge channel first shows that this temperature is reached. The exact duration of the holding period is decided according to the nature of the load, particularly the time which must be allowed for this to become heated throughout to the temperature of the steam (see pp. 705, 709). During the early part of the holding period some residual air may gradually be displaced from the interior of a porous load; this air together with excess condensate collects in the discharge channel above the steam trap, cools to 120° C. or less, and so causes the trap to open momentarily and allow its escape. (A "near-to-steam" trap is essential, *i.e.* one which opens when the temperature falls by only 1° C. below that of pure steam.)

Since a pressure gauge is liable to become inaccurate, the steam-pressure regulator is ultimately adjusted so as to produce a thermometer reading of 121° C. after the completion of air discharge. This control by the thermometer in the discharge channel ensures that autoclaving is carried out at the correct temperature, and is greatly preferable to control by pressure readings. Any obstruction to the discharge of air and condensate is indicated by the temperature falling below 121° C. while the pressure remains at 15 lb. The discharge channel and trap must be kept clear and the removable strainer in the mouth of the discharge channel should be cleaned daily.

Cooling and Drying Period.—At the end of the holding period the supply of steam to the chamber is stopped, while that to the jacket is maintained. The steam left in the chamber begins to cool by loss of heat through the unjacketed door and its pressure falls accordingly. The management of this stage depends on whether drying of the load is required, as for wrapped apparatus or surgical dressings, or must be avoided, as for aqueous media in loosely stoppered containers. Details of the methods of cooling and drying are given in the section dealing with the sterilisation of these articles in detail.

High Pre-Vacuum Sterilisers

The most advanced surgical sterilisers are equipped with electrically driven pumps capable of exhausting the chamber to an almost perfect vacuum (*e.g.* to an absolute pressure of 20 mm. Hg or below). In effect this means removing more than 98 per cent. of the air initially present (Medical Research Council, 1959, 1964.) A high pre-vacuum is drawn before admission of steam to the chamber and the absence of air then enables the steam very rapidly to penetrate and heat up all parts of the interior of the load. *Even a tightly packed load is heated rapidly and uniformly to the sterilising temperature and this is the only method of sterilisation that can overcome the effects of bad packing or overloading of the steriliser.* This makes it feasible to employ a higher sterilising temperature for a shorter time, namely 134° C. for 3 minutes (*i.e.* jacket and chamber steam at 30 lb. per sq. in. gauge pressure). The total operation time is greatly shortened and damage to heat-sensitive materials through exposure to injurious air-steam mixtures or prolonged heating in the outer parts of the load, is avoided. Note, however, that the operating steam temperature need not always be as high as this. For many purposes a temperature of 121° C.–126° C. held for a longer period is perfectly satisfactory.

The chamber is loaded with as tight packing as desired and the vacuum drawn to remove all air from the chamber and load within 5–10 min. (Automatic control, *vide infra*, obviates the possibility of the evacuation being unduly prolonged, with resultant overdrying and superheating.) Steam is admitted to the chamber and heats the whole load to 134° C. within 2–3 min. The holding period is continued for 3 min. from the time the thermometer first reaches 134° C. The load is then dried within a few minutes by exhaustion of the chamber to a high vacuum with a water-sealed pump, and the vacuum is finally broken by admission of air through a filter. A specification is detailed in British Standard 3970 : Part 1 : 1966.

AUTOCLAVE CONTROLS AND STERILISATION INDICATORS

Automatic Process Control.—It is advantageous for the steriliser to be furnished with an automatic control system that carries through the whole sterilisation cycle, including the heating-up, holding, cooling and drying stages, according to a pre-selected scheme for the duration, temperature and pressure of each stage. After the chamber has been loaded and the process started, no further attention is required until the load is ready for removal. Apart from saving the time of a skilled operator, automatic control is a valuable safeguard against error due to negligence or distraction. A monitoring system ensures that if the temperature at any time falls below that selected, the operation will be repeated.

Recording Thermometer.—This desirable adjunct makes a graphic timed record of the temperature changes in the chamber discharge channel and thus, in the absence of automatic control, helps the operator to avoid errors in timing the holding period.

It has been emphasised (M.R.C. Report 1959) that a daily inspection of such a temperature record by a responsible person is of more value than more elaborate tests carried out at infrequent intervals.

Thermocouple Measurement of Load Temperature.—This is the method of discovering the heating-up time required for a given kind of load. A thermocouple is inserted deeply inside a test article in the autoclave chamber, *e.g.* a bottle of liquid or a pack of dressings, and its wire leads are carried out under the chamber door or through a leak-proof port to a potentiometer. The latter indicates the temperature inside the test article during the course of autoclaving.

These instrumental means of controlling the sterilising cycle in the autoclave are of the greatest value but there are occasions, even with a perfect steriliser, when a test of overall efficiency is desirable. Two methods are available, one using chemical indicators, the other spore indicators.

Chemical Indicators may be placed inside the load. Browne's steriliser control tubes contain a red solution which turns green when heated at 115° C. for 25 min. (type 1) or 15 min. (type 2), or at 160° C. for 60 min. (type 3). They must be stored at less than 20° C. to avoid deterioration and premature colour change. These indicators have the advantage of being readable immediately the test is done and Browne's tubes are generally accepted as being satisfactory.

Adhesive Tape.—The Bowie-Dick autoclave tape test for steam penetration used in conjunction with other tests yields valuable information (M.R.C. Report 1964).

Spore Indicators.—A preparation of dried bacterial spores is placed within the load in the autoclave and after autoclaving is tested for viability.

Bacillus stearothermophilus, a thermophile that requires to be cultivated at 55°–60° C., is a suitable test organism. Its spores are killed at 121° C. in about 12 min. Commercial spore preparations are available. Otherwise a culture grown aerobically on nutrient agar for 5 days is suspended in sterile water to a concentration of 1 million spores per ml. Small strips of filter paper are soaked in the suspension, dried at room temperature and placed in paper envelopes which are then sealed. A few of these packets are placed in different parts of the load and at least two spore papers should be placed at each site since in any spore preparation there may be a few spores of exceptional resistance. After autoclaving, the envelope is cut with sterile scissors and the strip transferred with sterile forceps to a tube or flask of "recovery medium", *e.g.* thioglycollate broth or cooked-meat medium; it is necessary to take rigorous precautions against contamination while making this transfer. The tube is incubated for 7 days at the appropriate temperature and then examined for growth. An unautoclaved spore strip is cultured as a positive control and an uninoculated tube of medium as a negative control. The results should be reported in terms of the degree of heat-resistance of the spore preparation used. This may be determined by holding small sealed tubes of the spore suspension for varying periods in a waterbath at 100° C. or in an oil-bath at higher temperatures, and then testing for viability by culture. Instead of spore strips, envelopes containing about 1 g. of dried earth may be used, since samples of earth almost always contain highly resistant spores. Such samples, however, are variable and less satisfactory; the spores they contain are often too resistant.

Recovery Media.—Bacteria and spores that have been damaged by heat, may require special cultural conditions to allow their recovery and growth. They may lie dormant for several days when placed in a culture medium, and incubation should be continued for at least a week to give them the opportunity of growing. Moreover, certain enriched media may permit their growth when ordinary media fail. Enrichment with yeast extract, starch, glucose, blood or milk has been found beneficial. Thioglycollate broth and cooked-meat medium are suitable for recovery of both aerobic and anaerobic bacteria.

The chemical or spore indicators are placed in the centre of the largest and most densely packed items of the load, and some near the bottom of the chamber where air tends to collect. The results may reveal the failure of some parts of the load to become adequately heated and thus draw attention to a fault in the construction, loading or operation of the steriliser. Successful tests, on the other hand, give no assurance that the steriliser and technique are reliable, since heating might yet be inadequate in other parts of the load or under different conditions of loading. The essential guarantee of sterilisation is that a properly designed and properly loaded autoclave be operated so as to show the correct sterilising temperature on the discharge-channel thermometer for the appropriate time.

STERILISATION BY RADIATION

Ultra-Violet Radiation

The ability of sunlight to kill bacteria is mainly due to the ultra-violet rays that it contains. Visible light at the violet end of the spectrum has a wave-length of 400 mμ (4000 Å, or Ångström units) and ultra-violet radiation is not markedly bactericidal until 330 mμ is reached. Thereafter the effectiveness of ultra-violet light as a sterilising agent increases with decrease in wave-length. The shortest ultra-violet rays in sunlight that reach the earth's surface in quantity have a wave-length of some 290 mμ but even more effective radiations, 240–280 mμ, can be produced by mercury vapour lamps.

In an attempt to reduce post-operative sepsis high intensity ultra-violet radiation has been applied to the operation area but elaborate precautions have to be taken to protect the skin and cornea from the highly irritant rays (Hart, 1942).

Ultra-violet rays from suitably shielded lamps have been used to reduce the number of bacteria in the atmosphere but for safety their intensity has to be restricted (Wells & Wells, 1942). There are, however, a number of reports that "curtains" of more intense ultra-violet light at the entrance to cubicles, through which personnel pass quickly and therefore avoid injury, are of value in reducing cross-infection (McMath & Hussein, 1960). (It should be noted that daylight passing through ordinary window glass has a significant effect in shortening the survival of pathogenic organisms in the dust on the floor and furniture in rooms.)

Ionising Radiation

Ionising radiations include high-speed electrons, X-rays and γ-rays (short X-rays). In adequate dose these radiations are lethal to all cells, bacteria included. Sterilisation by radiation is achieved in practice by the use of either high-speed electrons from a machine such as a linear accelerator or γ-rays from an isotope source such as Cobalt 60. Although available the necessary apparatus is much too expensive for installation in a hospital and it is worthwhile commercially only for the sterilisation of large amounts of pre-packed disposable items that are unable to withstand heat. These include plastic syringes and catheters. Darmady *et al.* (1961) investigated the efficiency of radiation sterilisation using a variety of vegetative and spore-bearing test organisms and found that a dose of 2·5 Mrad was adequate for producing sterility. Spores of *Bacillus pumilus* (E601) were recommended as a suitable test organism.

STERILISATION BY FILTRATION

It is possible to render fluids, including bacterial cultures, free from bacteria by passing them through special filters. The method is especially useful in making preparations of the soluble products of bacterial growth, such as toxins, and in sterilising liquids that would be damaged by heat, such as serum and antibiotic solutions. These filters have pores so small that ordinary bacteria are arrested. The British Pharmaceutical Codex test for bacteria-proof filters requires that efficient filters should be able to retain *Serratia marcescens*. This indicates an average pore diameter of 0·75 μ or less. It is possible to produce some types of filter with a smaller pore diameter and they are able to retain smaller microorganisms including many viruses. In fact, it is possible to estimate the size of viral particles by using filters of different pore diameter although this technique has been largely superseded. In general, however, "sterilising" filters must be regarded as rendering a liquid bacteria-free but *not* virus-free; for many laboratory purposes this is perfectly satisfactory but such fluids, *e.g.* serum "sterilised" by Seitz filtration, must *not* be regarded as safe for clinical use.

TYPES OF FILTER

The various types of filter used in bacteriological work are considered here, but some are clarifying filters and do not remove bacteria.

(1) Earthenware candles, *e.g.* Berkefeld, Chamberland.
(2) Asbestos and asbestos-paper disks, *e.g.* Seitz.
(3) Sintered glass filters.
(4) Cellulose membrane filters.

Berkefeld Filters

These are made from kieselguhr, a fossil diatomaceous earth found in deposits in Germany and other parts of the world. Filters made from this material are coarse—that is, have relatively large pores owing to the size of the granules forming the substance of the filter. They are made in three grades of porosity—namely V (viel) the coarsest, W (wenig) the finest, and N (normal) intermediate. Of these, the Berkefeld V is the one usually employed, and it should not pass a small organism such as *Serratia marcescens*.

A similar type to the Berkefeld is the Mandler filter, manufactured in the United States.

These filters can be sterilised by steaming or autoclaving. After use they should be brushed with a stiff nail-brush and then boiled in distilled water. Before sterilising again, distilled water should be run through them to show that they are pervious. When the pores of earthenware or porcelain filters become clogged with organic matter they should be heated to redness in a muffle furnace and allowed to cool slowly.

Chamberland Filters

These are made of unglazed porcelain and are produced in various grades of porosity. The finer grades will pass only certain viruses of extreme minuteness, such as the viruses of foot-and-mouth disease and of fowl plague. The most porous, L_1, allows many organisms to pass, being merely a clarifying filter. The next three, L_{1a}, L_2 and L_3, are comparable with the Berkefeld V, N and W candles respectively. The porcelain filters may be used for the removal of organisms from fluid cultures in order to obtain the bacterial toxin.

Seitz Filters

This type consists of a disk of an asbestos composition through which the fluid is passed. The disk is inserted into a metal holder that ensures a tight joint being made. After use the asbestos disk is discarded and a new one employed for each filtration. Various sizes for laboratory work are available. The large size of Seitz filter, with

14 cm. diameter disk, can be recommended for the sterilisation of large amounts of serum to be used in the preparation of media. The disks are supplied in three grades—termed clarifying (K), normal and "special EK". The normal and EK grade of disk do not allow the ordinary test bacteria, e.g. *Serr. marcescens*, to pass.

Similar disks are made in Britain, and are as reliable and efficient as the foreign ones. The grade GS corresponds to the EK, and the FCB to the K disks. These are supplied by A. Gallenkamp & Co. Ltd., London, and John C. Carlson, Ltd., Weir Mills, Mossley, Lancs.

The filter is loosely assembled with the asbestos disk in position and the delivery tube passed through a rubber bung when a filtering flask is used. The whole is wrapped in kraft paper and sterilised in the steamer or autoclave. The filtering flask is plugged and fitted with an air filter. When using Seitz filters it is advisable to moisten the disk with sterile saline and then screw down tightly the upper part of the metal on the softened asbestos before pouring in the liquid to be filtered.

Sintered Glass Filters

These are made of finely ground glass fused sufficiently to make the small particles adhere. A special grade for sterilisation purposes is manufactured by supporting a specially fine ("grade 5") filter on a coarser ("grade 3") layer, and is known as the "3/5" type. These filters are attached to the filtering apparatus and sterilised in the same way as the Seitz filter, but care must be taken that extremes of temperature are avoided. After use they are washed with running water in the reverse direction. They should be cleaned with warm sulphuric acid to which has been added a quantity of potassium nitrate, and not with sulphuric-acid-bichromate mixture.

Cellulose Membrane Filters

Two types of cellulose membrane filters are available: the older type (gradocol membranes) are composed of cellulose nitrate whereas the modern membrane filters consist of cellulose acetate.

Gradocol membranes.—Elford (1931) devised a technique for preparing collodion (nitro-cellulose) membranes of graded porosity which he termed *gradocol* membranes, since they are products of graded coagulation of collodion. Collodion films show two types of structure:

(a) *microgel*, which has a coarse structure visible microscopically, and
(b) *ultragel*, the structural elements of which are not resolvable by the microscope, but which is built up of particulate matter. Hitherto, these membranes, although uniform, had not been sufficiently permeable for filtration work.

The *gradocol* membranes possess the permeability of the microgel type, but have the ultragel structure and are very uniform in their porosity. They are made from an acetone solution of collodion diluted with an ethyl-alcohol-ether mixture to which are added varying amounts of amyl alcohol; 75 ml. of the mixture are poured into a shallow cell 20 cm. in diameter in a constant-temperature room (22·5° C.), allowed to evaporate for varying periods of one to three hours, and then washed over an extended period with distilled water. By varying the amount and composition of the collodion mixture, and the conditions of evaporation, permeable filters of average-pore size (APS) ranging from 3 μ down to 10 mμ or less have been prepared. It is possible to reproduce accurately at any time filters of any desired permeability and porosity. The technical details are elaborate and of extreme importance. It is recommended that gradocol membranes are sterilised by steaming. Autoclaving is too drastic since it alters the permeability of the membrane.

By means of these collodion membranes it has been possible to determine the size of many of the viruses.

Modern membrane filters.—These filters were first developed by the Millipore Filter Corporation in America where they are referred to as "millipore" filters. Similar filters made by Courtaulds Limited and marketed by Oxo Limited as "Oxoid" membrane filters have been available in this country since 1955. The filters consist of cellulose acetate and are composed of two layers, a basal layer with pores of 3–5 μ and an upper layer with pores of 0·5–1·0 μ in diameter. This structure gives a remarkable degree of porosity yet ensures that bacteria are trapped on the upper surface. The filters are effective in retaining *Serratia marcescens.* They withstand sterilisation by autoclaving at 121° C. and may be stored indefinitely in a dry condition. They are made in a variety of sizes from 1·7 cm. to 14 cm. and can be fitted into metal or glass holders.

Cellulose membrane filters have several advantages over the widely used Seitz asbestos filters. They are much less adsorptive and the rate of filtration is much greater. Also, bacteria retained on the surface of a membrane filter can be subsequently grown by placing the filter in contact with culture media when, after suitable incubation, visible colonies will develop. This technique, which can be made quantitative, has many varied applications (see p. 974).

Technique of Filtration

As fluids do not readily pass through filters by gravity, it is necessary to use positive or negative pressure. Suction is the most convenient method of filtration, the fluid being drawn through the filter into a sterile container, usually a "filtering flask", which is a conical flask of thick glass with a side-arm. Note, however, that negative pressure is unsuitable for filtering bicarbonate-buffered solutions.

The smallest negative pressure that produces satisfactory filtration should be used, commencing with a small pressure and gradually increasing it. A negative pressure of 100–200 mm. of mercury is usually sufficient.

When using a filter of the Berkefeld type, the earthenware "candle" is fitted by means of a screw and washers into a cylindrical glass mantle, and the metal tube of the filter passes through a rubber stopper which is fitted into the neck of the flask. The side-arm of the flask is connected with an exhaust pump by pressure tubing. The fluid is poured into the mantle and after filtration is collected into the flask. The necessary suction is obtained by the usual form of water pump or by a mechanical air pump. The negative pressure is estimated by means of an attached mercury or other type of manometer.

Similarly, when using other filters the metal tube may be inserted into a rubber bung which fits into a filtering flask.

A disadvantage of the filtering flask is that the filtered fluid has to be transferred later to another container, and where it is desired to store filtered fluids, *e.g.* serum or culture media, contamination may occur in the process. It has also been observed that rubber bungs are not resilient after one autoclaving and do not again fit satisfactorily so that it is necessary to tie the bung to the filter flask and seal the joints with wax.

As an alternative to a filtering flask a simple fitting attached to a screw-capped bottle can be recommended. It consists of a straight piece of metal tubing, 6–7 mm. external diameter, surrounded by a wider piece of tubing to which is fitted a side-arm. The tubes are fitted into a metal screw-cap furnished with a washer to secure an air-tight joint (figure 51). The fitting is made preferably of stainless steel. Any of the screw-capped bottles can be used according to the amount of fluid to be filtered. As several sizes of bottles may fit one size of screw-cap, a few different sizes of cap will cover a range from a few ml. up to 4 litres. The filter employed is connected to the top of the fitting by rubber pressure tubing.

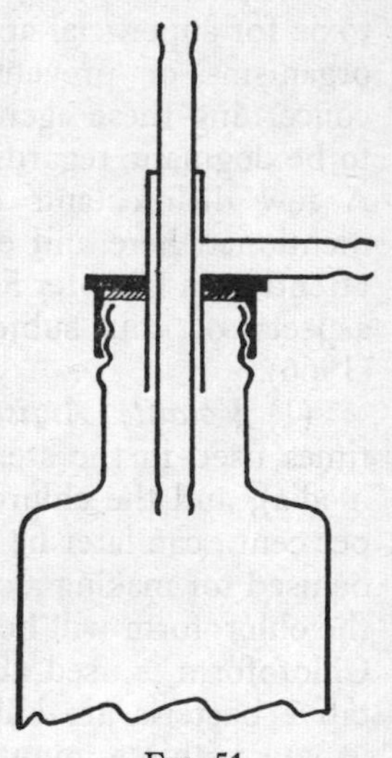

FIG. 51

One of the advantages of the metal screw-cap fitting is that when the filtrate has to be stored, *e.g.* toxin, serum, etc., it need not be removed from the container. An ordinary screw-cap for the bottle is wrapped in kraft paper and sterilised with the remainder of the apparatus. After filtration the filter and screw attachment are removed, the ordinary cap is taken from its sterile wrapper and screwed on. Where the filtrate is to be kept for some time a viskap over the screw-cap is recommended to exclude dust and obviate unauthorised opening.

Filtration of Small Amounts of Fluid

With the smaller sizes of filters, a small test-tube may be arranged inside the filtering flask so that the delivery tube of the filter projects into the open end of the tube and the filtered fluid is collected directly in the small tube instead of the flask itself.

Centrifugal Filter.—A small amount of fluid may be conveniently filtered with a simple filter holder (supplied by H. A. Jones, Beaumaris, Anglesey) carrying a sterile screw-topped ¼-oz. or 1-oz. bottle at either end. The fluid is placed in one bottle and the holder, which is fitted with either a Seitz filter pad (1·8 cm.), or an "Oxoid" membrane filter (1·7 cm.) is screwed on to the top of the bottle. The second bottle is screwed on to the other end of the holder and the assembly then placed in a bucket of a centrifuge so that the empty bottle will be outermost. Filter holders are now available that fit onto the end of a syringe so that the fluid to be sterilised is forced through the membrane by the syringe piston.

CHEMICAL METHODS OF DISINFECTION

Chemical 'sterilising' agents are widely used but few of them have any effect on spores. The terms *disinfectant* and *antiseptic* are generally applied to different types of substances. Disinfectants are potent but toxic preparations which are able to destroy pathogenic microorganisms but not necessarily resistant spores. They are suitable only for application to inanimate objects. Antiseptics are substances sufficiently non-toxic for superficial application to living tissue which either kill micro-organisms or prevent their growth. The mass of available data concerning these agents is often contradictory and it may be difficult to be dogmatic regarding the best preparation for a particular purpose. A few disinfectants and antiseptics with their particular uses are mentioned here and elsewhere in this chapter. They receive further attention in Chapter 53 and for comprehensive treatment of the clinical aspects of this subject the reader is referred to Williams *et al.* (1966).

(1) *Volatile Antiseptics*, e.g. *Chloroform.*—Chloroform is sometimes used in the sterilisation and preservation of serum (for culture media), and the chloroform, which is added in the proportion of 0·25 per cent., can later be removed by heating at 56° C. If the serum is to be used for making a coagulated serum medium (*e.g.* Löffler's medium) the chloroform will be removed by the heating applied for coagulation. Chloroform is used also for preserving culture media in bulk. Vegetative bacteria are killed by exposure to chloroform liquid or strong vapour within a minute or so. Plate cultures of vegetative bacteria are sometimes killed by exposure for a few minutes to the vapour of a little chloroform placed in the lid of the plate.

(2) *Antiseptics of the Phenol Group.*—Liquor cresolis saponatus (lysol) and cresol are powerful antiseptics. Their chief use in a laboratory is for sterilising surgical instruments and discarded cultures, and killing cultures accidentally spilt by the worker. Lysol is generally used in a 3 per cent. solution. Phenol, 0·5 per cent., or *p*-chloro-*m*-cresol, 0·1 per cent., is used for preserving sera and vaccines.

(3) *Metallic Salts or Organic Compounds of Metals.*—e.g. mercuric chloride (perchloride of mercury) is sometimes used as a disinfectant in a 1 in 1000 solution. "Merthiolate", a proprietary name for sodium

ethylmercurithiosalicylate, is used in a dilution of 1 in 10,000 for the preservation of antitoxic and other sera.

(4) *Formaldehyde.*—This irritant water-soluble gas is highly lethal to all kinds of microbes and spores, killing bacterial spores almost as readily as the vegetative forms. It is cheap, and non-injurious to cloth-fabrics, wood, leather, rubber, paints and metals, and can thus be used to disinfect rooms, furniture and a wide variety of articles liable to damage by heat (*e.g.* woollen blankets and clothing, shoes, respirators, hairbrushes, gum-elastic catheters). It is applied as an aqueous solution or in gaseous form (Monthly Bull. Ministr. Hlth. Lab. Serv., 1958).

Disinfection with Aqueous Formaldehyde Solution.—Commercial "formalin" is a 40 per cent. (w/v) solution of formaldehyde in water containing 10 per cent. methanol to inhibit polymerisation. A dilution containing 5 or 10 per cent. formaldehyde in water is a powerful and rapid disinfectant when applied directly to a contaminated surface.

Bacterial cultures and suspensions are commonly killed and fixed by addition of formaldehyde to a concentration of 0·04–1·0 per cent., *e.g.* for preservation prior to counting or other measurements, and in preparation of a killed vaccine or agglutinable suspension.

Cleaned metal instruments may be sterilised by overnight immersion in a borax-formaldehyde solution (sodium tetraborate, 50 g. formaldehyde, 4 per cent. in water, 1000 ml.) or by using glutaraldehyde ("Cidex").

Disinfection by Formaldehyde Gas.—Gaseous disinfection is required for articles that cannot be wetted completely with solution, or are damaged by wetting, but care is required to provide the proper conditions for action of the gas. Thus, the atmosphere must have a high relative humidity, over 60 per cent. and preferably 80–90 per cent., and a temperature of at least 18° C. Moreover, the materials must be arranged to allow free access of the gas to all infected surfaces, since its penetration into porous fabrics is slow.

The gas is liberated by spraying or heating formalin, or by heating solid paraformaldehyde. When spraying cold formalin, an equal volume of industrial spirit (ethanol) may be added to prevent polymerisation. The best method is by boiling 1 part formalin diluted with 2 parts of water (Beeby, Kingston & Whitehouse, 1967). Because of the tendency of the gas to polymerise to paraformaldehyde, the maximal vapour concentration attainable at 20° C. is about 2·0 mg. per litre of air; it is desirable to achieve this concentration. Higher concentrations, which may be potentially explosive, are attainable at higher temperatures. After disinfection, the article may contain sufficient paraformaldehyde to give off irritant vapour over a long period; this paraformaldehyde can be neutralised by exposure to ammonia vapour.

Small articles, such as instruments, shoes and hair-brushes, are disinfected by exposure for at least 3 hr. to formaldehyde gas in an air-tight cabinet of metal or painted wood. The gas is introduced into the air in the cabinet by boiling formalin in an electric boiler to the extent of 50 ml. of 40 per cent. formaldehyde per 100 cu. ft. of air space.

Blankets and the surfaces of mattresses are disinfected similarly in a large cabinet, where they are hung unfolded; to allow for absorption by the fabric, a much greater amount of formalin is used, namely 500 ml. per 100 lb. of fabrics. The vapour is finally vented to the open air.

An efficient process of sterilising articles using formaldehyde and steam at 80° C. (i.e. at subatmospheric pressures) has been described (Alder, Brown & Gillespie, 1967). Penetration is good and most fabrics, plastics and instruments are unharmed.

(5) *Ethylene Oxide.*—This gaseous disinfectant is also highly lethal to all kinds of microbes and spores, but is capable of much more rapid diffusion into dry, porous materials. It is of particular value for sterilising articles liable to damage by heat, *e.g.* plastic and rubber articles, blankets, pharmaceutical products and complex apparatus such as heart-lung machines (Kelsey, 1961). It is a colourless liquid, boiling point 10·7° C. Above this temperature it is a moderately toxic gas which forms an explosive mixture when more than 3 per cent. is present in air. A non-explosive mixture, however, of 10 per cent. ethylene oxide in carbon dioxide, or in halogenated hydrocarbon can be employed for sterilisation. It is lethal to bacteria and viruses, and kills spores almost as easily as vegetative cells. The sterilisation time depends, among other factors, on the temperature of the reaction and the relative humidity, which ideally should be between 20 and 40 per cent. The test organism commonly used is *Bacillus subtilis* var. *globigii.* Desiccated organisms are difficult to kill especially if they have been dried on to a hard surface such as glass or plastic. Objects to be sterilised are placed in a cabinet from which the air has been removed by drawing a high vacuum, and a non-explosive mixture containing ethylene oxide is then introduced to a pressure of 5–30 lb. per sq. in. above atmospheric pressure. The cabinet should be maintained at 45°–55° C. and water introduced, if necessary, to give a relative humidity of 30 per cent. After exposure for several hours or overnight, the gas is removed by drawing a high vacuum.

An alternative system using pure ethylene oxide at subatmospheric pressure has been described (Weymes, 1966).

SOME SPECIAL APPLICATIONS OF STERILISING METHODS IN LABORATORY AND MEDICAL PRACTICE

Autoclaving of Aqueous Solutions and Culture Media

The autoclaving of aqueous solutions and culture media must be managed in such a way that the exposure to heat is sufficient for sterilisation, but not so excessive or prolonged as to damage heat-sensitive ingredients. Culture media vary in heat sensitivity. Some, such as gelatin media, will not stand autoclaving and are sterilised by intermittent steaming at 100° C. Many other media can withstand autoclaving at 121° C. for 15 min., but are spoiled if heated at this temperature for 30–45 min., or if, after a 15-min. exposure, they are cooled so slowly as to be maintained above 100° C. for a further 30–60 min. Thus, sugars such as glucose, maltose and lactose may be partially decomposed to form acids, peptones may be broken down, and agar, especially in acid media, may lose its ability to form a firm gel. The media should therefore be autoclaved for the minimum period sufficient for sterilisation and then cooled as rapidly as possible (*vide infra*). Bottles of media should be of such a size that their whole contents are used on one occasion, so as to avoid the need for repeated sterilisation or melting. Agar medium should be sterilised when first made and melted, to avoid the extra heating needed to melt it on another occasion.

An exposure of the microbes to 121° C. for 10–12 min. is generally thought sufficient for sterilisation. The holding period of sterilisation, which is timed to begin when the chamber steam first reaches 121° C. at 15 lb. pressure, must include not only this 10–12 min. but also a time sufficient for the bottles, tubes, etc., and their contents to become heated up to the same temperature as the steam. The length of the heating-up period depends on the nature of the container, the volume of its contents and the mode of operation of the autoclave. Thus, it might be only 1–2 min. for 10-ml. volumes in test-tubes loosely placed to allow free circulation of steam, and as much as 45 min. for a flask of 9 litres. Ideally, the exact time should be determined by trial for the particular kind of container and volume of contents; the autoclave is fitted with a thermocouple and this is inserted in a test container to reveal its temperature throughout the course of autoclaving. In general, the following are recommended as the total holding periods in steam at 121° C.: 12 min. for 10-ml. volumes in loosely packed test-tubes, 15 min. for 10-ml. volumes in tubes tightly packed in wire baskets, 15 min. for volumes up to 100 ml. in bottles or flasks, 20–25 min. for 500-ml. volumes, 25–30 min. for 1000-ml. volumes and 35–45 min. for 2000-ml. volumes. It is a bad practice to autoclave large and small volumes in the same load, since with the same holding period (*e.g.* 20 min.) the former (*e.g.* 2000 ml.) may not be sterilised, yet the latter (*e.g.* 10 ml.) be damaged by overheating.

The bottles, tubes, etc., should not be filled to more than 75–80 per cent. of their capacity lest the contents overflow on expansion during heating. The containers may be loosely stoppered, *e.g.* with cotton-wool plugs or loosely applied screw-caps, or else hermetically sealed, *e.g.* sealed ampoules and bottles with tightly applied screw-caps. In sealed containers the aqueous content provides the conditions for moist-heat sterilisation and the presence of some air does not interfere with this. Hermetic sealing is an advantage in preventing loss of water from the contents by evaporation or violent boiling during the cooling period when the steam pressure is being reduced. It also makes possible the autoclaving of solidified egg medium without disruption by bubble formation. However, except for the smallest bottles, the tight application of a screw-cap increases the liability to breakage during autoclaving and makes cooling-down slower.

For these reasons, it is usual to autoclave aqueous media in containers stoppered with cotton-wool, with loose metal caps or with screw-caps which are loosened slightly. This practice necessitates careful management of the cooling period. When the steam supply to the chamber is stopped at the end of the holding period, the steam already in the chamber gradually cools and diminishes in pressure. This induces evaporation of water from the medium in the container and escape of the vapour through the loose stopper. The evaporation is the main means of cooling of the containers and contents. With the correct management the loss of water from the medium is only 3–5 per cent. It is therefore usual to prepare aqueous media and solutions for autoclaving by adding an extra 5 per cent. of distilled water, so that their concentration will be correct after the autoclaving. The cooling process should be managed in such a way that the chamber pressure diminishes gradually from 15 lb. per sq. in. to atmospheric pressure in the course of 10–30 min., the optimal time varying with the volume of medium per container (15–20 min. is usually most satisfactory). The rate at which the chamber steam spontaneously cools and loses pressure, *i.e.* without opening of the chamber discharge valve, varies with the type of autoclave, the load and other conditions. The reduction to atmospheric pressure may occur in the desired time (*e.g.* 15–20 min.), or may take up to an hour or longer. The slower cooling is undesirable since it may result in damage to heat-sensitive materials. If necessary, therefore, the chamber discharge valve should be opened slightly so as to bring about a gradual reduction to atmospheric pressure over the proper period of time. Too rapid a reduction must be avoided, since the media would then boil explosively. Some modern autoclaves, specially designed for sterilising aqueous media, incorporate a device which effects rapid cooling without violent boiling; this may involve the replacement of chamber steam with air at the same pressure, or spraying of the load with condensate at a temperature slightly below that of the steam.

When the pressure gauge shows that the steam in the chamber has reached 0 lb. per sq. in. (atmospheric pressure), air is at once admitted into the chamber, through the air inlet and filter if available, or through the chamber discharge tap, or by opening the chamber door slightly. If this is not done until the pressure has fallen below atmospheric, more water will be lost by evaporation from the containers. When sufficiently cool, *e.g.* below 70° C., the containers are removed from the autoclave and their screw-caps tightened firmly.

Autoclaving in "Free Steam".—When a Koch or Arnold steamer is not available, an autoclave may be used to sterilise culture media at a temperature of 100° C., or just over. The door of the chamber is tightly closed, the steam supply turned on and the air expelled through the open discharge tap. After expulsion of the air, the steam supply is adjusted so that an adequate amount continues to escape through the open tap, and a pressure of 1–2 lb. (above atmospheric) is maintained in the chamber during the holding period; this may be less than in the ordinary steamer (*e.g.* 60 min.).

Sterilisation of Bottled Fluids

Hydrated fluids, as used for therapeutic intravenous infusions, can be sterilised in a relatively simple manner because any contaminating bacteria will already be moist and their destruction merely necessitates heating the fluid in each container to the appropriate temperature and holding it there for the appropriate time viz. 121° C. for 12 min. or 115° C. for 30 min. (M.R.C. Report, 1964). Unduly prolonged exposure periods are to be avoided since deterioration of the solutions may result. Water itself should be sterilised in this way as it is the only safe method of preparing and handling sterile water for use in operating theatres and elsewhere. For sterilising bottled fluids a gravity displacement autoclave is satisfactory. It does not need to be jacketed and it does not require a vacuum-producing apparatus. The autoclaves employed are often large and heat "layering" may be present. The rate and evenness of heating can be improved by introducing steam through a number of inlets so that turbulence of the steam/air mixture is produced (Wilkinson & Peacock, 1961). Excessive breakage, the result of heating or cooling the bottles too quickly, has to be avoided and the process is a slow one. However, devices are being developed to give more rapid cooling and shorten the whole cycle of sterilisation (British Standard 3970 : Part 2 : 1966).

Sterilisation of Empty Bottles and Impervious Containers

If empty and dry containers are to be autoclaved, they must not be tightly stoppered, since steam would be excluded and sterilisation by moist heat impossible. They should be placed on their sides in the autoclave to allow a horizontal path for the entry of steam and escape of air. If unstoppered, they will be sterilised quickly, but if stoppered even loosely, as with cotton-wool or a loosened screw-cap, the displacement of air is slow and the holding period at 121° C. should be extended to at least 30 min. Because of the uncertainty of air displacement from stoppered empty containers, it is better to sterilise them in the hot-air oven.

The disadvantage of dry heat sterilisation, however, is that the liner inside the screw-cap is usually made of rubber which perishes at the high temperatures (160° C.) employed but this problem can be overcome by using liners made of silicone rubber (available from ESCO (Rubber) Ltd., Seal Street, London, E.8). Although expensive, silicone rubber is able to withstand repeated exposures in the hot air oven and being more porous than ordinary rubber the caps may be screwed down tightly without the risk of the bottle exploding during sterilisation.

Sterilisation of Wrapped Dry Goods and Surgical Dressings

Dry porous goods such as paper- or cloth-wrapped apparatus, and surgical linen and dressings, require special attention in autoclaving, firstly to ensure the complete displacement of air from their interior by steam, and secondly to dry them before removal from the autoclave (for much detailed information consult the M.R.C. Report, 1964).

In conventional sterilisers the air is removed by the *gravity displacement method*, being driven downwards through the load by the lighter steam accumulating above it. This method requires that the load be carefully packed so that adequate spaces are left for circulation of steam between the packs and that a free downward movement of air is possible through the materials of each pack. Dry materials must not be enclosed in sealed impervious containers which prevent the entry of steam and escape of air. Glass and metal containers are left open or covered only loosely, and placed on their sides. Metal drums and caskets must be provided with air ports and these must not be obstructed by the contents being packed against them. The ports must always be fully open during sterilisation and the container so positioned in the autoclave that steam can flow through freely from top to bottom via the open vents. Formerly, dressing drums were round, but rectangular caskets, much more easy to pack and handle, are now being introduced. It must be stressed that a drum which can only be closed with difficulty is grossly overpacked. In many ways it is preferable to pack materials in a wrapper of porous cloth or paper, since this allows a much freer passage of air and steam. For surgical packs, a wrapping of at least two layers of cloth or paper is recommended. A single layer is not satisfactory because dust on the outside can contaminate the contents when the pack is opened. A paper wrapping is commonly used for small articles of laboratory apparatus (see Maintenance of Sterility).

Surgical dressings and other cloth articles should be arranged in packs no bigger than 12 × 12 × 20 inches, and these should be placed on edge in the autoclave so that the layers of cloth are vertical. Rubber gloves are powdered and packed loosely in muslin wraps, with pads of muslin in the palm and folds to allow access of steam to all parts. In an attempt to minimise deterioration it used to be customary to autoclave rubber gloves at 5 to 10 lb. pressure for a short period of time. Such exposures do *not* guarantee sterility and gloves should be autoclaved at the same temperature as other packaged goods. Treatment in a high-pressure, high-vacuum steriliser requires only a brief exposure at 130°–134° C. and this probably combines safety with minimum deterioration (M.R.C. Report 1964). Tubing is wetted inside with water just before placing in the autoclave. Instruments and syringes must be free from oil and grease, jointed instruments open, and syringes either disassembled or else moistened internally with water. The autoclave chamber must not be overloaded nor the perforated tray removed to make more room.

Vacuum Removal of Air.—The venturi vacuum device that is commonly incorporated in autoclaves to assist drying can draw a partial vacuum only and remove no more than a third to a half of the air from the chamber. This vacuum is sometimes applied before the admission of steam, but the partial evacuation of air is of little value. Sometimes this vacuum is drawn two or more times, steam being admitted between each vacuum. In the case of textiles such repeated evacuation merely produces a "breathing" motion of the same air inside the material. In fact, if prolonged, the result of this type of vacuum may be overdrying and injurious superheating of the load. On the other hand, vacuum removal of more than 98 per cent. of the air is employed to great advantage in modern "high pre-vacuum" sterilisers. The high pre-vacuum contributes to the efficient steam sterilisation of dressings, helping to produce a dry sterile load in the shortest possible time without causing damage (Fallon, 1961). It should be emphasised that this method is the only one which overcomes the effects of bad packing and overloading.

Avoidance of Damage by Superheating.—Cloth and rubber articles are liable to be damaged by excessive heating. When very dry cloth is first exposed to steam, it adsorbs and condenses an excessive amount of it and receives the corresponding excess of latent heat; this may raise its temperature to 25°–100° C. above that of the autoclave. Freshly laundered fabrics contain sufficient moisture to prevent this and so should not be stored overlong in a place of low humidity before being sterilised, nor be subjected to drying by pre-heating in the steriliser or a prolonged application of vaccum. Heating in steam mixed with some air is more damaging than heating in pure steam, especially in the case of rubber articles.

The Duration of the Holding Period at 121° *C.*—The holding period is timed as beginning when the discharge-channel thermometer first indicates 121° C. All free air has then been displaced from the chamber, but some still remains trapped in the interior of the porous load. The further time required for the steam to penetrate all parts, displace the air and heat the load throughout to 121° C., may extend to 30 min. or even longer. This "steam penetration time" must be added to the "sterilising time" of 12 min. in computing the holding period. The following are generally recommended as the total holding times at 121° C.: 15–20 min. for muslin- or paper-wrapped instruments, rubber gloves and open metal or glass containers; 30 min. for muslin- or paper-wrapped packs of surgical linen and dressings, wrapped syringes, and loosely stoppered metal or glass containers; 45 min. for metal surgical dressing drums with muslin liners. The holding period is much shorter when a high pre-vacuum steriliser is employed. Once the pre-sterilisation vacuum has been drawn, heating up and full penetration by steam of a load of textiles firmly packed in dressing drums will be accomplished in 3 min. and the sterilisation time is also shorter, *e.g.* 3 min. at 135° C. (see table, p. 710).

Drying of the Load.—The load is dried during the cooling period. The supply of steam at 121° C. is maintained in the jacket, while that to the chamber is cut off. The chamber steam is allowed to escape rapidly through the discharge tap until zero gauge pressure is reached. The moisture of the load is then evaporated by the residual heat of the articles and radiant heat from the jacketed walls of the chamber. The drying is assisted to completion by the removal of vapour from the chamber. The venturi device is used to suck warmed, filtered air into and through the chamber; this carries away the vapour and dries the load in 15–25 min. The air allowed into the chamber must be drawn through an efficient filter to free it from dust-borne bacteria which otherwise might enter the sterilised packages.

Without the concurrent admission of air, the application of the partial vacuum (15 in. Hg. or less) obtainable by the venturi device is quite inadequate to effect drying. Alternatively as long as the load is not wet from inadequately dried steam the attaining of a vacuum of 20 in. Hg. or more should be sufficient to achieve drying since water retained in the load will "boil off" more rapidly at this reduced chamber pressure. Filtered air is still required, however, to break the vacuum before the steriliser is opened. Thus in a modern high pre-vacuum autoclave the drying period is very short. The table shows how the overall process time for a load of surgical dressings is greatly reduced by employing a high pre-vacuum autoclave (Bowie, 1958).

Process Time in a 9 cu. ft. Gravity Displacement Steriliser (LOAD-*Dressings packed loosely in caskets*)		Process Time in a 9 cu. ft. High Pre-Vacuum Steriliser (LOAD-*Dressings firmly packed in caskets*)	
Stage	*Time (min.)*	*Stage*	*Time (min.)*
Time for thermometer to indicate 121° C. (250° F.)	10	Time to draw pre-sterilisation vacuum	7
Estimated penetrating and heating-up time	27	Time for thermometer to indicate 134° C. (273° F.) (includes steam penetration and heating-up time.)	3
Sterilisation holding period	12	Sterilisation holding period	2
Safety margin	6	Safety margin	1
Vacuum drying period	25	Vacuum drying period	3
		Breaking vacuum	1
Total	80	Total	17

Comparison of process times in a gravity displacement and a high pre-vacuum steriliser (after Bowie, 1958).

Sterilisation of Surgical Instruments

Boiling is effective only when 2 per cent. sodium carbonate or a germicide has been added to the water and there is always the risk of recontamination when the instruments are being washed before use to free them from these substances. Moreover, there may be a tendency to shorten the process in order to please the waiting surgeon. As a result the use of small pressure sterilisers that will ensure the safety of unwrapped instruments and bowls is to be preferred. Such autoclaves can be of simple design and since heating up and penetration are instantaneous the process time is short, especially if the steriliser can be operated at 132°–134° C. or at 150° C.

Heat is said to blunt sharp instruments but this effect is mainly due to oxidation and damage should not be caused by pure steam. The only established chemical sterilising agents are ethylene oxide and formaldehyde and they can be used to sterilise instruments such as scalpels. Complex pieces of apparatus like cystoscopes, which cannot withstand heat even at 100° C., may often be rendered safe for their particular purposes by removing all vegetative organisms including *Mycobacterium tuberculosis*. Pasteurisation at 75° C. or treatment with chlorhexidine preferably in 75 per cent. ethanol can be recommended for this purpose.

Sterilisation of Syringes

As syringes play an important part in the work of bacteriological laboratories and hospital wards, particular attention must be given to their use, care and sterilisation. Sterilisation by heat is the method of choice and chemical agents are in general unsatisfactory.

It is recommended that all-glass syringes should be used in preference to the glass-metal syringe of the "Record" type, over which they have many advantages. The glass-metal type is more difficult to clean, and is more likely to break on heating owing to the difference of expansion of glass and metal. It cannot be sterilised when assembled and is more difficult to keep sterile until ready for use. The solder uniting the glass and metal parts may melt in the hot-air oven, and may even do so in the autoclave. Syringes are now available, however, with cement at the glass-metal junction that will withstand 200° C. Syringes of 5 ml. capacity and upwards should have excentric nozzles. The needles should be of stainless steel of the best quality. The mounts of the needles must fit accurately to the nozzle of the syringe.

All-glass Syringes.—Before being put into use, new syringes must be well washed in soap and water with a test-tube brush or burette brush according to size. After washing in clean, warm water, both barrel and piston are dried.

In a laboratory it is convenient to have the syringes assembled, wrapped and sterilised, ready for use, and to have a supply of these sterilised syringes always on hand. When this service is not available, all-glass syringes may be sterilised just before use by boiling in a fish kettle or saucepan. If the tap water is hard it is best to use distilled water. The syringe is dismantled and the barrel and piston are placed in cold water, which is brought to the boil and kept boiling for not less than 5 min. The perforated tray is removed from the steriliser, the water poured off and the tray returned to the steriliser, which is covered immediately. When *dry* and cool enough, the barrel and piston are assembled with sterile forceps or clean, dry fingers, touching only the outside of the barrel and the top of the piston. The sterile syringe should be used immediately and not placed in stock "sterile" water or alcohol. The needle should be boiled at the same time, and it is an advantage to thread it through a piece of lint to protect the point. The needle is affixed to the nozzle by means of sterile forceps.

It is much better, however, to sterilise all-glass syringes in the hot-air oven as follows. New syringes are cleaned as above in soap and water, washed and dried. The piston is lightly smeared with liquid paraffin or silicone fluid, the lubricant being well rubbed into the ground glass, inserted into the barrel, and moved backwards and forwards several times so that the syringe works evenly and smoothly. Excess of lubricant is to avoided. The assembled syringe is placed in a stout glass tube of such diameter that the barrel of the syringe fits loosely and the flange rests on the top of the tube. The tube should be of such length that it accommodates the syringe with needle fitted. The tube containing the syringe is then wrapped in clear transparent cellophane or similar material, a strip of material of the following sizes being used: for 1-ml. and 2-ml. syringes 3 in. × 9 in., for 5-ml. 4 in. × 11 in., for 10-ml. and 20-ml. 5 in. × 14 in. The cellophane is rolled in a spiral fashion round the tube, commencing at the bottom with a fold and turn-in, and finishing above the piston of the syringe with a firm twist. If cellophane is not available, kraft paper can be used, but the disadvantage of this is that the syringe cannot be seen, and relevant information, *e.g.* size of syringe, etc., must be written in pencil on the paper. Alternatively the syringe may be packed in a metal tube, usually made of aluminium and sealed with a foil cap.

The assembled and wrapped syringe is sterilised in the hot-air oven at 160° C. (± 2° C.) for not less than 1 hr. Under these conditions the cellophane turns slightly brown, indicating to the user that the syringe may be controlled with a Browne's tube (type 3).

Needles are sterilised in 3 in. × ½ in. test-tubes plugged with cotton-wool. In order to protect the point of the needle, a piece of 5-mm. glass tubing 2 in. long is placed in the tube and the point of the needle passed down it so that the mount of the needle rests on the tubing. The cotton-wool plug keeps the needle in place. The tubes with contained needles are individually wrapped in cellophane and sterilised as above at 160° C. for 1 hr.

When large numbers of syringes have to be handled some form of conveyor oven has many advantages. The assembly consists of a heated insulated tunnel through which a metal moving belt carried the articles to be sterilised. This enables a continuous and large output of material and should ensure standard heat treatment. Such an apparatus, with a series of infra-red projectors which produce rapid heating of the moving load, has been described by Darmady *et al.* (1957).

Sterilisation in the autoclave is only possible if steam is able to penetrate to every surface of the syringe. In practice this means that the piston must not be smeared with lubricant and if packed in an impervious container this must not be sealed until *after* the syringe has been sterilised. Assembled syringes may be sterilised in a high pre-vacuum autoclave, but in a gravity-displacement steriliser the syringe must be dismantled otherwise air discharge would be inefficient.

After the syringe has been used, *e.g.* for blood culture, aspiration, etc., it is *immediately* washed out in a cold solution of 2 per cent. lysol, which should always be ready for the purpose. Blood must never be allowed to clot in the syringe, otherwise it will be difficult to remove the piston. Hot fluid must not be used, otherwise it will coagulate the protein and the piston will stick. If the needle has been removed before the blood, etc., is expelled, it must immediately be cleaned after the syringe has been washed out by affixing it to the syringe again and washing it through with the lysol solution. After washing, syringe and needle are returned to the tube in which they were sterilised.

Before re-sterilising, the syringe is thoroughly cleaned in soapy water, a brush being used, then washed in clean, warm water and dried. If it is to be sterilised by dry heat it is finally lubricated with liquid paraffin, before assembly.

The needle is washed in warm water, the bore of the needle cleared with a stilette, and the mount of the needle cleaned with a piece of cotton-wool on a swab-stick to remove any blood, etc. After washing it with warm water it is run through with alcohol and allowed to dry. Before being sterilised the point is touched up on a fine Arkansas slip-stone (size 4 in. × 1¼ in.), lubricated with thin machine oil or liquid paraffin, and examined with an 8 × hand-lens to see that the point is really sharp. It is then run through with the stilette, washed in alcohol and dried.

Glass-Metal ("Record") Syringes.—These cannot be sterilised as above described because the solder-cement joining the glass and metal parts together may melt in the hot-air oven. Moreover, they cannot be sterilised, while assembled, by any heat method as the unequal expansion of glass and metal causes cracking of the barrel. In order to sterilise Record type syringes they must be taken apart. The Record type syringe is usually sterilised by boiling for 5 min. as described above for all-glass syringes. Alternatively, the piston and barrel can be wrapped separately in kraft paper and sterilised in the autoclave, although it should be noted that the solder-cement in some makes may melt even at this temperature.

Glass-metal syringes are washed out immediately after use as described above, and the needles are cleaned and sharpened as for all-glass syringes.

Disinfection of Rooms

Fumigation with gaseous disinfectants was at one time commonly performed after a room had been occupied by a patient with an infectious disease. Sulphur dioxide, generated by burning sulphur, was the popular agent for this purpose but it is effective only if the relative humidity is 60 per cent. or more.

Terminal disinfection is now practised only if the environment has been contaminated with the organisms of a serious infectious disease such as anthrax, smallpox or tuberculosis and formaldehyde is generally used.

Disinfection of Rooms by Spraying Formalin (Jack, 1952, 1954).—This is probably the most effective means of disinfecting the interior and furniture of a room. The room is first well sealed by covering cracks, ventilators, fireplaces, etc., with brown paper and adhesive tape. An operator protected by an efficient anti-gas respirator thoroughly moistens all surfaces of the walls, floor and furniture with a spray of 10 per cent. formaldehyde solution (1 volume of formalin and 3 volumes of water), and finally saturates the atmosphere by spraying undiluted formalin to the extent of 1 litre per 1000 cu. ft. The room is closed by sealing the door and left for 24 hr. A basin of ammonia solution is then introduced and left to evaporate for several hours (1 litre SG 880 ammonia solution mixed with 1 litre of water per litre of 40 per cent. formaldehyde used). This neutralises the formaldehyde and paraformaldehyde, and the excess ammonia is readily removed by ventilation.

Disinfection of Rooms with Formaldehyde Vapour.—The room is sealed as described above and heated, if necessary, to above 18° C. Formalin is boiled within the room in an electric boiler having a safety plug which kicks out when the vessel boils dry and a time switch set to cut off the current just prior to this; 500 ml. of 40 per cent. formaldehyde plus 1000 ml. water are boiled per 1000 cu. ft. of air space. The room is kept sealed for 4–24 hr. and an operator wearing a respirator then introduces a cloth soaked in ammonia solution (250 ml. per litre of formalin used). This is left for 2 hr. to neutralise the formaldehyde.

Disinfection of Bedclothes

The bedding of a patient or carrier is liable to become heavily contaminated with pathogenic bacteria such as *Staph. aureus* and *Strept. pyogenes*, and, when disturbed, liberates large numbers of these into the air. Cotton and linen sheets, and blankets made from cotton or some synthetic fibres (Calnan, 1959), may be sterilised by boiling during laundering and it has been recommended that these blankets replace the conventional woollen ones which shrink on boiling. High temperature laundering of woollen blankets sufficient to destroy vegetative bacteria is feasible, however, if a slightly acid detergent mixture is used. Alternatively steam at subatmospheric pressure may be used to disinfect bedding (Alder, 1966). Woollen blankets can be rendered safe by exposure to suitable chemical agents. Treatment with gaseous disinfectants such as formaldehyde vapour or ethylene oxide is effective but requires special equipment. Simpler methods include impregnation of the blankets with either quaternary ammonium disinfectants or synthetic phenolic compounds (Larkin *et al.*, 1961). Application of oil to the blankets in the last stage of the laundering process reduces the subsequent scatter of organisms.

Disinfection of Skin

The bacterial flora of the skin may be divided into the resident flora and the transient flora. The resident flora consists of bacteria that grow in the glands and hair follicles of the skin and it is very difficult to remove entirely. However, it is composed mainly of harmless commensal organisms such as *Staph. albus* and corynebacteria. Sometimes it includes *Staph. aureus*. The transient flora, made up of bacteria acquired from the environment, often contains potential pathogens. The first step in skin disinfection is thorough washing and scrubbing in warm water with soap or some other surface-tension reducing agent, *e.g.* a disinfectant cationic detergent such as cetrimide ("Cetavlon") or benzalkonium chloride ("Roccal"). A prolonged general reduction in skin flora can be achieved by the repeated and exclusive use of a detergent containing 2 to 3 per cent. hexachlorophene. After the skin is washed, it may be rinsed in 70 per cent. ethanol, which dries rapidly and has a transient bactericidal effect. The action of the alcohol is slightly improved by the addition of 0·5 per cent. chlorhexidine.

Where strict asepsis is required, as in surgery, it is necessary to wear sterile rubber gloves which are impervious to the organisms on the skin. As there is always a danger of the gloves being perforated during use, it is important before donning them to remove as many of the bacteria from the hands as possible. This may be done as above. The addition of neomycin and bacitracin to the glove powder will reduce substantially the number of live bacteria deposited inside surgical gloves during use. Since the operator's hands may have to be disinfected repeatedly it is essential that non-irritant agents are employed, but when only a single application is required, as in preparing the skin of a patient or animal for incision or puncture, stronger disinfectants may be used. Recently however, it has been shown that 0·5 per cent. chlorhexidine in 70 per cent. ethanol is as effective a disinfectant as 1 per cent. iodine in alcohol and its use is free from the risks of sensitisation and irritation. Iodine compounds have some sporicidal action and this is of special value when cleansing sites which may have been contaminated with clostridia; an iodophor (*e.g.* "Betadine") may be used for this purpose. For further details see Lowbury (1961).

MAINTENANCE OF STERILITY

Once articles have been rendered sterile it is essential that they are handled and stored in such a way as to prevent recontamination before they are used.

Test Tubes and Flasks.—The interiors of test-tubes, flasks, bottles, etc., must be carefully protected from bacterial contamination due to access of air, dust, etc., before and after the addition of medium and during the subsequent cultivation of organisms. This has usually been done by means of cotton-wool stoppers. These should be 1¼–1½ in. long, ¾–1 in. being inserted into the mouth of the tube, etc., and the remainder projecting. They should fit firmly, but not so tightly as to render their removal difficult.

The stoppers should be made from long-fibre cotton-wool which is free from short broken fibres and dust. Non-absorbent cotton is preferable, because, after steaming, plugs tend to remain moist, and if the medium is to be kept for any length of time and absorbent wool is used, moulds will grow through the stopper and contaminate the medium. A sufficient amount of cotton-wool (*vide supra*) should be forced into the tube with a rod or pair of forceps, but should not be twisted in, as creases are formed along the sides of the glass and create channels for contaminating organisms.

Instead of the ordinary roll of cotton-wool being used, it is recommended that the non-absorbent wool be obtained in the form of a long thin ribbon known as "rope wool" or "neck wool" of the type used by hairdressers. It is kept in a tin container with a hole in the lid, and the appropriate amount of wool for the stopper is easily obtained without waste.

When tubes or flasks have to be stored for some time the stoppers or tops of the crates or boxes should be covered with sterile kraft paper, kept in place by means of fine string or a rubber band. Sterile rubber stoppers may, in some cases, be used instead of cotton-wool, particularly where the contents of the flask or tube have to be kept a considerable time, as in the case of immune sera; this also applies to vessels that have to be transported by post or by messenger.

Slip-on aluminium caps of various patterns are available for use instead of cotton-wool plugs, for the stoppering of test tubes. They have the advantage of protecting the rim of the tube from airborne dust and their use thus makes unnecessary the conventional "flaming" of the mouth of the tube on each occasion of its opening. These caps should be used for cultures of delicate organisms that are affected by toxic volatile substances liberated from cotton-wool during the process of sterilisation.

Screw-capped Bottles.—Flasks for storing culture media have now been replaced by screw-capped bottles of 3-, 5- and 10-oz. capacity, while the smaller bottles of ¼-, ½- and 1-oz. capacity may be employed instead of test-tubes.

Petri Dishes.—Each individual dish should be wrapped in kraft paper before sterilisation, and kept in the paper until used. For a 4-in. dish the size of paper should be 12 in. square. The dishes may also be sterilised (unwrapped) and kept in metal boxes.

Pipettes.—1-ml. and 10-ml. graduated pipettes should be wrapped in a long strip of kraft paper, which is wound round them in a spiral manner before sterilising in the hot-air oven. Bulb pipettes (10 ml., 50 ml., etc.) are also covered with kraft paper. Under these conditions pipettes remain sterile in their wrappers for considerable periods of time. Alternatively they may be sterilised and stored in suitable canisters.

Capillary pipettes are sterilised in large test-tubes 15 in. × 2½ in., having a gauze or cotton-wool stopper, or in metal boxes. The former method is preferable. Alternatively, 8-in. lengths of 5-mm. glass tubing are plugged with cotton-wool at both ends, wrapped in batches of a dozen in kraft paper, sterilised and stored. When capillary pipettes are required, the middle of the tubing is heated in a Bunsen or blowpipe and pulled out, the ends of the two pipettes being sealed in the making.

Ampoules are sterilised in the hot-air oven with the necks sealed, and are kept in metal boxes. If unsealed ampoules are used, they should be plugged with cotton-wool before sterilisation.

It must be emphasised that a wrapping of kraft paper or double-thickness muslin is effective in excluding contaminating bacteria *only when it is dry*. If the wrapped articles are sterilised in an autoclave instead of a hot-air oven, they must be dried before placing on an unsterile surface.

Surgical Dressings.—The M.R.C. Report (1959) points out that a load sterilised in the autoclave may become contaminated during removal from the steriliser, in transport or during subsequent storage. It is essential that metal dressing drums should have tightly fitting lids and a protective lining that will cover the ports inside the drums. Wrapped packs on removal from the autoclave should not at once be placed on a cold flat surface, since residual moisture will condense on this, make damp the fabric or paper wrapping, and so permit the entry of contaminating bacteria. Alder and Alder (1961) measured the re-contamination rate of dressings wrapped in different materials. They concluded that paper was more efficient than either calico or balloon cloth and that one layer of any of these materials was better than two layers of muslin. Crepe paper is usually preferred to kraft paper because it drapes better and it is always advisable to use a double layer in case the outer covering becomes torn. As an extra precaution the double-wrapped packs may be enclosed in rigid or semi-rigid containers such as cardboard cartons. The shelf life after sterilisation of dressings packaged in this way is several weeks and this period can be prolonged if storage conditions are good.

Pre-sterilised materials.—Disposable syringes, catheters and needles sterilised by gamma radiation or ethylene oxide gas are usually marketed in plastic or paper envelopes. It must be emphasised that a high standard of packaging is necessary if such pre-sterilised products are to remain sterile. Particular attention must be paid to the sealing of the container.

CENTRAL STERILE SUPPLY IN HOSPITALS

The supply of sterile articles from a central source in a hospital has evolved in the last few years as a development of central sterile syringe services. Central sterile supply departments (CSSD) have now been widely introduced. The need for them in hospitals in Great Britain became apparent when current sterilising practice was critically examined (Nuffield Provincial Hospitals Trust Report, 1958).

The advantages of Central Sterile Supply are many. These departments should be expertly supervised by a specially trained senior member of the nursing staff or a pharmacist who is responsible to a special medical committee and they should be staffed by technicians and orderlies familiar with modern sterilising methods. This frees nurses from routine repetitive tasks such as cleaning syringes, making swabs and packing dressing drums and allows them to spend more time looking after their patients. Also, because of the centralisation, expensive automatically controlled equipment can be used intelligently and economically to ensure the efficiency of sterilising procedures. A hospital requires a much smaller number of autoclaves when the great potential output of a high pre-vacuum steriliser (about 3 to 5 times that of a gravity displacement instrument of the same cubic capacity) can be fully utilised. No sterilisation is done in wards or departments and theatres sterilise only their own bowls and instruments. As a result space is vacated and the old sterilising rooms can become much-needed dressing rooms or isolation cubicles. The CSSD provides a number of different dressing and instrument packs and the contents of each pack should be used at the time it is opened. This eliminates bulk packs which are entered on a number of occasions and so increases the safety of many ward and theatre procedures.

A hospital may have its own CSSD or a number of hospitals in a given area may be supplied from one department. Sterilisation is effected by heat and the basic equipment is hot air ovens (probably a conveyor-belt oven) and autoclaves (usually of high pre-vacuum type). Apparatus for sterilisation by gamma radiation is too expensive for a CSSD but it may be an economy to issue commercially prepared disposable articles such as needles and syringes which have been sterilised in this way. The CSSD is organised in three separate sections, "dirty", "clean" and "sterile". Apparatus and materials returned dirty which have to be used again, such as syringes and rubber gloves, are first of all cleaned. These pass to the next section along with freshly laundered fabrics where packing of all clean materials is carried out. Sterilisation is the third phase followed by careful storage of the sterile materials prior to distribution. For further details see Griffin *et al.* (1962) and Welch (1961).

PREPARATION OF BACTERIAL VACCINES

The method to be described refers mainly to the preparation of vaccines on a small scale, such as *autogenous vaccines*—*i.e.* consisting of the organism or organisms isolated from a particular patient and used for the treatment of the case. Therapeutic vaccines are now little used and have been superseded by chemotherapeutic and antibiotic substances in the treatment of bacterial infections.

In preparing stock bacterial vaccines for prophylactic use, *e.g.* typhoid-paratyphoid (TAB) vaccine, it is essential that the strains used should be carefully selected, as pathogenic bacteria when maintained in laboratory culture for any length of time may undergo variation in antigenic characters and so lose their specific immunising properties.

The organism must be isolated in pure culture, and then several cultures are made on appropriate solid medium so as to yield sufficient growth after twenty-four to forty-eight hours' incubation, according to the amount of vaccine to be prepared and the abundance of the growth on the particular medium. The growth is emulsified in sterile saline solution (0·85 per cent. sodium chloride) so as to form a fairly dense suspension. This should be free from fragments of medium; if present, they can be removed by centrifuging the suspension for two or three minutes or by allowing them to sediment by gravity and then decanting the supernatant fluid. The bacterial suspension must be rendered as uniform as possible by shaking in a tube or bottle with glass beads. A special shaking machine is generally used for this purpose. *All manipulations involved in preparing the suspension must be carried out with strict precautions to avoid contamination.*

Standardisation

It is necessary at this stage to estimate the *approximate* number of bacteria per ml. of the suspension. Various methods are available for this purpose; the turbidity of the suspension may be compared with standard opacity tubes or the bacteria themselves may be counted in a haemocytometer.

Sterilisation of the Bacterial Suspension

The suspension is sterilised at relatively low temperatures, *e.g.* 60° C. for 1 hr. in a waterbath.

The *vaccine bath* consists of a metal container, heated either by gas or electricity, and may have an agitator to ensure even distribution of the heat. The bath is fitted with a suitable removable rack for holding the tubes, while the lid has a hole into which a thermometer is placed. The bath is maintained at a constant temperature, usually 60° C., by means of a thermostatic control, which is either a "capsule", similar to that in an incubator, or a bimetallic device. When the temperature rises above the desired level, the thermostatic control diminishes the gas supply or cuts off the electricity. When the temperature falls the heating is resumed. By means of an adjusting screw, the temperature can be regulated to $\pm$ 1° C. of that required. All waterbaths should be inspected at weekly intervals and any loss of water, due to evaporation, etc., restored. To ascertain whether the organisms have been killed, several loopfuls are transferred to a tube of *suitable* medium and incubated for 48 hr. (For further sterility tests, *vide infra.*)

Preparation of the Vaccine for Administration

Any series of doses consisting of a certain number of organisms (computed in millions) can be prepared in volumes of 1 ml. by making appropriate dilutions in carbol-saline (0·85 per cent. sodium chloride + 0·5 per cent. phenol) from the original standardised suspension. Graduated pipettes, as used in serological work, are employed for the purpose. The dilutions are made in sterile tubes and each dose is transferred to a sterile vaccine ampoule which is then sealed.

The most convenient method of supplying the vaccine for actual use is to prepare, from the stock suspension, concentrations of 50, 100, 500 or 1000 million organisms per ml. (according to the doses required) in quantities of 20 ml. The dilutions are placed in 25-ml. "vaccine bottles" with special tightly fitting thick rubber caps which are covered with a layer of paraffin wax, or in 1-oz. bottles with perforated screw-caps, like that of the blood-culture bottle, and covered with a viskap before issue. The required dose can be obtained by puncturing the cap with the hypodermic syringe, and withdrawing the appropriate amount.

When a vaccine representing more than one type of organism is required, *e.g.* from mixed infections, pure cultures of each organism must be obtained and separate standardised suspensions prepared. Appropriate concentrations of each are then combined in the final preparation.

In preparing dilutions from the stock vaccine all manipulations, etc., must be carried out with strict precautions to prevent contamination. Pipettes, tubes, ampoules, bottles, caps, etc., must be absolutely sterile.

Before supplying the diluted vaccine it is essential to carry out further sterility tests with the contents of two of the ampoules, or 2-ml. withdrawn from the bottled vaccine with a syringe. One-half of this sample is tested for aerobic organisms and one-half for anaerobes by appropriate cultural methods.

Earlier regulations under the Therapeutic Substances Act applicable to the manufacture for sale of various therapeutic substances laid down the following sterility tests which may be adopted in the case of bacterial vaccines preserved with a phenolic antiseptic:—

"*The tests shall be made on fluid media, the quantity of medium contained in each tube or other vessel used in the test being such as to secure that any phenolic antiseptic present in the sample is diluted to less than* 0·01 *per cent. In the case of a test for aerobic organisms the medium shall consist either of a meat extract with the addition of* 1 *per cent. of peptone, or of such an equivalent as can be prepared by the tryptic digestion of muscle. After the final sterilisation the hydrogen-ion concentration of the medium shall be between the limits represented by pH*=7·2 *and pH*=7·8. *In the case of a test for anaerobic organisms the medium shall consist of a nutrient broth similar to that used in testing for aerobic organisms, with the addition of heat-coagulated muscle of an amount sufficient to occupy a depth of not less than* 1 *centimetre at the bottom of the tube. After the final sterilisation the hydrogen-ion concentration of the medium shall be between the limits represented by pH*=7·2 *and pH*=7·8. *Before the test inoculation the medium shall be heated to* 100° *C. for a period sufficient to free it completely from dissolved oxygen, and then cooled to* 37° *C. or lower. The inoculated tubes shall be incubated at* 37° *C. for five days. . . .*"

If a vaccine has been prepared from an organism which does not grow readily in ordinary media, a similar test must be carried out with media specially suitable for the growth of the particular organism, or the vaccine may be tested by injection of an animal of a species known to be susceptible to infection by that organism.

For details of the present requirements in the application of sterility tests to therapeutic substances and the methods to be used, reference should be made to the latest Therapeutic Substances Regulations.

TESTING OF SURGICAL CATGUT FOR STERILITY

The following method was prescribed in the earlier Therapeutic Substances Regulations (Therapeutic Substances Act) and has been extensively used.

"... The sample shall, when practicable, be the contents of at least one whole container or packet ...

(*a*) the container or packet shall be opened and the sample removed with aseptic precautions;

(*b*) after all the adherent fluid has been drained off as completely as possible, the sample shall be placed entire in a test-tube at least 3·5 cm. in diameter and 17·5 cm. in length and containing 50 ml. of sterile distilled water. This tube shall then be closed by some method which will preclude the access of bacteria, and be placed in an incubator at 37° C. for 24 hr.;

(*c*) after this incubation, the sample shall be aseptically transferred to a similar tube containing a solution of 1 per cent. of sodium thiosulphate and 1 per cent. of crystallised sodium carbonate in distilled water, the tube and solution having been previously sterilised in the autoclave. In this solution the sample shall again be incubated for 24 hr. at 37° C.;

(*d*) after the second incubation the sample shall again be removed aseptically and, without further washing, shall be examined for the presence of living bacteria and their spores.

The sterility tests shall be carried out ... by placing the sample in a tube at least 3·5 cm. in diameter and 17·5 cm. in length, containing not less than 50 ml. of a culture medium prepared by dissolving 0·2 per cent. of prepared agar-agar in a nutrient bacteriological broth ... the broth may preferably be made by the digestion of meat with trypsin (Douglas's broth or Hartley's modification thereof) ... the mixture being sterilised in the autoclave; ...

(*e*) The tubes of culture medium containing the sample shall be incubated at 37° C. for twelve days and examined daily for the growth of bacteria;

(*f*) if no such growth is detected during this period, the batch from which the sample was drawn shall be treated as free from living bacteria and their spores, and as having passed the test; ..."

An *alternative culture medium* which has been used is the cooked-meat medium with 30 ml. of broth added to each tube (these being 6 × 1 in.). Before transferring the catgut to the medium from the thiosulphate solution it is placed in a tube of sterile distilled water for a few hours. Meat medium has been found to be particularly valuable for obtaining growths of sporing anaerobic bacilli from catgut, and also serves very well for the detection of other organisms that may occur as contaminants in catgut.

It should be emphasised that in all the manipulations of the catgut sample in the above specified processes, care is required to exclude extraneous contamination and it is advisable to carry out these manipulations under an inoculating hood, or with the aid of a similar apparatus, to prevent aerial contamination.

For details of present requirements in the application of sterility tests to Surgical Catgut reference should be made to the latest Therapeutic Substances Regulations (1957).

FURTHER READING

RUBBO, S. D. & GARDNER, J. F. (1965). *A Review of Sterilisation and Disinfection.* London: Lloyd-Luke Ltd.

REFERENCES

ALDER, V. G. & ALDER, F. I. (1961). Preserving the sterility of surgical dressings wrapped in paper and other materials. *J. clin. Path.*, **14**, 76.

ALDER, V. G., BROWN, A. M. & GILLESPIE, W. A. (1966). Disinfection of heat-sensitive material by low-temperature steam and formaldehyde. *J. clin. Path.*, **19**, 83.

BEEBY, M. M., KINGSTON, D. & WHITEHOUSE, C. E. (1967). Experiments on terminal disinfection of cubicles with formaldehyde. *J. Hyg.* (*Camb.*), **65**, 115.

BOWIE, J. H. (1955). Modern apparatus for sterilisation. *Pharm. J.*, **174**, 473.

BOWIE, J. H. (1958). The nurse, steam and the engineer. *Hosp. Engr.*, **12**, 158, 182.

CALNAN, J. S. (1959). Clean blankets, new boilable bedcover. *Lancet*, **i**, 300.

DARMADY, E. M., HUGHES, K. E. A. & TUKE, W. (1957). Sterilization of syringes by infra-red radiation. *J. clin. Path.*, **10**, 291.

DARMADY, E. M. & BROCK, R. B. (1954). Temperature levels in hot-air ovens. *J. clin. Path.*, **7**, 290.

DARMADY, E. M., HUGHES, K. E. A., BURT, M. M., FREEMAN, B. M. & POWELL, D. B. (1961). Radiation sterilisation. *J. clin. Path.*, **14**, 55.

ELFORD, W. J. (1931). A new series of graded collodion membranes suitable for general bacteriological use, especially in filterable virus studies. *J. Path. Bact.*, **34**, 505.

FALLON, R. J. (1961). Factors concerned in the efficient steam sterilization of surgical dressings. *J. clin. Path.*, **14**, 505.

GRIFFIN, S. G., NIXON, F. M., SANFORD, D. A. & WILSON, J. F. (1962). Hospital central sterile supply. *Brit. med. J.*, **ii**, 912.

HART, D. (1942). The importance of air-borne pathogenic bacteria in the operating room: a method of control by sterilization of the air with ultra-violet radiation, p. 186 in *Aerobiology*, ed. F.R. Moulton. Washington D.C.: American Association for Advancement of Science.

HOWIE, J. W. & TIMBURY, M. C. (1956). Laboratory tests of operating-theatre sterilisers. *Lancet*, **ii**, 669.

JACK, R. P. (1952 and 1954). *City of Edinburgh Public Health Reports.*

KELSEY, J. C. (1961). Sterilization by ethylene oxide. *J. clin. Path.*, **14**, 59.

LARKIN, I. M., BRIDSON, E. Y., GRIEVE, W. S. M. & GIBSON, J. W. (1961). Disinfection of hospital blankets with synthetic phenolic compounds. *J. clin. Path.*, **14**, 80.

LOWBURY, E. J. L. (1961). Skin disinfection. *J. clin. Path.*, **14**, 85.

MCMATH, W. F. T. & HUSSAIN, K. K. (1960). Investigation of U.V. radiation in the control of chicken-pox cross-infection. *Brit. J. clin. Pract.*, **14**, 19.

MEDICAL RESEARCH COUNCIL (1964). Working party's report on sterilisation by steam under increased pressure. *Lancet*, **2**, 193.

MINISTRY OF HEALTH (1958). The practical aspects of formaldehyde fumigation. *Mth. Bull. Minist. Hlth. Lab. Serv.* **17**, 270.

NUFFIELD PROVINCIAL HOSPITALS TRUST (1958). *Present Sterilizing Practice in Six Hospitals.*

WELCH, J. D. (1961). The organization of central sterile supply departments. *J. clin. Path.*, **14**, 69.

WELLS, W. F. & WELLS, M. W. (1942). Air-borne infection as a basis for a theory of contagion. In *Aerobiology*, p. 99. American Association for Advancement of Science.

WEYMES, C. (1966). Sterilisation with Ethylene Oxide at Sub-Atmospheric Pressure. *Brit. Hosp. J. and Social Science Review*, 1745.

WILKINSON, G. R. & PEACOCK, F. G. (1961). Improvement of heating of bottled fluids during autoclave sterilisation using low pressure steam. *J. Pharm. Pharmacol.*, **13** (Supplement), 72 T.

WILLIAMS, R. E. O., BLOWERS, R., GARROD, L. P. & SHOOTER, R. A. (1966). Chapter XIX. Sterilisation or disinfection by chemicals. In *Hospital Infection*, p. 311. London: Lloyd-Luke Ltd.

CHAPTER 47

CULTIVATION OF MICROORGANISMS

CULTURE MEDIA

ONLY in exceptional cases can the identity of a microorganism be established by its morphological characters. It is therefore essential to obtain a culture by growing the organism in an artificial culture medium, and if more than one species or type of organism are present, each requires to be carefully separated or isolated in pure culture. In this process there are three distinct operations:

(i) The preparation of a suitable culture medium.

(ii) The initial removal of other organisms from the medium and its containers by sterilisation. Bacteria are ubiquitous and are present in the material and on the articles used for making media. These contaminating organisms must be destroyed or removed so that the culture medium is rendered sterile.

(iii) The cultivation of the organism and its isolation from others present in the material to be examined. Techniques for the separation of mixed cultures are described in the next chapter and the general subject of bacterial nutrition and conditions for growth has been dealt with in Chapter 3.

LIQUID AND SOLID MEDIA

There are two broad groups of media, liquid and solid. Many liquid media containing different nutrients have been devised and most bacteria will grow in at least one of them. However, liquid media have two disadvantages. Growths usually do not exhibit specially characteristic appearances in them and, except when they are designed for a particular biochemical test, they are of only limited use in identifying species. Also, organisms cannot be separated with certainty from mixtures by growth in liquid media. If liquid media are madc solid (gelatinous) these disadvantages are overcome. On solid media the appearances exhibited by the colonies of different bacteria are useful in identification; and solid media are almost indispensable for the isolation of pure cultures. It is only occasionally that organisms can be grown directly from the body in pure culture so that solid media are almost always needed for the examination of pathological specimens.

Gelatin was used by the early bacteriologists to make the first solid media; pieces of potato impregnated with nutrient solutions can be used as solid media; serum or egg can be coagulated by heating in an inspissator to make media solid; but agar is most commonly used for this purpose.

Agar-agar, or "agar" for short, is derived from certain seaweeds. In watery solutions it gives a firm gel that remains unmelted at all incubation temperatures and that is generally bacteriologically inert, being decomposed or liquefied only by a few varieties of marine bacteria. In these respects it is more suitable than gelatin; a 15 per cent. solution of gelatin melts at 24° C. and gelatin is decomposed by many proteolytic bacteria. Agar does not add to the nutritive properties of a medium and a suitable agar should be free from growth-promoting as well as growth-inhibiting substances.

The melting and solidifying points of agar solutions are not the same. At the concentrations normally used, most bacteriological agars melt at about 95° C. and solidify only when cooled to about 42° C. The ability of agar to be melted is an advantage compared with the inability of serum or egg to be melted, and the low solidifying point of agar allows heat-sensitive nutrients to be added to it in the molten state at temperatures as low as 45° C.

CONTAINERS FOR MEDIA AND CULTURES

Flasks stoppered with cotton-wool, test-tubes stoppered with cotton-wool or with slip-on metal caps, and screw-capped bottles of different capacity and shape can be used as containers for media and cultures. Metal caps are satisfactory provided the medium is stored not longer than a few weeks and they are economical because they can be used repeatedly. Cotton-wool plugs must be discarded after each use but they have the advantage that medium can be stored longer. Air passing into the tubes as a result of changes in temperature or pressure, as when cultures are incubated anaerobically, is filtered through the wool; such protection is not provided by metal caps. Screw-capped bottles are air-tight and thus do not allow their contents to dry out during storage. Media in bottles need not be stored in a cold room and can be kept almost indefinitely. Bottles are particularly valuable in large laboratories where culture media are prepared in quantity for distribution.

Screw-capped bottles are made of clear white flint glass, the neck having an external screw thread. The caps are made of aluminium and each has a rubber washer 3 mm. thick, of special rubber that is not inhibitory to bacterial growth. A list of bottles that covers practically all needs is given. With the exception of the 2-oz. squat bottle, these are made by United Glass, Ltd., and may be bought only from retailers. The 4-oz. is the standard blood culture bottle and perforated caps may be obtained for these. The 2-oz. squat is suitable for specimens of sputum. The 40- and 20-oz. rounds are also used for intravenous solutions such as saline and glucose saline.

Glassware must be thoroughly cleaned before use for culture media and new glassware requires special treatment to remove free alkali (page 862). Most of the bottles listed are supplied cleaned and washed by a special process. The rubber washers have been well boiled and the caps already fitted. No further treatment is necessary before they are used. This saving of time is of especial value where large quantities of culture media are produced. The cardboard cartons in which the bottles are supplied keep them clean during storage, either empty or containing medium, and are useful for dispatching medium. When bottles are cleaned for re-use the old caps and washers should be discarded and replaced with new caps and washers. If undamaged caps are to be re-used they should be thoroughly washed and dried, care being taken to see that there is no moisture between the washer and the cap, since this can interfere with sterilisation.

Copper salts are inimical to the growth of many organisms and copper utensils should not be used for the preparation of media. Heavily tinned copper articles are safe to use, but if the tinning shows signs of wear the article must be re-tinned.

Bottle	Capacity in ml.	Cap	Washer
1 gallon, narrow mouth .	4600	Special, to fit	"Compo" cork and "resistol"
80 oz. round . . .	2400	KN 31	Rubber
40 oz. round . . .	1190	KN 31	Rubber
20 oz. round . . .	600	KN 31	Rubber
10 oz. round . . .	290	KN 350	Rubber
5 oz. round . . .	140	KN 350	Rubber
1 oz. round (H 53), McCartney . . .	28	KN 135	Rubber
½ oz. round . . .	15	KN 132	Rubber
¼ oz. round, bijou . .	6	KN 132	Rubber
1 oz. Universal container .	28	KN 86	Rubber
8 oz. medical flat . .	236	KN 350	Rubber
6 oz. medical flat . .	180	KN 349	Rubber
4 oz. medical flat . .	125	KN 349	Rubber
3 oz. medical flat . .	85	KN 359	Rubber
2 oz. medical flat . .	60	KN 359	Rubber
1 oz. medical flat . .	33	KN 347	Rubber
2 oz. squat (J1/2)[1] . . .	65	2 in.	Cardboard or rubber

[1] The 2-oz. squat bottle, and a range of squat forms from 1-16 oz. capacity with aluminium screw-caps, are obtainable from Solmedia Ltd., 31, Orford Road, London, E.17.

FORMS IN WHICH LIQUID AND SOLID MEDIA ARE USED

Tubing and bottling of liquid media

Liquid media may be distributed in test-tubes with slip-on metal caps or cotton-wool plugs, the tubes being about half-filled. If bottles are to be used, broth or peptone water in 2·5 ml. amounts and fermentation media in 3 ml. amounts may be distributed in bijou bottles. Media required in 5 or 10 ml. amounts may be put in 1-oz. bottles and 50 to 100 ml. amounts of media in 3- or 5-oz. bottles. It is convenient to store liquid media in 250 ml. amounts in 10-oz. bottles but larger amounts in larger bottles may be desired.

Tubing, bottling and pouring plates of solid media

Solid media may be distributed in test-tubes with slip-on metal caps or cotton-wool plugs. The shape in which the medium is allowed to solidify depends on the method of inoculation for which it is to be used. The commonest shape is the "slope" or "slant", which provides a large surface area of medium for inoculation. For $6 \times \frac{5}{8}$ in. test-tubes, 5 ml. of medium is sufficient and it is allowed to set at such an angle that there is a thick butt at the bottom (Fig. 52). When a large number of tubes of agar have to be sloped, special trays that allow the tubes to be laid at the correct angle are useful and, moreover, the tubes can be stacked one upon another so that very little bench space is required during solidification. After cooling, fresh agar slopes contain "water of condensation" at the foot of the tube, and the tubes should be stored and handled in the vertical position to prevent the liquid from flowing over the surface of the medium or entering the cotton-wool plug or metal cap.

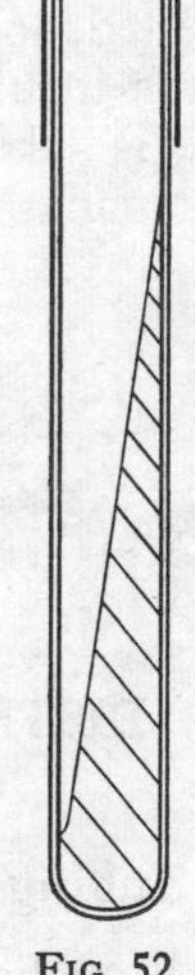

FIG. 52

Slope of solid medium in test-tube. A cotton-wool plug may be used instead of the slip-on metal cap illustrated here.

If the medium is to be used for a "stab" or "shake" culture the test-tube is half filled with the medium, which is allowed to solidify in the upright position. The most frequent use of media solidified with gelatin is as a stab culture.

Screw-capped bottles can be substituted for test-tubes. The amounts of medium for slopes in 1-oz. and bijou bottles are 5 ml. and 2·5 ml. respectively. The medium may be allowed to set at an angle to form a butt as in test-tubes, but it is easier to inoculate with a loop if it is parallel to the side of the bottle (Fig. 53). For stab or shake cultures 1-oz. bottles are half-filled with medium.

Agar media stored in 4-, 6- or 8-oz. medical flat bottles melt much more quickly than agar in 3-, 5- or 10-oz. round bottles.

Where a large surface is necessary as in the separation of organisms from mixtures the medium is allowed to solidify in the form of a thin layer in a Petri dish. Solid media in Petri dishes are often called "plates". For a dish of $3\frac{1}{2}$ in. (88 mm.) diameter, 14 ml. of medium is usually ample and it is convenient to store 100 ml. amounts in 4- or 5-oz. screw-capped bottles, sufficient for seven plates. The melted medium is poured into the dishes on a flat surface and the dishes are left undisturbed until the medium has set. In separating organisms from mixed cultures by plating, it is essential

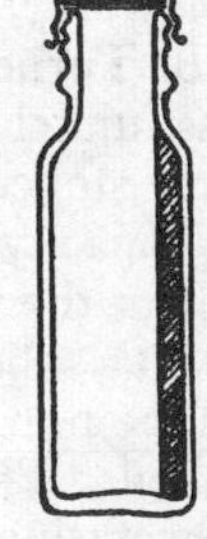

FIG. 53

Slope of solid medium in screw-capped bottle.

that the surface of the medium should be dry. When plates have been poured, the steam from the hot liquid condenses on the surface of the medium and this moisture is undesirable. It is removed by drying the poured and set plates in a warming or drying cabinet at 37° C. for 1 hr., or at 65° C. for 15 to 30 min., depending on the medium. Suitable cabinets are available from manufacturers of food catering equipment. A bacteriological incubator may be used, but this is less efficient since it is not provided with a means of escape for the moist air. The lid of the dish is first laid down; the portion containing the medium is then inverted, so that the surface of the medium is downwards and placed in the incubator with the free edge resting on the lid (Fig. 54). If care is taken to avoid disturbing dust, there is very little risk of contamination of the medium by air organisms.

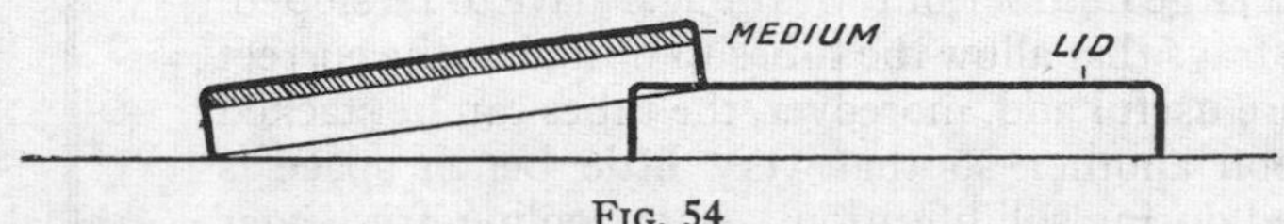

FIG. 54
The drying of an agar plate before inoculation.

DISTRIBUTION OF MEDIA INTO TUBES, BOTTLES AND PLATES

Tubing and bottling of media without sterile precautions

All media are distributed as liquids, gelatin and agar media being melted, and serum and egg media being distributed before they are solidified by heat. For safety it is usual to cool melted agar media to 55° C. before distribution.

Most media are tubed or bottled without sterile precautions being taken. Clean but unsterile glassware is used, and the medium and container together are subsequently sterilised by heat. A suitable apparatus is a 6-in. glass funnel, fixed in a burette stand, with a short length of rubber tubing and a glass delivery nozzle fitted to the stem and controlled by a pinchcock.

However, an automatic filler devised by T. H. Ayling and supplied by R. B. Turner & Co., London, can be recommended. It consists of a glass funnel 7 in. in diameter, connected with rubber tubing to a metal 3-way stopcock which in turn is connected to an all-glass syringe of 15 ml. capacity (Fig. 55). The syringe is of the three-piece type, but without the nozzle, and the plunger is hollow, as the head of liquid will not lift a solid glass piston. The barrel is graduated to 15 ml. by 0·5 ml., and the numbers are so engraved as to be readable when the syringe is vertical. The syringe is connected to the stopcock by means of a metal screw fitting. A clamp secures the lower end of the syringe. The amount of fluid delivered is determined by the adjustable screw. The action of the filler is simple. The head of medium in the funnel forces up the plunger until it is stopped by the adjustable screw. The handle of the stopcock is then turned and the syringe empties itself under the weight of the plunger. Air bubbles in the syringe are removed by first filling the apparatus, and emptying and filling the syringe two or three times, manipulating the piston by hand while this is being done. The adjustable screw is then turned to deliver the correct amount. If a smoothly working syringe is used, very little head of pressure is necessary, and the height need not be greater than 18 inches. Once set, the accuracy of the filler is much greater than that of an ordinary pipette, and media can be tubed with great rapidity. It works equally well with melted agar or gelatin, provided that fresh hot supplies are available, and the syringe and stopcock are washed out immediately after use.

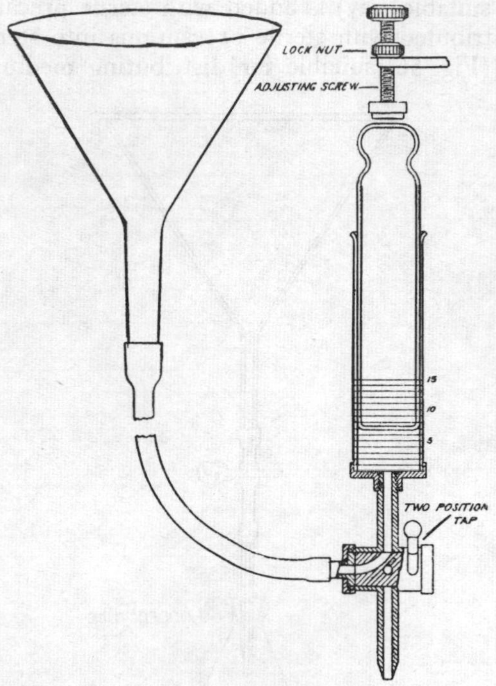

Fig. 55

Automatic filler for dispensing media without sterile precautions.

An electrically driven automatic dispenser designed by Struer can be obtained from Camlab (Glass) Ltd., Cambridge. With it, measured volumes from 0·2 to 20 ml. can be delivered at any chosen rate, or individually at the touch of a foot pedal, and media may be dispensed under sterile conditions.

Pouring of plates, and tubing and bottling of media with sterile precautions

Plates are always poured with sterile precautions. Bulk medium is prepared sterile and is poured into sterile Petri dishes. Care must be taken to avoid contamination from the air during pouring. It is desirable to pour plates on a bench in a small room free from draughts and preferably with ultraviolet radiation to reduce the number of bacteria in the air. Alternatively, an inoculation hood or cabinet, as described on p. 796 may be used. To reduce water of condensation on the Petri dish lids, the medium should be cooled to 52° C. before pouring.

Sterile precautions for tubing and bottling media are necessary if an ingredient of the medium is heat-labile, for example, certain sugars used in fermentation test media (see p. 813). The ingredients that are stable to heat are prepared and sterilised, the unstable ingredient (previously sterilised in a suitable way) is added with sterile precautions and the medium is distributed with sterile precautions into sterile containers. An apparatus (Fig. 56) suitable for distributing medium with sterile

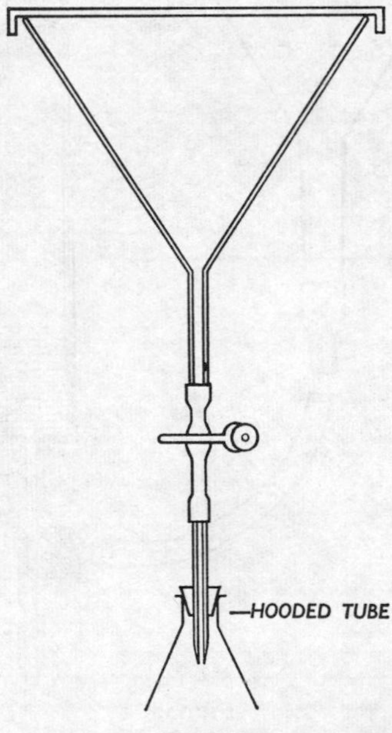

FIG. 56
Apparatus for dispensing media with sterile precautions.

precautions is a hooded tube attached by means of rubber tubing and a pinchcock to a funnel covered with a large Petri dish lid. The whole apparatus is wrapped in paper and sterilised. The Petri dish lid protects sterile medium in the funnel and the hood protects the medium as it is distributed to sterile tubes or bottles.

Alternatively the heat-stable part of the medium may be distributed into clean glassware without sterile precautions and then be sterilised. The sterile unstable ingredient, for example, a sugar, can later be added from a sterile graduated pipette or an apparatus incorporating a filter, a siphon and a hooded pipette (Fig. 57).

Apparatus for dispensing small quantities of sterile ingredients

A special stainless-steel metal fitting is adapted to a 10-oz. bottle with a screw neck. It consists of a straight piece of tube (A), with a curved side-arm (B); around this is a slightly wider tube (C), with a side-arm

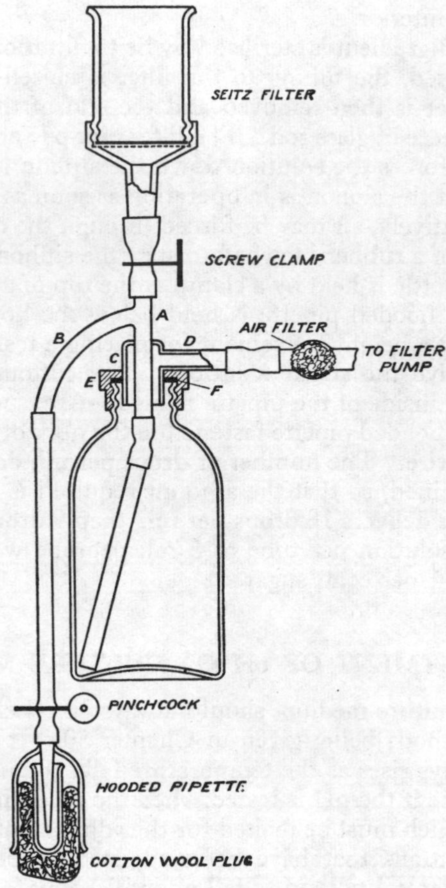

Fig. 57
Apparatus for adding small quantities of sterile ingredients to media.

(D), fitted to a screw-cap (E) which screws on to the bottle, a rubber washer (F) ensuring an air-tight joint. To the upper end of tube A is connected a Seitz filter by means of a short piece of pressure tubing furnished with a screw-clamp, and attached to the lower end by means of a short piece of rubber tubing is a glass tube, 5 mm. in diameter, reaching to the bottom of the bottle. To the side-arm B is connected a piece of rubber tubing furnished at the other end with a pinchcock and hooded pipette. The hooded pipette is closed with a cotton-wool stopper containing a small glass test-tube to cover the delivery tube. The side-arm D is connected with pressure tubing to a cotton-wool air filter, the other end of which is to be attached to a filter pump. The joints are bound with tinned copper wire and the whole apparatus, as figured, is wrapped in kraft paper. If silicone rubber is used for all the fittings it can be sterilised in the hot air oven. Otherwise it must be autoclaved with a little water (a few drops) in the bottle to provide steam to drive out air from the interior.

The unstable ingredient is sterilised by Seitz filtration and, before the pressure is released, the tubing to the filter is closed with the screw-clamp. The filter is then removed and the end of the rubber tubing plugged with a piece of glass rod. The filter pump is now disconnected; the air pressure forces the solution down the siphon tube as far as the pinchcock so that the siphon is in operation as soon as the pinchcock is opened. Alternatively, air may be forced through the cotton-wool filter on D by means of a rubber blowball to start the siphon action. In use, the neck of the bottle is held by a clamp at the top of a tall retort stand. The stem of the hooded pipette is held below the bottle by means of another clamp, at a height convenient for placing a test-tube (or bottle) under it to receive the sterile solution. The cotton-wool stopper is removed and the inside of the pipette flamed. After use, the stopper is replaced and the hooded pipette fastened to the neck of the bottle with a piece of copper wire. The number of drops per ml. delivered from the pipette is determined, so that the amount required is easily estimated. Thus, if a pipette delivers 18 drops per ml., then 9 drops (0·5 ml.) of 10 per cent. sugar solution per tube of 5 ml. peptone water gives a final concentration of 1 per cent. sugar.

ADJUSTMENT OF pH OF CULTURE MEDIA

The pH of a culture medium should always be checked and adjusted if necessary, methods being given in Chapter 50. It should be noted that the pH always rises as the temperature falls and allowance for this rise must be made if the pH is tested when the medium is hot, as is the case with agar which must be melted for the adjustment of pH. During autoclaving, solutions that have been adjusted to be a little on the alkaline side of neutrality tend to fall about 0·1 unit.

STERILISATION OF PREPARED MEDIA

The choice of method to be used to sterilise a medium depends on whether or not the ingredients are decomposed by heat. If autoclaving will not damage the medium, it is the best method of sterilisation, and its application was discussed in Chapter 46 (p. 704).

The sterilisation time at a particular temperature is the sum of the heat penetration time, which is variable, and the holding time, which is constant for each temperature. The heat penetration time, and consequently the sterilisation time, varies greatly with the volume of medium and also with the container. For test tubes containing 10 ml. of medium, a sterilisation time of 15 min. at 121° C., or 35 min. at 115° C., is required. McCartney bottles containing 10 ml. of medium require 20 min. at 121° C. Larger amounts of medium require longer sterilisation times and so do small amounts of medium in large containers. Sterilisation times at 121° C. given in this chapter are based on the following table. Molten agar requires the same sterilisation time as liquid media; but if agar is solid, 5 to 10 min. must be added for melting.

Volume of medium	Container	
	Flask	Bottle
10 ml.	15 min.	20 min.
100 ml.	20 min.	25 min.
500 ml.	25 min.	30 min.
1 l.	30 min.	40 min.

Sterilisation times at 121° C.

Tubes and bottles of medium must be put in the autoclave so that steam has free access to them. Wire crates are suitable holders, but tins are unsuitable unless holes have been punched in them. Care must be taken that bottles of medium are not packed tightly in a holder, otherwise breakages will occur.

Sometimes lower temperatures, such as 115° C., for times ranging from 10 to 20 min. are recommended for "sterilisation" of media containing ingredients that are not very stable to heat. These conditions are not strictly reliable for sterilisation and should be used only for media distributed in small quantities. They are usually satisfactory because it is unlikely that many heat-resistant spores would be present in media prepared under clean conditions.

Steaming at 100° C., either for a long time, *e.g.* 90 min., on one occasion or for shorter times on several occasions, is not a sure way of sterilising media. Spores are not necessarily destroyed at 100° C. and will not be destroyed by successive heatings at 100° C. unless they are incubated in the intervening periods under conditions in which they will germinate to yield heat-sensitive vegetative organisms.

If any of the ingredients of a medium are liable to be spoiled by autoclaving, the complete medium should not be sterilised by heat. In such cases, it is usual to autoclave the heat-resistant ingredients of the medium and to add the sterile heat-sensitive ingredients with sterile precautions. Some heat-sensitive ingredients such as blood, serum or egg-yolk can be obtained sterile from natural sources. Others must be sterilised by filtration through a bacterial filter (Chapter 46, p. 697).

Some media that cannot be autoclaved contain ingredients that are inhibitory to the most probable contaminants. These media are sometimes prepared without the sterilisation of some ingredients, reliance being placed on the inhibitors to suppress contaminants. The method is usually successful but must always be regarded as less than ideal.

INSPISSATION OF SERUM AND EGG MEDIA

The serum in Löffler's medium and the egg in media such as Löwenstein-Jensen medium are usually solidified in an apparatus called an inspissator. It consists of a water-jacketed copper box, the temperature of which can be regulated automatically. The serum or egg medium is tubed and placed in special racks, so that the tubes are at the correct angle for forming slopes. The temperature used is between 75° and 85° C. At this temperature the protein is completely solidified, but the temperature is not so high as to cause bubbles of steam to disrupt the surface of the medium. As medium in tubes is apt to dry if kept in the inspissator for any time, a small opening should be present in the inner wall communicating with the top of the water-chamber above the level of the water. Water vapour can enter the interior of the inspissator and the medium is kept moist. Electric inspissators without a water-jacket do not yield such satisfactory media if tubes with cotton-wool stoppers are used.

VARIETIES OF CULTURE MEDIA

1. *Defined synthetic media.* Chemically defined media are used for various experimental purposes. They are prepared exclusively from pure chemical substances and their exact composition is known. The ingredients should be of analytical reagent quality and are dissolved in distilled or demineralised water.

Simple synthetic media contain a carbon and energy source such as glucose or lactic acid; an inorganic source of nitrogen, usually in the form of ammonium chloride, phosphate or sulphate; and various inorganic salts in a buffered aqueous solution. They provide the basic essentials for the growth of many non-parasitic heterotrophs, but they will not support growth of most kinds of parasitic bacteria. *Complex synthetic media* incorporate, in addition, certain amino acids, purines, pyrimidines and other growth factors. They can therefore be used for the growth of more exacting bacteria.

2. *Routine laboratory media.* The majority of organisms to be studied in medical bacteriology are either pathogens or commensals of the human body, and in order to obtain suitable growths the artificial culture medium should provide nutrients and a pH (about 7·2) approximating to those of the tissues and body fluids. For routine purposes many of these requirements are supplied by aqueous extracts of meat and the products of digestion of protein.

Basal media such as nutrient broth and peptone water are simple routine laboratory media. *Enriched media* are prepared to meet the nutritional requirements of more exacting bacteria by the addition of substances such as blood, serum and egg to a basal medium. *Selective media* contain substances that inhibit or poison all but a few types of bacteria. They facilitate the isolation of particular species from a mixed inoculum. If a liquid medium favours the multiplication of a particular species, either by containing enrichments that selectively favour it or inhibitory substances that suppress competitors, cultures from mixed inocula are called *enrichment* cultures. These cultures fail to indicate the proportion of the species present in the inoculum. *Indicator media* incorporate some substance that is changed visibly as a result of the metabolic activities of particular organisms. Combinations of enriched media with selective agents and indicator systems are frequently used in the diagnostic laboratory.

COMMON INGREDIENTS OF CULTURE MEDIA

Information on the preparation and composition of commercial products used in culture media is given in a report edited by Sykes (1956).

Water.—Tap water is often suitable for culture media, particularly if it has a low mineral content, but if the local supply is found unsuitable, glass-distilled or demineralised water must be used instead. Small amounts of copper are highly inhibitory to bacterial growth so that copper-distilled water cannot be used for media. Suitable demineralisers are manufactured by the Permutit Co. Ltd., Chiswick, London.

Agar.—Agar is prepared in several countries from a variety of seaweeds, *Gelidium*, *Eucheuma*, *Pterocladia* and others, the weed being dried, extracted by hot-water processes, clarified, dried and finally supplied as the dried strands or as a powder. There are considerable differences in the properties of the agars manufactured in different places, and even between different batches from the same source. Japanese and New Zealand agars are the most generally used. Japanese agar yields a gel of suitable firmness at a concentration of about 2 per cent., and New Zealand agar at about 1·2 per cent. The exact concentration to be used may require some adjustment according to the batch of agar and also according to the other constituents of the medium. *In the formulae for media given in this book, the amount of agar is stated as for Japanese agar powder: if New Zealand agar is used, the amount will be barely two-thirds as much.*

The chief component of agar is a long-chain polysaccharide, mainly composed of d-galactopyranose units. It also contains a variety of impurities including inorganic salts, a small amount of protein-like material and sometimes traces of long-chain fatty acids which are inhibitory to growth. The minerals present are mainly magnesium and calcium, and agar is thought to exist as the magnesium or calcium sulphate esters of the polysaccharide.

In preparing agar media, the appropriate amount of agar powder or fibre is added to the liquid medium and dissolved by placing the mixture in a steamer at 100° C. for 1 hr.

Most agars dissolve to give a clear solution but sometimes it is necessary to filter off particulate impurities and, possibly, excess phosphates from the nutrient liquid. The hot agar solution, preferably first adjusted to pH 8·0 and held at 100° C. for 30 min. to precipitate phosphates, is filtered before it can cool and is re-adjusted to pH 7·4. For smaller amounts a hardened filter paper that is rapid in passing fluid and strong when wet, is used. A recommended grade is "Hyduro" 904½, supplied by J. Barcham Green, Ltd., Maidstone, England. For larger amounts, paper pulp or cellulose wadding enclosed in muslin is better, a fresh filter being prepared on each occasion. A suitable paper pulp is "White Heather" brand or T. B. Ford's filter pulp, both of which are sold in slabs. A suitable cellulose wadding is "Cellosene" supplied in sheet form by Robinson & Sons, Ltd., Chesterfield. A porcelain Buchner-type filter funnel with a flat perforated platform about 10 in. in diameter is convenient for 5–10 litre quantities. Place two 10 in. disks of cellulose wadding, one on top of the other, on a 24-in. square of muslin and fold over the excess muslin to enclose them completely. Invert the disk-like bundle and press it into position on the platform of the filter, ensuring a good fit at the edges. Pour some hot water through the filter and then heat it at 100° C. in the steamer at the same time as the agar solution, so that it is hot at the time of its use. Without allowing any time for cooling, pour the whole of the hot agar solution quickly through the filter without assistance by suction. If a large Buchner funnel is not available, quantities up to five litres may be filtered using a 10-in. conical glass funnel, the lower third of which is filled with pebbles or glass beads to form a supporting platform for the filter material. Paper pulp or cellulose wadding wrapped in muslin to form a bundle about 2 in. deep is pressed into position on the platform and fitted closely to all sides of the filter funnel. Moist pulp may be superimposed to ensure that the filter is not leaky.

Agar can be added to any nutrient liquid medium if the advantages of a solid medium are desired. Nutrients that are not damaged by autoclaving may be added to the medium before dissolving the agar. Such media can be sterilised and allowed to set for storage, being remelted in the steamer before use. However, nutrients that are damaged by autoclaving must be prepared sterile, separately from the agar base. The sterilised agar base can be melted in the steamer and cooled to about 45–50° C. before adding any heat-labile ingredients, but once these are added the medium must at once be distributed for its final use because it cannot be remelted without damaging the heat-sensitive ingredients.

Agar is hydrolysed to products that do not solidify on cooling if it is heated at a low pH. Agar usually does not alter the pH of the medium to which it is added but if it contains free acid this must be neutralised before it is autoclaved. For media whose pH is about 5, such as those for lactobacilli and fungi, heating should be reduced to a minimum after the agar is in an acid solution. After autoclaving, the medium may be allowed to solidify in bulk but it should be remelted with as little heating as possible and then be wholly distributed for its final use; it should not be partly used, allowed to solidify and later heated a third time.

Peptone.—Peptone consists of water-soluble products obtained from lean meat or other protein material, such as heart muscle, casein, fibrin or soya flour, by digestion with, mainly, the proteolytic enzymes, pepsin, trypsin or papain. The important constituents are peptones, proteoses, amino acids, a variety of inorganic salts, including phosphates, potassium and magnesium, and certain accessory growth factors, including nicotinic acid and riboflavin. Peptone is supplied as a golden granular powder with a low moisture content, preferably under 5 per cent., and usually a slightly acid reaction, giving a pH between 5 and 7 in a 1 per cent. solution. It is hygroscopic and soon becomes sticky when exposed to air; stock bottles should therefore be kept firmly closed and weighing of loose powder rapidly completed. According to the starting materials and mode of preparation, the brands of peptone supplied by different manufacturers show appreciable differences in composition and growth-promoting properties; moreover, variations may occur between different batches of one brand.

The essential requirements of a good peptone have not yet been fully defined, but include the ability to support the growth of moderately exacting bacteria from small inocula (e.g. *Staph. aureus*, *Strept. pyogenes* and *Sh. dysenteriae* type 1), the absence of fermentable carbohydrates, a low content of contaminating bacteria and a very low content of copper. Apart from the standard grades of bacteriological peptone, some manufacturers supply special grades of peptone recommended for particular purposes, *e.g.* "Neopeptone", "Proteose peptone", mycological peptone, etc.

The analysis of a suitable bacteriological peptone (Oxoid) has been supplied by the makers as follows:

Total nitrogen	14·5 per cent.
Total proteose nitrogen (sat. $ZnSO_4$) .	1·9 per cent.
Primary proteose nitrogen (half-sat. $ZnSO_4$)	0·14 per cent.
Amino acid nitrogen (formol titration) .	1·7 per cent.
Tryptophane	1·2 per cent.
Ash	5·5 per cent.
Chloride	1·0 per cent.
Phosphate (as P_2O_5)	1·3 per cent.
Calcium	0·13 per cent.
Magnesium	0·07 per cent.
Copper	0·0010 per cent.
Iron	0·0075 per cent.
Zinc	0·0025 per cent.
Sulphur (total)	0·68 per cent.
Ether-soluble extract	0·03 per cent.
Nicotinic acid	75 μg. per g.
Riboflavin	50 μg. per g.
Carbohydrate (fermentation test) . .	nil
Moisture	less than 5 per cent.
pH of a 1 per cent. solution . . .	5·9 to 6·1
(Indole production test, good reaction)	

Casein Hydrolysate.—This consists largely of the amino acids obtained by hydrolysis of the milk protein, "casein". It also contains phosphate and other salts, and certain growth factors. Hydrolysis is effected either with hydrochloric acid, when the product is neutralised with sodium carbonate and so becomes very rich in sodium chloride, or with a proteolytic enzyme (trypsin). The acid hydrolysate is the poorer nutritionally because tryptophane is largely destroyed during the hydrolysis and some other amino acids are reduced in amount; tryptophane must therefore be added to the medium to make it suitable for tryptophane-requiring bacteria. The more expensive enzymic hydrolysate contains abundant tryptophane and the full range of amino acids, and does not require such supplementation. Casein hydrolysate may be substituted for peptone in broth and other media. It is of particular use in experimental work where a nearly defined medium is required, since its composition is more constant and more fully known than that of other peptones. Thus it may be added to a minimal synthetic medium to render it suitable for growth of exacting bacteria.

Meat Extract.—A commercially prepared meat extract known as Lab-Lemco is used as a substitute for an infusion of fresh meat. Meat extract is manufactured by a method derived from that invented by Liebig. Finely divided lean beef is held in boiling water for a short time while its readily soluble constituents pass into solution and form the unconcentrated extract. This is freed of excess fat and then concentrated by evaporation to a dark viscid paste containing 70–80 per cent.of solids. The product contains a wide variety of water-soluble compounds, including protein degradation products, *e.g.* gelatin, albumoses, peptones, proteoses and amino acids, and other nitrogen compounds such as creatine, creatinine, carnosine, anserine, purines and glutathione (total N about 10 per cent.); it also contains many mineral salts (KH_2PO_4 and NaCl most abundantly), accessory growth factors (*e.g.* thiamine, nicotinic acid, riboflavine, pyridoxine, pantothenic acid and choline) and certain amounts of carbohydrates. The required quantity of the sticky extract is conveniently weighed on a piece of clean paper and put with the paper into the water for solution; the paper is subsequently removed from the broth.

Yeast Extract.—Commercial yeast extract is prepared from washed cells of brewers' or bakers' yeast. These are allowed to undergo autolysis, which is initiated by mild heating (*e.g.* at 55° C.) or, in some cases, are hydrolysed with hydrochloric acid or a proteolytic enzyme. After removal of the cell walls by filtration or centrifugation, the extract is evaporated to a thick dark paste containing about 70 per cent. of solids. It contains a wide range of amino acids (amounting to nearly 50 per cent. of its mass), growth factors (especially of the vitamin B group) and inorganic salts (particularly potassium and phosphate); over 10 per cent. of carbohydrates are present, including glycogen, trehalose and pentoses. Yeast extract is used mainly as a comprehensive source of growth factors and may be substituted for meat extract in culture media.

Blood.—Blood for use in media must be collected with aseptic precautions adequate to exclude bacterial contamination and preserve the blood in its original sterile condition. Any attempt to sterilise blood by heat would lead to disintegration of the cells, coagulation of cell and serum proteins, and denaturation of the red haemoglobin to brown derivatives. It must be rendered non-coagulating by defibrination or by the addition of citrate or oxalate; the former is recommended because it involves no additive that might alter the nutritive properties of the medium.

Sterile horse blood can be obtained commercially, defibrinated from Evans Medical Supplies Ltd., Liverpool, and oxalated from Burroughs Wellcome Ltd. Alternatively blood may be collected from rabbits and other laboratory animals, sheep, oxen and horses at the abattoir, or from man.

Small amounts of blood may be obtained from rabbits, up to 20–30 ml. from the ear vein and about 50 ml. per kg. body weight by cardiac puncture. The procedures for withdrawing blood aseptically in these ways are described on p. 1008. The blood should be collected into a sterile bottle containing glass beads; as soon as this is half full, it is stoppered and shaken for 5 min. to separate the fibrin.

Very large quantities of sterile blood are obtained from sheep or horses. A cannula or wide-bore needle is inserted into the external jugular vein. If a sheep is selected, the wool is clipped from the side of the neck and the part shaved. Contamination can be minimised by placing a bag made of waterproof material over the head of the animal. It is best to use a cannula connected with rubber tubing to a screw-capped bottle containing glass beads or anticoagulant, the whole being enclosed in kraft paper and sterilised. The vein may be made prominent by pressure on the lower part of the side of the neck. The skin over the vein is carefully sterilised with soap and water and then alcohol. The cannula is inserted into the vein and the requisite amount of blood removed. Horses are treated similarly except that it is advisable to make a small incision with a sharp knife in the skin over the vein. The cannula is then more easily introduced.

For defibrination, a bottle containing glass beads is half filled with the blood, stoppered at once and shaken continuously for 5 min. Oxalated blood is prepared by bleeding the animals into bottles containing 10 ml. of a 10 per cent. solution of neutral potassium oxalate per litre of blood.

The sterile blood is immediately distributed in 5 or 10 ml. amounts in sterile ½-oz. screw-capped bottles and stored in the refrigerator. It will keep for up to two months. It must not be allowed to freeze or the corpuscles may be lysed.

Fildes' Peptic Digest of Blood.—Peptic digestion of blood liberates nutrients from red cells. Fildes' digest is prepared as follows:

Sodium chloride, NaCl, 0·85 per cent. aqueous	150 ml.
Hydrochloric acid, HCl, pure	6 ml.
Defibrinated sheep blood	50 ml.
Pepsin (B.P. granulated)	1 g.
Sodium hydroxide, NaOH, 20 per cent. aqueous	About 12 ml.
Chloroform	0·5 ml.

In a stoppered bottle, mix the saline, acid, blood and pepsin. Heat at 55° C. for 2–24 hr. Add sodium hydroxide until a sample of the mixture diluted with water gives a permanganate red colour with cresol red indicator. Add pure hydrochloric acid drop by drop until a sample of the mixture shows almost no change of colour with cresol red but a definite red tint with phenol red. It is important to avoid excess of acid. Add chloroform and shake the mixture vigorously.

This peptic digest of blood keeps well for months.

Serum.—Serum for use in media need not be collected with aseptic precautions because it can be Seitz-filtered to sterilise it. Sterile horse serum can be obtained commercially.

If serum is to be collected without aseptic precautions, a wide-mouthed stoppered bottle is taken to the abattoir at a time when animals, preferably sheep, are being killed. After the neck vessels have been severed, the blood is allowed to flow for a short time and then the stream from the carotid artery is allowed to spurt directly into the bottle. When filled, the bottle is stoppered and returned carefully to the laboratory. The clot is then separated from the sides of the bottle by means of a stiff wire. The blood is kept overnight in the refrigerator and the clear serum is then pipetted off. At some abattoirs serum is prepared in bulk from blood allowed to coagulate in open trays; this is liable to greater bacterial contamination, but may be used when large quantities are required.

Serum may also be prepared from unsterile defibrinated or oxalated blood which does not clot on standing. It is stored overnight in the cold to allow settling of the corpuscles, and the serum or plasma is siphoned off into a Winchester quart bottle. Plasma requires warming to about 37° C., the addition of 22·5 ml. of a 4 per cent. solution of calcium chloride per litre and shaking, preferably on a machine, until the fibrin has separated.

Serum is sterilised by filtration through a Seitz filter using a sterilising grade of Ford's Sterimat asbestos-cellulose disk, and may be stored at 3–5° C. in the refrigerator until required for use. It is convenient to store serum in a large sterile screw-capped bottle of 1–5 litres capacity, fitted with siphon delivery tube and hooded pipette, as described on p. 730.

Small quantities of serum may be prepared without filtration from sterile rabbit blood. The blood is collected into a sterile container and allowed to clot. Free contraction of the clot is assisted if the container is lined with agar; 10 ml. of melted 1·5 per cent. agar in physiological saline (0·85 per cent. NaCl) is spread inside an 8 × 1 in. boiling tube by rotating the tube until the agar sets as a thin layer. When the blood is fully coagulated the serum is removed with a sterile pipette. It may require centrifuging to remove any remaining red cells. It can be stored in sterile screw-capped bottles, preferably fresh but it can be heated at 56° C. for 1 hr. without being coagulated.

FORMULAE FOR THE PREPARATION OF CULTURE MEDIA

DEHYDRATED CULTURE MEDIA

Culture media are available in dehydrated form from commercial firms. These are especially convenient for small laboratories where facilities for medium making are inadequate. The dehydrated medium is dissolved in water according to the directions supplied, and the resulting preparation is tubed or bottled and sterilised in the usual way. While such media are satisfactory for most purposes, they are not equal in quality to freshly made culture media, particularly those made from fresh meat.

SYNTHETIC MEDIA

Minimal Medium of Davis and Mingioli and its Variants

This medium is suitable for growth of a wide variety of bacteria for research purposes.

Basal medium

Glucose, sterile 10 per cent. solution	20 ml.
Dipotassium hydrogen phosphate, K_2HPO_4	7 g.
Potassium dihydrogen phosphate, KH_2PO_4	3 g.
Sodium citrate, $Na_3C_6H_5O_7.2H_2O$	0·5 g.
Magnesium sulphate, $MgSO_4.7H_2O$	0·1 g.
Ammonium sulphate, $(NH_4)_2\ SO_4$	1 g.
Agar, if required	20 g.
Distilled water to	1 l.

Trace element solution

Ferrous sulphate, $FeSO_4.7H_2O$	0·5 g.
Zinc sulphate, $ZnSO_4.7H_2O$	0·5 g.
Manganese sulphate, $MnSO_4.3H_2O$	0·5 g.
Sulphuric acid, H_2SO_4, 0·1 *N*	10 ml.
Distilled water	1 l.

Since glucose is partly decomposed when autoclaved in the presence of phosphate, it is added as a sterile solution after the remainder of the medium has been autoclaved.

Essential minerals other than those in the basal medium are likely to be present in sufficient amounts contaminating agar, water and other ingredients. If necessary, 5 ml. of the trace element solution and also 1 ml. of a 1 per cent. calcium chloride solution may be added per litre of medium.

The large phosphate content is required to buffer the acid that is formed by fermentation of glucose, the mixture shown giving a pH of 7·1. If it is required that the phosphate content of the medium should below, a citrate or bicarbonate buffer may be used. Thus a pH of 7·1 is obtained by incorporation of 0·3 per cent. of $NaHCO_3$ in the medium and incubation of the culture in an atmosphere containing 20 per cent. (v/v) of carbon dioxide.

Other sugars may be substituted for the glucose. The citrate may be omitted. Particular amino acids or growth factors may be added, or a mixture of the essential amino acids in the form of a vitamin-free casein hydrolysate, to give a nearly defined medium.

NUTRIENT BROTH

This is the basis of most media used in the study of the common pathogenic bacteria. There are three types of nutrient broth; meat infusion broth consisting of a watery extract of lean meat to which peptone is added; meat extract broth prepared as a mixture of commercial peptone and meat extract; and digest broth consisting of a watery extract of lean meat that has been digested with a proteolytic enzyme so that additional peptone need not be added.

MEAT INFUSION BROTHS

These are good broths but the amount of peptone in them makes them expensive compared with digest broths.

Standard Meat Infusion Broth

Lean meat, ox heart or beef	500 g.
Water	1 l.
Peptone	10 to 20 g.
Sodium chloride, NaCl	5 g.

The type of meat used is an important factor in determining the quality of the broth. It should be fresh, not frozen. Horse flesh is cheap, but is usually not so fresh, and, coming from older animals, is more fibrous than beef. In addition it contains a higher percentage of fermentable sugar which may make the broth unsuitable for many purposes, such as the preparation of toxins.

Carefully remove all fat from the meat and mince it as finely as possible. Add the minced meat to the water and extract for 24 hr. in the cold, for example in the refrigerator, then strain through muslin and express the meat residue. The extract is bright red and often has a thin surface layer of fat which can be removed by skimming with a piece of filter paper. Boil for 15 min. or steam at 100° C. for 2 hr. The extract becomes brown and turbid because haemoglobin is altered and soluble proteins are coagulated. Filter. If filtration is done when the medium is hot, use a hardened filter paper as recommended for agar. The extract should be clear and light yellow in colour. Add the peptone and salt and dissolve by heat. Filter. The reaction of the broth will be acid because of lactic acid from the meat. Adjust to the desired pH, usually 7·5, which will give a final pH of 7·4, distribute to tubes or bottles and sterilise by autoclaving at 121° C. for 15 min.

Wright's (1933) Meat Infusion Broth

This differs from ordinary meat infusion broth in that veal is used and the peptone and salt are present when the meat is extracted. A little (0·15 per cent.) glucose is added and the medium is especially good for the cultivation of the pneumococcus, although anaerobes such as the tetanus bacillus do not grow well in it.

MEAT EXTRACT BROTHS

These broths are the easiest and quickest to prepare. They can be varied widely but are usually less nutritive than infusion or digest broths. They are good for the preservation of stock cultures.

Standard Meat Extract Broth

Peptone	10 g.
Meat extract (Lab-Lemco)	10 g.
Sodium chloride, NaCl	5 g.
Water	1 l.

Mix the ingredients and dissolve them by heating briefly in the steamer. When cool, adjust the pH to 7·5–7·6. A precipitate of phosphates may appear and this may be removed by filtration through filter paper. If clarity of the broth is essential, the mixture should be adjusted to pH 8·0, heated at 100° C. for 30 min. to precipitate most of the phosphates, cooled, filtered and finally adjusted to pH 7·5. Distribute in tubes or bottles and sterilise by autoclaving at 121° C. for 15 min.

The medium should be clear. The presence of a deposit, generally of phosphates, does not interfere with the nutrient value of the medium, but it may hinder the recognition of slight bacterial growth indicated by a developing turbidity.

Modifications of Meat Extract Broth

The formula for meat extract broth may be varied. With less exacting bacteria, 0·5 per cent. of peptone and 0·3 per cent. of meat extract are sufficient, and if the peptone is of high quality it may be possible to omit the meat extract. Sodium chloride can be omitted without reducing the nutritive value of the medium, but then the broth is hypotonic enough to lyse red cells and is unsuitable as a base for blood agar.

Sometimes meat extract is replaced by yeast extract, or peptone is replaced by either casein hydrolysate or soya hydrolysate.

DIGEST BROTHS

Digest broths are economical and are good for obtaining luxuriant growths of exacting organisms. However, cultures tend to die out rapidly in them. The proteolytic enzyme used may be varied. Trypsin obtained from pancreas, and papain (Asheshov, 1941) obtained from paw-paw may be used, attention being paid to the optimum temperature and pH for activity of the enzyme.

Hartley's Broth

Trypsin is the proteolytic enzyme used to prepare this medium.

Pancreatic extract (Cole and Onslow)

Fresh pig pancreas	500 g.
Water	1500 ml.
Absolute alcohol or methylated spirit (see p. 644)	500 ml.
Concentrated hydrochloric acid, HCl . .	About 2 ml.

Remove the fat from the pancreas, mince it and mix it with the water and alcohol. Shake the mixture thoroughly in a large stoppered bottle and allow it to stand for three days at room temperature, shaking occasionally. Strain through muslin and filter through paper. Measure the volume of the filtrate and add 0·1 per cent. hydrochloric acid. This causes a cloudy precipitate which settles in a few days and can be filtered off, although this is not essential.

This extract keeps for about two months in stoppered bottles in the cold. If used at once there is no need to add acid, whose action is to retard the slow deterioration of the trypsin.

Preparation of complete medium

Lean meat, ox heart, or beef	1500 g.
Water	2500 ml.
Sodium carbonate, Na_2CO_3, 0·8 per cent. solution	2500 ml.
Pancreatic extract	50 ml.
Chloroform	50 ml.
Concentrated hydrochloric acid, HCl . .	40 ml.

Mix the meat and water and heat them in the steam steriliser until a temperature of 80° C. is reached. Add the sodium carbonate, cool to 45° C. and add the pancreatic extract and chloroform. Incubate the mixture at 37° C. for 6 hr. or 45° C. for 3 hr., stirring frequently. When digestion is complete, add the acid, steam at 100° C. for 30 min. and filter. The broth is stored in an acid condition in one-gallon screw-capped bottles with 0·25 per cent. of chloroform. Shake vigorously and frequently in the next two or three days. Store in a cool, dark place.

For use, adjust to pH 8·0 with normal caustic soda and steam at 100° C. for 1 hr. to precipitate phosphates. Filter while hot and allow to cool. Adjust the reaction to pH 7·6, distribute, and autoclave at 115° C. for 20 min.

Horse Flesh Digest Medium

This medium is a pancreatic digest of horse meat enriched by the addition of peptone and sterilised by Seitz filtration to preserve heat-sensitive substances. It is specially suitable for cultivating haemolytic streptococci when an abundant growth is required.

Horse flesh	900 g.
Water	3500 ml.
Sodium carbonate, Na_2CO_3	12 g.
Pancreatin	17·5 g.
Concentrated hydrochloric acid, HCl . .	20 ml.
Peptone, high quality	35 g.
Calcium chloride, $CaCl_2$	4·4 g.
Sodium bicarbonate, Na_2HCO_3 . . .	7 g.

Mince the meat and mix it with 1500 ml. of cold water, raising the temperature to 80° C. Add the remainder of the cold water and the sodium carbonate. Adjust the pH to 8·0, add the pancreatin and keep the mixture at 56° C. for 6 hr. Add the acid, boil at 100° C. for 30 min. to arrest digestion and filter. Add the peptone, adjust the pH to 8·0, add the calcium chloride, steam and filter when cold. Add the sodium bicarbonate and filter through a Seitz filter.

Store in bottles, first incubated at 37° C. to test for sterility.

NUTRIENT AGAR

Standard Nutrient Agar

Nutrient agar is nutrient broth solidified by the addition of agar. It should be noted that nutrient agar is frequently referred to as "agar", the context making clear that the agar-broth mixture is meant and not the pure, non-nutritive agar itself. Japanese agar yields a gel of suitable firmness at a concentration of about 2 per cent. and New Zealand agar at about 1·2 per cent.

Semi-Solid Agar

For special purposes agar is added to media in concentrations that are too low to solidify them. At 0·2–0·5 per cent. it yields a semi-solid medium through which motile, but not non-motile, bacteria may spread (see p. 835). At 0·05–0·1 per cent. it prevents convection currents and retards the diffusion of air into media used for anaerobic and microaerophilic organisms.

Concentrated Agar

If agar is added to media in concentrations greater than that necessary for solidification, "spreading" bacteria such as *Pr. vulgaris* and *Cl. tetani* will grow as discrete colonies. The necessary concentration must be determined by experiment but 6 per cent. of Japanese agar and 4 per cent. of New Zealand agar are usually satisfactory.

Concentrated agar takes longer to dissolve and to cool and is more difficult to handle than agar at ordinary concentrations.

STANDARD BASAL MEDIUM

CYLG medium

In this modification (Marshall and Kelsey, 1960) of the CCY medium of Gladstone and Fildes (1940) yeast autolysate and casein digest replace the meat extract and peptone of broth. It is a good nutrient medium, cheap and easy to prepare, versatile in use and as fully defined as possible in terms of known nutritional factors.

Inorganic salt solution

Magnesium sulphate, $MgSO_4.7H_2O$	4 g.
Manganese sulphate, $MnSO_4.4H_2O$	0·4 g.
Ferrous sulphate, $FeSO_4.7H_2O$	0·4 g.
Water	100 ml.
Sulphuric acid, 10 N H_2SO_4	2 drops

Dissolve the salts and acidify them.

Concentrate for storage

Casein digest (Oxoid Tryptone)	10 g.
Yeast autolysate (Marmite)	5 g.
Sodium glycerophosphate	10 g.
Potassium lactate, 50 per cent. w/w	10 ml.
Inorganic salt solution	5 ml.
Water to	100 ml.

Dissolve the ingredients. Filter. The concentrate can be stored in this form at room temperature without autoclaving provided a volatile preservative is added; 3–4 ml. per litre of carbon tetrachloride/toluene (1 : 1, v/v) is recommended.

Sterile glucose solution

Glucose	20 g.
Water	100 ml.

Dissolve and autoclave at 121° C. for 20 min. at a pH not greater than 7. Adding a drop of phosphoric acid ensures that the solution is not alkaline.

Double strength agar

Agar	40 g.
Water	1 l.

Dissolve the agar, filter if necessary and distribute 100 ml. amounts in 200 ml. bottles. Autoclave at 121° C. for 25 min.

Preparation of complete CYLG liquid medium

Concentrate	100 ml.
Water	900 ml.
Sterile glucose solution	10 ml.

Dilute the concentrate with water, autoclave it at 121° C. for 30 min. and add the glucose with sterile precautions.

Preparation of complete solid medium

Concentrate	20 ml.
Water	80 ml.
Double strength agar	100 ml.
Sterile glucose solution	2 ml.

Melt the agar, add the concentrate and water, autoclave at 121° C. for 20 min. and add the glucose with sterile precautions.

Preparation of supplemented CYLG media.—Additional ingredients such as blood or serum can replace part of the water when the concentrate is diluted. For MacConkey-type media, solutions of ingredients such as lactose, bile salts and neutral red replace some of the water, and glucose is omitted.

CARBOHYDRATE-FREE BASAL MEDIUM

Peptone Water

This medium is used chiefly as the basis for sugar fermentation media (see Chap. 48), since broth may contain a small amount of sugar derived from meat and it is essential that the basal medium to which various carbohydrates are added for fermentation tests should be free from natural sugars. It is also used to test the formation of indole.

Peptone	10 g.
Sodium chloride, NaCl	5 g.
Water	1 l.

Dissolve the ingredients in warm water, adjust the pH to 7·4–7·5 and filter. Distribute as required and autoclave at 121° C. for 15 min.

ENRICHED CULTURE MEDIA FOR GENERAL USE

Any additional enrichment may be added to nutrient broth or nutrient agar. Some of these enriched media are described here.

Blood Agar and Broth

Blood agar is widely used in medical bacteriology. It is especially suitable for the gonococcus, the haemophilic group of bacteria and other delicate pathogens. In addition to being an enriched medium, it is an indicator medium showing the haemolytic properties of bacteria such as *Strept. pyogenes*. It is generally poured as plates.

The medium is prepared by adding sterile blood to sterile nutrient agar that has been melted and cooled to 55° C. The appropriate amount of blood can be poured from a screw-capped bottle. No pipette is necessary as the screw cap keeps the lip of the bottle sterile.

The concentration of blood may be varied from 5 per cent. up to 50 per cent. for special purposes. Ten per cent. is the most usual concentration. Either human or animal blood may be used. Horse blood is the commonest.

A fairly thick layer of medium is required to prevent excessive drying during incubation and if this consists entirely of 10 per cent. blood agar, the medium is almost opaque when viewed by transmitted light and haemolysis is difficult to see. Double-layer blood agar overcomes this difficulty. A thin layer of melted nutrient agar, about 7 ml. for a 4-in. Petri dish, is poured and allowed to set. Then a similar thin layer of 10 per cent. blood agar is poured on top of the first layer. Any bubbles caused by the mixing of the blood and agar can easily be removed by drawing a Bunsen flame quickly across the surface of the medium in the dish.

Nutrient broth to which 5 to 10 per cent. of blood has been added with sterile precautions is occasionally used as an enriched liquid medium.

Heated Blood Agar ("*Chocolate Agar*")

This medium is suitable for *H. influenzae* and other organisms such as the pneumococcus. During heating the red cells are ruptured and nutrients are liberated.

It is prepared by heating 10 per cent. of sterile blood in sterile nutrient agar. Melt the agar, cool it in a waterbath at 75° C., add the blood and allow the medium to remain at 75° C., mixing the blood and agar by gentle agitation from time to time until the blood becomes chocolate-brown in colour, within about 10 min. Then pour as slopes or plates.

An alternative method of preparing plates of heated blood agar (Naylor, 1961) involves the heating of already poured and set plates of ordinary blood agar. The blood agar plates are held in an incubator or hot air oven at 55° C. for 1–2 hr. The exact time of heating required for "chocolating" depends on the conditions of heating and is determined by trial. Colonies of *H. influenzae* on this medium are larger than on medium heated at 75° C. and it is more conveniently prepared.

Serum Agar and Broth

Serum agar can be used to grow the more highly exacting pathogens. It is generally used as slopes.

It is prepared by adding 10 per cent. of sterile serum to sterile nutrient agar that has been melted and cooled to 55° C. In an emergency, a useful but less satisfactory serum medium can be made by running a few drops of sterile serum over the surface of a nutrient agar slope or plate.

Serum broth is frequently used for liquid medium cultures of the more highly exacting pathogens. It is prepared by adding 10 per cent. of sterile serum to sterile nutrient broth.

Sterile hydrocele fluid or ascitic fluid may be used instead of serum.

Fildes' Agar and Broth

Fildes' peptic digest of blood is added to nutrient broth or agar in the proportion of 2 to 5 per cent. after heating at 55° C. for 30 min. to remove the chloroform. It stimulates the growth of *Haemophilus* and *Cl. tetani* and the toxin production of *Cl. welchii.*

Glucose Agar and Broth

Glucose added to nutrient media promotes luxuriant growth of many organisms. It also acts as a reducing agent, and glucose agar is used for deep stab and shake cultures of anaerobes.

If glucose is added before autoclaving the medium, some darkening of it may occur. It is better to prepare a 20 per cent. solution of glucose separately, add a drop of phosphoric acid to ensure that the pH is not more than 7·0, and autoclave at 115° C. for 20 min. The sterile glucose can then be added with sterile precautions to the sterile basal medium.

Concentrations of 0·1, 0·25 and 1·0 per cent. glucose are used. One per cent. is the commonest.

p-Aminobenzoic Acid in Culture Media

There may be enough sulphonamide in the blood stream of patients treated with sulphonamide compounds to prevent the growth of bacteria when blood culture is carried out. As the sulphonamide is antagonised by *p*-aminobenzoic acid (p. 892), its addition to the medium will prevent the bacteriostatic action of the sulphonamide. It has also been found valuable in media for the isolation of pathogenic cocci. Even if no sulphonamide has been administered, *p*-aminobenzoic acid improves the nutritive qualities of the medium.

p-aminobenzoic acid is added in the proportion of 5 to 10 mg. per 100 ml. of medium. It is stable and withstands autoclaving.

MEDIA FOR THE CULTIVATION OF STAPHYLOCOCCI

Milk Agar

On this medium (Christie and Keogh, 1940) large characteristic colonies of staphylococci appear within 24 hr. Pigmentation is particularly marked and easily recognised against the opaque white background; this facilitates recognition of weakly aureus colonies.

Fresh milk	100 ml.
Sterile nutrient agar, containing 3 per cent. agar .	200 ml.

Heat the milk to 60° C., shake it, then sterilise it by autoclaving at 121° C. for 20 min. Repeated sterilisation should be avoided as this causes caramelisation with alteration of colour. Suitable sterilised milk may be obtained commercially.

Melt the agar, cool to 56° C., mix with the milk and pour plates or make slopes.

Glycerol Monoacetate Agar

This medium (Jacobs, Willis and Goodburn, 1964) is an alternative to milk agar for the examination of clinical specimens, particularly nose swabs, for staphylococci. On it, colonies of coagulase-positive staphylococci are always orange, yellow or buff whereas coagulase-negative strains are usually porcelain-white. There is maximum differentiation after 48 hours' incubation. Colonies from this medium give brisk and coarse clumping in the slide coagulase test.

Heart infusion broth (Bacto)	100 ml.
Glycerol monoacetate (BDH)	1 g.
Agar	2 g.

Dissolve the agar in the broth by steaming at 100° C., add the glyceride and autoclave at 121° C. for 15 min. Cool to 50-55° C., mix thoroughly to ensure even distribution of the glyceride and pour plates immediately.

The use of heart infusion base is essential. Overheating of the medium must be avoided; it cannot be allowed to solidify and then be remelted.

Salt Media

Staphylococci grow in sodium chloride concentrations that are high enough to be inhibitory to many other bacteria (Hill & White, 1929; Fairbrother & Southall, 1950). Salt has been used in selective media for isolating *Staph. aureus* when these organisms are likely to be present in small numbers, as in faeces.

Salt Cooked Meat Broth.—This is the most satisfactory salt liquid medium. It is less inhibitory to staphylococci than meat extract or digest broth containing increased salt and enables very small numbers to be detected. It is prepared in the same way as cooked meat broth except that 10 per cent. of sodium chloride is added to the peptone infusion broth.

Salt Milk Agar.—Besides being selective, salt in this medium has been regarded as increasing chromogenesis. The medium is prepared in the same way as milk agar excepting that 8–10 per cent. of sodium chloride is added.

Salt Glycerol Monoacetate Agar.—For isolating staphylococci from sources such as blankets and dust, 5 per cent. of sodium chloride may be added before the glyceride.

Polymyxin Agar

Lithium chloride and tellurite (Ludlam, 1949) have been used in a selective medium for *Staph. aureus*. More recently it has been found that coagulase-positive strains of staphylococci grow well on nutrient agar containing concentrations of polymyxin that inhibit coagulase-negative strains (Finegold & Sweeney, 1961). Polymyxin also inhibits coliform bacilli. Growth and pigment production by *Staph. aureus* are optimal after 24 hours' incubation and at this time growth of other organisms is minimal. Cycloheximide (Actidione), 400 μg. per ml., may be added to inhibit fungi in cultures from air, dust and clothes.

Nutrient agar	1 l.
Polymyxin B (Burroughs Wellcome) . . .	75 units

Melt the agar, add the polymyxin and autoclave at 121° C. for 30 min. Pour plates.

MEDIA FOR THE CULTIVATION OF *STREPT. PYOGENES*

Crystal Violet Blood Agar

The addition of a low concentration (1 in 500,000, *i.e.* 0·0002 per cent.) of crystal violet to blood agar inhibits the growth of some bacteria, notably staphylococci, while allowing the growth of *Strept. pyogenes*. Crystal violet blood agar is therefore a selective medium for *Strept. pyogenes*.

Sterile nutrient agar	90 ml.
Sterile horse blood	10 ml.
Crystal violet, 1 in 1000 aqueous solution . .	0·2 ml.

Melt the agar, cool to 50° C., add the blood and crystal violet and pour plates.

Todd-Hewitt Meat Infusion Broth

This glucose broth is used for typing *Strept. pyogenes* (Diagnostic Procedures and Reagents, 1950). The pH of the medium is high (7·8) and it contains 0·2 per cent. glucose.

MEDIA FOR THE CULTIVATION OF CORYNEBACTERIA

Hoyle's Medium

This medium (Hoyle, 1941) is satisfactory for routine examination of throat swabs for the diphtheria bacillus. Type differentiation on colonial morphology is not as good as on other media. It is a medium for isolation rather than typing of diphtheria bacilli.

Agar base

Meat extract (Lab-Lemco)	10 g.
Peptone (Difco proteose, or Evans)	10 g.
Sodium chloride, NaCl	5 g.
Agar	20 g.
Water	1 l.

Dissolve the ingredients and adjust the pH to 7·8. Distribute in 100 ml. quantities in screw-capped bottles and autoclave at 121° C. for 25 min.

Laked horse blood.—Sterile horse blood may be laked by freezing and thawing four times and then stored in the cold, preferably frozen.

It is more simple and convenient to lake with saponin (Young, 1942). Prepare 10 per cent. saponin (white) in water and sterilise it in the autoclave at 115° C. for 30 min. Incubate the blood for 15 min., add 0·5 ml. saponin solution for each 10 ml. blood and invert the bottle gently several times to ensure thorough mixing, avoiding the formation of bubbles. Replace the blood in the incubator for a further 15 min. when it should have an "inky" black appearance. It will keep for several months in the refrigerator.

Tellurite solution

Potassium tellurite, K_2TeO_3	0·7 g.
Water	20 ml.

Dissolve, autoclave at 115° C. for 20 min. and store in a tightly stoppered bottle in the dark.

Preparation of complete medium

Agar base	200 ml.
Laked blood	10 ml.
Tellurite solution	2 ml.

Melt the agar and cool it to 55° C., add the blood and tellurite and pour plates.

Anderson's Medium

This medium can be recommended for the provisional detection of *C. diphtheriae* from throat swabs in 24 hr. (Anderson, 1944). It is selective and preserves the microscopic morphology of *C. diphtheriae* but type-specific colonial morphology is not elicited.

Agar base

Meat extract (Lab-Lemco)	5 g.
Peptone (Parke, Davis & Co.)	10 g.
Sodium chloride, NaCl	5 g.
Agar	25 g.
Water	1 l.

Dissolve the ingredients and adjust the pH to 7·6. Distribute in 100 ml. quantities in bottles and autoclave at 121° C. for 25 min.

Glycerolated blood tellurite mixture

Sterile defibrinated sheep blood	14 ml.
Sterile glycerol	6 ml.
Sterile tellurite solution, 1 per cent. aqueous	4 ml.

Sterilise the glycerol in a hot air oven at 160° C. for 60 min. and the tellurite solution by autoclaving at 115° C. for 20 min. Mix the ingredients in a sterile flask, incubate for 1–2 hr. at 37° C., then refrigerate. Haemolysis is complete after 24 hr. The mixture keeps well in the refrigerator.

A one per cent. solution of good quality tellurite is sufficient but up to two per cent. of some batches is necessary.

Preparation of complete medium

Agar base	100 ml.
Glycerolated blood tellurite mixture	24 ml.

Melt the agar, cool to 45° C., add the blood and tellurite and pour plates.

Downie's Medium

The classical medium for the typing of *C. diphtheriae* is McLeod's medium (Anderson, Happold, McLeod and Thomson, 1931) which is a chocolate agar medium made from a meat infusion broth sterilised by filtration to avoid heating, rabbit blood and tellurite. Downie's medium is easier to prepare and has been used to give good differentiation of the types of *C. diphtheriae* on colonial morphology without interfering with microscopic morphology.

Nutrient agar	100 ml.
Sterile defibrinated blood	10 ml.
Sterile tellurite solution, 4 per cent. aqueous	1 ml.

The effectiveness of the medium depends on the quality of the nutrient agar. A digest broth agar may be satisfactory or may require the addition of 1 per cent. peptone.

The potassium tellurite solution is prepared as for Hoyle's medium. Double layer plates are poured, a layer of nutrient agar being covered by a layer of blood tellurite agar.

Löffler's Serum Medium

This medium is especially useful for cultivation of the diphtheria bacillus, producing luxuriant growth in 12 to 18 hr. with characteristic staining of the organism by Neisser's and Albert's methods. It is also used to show proteolytic properties particularly of *Clostridium* species.

Sterile ox, sheep or horse serum	300 ml.
Nutrient broth	100 ml.
Glucose	1 g.

Dissolve the glucose in the broth and autoclave at 115° C. for 20 min. Add the glucose broth to the serum with sterile precautions and distribute in sterile test tubes or in 2·5 ml. amounts in sterile ¼-oz. bottles. To inspissate, tubes are laid on a sloped tray but bottles are laid flat with the caps tightly screwed on. The temperature is then slowly raised to 80–85° C. and maintained for 2 hr., when the serum coagulates to a yellowish-white solid.

If an inspissator is not available, the serum may be coagulated by placing the slanted tubes at the top of a steam steriliser, where the temperature is a little below 100° C., for 5–7 min. Overheating causes expansion of air bubbles and the formation of steam from the fluid droplets in the partially solidified material, leading to disruption of the medium.

Inspissated medium should be allowed to cool before being handled. Medium in screw-capped bottles can be stored for a long period of time.

MEDIA FOR THE CULTIVATION OF LACTOBACILLI

DeMan, Rogosa and Sharpe's (1960) Medium

This is a non-selective medium that supports good growth of lactobacilli. Slightly modified, it serves as a basal medium for fermentation tests and made with agar, it can be used as a plating medium.

Peptone (Oxoid)	10 g.
Meat extract (Lab-Lemco)	10 g.
Yeast extract	5 g.
Glucose	20 g.
Tween 80 (Polyoxyethylene sorbitan mono-oleate)	1 ml.
Dipotassium hydrogen phosphate, K_2HPO_4	2 g.
Sodium acetate, $CH_3COONa.3H_2O$	5 g.
Triammonium citrate	2 g.
Magnesium sulphate, $MgSO_4.7H_2O$	200 mg.
Manganese sulphate, $MnSO_4.4H_2O$	50 mg.
Water	1 l.

Dissolve the ingredients, distribute and autoclave at 121° C. for 15 min. The pH lies between 6·0 and 6·5 after sterilisation.

Tomato Juice Agar

Hadley's Modification of Kulp and White's Medium.—In the formula given here, Hadley's (1933) medium is further modified by replacing peptonised milk with casein hydrolysate. Tomato juice provides growth factors and a pH of 5·0 makes the medium selective for lactobacilli. The medium can be used for counts of lactobacilli in saliva.

Peptone	1 g.
Casein hydrolysate	1 g.
Tomato juice	40 ml.
Agar	2 g.
Water	60 ml.

The tomato juice sold as a beverage is not suitable. Juice must be expressed from canned whole tomatoes.

Dissolve the peptone and casein hydrolysate in the tomato juice, heating gently and taking care to avoid overheating. Adjust to pH 5·0 with lactic acid. Dissolve the agar in the water and mix both solutions while they are hot. Filter through a thin layer of absorbent cotton-wool, distribute in 100-ml. amounts and autoclave at 115° C. for 10 min.

On cooling, the tomato tends to flocculate. On remelting the medium the bottle must be inverted several times until the tomato goes into suspension. At pH 5·0, agar tends to be hydrolysed on heating and repeated melting of a batch of this medium should be avoided.

MEDIA FOR THE CULTIVATION OF MYCOBACTERIA

Löwenstein-Jensen Medium

As prescribed by the International Union against Tuberculosis (IUT).

This medium (Jensen, 1955) has been modified from the original Löwenstein-Jensen medium by omitting starch, which makes it more difficult to prepare and is unnecessary for the growth of tubercle bacilli. Malachite green suppresses the growth of organisms other than mycobacteria. The medium is recommended for the isolation of the human type of the tubercle bacillus whose growth is enhanced by glycerol, and for drug sensitivity tests. Colonial morphology on this medium allows the differentiation of human and bovine types.

Mineral salt solution

Potassium dihydrogen phosphate, KH_2PO_4 anhydrous	2·4 g.
Magnesium sulphate, $MgSO_4$	0·24 g.
Magnesium citrate	0·6 g.
Asparagine	3·6 g.
Glycerol	12 ml.
Water	600 ml.

Dissolve the ingredients by heating. Autoclave at 121° C. for 25 min. to sterilise. This solution keeps indefinitely and may be stored in suitable amounts.

Malachite green solution.—Prepare a 2 per cent. solution of malachite green in sterile water with sterile precautions by dissolving the dye in the incubator for 1–2 hr. This solution can be stored indefinitely and should be shaken before use.

Preparation of complete medium

Mineral salt solution	600 ml.
Malachite green solution	20 ml.
Beaten egg (20 to 22 hens' eggs, depending on size)	1 l.

All utensils used to prepare the complete medium must be sterile. The eggs must be fresh, *i.e.* not more than four days old. Wash them thoroughly in warm water with a brush and a plain alkaline soap, such as Windsor soap, and rinse in running water for 30 min. Drain off the water and allow the eggs to dry covered with paper until the following day. Alternatively, to save time, the washed and rinsed eggs may be dried by sprinkling them with methylated spirit and burning it off. The risk is that wet shells lead to contamination of the egg. Before handling the clean, dry eggs, scrub the hands and dry them. Crack the eggs with a sterile knife into a sterile beaker and beat them with a sterile egg whisk. There is no need to filter the beaten egg. Mix the complete medium, distribute it in 5 ml. amounts in sterile 1 oz. (McCartney) bottles and screw the caps tightly on. Lay the bottles horizontally in the inspissator and heat at 75°–80° C. for 1 hr. Since the medium has been prepared with sterile precautions this heating is to solidify the medium, not to sterilise it.

The medium will keep for some months in screw-capped bottles, but if slopes are made in test tubes they must be stored in the cold and used within a month.

Stonebrink's Medium

This medium (Stonebrink, 1957) is particularly suitable for the isolation of bovine strains of the tubercle bacillus. It does not contain glycerol, which has no effect on or may even be inhibitory to the growth of the bovine type. The medium may also be used for the isolation of human strains that are drug-resistant and difficult to grow. It should be used for specimens other than sputa and for sputa if the tubercle bacillus is highly resistant. It is unsuitable for drug sensitivity tests.

Mineral salt solution

Potassium dihydrogen phosphate, KH_2PO_4 anhydrous	7 g.
Disodium hydrogen phosphate, $Na_2HPO_4.2H_2O$	4 g.
Sodium pyruvate	12·5 g.
Water	1 l.

Dissolve the salts and autoclave at 121° C. for 30 min. This solution keeps indefinitely.

Malachite green solution.—This is a 2 per cent. solution prepared as for Löwenstein-Jensen medium.

Preparation of complete medium

Mineral salt solution	1 l.
Malachite green solution	40 ml.
Beaten egg	2 l.

Prepare the beaten egg, mix and dispense the medium with sterile precautions and inspissate it as for Löwenstein-Jensen medium.

Dorset's Egg Medium

This simple egg medium is suitable for the growth of laboratory strains of tubercle bacilli. In an emergency it may be used for isolations, when it would be advisable to add malachite green, but the more enriched media yield the greatest number of positive cultures from primary inoculations of specimens from human and animal infections.

Beaten egg (2 or 3 hens' eggs, depending on size)	75 ml.
Sterile broth	25 ml.
Malachite green solution, 2 per cent. (if for isolation of tubercle bacilli)	1·25 ml

Prepare the beaten egg, mix and dispense the medium with sterile precautions as for Löwenstein-Jensen. If an inspissator is not available the medium may be solidified in about 20 min. on the top of the steam steriliser but it is better to heat at a lower temperature for a longer time.

Liquid Media for *M. tuberculosis*

Various liquid media may be used for growing tubercle bacilli for special purposes. For example, Ives and McCormick (1956) recommend a medium for culturing tubercle bacilli from pleural fluid. Other liquid media include Kirchner's (1932), Youman's (1944) and Dubos's (Medical Research Council, 1948) media. Note that the casein hydrolysate for Dubos's medium is already a 20 per cent. solution and should not be diluted further.

Smith's Medium

This medium (Smith, 1953) is suitable for the growth of Jöhne's bacillus. Essentially it is Dubos's medium with the addition of an alcoholic extract of *Mycobacterium phlei* and solidified with agar. For isolations from the intestinal mucosa Actidione and chloramphenicol may be added to inhibit contaminants (Brotherston, Gilmour and Samuel, 1961).

MEDIA FOR THE CULTIVATION OF CLOSTRIDIA

Cooked Meat Broth

The original medium is known as "Robertson's bullock-heart medium", but the following modification of Martin and Lepper is recommended. It is suitable for growing anaerobes in air and also for the preservation of stock cultures of aerobic organisms. The inoculum is introduced deep in the medium in contact with the meat.

Cooked Meat

Fresh bullock's heart	500 g.
Water	500 ml.
Sodium hydroxide, 1 *N* NaOH	1·5 ml.

Mince the heart, place in the alkaline boiling water and simmer for 20 min. to neutralise the lactic acid. Drain off the liquid through a muslin filter and, while still hot, press the minced meat in a cloth and dry partially by spreading it on a cloth or filter paper. In this condition it can be introduced into bottles without soiling them.

Peptone Infusion Broth

Liquid filtered from cooked meat	500 ml.
Peptone	2·5 g.
Sodium chloride, NaCl	1·25 g.

Steam at 100° C. for 20 min., add 1 ml. pure hydrochloric acid and filter. Bring the reaction of the filtrate to pH 8·2, steam at 100° C. for 30 min. and adjust reaction to pH 7·8.

Preparation of complete medium.—Place meat in each 1-oz. bottle to a depth of about one inch and cover with about 10 ml. broth. Autoclave at 121° C. for 20 min. After sterilisation, the pH of the broth over the meat is about 7·5. If test-tubes are used the surface of the medium may be covered with a layer of sterile liquid paraffin ½-in. (1 cm.) deep, but this is not essential.

A tall column of meat is essential because conditions are anaerobic only where there are meat particles. There need be only sufficient broth to extend about ½ in. above the meat.

Thioglycollate Broth

The addition of sodium thioglycollate to liquid media was shown by Brewer (1940) to prolong the time that anaerobic conditions are maintained after sterilisation, and anaerobes can be grown in tubes like aerobic organisms. The addition of a small amount of agar prevents convection currents and assists in maintaining anaerobiosis. Methylene blue or resazurin acts as an oxidation-reduction potential indicator. It should be decolourised except in the surface layer.

Any nutrient broth can be made anaerobic in this way. The formula for the thioglycollate medium prescribed in the United States Pharmacopeia for sterility tests is given here.

Yeast extract, water soluble	5·0 g.
Casein hydrolysate, pancreatic digest	15·0 g.
Glucose	5·5 g.
L-cystine	0·5 g.
Agar	0·75 g.
Sodium chloride, NaCl	2·5 g.
Sodium thioglycollate	0·5 g.
Resazurin sodium solution, 1 in 1000, freshly prepared	1·0 ml.
Water	1 l.

Dissolve the ingredients other than thioglycollate and resazurin by steaming at 100° C. Add the thioglycollate and adjust the pH to 7·3. If there is a precipitate, heat without boiling and filter hot through moistened filter paper. Add the resazurin solution, mix thoroughly, distribute and sterilise at 121° C. for 15 min. Cool at once to 25° C. and store in the dark, preferably between 20° and 30° C. Do not use the medium if it has evaporated enough to affect its fluidity. If more than the upper third is pink in colour, anaerobic conditions may be restored once only by steaming at 100° C. for a few minutes.

Lowbury and Lilly's (1955) Medium

This is both a selective and an indicator medium for *Cl. welchii.* It contains Fildes' peptic digest of blood to stimulate the production of lecithinase by *Cl. welchii*, human serum to indicate lecithinase production and neomycin to inhibit lecithinase-producing aerobic sporing bacilli. The concentration of agar is high to prevent the swarming of Proteus. Double layer medium allows a clearer demonstration of lecithinase reactions.

Agar base

Agar, New Zealand (Davis)	50 g.
Peptone water (Evans peptone)	1 l.

This agar base autoclaved at 121° C. for 30 min. is used for the lower layer of the medium and as basal medium for the upper layer.

Preparation of complete medium

Agar base	100 ml.
Fildes' peptic digest of sheep blood	6·5 ml.
Human serum, sterile	40 ml.
Neomycin sulphate (Upjohn), sterile aqueous solution: 10,000 μg. per ml.	1·5 ml.

The serum may be prepared by treating plasma with 5 per cent. of sterile 10 per cent. calcium chloride at 37° C. Heat the Fildes' digest at 55° C. for 30 min., melt the agar base and cool it to 56° C. Add the remaining ingredients and pour the medium as the upper layer of double layer plates on a layer of agar base. The final concentration of neomycin in the upper layer is 100 μg. per ml.

Spread 250 international units of *Cl. welchii* antitoxin over half of each agar surface.

Willis and Hobbs' (1959) Medium

This medium for the isolation of clostridia is a lactose egg-yolk milk agar made selective for various clostridia, particularly *Cl. welchii*, by the addition of neomycin. The recommended concentration of 250 μg. neomycin sulphate per ml. may inhibit some clostridia, usually inhibits strains of *Bacillus* and *Staphylococcus*, and greatly reduces the growth of coliform bacilli. Nagler-positive organisms produce zones of opalescence that can be specifically inhibited by the appropriate antiserum spread over half the medium in a plate and dried-in before inoculation. Some clostridia produce a "pearly layer". Lactose fermentation is indicated by a pink halo in the medium around the colony and proteolysis by a clearing of the milk in the medium.

Egg yolk suspension.—Break eggs with precautions to keep their contents sterile, as described for Löwenstein medium, at the same time separating the yolks from the whites. Discard the whites and dilute the yolks with an equal volume of sterile 0·9 per cent. sodium chloride solution.

Sterile stock milk.—Remove the cream from ordinary milk by centrifuging. Sterilise the skimmed milk by autoclaving at 121° C. for 15 min.

Basal medium

Agar (New Zealand)	4·8 g.
Lactose	4·8 g.
Neutral red, 1 per cent. solution	1·3 ml.
Meat infusion broth, pH 7	400 ml.
Egg yolk suspension	15 ml.
Milk	60 ml.

Dissolve the agar and lactose in the neutral red and broth by steaming, and sterilise at 121° C. for 25 min. Cool to 50–55° C. and add the egg yolk and milk. Pour plates.

Possible additions to basal medium

Neomycin sulphate (Upjohn)	250 μg. per ml.
Sodium thioglycollate	0·1 per cent.

Stock sterile solutions of neomycin may be stored in the refrigerator with little loss of potency. The antibiotic is not decomposed by heating at 60° C. for 20 min. Thioglycollate may assist the growth of the stricter anaerobes.

Either or both of these reagents may be added at the same time as the egg yolk and milk.

Ellner's (1956) Medium

This medium is used to induce spore formation in *Cl. welchii.* Anaerobiosis may be ensured by heating at 100° C. for 10 min. and cooling just prior to inoculation. It is important that the inoculum should be adequate; 0·5 ml. of an actively growing 4–12 hr. meat broth culture should be introduced with a pipette into the bottom of the tube of medium. Incubation is in an anaerobic jar at 37° C.

Peptone (*e.g.* Proteose peptone, Difco)	10 g.
Yeast extract	3 g.
Soluble starch	3 g.
Magnesium sulphate, $MgSO_4$	0·1 g.
Potassium dihydrogen phosphate, KH_2PO_4 . .	1·5 g.
Disodium hydrogen phosphate, $Na_2HPO_4.12H_2O$.	67 g.
Water	1 l.

Steam briefly at 100° C. to dissolve, adjust to pH 7·8 with sodium hydroxide, dispense in tubes and autoclave at 121° C. for 15 min. Tubes should be half to two-thirds full.

Alkaline Egg Medium

This medium promotes spore formation by clostridia. Clostridia remain viable in it for years.

Egg yolk	1
Egg whites	2
Sodium hydroxide, 1N NaOH	6 ml.
Water to	500 ml.

Beat the yolk and whites, add the sodium hydroxide and water. Heat slowly to 95° C. for 1½ hr., filter through cotton-wool and distribute. Sterilise by autoclaving at 121° C. for 15 min.

MEDIA FOR THE CULTIVATION OF ENTEROBACTERIA

MacConkey's Agar

This is a useful medium for the cultivation of enteric bacteria. It contains a bile salt to inhibit non-intestinal bacteria and lactose with neutral red to distinguish the lactose-fermenting coliforms from the non-lactose-fermenting salmonella and dysentery groups.

Peptone	20 g.
Sodium taurocholate, commercial	5 g.
Water	1 l.
Agar	20 g.
Neutral red solution, 2 per cent. in 50 per cent. ethanol	About 3·5 ml.
Lactose, 10 per cent. aqueous solution	100 ml.

Dissolve the peptone and taurocholate (bile salt) in the water by heating. Add the agar and dissolve it in the steamer or autoclave. If necessary, clear by filtration. Adjust the pH to 7·5. Add the lactose and the neutral red, which should be well shaken before use, and mix. Heat in the autoclave with "free steam" (*c.* 100° C.) for 1 hr., then at 115° C. for 15 min. Pour plates.

The medium should be a distinct reddish-brown colour. If it is acid, it assumes a rose-pink colour. When the medium is stored for any length of time the neutral red indicator tends to fade. To overcome this the medium is made up and stored without neutral red, indicator being added and thoroughly mixed before pouring plates.

Teepol Lactose Agar

Jameson and Emberley (1956) described this medium as a substitute for MacConkey's agar. Teepol (Shell Chemicals Ltd.), which is a detergent containing sodium and potassium salts of alkyl sulphates with chains of 8–18 C atoms, is used in place of sodium taurocholate as the selective agent for enterobacteria; it has the advantages of being much cheaper and more reliable in its properties.

Eupeptone No. 2 (Allen & Hanburys)	20 g.
Lactose	10 g.
Sodium chloride NaCl	5 g.
Teepol	1 g.
Bromothymol blue (1 in 500 solution)	25 ml.
Agar (New Zealand, Davis)	9 g.
Water	1 l.

Adjust to pH 7·5 and sterilise at 115° C. for 15 min.

Colonies of lactose-fermenting *Esch. coli* organisms are *pale cream* in colour and are usually large and opaque. Colonies of salmonellae and shigellae are *pale green* and less opaque.

Brilliant Green MacConkey Agar

Brilliant green is inhibitory to *Esch. coli* and renders the medium selective for salmonella organisms.

The medium is prepared as MacConkey's agar but with the addition of 0·04 g. brilliant green per litre.

Desoxycholate Citrate Agar (DCA)

This modification by Hynes of Leifson's medium is particularly suitable for the isolation of the dysentery bacilli, the salmonella food-poisoning group and *S. paratyphi B*. It is not quite so selective for *S. typhi*, though superior to MacConkey's medium.

Neutral red lactose agar

Meat extract (Lab-Lemco)	20 g.
Peptone (Difco proteose or Evans)	20 g.
Agar	90 g.
Neutral red solution, 2 per cent. in 50 per cent. ethanol	5 ml.
Lactose	40 g.
Water	4 l.

Dissolve the meat extract in 200 ml. water over the flame. Make just alkaline to phenolphthalein with 50 per cent. sodium hydroxide, boil at 100° C. and filter. Adjust the pH to 7·4, make up the volume to 200 ml. and add the peptone. Dissolve the agar in 3700 ml. water by steaming at 100° C. for 1 hr. Filter if necessary. Add the meat extract and peptone solution and mix. Add the neutral red and lactose, mixing again. Bottle in accurate 100 ml. lots and heat in the autoclave with "free steam" at *c.* 100° C. for 1 hr. and then at 115° C. for 15 min.

Solution A

Sodium citrate, Analar, $Na_3C_6H_5O_7.2H_2O$	17 g.
Sodium thiosulphate, Analar, $Na_2S_2O_3.5H_2O$	17 g.
Ferric ammonium citrate, green scales	2 g.
Sterile water	100 ml.

Solution B (bile salt)

Sodium desoxycholate	10 g.
Sterile water	100 ml.

Prepare these solutions with sterile precautions, heating at 60° C. for 1 hr. to facilitate solution.

Preparation of complete medium

Neutral red lactose agar	100 ml.
Solution A	5 ml.
Solution B	5 ml.

Melt the agar and add solutions A and B in this order, using separate sterile pipettes and mixing well between. Pour plates *immediately* and dry the surface. The medium is pale pink in colour and should be quite clear.

The medium should be poured and cooled as soon as possible after the addition of the desoxycholate, otherwise it tends to become very soft. The desoxycholate must be pure and samples should be tested with known positive specimens before purchase is made.

Wilson and Blair's Medium

The use of this medium (Wilson, 1938) depends on the reduction of sulphite to sulphide in the presence of glucose by *S. typhi* and *S. paratyphi B*, yielding black colonies, and the inhibition of *Esch. coli* by brilliant green and by bismuth sulphite in the presence of an excess of sodium sulphite.

Bismuth sulphite glucose phosphate mixture

Bismuth ammonio-citrate, scales	30 g.
Sodium sulphite, Na_2SO_3	100 g.
Disodium hydrogen phosphate, $Na_2HPO_4.12H_2O$	100 g.
Glucose, commercial	50 g.
Sterile water	1 l.

With sterile precautions dissolve the bismuth ammonio-citrate in 250 ml. boiling water, and the sodium sulphite in 500 ml. boiling water. Mix the solutions and while the mixture is boiling add the sodium phosphate crystals. When this mixture is cool add the glucose dissolved in 250 ml. boiling water and cooled. This mixture will keep for months.

Iron citrate brilliant green mixture

Ferric citrate, brown scales	2 g.
Brilliant green	0·25 g.
Sterile water	225 ml.

With sterile precautions mix solutions of the ferric citrate in 200 ml. water and the brilliant green in 25 ml. water. This mixture will keep for months.

Preparation of complete medium

Sterile 3 per cent. nutrient agar	100 ml.
Bismuth sulphite glucose phosphate mixture	20 ml.
Iron citrate-brilliant green mixture	4·5 ml.

Melt the agar and cool to 60° C. Add the other ingredients with sterile precautions and pour plates.

Tetrathionate Broth

The tetrathionate in this liquid medium inhibits coliform bacilli while permitting bacilli of the typhoid-paratyphoid group to grow freely; thus, an enriched culture of the latter can be obtained from faeces and sometimes an almost pure growth. However it permits the growth of *Proteus* spp.

Thiosulphate solution

Sodium thiosulphate, $Na_2S_2O_3 . 5H_2O$ . . .	24·8 g.
Sterile water to	100 ml.

Mix the salt and water with sterile precautions and steam at 100° C. for 30 min. It is a 1 *M* solution.

Iodine solution

Potassium iodide, KI	20 g.
Iodine, I	12·7 g.
Sterile water to	100 ml.

With sterile precautions dissolve the potassium iodide in about 50 ml. of warm water, add the iodine and make up to a final volume of 100 ml. This gives a normal or 0·5 *M* solution.

Preparation of complete medium

Calcium carbonate, $CaCO_3$	2·5 g.
Nutrient broth	78 ml.
Thiosulphate solution	15 ml.
Iodine solution	4 ml.
Phenol red, 0·02 per cent. in 20 per cent. ethanol .	3 ml.

Add the calcium carbonate to the broth and sterilise it by autoclaving at 121° C. for 20 min. When cool, add the thiosulphate, iodine and phenol red solutions with sterile precautions. Distribute in 10 ml. amounts in sterile screw-capped bottles. Even in the refrigerator, tetrathionate broth does not keep for more than a few weeks. It is convenient to keep stock solutions and prepare the complete medium as required (Knox, Gell and Pollock, 1942).

Kauffmann-Müller Tetrathionate Broth

This medium is more selective than the original tetrathionate broth because the brilliant green in it checks the growth of *Proteus* spp.

Thiosulphate solution

Sodium thiosulphate, $Na_2S_2O_3 . 5H_2O$ . . .	50 g.
Sterile water	100 ml.

Mix the salt and water with sterile precautions and steam at 100° C. for 30 min.

Iodine solution

Potassium iodide, KI	25 g.
Iodine, I	20 g.
Sterile water	100 ml.

With sterile precautions dissolve the potassium iodide and add the iodine.

Ox bile solution

Desiccated ox bile	0·5 g.
Water	5 ml.

Dissolve with sterile precautions.

Preparation of complete medium

Nutrient broth, pH 7·4	90 ml.
Calcium carbonate, $CaCO_3$	5 g.
Brilliant green, 1 in 1000 aqueous	1 ml.
Thiosulphate solution	10 ml.
Iodine solution	2 ml.
Ox bile solution	5 ml.

Add the calcium carbonate to the broth and sterilise it by autoclaving at 121° C. for 20 min. When cool, add the other solutions and distribute aseptically in approximately 10 ml. amounts. Heat once in the steamer at 100° C. for 10 min.

Selenite F Broth

The selenite in this medium (Leifson, 1936) serves the same purpose as tetrathionate in tetrathionate broth and has been preferred to it (Hobbs & Allison, 1945).

Sodium acid selenite, $NaHSeO_3$	4 g.
Peptone	5 g.
Lactose	4 g.
Disodium hydrogen phosphate, $Na_2HPO_4 . 12H_2O$	9·5 g.
Sodium dihydrogen phosphate, $NaH_2PO_4 . 2H_2O$	0·5 g.
Sterile water	1 l.

Dissolve the ingredients with sterile precautions and distribute the yellowish solution in 10 ml. amounts in sterile screw-capped bottles. Steam at 100° C. for 30 min. Excessive heat is detrimental to the medium and autoclaving must not be used to sterilise it. A slight amount of red precipitate may form but this does not interfere with the action of the medium. The pH of the medium should be 7·1 and the phosphates may be varied slightly if necessary to attain this.

Salts of selenium are very toxic for animals and man and must be handled with some care. Some organic compounds of selenium and hydrogen selenide are volatile and toxic if inhaled.

MEDIA FOR THE CULTIVATION OF VIBRIOS

The classical vibrio media are Dieudonné's (1909) alkaline blood agar and Aronson's (1915) sucrose dextrin agar. New media utilise the ability of vibrios to split gelatin with the production of haloes around colonies on solid agar media containing gelatin.

Monsur's Medium

This medium is for the isolation of cholera and other vibrios either from rectal swabs and stool specimens or from other contaminated sources. A similar fluid medium is used for enrichment or preservative purposes (see Monsur, 1963); this is the "Bile peptone transport medium" described on p. 782. The potassium tellurite in these media is highly inhibitory to most coliform bacilli although *Proteus* species grow as small colonies.

Bile salt gelatin agar

Trypticase (Baltimore Biological Laboratories) or Bactotryptone	1 g.
Sodium chloride, NaCl	1 g.
Sodium taurocholate	0·5 g.
Sodium carbonate, Na_2CO_3	0·1 g.
Gelatin (Difco)	3 g.
Agar	1·5 g.
Water	100 ml.

It is thought essential to use the Difco brand of gelatin. Dissolve the ingredients by steaming and adjust the pH to 8·5 with sodium hydroxide. Sterilise by autoclaving at 121° C. for 20 min.

Potassium tellurite solution.—Prepare a 0·5 per cent. solution in water and autoclave at 115° C. for 20 min. This solution keeps indefinitely.

Preparation of complete medium

Bile salt gelatin agar	100 ml.
Potassium tellurite solution, K_2TeO_3, 0·05 per cent.	1 ml.

Make a 1 in 10 dilution of the stock potassium tellurite solution with sterile precautions and add it to the melted and cooled agar medium. The final pH of the medium must be 8·5 to 9·2. Pour plates.

This medium should be used when fresh because its pH tends to fall on keeping.

Gelatin Agar

This medium is complementary to Monsur's medium. It is unsuitable as the sole medium for primary isolation of cholera vibrios because it is not inhibitory to coliform bacilli. It is used to provide a semi-quantitative assessment of the numbers of vibrios that are being excreted.

Trypticase (Baltimore Biological Laboratories)	1 g.
Sodium chloride, NaCl	1 g.
Gelatin (Difco)	3 g.
Agar	1·5 g.
Water	100 ml.

It is thought essential to use the correct brands of trypticase and of gelatin. Dissolve the ingredients by steaming. The pH should be 7·2–7·4. Autoclave at 121° C. for 20 min. to sterilise, and pour plates.

MEDIA FOR THE CULTIVATION OF BRUCELLA

Liver infusion agar (Huddleson, 1939) has been used to grow brucellae but some infusions can be inhibitory and lead to differences in the quality of different batches of medium. Serum dextrose agar or Albimi agar are to be preferred.

Serum Dextrose Agar with Added Antibiotics

This medium (Jones & Morgan, 1958) containing antimicrobial agents is good for isolating even very fastidious strains of *Br. abortus*. The antimicrobial substances may be omitted if cultures are being made from uncontaminated sources.

Bacitracin solution (2000 units per ml.).—Bacitracin is supplied in vials containing 500,000 units. Dissolve the contents of one vial in 250 ml. of sterile water. Store at 4° C., but this solution will not keep for more than one week.

Polymyxin B solution (5000 units per ml.).—Polymyxin B is supplied in bottles containing 500,000 units. Dissolve the contents of one bottle in 100 ml. of sterile water. Store in a deep freeze at −20° C. or in the ice chamber of a refrigerator.

Actidione solution (10 mg. per ml.).—Actidione is supplied in 4 g. bottles. It is important to dissolve this amount of powder in 20 ml. of acetone and dilute to 400 ml. with sterile water. Store at 4° C.

Dextrose solution (25 per cent.)

Dextrose	12·5 g.
Water	50 ml.

Prepare the solution and sterilise it by Seitz filtration.

Preparation of complete medium

Agar	15 g.
Peptone	10 g.
Sodium chloride, NaCl	5 g.
Meat extract	5 g.
Water	1 l.
Sterile inactivated horse serum	50 ml.
Dextrose solution, 25 per cent.	40 ml.
Bacitracin solution, 2000 units per ml.	12·5 ml.
Polymyxin B solution, 5000 units per ml.	1·2 ml.
Actidione solution, 10 mg. per ml.	10 ml.

Dissolve the first four ingredients by gentle heating, adjust to pH 7·5 and autoclave at 121° C. for 30 min. Cool to 52° C. and add the remaining ingredients, mixing well to ensure even distribution of the antimicrobial agents. Pour plates, this amount of medium making about

50 plates. Cooling to 52° C. will reduce water of condensation on the lids.

It is best to use freshly prepared medium because Actidione is unstable. However plates can be stored for a week in the refrigerator with the lids uppermost, either in a container with a lid or in a wire tray covered with a sheet of polythene. Before use, plates should be incubated overnight with the medium uppermost, but in an emergency plates with lids partly opened may be dried for 1 hr. in the incubator. It is important that the surface of the medium be dry to discourage dissociation.

Albimi Agar (Joint FAO/WHO, 1958)

This selective medium is an alternative to serum dextrose agar for isolating brucellae but is not so suitable for fastidious strains. By raising the agar concentration to 2·5 or 3 per cent. of the final medium its selectivity is increased and the possibility of overgrowth by Proteus is reduced. Albimi agar is manufactured by Albimi Laboratories, Brooklyn, N.Y. It has the advantage of not requiring the addition of serum.

Ethyl violet solution (1 in 1000).—The concentration is calculated on the basis of the pure dyestuff and not on the weight of the product as supplied.

Bacitracin, polymyxin B and Actidione solutions are prepared as for serum dextrose agar.

Preparation of complete medium

Albimi agar	1 l.
Ethyl violet solution, 1 in 1000	1·25 ml.
Bacitracin solution, 2000 units per ml.	12·5 ml.
Polymyxin B solution, 5000 units per ml.	1·2 ml.
Actidione solution, 10 mg. per ml.	10 ml.

Prepare and sterilise the Albimi agar in accordance with the manufacturer's instructions. Cool to 52° C. and add the remaining ingredients. Mix the medium, pour, store and dry plates as for serum dextrose agar.

MEDIA FOR THE CULTIVATION OF BORDETELLA

Bordet-Gengou Medium

This modification has given good growth of *Bord. pertussis*. Peptone was not included in the original Bordet-Gengou medium and may be omitted. Some brands of peptone are markedly inhibitory to the growth of *Bord. pertussis* probably due to their content of colloidal sulphur or sulphide. The medium can be made more selective for *Bord. pertussis* by adding 0·25 units penicillin per ml. Lacey (1954) has described an even more selective medium containing a diamidine, sodium fluoride and penicillin.

Glycerol potato agar

Potato slices	250 g.
Sodium chloride, NaCl	9 g.
Water	2 l.
Agar	45 g.
Glycerol	20 ml.
Proteose peptone (Difco)	20 g.

Clean and pare potatoes, and cut them into thin slices. Boil the slices with the salt in 500 ml. of water until they fall to pieces. Make up the water lost in boiling, filter through linen and adjust to pH 7. Dissolve the agar in 1500 ml. of water by heat and add the potato extract, glycerol and peptone. Distribute in bottles and heat in the autoclave with "free steam" at *c.* 100° C. for 1 hour, then at 115° C. for 10 min. Store until required.

Preparation of complete medium

Glycerol potato agar	2 volumes
Sterile defibrinated horse blood	1 volume

Melt the agar in the steamer for 1 hr., inverting the bottle several times. Place in the water bath at 55° C. for about 5 min. until the temperature of the agar has dropped to about 65° C. Warm the blood slightly by placing it in the 55° C. bath for 2–3 min. Mix the blood and the agar thoroughly and pour plates. The layer of agar should be thick, about 30 ml. of medium per 4 in. Petri dish. The plates should not be dried in the incubator, but should be stored at once in the refrigerator, and may be used up to two or three days after preparation.

Colindale Modification of Bordet-Gengou Medium

This medium is easier to prepare than the original Bordet-Gengou medium because starch is used in place of a preparation from potato slices. Also the brand of peptone used appears to be better for growth of *Bordetella*. The penicillin and diamidine (M & B 938) make it more selective for *Bordetella*.

Glycerol starch agar

Peptone (Bengers or Evans)	10 g.
Sodium chloride, NaCl	5 g.
Glycerol	10 ml.
Starch (Soluble BDH)	2·5 g.
Water	1 l.
Agar (Davis)	11 g.

Dissolve the ingredients, except the agar, in the water and adjust to pH 7·8. Add the agar. Check the pH which should be 7·5–7·6. Distribute in 200 ml. quantities and autoclave at 115° C. for 10 min.

Preparation of complete medium

Glycerol starch agar	200 ml.
Penicillin (50 units per ml.)	1·5 ml.
M & B 938 (0·1 per cent. solution) . . .	0·9 ml.
Sterile defibrinated horse blood	100 ml.

Melt the agar in the steamer at 100° C., cool to 40–45° C. Warm the blood to 37° C. and add all the ingredients. Mix thoroughly and pour not more than 10 plates from this quantity of medium. Store in the refrigerator. A short (10–15 min.) period of drying *may* be necessary but only when the plates are freshly poured.

M & B 938 is 4 : 4 diamido-diphenylamine-hydrochloride.

MEDIUM FOR THE CULTIVATION OF HAEMOPHILUS

Levinthal's Medium

For this medium the contents of red cells are liberated by heat to improve on blood agar for the cultivation of *Haemophilus* species.

Sterile nutrient agar	100 ml.
Sterile rabbit or human blood	5 ml.

Melt the agar, add the blood and heat the mixture in boiling water. Allow the deposit to settle and distribute the clear supernatant.

MEDIA FOR THE CULTIVATION OF FUNGI

Media for the isolation of pathogenic fungi are designed to be inhibitory to bacterial contaminants. Sabouraud's glucose peptone medium, tellurite malt agar and penicillin streptomycin agar are described here. Sabouraud's medium is generally preferred for the ringworm fungi and penicillin streptomycin blood agar for the systemic fungi.

Malt agar is a general purpose medium for the cultivation of fungi. Corn meal agar, zein agar and rice starch agar are designed to induce the formation of chlamydospores in *Candida* species. A preservation medium (p. 780) and two liquid media also are described.

Agar is hydrolysed by heat at a low pH and acid media for fungi are not heated above 115° C. After autoclaving, the medium may be allowed to solidify in bulk but it should be remelted only once and then with a minimum of heating. The high concentration of sugar in some media for fungi is another reason for avoiding overheating and repeated heating, because heat tends to char sugar.

Sabouraud's Glucose Agar and Broth

The low pH and high sugar content of this medium make it particularly selective for fungi as against bacterial contaminants. The agar medium is suitable for the primary isolation of fungi from clinical material.

Glucose	40 g.
Peptone	10 g.
Agar	20 g.
Water	1 l.

A suitable peptone is Oxoid mycological peptone supplied by Oxo Ltd. (Medical Dept.), London, E.C.4. For broth, the agar is omitted.

Dissolve the ingredients in the steamer or autoclave. Filter through cotton gauze and adjust to pH 5·4. Dispense in stock bottles or in tubes. Autoclave at 115° C. for 15 min.

Tellurite Malt Agar

Like Sabouraud's medium, this has a low pH and high sugar content. In addition it contains tellurite to inhibit bacteria.

Malt extract is prepared commercially by extracting the soluble materials from sprouted barley in water at about 55° C. The liquor is strained and concentrated by evaporation at a temperature below 55° C. to yield a brown viscous material. It consists mainly of maltose (about 50 per cent.), starch, dextrins and glucose, and contains about 5 per cent. of proteins and protein breakdown products, and a wide range of mineral salts and growth factors, such as thiamine, nicotinic acid, riboflavine, biotin, pantothenic acid, pyridoxine, folic acid and inositol. For use in mycological media it must not contain added sugar or cod-liver oil.

Basal medium

Malt extract	40 g.
Agar	20 g.
Water	1 l.

Dissolve the malt extract and agar by steaming, filter through cotton gauze, adjust to pH 5·4 and distribute in 100 ml. amounts in stock bottles. Autoclave at 115° C. for 15 min.

Potassium tellurite solution

Potassium tellurite, K_2TeO_3	0·5 g.
Water	25 ml.

Dissolve the salt, autoclave at 115° C. for 20 min. and store in a tightly stoppered bottle in the dark.

Preparation of complete medium

Basal medium	100 ml.
Potassium tellurite solution	1·8 ml.

Melt the basal medium, cool to 55° C., add the tellurite solution and distribute as desired.

The final concentration of tellurite is 0·036 per cent.

Penicillin Streptomycin Blood Agar

This medium is used for selective cultivation of yeasts and certain dimorphic fungi.

Nutrient agar	90 ml.
Blood	10 ml.
Penicillin	300 units
Streptomycin	300 μg.

Prepare solutions of penicillin and of streptomycin from sterile antibiotics with sterile precautions. Melt the sterile nutrient agar, cool it to 55° C. and add the sterile blood and the appropriate amounts of the antibiotic solutions. Distribute as desired.

Malt Agar

This medium is extensively used for the cultivation of saprophytic as well as parasitic yeasts and fungi, its high sugar content making it very suitable for this purpose. It is the best medium for highly exacting strains of fungi.

It is the basal medium described for tellurite malt agar (p. 771).

Corn Meal Agar

This medium (Benham, 1931) is used to investigate a yeast-like culture for the production of mycelium and chlamydospores. In the case of *Candida albicans* the appearance of the chlamydospores is diagnostic. Their production is favoured because the medium is poor in nutrients.

Corn meal (ground yellow maize)	40 g.
Agar	20 g.
Water	1 l.

Heat the corn meal in the water at about 60° C. for one hr. Filter through filter paper or gauze. Add water to bring the volume back to one litre. Add the agar and steam or autoclave to dissolve it. Filter. Autoclave at 121° C. for 30 min. The pH is about 6·8, requiring no adjustment.

Zein agar

Zein is the basic protein of corn meal and is a very effective substitute for corn meal in inducing the formation of chlamydospores by *Candida albicans*. Zein agar (Reid, Jones & Carter, 1953) has the advantage over corn meal agar of being clear, thus facilitating the search for the spores, and in giving more rapid and profuse formation of chlamydospores (within 24 hr.) because of the absence of reducing sugar. Zein may be obtained from Brown and Polson, Ltd., London.

Zein	40 g.
Agar	15 g.
Water	1 l.

Heat the zein in the water at 60° C. for 1 hr. Filter through gauze and coarse filter paper, and make up to original volume with distilled water.

Add agar and steam at 100° C. for 30 min. If necessary, adjust pH to 7·3–7·6 (adjustment is usually unnecessary). Sterilise by autoclaving at 121° C. for 15 min.

Rice Starch Agar

Like corn meal agar, this medium (Taschdjian, 1957) is used to stimulate mycelium and chlamydospore formation by *Candida albicans*. Rice flour is more easily obtained than American household yellow corn meal.

Rice flour	10 g.
Agar	15 g.
Tween 80	10 ml.
Water	1 l.

Bring the water to the boil and sprinkle in the rice flour. Boil for 30 sec., stand for a few seconds and filter through cotton gauze. Add water to re-adjust the volume to one litre. Add the agar and Tween 80 and autoclave at 121° C. for 30 min.

Malt Extract Broth

Malt extract	17 g.
Peptone (Oxoid mycological peptone)	3 g.
Water	1 l.

Dissolve the ingredients, adjust to pH 5·4, distribute and autoclave at 115° C. for 15 min.

MEDIA FOR THE CULTIVATION OF SPIROCHAETES

Of the three genera of spirochaetes, *Leptospira*, *Treponema* and *Borrelia*, only *Leptospira* will grow readily in culture media. Noguchi's (1912) medium is chiefly of historical interest but it has been used for isolating some pathogenic borreliae and for growing strains of *Treponema* that are probably non-pathogenic.

Other better media are available for cultivating *Leptospira*. These are usually liquid because the organisms do not grow readily on the surface of solid media. A semi-solid medium is less readily evaporated and may be of special value in the tropics.

LEPTOSPIRA MEDIA

Modified Korthof's Medium

Blood serum is an essential constituent of all leptospira media and a source of suitable serum must be established. Choice of a suitable peptone is also necessary for Korthof's medium because different batches, even of the same brand of peptone, vary in their growth-promoting abilities. Witte peptone and Difco neopeptone are recommended but any good brand is likely to be suitable. A preliminary test should be made of each new batch before taking it into use. With precautions as to serum and peptone this modified medium (Alston & Broom, 1958) is good for the cultivation of *Leptospira*.

All glassware must be perfectly clean and free from any trace of soap or other detergent since these are lethal to spirochaetes. After the usual cleaning it should be thoroughly rinsed, preferably by soaking for 24 hr. in a phosphate buffer solution at pH 7·6 (see Stuart's medium) and then rinsing in distilled water.

Peptone salt solution

Peptone	0·8 g.
Sodium chloride, NaCl	1·4 g.
Sodium bicarbonate, $NaHCO_3$	0·02 g.
Potassium chloride, KCl	0·04 g.
Calcium chloride, $CaCl_2$	0·04 g.
Potassium dihydrogen phosphate, KH_2PO_4	0·24 g.
Disodium hydrogen phosphate, $Na_2HPO_4 . 2H_2O$	0·88 g.
Distilled water	1 l.

Steam the ingredients at 100° C. for 20 min. and filter through Chardin-type or double thickness Whatman No. 1 paper. The pH should be approximately 7·2. Bottle in 100 ml. amounts and autoclave at 115° C. for 15 min.

Blood serum.—Rabbit serum is generally found the most satisfactory though the sera of some larger animals such as sheep, horse or new-born calf have been used successfully. Individual rabbit sera may be inhibitory to leptospires because of agglutinins or other agents. For this reason the sera of several rabbits should be tested individually for agglutinins or by making separate trial batches of medium from each serum. The suitable animals are retained to supply serum as required. Blood is collected from an ear vein or, preferably, by cardiac puncture and allowed to clot. The serum is pipetted off, inactivated by heating at 56° C. for 30 min. and sterilised by Seitz filtration.

"*Haemoglobin*" *solution.*—To the blood clot after removal of the serum add an equal volume of distilled water and freeze and thaw repeatedly to haemolyse the corpuscles. Sterilise by Seitz filtration.

Preparation of complete medium

Peptone salt solution	100 ml.
Sterile blood serum	8 ml.
Sterile "haemoglobin" solution	0·8 ml.

Mix the ingredients with sterile precautions. Distribute the medium in 2–3 ml. amounts in sterile screw-capped bijou bottles (p. 730). Test for sterility by incubating at 37° C. for 2 days and at 22° C. for 3 days.

Modified Stuart's Medium

Stuart's (1946) medium does not contain peptone and therefore is not subject to variations in peptones. It contains phenol red to confirm the pH of the medium and as an indicator of contaminants which tend to increase the acidity. Bryan's (1957) modification is described here.

All glassware must be specially cleaned as for Korthof's medium.

Stock solutions

L-asparagine (dextro-rotatory)	1·3 per cent.
Ammonium chloride, NH_4Cl	0·54 per cent.
Magnesium chloride, $MgCl_2 . 6H_2O$	2·03 per cent.
Sodium chloride, NaCl	0·58 per cent.
Thiamine hydrochloride	0·1 per cent.
Phenol red	0·02 per cent.

Prepare the stock solutions with distilled water and sterilise them by autoclaving at 115° C. for 15 min. The salt solutions are 0·1 *M.*

Phosphate buffer solutions

Potassium dihydrogen phosphate, KH_2PO_4 (A)	9·078 g. per l.
Disodium hydrogen phosphate, $Na_2HPO_4 . 2H_2O$ (B)	11·876 g. per l.

Prepare the solutions in distilled water and sterilise them by autoclaving at 121° C. for 30 min. A buffer solution of pH 7·6 contains the solutions in the proportion of 2·6 ml. of A to 17·4 ml. of B.

Blood serum.—Serum is prepared as for Korthof's medium (p. 774).

Preparation of complete medium

L-asparagine solution	2 ml.
Ammonium chloride solution	10 ml.
Magnesium chloride solution	4 ml.
Sodium chloride solution	66 ml.
Thiamine hydrochloride solution	0·4 ml.
Phenol red solution	10 ml.
Distilled water	91 ml.
Phosphate buffer, pH 7·6	16 ml.
Sterile inactivated rabbit serum	20 ml.

Mix all ingredients except the rabbit serum and steam at 100° C. for 30 min. to drive off dissolved carbon dioxide. Autoclave at 115° C. for 15 min. Add the serum with sterile precautions, distribute and test for sterility as for Korthof's medium. If the pH is correct the medium is an amber colour.

To obtain satisfactory results a large inoculum, about 10 per cent. of previous culture introduced with a Pasteur pipette, is used.

Dinger's Modification of Noguchi's Medium

This semi-solid medium (Wolff, 1954) is slower to evaporate than liquid media, especially in the tropics. Subcultures can be made less frequently so that virulence is maintained longer.

Nutrient agar, 3 per cent.	6 ml.
Distilled water	100 ml.
Sterile inactivated serum	10 ml.

Mix the agar and water and sterilise by autoclaving at 121° C. for 20 min. Add the serum with sterile precautions, distribute and test for sterility as for Korthof's medium.

MEDIA FOR THE CULTIVATION OF ENTAMOEBAE

The standard medium for the isolation of *Entamoeba histolytica* from faeces is that of Dobell and Laidlaw (1926) but Balamuth's (1946) medium is an improvement on it and is suitable for the cultivation of all other entamoebae from faeces.

Balamuth's Medium

1*M phosphate buffer*, *pH* 7·5

Dipotassium hydrogen phosphate, K_2HPO_4, 174 g. per l.	8·6 ml.
Potassium dihydrogen phosphate, KH_2PO_4, 136 g. per l.	1·4 ml.

It is convenient to keep separate stock solutions of the two salts and to mix them before use.

Stock solution of liver extract

Liver extract	5 g.
Water	100 ml.

Dissolve by boiling, filter and autoclave at 121° C. for 20 min.

Preparation of complete medium

Dehydrated egg yolk	36 g.
Sodium chloride, NaCl, 0·8 per cent. aqueous	About 150 ml.
Phosphate buffer, *M*/15 at pH 7·5	125 ml.
Liver extract, 5 per cent. aqueous	25 ml.
Rice starch, sterile	(1 loopful per 7–10 ml.)

Mix the egg yolk with an equal volume of water and add 125 ml. of saline. Stir vigorously with a rotary beater or in a Waring blender. Heat in a covered double boiler for 20 min. after the temperature of the infusion reaches 80° C. Make up the loss from evaporation with water, about 20 ml. being required. Express the extract through a double layer of muslin to yield about 100 ml. of yellowish fluid. Make up the volume to 125 ml. with saline. Autoclave at 121° C. for 20 min. The yellowish sediment may be removed by cooling below 10° C. and filtering but this is not essential.

Add phosphate buffer diluted from $1M$ to $M/15$. Add liver extract, dispense in tall test tubes and autoclave. Make sure that the rice starch is thoroughly dry and sterilise it by dry heat at 160° C. for 1½ hr. Dispense the medium in 7 to 10 ml. amounts in ordinary tubes and add a loopful of sterile rice just before use. The final pH is 7·3.

Jones's Medium

This medium (Jones, 1946) is best for routine passage of entamoeba cultures. It is easy to prepare and all amoebae grow in it.

Buffer saline solution, pH 7·2

Disodium hydrogen phosphate, Na_2HPO_4, anhydrous 9·48 g. per l.	375 ml.
Potassium dihydrogen phosphate, KH_2PO_4, 9·08 g. per l.	125 ml.
Sodium chloride, NaCl, 0·9 per cent.	2,250 ml.

Preparation of complete medium

Yeast extract, autolysed, 1 per cent.	100 ml.
Buffer saline solution, pH 7·2	850 ml.
Sterile horse serum	50 ml.
Rice starch, sterile	3 g.

Mix the yeast extract and saline. Sterilise by autoclaving at 121° C. for 30 min. Sterilise the rice starch as for Balamuth's medium. Add the serum and starch and distribute the medium with sterile precautions.

A suitable autolysed yeast extract is made by Marmite Limited, London.

Diamond's Medium

This medium (Diamond, 1960) is suitable for axenic cultures of entamoebae. It is clear and free from gross particulate matter; it is easily prepared and supports the growth of a large number of parasites.

Trypticase (BBL) or tryptone	2 g.
Yeast extract (BBL)	1 g.
Maltose	0·5 g.
L-cysteine hydrochloride	0·1 g.
L-ascorbic acid	0·02 g.
Potassium dihydrogen phosphate, KH_2PO_4	0·08 g.
Dipotassium hydrogen phosphate, K_2HPO_4	0·08 g.
Water	90 ml.
Horse or sheep serum, sterile, inactivated at 56° C. for 30 min.	10 ml.

Dissolve the dry ingredients in water. Adjust to pH 7·0 to 7·2 with N sodium hydroxide. Autoclave at 121° C. for 10 min. Cool. Add the serum and distribute in 10 ml. aliquots to sterile screw-capped bottles with sterile precautions. Store at 4° C. till used.

Subculture 1 ml. to each bottle of fresh medium and incubate at room temperature, not below 25° C.

MEDIUM FOR CULTIVATION OF *TRICHOMONAS VAGINALIS*

Modified CPLM Medium

Media for *T. vaginalis* must provide a carbohydrate energy source; inorganic phosphate; proteolysed tissue to provide the so-called pancreatic "s" factor, amino acids, nucleic bases and possibly B vitamins; and serum to provide pantothenic acid, linoleic acid and other less well-defined nutrients. Johnson and Trussell (1943) recommended CPLM (cysteine-peptone-liver infusion-maltose) medium and the following modification of it (Smith, 1964) has been found satisfactory. Agar has been omitted from this modification because it complicates handling of the medium and of cultures in it. Methylene blue is omitted also. Phosphate as such is not added because there is sufficient of it in other ingredients.

This medium supports growth from a single protozoon under strictly anaerobic conditions, the maximum population of 1–3 × 10^6 organisms per ml. being reached in 5–7 days at 37° C. Under aerobic conditions, massive inocula are required. *T. vaginalis* is an anaerobe and contains no catalase.

Basal Medium

Peptone	32 g.
Maltose	1·6 g.
Liver digest (Panmede)	20 g.
Cysteine hydrochloride	2·4 g.
Ringer's solution, ¼ strength	1 l.
Sodium hydroxide, NaOH, 1*N*	About 9 ml.

The brand of peptone is not important. Panmede ox liver digest obtainable from Paines and Byrne Ltd., Greenford, Middlesex, can be replaced by 32 per cent. of any brand of liver infusion made according to the manufacturer's instructions. Cysteine is not essential when cultures are incubated anaerobically but it assists the maintenance of anaerobiosis.

Dissolve the ingredients by shaking. Adjust the pH to 6·0 with sodium hydroxide, steam at 100° C. for 30 min. and filter off the fine grey precipitate with Whatman's No. 1 or coarse paper. Bottle in 90 ml. lots and autoclave at 115° C. for 10 min.

This medium keeps for several weeks.

Penicillin streptomycin solution

Penicillin	1 × 10^5 units
Streptomycin	0·1 g.
Sterile water	10 ml.

Dissolve the sterile antibiotics with sterile precautions. The solution contains 10^4 units of penicillin and 10^4 μg. streptomycin per ml. It will keep up to 10 days in the refrigerator.

Nystatin solution

Nystatin	5×10^4 units
Sterile water	10 ml.

Suspend the sterile antibiotic in the water. The suspension contains 5×10^3 units per ml. It keeps in the refrigerator at less than 10° C. but is rapidly destroyed at 37° C.

Preparation of complete medium

Basal medium	90 ml.
Sterile inactivated horse serum	10 ml.
Penicillin streptomycin solution	1 ml.
Nystatin solution	1 ml.

Before use, add the serum and antibiotics and distribute in suitable aliquots with sterile precautions. Serum from human, calf, ox, sheep or rabbit may be used. The addition of antibiotics is unnecessary for routine subcultures but is essential for clinical diagnostic cultures and for isolating axenic cultures. Nystatin can be omitted unless yeast or fungal contaminants are suspected.

MEDIUM FOR THE CULTIVATION OF LEISHMANIAE AND TRYPANOSOMES

The classical medium for the cultivation of trypanosomes and leishmaniae is NNN medium, a solid medium devised by Novy and MacNeal (1904) and modified by Nicolle (1908). The following medium (Tobie, von Brand & Mehlman, 1950) differs from it in that it consists of two phases, blood agar and Locke's solution. Trypanosomes incubated at 26° C. grow dispersed in the liquid and reach 20×10^6 per ml. in 10 to 14 days. They develop only to the proventricular stage. If the uninoculated medium is kept for six days the overlying liquid can be drawn off and used as a liquid medium. In it trypanosomes reach 9×10^6 per ml. in 8–10 days.

Solid Phase

Basal medium

Meat extract (Bacto-beef, Difco)	1·5 g.
Peptone (Bacto-peptone, Difco)	2·5 g.
Sodium chloride, NaCl	4 g.
Agar (Bacto-agar, Difco)	7·5 g.
Water	500 ml.

Dissolve the ingredients, adjust the pH to 7·2–7·4 with sodium hydroxide and autoclave at 121° C. for 25 min.

Citrated blood.—Whole rabbit blood containing 0·5 per cent. of sterile sodium citrate is inactivated at 56° C. for 30 min. Human blood can be used, but the blood of different donors varies in suitability.

Preparation of complete medium

Basal medium	75 ml.
Blood	25 ml.

Melt the basal medium, cool to 45° C., add the blood and distribute in 5 ml. amounts in sterile test-tubes or 25 ml. amounts in sterile flasks. Keep test-tubes in a slanted position and flasks upright until the medium has solidified.

Liquid Phase

Sodium chloride, NaCl	8 g.
Potassium chloride, KCl	0·2 g.
Calcium chloride, $CaCl_2$	0·2 g.
Potassium dihydrogen phosphate, KH_2PO_4 . .	0·3 g.
Glucose	2·5 g.
Water	1 l.

Dissolve the ingredients and autoclave at 121° C. for 15 min. With sterile precautions add 2 ml. to test-tubes and 10–15 ml. to flasks containing the solid medium.

MEDIA FOR PRESERVATION OF CULTURES

Egg Saline Medium

This modification of Dorset's egg medium, in which the broth is replaced by saline and no malachite green is added, is good for preserving cultures of Gram-negative cocci and bacilli.

Beaten egg	75 ml.
Sodium chloride, NaCl, sterile 0·85 per cent. solution	25 ml.

Prepare the beaten egg, mix and dispense the medium with sterile precautions as for Löwenstein-Jensen medium. Bijou bottles containing 2–3 ml. of medium may be used. Inspissate in a slanted position at 75–80° C. for 1 hr.

If the medium has been prepared without sterile precautions it can be allowed to cool for a few hr. after inspissation and then autoclaved at 121° C. for 15 min. with the screw-caps tightened. If the screw-caps are loose, some of the slants may be disrupted by bubbles of steam.

Fungus Preservation Medium

This is used to prevent pleomorphic variation in stock cultures of ringworm fungi.

Peptone	30 g.
Agar	20 g.
Water	1 l.

Dissolve the ingredients, filter through cotton gauze, adjust to pH 5·4, distribute and autoclave at 115° C. for 15 min.

TRANSPORT MEDIA

When the patient is not close to the bacteriological laboratory there is a risk that the pathogen in a bacteriological specimen may not survive or may be overgrown by non-pathogens during the time it takes to transport the specimen to the laboratory. Some media have been devised to protect pathogens during such a delay.

Pike's Medium

This medium (Pike, 1944) is used to preserve *Strept. pyogenes*, pneumococci and *H. influenzae* in nose and throat swabs (Holmes & Lermit, 1955; Masters, Brumfitt, Mendez & Likar, 1958). It is blood agar containing 1 in 1,000,000 crystal violet and 1 in 16,000 sodium azide distributed as for stab cultures in tubes or bottles.

Stuart's (1959) Transport Medium

This soft agar medium is used to maintain the viability of gonococci on swabs during their transmission through the post to a laboratory.

It is essential that the distilled water used in the medium be free from chlorine. To ensure this, it should be passed through an ion-exchange resin column before use.

Anaerobic salt solution

Thioglycollic acid (Difco)	2 ml.
Sodium hydroxide, 1*N* NaOH	12–15 ml.
Sodium glycerophosphate, 20 per cent. aqueous .	100 ml.
Calcium chloride, $CaCl_2$, 1 per cent. aqueous .	20 ml.
Distilled water	900 ml.

Mix the ingredients, adding sufficient sodium hydroxide to bring the pH to 7·2.

Agar solution

Agar	6 g.
Distilled water	1 l.

Dissolve by steaming.

Preparation of complete medium

Anaerobic salt solution	900 ml.
Agar solution	1 l.
Methylene blue, 0·1 per cent. aqueous . . .	4 ml.

Melt the agar and add the salt solution. Adjust the pH to 7·3–7·4. Add the methylene blue and distribute in bijou bottles, filling nearly to capacity. Autoclave at 121° C. for 15 min. and immediately tighten caps. When cool, the medium should be colourless.

Preparation of swabs.—Make neat swabs of absorbent cotton-wool on applicator sticks and boil 5 min. in 0·07 *M* phosphate buffer at pH 7·4. Shake off excess moisture and immerse in a 1 per cent. watery suspension of *finely powdered* charcoal, such as BDH activated charcoal, twirling until the cotton-wool is black. Shake off excess moisture, place in test-tubes, plug these with cotton-wool, dry in oven and sterilise in oven at 160° C. for 1½ hr.

Glycerol Saline Transport Medium for Enteric Bacilli

If there is likely to be a delay of some hours before specimens of faeces for culture reach the laboratory this transport medium prevents other intestinal organisms from overgrowing the enteric fever bacilli.

Glycerol	300 ml.
Sodium chloride, NaCl	4·2 g.
Disodium hydrogen phosphate, Na_2HPO_4, anhydrous	10 g.
Phenol red, 0·02 per cent. aqueous	About 15 ml.
Water	700 ml.

Dissolve the sodium chloride in the water and add the glycerol. Add the phosphate and steam to dissolve it. Then add enough phenol red to give a purple-pink colour, judged by pouring a small quantity of the solution into a Universal container. Distribute in 6 ml. amounts in Universal containers and autoclave at 115° C. for 20 min.

The fluid should not be used if it becomes acid, indicated by a change in colour to yellow.

Bile Peptone Transport Medium

This medium is useful for field work in hot climates where cholera may occur. Rectal swabs of faeces may be inoculated into the medium which is then returned to the base laboratory. Subcultures to Monsur's medium should be made within 6 hr. if possible. If this is impracticable it should be subcultured to Monsur's medium immediately on return to the base laboratory and then incubated at 37° C. overnight and sub-cultured again the next day.

Trypticase or any good peptone	1 g.
Sodium chloride, NaCl	1 g.
Sodium taurocholate	0·5 g.
Water	100 ml.

Dissolve the ingredients, adjust to pH 8·5 with sodium hydroxide, distribute into bottles and autoclave at 121° C. for 15 min.

In order to make this medium more selective for vibrios, sterile potassium tellurite solution may be added after autoclaving to give a final concentration of 1 in 200,000 as for Monsur's medium. The medium is slightly turbid. It should not be kept longer than two weeks.

MEDIA FOR THE EXAMINATION OF MILK AND WATER

Yeast Extract Agar

This is a nutrient agar in which yeast extract replaces meat extract. It is employed particularly for making plate counts of the viable bacteria in drinking water. The formula given is that prescribed by the Ministry of Health in a Report on Public Health and Medical Subjects (1934).

Yeast extract	3 g.
Peptone	5 g.
Agar, shredded or powdered	15 g.
Water	1 l.

The recommended brand of yeast extract is "Yeastrel", supplied by the Brewer's Food Supply Co. Ltd., Edinburgh. Dissolve the yeast extract and peptone in the water at 100° C., cool to room temperature and adjust to pH 7·4. Place the agar if shredded in a muslin bag, wash in running water for 15 min. and express excess moisture before adding it to the broth. Autoclave at 121° C. for 20 min. and filter hot through paper pulp. Test the pH of the filtrate at 50° C. and adjust to pH 7·0 to give a final pH of 7·2 when cool. Distribute in 10 ml. amounts and sterilise by autoclaving at 121° C. for 20 min.

Yeast Extract Milk Agar

This medium is used for making plate counts of viable bacteria in milk supplies and rinse waters from dairy and food utensils. It is the medium specified by the Secretary of State for the examination of milk supplies in Scotland under the Milk (Special Designations) (Scotland) Order, 1951. The medium is prepared in the same way as yeast extract agar, but 10 ml. of fresh or spray-dried, skim or whole milk is added per litre of broth at the same time as the washed agar is added.

MacConkey Bile-Salt Lactose Peptone Water

This medium is used for detecting the presence of coliform organisms in water and milk.

Single strength

Sodium taurocholate (commercial)	5 g.
Peptone (any good make)	20 g.
Sodium chloride, NaCl	5 g.
Lactose	10 g.
Bromocresol purple, 1 per cent. solution in ethanol	1 ml.
or Neutral red, 1 per cent. aqueous solution . .	5 ml.
Water	1 l.

Dissolve the bile salt, peptone and sodium chloride, steam for 2 hr., cool and transfer to the refrigerator overnight. Add the lactose and when dissolved filter cold through Chardin filter paper. Adjust the reaction to pH 7·4 and add the indicator. Distribute in 5 ml. amounts in 1-oz. bottles or $6 \times \frac{5}{8}$ in. test-tubes with Durham tubes and autoclave at 115° C. for 15 min.

Double strength.—Make as above, but with double the amounts of the ingredients, except water. Distribute in 50 ml. amounts in 5-oz. bottles using $3 \times \frac{3}{8}$ in. test-tubes as Durham tubes, and in 10 ml. amounts in 1-oz. bottles using $2 \times \frac{1}{4}$ in. Durham tubes.

Brilliant Green Bile Broth

This medium is used in the differential coliform test of water supplies to eliminate false positives due to anaerobes.

Ox bile.—Fresh ox bile may be used. Otherwise dissolve 20 g. dehydrated ox bile in 200 ml. water and adjust the pH to 7·0–7·5.

Preparation of medium

Peptone	10 g.
Ox bile	200 ml.
Lactose	10 g.
Brilliant green, 0·1 per cent. aqueous solution	13 ml.
Water to	1 l.

Dissolve the peptone in 500 ml. water, add the ox bile and lactose. Adjust the pH to 7·4. Add the brilliant green solution and water to make up 1 l. Distribute in 5 ml. quantities in $6 \times \frac{5}{8}$ in. tubes with Durham fermentation tubes. Autoclave at 115° C. for 15 min.

Sodium Azide Medium

This medium (Hannay and Norton, 1947) is used for the isolation of *Strept. faecalis* from water.

Peptone	10 g.
Sodium chloride, NaCl	5 g.
Dipotassium hydrogen phosphate, K_2HPO_4	5 g.
Potassium dihydrogen phosphate, KH_2PO_4	2 g.
Glucose	5 g.
Yeast extract (Yeastrel)	3 g.
Sodium azide, NaN_3	0·25 g.
Bromocresol purple, 1·6 per cent. solution in ethanol	2 ml.
Water	1 l.

Dissolve the ingredients. The medium has a pH of 6·6–6·8 and no adjustment is necessary. Distribute in 5 ml. quantities in tubes. For use with inocula of 10 or 50 ml. of water, a medium of double this strength is prepared and distributed in 10 and 50 ml. quantities. Sterilise in the autoclave at 121° C. for 15 min.

IDENTIFICATION OF MEDIA

It is necessary to identify a culture medium after it has been made and, as media such as the kinds of nutrient agar and the different sugar media are similar in appearance, it is essential to have some simple but reliable system of marking. Gummed labels are generally unsatisfactory especially as they become detached in the steamer when solid media are melted. Colours, either alone or in combination, are good for distinguishing media. It is better to use a few outstanding colours alone or in combination if necessary, rather than different shades of a colour; thus, green, irrespective of the shade, whether it be light or dark, yellowish green or bluish green, always indicates glucose. The colour may be indicated with coloured cotton-wool; or with cellulose paint applied to the caps of screw-capped bottles or applied as a small patch on glassware; or with coloured beads.

Coloured cotton-wool can be used for tubes and flasks. Some other system is needed for screw-capped bottles and tubes with metal caps. The cotton-wool colour range does not include gold and silver for which there are paints.

Cellulose paint on the caps is the best method for small screw-capped bottles and tubes with metal caps. Coloured beads are good for large bottles. Ordinary opaque glass beads, 6–7 mm. in diameter are suitable, but clear glass beads are not. Before use the beads are boiled twice in distilled water and dried in the incubator. The appropriate bead is dropped into the bottle before it is filled. Owing to the convexity of the bottom of the bottle, the bead remains to one side and is very easily recognised no matter what type of culture medium is used. On tilting the bottle for pouring, the bead comes to rest on the shoulder and remains in this position, even when the bottle is almost completely inverted.

It is recommended that a standard colour scheme be adopted and the following system is suggested, as it is already widely used.

Nutrient broth and agar from dehydrated stock	White
Infusion broth and agar	Yellow
Meat extract broth and agar	Brown
Digest broth and agar	Black
Fildes' broth and agar	Black/white
Casein yeast lactate (CYL) concentrate (Marshall and Kelsey)	Brown/white
Complete CYLG medium (Marshall and Kelsey)	Brown/green
Peptone water	White
Salt cooked meat broth	Orange
Serum broth and agar	Blue/white
Glucose broth and agar	Green
Crystal violet blood agar	Red/blue
MacConkey's liquid medium. Single strength	1 red spot

MacConkey's liquid medium. Double strength	2 red spots
MacConkey's agar medium	Red
Desoxycholate citrate agar (DCA)	Red/orange
Tomato juice agar	Red/yellow
Sabouraud's medium	Light blue
Distilled water	White
Normal saline (0·85 per cent.)	Dark blue
Glucose in saline	Blue/green
Saline agar bleeding tubes	White

Media for Biochemical Tests

Citrate	Orange/white
Craigie tubes	White
Decarboxylase—Arginine	Pink
Lysine	White
Ornithine	Blue
Control	Black
Gillies' I and II	White
Gluconate	Green/yellow
Glucose phosphate for V.P. test	Green/orange
H_2S broth	Blue/brown
Malonate—Phenylalanine (combined medium of Shaw and Clarke)	Blue/green
Nitrate broth	Brown/red
Nitrite broth	Brown/yellow
Nutrient gelatin	Blue
Organic acids—Citrate	Orange/white
Mucate	Mauve
Dextro-tartrate	Red/black
Laevo-tartrate	Brown/black
Meso-tartrate	Mauve/black
Phenylalanine agar	Pink
Plasma broth	Green/white
Urea	Mauve

Fermentation Media ("Sugars")

Where colours are mentioned for which there is no coloured cotton-wool, a small patch of cellulose paint is placed on the tube itself.

Adonitol	Silver	Fructose (laevulose)	Yellow
Aesculin	Brown		
Arabinose	Black and yellow	Galactose	Mauve and white
Dextrin	Red and mauve	Glucose	Green
Dextrose	(see Glucose)	Glycerol	Brown and white
Dulcitol	Pink	Glycogen	Blue and yellow
Erythritol	Black and red	Inositol	Gold

Inulin	Yellow and white	Salicin	Pink and white
Lactose	Red	Sorbitol	Black and blue
Maltose	Blue and white	Starch	Yellow and mauve
Mannitol	Mauve	Sucrose (saccharose)	Blue
Mannose	Black and green		
Raffinose	Red and white	Trehalose	Mauve and green
Rhamnose	Black and pink	Xylose	Red and green

REFERENCES

ALSTON, J. H. & BROOM, J. C. (1958). *Leptospirosis in Man and Animals.* p. 303. Edinburgh: Livingstone.

ANDERSON, J. S., HAPPOLD, F. C., MCLEOD, J. W. & THOMSON, J. G. (1931). On the existence of two forms of diphtheria bacillus—*B. diphtheriae gravis* and *B. diphtheriae mitis*—and a new medium for their differentiation and for the bacteriological diagnosis of diphtheria. *J. Path. Bact.*, **34**, 667.

ANDERSON, P. M. (1944). A simple medium for the detection of *Corynebacterium diphtheriae. Med. J. Aust.*, **1**, 213.

ARONSON, H. (1915). Eine neue Methode der bakteriologischen Choleradiagnose. *Dtsch. med. Wschr.*, **41**, 1027.

ASHESHOV, I. N. (1941). Papain digest media and standardisation of media in general. *Canad. J. publ. Hlth.*, **32**, 468.

BALAMUTH, W. (1946). Improved egg yolk infusion for cultivation of *Entamoeba histolytica* and other intestinal protozoa. *Amer. J. clin. Path.*, **16**, 380.

BENHAM, RHODA W. (1931). Certain monilias parasitic on man. Their identification by morphology and by agglutination. *J. Infect. Dis.*, **49**, 183.

BREWER, J. H. (1940). Clear liquid mediums for the "aerobic" culture of anaerobes. *J. Amer. med. Ass.*, **115**, 598.

BROTHERSTON, J. G., GILMOUR, N. J. L. & SAMUEL, J. MCA. (1961). Quantitative studies of *Mycobacterium johnei* in the tissues of sheep. *J. comp. Path. Therap.*, **71**, 286.

BRYAN, H. S. (1957). Studies on leptospirosis in domestic animals. *Vet. Med.*, **52**, 111.

CHRISTIE, R. & KEOGH, E. V. (1940). Physiological and serological characteristics of staphylococci of human origin. *J. Path. Bact.*, **51**, 189.

DE MAN, J. C., ROGOSA, M. & SHARPE, M. E. (1960). A medium for the cultivation of lactobacilli. *J. appl. Bact.*, **23**, 130.

Diagnostic Procedures and Reagents (1950). 3rd ed., p. 44. New York: American Public Health Association.

DIAMOND, L. S. (1960). The axenic cultivation of two reptilian parasites, *Entamoeba terrapinae* Sanders and Cleveland, 1930, and *Entamoeba invadens* Rodhain, 1934. *J. Parasit*, **46**, 484.

DIEUDONNÉ, A. (1909). Blutalkaliagar, ein Elektivnährboden für Choleravibrionen. *Zbl. Bakt. I. Abt. Orig.*, **50**, 107.

DOBELL, C. & LAIDLAW, P P. (1926). On the cultivation of *Entamoeba histolytica* and some other entozoic amoebae. *Parasitology*, **18**, 283.

ELLNER, P. D. (1956). A medium promoting rapid quantitative sporulation in *Clostridium perfringens. J. Bact.*, **71**, 495.

FAIRBROTHER, R. W. & SOUTHALL, J. E. (1950). The isolation of *Staphylococcus pyogenes* from faeces. *Mth. Bull. Minist. Hlth Lab. Serv.*, **9**, 170.

FINEGOLD, S. M. & SWEENEY, E. E. (1961). New selective and differential medium for coagulase-positive staphylococci allowing rapid growth and strain differentiation. *J. Bact.*, **81**, 636.

GLADSTONE, G. P. & FILDES, P. (1940). A simple culture medium for general use without meat extract or peptone. *Brit. J. exp. Path.*, **21**, 161.

HADLEY, F. P. (1933). A quantitative method for estimating *Bacillus acidophilus* in saliva. *J. dent. Res.*, **13**, 415.

HANNAY, C. L. & NORTON, I. L. (1947). Enumeration, isolation and study of faecal streptococci from river water. *Proc. Soc. appl. Bact.*, **1**, 39.

HILL, J. H. & WHITE, E. C. (1929). Sodium chloride media for the separation of certain Gram-positive cocci and Gram-negative bacilli. *J. Bact.*, **18**, 43.

HOBBS, BETTY C. & ALLISON, V. D. (1945). Studies on the isolation of *Bact. typhosum* and *Bact. paratyphosum B. Mth. Bull. Minist. Hlth Lab. Serv.*, **4**, 12 and 63.

HOLMES, M. C. & LERMIT, A. (1955). Transport and enrichment media in the isolation of haemolytic streptococci from the upper respiratory tract. *Mth. Bull. Minist. Hlth Lab. Serv.*, **14**, 97.

HOYLE, L. (1941). A tellurite blood-agar medium for the rapid diagnosis of diphtheria. *Lancet*, **1**, 175.

HUDDLESON, I. F. (1939). *Brucelloses in Man and Animals*. p. 13. New York: Commonwealth Fund.

IVES, J. C. J. & MCCORMICK, W. (1956). A modification of Sula's method for the cultivation of tubercle bacilli from pleural fluid. *J. clin. Path.*, **9**, 177.

JACOBS, S. I., WILLIS, A. T. & GOODBURN, G. M. (1964). Pigment production and enzymatic activity of staphylococci: the differentiation of pathogens from commensals. *J. Path. Bact.*, **87**, 151.

JAMESON, J. E. & EMBERLEY, N. W. (1956). A substitute for bile salts in culture media. *J. gen. Microbiol.*, **15**, 198.

JENSEN, K. A. (1955). Second Report of the Sub-Committee of Laboratory Methods of the International Union against Tuberculosis. *Bull. int. Un. Tuberc.*, **25**, 89.

JOHNSON, G. & TRUSSELL, R. E. (1943). Experimental basis for the chemotherapy of *Trichomonas vaginalis* infestations I. *Proc. Soc. exp. Biol.* (*N.Y.*), **54**, 245.

Joint FAO/WHO Expert Committee on Brucellosis. Third Report (1958). Annex 10. Selective media for the culture of *Brucella* from potentially contaminated samples. *Wld Hlth Org. techn. Rep. Ser.*, No. 148, 50.

JONES, L. M. & MORGAN, W. J. B. (1958). A preliminary report on a selective medium for the culture of *Brucella*, including fastidious types. *Bull. Wld Hlth Org.*, **19**, 200.

JONES, W. R. (1946). The experimental infection of rats with *Entamoeba histolytica*, with a method for evaluating the anti-amoebic properties of new compounds. *Ann. trop. Med. Parasit.*, **40**, 130.

KIRCHNER, O. (1932). Die Leistungsfähigkeit der Tiefenkultur des Tuberkelbazillus bei Verwendung besonders geeingneter flüssiger Nährboden. *Zbl. Bakt. I. Abt. Orig.*, **124**, 403.

KNOX, R., GELL, P. G. H. & POLLOCK, M. R. (1942). Selective media for organisms of the Salmonella group. *J. Path. Bact.*, **54**, 469.

LACEY, B. W. (1954). A new selective medium for *Haemophilus pertussis*, containing a diamidine, sodium fluoride and penicillin. *J. Hyg.* (*Lond.*), **52**, 273.

LEIFSON, E. (1936). New selenite enrichment media for the isolation of typhoid and paratyphoid (Salmonella) bacilli. *Amer. J. Hyg.*, **24**, 423.

LOWBURY, E. J. L. & LILLY, H. A. (1955). A selective plate medium for *Cl. welchii*. *J. Path. Bact.*, **70**, 105.

LUDLAM, G. B. (1949). A selective medium for the isolation of *Staph. aureus* from heavily contaminated material. *Mth. Bull. Minist. Hlth Lab. Serv.*, **8**, 15.

MARSHALL, J. H. & KELSEY, J. C. (1960). A standard culture medium for general bacteriology. *J. Hyg.* (*Lond.*), **58**, 367.

MASTERS, P. L., BRUMFITT, W., MENDEZ, R. L. & LIKAR, M. (1958). Bacterial flora of the upper respiratory tract in Paddington families, 1952-4. *Brit. med. J.*, **1**, 1200.

MEDICAL RESEARCH COUNCIL (1948). Specific laboratory tests in streptomycin therapy of tuberculosis. *Lancet*, **2**, 862.

MONSUR, K. A. (1963). Bacteriological diagnosis of cholera under field conditions. *Bull. Wld Hlth Org.*, **28**, 387.

NAYLOR, P. G. D. (1961). An improved method for the preparation of "chocolate" agar. *J. med. Lab. Technol.*, **18**, 275.

NICOLLE, C. (1908). Culture du parasite du bouton d'Orient. *C. R. Acad. Sci.* (*Paris*), **146**, 842.

NOGUCHI, H. (1912). The pure cultivation of *Spirochaeta duttoni*, *Spirochaeta kochi*, *Spirochaeta obermeieri* and *Spirochaeta novyi*. *J. exp. Med.*, **16**, 199.

NOVY, F. G. & MACNEAL, W. J. (1904). On the cultivation of *Trypanosoma brucei*. *J. infect. Dis.*, **1**, 1.

PIKE, R. M. (1944). An enrichment broth for isolating haemolytic streptococci from throat swabs. *Proc. Soc. exp. Biol.* (*N.Y.*), **57**, 186.

REID, J. D., JONES, MURIEL M. & CARTER, EVELYN B. (1953). A simple, clear medium for demonstration of chlamydospores of *Candida albicans*. *Amer. J. clin. Path.*, **23**, 938.

Rep. publ. Hlth med. Subj., Lond., No. 71 (1934). The bacteriological examination of water supplies. p. 30. London: H.M. Stationery Office.

SMITH, H. W. (1953). Modifications of Dubos's media for the cultivation of *Mycobacterium johnei*. *J. Path. Bact.*, **66**, 375.

SMITH, K. (1964). Personal communication.

STONEBRINK, B. (1957). Tubercle bacilli and pyruvic acid. *Proc. Tuberc. Res. Coun.*, **44**, 67.

STUART, R. D. (1946). The preparation and use of a simple culture medium for leptospirae. *J. Path. Bact.*, **58**, 343.

STUART, R. D. (1959). Transport medium for specimens in Public Health bacteriology. *Publ. Hlth Rep.* (*Wash.*), **74**, 431.

SYKES, G. (1956). Constituents of Bacteriological Culture Media. *Report of the Society for General Microbiology*. Cambridge University Press.

TASCHDJIAN, CLAIRE L. (1957). Routine identification of *Candida albicans*: current methods and a new medium. *Mycologia*, **49**, 332.

TOBIE, E. J., von BRAND, T. & MEHLMAN, B. (1950). Cultural and physiological observations on *Trypanosoma rhodesiense* and *Trypanosoma gambiense*. *J. Parasit.*, **36**, 48.

WILLIS, A. T. & HOBBS, G. (1959). Some new media for the isolation and identification of clostridia. *J. Path. Bact.*, **77**, 511.

WILSON, W. J. (1938). Isolation of *Bact. typhosum* by means of bismuth sulphite medium in water- and milk-borne epidemics. *J. Hyg.* (*Lond.*), **38**, 507.

WOLFF, J. W. (1954). *The Laboratory Diagnosis of Leptospirosis*. p. 23. Springfield: Thomas.

WRIGHT, H. D. (1933). The importance of adequate reduction of peptone in the preparation of media for the pneumococcus and other organisms. *J. Path. Bact.*, **37**, 257.

YOUMANS, G. P. (1944). Subsurface growth of virulent human tubercle bacilli in a synthetic medium. *Proc. Soc. exp. Biol.* (*N.Y.*), **57**, 122.

YOUNG, M. Y. (1942). Diphtheria diagnosis with Hoyle's medium. Saponin and sodium-dioctyl-sulpho-succinate as haemolysing agents in the preparation of the medium. *J. Path. Bact.*, **54**, 253.

CHAPTER 48

CULTIVATION OF MICROORGANISMS

USE OF CULTURE MEDIA

GENERAL methods of culture and preservation of microorganisms are described here. Special methods applicable for particular purposes are referred to elsewhere, in the appropriate sections.

PERSONAL PRECAUTIONS IN BACTERIOLOGICAL LABORATORY WORK

It is essential to wear an overall while at work. If any material containing pathogenic organisms drops on the bench, floor, clothes, apparatus, etc., it should be sterilised at once with 3 per cent. lysol or a 0·1 per cent. solution of mercuric chloride. If the hands become contaminated they should be disinfected in a basin of dilute lysol or mercuric chloride solution, and workers should make it a rule always to wash the hands thoroughly after completing any bacteriological work and particularly when leaving the laboratory.

It must be emphasised that in the laboratory labels must never be licked. There is always a grave risk of infection by this habit. Labels should be moistened either by a drop of water on the finger or by a pledget of wet cotton wool.

It is recommended that the worker refrains from smoking, particularly when dealing with cultures or infective material. No food should be consumed in a bacteriological laboratory.

Precautions to be taken in carrying out special methods are referred to later.

Bacteriological and pathological laboratory workers should consult the Report (1958) on precautions against tuberculous infection in the diagnostic laboratory. This deals with the risk of tuberculous infection associated with work on material containing tubercle bacilli, not only in the laboratory but also in the animal house and post-mortem room; it summarises the precautions to be taken in the course of such work to avoid accidental infection. It is emphasised that no protective face mask less complex and uncomfortable than the Service type gas mask will give useful protection against the inhalation of infected, airborne particles. When work is done with dangerous pathogens, such as the tubercle bacillus, it is recommended that the procedures are carried out in a protective "inoculation cabinet", which is specially ventilated and contains an ultraviolet lamp for disinfection after use (see p. 796).

SEPARATION OF MIXED CULTURES AND ISOLATION OF PURE CULTURES

Isolation of Pure Cultures.—Most studies and tests of the physiological, immunological and other characters of bacteria are valid only when made on a *pure culture*, i.e. an isolated growth of a single strain free from mixture and contamination with other bacteria. For this reason, in the diagnostic examination of mixed infective material, an essential preliminary is the isolation of the pertinent organism in a pure culture. This is normally achieved by the method of "plating out" on a solid culture medium. The solid medium most used is *nutrient agar*, a preparation of nutrient broth jellified by addition of the polysaccharide "agar-agar" (p. 735); it is usually dispensed as a flat layer in a shallow "Petri" dish. The infected material is inoculated on the surface of this and spread out very thinly. Where the bacteria are deposited singly at sufficient distance from each other (*e.g.* 1 cm.), the whole progeny of each accumulates locally during growth to form a discrete mass, or *colony*, which is readily visible to the naked eye (*e.g.* 0·5–5 mm. diam.). Each colony constitutes a pure culture, since it consists exclusively of the descendants of a single cell; it may be "picked" with a sterile inoculating wire to prepare a pure subculture in a fresh medium. Occasionally a mixed colony is formed from two bacteria that have been inoculated close together on the agar, and this must be avoided. The maintenance of pure cultures necessitates the use of properly sterilised media, containers and instruments, and continuous covering against the deposition of dust-borne bacteria from the air; during inoculation, the culture medium should be uncovered only for a few seconds.

The several techniques available for the isolation of pure cultures are:—

1. By Plating Out.—In most cases the method shown in Fig. 58 is employed.

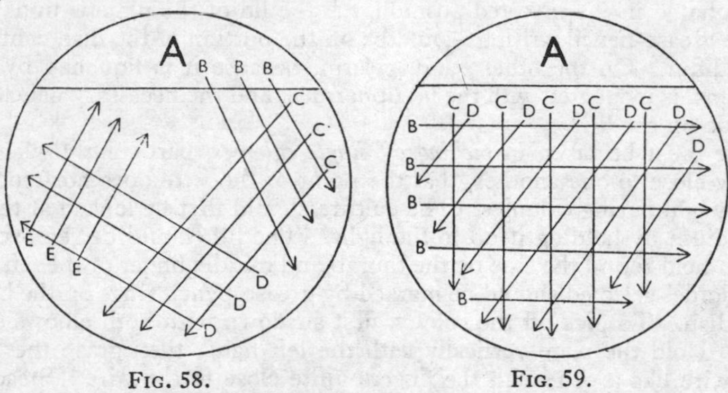

Fig. 58. Fig. 59.

A wire loop, sterilised by heating in a Bunsen flame, and then allowed to cool, is charged with the bacterial mixture, pus or other pathologic material and smeared thoroughly over area A to give a well-inoculum. The loop is resterilised and then drawn from the well-inoculum in two or three parallel lines on to the fresh surface of the medium (B, B, B); this process is repeated as shown in the Figure, care being taken to sterilise and then cool the loop between each sequence. At each step the inoculum comprises the most distal part of the immediately preceding strokes.

When selective media are being employed, *e.g.* DCA, they can be more heavily inoculated (Fig. 59). Several loopfuls of the specimen are used to spread the well-inoculum (A); the loop is resterilised in a flame, recharged by rubbing it over area A, and then used to inoculate the remainder of the plate by successive parallel strokes, B, C and D, drawn in the directions indicated in the diagram. Using this method with selective media a heavy inoculation can be made with the resulting colonies well separated except, of course, in the well-inoculum.

An alternative method for Petri dishes is to employ a spreader. This is made by bending a piece of glass rod, 3 mm. diameter, at a right angle in the blowpipe flame, the short limb, used for spreading, being 1 in. long. Spreaders may be sterilised in the hot air oven, a number being packed in a metal tin with a "press-on" lid loosely applied. Alternatively, a sterile capillary pipette held horizontally may be heated about ½ in. from its lip in the pilot flame of a Bunsen burner. As the glass softens, the end of the pipette bends at right angles making a spreader. A small amount of the bacterial mixture is placed on the plate with an inoculating loop or capillary pipette. By means of a sterilised spreader the material is evenly distributed over the surface. The spreader is then transferred to a second plate, which is similarly inoculated. Thus the medium in the second dish is inoculated merely with the organisms carried over by the spreader from the first.

By these methods the bacteria are gradually wiped off the wire or spreader so that they are ultimately deposited singly. Generally from each individual organism an isolated colony will grow; a single colony may be subcultured on fresh media and so yield a pure growth. If there is any doubt as to whether a pure colony has been obtained for picking, the colony should be replated immediately on a fresh plate and a single colony picked from this second plating. *In order to ensure separation, the surface of the medium must be dry* (see p. 728).

Plate cultures should have the nature of the material, and also the date, written on the glass of the Petri dish by means of a grease pencil. Agar plates are incubated in the inverted position, *i.e.* the lid of the plate is underneath and the grease-pencil writing should be on the portion of the dish containing the medium. On the other hand, gelatin, because it is liquefied by many organisms, is incubated with the lid uppermost and the necessary pencil notes are made on the lid.

Care must be taken in *picking off single colonies*, particularly when they are very close to one another, that the point of the wire does not touch any of the neighbouring colonies. The culture should first be looked at through the medium by holding it up to the light. The lid should be removed and the dish held round the side by the thumb and middle finger of the left hand. The colonies selected should be marked by grease-pencil rings on the bottom of the dish. To pick off the colony, first sit down with both elbows on the bench. Hold the plate vertically with the left hand, then grasp the holder of the wire like a pen, with the fingers quite close to the wire. Steady the right hand by placing the little finger on the left thumb in the way artists support the hand when painting. The selected colony is then easily removed without touching the others. Lay the plate on the bench, withdraw the right hand to the other end of the holder and inoculate the required medium in the manner previously described.

Plate Culture Microscope.—Several makers produce low-power binocular magnifiers which are extremely useful for examining plate cultures of organisms; they have a long working distance so that a colony can also be picked off the plate while using the instrument. When dealing with bacteria forming small delicate colonies, or where the colonies of the desired organism are few in number, the low-power binocular is invaluable. A magnification of ten diameters is useful for general work, but with interchangeable eye-pieces and objectives, magnifications from six to thirty diameters are available.

2. By Plating Decimal Dilutions of the Inoculum.—A series of tubes or bottles of melted agar or gelatin are inoculated with successive decimal dilutions of the infected material and then the medium in each tube is poured into a Petri dish and allowed to solidify. By dilution, the bacteria are separated from one another, and on incubation the resulting colonies are distributed

singly throughout the solid medium. A colony may be picked for subculture by pricking through the agar to it with the point of an inoculating wire.

3. By Heating and Subsequent Plating.—This method is employed when the organisms to be obtained in pure culture are more resistant to heat than the remainder of the bacteria present. The method applies especially to spore-bearing organisms, such as the clostridia, the spores of which survive the heating. The mixture of bacteria is heated to 65° C. for half an hour and then plated. From the spores, individual colonies develop, and these may then be picked off.

4. By Shake Culture in Tubes.—This method is sometimes used in the separation of anaerobic organisms.

5. By the Use of Selective Media.—Media such as desoxycholate-citrate-agar for the *Salmonella* and *Shigella* groups, Dieudonné's for the cholera vibrio, the tellurite media for the diphtheria bacillus, etc., have been devised so that the majority of the organisms other than those for which the media are used will not grow, and the isolation of pure cultures is thus facilitated.

6. By Animal Inoculation.—Advantage is taken of the fact that laboratory animals are highly susceptible to certain organisms—for example, the mouse to the pneumococcus. If a mixture of organisms containing the pneumococcus, *e.g.* sputum, be inoculated subcutaneously into a mouse, the animal dies of pneumococcal septicaemia in 24–36 hr., and from the heart blood the organism can be obtained in pure culture. Similarly the tubercle bacillus can be isolated from contaminating organisms by inoculation of a guinea-pig. The tubercle bacillus is found in a pure state in the resulting lesions.

INOCULATION OF CULTURE MEDIA

According to the nature of the medium and the inoculum, various methods are employed for inoculation, and the following instruments are commonly used:

Wire Loop.—The original type of inoculating wire was of platinum, No. 23 SWG, 2½ in. long, but, owing to the high cost of platinum, "Nichrome" or "Eureka" resistance wire, No. 24 SWG, is now generally used. One end of the wire is fused into a glass rod, or inserted into a special aluminium holder. The other end is bent in the form of a loop, 2 mm. internal diameter, care being taken that the loop is flat and completely closed.

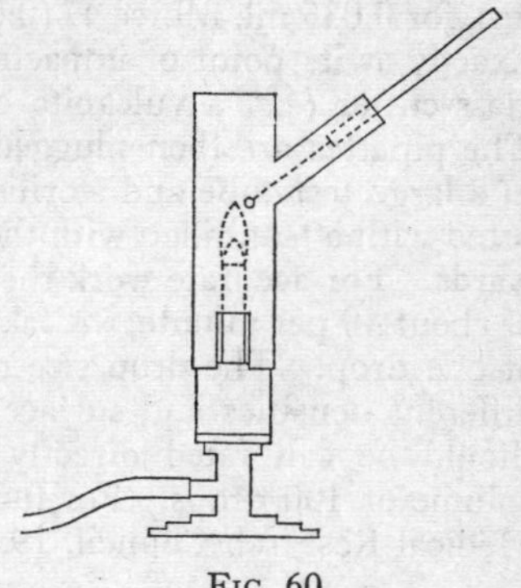

Fig. 60.

The wire is sterilised by holding it vertically in a Bunsen flame so that the whole length becomes red-hot at the same time. A wire charged with certain growths, *e.g.* of the tubercle bacillus, should be sterilised slowly in the cooler part of the flame, or a hooded Bunsen burner should be used (see diagram), as particles of unsterilised culture may "spurt" from the wire on to the bench. The loop is the most useful of the inoculating wires. It takes up a considerable amount of solid culture, or a large drop of fluid.

Straight Wire.—This is similar to the foregoing, but without the loop. It is used for stab cultures, and also for picking off single colonies.

Long Straight Wire.—A wire 4½ in. long mounted on a holder is employed for deep-stab inoculation when working with anaerobes.

Thick Wire, particularly with a loop, is very useful on account of its rigidity for lifting thick viscid sputum and tenacious growths.

Scalpel.—This instrument, sterilised by flaming, is used for making inoculations with scrapings from tissues and ulcers, etc.

STERILE PIPETTES.—Bulb pipettes (10–100 ml.) are used when large amounts of fluid inoculum have to be added to a medium, and graduated 1-ml. or 10-ml. pipettes when the inoculum is between 0·1 and 10 ml. These pipettes are stoppered with a cotton-wool plug in their upper end to guard against contamination of their interior or accidental aspiration of their contents. Because of the danger of infection, they should not be placed directly in the mouth, but should be operated either with a rubber teat or with a glass mouthpiece which is attached by a length of rubber tubing and sterilised by flaming (see p. 911 for details).

STERILE CAPILLARY PIPETTES.—These are made by heating the middle of a piece of glass tubing, 5 mm. bore and 20 cm. long, and when melted pulling out the two halves; the capillary formed in the middle is broken after cooling and two pipettes are thus obtained. The capillary ends, which should not be too thin, are sealed in the flame, and the other ends are plugged with cotton-wool. They are placed in a large test-tube (*e.g.* 8 × 1½ in.), which is then stoppered with cotton-wool, or covered with paper or aluminium foil, and sterilised with dry heat. Before use, the tip of the capillary portion is broken off and a rubber teat fitted to the other end. An alternative method is to prepare the 8-in. lengths of glass tubing with cotton-wool plugs in each end, wrap them in bundles of 8–10 in kraft paper, sterilise in the hot-air oven, and draw the capillaries in a flame just before they are required for use. These pipettes are very useful in many bacteriological manipulations.

CAPILLARY PIPETTES DELIVERING MEASURED DROPS.—Small measured volumes are conveniently delivered with sterile capillary pipettes that have been prepared to give drops of a known volume. The pipettes are drawn from glass tubing as described above. When cool, the capillary is inserted into the appropriate hole of a Morse drill gauge and pressed through until it engages. For water drops of 0·020 ml. the hole used is Morse 59 (*i.e.* 0·041 in. diameter), for 0·025 ml. Morse 55 (0·052 in.), for 0·030 ml. Morse 52 (0·063 in.), for 0·035 ml. Morse 47 (0·078 in.) and for 0·040 ml. Morse 43 (0·089 in.). Exactly at its point of impaction in the hole, the capillary is scored with a glass-cutter (*e.g.* a vulcanite carborundum disk), and broken off squarely. The pipettes are then plugged in their wide end with cotton-wool, packed in a large test-tube and sterilised in the hot air oven. In use the pipette is fitted with a teat, filled with the liquid and held vertically with the tip downwards. For accurate work the drops should be expelled at the constant rate of about 40 per minute, *i.e.* taking about 1½ seconds for the gradual expulsion of one drop. The drop size may differ slightly in the case of liquids with different densities and surface tensions from that of water, and the pipette should be calibrated directly for the particular liquid by measuring the volume of 100 drops. For further details consult *A System of Bacteriology*, Medical Research Council, 1931, vol. 9, pp. 174-83.

Technique of Inoculating Medium in Tubes

The following routine methods are recommended.

Inoculation of one "slope" from another.—The two tubes are firmly held at their lower ends between the thumb and first two fingers of the left hand, with the sloped surface of the medium towards the worker. The tube containing the growth should be on the left and the uninoculated tube on the right. With the right hand loosen the cotton-wool stoppers by rotating them in the mouths of the tubes so that they may be removed easily. Take the holder of the inoculating wire at its end between the thumb and first two fingers of the right hand (as in holding a pen). Sterilise the wire by holding it vertically in the Bunsen flame. Remove the stopper of the tube from which the inoculation is to be made, with the crooked third finger of the right hand, and flame the mouth of the tube. Pass the wire into the tube and touch a portion of the medium free from growth to ascertain if the wire is sufficiently cool. If too hot, the wire will melt the agar, causing a furrow, and might, of course kill the organisms in removing the growth. When the wire is cool, the growth is scraped from the surface, care being taken not to wound the agar. Withdraw the wire, remove the stopper from the other tube with the crooked little finger and flame the mouth of the tube. Insert the wire charged with the growth and lightly smear the surface of the agar. Withdraw the wire and sterilise it, flame the mouths of the tubes and replace the stoppers. The nature of the inoculated material and also the date should be written on the tube by means of a grease pencil, or on a gummed label which is then affixed to the tube.

For *stab cultures*, the tubes are held similarly and the straight wire charged with bacterial growth is plunged into the centre of the medium, care being taken to withdraw the wire in the same line to avoid splitting of the medium.

For *shake cultures*, agar or gelatin medium in tubes is inoculated in the melted condition at a temperature that keeps the medium fluid but is not *immediately* lethal to the organisms inoculated, *e.g.* 45°–50° C. The contents of the tubes are mixed by rotation between the palms of the hands and then poured at once into a Petri dish, or left to solidify in the tube so that colonies may develop in the depth of the medium, as when separating anaerobes.

In *inoculating a fluid medium*, such as broth, from a solid culture, the tube should be inclined almost to the horizontal and the growth on the loop deposited on the wall of the tube just above the surface of the liquid at the lower end of the tube. On returning the tube to the vertical position the inoculum is below the surface of the broth.

Technique of Inoculating Medium in Screw-Capped Bottles

When inoculating medium in screw-capped bottles, essentially the same procedure is carried out as for tubes. Before the bottles are held in the hand it is advisable to loosen the screw cap, as this is often tightly screwed. If the caps are very tight they can easily be loosened by means of a bored-out rubber bung, a section of which is shown in the figure. A bung about 2 inches across is suitable, and by means of a cork-borer a number of holes are bored in a slanting direction round a diameter of $1\frac{1}{4}$ inches, so that the whole centre is removed, leaving a conical-shaped cavity. It is preferable to have the wall ridged, as it grips the cap more easily. The bung can be held in the hand, or suitably mounted just below the edge of the bench.

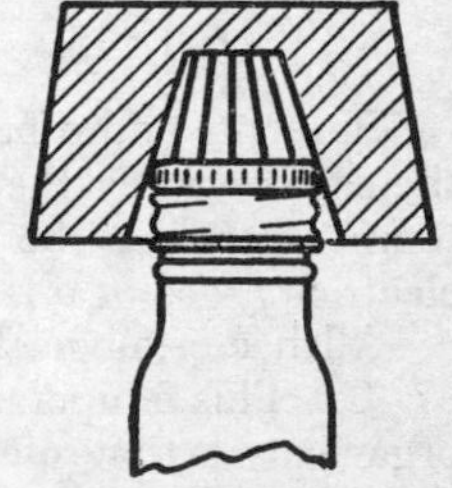

Fig. 61.

For *inoculation*, the bottles are held exactly as test-tubes, and the cap is held in the same way as the cotton-wool stopper. The bottles are then unscrewed from the cap, the wire is introduced and the inoculation made. The cap is now loosely screwed on, and when the bottle is ready for the incubator the screw-cap is tightened if considered necessary.

Inoculation Hood or Cabinet

It is advisable, as far as possible, to carry out certain inoculation procedures under a hood in order to minimise the chances of aerial contamination.

A suitable size of hood is 5 ft. wide, 5 ft. deep, 7 ft. 6 in. high. It fits over the bench to form a completely enclosed chamber and is entered by a sliding (not swing) door. All sides above the bench level consist of windows. Ventilation is secured by two holes in the roof; from the top of each is attached a vent pipe 3 in. wide and 18 in. long, and turned at right angles. The bench on which the hood is fitted should have a gas supply for the Bunsen burner, and it is convenient to have a pipe from the roof 3 in. in diameter with a funnel-shaped opening situated 24 in. above the bench top, under which the Bunsen burner is placed so that the gas fumes are led directly away. The hood may be lighted by an electric lamp suspended from the roof.

The table under the hood is covered by a towel soaked in 1 : 1000 mercuric chloride solution, so that any organisms deposited in dust are destroyed. The advantage of the hood depends on the relative absence of dust and air currents, which are likely to produce contamination of medium, etc., exposed in the process of inoculation. The inoculating hood may be used with advantage in the preparation of blood agar plates and other highly nutritive media, and in conducting autopsies on animals under aseptic conditions.

A more simple inoculation box which is movable can easily be constructed as shown in the figure (Fig. 62). The frame is made of wood and it has a sloping glass window in front, and two apertures whereby the hands and arms can be inserted to carry out the necessary manipulation of the cultures. A convenient size is 3 ft. wide, 2 ft. deep and 3 ft. high.

Protective inoculation cabinet.—When work is done with dangerous pathogens, such as the tubercle bacillus, it is advisable that procedures are carried out in a cabinet fitted with a ventilation system that does not allow contamination of the laboratory air and an ultraviolet lamp that can be used to disinfect the cabinet after the work is finished. A suitable cabinet has been described by Williams and Lidwell (1957). Convenient cabinets are available commercially, e.g. the "Bassaire" cabinet supplied by John Bass Ltd., Crawley, Sussex. These "protective" cabinets are also quite suitable for carrying out 'dust-free" inoculations and other procedures.

INCUBATION

Students and others commencing work in a laboratory should familiarise themselves with the mechanism of the incubator, whereby any desired temperature may be constantly maintained. Incubators may be heated by electricity, gas or oil, according to the facilities of the laboratory.

All bacteriological laboratories have one or more incubators working at 37° C. This temperature, which is the optimum for practically all pathogenic organisms, is that referred to when speaking of incubation without mentioning the temperature.

Some laboratories have a warm room heated by gas or electricity, and kept at 37° C., in which large quantities of material can be incubated. The room has a regulating mechanism similar to the ordinary incubator to keep the temperature constant, and if electrically heated it should be fitted with a device to cut off the current for the room at the main switch if the temperature rises above 40° C.

Other temperatures for incubation are 30° C., used for cultivating staphylococci and leptospirae, 25–28° C., used for many fungi, and 22° C. ("cool incubator"), used for certain fungi and for gelatin cultures. (Gelatin medium melts at about 24° C.).

In order to prevent drying of the medium in test-tubes when prolonged incubation is necessary, as in the cultivation of the tubercle bacillus, the mouths of the tubes are sealed with paraffin wax, or covered with special rubber caps. Under these circumstances, however, we strongly advise that screw-capped bottles should be used instead of test-tubes.

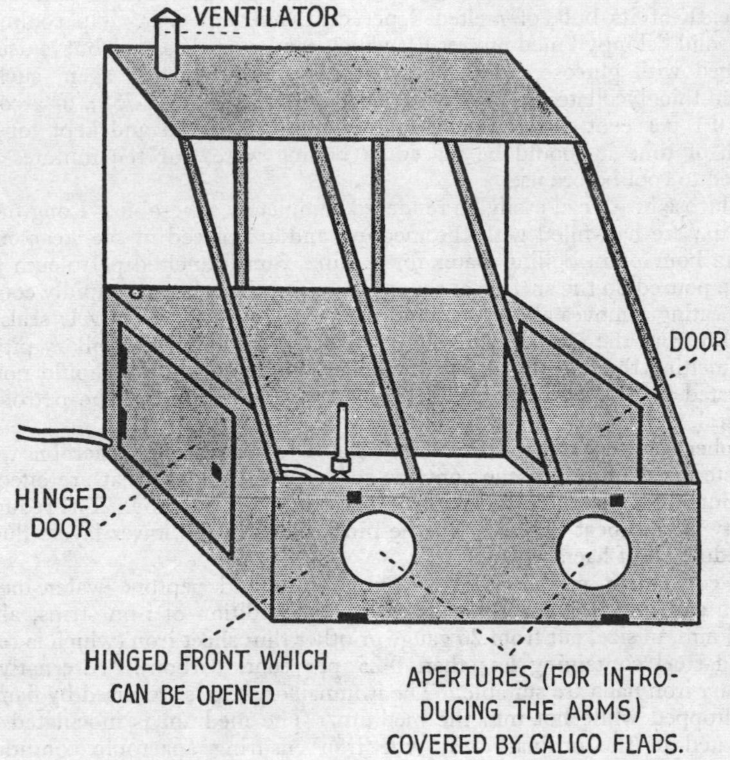

FIG. 62.

METHODS OF ANAEROBIC CULTURE

Obligate anaerobes are defined as organisms that will grow only in the absence of free oxygen. The method usually employed to establish anaerobic conditions is to remove oxygen from the atmosphere surrounding the culture; the oxygen is sometimes replaced by an inert gas.

The simplest method of securing anaerobiosis is by growing the organisms in solid medium. Deep agar tubes are convenient and efficient for the purpose. The addition of 0·5 per cent. glucose to the medium is of value, particularly when cultivating the saccharolytic group of anaerobes. Glucose acts as a reducing agent, and further serves as a suitable pabulum for bacterial growth. The agar may be inoculated when solid by means of a long straight wire. The colonies develop best in the depth of the tube, becoming fewer and smaller towards the surface. No growth is usually noted in the top half-inch of the medium. An alternative method is to melt the agar, cool it to 45° C. and introduce the inoculum by means of a capillary pipette. The contents of the tube are mixed by rotation between the palms of the hands. The agar is then rapidly solidified by placing the tube in cold water. The colonies develop in the deep portions of the tube, usually separated from one another.

A convenient method is the use of semi-solid agar medium. A fluid medium, *e.g* nutrient broth, is heated in boiling water and to it is added one-tenth of its bulk of melted 2 per cent. nutrient agar. On cooling, a semi-solid "sloppy" medium results which can be used as it is, but is usually enriched with glucose, 0·5–1 per cent., or other reducing agent such as sodium thioglycollate, 0·1 per cent. (Brewer's medium, p. 758), or ascorbic acid, 0·1 per cent. If the semi-solid medium is tubed and kept for any length of time it should be placed in boiling water for ten minutes and allowed to cool before use.

Glucose broth can easily be rendered completely anaerobic. Long tubes, $8 \times \frac{1}{2}$ in., are half-filled with the medium and are placed in the steamer for half an hour or in boiling water for 5 min. Sterile melted petroleum jelly is then poured on the surface of the medium and the tubes are rapidly cooled. The heating removes all oxygen, and the petroleum jelly effectively seals the medium from the air. Inoculation is made by means of a capillary pipette after melting the petroleum jelly. Gas-producing anaerobes should not be cultivated in this medium, as the gas formed will force out the petroleum jelly seal.

Robertson's cooked-meat medium is also very useful for anaerobic work. The sterilised muscle tissue contains reducing substances that are effective in maintaining anaerobic conditions at the bottom of the tube. The reducing activity of the meat is shown by the pink colour in the lower layers due to the reduction of haematin.

A convenient method of converting broth and peptone water media, gelatin and milk for anaerobic use is by the addition of iron strips, about 25×3 mm. in size, cut from 26 gauge or other thin sheet iron (which is really a mild steel containing less than 0·25 per cent. carbon). Alternatively, ordinary iron nails are suitable. The iron nail or strip is sterilised by flaming and dropped while hot into the medium. The medium is inoculated and incubated in the ordinary way, the iron ensuring anaerobic conditions. Sugar reactions may be noted and tests for indole may be carried out after 24–48 hours' incubation. The results should be read before the heavy deposit of iron hydroxide masks the reaction, but this is minimal if the iron is completely immersed in the medium.

McIntosh and Fildes' Jar

To grow anaerobes on the surface of solid media it is necessary to provide an atmosphere free from oxygen. This is achieved by the use of McIntosh and Fildes' jar or a modification of it.

The principle is that spongy palladium or spongy platinum acting as a catalytic agent causes the slow combination of hydrogen and oxygen to form water.

The jar itself (8×5 in.) should be made of metal, and has a tight-fitting lid that can be clamped down. Glass jars have been used in the past but, as explosions occasionally occur, their use is not justified. The lid is furnished with two tubes and taps, so that hydrogen may be introduced into the jar. Suspended from the lid by means of two stout wires, which are connected to terminals, is a small grooved porcelain spool around which is wound a fine coil of resistance wire, the ends of which are connected to the two wires supporting the spool. Around the spool is wrapped a layer of palladinised asbestos. When an electric current is passed through the resistance wire on the spool the spongy palladium is heated. The spool is surrounded with wire gauze which, on the principle of the Davy lamp, prevents an explosion of the hydrogen and oxygen mixture. The electric terminals must be connected to the mains through an appropriate resistance, such as the rheostat supplied for the purpose by certain manufacturers.

Petri dishes or tubes are placed inside the jar, and also an indicator to show that anaerobiosis is maintained. The Petri dishes are placed in the usual way with medium uppermost and lid downwards. It is advantageous to separate the lid from the rim of the dish about 1 mm. by the insertion between them of a bent pin or fragment of blotting-paper; this prevents sealing of the lid by condensed moisture.

The rim of the jar is smeared with petroleum jelly and the lid clamped firmly in place. One tap is closed and the other connected with rubber pressure tubing to a water-pump or mechanical pump. This is used to evacuate at least three-quarters of the air from the jar, preferably reducing the remaining content to less than 60 mm. Hg absolute pressure. Evacuation of most of the air from the jar before admitting the hydrogen prevents trapping of oxygen in Petri dishes and tubes that are too tightly closed. The tap is then tightly closed and the other tap connected with rubber tubing to a hydrogen supply. Hydrogen is allowed to pass into the jar through a small wash bottle until the jar is full. The electric current is now switched on so that the palladinised asbestos may be heated. The combination of hydrogen and oxygen takes place quietly in the jar. Water is formed, and more hydrogen enters to take the place of the hydrogen and oxygen consumed. When hydrogen stops bubbling into the jar, usually within 20 min. or so, the tap is closed and the hydrogen and electricity supplies disconnected. The jar is placed in the incubator, and an indicator tube containing methylene blue (see below) should remain colourless, showing that complete anaerobiosis is established.

Simple Form of McIntosh and Fildes' Jar

Another form of the catalyst for a McIntosh and Fildes' jar allows the jar to be set up more quickly and may be prepared inexpensively. It is active at room temperature and does not require heating electrically.

The catalyst is made by dissolving one gram of palladium chloride in 10 ml. of distilled water containing a few drops of concentrated hydrochloric acid; 1·5 g. of asbestos wool is saturated with this solution and dried. The asbestos is teased out as finely as possible and heated in a smoky flame until black, and then roasted in the outer part of a Bunsen flame till the black material vanishes. The catalytic activity of the preparation may be tested by directing a fine jet of hydrogen on to it, when the asbestos should glow and ignite the gas. This amount of catalyst is sufficient for about 6 capsules made by spreading palladinised asbestos in a thin layer, $1\frac{1}{2}$ inches square, on one half of a sheet of 30–40 mesh brass or copper gauze, $1\frac{5}{8} \times 3\frac{1}{4}$ in., folding over the other half and turning in the edge of the two layers. The capsules should be stored in a dry place, preferably in a desiccator. Moisture deposited on the surface inhibits catalytic activity; it is removed before each use by heating the capsule in the outer part of a Bunsen flame. Inactive palladium sulphide may be formed from hydrogen sulphide evolved by cultures in the jar. When this happens, it is best to discard the capsule.

Place the cultures and an indicator tube into an airtight container fitted with an inlet tap and a capsule in a clip under the lid. Seal the lid by pressing plasticine between its edge and the jar rim. Connect the tap to a pump and pressure gauge, and exhaust two-fifths of the air from the jar (*i.e.* to about 450 mm. Hg absolute pressure); ensure that the jar is not leaking at this stage. Close the tap, connect to the hydrogen supply via a small wash-bottle and open the tap to let the jar fill with hydrogen. After the initial inrush of hydrogen there is a pause followed by a secondary bubbling as hydrogen is drawn through the wash-bottle into the jar to replace the hydrogen and oxygen that have combined due to the action of the catalyst; this second intake is evidence that the catalyst is active. When it has occurred, close the tap and transfer the jar to the incubator, where the catalysed combustion will continue, the volume of hydrogen now in the jar being sufficient to utilise all the remaining oxygen.

There is no need to wait further until hydrogen completely stops bubbling into the jar and this, in addition to the avoidance of electrical equipment and connections, is a great advantage in comparison with the use of jars with electrically heated catalysts.

An anaerobic jar which operates with a catalyst active at room temperature is commercially available.[1] This jar is provided with a capsule containing a semi-solid indicator of anaerobiosis fitted externally to a side arm.

Hydrogen Supply

A hydrogen supply may be obtained from a Kipp's apparatus by the action of sulphuric acid on zinc. The gas must be purified by passing through three wash-bottles containing: (1) 10 per cent. solution of lead acetate, to remove sulphuretted hydrogen; (2) 10 per cent. solution of silver nitrate, to absorb arseniuretted hydrogen; and (3) a mixture of pyrogallic acid and caustic soda, to remove oxygen.

It is more convenient, however, to obtain hydrogen from a cylinder containing the compressed gas. The commercial hydrogen so obtained is suitable for use in the various anaerobic apparatus employed. The hydrogen cylinder cannot be connected directly to the McIntosh and Fildes' jar, as the pressure is too great. It should be fitted with a reducing valve to deliver hydrogen at a constant pressure (*e.g.* 2–3 lb. per square inch) which can be predetermined or altered at will. The gas is then passed through a small wash-bottle containing water in order that its rate of flow may be observed, and to detect when no further hydrogen is drawn into the anaerobic jar—a state which is reached when all the oxygen in the jar has combined with hydrogen.

A very simple alternative method is to attach an ordinary football bladder to the hydrogen cylinder. The gas is turned on and the bladder inflated. The gas is then turned off and the tube of the bladder closed by a screw clamp, and removed from the cylinder. The inflated bladder is connected by its tube to the anaerobic jar via a wash bottle (See diagram, p. 801). The wash bottle shows when hydrogen is flowing into the jar. Since the flow can be

[1] Baird & Tatlock Ltd., Chadwell Heath, Essex, England.

judged from the change in the size of the bladder, the wash bottle can be omitted and the bladder be attached directly to the jar.

Indicator of Anaerobiosis

The indicator of anaerobiosis consists of a mixture in a cotton-wool plugged test-tube of equal volumes of (*a*) 0·1 *N* NaOH 6 ml., water to 100 ml., (*b*) 3 ml. ½ per cent. watery methylene blue, water to 100 ml., (*c*) glucose 6 grams, water to 100 ml., and a small crystal of thymol; the mixture is boiled until it becomes colourless and is at once placed in the jar. This indicator, when in the jar, should remain colourless except for a slight tinge of blue at the top, which disappears during incubation.

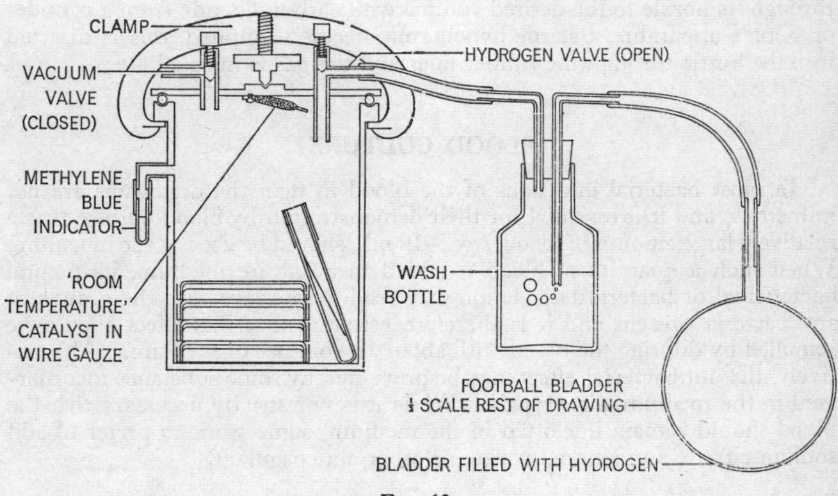

FIG. 63.

CULTIVATION IN AN ATMOSPHERE WITH ADDED CARBON DIOXIDE

Certain organisms will grow only when carbon dioxide is added to the atmosphere surrounding them, e.g. *Br. abortus*, and some grow better in such atmospheres than in ordinary air, *e.g.* pneumococcus, etc. A convenient method is to use tin containers, size 8 × 10 in., with press-on lids, and capacity of about 3½ litres.[1] The carbon dioxide is generated in the tin itself from marble and hydrochloric acid. The cultures, either in Petri dishes (enclosed in a simple wire basket) or in tubes, are placed in the tin together with an open tube, 8 × 1 in., containing 10 ml. (excess) of 2 *N* hydrochloric acid. A marble chip of about 0·7 g. (weight need only be approximate) is dropped into the acid and the lid pressed on. (*Note*—1 g. $CaCO_3$ treated with 10 ml., or more, of 2 *N* HCl liberates 224 ml. CO_2 at normal temperature and pressure.) The slight increased pressure of the carbon dioxide is of no consequence. If the cultures are carefully removed and fresh ones added immediately there is no need to renew the marble and acid.

[1] Obtainable from A. Gallenkamp & Co., Ltd., London.

In using such closed containers there is a tendency for moisture to collect on the lid of the Petri dish. The same occurs in anaerobic jars. It is recommended, therefore, before incubating to place in the lid of the dish a square piece of filter- or blotting-paper of such a size that it is just held in position by its four corners, *e.g.* for the usual 4-in plate, a 3-in. square. The paper should not fill the top of the dish, as it would, when wet, act as a seal and prevent the access of carbon dioxide to the inside of the dish.

For larger proportions of carbon dioxide an anaerobic jar may be used. Air is withdrawn by means of a filter pump and replaced by carbon dioxide from a Kipp's apparatus or cylinder, as described above for hydrogen.

A measured volume of carbon dioxide may be added to a culture in liquid or on solid medium in a bottle which is tightly sealed by a perforated metal screw-cap with an unperforated thick rubber liner. A syringe is filled through its nozzle to the desired volume with carbon dioxide from a cylinder or Kipp's apparatus, a sterile hypodermic needle is applied, this is inserted into the bottle through the rubber liner and the gas is injected.

BLOOD CULTURE

In most bacterial infections of the blood in man the organisms are not numerous, and it is essential for their demonstration by blood culture that a relatively large amount of blood, *e.g.* 5–10 ml., should be used as the inoculum. When such a quantity of blood is added to a culture medium, its natural bactericidal or bacteriostatic action may readily interfere with the growth of any bacteria present and it is therefore essential that this effect should be annulled by diluting the blood with about 10 volumes of medium. Alternatively, the antibacterial effect may be prevented by some substance incorporated in the medium, *e.g.* trypsin. While it is not strictly necessary that the blood should remain unclotted in the medium, some workers prefer to add sodium citrate, ammonium oxalate or other anticoagulant.

Requisites

(1) A 10-ml. " all-glass" syringe (with a firmly fitting needle) sterilised in the hot air oven as described on p. 709 should be used.

If a syringe that will not withstand heating at 160° C. is used it must be sterilised by boiling in water for 15 min.; the syringe must not come into contact with any antiseptic; it should not be removed from the steriliser until it is immediately required, and the parts should be taken out of the steriliser and fitted together with the aid of forceps so that the needle, nozzle and piston are not touched by the fingers. Extraneous bacterial contamination of blood specimens is more frequent when the syringes are sterilised by boiling (*e.g.* 10 per cent. of specimens contaminated) than when they are sterilised in the hot air oven (*e.g.* 1 per cent. contaminated). The syringes are liable to be contaminated with non-sporing bacteria while being assembled after their removal from the boiling water (p. 686).

(2) Gauze or cotton-wool, bandage, antiseptic (*e.g.* 2 per cent. iodine in 70 per cent. alcohol or 5 per cent. carbolic acid in water), methylated spirit, collodion, dissecting forceps, Bunsen burner or spirit lamp.

(3) 50 ml. sterile digest broth (*e.g.* Hartley's, p. 744) in a stoppered flask, or preferably the special blood culture bottle described later. (0·2 per cent. sodium citrate or 1·0 per cent. ammonium oxalate may be incorporated in the medium.)

Withdrawal of Blood.—The blood is drawn by vein puncture. The skin of the patient's arm at the bend of the elbow is *thoroughly sterilised* by first washing with soap and water, then applying spirit and finally treating with the iodine solution. Alternatively, the skin is rubbed with 5 per cent. carbolic acid solution and a gauze swab soaked in the solution is then applied to the skin over the vein and held in position for 2–3 min. Thorough disinfection is necessary to obviate contamination of the culture with skin organisms—*e.g.* staphylococci. Several turns of a bandage are applied round the upper arm about the middle of the biceps to render the veins turgid, or a piece of rubber tubing firmly, but not too tightly, wound once round the arm and clipped with pressure forceps provides a convenient and easily released tourniquet for the purpose. The turgescence of the veins can be increased by the patient's alternately opening and clenching the hand. The needle of the syringe is inserted into a prominent vein and 5–10 ml. of blood are drawn into the syringe. The tourniquet is then released. The needle is now withdrawn from the vein and detached from the syringe by means of forceps so that the nozzle is not touched by the fingers. The flask of broth is unstoppered and the mouth of the flask flamed. The blood is added to the broth and the flask re-stoppered. The blood and broth are thoroughly mixed by rotation of the flask. These operations are all done at the bedside. A spirit lamp may be used for flaming. The flask is incubated at 37° C.

The patient should raise the arm after blood has been withdrawn and firm pressure should be applied to the site of the puncture to obviate haematoma formation. (*Note*—Carbolic acid is irritant on prolonged contact with skin; when it has been used to disinfect the skin, it should be removed by sponging with water as soon as the specimen has been taken.)

The syringe and needle should be washed out at once with 2 per cent. lysol solution. The puncture wound may be dressed with gauze or cotton wool, and collodion.

When the flask has to be transported some distance to the laboratory it is essential to stopper it with a rubber bung which has been sterilised by boiling, and inserted into the flask with flamed forceps, but under these circumstances a blood culture bottle should be used (*vide infra*).

Special Media for Blood Culture.—"Liquoid" (sodium polyanethol sulphonate), 0·05 per cent., is of value in annulling the natural bactericidal action of blood.

In patients on sulphonamide therapy, there may be enough sulphonamide in the blood to prevent the growth of bacteria when blood culture is performed. The addition of 5 mg. of *p*-aminobenzoic acid per 100 ml. of broth will prevent the bacteriostatic action of the drug. The *p*-aminobenzoic acid is stable and withstands autoclaving.

If the patient is being treated with penicillin when blood culture is attempted, penicillinase should be incorporated in the medium. A 1·0 ml. volume of the preparation, supplied by Wellcome Laboratories, Beckenham, England, will inactivate 100,000 units of penicillin, but proportionately more is required for lower levels of penicillin. For blood culture work, it is recommended that a suitable dilution containing 0·01 ml. of this penicillinase solution should be added per 100 ml. of sterile broth, with aseptic precautions.

The addition of 0·2 per cent. sodium citrate and 0·1 per cent. white saponin (B.D.H.) to broth produces saponin broth in which blood does not clot and is promptly lysed. Saponin broth should be sterilised by intermittent steaming. It is favoured by some workers for the isolation of *Streptococcus viridans*, which may be slightly sensitive to Liquoid.

Broth containing 0·1–0·5 per cent. glucose is recommended for the isolation of pneumococci and streptococci from the blood. Glucose broth plus one part of filtered Liquor trypsini Co. (Allen & Hanburys) to 10 parts of the medium also may be used for the pyogenic cocci.

In suspected cases of enteric fever, a 5 ml. volume of the patient's blood may be added to 50 ml. of broth containing 0·5 per cent. of sodium taurocholate as a selective agent.

To obtain the best general results, a range of media should be used. The routine inclusion of an anaerobic medium, such as cooked-meat broth, is recommended because anaerobes, *e.g.* certain streptococci and *Cl. welchii*, may otherwise be missed. Since this medium also serves for the growth of aerobes, it is an excellent general purpose medium for blood culture.

Quantitative counts of bacteria in the blood are sometimes useful in differentiating between bacteriaemia and septicaemia or for prognostic purposes. A simple procedure is to inoculate 1·0 ml. amounts of blood into several tubes of melted agar and make pour plates either at the bedside or from unclotted blood in Liquoid in the laboratory.

Special procedures or culture media for certain suspected infections, *e.g.* brucellosis, leptospirosis, are described in the appropriate chapters.

Blood Culture Bottle.—Instead of using a flask of broth with a cotton-wool or rubber stopper, as described above, the following container is much more simple and convenient, especially when the patient is some distance from the laboratory.

It consists of a 3 oz. round bottle or a 4 oz. (120 ml.) "medical flat" bottle, with a screw cap, similar to that used for storing nutrient agar, etc., in 50 ml. amounts (p. 726). A hole is punched out of the cap and the rubber washer re-inserted. In order to protect the surface of the cap and the exposed portion of the rubber washer from contamination before use, the cap and neck of the bottle are covered with a "viskap",[1] such as is used for perfume bottles. This is a cellulose preparation which is slipped on moist and allowed to dry. In so doing the viskap shrinks, moulding itself tightly to the cap and neck of the bottle.

The apparatus is fitted up as follows. The bottles are supplied in a carton already washed, cleaned and capped, so that no further preparation is required. The rubber washer is removed, a $\frac{5}{16}$-in. hole punched out of the centre of the cap by means of a hollow punch, and the rubber washer re-inserted. The medium in the bottle is a matter of choice, and the following range is useful. The different types are recognised by the colour of the viskap and the glass bead in the bottle:

(1) plain broth (white cap and bead). To this can be added saponin 0·1 per cent., or Liquoid 0·05 per cent., if required;
(2) broth+0·1 per cent. glucose (green cap and bead);
(3) glucose broth as in (2) *plus* 5 mg. per cent. *p*-aminobenzoic acid (*e.g.* for pneumococci and streptococci);
(4) broth+0·5 per cent. sodium taurocholate (yellow cap and bead (for enteric fever)).

The size of the viskap is No. 2 semi-opaque cut $1\frac{3}{8}$ in. The top of the viskap is coloured with cellulose paint. The bead is to identify the medium on its return to the laboratory. If beads are not available a small dab of coloured paint is placed on the shoulder of the bottle. If large numbers of bottles are used, coloured labels are preferable and they obviate the use of coloured beads or painted caps.

[1] Made by the Viscose Development Co., Ltd., Woldham Road, Bromley, Kent.

50 ml. of the medium is placed in the bottle, the appropriately coloured bead added, and the perforated cap with rubber washer firmly screwed on. The bottle is now sterilised in the autoclave for 15 min. at 121°C. (15 lb. pressure). When the bottle is cool the viskap is at once slipped on. Viskaps dry in a few hours and mould themselves to the cap and neck of the bottle. The broth can be stored without deterioration.

For use, the bottle is taken to the bedside of the patient. Just before the vein is punctured the viskap is removed. Blood (5 ml.) is now withdrawn from the vein, with the usual precautions, and immediately afterwards the needle is passed through the rubber washer and the blood is expelled into the medium. The needle is withdrawn and the puncture in the washer seals itself. The bottle is shaken to mix blood and broth, and sent to the laboratory for incubation. It is advisable to wipe the exposed portion of the washer with a little antiseptic (*e.g.* alcohol), in order to remove any infective material at the site of the puncture. If more blood than 5 ml. is removed, further bottles are inoculated with successive 5 ml. amounts.

When the culture is examined after incubation, the screw cap is removed in the ordinary way.

It has been shown that, particularly with blood cultures in flasks, incubation in an atmosphere containing 5 per cent. carbon dioxide is an advantage.

"Clot" Culture.—When blood samples from suspected enteric fever have been submitted for the Widal test (p. 909) it is useful as a routine to cultivate the clot after the serum has been removed. If blood is taken in the early stages of the disease the Widal reaction may be negative, but blood culture will probably be positive. Moreover, enteric organisms may be present in the blood stream at any time throughout the illness, and isolation of the causative organism is the most satisfactory form of diagnosis.

If it is known that the blood has been withdrawn with strict aseptic precautions, the clot may be placed in a wide tube (8 × 1 in.) half filled with broth, or in a wide-mouth screw-capped bottle (8-oz. pot) containing 80 ml. of broth. Where, however, there is any doubt as to the presence of contaminating organisms, and this is always a possibility when specimens of blood are sent to the laboratory from a distance, the clot should be transferred directly to a tube of sterile ox bile. After incubation overnight the bile culture is examined for enteric organisms in the usual manner.

A method of clot culture with streptokinase has been recommended (Watson, 1955). Take blood from the arm vein in the usual way and allow 5 ml. quantities to clot in sterile screw-capped Universal containers (p. 726). Remove the separated serum and add to each bottle 15 ml. of 0·5 per cent. bile-salt broth containing 100 units per ml. of streptokinase. The streptokinase causes rapid clot lysis with release of bacteria trappen in the clot. The cultures are then incubated.

Examination of Blood Culture.—After incubation for 18–24 hr., films are made from the blood broth mixture and stained by Gram's method. If organisms are noted, subinoculations are made on a plate of a suitable medium by successive strokes with a charged loop. The subcultures are incubated and the organisms developing are identified as far as possible by their microscopic characters and colony appearances. If further investigations are required for accurate identification, single colonies are picked off on to slopes and the resulting cultures are studied.

Where an infection with the enteric group is suspected, it is convenient to plate directly from the blood culture on to MacConkey's medium to obtain the characteristic colonies on this medium.

Even when no organisms can be detected in films from the primary blood culture, it is advisable to make subinoculations. Scanty organisms may not be observed but these may develop colonies in subculture.

If no result is obtained after 24 hours' incubation, the blood broth should be incubated continuously for at least four days, films and subinoculations being made each day. If brucellosis is suspected, cultures should be incubated for three weeks before being discarded as negative.

THE AGAR BLOCK METHOD OF ØRSKOV FOR STUDYING THE MORPHOLOGY OF GROWING BACTERIAL CULTURES

This method has been applied by Ørskov (1923) and others for the morphological study of *Actinomyces* and it allows the maintenance of living cultures under continuous observation.

Cubes of suitable size are cut out of an agar plate by means of a sterilised knife. These cubes should not exceed 3–4 mm. in thickness. They are transferred with the knife to a sterilised microscope slide. The agar is now inoculated with the organism by a fine stroke. With first a low-power objective the stroke is defined and then with a higher power an area is found where the bacteria lie sufficiently scattered. With a suitable lamp and objective and closing down of the diaphragm young bacteria appear as strongly refractile and well-defined bodies. The area is then registered by means of the vernier scales on the mechanical stage. The slide is removed and placed in a Petri dish with a piece of moist filter paper in the bottom, and the dish is incubated at a suitable temperature. The selected area is then examined at intervals and the changing features observed. In this way the development of individual bacteria can be studied and also that of colonies at each stage. (A microscope incubator, heated electrically, by means of which a colony can be observed microscopically throughout its period of growth is also very convenient for these and similar studies.)

DISPOSAL OF CULTURES

Cultures to be discarded should be killed by heat or antiseptics before the container is cleaned for re-use.

In the case of non-sporing organisms, it is sufficient to remove the cotton-wool plugs and immerse the tubes and plugs in a large basin of 3 per cent. lysol or cresol.

When screw-capped bottles are used the cap is completely unscrewed and both it and the bottle placed in the lysol solution.

Petri dish cultures are also similarly immersed in lysol solution.

Cultures of the tubercle bacillus and sporing organisms, such as Cl. tetani, B. anthracis, etc., must be sterilised by autoclaving.

COLD STORAGE

It is essential to have some form of cold storage in the laboratory for the preservation of blood, serum, culture media, cultures, vaccines, etc.

Mechanical refrigeration is now universally used, and refrigerators are available in a large number of sizes from 1½ cubic feet capacity to cold storage rooms of several thousand cubic feet. For the smaller laboratory one of the domestic refrigerators of 4–7 cubic feet capacity is suitable, while larger laboratories require a correspondingly larger instrument, or an insulated cold room with the refrigerating plant outside. Mechanical refrigerators can be obtained to work with electricity, gas or oil, and most of them have provision for making small quantities of ice. The temperature should be maintained between 4°–5° C. (39°–41° F.). It should never be so low as to cause freezing, as this may be detrimental to vaccines, bacterial suspensions, red cells and certain sera containing a preservative.

It should be noted that with the domestic type of refrigerator an accumulation of ice, due to freezing of water vapour, surrounds the freezing unit, and at intervals (about 10–14 days) it is necessary to "de-frost" to remove this ice. The contents of the refrigerator are removed, the current (or gas) turned off and the doors opened. The melted water from the ice is caught in a suitable receptacle. When the ice is melted the interior of the refrigerator is wiped with a cloth, the contents replaced, and the refrigerating unit started again.

It is convenient also to have a refrigerator working at low temperatures for the preservation of sera, viruses, etc., and one of the commercial type of "deep freeze" refrigerators working at −10° to −40° C. is suitable for this purpose.

PRESERVATION OF CULTURES

Bacterial species vary greatly in the ability of their cultures to remain alive after the completion of growth (*e.g.* after twenty-four hours at 37° C.). Some species such as *Neisseria gonorrhoeae* and *Streptobacillus moniliformis* are poorly viable and their cultures usually die out within a few days, whether kept at 37° C., at room temperature or at 4°–5° C.; thus, they must be subcultivated every two to four days for maintenance in the laboratory. Other species are much hardier, especially sporing species which may remain viable for many years. There are also many non-sporing species (*e.g.* enterobacteriaceae) whose cultures, under suitable conditions, commonly remain viable for several months and often for as much as a few years. Their prolonged preservation requires the following: (1) that drying of the culture is prevented by hermetic sealing of the tube or bottle with a screw cap and new rubber liner, or with a cotton-wool plug soaked in paraffin wax, (2) that the culture is stored in the dark, and either at room temperature or in a refrigerator at 4°–5° C., but not at 37° C., and (3) that the culture be grown on a suitable "preservation medium", *e.g.* on a slope of coagulated egg medium, though nutrient agar stab cultures are also generally satisfactory. It is desirable that at least a moderate proportion of the cells in the culture should remain alive; if only a few survive, these may be exclusively resistant mutants, all cells of the original type being lost. Frequent subcultivation also tends to replace the original type by mutants and must therefore be avoided as far as possible. Specific recommendations for the short term preservation of bacterial cultures have been made by Stokes (1962).

Egg Medium for preservation of cultures

Egg medium is recommended for the prolonged storage of cultures at room temperature (below 20° C.). Organisms of the enterobacteria group may be kept alive on this medium for several years without subcultivation; they survive longer than on nutrient agar, and are less liable to vary to the "rough" state (p. 89). The culture is grown overnight at 37° C. and the screw cap of the bottle is firmly tightened before storing in a dark cool cupboard. Survival is dependent on the culture not being allowed to dry out.

PRESERVATION OF CULTURES AND SERA BY FREEZE-DRYING *IN VACUO*

When dried and kept in the dry state under suitable conditions, bacterial cultures and virus suspensions may remain viable for several years, and antisera may be preserved without appreciable loss of antibody potency. If such materials are dried from the liquid state, a high salt concentration is produced in the later stages of drying, which causes denaturation of proteins, death of organisms and deterioration of serum. This is largely avoided by the "freeze-drying", or "lyophile" method, in which the culture or serum is dried rapidly *in vacuo* from the frozen state (see Harris, 1954). The material is frozen by a suitable method (*vide infra*) and then dried by sublimation of the ice. The sublimation is effected by exposure to an atmosphere of very low pressure (*e.g.* 0·01 mm. Hg or less) which is dried by a chemical desiccant or refrigerated condenser. The dried material is preserved *in vacuo* in hermetically sealed ampoules which are stored in the dark, either at room temperature or, preferably, in a refrigerator at 4°–5° C. This is a convenient means of preserving stock strains of bacteria, guinea-pig complement serum and samples of antisera required for reference or standardisation purposes. On a larger scale, it is used for preserving therapeutic antisera, human plasma, antibiotics and vaccines.

Freezing must be very rapid, with the temperature lowered to well below 0° C. (*e.g.* to −20° C.), since slow freezing would prolong exposure to the denaturing influence of the suspending salt solution as it was concentrated to its eutectic level by the formation of pure ice crystals. The liquid should be frozen in a shallow layer with a large surface available for evaporation. Two methods of freezing are available: (1) *prefreezing*, i.e. before the drying process is begun, and (2) *evaporative freezing*, effected during the first stage of the drying process.

Prefreezing is generally employed for large volumes. The liquid is frozen as a layer, or "shell", lining the walls of the bottle, either by rotating the bottle while immersed nearly horizontally in a bath of ethyl alcohol and solid carbon dioxide, or of refrigerated coolant, or by spinning the bottle on its vertical axis in a current of refrigerated air.

Evaporative freezing is conveniently employed for the smaller quantities that generally suffice for laboratory purposes. The liquid is quickly frozen by the withdrawal of latent heat during its initial rapid evaporation when exposed to the vacuum applied for drying. Precautions must be taken against frothing and spilling during desolution of the atmospheric gases; the "centifrugal" and "degassing" methods have been developed for this purpose.

Greaves's Centrifugal Method of Freeze-Drying.—This is a most convenient method for preserving a number of cultures. Frothing is prevented by centrifuging the liquid during the first stage of evacuation and drying, until freezing is complete. A suitable centrifugal freeze-dryer[1] consists of a glass bell-jar and metal chamber containing the centrifuge and trays of desiccant for the primary drying, a manifold for the secondary drying, a rotary oil-sealed pump capable of drawing a vacuum below 0·04 mm. Hg

[1] Supplied by Edwards High Vacuum Ltd., Crawley, Sussex.

and a Pirani-type pressure gauge. The liquid cultures or suspensions (see p. 809) are dried in special hard-glass tubes or ampoules with a stem bore of 6 mm. The procedure is as follows.

(1) Place in each ampoule a small strip of filter paper on which has been typed the number designating the culture to be introduced. Plug the ampoules with cotton-wool and sterilise in the autoclave. With a sterile capillary pipette, put 0·25–0·5 ml. of liquid culture into each small "ampoule" (tube type) and up to 2·5 ml. into each of the larger ampoules. Discard the original sterility plug and insert a fresh, *loose* plug of sterile cotton-wool, pressing it wholly within the stem of the ampoule.

(2) Prepare the chamber for primary drying by charging the metal desiccant trays with fresh phosphorus pentoxide to the extent of at least 3 grams (about 10 ml.) of powder per ml. of water to be absorbed. (*Note*—Phosphorus pentoxide is corrosive and care must be taken to avoid spilling it on the skin, clothing or freeze-dryer. After each use of the dryer, the expended desiccant must be washed from the trays with an excess of water, taking care to avoid the corrosive fumes evolved, and the trays are then thoroughly dried. The makers' instructions must be followed for cleaning the apparatus and removing spilt powder, which may interfere with the working of the centrifuge motor.)

(3) *Primary Drying*.—Place the ampoules in the nearly vertical holes of the constant speed centrifuge. Cover the centrifuge with the bell-jar and press this firmly into position on the sealing ring of the base plate. (The contact surfaces are previously cleaned with ether and lightly smeared with high-vacuum grease.[1]) While pressing down the jar, switch on first the centrifuge and then the rotary pump. Observe the rapid fall of pressure on the Pirani gauge. When a low pressure of about 0·1 mm. Hg has been achieved in two to five minutes, it can be assumed that the material is frozen as a thin layer on the outer wall of the ampoule. *Immediately switch off the centrifuge to avoid overheating*. Leave the rotary pump running for a period sufficient to complete the primary drying: about three hours for 0·25 ml. volumes, six hours for 0·5 ml. volumes and eight hours for 2·5 ml. volumes. Then isolate the chamber, switch off the pump and leave the chamber evacuated until ready to remove the ampoules for the secondary drying. The ampoules must not be exposed to sunlight, nor, for more than a few hours, to weak daylight; if necessary, cover the apparatus to shield the ampoules from the light.

(4) Open the chamber air-release valve, lift the bell-jar and remove the ampoules. Draw out the stem of the ampoule to form a thin capillary neck near the open end. First flame the opening and press the loose cotton-wool plug about 2¼ in. (5·7 cm.) down the stem. While rotating the ampoule, heat the stem in a small gas flame at about 1¼ in. (3·2 cm.) from its open end, until the glass walls have softened and nearly doubled in thickness. Remove the ampoule from the flame and stretch it to form a capillary neck of about 2 mm. external diameter and 1 mm. bore. When cool, apply the open end to one of the rubber adaptors on the manifold used for the secondary drying; the manifold is placed so that the ampoules lie horizontally. Any adaptors not in use must be sealed by application of an empty ampoule.

(5) *Secondary Drying*.—Remove the expended desiccant from the trays and replace with fresh phosphorus pentoxide powder. Press the bell-jar into position, close the air-release valve and switch on the pump. Leave the

[1] Edwards High Vacuum Ltd., supply Apiezon " M " grease for glass joints and "N" grease for glass-metal and glass-rubber joints.

pump running for a sufficient period to ensure complete drying, *e.g.* 6–18 hr. Test the ampoules for vacuum tightness by briefly passing a high frequency vacuum tester near the surface of the glass; a satisfactory vacuum is indicated by a blue-violet glow, failure of vacuum by long streaky discharges or absence of glow, and cracks in the glass by bright sparking. The Pirani gauge should show that a pressure as low as 0·01 mm. Hg is reached.

(6) Seal the ampoules while they are attached to the manifold with the pump running. Heat the capillary neck with a small gas flame; when the glass is melted, pull gently and allow the flame to sever the thin filament so formed. When all the ampoules are sealed and set aside, open the air-release valve and switch off pump and Pirani gauge. After standing for half an hour, lay the ampoules on a metal surface and retest them for vacuum with the high-frequency tester; discard any not showing the blue-violet glow.

Freeze-Drying by the Degassing Method using a Laboratory Desiccator and High-Vacuum Pump.—By this method, small volumes of culture may be freeze-dried with simple apparatus. From 0·25 ml. to 2·5 ml. of liquid culture is pipetted into a sterile glass tube or ampoule (stem bore 6 mm.) which is then stoppered with a *loose* cotton-wool plug. The ampoule is placed in a glass desiccator jar over phosphorus pentoxide and is supported in a sloping position so that its contents form a thin layer on one side. The rim of the desiccator jar is smeared with vacuum grease and the lid pressed firmly into position. A tap in the desiccator lid is connected with rubber pressure tubing through a drying column of calcium chloride to a high-vacuum pump (*e.g.* Hyvac pump), all joints being sealed with vacuum grease (footnote, p. 809). The desiccator tap should be a three-way tap which will allow air to be admitted independently to the desiccator or the pump.

Start the pump and exhaust the desiccator only until the liquid is seen to bubble slightly, and then maintain at this pressure for 20–30 min. until the gentle degassing is complete. To do this, close the desiccator tap, admit air to the pump and switch off pump. If bubbling of the culture is marked, admit a very little air into the desiccator jar. When degassing is complete, reconnect the jar to the pump and rapidly exhaust it to high vacuum; the liquid in the ampoule is seen to freeze suddenly within a minute or so. Leave the pump running for about 1 hr., then close the tap, switch off the pump and leave for 18–24 hr. in the dark for drying to continue in the evacuated jar. Finally remove the ampoule from the desiccator, press the cotton-wool plug about 2¼ in. down the stem, heat the stem in a small gas flame at about 1¼ in. from its open end and draw it there to form a capillary neck about 2 mm. diameter (see p. 809). Attach the mouth of the ampoule stem to the rubber tubing leading to the vacuum pump and evacuate the ampoule to high vacuum for about one minute. Seal the ampoule by melting and severing the capillary neck in a small flame.

Cellophan Method of Freeze-Drying (Rayner, 1943).—Moderate quantities of agglutinating sera and guinea-pig complement serum may be preserved by this method. Disks of waterproof cellophan 2¾ in. in diameter are placed over upturned lids of about 2 in. diameter, *e.g.* the lids of 2-oz. waxed cardboard (sputum) cartons. The disks are sterilised individually in Petri dishes in the hot air oven and placed on the waxed cardboard lids by means of sterile forceps. The serum is pipetted in 1–5 ml. amounts on to the cellophan disks. These are stacked in a desiccator over phosphorus pentoxide, and this is exhausted by means of a Hyvac pump. The serum rapidly freezes solid and dries in a short time, but is left overnight in the desiccator. The dried serum is detached quite easily by crumpling the cellophan, and is then placed in sterile $6 \times \frac{5}{8}$ in. test-tubes. These are heated above the middle and constricted to a capillary neck about 2 mm. in diameter. They are placed in the desiccator, which is again evacuated and left overnight. Finally, the tubes are connected individually to the Hyvac pump, evacuated to high vacuum and sealed by melting and severing the neck with a flame.

Suspending Media for Freeze-Drying of Bacteria

The survival of bacteria on freeze-drying is greatly influenced by the nature of the medium in which they are suspended. Nutrient broth containing 1 per cent. of peptone and meat extract is a satisfactory medium for the most resistant organisms, *e.g. Strept. pyogenes* and *Staph. aureus*, and the moderately resistant, *e.g.* enterobacteriaceae and brucellae. Broth cultures of these may be dried directly.

Special protective suspending media are necessary for the poorly resistant organisms such as *Neisseria gonorrhoeae*, *Vibrio cholerae* and *Haemophilus influenzae*. Organisms from a fresh culture are suspended to a high density (*e.g.* equivalent to Brown's opacity standard No. 4, p. 873) in the sterile suspending medium just prior to freeze-drying. Various media have been advised, most of which contain sugar, peptone and a colloid (*e.g.* protein or dextran). Skimmed milk, containing lactose and protein, has been used with success. The most generally recommended at present is a serum broth containing 7·5 per cent. glucose; this is prepared as the following mixture:

Nutrient broth with 30 per cent. glucose . .	1 volume
Sterile inactivated serum (*e.g.* commercial sterile horse serum)	3 volumes

REFERENCES

HARRIS, R. J. C. (1954). *Biological Applications of Freezing and Drying.* New York: Levin and Munksgaard.

ØRSKOV, J. (1923). *Investigations into the Morphology of the Ray Fungi*, Copenhagen.

RAYNER, A. G. (1943). A simple method for the preservation of cultures and sera by drying. *J. Path. Bact.*, **55**, 373.

REPORT (1958). Precautions against tuberculous infection in the diagnostic laboratory. Tomlinson *et al.*, *Mth. Bull. Minist. Hlth Lab. Serv.*, **17**, 10.

STOKES, E. JOAN (1962). *Short Term Preservation of Bacterial Cultures.* Association of Clinical Pathologists: Broadsheet No. 40 (New Series).

WATSON, K. C. (1955). Isolation of *Salmonella typhi* from the blood stream. *J. Lab. clin. Med.*, **46**, 128.

WILLIAMS, R. E. O. & LIDWELL, O. M. (1957). A protective cabinet for handling infective material in the laboratory. *J. clin. Path.*, **10**, 400.

CHAPTER 49

TESTS EMPLOYED IN BACTERIAL IDENTIFICATION

In this chapter a number of "biochemical" tests and a few miscellaneous tests, used generally in the identification of microorganisms, are described. Tests used specifically for the identification of a particular organism are described elsewhere in the appropriate section dealing with that organism.

It should be realised that many of the tests described in this chapter are not "all-or-none" tests; some distinguish between organisms that differ in the rate with which they carry out a particular reaction. It is therefore important to use a method of test that is suitably poised to differentiate the organisms under consideration. For many of the tests given here, a large number of variations have been developed in different laboratories. In these cases, it has been difficult to make a choice of a method and in some instances we have described more than one test for a given reaction. The results obtained with variations on a particular test may not be comparable and it is essential to bear this in mind. Moreover, there may be considerable variation in the commercially available preparations of the reagents used. For example, the tryptophane content of peptone varies considerably according to the mode of preparation and this markedly influences its value as a substrate in the indole test.

Unfortunately many routinely used tests are not yet standardised, but a start has been made by various organisations. For example, the International Committee on Bacteriological Nomenclature have published recommended biochemical methods for the group differentiation of the *Enterobacteriaceae* (Report, 1958) and much use has been made of these proposals in this chapter.

Diagnostic tables showing the biochemical reactions identifying many genera and species of pathogenic and saprophytic bacteria are given by Cowan and Steel (1961).

Preparation of inoculum for test media

The validity of the identification of an unknown bacterial culture by its reactions in a range of biochemical tests depends absolutely on the use of a *pure* culture of the bacterium for inoculation of the test media. Single, well-separated colonies grown on a primary diagnostic plate that has been inoculated with material containing a mixture of bacterial species, e.g. sputum or faeces, are usually but not always pure. A small proportion of the colonies are likely to be contaminated with a minor admixture of bacteria of another kind, e.g. an anaerobic or other exacting species that does not grow well under the conditions of culture in the primary plate. If such a colony is accidentally picked and the test media are inoculated either directly from it or from an immediate slope or broth subculture of it, the contaminating bacteria may grow out selectively in some of the media and give false results.

It is recommended, therefore, that the chosen colony should first be plated out on an unselective culture medium and that a well-isolated colony on the secondary plate should be used as the inoculum for the tests. This precaution is often omitted in medical diagnostic bacteriology, where speed in obtaining results is important. The results are then not fully reliable and if they are unexpected a freshly purified inoculum culture should be prepared and the tests be repeated.

If a larger number of test media have to be inoculated than can conveniently be done from a single colony, the colony should first be subcultured on an agar slope, or in a tube of broth, and this subculture should be used to inoculate the test media. The subculture can then be preserved for making confirmatory or other different tests on subsequent days. It is an unsound practice to use another, apparently similar colony on the primary plate to provide inocula for additional tests.

Controls for tests

The sterility of each batch of test medium should be confirmed by incubating one or two uninoculated tubes of the batch along with the inoculated tests. If the uninoculated tubes show evidence of bacterial growth, the tests and the remainder of that batch of medium should be discarded.

Control tests are also made to confirm that the test media have been made up correctly and that they are used and observed under the proper conditions. One tube of each batch of test medium is inoculated with a stock culture of a bacterium known to give a positive reaction and another tube with a stock culture known to give a negative reaction. These positive and negative controls are incubated and examined along with the tests.

TESTS FOR CARBOHYDRATE METABOLISM

Bacteria differ widely in their ability to metabolise carbohydrates and to use them as a source of carbon and energy. Knowledge of the range of sugars that can be broken down and the nature of the attack (whether by fermentation or oxidation) provides a very valuable aid to diagnosis.

Metabolism of a carbohydrate, particularly anaerobic breakdown or fermentation, usually results in the production of acids. Gas is also commonly produced. The most convenient method of demonstrating such metabolism, therefore, is to test a culture for acid production, with or without gas production, in a medium in which a specific carbohydrate is provided as a potential substrate. There is a wide difference in the products of breakdown during fermentation; these can also be tested for and their nature ascertained for diagnostic purposes.

Carbohydrates may be altered when exposed to normal heat-sterilisation temperatures. They may also be altered when heated in the presence of other ingredients of culture media, *e.g.* peptone, phosphate, and they are particularly susceptible to heat in an alkaline environment.

For these reasons, we recommend that the basal ingredients of sugar fermentation media should be heat-sterilised before the sugar is added. A solution of the sugar should then be sterilised and the requisite amount subsequently added to the sterile basal medium.

If a sugar solution is to be sterilised by heat, the prior addition of one or two drops of phosphoric acid will ensure that the solution is not alkaline. In general, tyndallisation (intermittent steaming) is less likely to alter the sugar than autoclaving at 121° C., but the important point is to sterilise the sugar separately from the other ingredients. Sterilisation of sugar solutions by filtration is recommended.

Method to Distinguish between Aerobic and Anaerobic Breakdown of Carbohydrates

This method (Hugh & Leifson, 1953) depends upon the use of a solid tubed medium containing the carbohydrate together with a pH indicator. If acid is produced only at the surface of the medium, where conditions are aerobic, the attack on the sugar is oxidative. If acid is found throughout the tube, including the lower layers where conditions are anaerobic, the breakdown is fermentative.

Medium

Peptone	2·0 g.
Sodium chloride, NaCl	5·0 g.
Dipotassium hydrogen phosphate, K_2HPO_4	0·3 g.
Bromothymol blue (1 per cent. aqueous solution)	3 ml.
Agar	3 g.
Water	1 l.

The pH is adjusted to 7·1 before adding the bromothymol blue and the medium is autoclaved at 121° C. for 15 min. The carbohydrate to be added is sterilised separately and added to give a final concentration of 1 per cent. The medium is then tubed to a depth of about 4 cm.

Method.—Duplicate tubes of solidified medium are inoculated by stabbing, one tube is promptly covered with a layer of sterile melted petroleum jelly (yellow soft petroleum) to a depth of 5–10 mm. and both are incubated for up to 30 days. Fermenting organisms (*Enterobacteriaceae*, *Aeromonas*, *Vibrio*) produce an acid reaction throughout the medium in the covered (anaerobic) as well as the open (aerobic) tube. Oxidising organisms (e.g. *Pseudomonas*, *Malleomyces*) produce an acid reaction in the open tube only; this begins at the surface and gradually extends downwards, and may appear only after an alkaline reaction has been present for several days. Organisms that cannot break down the carbohydrate aerobically or anaerobically (e.g. *Alcaligenes faecalis*) produce an alkaline reaction in the open tube and no change in the covered tube.

It should be noted that this medium may also be used for recording gas production and motility.

SUGAR MEDIA TO TEST FOR CARBOHYDRATE FERMENTATION

Media for determining the ability of a particular organism to ferment a particular sugar contain the following components:

(1) Suitable material to allow the growth of the organism under consideration. The nature of these materials depends upon the nutritional requirements of the organism.

(2) The carbohydrate. A large variety of sugars are used, *e.g.*

(a) *Monosaccharides*
Pentoses—Arabinose, xylose, rhamnose.
Hexoses—Glucose, fructose, mannose, sorbose, galactose.

(b) *Disaccharides*—Sucrose, maltose, lactose, trehalose, cellobiose.

(c) *Trisaccharides*—Raffinose.

(d) *Polysaccharides*—Starch, inulin, dextrin, glycogen.

(e) *Sugar alcohols*—Glycerol, erythritol, adonitol, mannitol, dulcitol, sorbitol, inositol.

(f) *Glycosides*—Salicin, coniferin, aesculin.

For some purposes, certain organic acids are used:—

(g) D-tartrate, L-tartrate, M-tartrate, citrate, and mucic acid.

(3) A suitable indicator that will change colour only as a result of the formation of acids during the fermentation of the sugar. A variety of indicators with a pK between pH 6 and 8 have been used.

(4) A small inverted tube (Durham's fermentation tube) is placed in each culture tube to detect gas. During the process of sterilisation the heat drives out the air from the inverted tubes which, when cool, should be completely filled with liquid and contain no air bubbles.

Sugar Medium 1. Peptone water base

Peptone	10 g.
Sodium chloride, NaCl	5 g.
Water	1 l.

The medium is adjusted to pH 7·2–7·3 and a previously sterilised solution of the fermentable carbohydrate (p. 813) is added in the proportion of 0·5 to 1·0 per cent. An indicator is incorporated to detect acid production. Various indicators are employed, including Andrade's indicator, phenol red, bromothymol blue, and bromocresol purple.

Indicators

Andrade's indicator is made by adding 1 *N* NaOH to a 0·5 per cent. solution of acid fuchsin until the colour just becomes yellow. It is used at a final concentration of 1 per cent. in the medium and it turns dark reddish pink if acid is produced. Andrade's indicator fades fairly rapidly when stored and should not be used unless the media can be utilised within a few months.

Phenol red is made up in a 0·2 per cent. solution prepared as described in the footnote on p. 848 except that the phenol red is ten times as strong. For use, 5 ml. of the 0·2 per cent. solution is added to each 100 ml. of medium. This indicator does not fade on storage and may be incorporated in bottled media that may not be used for some time. Phenol red turns yellow if acid is produced. (Phenol red is yellow at pH 6·8 and purple-pink at pH 8·4.)

Bromothymol blue is recommended as a useful indicator for sugar fermentation tests. It turns yellow in the presence of acid. It is best prepared and used as detailed in Sugar Medium 2. (Bromothymol blue is yellow at pH 6·0 and blue at pH 7·6.)

Bromocresol purple is used in the media at a final concentration of 0·005 per cent. It turns yellow in the presence of acid. (Bromocresol purple is yellow at pH 5·2 and violet-purple at pH 6·8.)

Preparation of sugar media

Peptone water with an indicator is tubed in 5 ml. amounts, the Durham fermentation tubes inserted, and the test-tubes are stoppered with coloured cotton-wool. They are then sterilised in the autoclave at 121° C. for 15 min. The sugars are made up separately in 10 per cent. solutions in distilled water, and are sterilised, preferably by filtration or in the steamer. The sterile sugars are kept conveniently in 10-oz. screw-neck bottles fitted with a siphon and hooded pipette. When required, 0·25 ml. of a 10 per cent. solution of sugar is added to each tube.

Sugar media containing sugars that are only occasionally required may be distributed in 3 ml. amounts into small screw-capped bottles of ¼-oz. capacity with a 19 mm. Durham tube. By this means the medium can be stored and transported without risk of contamination or alteration in the concentration of the ingredients. As a result of shaking during transit, air may enter the Durham fermentation tube, but it is easily removed by inverting the bottle, as the amount of fluid is such that the open end of the tube is below the surface. When the bottle has been inoculated the cap should be loosely screwed on to allow access of air. In order to identify the various sugar media the caps are painted with cellulose paint (see p. 785).

The various sugar media in tubes can be distinguished by having the cotton-wool stoppers of different colours. It is better to employ wool dyed in bulk rather than to colour white-wool stoppers with various stains.

Use of sugar media

Before inoculation, the tubes are inspected to confirm the absence of bubbles of gas from the Durham tubes. A tube of each medium is inoculated with a speck of solid culture (e.g. from a single colony) or a drop or loopful of a liquid culture or a suspension of a solid culture in saline. The inoculated tubes are incubated, generally aerobically and at

37° C., for the required period, and the presence or absence of an acid colour change and gas formation in the Durham tube is noted.

Fermentation reactions are commonly completed within a period of incubation of 24 hr. and the identification of many organisms is based on the results recorded at this time. It should be noted, however, that some organisms that fail to ferment a given sugar in 24 hr., will give "late" fermentation of the sugar if incubation of the test medium is prolonged. Such fermentation may take place after a period of incubation that varies, on different occasions of testing the same strain of organism, from as little as 2, to as much as 40 days. Late fermentation appears generally to be the result of a non-fermenting culture giving rise to a fermenting mutant. In cases where late, mutational fermentation may be significant for the identification of an organism, and in research investigations made in order to characterise organisms, the sugar tests should be incubated for 40 days and should be inspected daily; if fermentation occurs, the day on which it first appears is recorded.

Sugar Medium 2. Broth base

Meat extract	5 g.
Peptone	10 g.
Sodium chloride, NaCl	3 g.
Disodium hydrogen phosphate, Na_2HPO_4 . .	2 g.
Bromothymol blue indicator solution . . .	12 ml.
Distilled water	1 l.

The indicator solution recommended is as follows:

Bromothymol blue	1 g.
0·1 *N* NaOH	25 ml.
Distilled water	475 ml.

Dissolve the ingredients of the broth by steaming, adjust the pH to 7·2–7·3, add the appropriate amount of indicator, and tube in 5-ml. volumes with inverted Durham tubes. Sterilise by autoclaving at 121° C. for 15 min. To the sterile medium is added 0·5 per cent. of the test carbohydrate in sterile aqueous solution, *e.g.* 0·25 ml. of a 10 per cent. sugar solution.

Sugar Medium 3. Hiss's serum water

As certain pathogenic organisms—*e.g.* streptococcus, pneumococcus—will not grow well in ordinary sugar media, it is necessary for some fermentation tests to use a medium containing serum.

One part of serum is mixed with three parts of distilled water, and 5 ml. of a 0·2 per cent. solution of phenol red per 100 ml. of medium (p. 848) are added. The reaction of the medium is adjusted to pH 7·6 before the indicator is added and prior to sterilisation. Some samples of horse serum may give fallacious results and batches should be tested before use. Sheep or ox serum is suitable. (Some workers prefer to substitute 0·1 per cent. peptone water for the distilled water.) The various sugars are incorporated in the proportion of 1 per cent. This medium, if not acid, does not coagulate on heating. It is best sterilised by filtration but it may be sterilised by intermittent steaming—20 min. each day on three successive days. Alternatively, the mixture of serum, distilled water and indicator is sterilised in the steamer, and the appropriate amount of a sterile solution of the requisite sugar is added as described on p. 731.

Fermentation is indicated by the production of acid, which alters the indicator and causes coagulation of the medium.

The Hiss's serum water may be made up with indicator, but without any carbohydrate added. The medium is distributed in 2·5 ml. amounts in ¼-oz. bottles. The caps are tightly screwed on, and the whole batch is sterilised in the steamer for 20 min. on three consecutive days. When a batch of any particular carbohydrate medium is required, the requisite amount of sterile 10 per cent. sugar is added from the siphon-filter bottle described on p. 731. The caps are then painted with cellulose paint, to indicate the sugar used (p. 785). Alternatively, the rarer sugars in 10 per cent. aqueous solutions may be sterilised and stored in ½-oz. screw-capped bottles fitted with a perforated cap and rubber washer similar to blood-culture bottles. When the sugar solution is required it is withdrawn from the bottle by perforating the rubber aseptically with the needle of a sterile syringe.

Hiss's Serum-Water Starch Medium.—This medium, which is used for differentiating the gravis type of *C. diphtheriae*, does not keep well as the starch undergoes gradual hydrolysis forming glucose which is fermented by all types of *C. diphtheriae*. It is essential, therefore, to make up the starch solution only when required and add it to the serum water medium immediately before use. A convenient method sufficient for about 24 small bottles (holding about 3 ml. of medium) is as follows. Weigh out 0·15 g. of soluble starch and place it in a sterile universal container. Add 5 ml. distilled water, screw on the cap and shake vigorously. Place the bottle in a pan of water, bring to the boil, and boil for about 5 min., shaking at intervals to ensure that all the starch is in solution and the contents are homogeneous. When the starch solution is cool add 0·15 ml. with a sterile 1-ml. pipette, or five drops from a sterile capillary pipette, to each of the fermentation bottles. After the starch has been added, the medium should be used within a few weeks.

Sugar Medium 4. For nutritionally exacting organisms

This medium is recommended for fermentation tests for organisms such as the meningococcus and gonococcus.

Peptone	20 g.
Sodium chloride	5 g.
Distilled water	900 ml.

Dissolve by steaming for 30 min. Make just alkaline to phenolphthalein (pH 8·4) and steam for a further 30 min. Filter through a coarse filter paper and re-adjust the reaction to pH 7·6. Add 100 ml. digest broth of the same pH. Add 25 g. agar powder (*i.e.* 2·5 per cent.) and autoclave for 45 min. in "free steam" (100° C.), and thereafter 15 min. at 110° C. Filter through paper pulp and bottle in 100-ml. amounts with 2 ml. of 0·2 per cent. phenol red solution (made as described in the footnote on p. 848, except that the phenol red is ten times as strong) in each bottle. Sterilise by holding for 1 hr. in "free steam" (100° C.) followed by 5 min. at 110° C.

For use, 100 ml. of the agar are melted, cooled to 55° C., and to this are added 5 ml. sterile guinea-pig or rabbit (not horse) serum, and 10 ml. of a 10 per cent. sterile solution of the required sugar. (This gives a concentration of about 5 per cent. serum and 1 per cent. sugar.) The mixture is immediately distributed into sterile tubes or ¼-oz. bottles, allowed to solidify in the sloped position and tested for sterility by incubation.

The sugars generally used are glucose, lactose, sucrose and maltose. When the sugar is fermented by the organism and acid is formed, the colour of the medium changes from purple-pink to yellow.

Sugar Medium 5. Litmus Milk

This is used in testing for the fermentation of lactose and clotting of milk.

Fresh milk is steamed for 20 min. and then allowed to stand for 24 hr. in order that the cream may separate. The milk is siphoned off and litmus is added in the proportion of 2·5 per cent. of an alcoholic solution. The medium is distributed in 5-ml. amounts in screw-capped bottles or tubes and then sterilised by steaming for 20 min. on three successive days. If bulk-amounts (*e.g.* 250 ml.) are put up, it is advisable not to add the litmus solution until the milk is redistributed in smaller amounts, as the colour fades on storing.

Litmus solution.—Litmus granules 80 g., 40 per cent. ethanol 300 ml. Grind up the granules and place in a flask with 150 ml. of the ethanol and boil for one minute. Decant the fluid and add remainder of ethanol to the granules; then boil for one minute. Decant the fluid and add to the first quantity of the extract. Make up to 300 ml. with 40 per cent. ethanol and add 1 N HC1 drop by drop, shaking continuously till the fluid becomes purple. To test for correct reaction, take a tube of tap water and one of distilled water, boil both and add one drop of the solution to each; the tap water should be blue and the distilled water mauve.

Sugar Medium 6. Methyl Red Test

The methyl red test is employed to detect the production of sufficient acid during the fermentation of glucose and the maintenance of conditions such that the pH of an old culture is sustained below a value of about 4·5, as shown by a change in the colour of the methyl red indicator which is added at the end of the period of incubation.

Medium ("glucose phosphate peptone water")

Peptone	5 g.
Dipotassium hydrogen phosphate, K_2HPO_4	5 g.
Water	1 l.

Dissolve the materials, adjust the pH to 7·6, filter and sterilise at 121° C. for 15 min. Add glucose (sterilised separately by filtration) to a final concentration of 0·5 per cent. in tubes containing 5 ml. medium.

Method.—Inoculate the fluid medium lightly from a young agar slope culture and incubate at 37° C. for 48 hr. Add about five drops of the methyl red reagent (see below). Mix and read immediately. Positive tests are bright red and negative are yellow. If the results after 48 hr. are equivocal, the test should be repeated with cultures that have been incubated for 5 days. For some organisms, incubation at 30° C. for 5 days is preferable to incubation at 37° C. for 2 or 5 days.

Methyl red indicator solution

Methyl red	0·1 g.
Ethanol	300 ml.

Make up to a volume of 500 ml. with distilled water.

Voges-Proskauer Test

Many bacteria ferment carbohydrates with the production of acetyl methyl carbinol (CH_3 . CO . CHOH . CH_3) or its reduction product 2, 3 butylene glycol (CH_3 . CHOH . CHOH . CH_3). The substances can be tested for by a colorimetric reaction between diacetyl (CH_3 . CO CO . CH_3—formed during the test by oxidation of acetyl methyl carbinol or 2, 3 butylene glycol) and a guanidino group under alkaline conditions. This test is usually done in conjunction with the methyl red test since the production of acetyl methyl carbinol or butylene glycol usually results in insufficient acid accumulating during fermentation to give a methyl red positive reaction. An organism of the enterobacterial group is usually *either* methyl-red-positive and Voges-Proskauer-negative *or* methyl red-negative and Voges-Proskauer-positive.

Medium.—Glucose phosphate peptone water, as for the methyl red test.

Method 1 (O'Meara).—Incubate at 37° or 30° C. for 48 hr. only.

Add 0·5 ml. of O'Meara reagent (40 g. potassium hydroxide and 0·3 g. creatine in 100 ml. distilled water). Place tubes in a 37° waterbath for 4 hr. Aerate by shaking at intervals. A positive reaction is denoted by the development of an eosin-pink colour, usually in 2-5 min.

Method 2 (Barritt).—Incubate at 37° or 30° C. for 48 hr. Add 1 ml. of 40 per cent. potassium hydroxide and 3 ml. of a 5 per cent. solution of α-naphthol in absolute ethanol. A positive reaction is indicated by the development of a pink colour in 2-5 min., becoming crimson in 30 min. The tube can be shaken at intervals to ensure maximum aeration.

Sugar Medium 7. Eosin Methylene Blue Agar

With strongly fermenting organisms, sugar fermentation reactions can be observed in cultures on plates of an agar medium containing a sugar and an indicator dye. Fermenting colonies or streaks of growth become distinctively coloured and the method makes it possible to test several pure cultures on the same plate. If a mixture of fermenting and non-fermenting organisms is plated, the different kinds of colonies can be recognised and their relative numbers estimated. The following modification of eosin methylene blue agar is recommended for use with sugars in a concentration of 0·5 per cent.

Peptone (Oxoid L37)	3·0 g.
Dipotassium hydrogen phosphate, K_2HPO_4 . .	0·6 g.
Eosin yellow	0·4 g.
Methylene blue	0·065 g.
Agar (New Zealand, Davis)	10–12 g.
Water	1000 ml.

Adjust to pH 6·8 and sterilise at 121° C. for 15 min. As the medium cools, add 50 ml. of a separately sterilised 10 per cent. solution of the sugar to be tested and immediately pour the plates (15–20 ml. per 3½ in. plate).

Inoculate the plate to give well-separated streaks or spots of growth, or else plate out to give well-separated colonies. Incubate at 37° C. and examine after 24 and 48 hr. Colonies of fermenting organisms are red to opaque black. Colonies of non-fermenting ones are pale yellow and nearly transparent. Full development of the dark red colour may require incubation for 48 hr.

Sugar Medium 8. Desoxycholate Agar

This medium, which differs from Leifson's DCA in not containing ferric ammonium citrate, is less inhibitory to *Esch. coli*. It gives better differentiation of the reactions of crowded colonies than eosin methylene blue agar.

Peptone agar

Peptone	20 g.
Sodium chloride	5 g.
Sodium hydroxide (40 per cent. solution) . .	5 ml.
Agar	20 g.
Water	1000 ml.

Melt at 100° C., filter through paper pulp to remove phosphates, adjust to pH 7·4 and sterilise at 121° C. for 15 min.

Medium.—To 1000 ml. of melted peptone agar add in the following order:—

Sodium desoxycholate (10 per cent. solution) .	25ml.
Neutral red (1 per cent. solution)	2·7 ml.

Sugar (20 per cent. solution)	50 ml.
Tris (hydroxymethyl) aminomethane (1 per cent. solution)	50 ml.

Mix and at once pour in plates (*c.* 25 ml. per 3½ in. plate). Plates must be used soon after their preparation.

Note.—The solutions of neutral red, sugar and Tris are sterilised separately before use by autoclaving at 121° C. The desoxycholate solution is pasteurised by immersing the bottle in a waterbath at 60° C. for 1 hr. or by bringing momentarily to 100° C. On keeping, this solution tends to precipitate and it may have to be warmed to 60° C. to melt it before use.

For *Esch. coli*, dehydrocholic acid, which is less inhibitory to this organism, may be substituted for the desoxycholate.

After incubation for 24 or 48 hr. at 37° C., colonies of fermenting organisms are bright red and opaque. Those of non-fermenting organisms are pale and transparent.

Sugar Medium 9. Bitter Medium

This medium (Bitter, Weigmann & Habs, 1926) distinguishes only the reactions of *strongly* fermenting organisms, *i.e.* those giving marked fermentation within 5–10 hr. at 37° C. in the conventional peptone water media (sugar media 1 and 2, above). The Bitter reaction with xylose is observed in the "fermentation typing" of organisms such as *S. typhimurium* (*e.g.* Kallings and Laurell, 1957).

Medium

Peptone	0·05 g.
$Na_2HPO_4 \cdot 2H_2O$	0·5 g.
$(NH_4)_2SO_4$	1·0 g.
Sodium citrate	2·0 g.
Sodium chloride	2·0 g.
Water (distilled)	1000 ml.

Adjust to pH 7·1 and sterilise at 121° C. for 15 min. Before use, add 50 ml. of a separately sterilised 10 per cent. solution of the test sugar (*e.g.* xylose), giving a final concentration of 0·5 per cent. Tube to a depth of *c.* 6 cm. and steam at 100° C. for 30 min.

Method.—Inoculate with a loopful of a suspension of $1–4 \times 10^8$ bacteria per ml. prepared in saline solution from a 24-hr. agar slope culture. Incubate at 37° C. for only 20–22 hr. and then test by adding a few drops of a 0·5 per cent. solution of methyl red in ethanol. A red colour is positive, orange is doubtful and yellow is negative.

Organic Acid Fermentation Media

Fermentation reactions with certain organic acids are used in the identification and fermentation typing of salmonellae (Kauffmann, 1954).

Base Medium

Peptone (*e.g.* Bacto-peptone, Difco) . . .	10 g.
0·1 *N* NaOH	8·5 ml.
Bromothymol blue (1 in 500 solution, p. 817) . .	12 ml.
Distilled water	1000 ml.

Complete Media

Add to the base medium one of the following acids to the stated concentration:—

D-tartrate, *i.e.* sodium potassium tartrate, dextro-rotatory, 1 per cent.
L-tartrate, *i.e.* tartaric acid, laevo-rotatory, 0·5 per cent.
M-tartrate, *i.e.* tartaric acid, inactive, 0·5 per cent.
Citrate, *i.e.* sodium citrate, neutral powder, 1 per cent.
Mucate, *i.e.* mucic acid, 1 per cent.

Adjust the complete medium to pH 7·4 by the addition of 5 *N* NaOH, tube to a depth of *c.* 6 cm. and sterilise at 121° C. for 15 min. Take care to dissolve all the mucic acid before tubing.

Method.—Inoculate with a loopful of a 20-hr. broth culture and incubate for 14 days at 37° C. Observe the colour of the tests daily. Positive reactions are generally shown by a shift from blue to green or yellow after 1 or 2 days, followed by reversion to blue. After 14 days, add to each tube of tartrate and citrate medium 0·5 ml. of a half-saturated solution of neutral lead acetate[1] per 4 ml. medium; allow the tubes to stand undisturbed for a further 24 hr. at room temperature. A negative reaction is shown by the presence of a bulky precipitate occupying more than half the depth of the medium. A positive reaction is shown by a diminution in the volume of the precipitate so that, after settling, it occupies less than a quarter the depth of the medium.

An uninoculated tube of each medium is incubated along with the inoculated tubes to serve as a control. Lead acetate is added to this tube at 14 days and the amount of precipitate formed serves to indicate the result of a negative reaction.

Stern's Glycerol Reaction

This reaction is also used in the identification and fermentation typing of salmonellae. It depends on the ability of the organism to convert glycerol into an aldehyde product that re-colourises fuchsin-sulphite.

Stern's (1916) *Glycerol Fuchsin Broth*

Solution 1.—	Meat extract (Lab-Lemco) . .	10 g.
	Peptone	20 g.
	Water	1000 ml.
	Adjust to pH 8·0.	

[1] This does not seem to be critical. "Neutral" refers to the normal form of lead acetate of which about 40–60 g. dissolves in 100 ml. water at 15–25° C. if the pure salt is used, but absorbtion of CO_2 from the air makes the salt incompletely soluble.

Solution 2.—Saturated alcoholic solution of basic fuchsin (10 per cent.).

Solution 3.—Fresh 10 per cent. aqueous solution of anhydrous sodium sulphite.

Medium.—Mix 1000 ml. of solution 1, 2 ml. of solution 2, 16·6 ml. of solution 3 and 10 ml. of glycerol. Tube to a depth of *c.* 6 cm. and sterilise at 121° C. for 15 min.

Method.—Inoculate from a culture on agar and incubate at 37° C. for 7 days. Examine daily for the development of a deep red colour and note the day of its development. Usually the reaction is fully developed at 2 days. An uninoculated tube should be incubated as a control and this should remain uncoloured or become only faintly pink.

TESTS FOR PROTEINASES AND AMINO ACID BREAKDOWN

Tests for proteolysis

Gelatin Liquefaction

Proteolytic organisms digest proteins and consequently may liquefy gelatin and coagulated serum. Cultures in meat media cause blackening of the meat, decomposing it and reducing it in volume with the formation of foul-smelling products. Strongly proteolytic organisms will decompose gelatin, coagulated serum and cooked meat, whereas weakly proteolytic organisms may not attack the meat, and some not the coagulated serum. Thus, liquefaction of gelatin is a routinely used index of proteolytic activity useful in differentiating certain organisms, but a positive result may take many days to develop.

For bacteriological use an edible grade of gelatin is preferred, since this is free from preservatives and inhibitory amounts of heavy metals. Gelatin will not by itself support the growth of many pathogens and it is added to a liquid nutrient medium to produce a firm gel sometimes called "nutrient gelatin". The proportion of gelatin used varies, but 15 per cent. is a suitable average.

It is important that the gelatin medium should not be exposed to a high temperature for longer than recommended, otherwise it may be partially hydrolysed and will not solidify on cooling.

Medium—Nutrient gelatin.

Add 15 per cent. of gelatin to the required amount of nutrient broth (p. 742) and hold at 4° C. overnight.

Next day dissolve the gelatin at 45° C., adjust to pH 8·4, and steam for 10 min. Cool quickly to 45° C. and slowly add the beaten white of two eggs, or 10 g. egg albumin dissolved in 50 ml. water, or 50 ml. of serum, per litre of medium; this helps to clear the medium of colloidal particles. Steam for 30 min., stirring occasionally. Filter through paper pulp or filter paper. The reaction should be approximately pH 7·6, but may require a little adjustment. Bottle in 12 ml. amounts.

Sterilise by holding in the autoclave in free steam (100° C.) for 10 min. followed by 115° C. for 10 min. Remove from the autoclave as quickly as possible and keep at a low temperature.

The resulting medium is perfectly transparent when solid, and should be of firm consistency, yet not so stiff that it is split by the wire when inoculated.

Method.—A stab culture of the organism to be tested is made using an inoculum from an agar slope culture. Pathogenic bacteria are usually grown at 37° C. and negative tests may be observed for as long as 30 days. Gelatin at the concentration used melts at about 24° C. and is therefore fluid at 37° C. Liquefaction is tested for at intervals by removing the nutrient gelatin cultures from the incubator and holding them at 4° C. for 30 min. before reading the results.

Miscellaneous Tests for Proteolysis

A combined test for hydrogen sulphide production and gelatin liquefaction is described on p. 827.

If proteolytic organisms are grown on a buffered nutrient agar medium containing 0·4 per cent. of gelatin, 1·5 per cent. of agar, and 0·005 per cent. of glucose, zones of altered gelatin around the colonies can be demonstrated by flooding the medium with a 1 per cent. solution of tannic acid (zones become more opaque than the surrounding medium) or an acid solution of mercuric chloride (zones are rendered less opaque than the surrounding medium)—see Barer (1946).

A glucose-gelatin medium containing 12 per cent. of gelatin with 1 per cent. of glucose, and phenol red as an indicator of acid production, has been recommended by Willis & Hobbs (1959) who have also incorporated milk in a complex medium; proteolytic organisms show zones of clearing as a result of decomposition of milk protein in solid media containing milk. Certain organisms producing clotting of litmus-milk medium may proceed to decompose the clotted milk by proteolytic activity.

Liquefaction of Charcoal Gelatin Disks

The method of Kohn (1953) employing sterile disks or cubes of formaldehyde-denatured gelatin containing finely powdered charcoal is a very rapid and convenient test for proteolysis.

The sterile disk is picked from its bottle with a hot inoculating wire, to which it adheres, and is transferred into a newly inoculated or already grown culture in liquid medium. The culture is incubated with the disk for up to a week at 37° C. (The denatured gelatin does not melt at this temperature.) Liquefaction of the gelatin is shown by the settling of free carbon particles to the bottom of the medium and, later, by the complete disintegration of the disk.

If the disks are added to a culture that is already fully grown or to a dense suspension in peptone water of a young culture grown on agar, liquefaction may be observed after only a few hours' incubation at 37° C.

Lautrop (1956) has described a modification of the test for the demonstration of a special, calcium-dependent gelatinase present in certain organisms (e.g. *Salmonella abortus-bovis*, *S. schleissheim* and *S. texas*). Organisms grown at 22° C. on agar are suspended to high density in 3–4 ml. saline containing 0·01 *M* $CaCl_2$, a gelatin-charcoal disk is added and the test is incubated at 37° C. for up to 3 days.

Amino Acid Decarboxylase Tests

This test (see Møller, 1955) is based on the ability of some bacteria to decarboxylate an amino acid to the corresponding amine with the liberation of carbon dioxide. The production of these decarboxylases is induced by a low pH and, as a result of their action, the pH rises to neutrality or above.

Medium

Peptone	5 g.
Meat extract	5 g.
Glucose	0·5 g.
Pyridoxal	5 mg.
Bromocresol purple (1 in 500 solution)	5 ml.
Cresol red (1 in 500 solution)	2·5 ml.
Distilled water	1 l.

Dissolve the solids in water and adjust the pH to 6·0 *before* the addition of the indicators. This is the basal medium and to it is added the amino acid whose decarboxylation is to be tested. Divide the basal medium into four portions and treat as follows:

(1) Add 1 per cent. L-lysine[1] hydrochloride.
(2) Add 1 per cent. L-ornithine[1] hydrochloride.
(3) Add 1 per cent. L-arginine[1] hydrochloride.
(4) No additions (control).

Readjust the pH to 6·0 if necessary. Distribute 1 ml. quantities in small tubes containing sterile liquid paraffin to provide a layer about 5 mm. thick above the medium. Autoclave at 121° C. for 15 min.

Method.—Inoculate lightly through the paraffin layer with a straight wire. Incubate and read daily for four days.

The media first become yellow due to acid production during glucose fermentation; later, if decarboxylation occurs, the medium becomes violet. The control should remain yellow.

Hydrogen Sulphide Production Test

Some organisms decompose sulphur-containing amino acids to form hydrogen sulphide among the products. The hydrogen sulphide is usually tested for by demonstrating its ability to form a black insoluble ferrous salt.

[1] If the DL components are used, add 2 per cent. of the amino acid.

Medium

Meat extract	7·5 g.
Peptone	25 g.
Sodium chloride, NaCl	5 g.
Gelatin	120 g.
Distilled water	1 l.

Adjust the pH to 7·6, steam and filter. Sterilise in the autoclave for 10 min. in free steam and then at 115° C. for 10 min. Remove from the autoclave as quickly as possible and cool to about 55° C. Add 5 ml. of a freshly prepared 10 per cent. solution of ferrous chloride sterilised by filtration. Tube the medium in narrow tubes and seal with corks impregnated with paraffin wax.

Method.—Inoculate with a straight wire (½ in. deep) and incubate at 20° C. for at least 7 days. Inspect daily for blackening due to the production of H_2S.

This medium contains gelatin and may therefore also be used to test for gelatin liquefaction (see p. 884).

It should be noted that hydrogen sulphide can be produced by a very large number of bacteria, at least in small amounts. Therefore the test must be poised at a certain definite level of sensitivity such as that described above for use in group differentiation within the Enterobacteriaceae. Methods have been developed using lead acetate strips suspended over peptone water cultures; these may be of value in intragroup differentiation, but it must be realised that such methods have a different sensitivity from that described above, and therefore give different results.

Phenylalanine Deaminase Test

This test indicates the ability of an organism to deaminate phenylalanine with the production of phenylpyruvic acid which will react with ferric salts to give a green colour.

Medium

Yeast Extract	3 g.
DL-phenylalanine	2 g.
(or L-phenylalanine	1 g.)
Disodium hydrogen phosphate, Na_2HPO_4	1 g.
Sodium chloride, NaCl	5 g.
Agar	12 g.
Distilled water	1 l.

Adjust the pH to 7·4, sterilise by autoclaving at 121° C. for 15 min. and pour into tubes as long slopes.

Method.—Inoculate with a fairly heavy inoculum. Incubate for 4 hr. or, if desired, for up to 24 hr. at 37° C. Allow a few drops of a 10 per cent. solution of ferric chloride to run down over the growth on the slant. If the test is positive, a green colour will develop in the fluid and in the slant.

Indole Test

This test demonstrates the ability of certain bacteria to decompose the amino acid tryptophane to indole which accumulates in the medium. Indole is then tested for by a colourimetric reaction with *p*-dimethyl aminobenzaldehyde.

Medium for growth

Peptone (brand containing sufficient tryptophane)	20 g.
Sodium chloride, NaCl	5 g.
Distilled water	1 l.

Adjust the pH to 7·4. Sterilise by autoclaving at 121° C. for 15 min.

Method.—Inoculate medium and incubate for 48 hr. at 37° C. Sometimes a period of 96 hr. at 37° C. may be required for optimum accumulation of indole. Add 0·5 ml. Kovac's reagent and shake gently. A red colour indicates a positive reaction.

Kovac's Reagent

Amyl or isoamyl alcohol	150 ml.
p-Dimethyl-aminobenzaldehyde	10 g.
Conc. hydrochloric acid, HCl	50 ml.

Dissolve the aldehyde in the alcohol and slowly add the acid. Prepare in small quantities and store in the refrigerator. Shake gently before use.

MISCELLANEOUS TESTS

Urease Test

Bacteria, particularly those growing naturally in an environment exposed to urine, may decompose urea by means of the enzyme urease:

$$NH_2 . CO . NH_2 + H_2O \longrightarrow 2NH_3 + CO_2$$

The occurrence of this enzyme can be tested for by growing the organism in the presence of urea and testing for alkali (NH_3) production by means of a suitable pH indicator. An alternative method is to test for the production of ammonia from urea by means of Nessler's reagent.

Medium 1 (Christensen's medium)

Peptone	1 g.
Sodium chloride, NaCl	5 g.
Monopotassium dihydrogen phosphate, KH_2PO_4	2 g.
Phenol red (1 in 500 aqueous solution)	6 ml.
Agar	20 g.
Distilled water	1 l.

The pH is adjusted to 6·8–6·9 and the basal medium is sterilised by autoclaving at 121° C. for 15 min. When it has cooled to about 50°, a sterile solution of glucose is added to give a final concentration of 0·1 per cent., and 100 ml. of a 20 per cent. solution of urea previously sterilised by filtration is added. The medium is tubed as deep slopes. It may, however, be used in fluid form without agar.

Method 1

Inoculate heavily over the entire slope surface and incubate at 37° C. Examine after 4 hr. and after overnight incubation, no tube being ascribed negative until after 4 days' incubation. Urease-positive cultures produce a purple-pink colour due to a change in the colour of the indicator.

Medium 2 (Elek's test)

Prepare a substrate solution of pH 7·2 containing 2 per cent. urea as follows: Add 35 ml. of 0·2 *N* NaOH and 4 g. urea to 50 ml. of 0·2 *M* KH_2PO_4, and make up the volume to 200 ml. with ammonia-free distilled water. Sterilisation of this substrate is not necessary, and it can be stored in a stoppered bottle (with the stopper smeared with petroleum jelly) in the refrigerator. Freshly prepared substrate should be checked with a known urea-splitting organism, and for the test a negative control and an uninoculated blank must be included. The glassware must be scrupulously clean but not necessarily sterile.

Method 2

Emulsify sufficient of a 24-hour culture of the organism to be tested in 0·5 ml. of the substrate in a $3 \times \frac{3}{8}$ in. tube. The fluid should be distinctly opalescent. Place the tube in a water-bath at 37° C. for 3 hr. Remove the tube and add 0·1 ml. of Nessler's reagent, and a similar amount to the negative control and blank tubes. Read the result 3 min. after adding the Nessler's reagent. Both negative and control tubes must be absolutely colourless. A positive reaction is shown by a colour ranging from a pale but distinct yellow to a dark-brown precipitate. The time of incubation is important and should be strictly adhered to.

When isolated colonies are to be examined, the volume of substrate is reduced to 0·3 ml. and only one drop of Nessler's reagent used. Readings are taken 4–5 min. after nesslerisation.

Catalase Test

This demonstrates the presence of catalase, an enzyme that catalyses the release of oxygen from hydrogen peroxide.

One ml. of hydrogen peroxide solution, H_2O_2 (10 vol.), is poured over a 24–hr. nutrient agar slope culture of the test organism and the tube is held in a slanting position.

Alternatively, a small amount of the culture to be tested is picked from a nutrient agar slope, using a clean sterile platinum loop or a clean, thin glass rod (a sealed capillary tube may be used for this purpose), and this is inserted into hydrogen peroxide solution held in a small clean tube. Enough material may be picked from a single colony to give a reaction by this method.

The production of gas bubbles from the surface of the solid culture material indicates a positive reaction. It occurs almost immediately.

Oxidase Test

This test depends on the presence in bacteria of certain oxidases that will catalyse the transport of electrons between electron donors in the bacteria and a redox dye—tetramethyl-*p*-phenylene-diamine. The dye is reduced to a deep purple colour.

The test is used for screening species of *Neisseria*, *Alcaligenes*, *Aeromonas*, *Vibrio* and *Pseudomonas*, which give positive reactions (see Steel, 1961) and for the exclusion of the Enterobacteriaceae, all species of which give negative reactions.

Plate method.—Cultures are made on a suitable solid growth medium. A freshly prepared 1 per cent. solution of tetramethyl-*p*-phenylene-diamine dihydrochloride is poured on to the plate so as to cover the surface, and is then decanted. The colonies of oxidase-positive organisms rapidly develop a purple colour. If subcultures are required from the colonies, they should be made immediately; after 5 min. exposure to the reagent it may not be possible to subculture them.

Dry filter paper method.—Since the oxidase reagent is unstable and has to be freshly prepared for use, the following method is convenient. Strips of Whatman's No. 1 filter paper are soaked in a freshly prepared 1 per cent. solution of tetramethyl-*p*-phenylene-diamine dihydrochloride. After draining for about 30 sec. the strips are freeze-dried and stored in a dark bottle tightly sealed with a screw cap. The papers have a light purple tint and will keep for several months in an airtight container at room temperature. For use, a strip is removed, laid in a Petri dish and moistened with distilled water. The colony to be tested is picked up with a platinum loop and smeared over the moist area. A positive reaction is indicated by an intense deep-purple hue, appearing within 5–10 sec., a "delayed positive" reaction by colouration in 10–60 sec., and a negative reaction by absence of colouration or by colouration later than 60 sec.

Wet filter paper method.—A strip of filter paper is soaked with a little freshly made 1 per cent. solution of the reagent and then at once used by rubbing a speck of culture on it with a platinum loop. The result is read as for the dry filter paper method.

Note that the reagent must be freshly made and the bacterial growth must be transferred to the test paper with a clean *platinum* loop or a clean glass rod, since traces of iron will catalyse the reaction and give false positive results. If the colony is small it may be necessary to pick up material from several similar colonies in order to have sufficient to give a strong reaction. When testing colonies from MacConkey's medium, a pink-violet colour is due to carry-over from the media and is not a true oxidase reaction; the true reaction gives an intense purple hue. Dimethyl-*p*-phenylene-diamine oxalate, 1 per cent., may be used in place of the tetra-methyl-*p*-phenylene-diamine dihydrochloride in this paper-strip test.

Carbohydrate Utilisation Tests

Bacteria that are capable of growing on a simple, chemically defined medium (i.e. *prototrophic* bacteria), can readily be tested for their ability to use a given compound as their sole source of carbon and energy. A defined medium such as that of Davis and Mingioli (p. 741) is prepared with the test compound substituted for the normal carbon and energy source (*i.e.* glucose and citrate in Davis and Mingioli's medium). The medium is usually made with agar and poured in plates. The organism is inoculated lightly in a streak or by plating out. After a suitable period of incubation the plate is examined and the appearance of bacterial growth indicates that the bacterium has been able to utilise the test compound.

Growth is often slower on a defined medium than on the ordinary peptone-containing media and observations should be continued for up to 7 days during incubation at 37° C. Usually growth is well-developed at 2 days.

The inoculum for these tests should not be heavy and should not be made from a broth culture in case so large an amount of nutritive organic matter is carried over with the inoculum into the test medium as to support a visible amount of growth. Preferably the bacterium is first grown for 18–24 hr. on an agar slope. A small amount of this growth is suspended in sterile saline solution to give a suspension of about $1–5 \times 10^8$ bacteria per ml. and a small loopful of the suspension is used to inoculate the defined medium.

Bacteria that fail to grow on the simple defined medium when glucose and citrate are present as sources of carbon and energy generally do so because they require as additional nutrients one or more specific amino acids or vitamins; they are described as *auxotrophic*. Growth tests made on further defined media supplemented with single amino acids or vitamins, or different combinations of these, will enable the particular nutritional requirements of an auxotroph to be determined.

Citrate Utilisation Test

This is a test for the ability of an organism to utilise citrate as the sole carbon and energy source for growth and an ammonium salt as the sole source of nitrogen. Koser's liquid citrate medium or Simmons' citrate agar may be used.

Koser's Medium (modified)

Sodium chloride, NaCl	5·0 g.
Magnesium sulphate, $MgSO_4$	0·2 g.
Ammonium dihydrogen phosphate, $NH_4H_2PO_4$.	1·0 g.
Potassium dihydrogen phosphate, KH_2PO_4 . .	1·0 g.

Sodium citrate, $Na_3C_6H_5O_7 . 2H_2O$ . . . 5·0 g.
Distilled water . . . . 1 l.

The pH should be 6·8. The medium is sterilised by autoclaving at 121° C. for 15 min.

Simmons' Medium

Simmons' citrate medium is a modification of Koser's medium with agar and an indicator added. To each litre of Koser's medium is added 20 g. washed agar and 40 ml. of a 1 in 500 aqueous solution of bromothymol blue (see p. 817).

The medium is sterilised by autoclaving and is poured as slopes.

Method.—Inoculate from a saline suspension of the organism to be tested. Incubate for 96 hr. at 37° C.

The results are read as follows:

(1) Koser's citrate medium:

Positive = Turbidity, *i.e.* growth.
Negative = No turbidity.

A positive test should be subcultured into a second tube to eliminate false positives due to an excessive initial inoculum.

(2) Simmons' citrate medium:

Positive = Blue colour and streak of growth.
Negative = Original green colour and no growth.

Nitrate Reduction Test

This is a test for the presence of the enzyme nitrate reductase which causes the reduction of nitrate, in the presence of a suitable electron donor, to nitrite which can be tested for by an appropriate colourimetric reagent. Almost all enterobacteriaceae reduce nitrate.

Medium

Potassium nitrate, KNO_3 (nitrite-free) . . 0·2 g.
Peptone . . . . 5·0 g.
Distilled water . . . . 1 l.

Tube in 5 ml. amounts and autoclave at 121° C. for 15 min.

Method.—Inoculate and incubate for 96 hr.

Test reagent

Solution A. Dissolve 8·0 g. of sulphanilic acid in 1 l. of 5 *N* acetic acid.

Solution B. Dissolve 5·0 g. of α-naphthylamine[1] in 1 l. of 5 *N* acetic acid.

Immediately before use, mix equal volumes of solutions A and B to give the test reagent.

Add 0·1 ml. of the test reagent to the test culture. A red colour developing within a few min. indicates the presence of nitrite and hence the ability of the organism to reduce nitrate.

[1] Care must be taken to avoid inhaling α-naphthylamine powder when making up this solution.

Gluconate Test

This is a test for the ability of an organism to oxidise gluconates to the 2 keto-gluconate which subsequently accumulates in the medium (see Shaw & Clarke, 1955; Carpenter, 1961). The basis of the test is the change from gluconate, a non-reducing compound when tested with a suitable reagent, to 2 keto-gluconate, which is a reducing compound when so tested.

Medium

Peptone	1·5 g.
Yeastrel (Yeast extract)	1·0 g.
Dipotassium hydrogen phosphate, K_2HPO_4	1·0 g.
Potassium gluconate	40·0 g.
Distilled water	1 l.

The pH, after solution, should be 7·0. Distribute in 10 ml. quantities in screw-capped bottles and autoclave at 121° C. for 15 min.

Method.—Add 1 ml. of the medium aseptically into a clean, sterile tube. Inoculate and incubate at 37° C. for 48 hr. Then add 1 ml. of Benedict's reagent for reducing sugars and place the tube in a boiling water bath for 10 min. Alternatively add one "Clinitest reagent" tablet (Ames Co., Nuffield House, London, W. 1), in which case heating is unnecessary. Observe for the production of a coloured precipitate of cuprous oxide.

Positive result = green to orange precipitate.
Negative result = the blue colour of the reagent is unchanged.

Malonate Utilisation Test

This tests the ability of an organism to utilise sodium malonate.

Medium

Yeast extract	1 g.
Ammonium sulphate, $(NH_4)_2SO_4$	2 g.
Dipotassium hydrogen phosphate, K_2HPO_4	0·6 g.
Potassium dihydrogen phosphate, KH_2PO_4	0·4 g.
Sodium chloride, NaCl	2·0 g.
Sodium malonate	3·0 g.
Bromothymol blue	0·025 g.
Distilled water	1 l.

Adjust the pH to 7·4 if necessary. Sterilise by autoclaving at 121° C. for 15 min.

Method.—Inoculate from a young agar slope culture and incubate at 37° C. for 48 hr. Positive results are indicated by a change in colour of the indicator from green to blue due to the rise in pH consequent upon the utilisation of sodium malonate.

Combined Malonate Utilisation and Phenylalanine Deaminase Test

This combines the two tests already described (see Shaw & Clarke, 1955).

Medium

Ammonium sulphate, $(NH_4)_2SO_4$	2·0 g.
Dipotassium hydrogen phosphate, K_2HPO_4	0·6 g.
Potassium dihydrogen phosphate, KH_2PO_4	0·4 g.
Sodium chloride, NaCl	2·0 g.
Sodium malonate	3·0 g.
DL-phenylalanine	2·0 g.
Yeast Extract	1·0 g.
Distilled water	1 l.

Steam for 5 min. and filter through paper. Add 5 ml. of a 0·5 per cent. solution of bromothymol blue in absolute ethanol. Distribute in 10 ml. quantities and autoclave at 121° C. for 15 min.

Method.—Distribute aseptically in 1 ml. volumes in small sterile tubes. Inoculate, incubate overnight, and read results as follows:

(1) Malonate utilisation test.

Observe colour of medium.

Blue = positive.
Green = negative.

(2) Phenylalanine deaminase test.

Having recorded the result of the malonate test, acidify with a few drops of 0.1 *N* HCl until the colour of the medium becomes yellow. Add a few drops of a 10 per cent. aqueous solution of ferric chloride, shake and observe colour.

Dark green = positive.
Yellow-buff = negative.

Potassium Cyanide Test

This tests the ability of an organism to grow in the presence of cyanide.

Medium (Møller)

Peptone	3 g.
Sodium chloride, NaCl	5 g.
Potassium dihydrogen phosphate, KH_2PO_4	0·23 g.
Disodium hydrogen phosphate, $Na_2HPO_4 . 2H_2O$	5·64 g.
Distilled water	1 l.

Adjust to pH 7·6 if necessary. Sterilise by autoclaving at 121° C. for 15 min. and then refrigerate until totally chilled. To the cold medium add 15 ml. of a 0·5 per cent. solution of potassium cyanide, KCN (0·5 g. KCN dissolved in 100 ml. of sterile distilled water). Distribute in 1 ml.

amounts in sterile bijou bottles, seal tightly without delay and store at 4° C. The medium will keep for 4 weeks under these conditions.

Method.—Inoculate from a 24-hr. nutrient broth culture and incubate at 37° C. with the cap tightly screwed down to prevent air exchange. Observe after 24 hr. and 48 hr. for a positive result, *i.e.* turbidity produced by growth.

Niacin Test

This test is used in the differentiation of the mycobacteria. Tubercle bacilli of human type produce niacin (nicotinic acid) and this is detected using cyanogen bromide and aniline.

Reagents

Cyanogen Bromide.—A 10 per cent. aqueous solution is used. Cyanogen bromide liberates toxic fumes and should be stored in a dark-coloured well-stoppered bottle in the refrigerator. The solution should be prepared in a fume cupboard and stored in a refrigerator. It is made up once a fortnight.

Aniline.—A 4 per cent. (v/v) solution in 96 per cent. ethanol is used. The aniline should be redistilled if coloured. The solution can be stored in the refrigerator for at least a month.

Method.—Cultures of mycobacteria should be grown on slopes of a colourless medium, *e.g.* the oleic acid–albumin agar medium of Dubos and Middlebrook (1947) incubated at 37° C. At intervals up to 10 weeks a slope is removed from the incubator and to it is added 1 ml. of the cyanogen bromide solution, followed after five min. by 1 ml. of the aniline solution. The development of a yellow colour in the test fluid is regarded as positive. The yellow pigment of certain chromogenic strains does not diffuse from the colonies and so can be distinguished from a positive test. After the test has been read, a few ml. of 10 per cent. ammonia solution are added to the bottles to destroy the residual cyanogen bromide before submitting the cultures for sterilisation.

Detection of Motility by Cultivation in Semi-Solid Nutrient Agar

In semi-solid agar media, motile bacteria "swarm" and give a diffuse spreading growth that is easily recognised by the naked eye. Motility may thus be detected more easily than by the microscopical "hanging drop" method.

The exact optimal concentration of agar depends on the particular brand used and must be determined by trial; usually it is about 0·4 per cent. of Japanese agar or 0·2 per cent. of New Zealand agar. This is dissolved in nutrient broth or peptone water. It is important that the final medium should be quite clear and transparent. Dispense 10-ml. amounts in test tubes and leave to set in the vertical position. Inoculate with a straight wire making a single stab down the centre of the tube to about half the depth of the medium. Incubate under the conditions favouring motility. Examine at intervals, *e.g.* after 6 hr. and 1, 2 and 6 days when incubating at 37° C.

Non-motile bacteria generally give growths that are confined to the stab-line, have sharply defined margins and leave the surrounding medium clearly transparent. Motile bacteria typically give diffuse, hazy growths that spread throughout the medium rendering it slightly opaque. The outgrowth may reach the walls of the tube after a few hours and the foot of the tube after one or two days. It is best observed by contrast while there is still some transparent medium not yet invaded. With a non-motile strain that yields motile variants, a discrete line of growth is formed along the stab and diffuse outgrowths then fan out from one or two points. Sharply defined finger-like outgrowths may be given by some kinds of poorly motile bacteria, and also by some kinds of non-motile bacteria, apparently by their "falling" through clefts in the medium; these doubtful cases may be resolved by use of the "hanging drop" method.

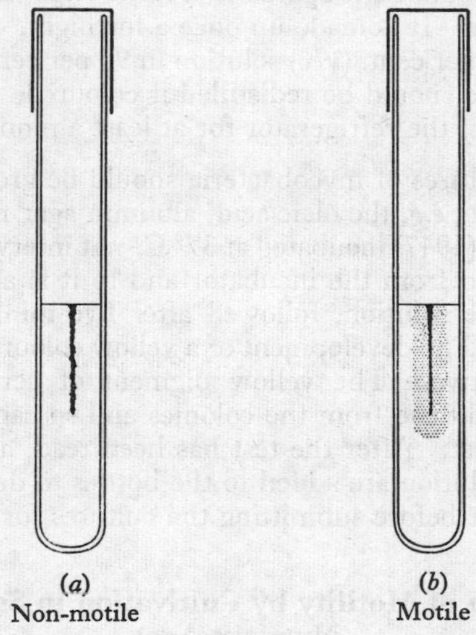

FIG. 64

Diagram showing growth of a non-motile organism (*a*) restricted to the stab line in semi-solid nutrient agar. The diffuse growth, or "swarm", of a motile organism (*b*) extends as a zone of turbidity from the stab line.

Composite Media for Preliminary Identification of Enterobacteria

The following modification of Kohn's method (Gillies, 1956) is a reliable substitute for the conventional method described on p. 243 to determine the biochemical identity of non-lactose-fermenting colonies prior to confirmation by serological typing.

Method

Composite medium I

Beef extract	2 g.
Proteose peptone No. 3 (Difco)	15 g.
Yeast extract	2 g.
Glucose	1 g.
Mannitol	10 g.
Agar	16 g.
Indicator mixture	26·5 ml.
Distilled water	1 l.

Adjust pH to 7·2

After autoclaving at 115° C. for 15 min. and cooling to 60° C., 50 ml. of a 20 per cent. urea solution sterilised by filtration are added and the medium is distributed aseptically in sterile test-tubes to a depth of 6·5 cm. and allowed to solidify in a sloped position so as to provide a butt of 2·5 cm.

Indicator mixture. Three separate 0·2 per cent. indicator solutions are made up.

Indicator	*grams*	*ml.* 0·05 *N* NaOH	*Add ml. water*
Bromothymol blue	0·20	6·4	100
Cresol red	0·20	10·6	100
Thymol blue	0·20	8·6	100

The final indicator is obtained by mixing the individual solutions in the following proportions:

Bromothymol blue	12·5 ml.
Cresol red	4 ml.
Thymol blue	10 ml.

Composite medium II

Agar	3 g.
Bacto-peptone (Difco)	10 g.
Tryptone (Difco)	10 g.
Sodium chloride, NaCl	5 g.
Disodium hydrogen phosphate, Na_2HPO_4, $12H_2O$	0·25 g.
Sucrose	10 g.
Salicin	10 g.
Bromothymol blue	0·01 g.
Sodium thiosulphate, $Na_2S_2O_3$, $5H_2O$	0·025 g.
Distilled water	1 l.

Adjust pH to 7·4

The medium is distributed into test-tubes in 8 ml. amounts, autoclaved at 121° C. for 15 min. and allowed to set with the tubes in the vertical position.

Lead acetate papers. Strips (5 mm. × 50 mm.) of filter paper are impregnated with saturated lead acetate solution and dried in an oven at 70° C. *Indole test papers* are similarly impregnated with the following solution:

p-dimethyl-aminobenzaldehyde	5 g.
Methanol	50 ml.
o-phosphoric acid	10 ml.

and are dried at 70° C. for a minimum period.

The two media are inoculated with a long straight wire charged from colonies of the organism to be identified; medium I is inoculated by both smearing the slant and then stabbing to the base of the butt; medium II is then inoculated by a single stab into its upper ½ inch; finally, the two test papers are suspended above the latter medium and held by the cotton-wool stopper.

Identifying Patterns of Organisms by the Composite Media
(18 hr. incubation at 37° C.)

Organism	Fermentation of		Urease production	Fermentation of Sucrose/Salicin	Motility	Production of H_2S	Formation of Indole
	Glucose	Mannitol					
S. typhi	⊥	⊥	−	−	+	+	−
Other salmonellae	+	⊥	−	−	+	V	−
Sh. sonnei	⊥	⊥	−	−	−	−	−
Sh. flexnerii	⊥	⊥	−	−	−	−	+
Sh. schmitzi	⊥	−	−	−	−	−	+
Proteus group	(−)	(−)	+	V	+	V	V

Key to table: Fermentation tests + = acid and gas produced.
⊥ = acid only for glucose; acid for mannitol (gas production not observable).
− = no reaction.
V = variable.
Other tests + = positive.
− = negative.
V = variable.
(−) = apparent negative reaction.

Results

In medium I the fermentation of glucose is indicated by the butt changing from deep green to yellow and that of mannitol by the development of a yellow slant. Urease production produces a deep blue colour throughout the medium. Gas production appears in varying degrees from a slight splitting along the wire track to disruption of the medium. In medium II, fermentation of sucrose or salicin or both changes the medium from light blue to yellow and accompanying gas production causes bubbles to form. Non-motile organisms grow only along the line of inoculation, whereas motile species show either a diffuse even growth spreading from the inoculum or more rarely localised outgrowths which are usually fan-shaped or occasionally nodular. H_2S production causes blackening of the lead acetate paper and the formation of indole gives a red colour in the yellow test paper.

Tests for Lecithinase

Certain bacteria produce enzymes (lecithinases or phospholipases) that split lipoprotein complexes in human serum and hen egg-yolk and produce opalescence or turbidity when grown in media containing these substrates. When the reaction is produced with egg-yolk it is sometimes referred to as the lecithovitellin reaction.

Tube Test

Medium.—Mix equal parts of a digest broth and sterile human serum (from clotted blood). Egg-yolk suspension, 10 per cent. v/v in physiological saline, is recommended in place of the serum. A sterile egg-yolk broth is obtainable commercially (Oxoid, Southwark Bridge Road, London, S.E.1).

Method.—Aliquots of the substrate medium are dispensed aseptically in sterile cotton-wool stoppered tubes. One tube is inoculated with a drop of fluid culture or a colony picked from a plate culture. One tube is left uninoculated as a negative control. A positive control may be inoculated with a known lecithinase-producing organism, and a further control may include the test organism and antitoxin to the specific lecithinase, e.g. *Cl. welchii* alpha antitoxin if *Cl. welchii* is the test organism (p. 314). Note that in some cases the enzyme is dependent upon divalent cations and may be inhibited by sequestering agents or buffers containing calcium-binding salts.

The tubes are incubated under conditions suitable for growth of the species involved and examined for turbidity daily up to five days. A positive reaction usually develops within 24–48 hr. and is indicated by the development of pronounced turbidity with a yellowish curd on the surface of the culture substrate mixture, the effect being absent from the negative control and antitoxin tube. A modification of this method may be used for testing culture filtrates or centrifuged supernates for lecithinase activity using an incubation time of 1 hr. These tests are more easily read after storage overnight at 4° C. when sufficient time has elapsed for the curd to rise to the surface of the mixture in a positive test.

Plate Test

Medium.—Egg-yolk agar is prepared by separating hen egg-yolks from the whites aseptically and mixing the yolks with an equal volume of sterile physiological saline. The mixture is then added, in the proportion of 5–10 per cent. (v/v), to sterile molten digest agar base at 55° C. and plates are poured immediately after mixing. (A sterile concentrated egg-yolk emulsion may be obtained from the Oxoid division of Oxo Ltd.)

Method.—Lecithinase-producing colonies grown on this medium are surrounded by wide zones of opalescence which are readily apparent through being much more opaque than the only slightly opaque egg-yolk agar (see also p. 759 and p. 314 for combined media and technique of antitoxin neutralisation). It should be noted that lipolytic organisms also produce opalescence in some lecithin-containing media, including egg-yolk agar (Willis, 1960). The opalescence is weaker than that due to lecithinase and the zones of opalescence are smaller, being more or less confined to the medium under the colonies.

Tests for Lipase

Culture on Tributyrin Agar

Medium

Peptone	5 g.
Yeast extract	3 g.
Tributyrin (glycerol tributyrate)	10 g.
Agar	20 g.
Water	1000 ml.

The medium is prepared so that the tributyrin forms a stable emulsion in the nutrient agar and the pH is adjusted to 7·5. For exacting organisms the medium may be enriched by addition of 5 per cent. of Fildes' extract of red cells before plates are poured (Willis, 1960).

Method.—Inoculate and incubate plates under appropriate conditions. Examine by transmitted light. Colonies of lipolytic organisms are surrounded by wide zones of clearing. The natural opacity of the medium is due to the presence of the micro-droplets of tributyrin and lipolytic organisms convert these into water-soluble butyric acid, so removing the opacity.

Culture on Egg-yolk Agar

Medium.—This may be as described above under Tests for Lecithinase or it may be the medium enriched with Fildes' extract described by Willis (1960). It is poured in plates immediately after the egg-yolk has been added and mixed in.

Method.—Inoculate and incubate under appropriate conditions and examine by reflected light. Lipolysis is indicated by the formation of a thin, iridescent "pearly layer" overlying the colonies and a "confined" opalescence in the medium underlying them (seen best when the colonies are scraped off).

Next flood the plate with a saturated aqueous solution of copper sulphate, stand for 20 min., drain off the excess solution and dry the plate in the incubator for a short while. When the plate is now examined, the pearly layer and the opalescence in the medium are both stained bright greenish-blue, indicating that they consist of free fatty acids that have been liberated by hydrolysis of the fats in the egg-yolk.

Test for Hyaluronidase

Hyaluronidase catalyses the hydrolysis of hyaluronic acid; it attacks the intercellular cement substance in tissues and acts as a "spreading factor". Hyaluronidase activity in bacterial culture filtrates can be demonstrated by a modification of the ACRA test (Burnet, 1948). A solution containing hyaluronic acid derived from synovial fluid is mixed with congo red. When a drop of this mixture falls into acid alcohol it produces a characteristic appearance. Progressive reduction of the amount of hyaluronic acid in the mixture, either by prior dilution or by snzymatic activity, leads to progressive changes in the pattern produced when a drop falls into acid alcohol. For an account of the procedure and details of factors influencing the test, the paper by Oakley and Warrack (1951) should be consulted.

Tests for Deoxyribonuclease

The enzyme deoxyribonuclease attacks DNA present in the nuclei of leucocytes and influences their subsequent affinity for Romanowsky stains such as Jenner's. The enzyme also digests DNA present in tissues, *e.g.* horse spleen, and reduces the viscosity of solutions of semi-purified DNA extracts. The nucleic acid is precipitated by alcohol as a fibrous mass before but not after enzymatic decomposition. There are three tests for deoxyribonuclease activity and they are based on the above observations.

Slide Test (Warrack, Bidwell & Oakley, 1951)

Substrate.—Rabbits are bled into 1·6 per cent. sodium oxalate, the leucocytes concentrated by centrifugation and resuspended in oxalated rabbit plasma, and trial films made. The concentration of leucocytes is adjusted to give 15–20 per $\frac{1}{12}$ in. objective field. Films are made in a standard manner on slides 7·5 × 1·2 cm., dried in the air and fixed in methanol.

Test.—The deoxyribonuclease activity of a culture filtrate is demonstrated as follows: A numbered slide bearing a fixed film is gently placed in each of a series of 4-ml. volume doubling dilutions of the culture filtrate so that half of each film is submerged. After incubation in this position at 37° C. for 18 hr., along with appropriate control tests, the slides are removed, rinsed with distilled water and stained with Jenner's stain. Each film is then examined microscopically, using the oil-immersion objective, and the half of each slide that was not immersed acts as a control for the number of intact leucocytes per field and for the efficiency of staining.

If the concentration of deoxyribonuclease is high, no stained leucocytes may be seen in the treated film. The first stage of action is reduction in nuclear staining of lymphocytes, progressing to production of unstained ("ghost") nuclei which are sharply demarcated from the surrounding faintly stained cytoplasm. Polymorphs are next affected and finally eosinophils are attacked.

OTHER TESTS FOR DEOXYRIBONUCLEASE.—A modification of the ACRA test of Burnet (1948) devised by Oakley and Warrack (1951), and the alcohol precipitation test (McCarty, 1949), may also be used to assess deoxyribonuclease activity.

Tests for Direct Bacterial Haemagglutinin

Adhesiveness for animal cells is commonly indicated by a tendency of certain bacteria to adhere to and bind together red blood cells and thus cause "direct bacterial haemagglutination". The bacterial haemagglutinin may be a fixed part of the bacterial surface (see *fimbriae*, p. 24) and this type of haemagglutinin is accordingly described as "non-diffusible". A few bacterial species produce a soluble or "diffusible haemagglutinin" which diffuses into the surrounding medium and, though reacting with red cells, cannot bind the bacteria to these or to other substrates.

TILE TEST FOR FIMBRIAL HAEMAGGLUTININ.—Red cells separated from fresh citrated guinea-pig blood are washed twice in physiological saline and made up to a 3 per cent. (v/v) suspension in fresh saline. A nutrient broth culture of the test organism is centrifuged to deposit the bacilli. After removal of the culture supernatant, the bacillary deposit is resuspended in the small amount of fluid remaining. A drop of the dense bacillary deposit is mixed with an equal drop of the red cell suspension in a depression on a white tile at 3–5° C., and the tile is then rocked gently for 5 min. while it is warming to room temperature. In the case of most fimbriate organisms tests made at room temperature (15–20° C.) without chilling the tile are entirely satisfactory. A few organisms, however, give haemagglutination at 3–5° C. but not at higher temperatures.

The haemagglutination produced by fimbriate organisms is seen with the naked eye and usually develops as a coarse clumping within a few seconds. Weakly active cultures produce a fine granularity within 2–3 min. Very poorly haemagglutinating cultures may show positive reactions only if mixing is continued for up to 30 min.

Inhibition of Fimbrial Haemagglutination with Mannose.—The incorporation of a small drop of a 2 per cent. solution of D-mannose in the haemagglutination mixture (final mannose concentration 0·5 per cent.) specifically inhibits fimbrial haemagglutination (see Duguid & Gillies, 1957).

TUBE TEST FOR SOLUBLE HAEMAGGLUTININ.—To doubling dilutions of the test culture supernatant in physiological saline (0·5 ml. volumes), 0·5 ml. aliquots of a 1 per cent. (v/v) red cell suspension in saline are added. The tubes are shaken and allowed to stand at room temperature for 1–2 hr. The red cells settle into a characteristic pattern at the foot of each tube and this is conveniently viewed in a mirror. In the absence of haemagglutinin, the red cells form a dense central button. In the presence of soluble haemagglutinin, the red cells fall in a reticulum and this covers the base of the tube. The patterns are very similar to those described by Salk (1944) for myxovirus haemagglutination.

REFERENCES

BARER, GWENDOLINE (1946). The rapid detection of gelatin-liquefying organisms. *Mth. Bull. Minist. Hlth. Lab. Serv.*, **5**, 28.

BITTER, L., WEIGMANN, F. & HABS, H. (1926). Bestimmung der gebildeten Säuremenge zur unterscheidung verwandter Baklerien Rhamnosereaktion zur Differenzierung von Paratyphus B and Brestaubakterien. *Münsch. med. Wschr.*, **73**, 940.

BURNET, F. M. (1948). The mucinase of *V. cholerae. Austr. J. exp. biol. med. Sci.*, **26**, 71.

CARPENTER, K. PATRICIA (1961). The relationship of the Enterobacterium A 12 (Sachs) to *Shigella boydii* 14. *J. gen. Microbiol.*, **26**, 535.

COWAN, S. T. & STEEL, K. J. (1961). Diagnostic tables for the common medical bacteria. *J. Hyg., Camb.*, **59**, 357.

DUBOS, R. J. & MIDDLEBROOK, G. (1947). Media for tubercle bacilli. *Amer. Rev. Tuberculosis*, **56**, 334.

DUGUID, J. P. & GILLIES, R. R. (1957). Fimbriae and adhesive properties in dysentery bacilli. *J. Path. Bact.*, **74**, 397.

GILLIES, R. R. (1956). An evaluation of two composite media for preliminary identification of shigella and salmonella. *J. clin. Path.*, **9**, 368.

HUGH, R. & LEIFSON, E. (1953). The taxonomic significance of fermentative versus oxidative metabolism of carbohydrates by various Gram negative bacteria. *J. Bact.*, **66**, 24.

KALLINGS, L. O. & LAURELL, ANNA-BRITA (1957). Relation between phage types and fermentation types of *Salmonella typhimurium. Acta. path. microbial. scand.*, **40**, 328.

KAUFFMANN, F. (1954). *Enterobacteriaceae*, 2nd edition. Copenhagen: Munksgaard.

KOHN, J. (1953). A preliminary report of a new gelatin liquefaction method. *J. clin. Path.*, **6**, 249.

LAUTROP, H. (1956). Observations on gelatin-liquefying strains of the Salmonella group. *Acta. path. microbiol. Scand.*, **39**, 370.

MCCARTY, M. (1949). The inhibition of streptococcal desoxyribonuclease by rabbit and human antisera. *J. exp. Med.*, **90**, 543.

MØLLER, V. (1955). Simplified tests for some amino acid decarboxylases and for the arginine dihydrolase system. *Acta path. microbiol. scand.*, **36**, 158.

OAKLEY, C. L. & WARRACK, G. HARRIET (1951). The ACRA test as a means of estimating hyaluronidase, deoxyribonuclease and their antibodies. *J. Path. Bact.*, **63**, 45.

REPORT (1958). Recommended methods for group differentiation with the enterobacteriaceae. *Int. Bull. Bact. Nomen. Tax.*, **8**, 53.

SALK, J. E. (1944). A simplified procedure for titrating hemagglutinating capacity of influenza-virus and the corresponding antibody. *J. Immunol.*, **49**, 87.

SHAW, CONSTANCE & CLARKE, PATRICIA H. (1955). Biochemical classification of *Proteus* and Providence cultures. *J. gen. Microbiol.*, **13**, 155.

STEEL, K. J. (1961). The oxidase reaction as a taxonomic tool. *J. gen. Microbiol.*, **25**, 297.

STERN, W. (1916). Studien zur Differenzierung der Bakterien der Coli-Typhus Gruppe mittels gefärbter flüssiger Nährölien. Beitrage zur Biologie des Bakterien gruppe Paratyphus-B. enteritidis. *Cbl. Bakt.*, (1), **78**, 481.

WARRACK, G. HARRIET, BIDWELL, ETHEL & OAKLEY, C. L. (1951). The beta-toxin (deoxyribonuclease) of *Cl. septicum. J. Path. Bact.*, **63**, 293.

WILLIS, A. T. (1960). The lipolytic activity of some clostridia. *J. Path. Bact.*, **80**, 79.

WILLIS, A. T. & HOBBS, G. (1959). Some new media for the isolation and identification of clostridia. *J. Path. Bact.*, **77**, 511.

CHAPTER 50

PHYSICAL AND CHEMICAL METHODS: I

pH BUFFERS, OXIDATION-REDUCTION POTENTIALS, STANDARD SOLUTIONS, THE PREPARATION OF GLASSWARE

pH IN MICROBIOLOGY

MICROORGANISMS, in common with other living organisms, are very susceptible to changes in the acidity or alkalinity of the surrounding medium. This is true with regard to both growth and survival. Whilst many bacteria show vigorous growth within a fairly wide range of acidity or alkalinity, there are others that require the "reaction" of the medium to be adjusted within narrow limits before multiplication takes place. Moreover, all microorganisms have a particular "reaction" at which growth is optimal. In order, therefore, to secure the best growth, particularly of highly parasitic organisms, it is necessary that the adjustment of the "reaction" should be made as accurately as possible. For this purpose, it is necessary to become familiar with the factors determining this "reaction", with the mode of its expression and with the methods used for its estimation.

The Meaning of the pH Scale

Pure water is very slightly dissociated into an equal number of hydrogen ions and hydroxyl ions.

$$H_2O \rightleftharpoons H^+ + OH^-.$$

According to the law of mass action, the following formula will hold at equilibrium (the square brackets refer to the molar concentrations):

$$K = \frac{[H^+]\,[OH^-]}{[H_2O]}.$$

But the amount of water ionised will be extremely small, so that the concentration of unionised water, $[H_2O]$, is virtually constant. Therefore, at equilibrium, the product of the concentration of hydrogen ions and hydroxyl ions will be a constant, which is termed the ion product of water K_w, *i.e.*

$$K_w = [H^+]\,[OH^-].$$

From conductivity measurements, it has been found that the concentration of hydrogen ions and hydroxyl ions in pure water at 22° C. is 10^{-7} gram ions per litre. Therefore K_w at 22° C. will be $1{\cdot}0 \times 10^{-14}$. At a given temperature and in dilute aqueous solutions, the product of the molar concentrations of hydrogen ions and hydroxyl ions will always be the same, *no matter what other substances are present.*

Consider what happens when an acid is added to water. The acid will dissociate, liberating hydrogen ions, the amount of which depends on the amount of acid added and on the degree of dissociation of the acid. A strong acid will be largely dissociated in dilute solutions while a weak acid will be largely undissociated, *e.g.*

$$HCl \rightleftharpoons H^+ + Cl^-$$
$$CH_3COOH \rightleftharpoons H^+ + CH_3COO^-.$$

As a result of the liberation of hydrogen ions caused by dissociation of the acid, the number of hydroxyl ions must be decreased in order to maintain the ion product of water at a constant value. Similarly, when an alkali is dissolved in water, it also undergoes dissociation and ionisation with the liberation of hydroxyl ions, the amount of these being proportional to the amount of alkali and its degree of ionisation, *e.g.*

$$NaOH \rightleftharpoons Na^+ + OH^-$$
$$NH_4OH \rightleftharpoons NH_4^+ + OH^-.$$

As a result of the liberation of hydroxyl ions, there must be a corresponding decrease in the number of hydrogen ions to keep the ionic product of water constant. It will be seen, therefore, that in spite of the fact that a solution may be alkaline, its reaction can still be expressed in terms of the hydrogen ions present, the stronger the alkali the smaller the concentration of hydrogen ions. A solution is *neutral* if $[H^+] = 10^{-7}$, a solution is *acid* if $[H^+]$ is greater than 10^{-7} and is *alkaline* if $[H^+]$ is less than 10^{-7}. Since $[H^+]$ can be measured with considerable accuracy, it is convenient to express acidity and alkalinity in terms of $[H^+]$. For reasons of practical convenience, $[H^+]$ is usually expressed as a logarithmic or pH scale.

The pH value of a liquid is defined as the logarithm of the reciprocal of the hydrogen-ion concentration, *i.e*

$$pH = \log \frac{1}{[H^+]}.$$

For neutral water, $pH = \log \frac{1}{10^{-7}} = 7.$

Two points should be borne in mind about the pH scale.

(1) Since it is a *logarithmic* scale, a change in one unit of pH is equivalent to a tenfold change in hydrogen-ion concentration, that is a tenfold change in acidity; thus a liquid of pH 5 is ten times more acid than one at pH 6, while a liquid of pH 9 is ten times more alkaline than one of pH 8.

(2) Since it is a *reciprocal* scale, the lower the pH, the greater will be the acidity. A pH value of less than 7 indicates an acid solution[1], and greater than 7 indicates an alkaline solution.

[1] 1 *N* HCl has an approximate pH value of 0,
0·1 *N* HCl has an approximate pH value of 1.
0·01 *N* HCl has an approximate pH value of 2.

IMPORTANCE OF pH MEASUREMENTS IN MICROBIOLOGY

Microorganisms are sensitive in varying degrees to the pH of the external environment. Although this is important for survival, it is even more important for growth, where there is an optimum, a maximum and a minimum pH. Media should be adjusted as far as possible to the pH optimal for the growth of the organism concerned. Most pathogenic bacteria have a fairly restricted pH range and grow best around pH 7·5, that is, at a slightly alkaline reaction. This may be a reflection of the fact that the pH of mammalian blood and tissues is of this order. For example, the pneumococcus has an optimum pH of 7·8, and a growth range between pH 7·3–8·3. On the other hand, commensal and saprophytic bacteria have a wider pH growth range. *Escherichia coli* has an optimum pH of 6·5, and a growth range between pH 4·4–7·8. Yeasts and fungi generally have an acid optimum and may grow at a pH of 2·0 or even lower. Not only should growth media be adjusted to the optimum pH, but all suspending fluids should be at a reaction giving the largest survival time (usually of the same order as the optimum pH).

METHODS USED IN pH MEASUREMENT

Two types of methods are generally employed for the measurement of pH in the laboratory. These depend either upon the use of pH indicator dyes or upon the use of electric pH meters.

Methods depending upon the use of pH indicator dyes

Indicator dyes are substances that will change in colour with variations in the pH of the solution in which they are dissolved. For example, phenol sulphone-phthalein (phenol red) is yellow in acid solution and red in alkaline solution. If alkali be gradually added to an acid solution containing phenol red, the change in colour will commence at pH 6·8, the yellow becoming redder until the final red is reached at pH 8·4; thus the "range" of the indicator is pH 6·8–8·4. Within this range, phenol red will have different colours for different pHs and this can be used to determine pH. The range of phenol red is particularly suitable for the adjustment of the pH of bacterial culture media. It must be emphasised that outside the range at which the colour is changing, an indicator can show only whether the solution is more acid or more alkaline than the indicator range. For example, phenol red is yellow at all pHs below 6·8 and is red at all pHs above 8·4. However, other dyes have their own different ranges in which colour change occurs, and there is now available a series of indicators which will cover the range from pH 1 to 11. The following are examples:

Indicator	*Range of pH*	*Colour change*
Thymol blue (acid range) .	1·2–2·8	red to yellow.
Bromophenol blue . .	2·8–4·6	yellow to violet.
Bromocresol green . .	3·6–5·2	yellow to blue.
Methyl red . . .	4·4–6·2	red to yellow
Litmus	4·5–8·3	red to blue.
Bromocresol purple . .	5·2–6·8	yellow to violet.
Bromothymol blue . .	6·0–7·6	yellow to blue.
Neutral red . . .	6·8–8·0	red to yellow.
Phenol red . . .	6·8–8·4	yellow to purple-pink.
Cresol red . . .	7·2–8·8	yellow to violet-red.
Thymol blue (alkaline range)	8·0–9·6	yellow to blue.
Phenolphthalein . .	8·3–10·0	colourless to red.
Thymolphthalein . .	9·3–10·5	colourless to blue.
B.D.H. "Universal" . .	3·0–11·0	red—orange—yellow —green—blue— reddish violet.

The simplest method of determining the pH of a solution is to use commercially available pH indicator papers. These papers are impregnated with an indicator that gives a change of colour over a specific or general range of pH. The paper can simply be dipped in the solution to be tested or, alternatively, a drop of the solution can be withdrawn by a wire loop or Pasteur pipette and placed on the paper. The resulting colour is compared with the chart supplied with the papers. One example of a good wide-range indicator is the "Universal Indicator" contained in test-papers supplied by Messrs. Johnson & Sons, Hendon, London, N.W.4. It must be emphasised, however, that these test-papers will only give, at the best, an approximate idea of the pH and the results should always be checked by a more accurate method.

The Comparator Method

The most convincing instrument of this type is the Lovibond Comparator (obtainable from British Drug Houses, Ltd.).

The comparator normally consists of a bakelite case with two holes at the top for tubes of standard bore and of colourless glass. Tube A contains water if the untreated "unknown" solution is colourless, but some of the untreated "unknown" if it is coloured. The hinged door of the case holds a rotatable disk containing a series of standard coloured glasses corresponding to various pH values and each glass can be brought in front of tube A in turn and viewed through aperture A.

It is possible to obtain disks for various indicators and the appropriate one can be inserted in the comparator. A solution of the indicator is added to tube B, which contains the unknown solution, and the disk is rotated until a match is obtained. The pH is then read in the aperture at the bottom of the apparatus. If the "unknown" is in the middle of the range of the indicator selected, it is possible to obtain a value accurate to within 0·1–0·2 pH units.

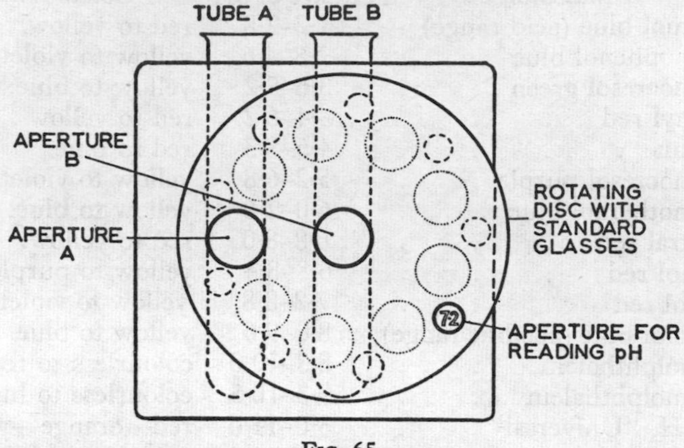

FIG. 65

Adjustment of pH of Nutrient Media

One of the commonest uses for a comparator in a bacteriological laboratory is in the adjustment of the pH of standard culture media. As an example, the adjustment of nutrient broth to pH 7·5 using phenol red will be considered. For this purpose, the following are required in addition to the Lovibond comparator with a phenol red disk.

(1) A solution of phenol red, 0·01 per cent.,[1] in distilled water.

(2) 0·05 *N* NaOH made up as follows:

500 ml. 0·1 *N* NaOH
91 ml. 0·01 per cent. phenol red
distilled water to 1 litre.

The indicator is incorporated into the standard alkali solution, so that when the medium is titrated, the actual concentration of the dye always remains constant.

(3) A burette, preferably a microburette, measuring to 0·01 ml.

To tube A is added 5 ml. nutrient broth and to tube B 5 ml. nutrient broth + 0·5 ml. of 0·01 per cent. phenol red solution. The 0·05 *N* NaOH solution is run into tube B until the tint produced is midway between the standard glasses of pH 7·4 and 7·6. The average of the two readings is taken and this gives the amount of 0·05 *N* NaOH required to bring 5 ml. of broth to the correct pH. From this, one can calculate the amount of 1 *N* NaOH required to bring the total amount of broth to the correct pH.

When media adjusted in this way by the addition of alkali are sterilised, it is common to obtain a precipitate of phosphates so that the

[1] First prepare a stock 0·02 per cent. solution as follows. Weigh out 0·1 g. phenol red, add to this 10 ml. (accurately) of 0·1 *N* NaOH and 20 ml. of distilled water. Dissolve by gentle heat. Transfer the contents to a 500 ml. volumetric flask, washing out all the indicator into the flask. Now add accurately 10 ml. 0·1 *N* HCl, and fill up to the mark. The 0·01 per cent. solution of phenol red is made by diluting the stock solution with an equal part of distilled water.

medium has to be filtered again before use. It may be preferable, therefore, when making media in bulk to have the reaction slightly alkaline and to adjust it for use by the addition of acid. The medium is first adjusted to a pH of about 8·0 with NaOH and steamed for thirty minutes. The precipitated phosphates are filtered off. The medium is then adjusted back to pH 7·5, using acid. The titration is carried out in exactly the same way as described previously except that, instead of NaOH solution, 0·05 *N* HCl containing phenol red is employed, and the calculated amount of normal hydrochloric acid is added per litre to obtain the desired reaction.

The standardisation of a solid medium such as nutrient agar presents greater difficulty than in the case of fluid media. The medium may be titrated when liquid, but the exact determination is not easy to obtain with any degree of accuracy. It has been found that agar of good quality has very little effect on the reaction of the broth to which it is added, but the reaction of the finished agar should be controlled by titrating the melted medium and then comparing the colour *when cold*. We have found the following method satisfactory. Mix together 0·5 ml. of the melted agar, 4·5 ml. of hot (neutral) distilled water and 0·5 ml. of 0·01 per cent. phenol red solution; cool and compare with the standard tubes. Gelatin may conveniently be adjusted if the medium is liquefied and kept at about 37° C.

The Capillator Method

A knowledge of the pH of bacterial cultures and of the pH changes which they undergo is often of importance and is sometimes of practical value (*e.g.* in the differentiation of *Streptococcus agalactiae* from *Streptococcus pyogenes*). When only small quantities of culture are available, one of the best methods of pH determination is the use of the capillator. The "B.D.H. Capillator Outfit"[1] is available with indicators and cards to cover the range from pH 1·2–11·0. Alternatively, separate sets can be obtained for each indicator.

The technique is as follows. The pH is first approximately determined by the use of a universal indicator. This can be done in two ways.

(1) A small quantity of the microbial culture is withdrawn with a sterile Pasteur pipette and transferred to a white tile and an equal amount of indicator added. From the resulting colour of the mixture, the approximate pH can be obtained by comparison with the standard set of colours supplied with the indicator. The tile is appropriately sterilised after use with 3 per cent. v/v lysol solution.

(2) A universal pH test-paper can be used (see previously). After use the test-paper is destroyed by burning or is placed in disinfectant solution.

The pH is then determined more accurately, using a capillator and choosing an indicator that acts over the desired range. The capillator consists of a series of standard-sized capillary tubes filled with buffer

[1] For full details see catalogue, British Drug Houses, Ltd.

solutions and indicator. These tubes show the colours corresponding to different pH values over the whole range of the indicator, and the pH value corresponding to each colour is marked on the card. The capillator set is used as follows.

(*a*) A capillary tube, identical in diameter with those in the capillator, is fitted with a rubber teat and is used for withdrawing a tube full of indicator (supplied with the caplator set and of double the concentration occurring in the standard tubes). The indicator is then pipetted on to the small watch-glass provided.

(*b*) After washing, the same "pipette" is used to withdraw an equal volume of the microbial culture or unknown solution which is pipetted on to the same watch glass. If the culture is to remain uncontaminated, a sterile capillator pipette must be used.

(*c*) The two fluids are mixed on the watch-glass by sucking in and out of the pipette, and finally the tube is filled with the mixture.

(*d*) The prepared tube is compared in colour with the standards and the pH value thus obtained.

Errors due to the colour of the culture or fluid itself can be corrected by using a compensation cell. Care should be taken when working with pathogenic cultures, and the used capillary tubes should be dropped into lysol solution.

The pH Meter

The methods described above, although simple and requiring relatively cheap apparatus, are generally not accurate. They are also very laborious if large numbers of estimations have to be carried out. Further, they all assume that the colour of an indicator is influenced only by the pH of the solution. This is not always so, since the dissociation of an indicator can be influenced by substances such as salts, ethanol and proteins in solution. These errors may be quite appreciable, although in the choice of indicators listed previously those with large errors have been discarded. The only accurate method of measuring pH is by using a pH meter, and in laboratories where numerous routine determinations of pH are required, this apparatus is a necessary piece of laboratory equipment. It is easy and quick to use although care must be taken in its maintenance.

A pH meter consists of an electrode pair which is sensitive to hydrogen-ion concentration and an electrical circuit which measures the e.m.f. developed across the electrode pair. Almost all modern pH meters employ a glass electrode as it is easy to use and maintain, together with a calomel electrode as a standard. Only a brief description of the instrument and basic directions for its use can be given here. More detailed descriptions of theory can be found in appropriate textbooks and instructions are provided in the makers' pamphlets.

The e.m.f. developed between the glass electrode and the calomel electrode will depend upon the concentration of hydrogen ions and, hence, the pH. In order to measure this e.m.f., no current must flow in the electrode pair or the resultant chemical reactions at the cell boundaries will result in a "polarisation" of the electrodes so that the observed e.m.f. will be due to a combination of phenomena. For this reason, a high impedance circuit is used to detect the potential developed and a vacuum tube is used to drive the measuring meter. This meter can be a microammeter in a vacuum tube circuit as in most line-operated meters, or a null-type bridge circuit may be used as with battery-operated meters.

The following precautions should be observed in the use and maintenance of a pH meter to avoid damaging the instrument and to get an accurate pH value.

(1) Always exercise extreme care in handling the electrodes, particularly the glass electrodes which usually have a very thin glass bulb. Do not allow this glass bulb to touch the beaker in which the measurements are taking place, or any other hard surface.

(2) Before a series of pH measurements, ensure that the calomel electrode is filled with a solution of saturated KCl.

(3) Make sure the instrument has been given sufficient time to warm up as specified by the manufacturers.

(4) Make frequent standardisation of the meter against a standard buffer solution of known pH as near as possible to the pH to be measured.

(5) Between measurements, wash the electrodes with a stream of distilled water using a wash bottle.

(6) When a "drift" in the reading occurs, give the electrodes time to reach equilibrium. Gently stirring the solution often hastens equilibrium.

(7) Never remove the electrodes from the solution when the measuring circuit is closed.

(8) When the instrument is not in use, keep the electrodes immersed in water.

BUFFERS AND THEIR USES

Not only is it important to have the suspending fluids for microorganisms within a certain pH range, it is also important to keep the pH within the same range. Most microorganisms produce acids or alkalis as a result of their metabolic activities and these must be prevented from altering the pH of the environment too radically. For example, bacteria when grown on a medium containing a sugar generally produce acid intermediates or end-products (*e.g.* formic, acetic, propionic, butyric, or lactic acids). This is particularly true of fermentation under relatively anaerobic conditions. If these acidic products were allowed to accumulate in an unbuffered medium, the organism would soon be killed by the low pH produced.

It is, therefore, preferable and often essential to include buffers in culture media and in suspending fluids. These buffers tend to resist changes in hydrogen-ion concentration. They are usually formed by mixing a weak acid with its salt, although a weak alkali and its salt can also be used. Buffering action is due to the fact that a weak acid is only weakly dissociated while its salt with an alkali metal is strongly dissociated. Thus, whereas 0·1 *N* acetic acid is only 1·35 per cent. dissociated, 0·1 *N* sodium acetate is 97 per cent. dissociated. If hydrogen ions are added to such a buffer solution, they will react with the high concentration of salt anions to form unionised acids. This weak acid, once formed, does not tend to ionise appreciably and, at the same time, its ionisation is opposed by the high concentration of anions present. Therefore hydrogen ions have been added, but have been removed leaving the pH of the solution only slightly altered.

Generally speaking, the buffering power of a mixture of a weak acid and its salt is greatest when the two are present in equimolar proportions. From such mixtures, buffers can be prepared covering a range of about 1 pH unit on each side of the pH given by an equivalent mixture (the pK of a buffer). Outside this range, the buffering capacity falls off very rapidly. Although the concentration of the buffer determines its ability to resist changes in hydrogen-ion concentration, the actual pH given by a certain mixture is only slightly affected by dilution.

Buffers suitable for use with biological material should have a pK around the optimal for this material and ideally they should also be non-toxic and non-physiological, *i.e.* not react with or affect the living organism or the component of the living organism to be studied. In practice, however, most buffers with useful pKs around 7 are physiologically active, and allowance must be made for this.

The following is a list of suitable buffer systems for use in microbiology. It should also be noted that some components of the complex organic growth media commonly used in microbiology are also buffers. This is particularly true of amino acids and peptides which, as well as providing nutrients, act as important buffers.

PREPARATION OF BUFFERS

(1) Citrate Buffer

Stock Solutions

A: 0·1 *M* solution of citric acid (19·21 g. in 1000 ml.).

B: 0·1 *M* solution of sodium citrate (29·41 g. $C_6H_5O_7Na_3.2H_2O$ in 1000 ml.).

x ml. of *A*+*y* ml. of *B*, diluted to a total of 100 ml.

x	*y*	pH
46·5	3·5	3·0
43·7	6·3	3·2
40·0	10·0	3·4
37·0	13·0	3·6
35·0	15·0	3·8
33·0	17·0	4·0
31·5	18·5	4·2
28·0	22·0	4·4
25·5	24·5	4·6
23·0	27·0	4·8

20·5	29·5	5·0
18·0	32·0	5·2
16·0	34·0	5·4
13·7	36·3	5·6
11·8	38·2	5·8
9·5	40·5	6·0
7·2	42·8	6·2

(2) **Acetate Buffer**

Stock Solutions

A: 0·2 *M* solution of acetic acid (11·55 ml. in 1000 ml.).

B: 0·2 *M* solution of sodium acetate (16·4 g. of $C_2H_3O_2Na$ or 27·2 g. of $C_2H_3O_2Na.3H_2O$ in 1000 ml.).

x ml. of *A*+*y* ml. of *B*, diluted to a total of 100 ml.

x	*y*	pH
46·3	3·7	3·6
44·0	6·0	3·8
41·0	9·0	4·0
36·8	13·2	4·2
30·5	19·5	4·4
25·5	24·5	4·6
20·0	30·0	4·8
14·8	35·2	5·0
10·5	39·5	5·2
8·8	41·2	5·4
4·8	45·2	5·6

(3) **Citrate-Phosphate Buffer**

Stock Solutions

A: 0·1 *M* solution of citric acid (19·21 g. in 1000 ml.).

B: 0·2 *M* solution of dibasic sodium phosphate (28·39 g. of Na_2HPO_4 or 71·7 g. of $Na_2HPO_4.12H_2O$ in 1000 ml.).

x ml. of *A*+*y* ml. of *B*, diluted to a total of 100 ml.

x	*y*	pH
44·6	5·4	2·6
42·2	7·8	2·8
39·8	10·2	3·0
37·7	12·3	3·2
35·9	14·1	3·4
33·9	16·1	3·6
32·3	17·7	3·8
30·7	19·3	4·0
29·4	20·6	4·2
27·8	22·2	4·4
26·7	23·3	4·6
25·2	24·8	4·8

x	*y*	pH
24·3	25·7	5·0
23·3	26·7	5·2
22·2	27·8	5·4
21·0	29·0	5·6
19·7	30·3	5·8
17·9	32·1	6·0
16·9	33·1	6·2
15·4	34·6	6·4
13·6	36·4	6·6
11·4	38·6	6·8
9·1	40·9	7·0
6·4	43·6	7·2

(4) **Phosphate Buffer**

Stock Solutions

A: 0·2 *M* solution of monobasic sodium phosphate (31·2 g. NaH_2PO_4, 2 H_2O in 1000 ml.).

B: 0·2 *M* solution of dibasic sodium phosphate (28·39 g. of Na_2HPO_4 or 71·7 g. of $Na_2HPO_4.12H_2O$ in 1000 ml.).

x ml. of *A*+*y* ml. of *B*, diluted to a total of 200 ml.

x	*y*	pH
92·0	8·0	5·8
87·7	12·3	6·0
81·5	18·5	6·2
73·5	26·5	6·4
62·5	37·5	6·6
51·0	49·0	6·8
39·0	61·0	7·0
28·0	72·0	7·2
19·0	81·0	7·4
13·0	87·0	7·6
8·5	91·5	7·8
5·3	94·7	8·0

(5) **Barbitone (Veronal) Buffer**

Stock Solutions

A: 0·2 *M* solution of sodium barbitone (sodium diethyl barbiturate).

B: 0·2 *M* HCl.

50 ml. of *A*+*x* ml. of *B*, diluted to a total of 200 ml.

x	pH
1·5	9·2
2·5	9·0
4·0	8·8
6·0	8·6
9·0	8·4

12·7	8·2
17·5	8·0
22·5	7·8
27·5	7·6
32·5	7·4
39·0	7·2
43·0	7·0
45·0	6·8

Solutions more concentrated than 0·05 *M* may crystallise on standing, especially in the cold.

(6) **Tris (hydroxymethyl) aminomethane HCl (Tris HCl) Buffer**

Stock Solutions

A: 0·2 *M* solution of tris (hydroxymethyl) aminomethane (24·2 g. in 1000 ml.).

B: 0·2 *M* HCl.

50 ml. of $A + x$ ml. of *B*, diluted to a total of 200 ml.

x	pH
5·0	9·0
8·1	8·8
12·2	8·6
16·5	8·4
21·9	8·2
26·8	8·0
32·5	7·8
38·4	7·6
41·4	7·4
44·2	7·2

(7) **Boric Acid-Borax Buffer**

Stock Solutions

A: 0·2 *M* solution of boric acid (12·4 g. in 1000 ml.).

B: 0·05 *M* solution of borax (19·05 g. in 1000 ml.; 0·2 *M* in terms of sodium borate).

50 ml. of $A + x$ ml. of *B*, diluted to a total of 200 ml.

x	pH
2·0	7·6
3·1	7·8
4·9	8·0
7·3	8·2
11·5	8·4
17·5	8·6
30·0	8·8
59·0	9·0
115·0	9·2

(8) **Bicarbonate—CO_2 Buffer**

The pH of these buffers is markedly dependent on temperature. The following examples are for a temperature of 37° C.

	Concentration of CO_2 in gaseous phase		
	5%	10%	20%
Concentration of $NaHCO_3$ — 0·02 *M*	7·4	7·1	6·8
Concentration of $NaHCO_3$ — 0·05 *M*	7·8	7·5	7·2

(9) **Carbonate-Bicarbonate Buffer**

Stock Solutions

A: 0·2 *M* solution of anhydrous sodium carbonate (21·2 g. in 1000 ml.).

B: 0·2 *M* solution of sodium bicarbonate (16·8 g. in 1000 ml.).

x ml. of *A* + *y* ml. of *B*, diluted to a total of 200.

x	*y*	pH
4·0	46·0	9·2
9·5	40·5	9·4
16·0	34·0	9·6
22·0	28·0	9·8
27·5	22·5	10·0
33·0	17·0	10·2
38·5	11·5	10·4
42·5	7·5	10·6

Note.—These buffers are all made up to a final concentration of 0·1 *M* (with the exception of the bicarbonate-CO_2 buffers). The pH will not change appreciably on dilution. It should be noted, however, that there will be variation in the ionic strengths of the different buffers and of the same buffer at different pHs. If isotonic solutions are required, the concentration should be adjusted accordingly. All the buffers are given as a mixture of the sodium salts with the acid. Potassium salts may also be used.

OXIDATION-REDUCTION (REDOX) POTENTIALS

It has been stated previously that the oxidation-reduction conditions in a medium are very important in the growth of certain bacteria. Strict aerobes are able to grow only in presence of dissolved oxygen while strict anaerobes require reducing conditions and hence absence of dissolved oxygen. This may be related to the metabolic character of the organism, a strict aerobe obtaining its energy and intermediates only through oxidation involving oxygen as the ultimate hydrogen acceptor, a strict anaerobe utilising hydrogen acceptors other than oxygen while a facultative anaerobe can act in both ways. However, strict anaerobes may be actually poisoned by the presence of oxygen, possibly due to the production of toxic hydrogen peroxide which cannot be removed by catalase, or possibly due to the oxidation of certain essential groupings in the organism, *e.g.* the sulphydryl groups of proteins.

We may consider oxidising agents as substances capable of taking up electrons and reducing agents as substances able to part with electrons. It is therefore possible to determine the intensity level of oxidising or reducing conditions in a system by the net readiness of all the components in that system to take up, or part with, electrons. This ability is usually expressed as the oxidation-reduction (redox) potential of the system.

Redox potentials can be best measured by virtue of the fact that when an "unattackable" electrode is immersed in a solution, an electrical potential difference is set up between the electrode and the solution, and the magnitude of this potential depends on the state of oxidation or reduction of the solution. This electrode potential (or, more shortly E_h) can be measured in millivolts, and the more oxidised a system, the higher (or more positive) is the potential; in more reduced systems the potential is lower (or more negative). By measuring the electrode potential it is possible to determine and follow the reducing conditions in cultures at different periods and to grade different systems in order according to their state of oxidation or reduction. This measurement can usually be carried out by coupling up a potentiometer with an electrode pair of platinum electrode (the "unattackable" electrode) and a standard calomel electrode. The redox potential can then be measured by the millivolt scale provided on most commercial pH meters. It should be borne in mind that the redox potential of a system indicates the oxidation-reduction *intensity* of the system itself, and not its *capacity* to oxidise or reduce some other component or system. Further, it must be emphasised that for a microorganism, not only is the redox potential of the system important, but the factors contributing to this redox potential may be equally critical. Thus a substance capable of giving up or taking in electrons may not necessarily affect a microorganism unless it can spatially reach certain essential components of the cell. Further, a substance, like oxygen, which can actually be metabolised by the catalytic action of enzymes in the cell, may be important through this metabolism as well as through its direct contribution to the redox potential.

Although the redox potential of a bacterial culture may be measured accurately by electrical methods, an approximate idea of the state of reduction may sometimes be obtained by adding various special dyes (oxidation-reduction indicators) and observing by the colour changes how much they are reduced. Such changes are in intensity of colour, not changes from one colour to another, as is the case with the indicators used for the measurement of pH. It is found that the state of oxidation or reduction of any particular dye depends on the electrode potential, so that at any given pH value, if we know the electrode potential of the solution, we can calculate the degree of reduction of the dye. Conversely, and this is more important practically, if the percentage reduction of the dye has been observed colorimetrically the corresponding electrode potential can be determined. Different dyes are reduced over different ranges of potential; for instance, methylene blue at pH 7 is 95 per cent. in the oxidised condition at $E_h + 50$ mv., and 99 per cent. reduced at $E_h - 50$ mv., whilst neutral red is still 87 per cent. oxidised at -300 mv., and 87 per cent. reduced at -350 mv. Theoretically it should be possible by suitable choice of indicators to measure any range of E_h, but in practice experimental difficulties arise due to poising (this corresponds to the buffering effect in pH estimation), catalytic effects and the toxicity of the dyes used towards bacteria, etc. Colorimetric E_h determinations do not reach the degree of accuracy and convenience attained in the case of pH indicators.

A few examples will suffice to illustrate the results obtained when the electrode potential of growing bacterial cultures are measured. In a culture of *C. diphtheriae* the initial E_h of the medium, about $+300$ mv., falls gradually and reaches -200 mv. after some forty-eight hours' incubation, and the potential remains at this low level for some considerable time. With haemolytic streptococci, on the other hand, the potential falls from $+300$ mv. to -150 mv. in twelve hours, but then rises fairly rapidly, probably owing to the formation of hydrogen peroxide. In a dextrose broth culture of *Esch. coli*, in which gas formation occurs, the potential falls extremely rapidly, reaching -370 mv. after about one hour's incubation. The behaviour of staphylococci is roughly similar to that of *C. diphtheriae*, whilst pneumococci behave similarly to haemolytic streptococci. Strict anaerobes are unable to proliferate in ordinary aerobic culture media unless the E_h is lowered to some extent. This lowering of the E_h, or establishment of reducing conditions, may be effected in a variety of ways, such as removal of oxygen in an anaerobic jar or by means of a pyrogallol seal, or reduction may be effected by adding a reducing agent, *e.g.* thioglycollate.

Oxidation-reduction potentials and oxidation-reduction indicators are employed in the testing of sewage and sewage effluents, in cheese-making, in the keeping qualities of beer, etc. The metabolic activities of bacteria and other cells and tissues and the functioning of enzymes are followed by observing the reduction of methylene blue in Thunberg tubes. A commonly used application of this technique is in the grading of milk and testing the hygienic quality of milk samples. The milk samples are incubated under standard conditions with methylene blue, and the time of reduction is noted. Heavily contaminated milks show a rapid decolourisation, whilst with good quality milk there is a long lag period and reduction is slow (*vide* p. 981).

For full details of this important subject consult *Oxidation-Reduction Potentials in Bacteriology and Biochemistry*, by L. F. Hewitt, 6th edition, 1950 (E. & S. Livingstone Ltd., Edinburgh).

WATER

Tap water contains many impurities and is unsuitable for the preparation of defined culture media, for chemical solutions and for many other uses in the laboratory. These impurities can be largely removed by distillation or demineralisation.

Distilled Water

Normally distilled water is prepared in a commercial metal-lined still which will deliver it at the rate of ½-50 gallons per hour, depending on size. However, for some purposes this water is insufficiently pure, and it may be necessary to use an all-glass distillation apparatus which should be fitted with an efficient spray trap. It is often advisable to add a knife point of potassium permanganate and a few pellets of sodium hydroxide to the tap water before commencing distillation in order to oxidise steam volatile organic compounds which might otherwise be carried over into the distillate. For some experimental methods such as tissue culture it may be necessary to repeat the distillation in a glass still to give doubly glass distilled water.

It is useful to check the purity of distilled water at times by simple conductivity testers. Satisfactory distilled water should have a conductivity no greater than that given by 1·5 p.p.m. of NaCl, and preferably below 1·0 p.p.m.

Demineralised Water

Ion-exchange resins may be used to demineralise water. A simple apparatus consists of an anion and a cation exchanger in two columns of glass tubing about 2 m. tall and 3 cm. in diameter. A variety of resins are available for the purpose, *e.g.* Amberlite IR 120 (H) as the cation-exchange resin followed by Amberlite IRA 400 (OH) as the anion-exchange resin.[1] Tap water or distilled water is passed over each of the resins in turn. The columns must be periodically regenerated by rinsing with 10 per cent. aqueous HCl for the cation-exchanger and 10 per cent. aqueous NaOH for the anion-exchanger. After regeneration, the columns are rinsed with distilled water until the final product has a neutral reaction. Commercial demineralisers are available,[2] which have the advantage of being transportable and of requiring no external source of heat or electricity. Demineralised water should be equivalent to double glass-distilled water and should have a very low conductivity. However, it may carry dissolved organic compounds derived from the resins.

FLUIDS FOR CELL SUSPENSION AND DILUTION

A variety of fluids are used for the suspension of microorganisms, blood cells or tissue culture cells. These fluids should preserve, as far as possible, the cells in their original condition. The following points should be noted.

[1] Obtainable from British Drug Houses, Ltd.

[2] *E.g.* the "Portable Deminrolits" produced by the Permutit Co. Ltd., Gunnersbury Avenue, London, W.4.

(1) They should have an osmotic pressure nearly isotonic with the cell to be suspended. This is particularly true of mammalian cells (*e.g.* red blood corpuscles) where lysis readily occurs in non-isotonic media. Microorganisms are generally more resistant to changes in the external osmotic pressure, but suspension in water or very dilute salt solutions may cause loss of viability.

(2) Suspension fluids should preferably contain a buffer to keep the cells at their optimum pH.

(3) Certain ions may be necessary for the optimal maintenance of cells, particularly with mammalian cells. Moreover, they may be required for certain in-vitro reactions, *e.g.* agglutination, complement fixation, etc. In some cases a source of energy such as glucose may be required.

(4) Other additions may be made for specific purposes.

The following suspension and diluent fluids are commonly used. In all cases analytical grade reagents (when available) should be made up in distilled or demineralised water.

Physiological Saline

A solution of 0·85 per cent. NaCl in water. This solution is sometimes called normal saline, a term which should be discarded because of its chemical connotation. It is also often referred to as "saline". The solution has an osmotic pressure roughly equivalent to that of mammalian blood serum and can therefore be used for the suspension of blood cells as well as most microorganisms. However, the solution has no buffer present and it is recommended that phosphate-buffered saline be used as a general suspension fluid in the laboratory.

Buffered Salines

As stated previously, it is preferable to have a buffer present in a suspending fluid or diluent and a variety of solutions containing basically NaCl but with a buffer added have been proposed. They should all have a final osmotic pressure roughly equivalent to that of physiological saline. A series of solutions can be prepared by diluting standard buffer solutions of the required pH (see pp. 852-856) with physiological saline to a strength of 0·01 *M*. If a greater buffering power is required, the concentration of buffer must be increased and of saline decreased.

The following types of buffered saline are recommended for various purposes:

(a) *Phosphate buffered saline:*

NaCl	8·00 g./l.
K_2HPO_4	1·21 g./l.
KH_2PO_4	0·34 g./l.

This solution gives a pH of about 7·3 and also provides potassium and phosphate ions. It is a very useful general diluent and suspending fluid.

(b) *Azide saline.*—Sodium azide at a concentration of 0·08 per cent. is added to physiological saline or buffered saline. The azide acts as a preservative preventing microbial decomposition and is often used for the dilution of serum, etc.

(c) *Borate-calcium saline:*

NaCl	8·0	g./l.
$CaCl_2$	1·0	g./l.
H_3BO_3	1·2	g./l.
$Na_2B_4O_7.10H_2O$	0·052	g./l.

This solution gives a pH of about 7·3 and is used for haemagglutination experiments where calcium is required and phosphate should be absent.

(d) *Veronal-NaCl diluent:*

NaCl	8·5	g./l.
Barbitone (diethyl-barbituric acid)	0·575	g./l.
Sodium barbitone	0·20	g./l.
$MgCl_2.6H_2O$	0·168	g./l.
$CaCl_2$	0·028	g./l.

A stock solution concentrated ×5 is made up by dissolving 5·75 g. barbitone in 500 ml. hot distilled water. Add 85 g. NaCl and make up the volume to about 1400 ml. Dissolve 2·0 g. sodium barbitone in 500ml. distilled water and add it to the NaCl-barbitone solution. Make up to 2000 ml. Add 1·68 g. $MgCl_2.6H_2O$ and 0·28 g. $CaCl_2$. For use dilute 1 in 5 with distilled water.

This saline may be used for complement-fixation tests and gives more reproducible results than physiological saline. If glass tubes are used to contain the reaction mixtures, there may be some absorption of complement on to the glass surfaces. To reduce this absorption, add 0·1 per cent. inactivated rabbit serum, 0·1 per cent. gelatin or 0·1 per cent. bovine serum albumin.

Complex Suspending Media

More complex media are required for the suspension and dilution of microorganisms and other cells where optimum viability must be maintained. For example, in viable counts of many bacteria, physiological saline may be to some extent bactericidal and must be replaced by solutions containing other ions as well as a buffer. For these fluids, prepare the following solutions which are all isotonic with mammalian serum and can be mixed in any proportions. The mixtures, although of different composition, will remain isotonic.

To simplify preparation and handling, the first five solutions can be made up in concentrations five times those listed. They are stable for months when stored in the cold.

The Krebs-Ringer solutions seem to be the most generally useful for the suspension of mammalian cells and are also valuable for many bacteria. It is also possible to use Davis's minimal medium for bacterial suspension (see p. 741). If growth is to be avoided, leave out the nitrogen source (ammonium sulphate) or the carbon and energy sources (glucose and citric acid).

Suspending media for tissue culture work are described on p. 1029.

				Krebs-Ringer		
	g./l.	Ringer	Locke	Plain	Bicarbonate[2]	Phosphate
NaCl	9·0	100	100	100	100	100
KCl	11·5	4	4	4	4	4
$CaCl_2$	12·2	3	3	3	3	3
KH_2PO_4	21·1	—	—	1	1	—
$MgSO_4.7H_2O$ . . .	38·2	—	—	1	1	1
$NaHCO_3$	13·0	—	3	—	21	—
0·1 *M* phosphate buffer[1] pH 7·4		—	—	—	—	20

[1] 17·8 g. $Na_2HPO_4.2H_2O$ + 20 ml. 1 *N* HCl diluted to 1 l.
[2] The solution should be gassed with 5 per cent. v/v. CO_2 in O_2, air or N_2.

PREPARATION AND CLEANSING OF GLASSWARE

New Glassware

New glassware requires special attention because of the resistant spores which may be present in the straw and other packing material and also because it tends to give off free alkali which may be sufficient to interfere with the growth of certain organisms. Consequently it should be placed in 1 per cent. HCl overnight, washed in tap water and distilled water and autoclaved.

Screw-capped bottles (described later) are subjected to a special cleansing process by the makers whereby surface alkali is removed, and the above treatment is unnecessary. The bottles may be used without further treatment, as received from the manufacturers.

Cleansing of Glassware for General Laboratory Use

Glass containers with discarded cultures can be placed in 3 per cent. lysol after use or transferred directly to boiling soap solutions. Containers with tubercle bacilli or spore-bearing organisms such as *B. anthracis*, *B. subtilis* or *Cl. tetani* must be autoclaved. The discarded cultures and their containers are then boiled for one hour in a 5 per cent. solution of a good quality soft soap in either tap water (if it is sufficiently soft) or distilled or demineralised water (if the tap water is hard). The glassware is cleansed with a test-tube brush (or other suitable brush) and well rinsed in hot and cold water. Again, if the tap water is hard and contains a considerable amount of calcium salts, rinsing in distilled or demineralised water is necessary. The glassware is then allowed to drain and is dried in a hot-air oven or cabinet.

Washing of Tissue Culture Tubes

Since tissue cells are particularly sensitive to minute traces of toxic substances, meticulous care is essential in cleaning glassware for tissue cultures and it is preferable to use hard glass (*e.g.* Pyrex) tubes, flasks and containers. The following cleaning method has been found satisfactory.

(1) Autoclave with rubber bungs *in situ* after use.

(2) Remove bungs and rinse tubes in hot running tap water.

(3) Boil for twenty minutes in demineralised water in a boiler with soapflakes (one handful to about five gallons). Small tubes are boiled in an enamel basin on a gas-ring. (Rinse water from the demineraliser may be used for this purpose.)

(4) Brush the tubes as removed from boiler (preferably with a motor-driven nylon brush). Do this *while the tubes are hot* or serum remains.

(5) Rinse in hot running tap water or in demineralised water if the local water is hard.

(6) Transfer tubes into hot demineralised water containing an inorganic detergent. Thoroughly wash in this by emptying and filling. The following solution can be used:

Sodium hexametaphosphate	40 g.
Sodium metasilicate (technical) . .	360 g.
Demineralised water	1 gallon

Dissolve and allow to stand overnight. Dilute 1 in 100 before use.

(7) Rinse in hot running tap water at least four times.
Rinse three times in demineralised water.

(8) Drain and dry in drying cabinet.

(9) Dry-sterilise at 160° C. for three hours in racks with the tubes either metal-capped or covered with aluminium foil.

Rubber bungs should be treated as follows after autoclaving:

(1) Rinse in hot tap water.

(2) Boil for 20 min. in 20 per cent. $NaHCO_3$.

(3) Rinse in hot tap water.

(4) Boil for 20 min. in 20 per cent. HCl.

(5) Rinse in hot tap water.

(6) Pack in layers separated by lint in tins or glass containers and autoclave.

Cleaning of Glassware for Biochemical Work

(1) Remove any grease with petroleum. Wash with warm tap water.

(2) Place in dichromate-sulphuric acid cleaning solution for 12–24 hr.

(3) Remove, washing by rinsing in hot tap water at least four times and in distilled water twice.

(4) Dry in oven if the glassware is not used for accurate volumetric purposes.

Dichromate-Sulphuric Acid Cleaning Solution

Dissolve 63 grams of sodium (or potassium) dichromate by heating with 35 ml. water. Cool and add concentrated H_2SO_4 to 1 litre. Technical grade reagents may be used.

This fluid should be handled with care. Preferably rubber gloves and an apron should be worn. If clothes or skin are splashed with the fluid, they should be immediately washed in water, and any residual acid neutralised with sodium carbonate solution. This, in time, is washed off with water.

Cleaning of Pipettes

(1) If contaminated with infective material, discard the used pipette into a 3 per cent. v/v lysol solution and leave until convenient to wash. (The lysol solution is best contained in a rubber cylinder about 15 in. high and 4 in. in diameter. The points of the pipettes are not liable to be broken when dropped to the rubber bottom of the cylinder.)

(2) Rinse in tap water.

(3) If necessary, steep overnight in dichromate-sulphuric acid cleaning fluid.

(4) Wash with tap water in an automatic pipette washer.

(5) Connect the pipette to a water pump by rubber tubing and draw through distilled or demineralised water followed by acetone. Finally, suck through air until the internal surface is quite dry.

(6) If required, the top end of the pipette is plugged with cotton-wool; this is pressed entirely within the end of the pipette so that there are no protruding strands of cotton to prevent close fitting of a rubber teat or mouth-piece tube which may be later attached to operate the pipette.

(7) To sterilise the pipettes, pack them in copper cylinders with slip-on lids or in lengths of wide-bore glass tubing stoppered with cotton-wool. Place in a hot air oven at 160° C. for 60 min.

Note.—Accurately calibrated volumetric glassware should never be heated in an oven, since the expansion and contraction of the glass makes the graduations inaccurate. Such glassware should be kept separate from that intended for sterilisation.

CHAPTER 51

PHYSICAL AND CHEMICAL METHODS: II

CENTRIFUGES, PHOTOELECTRIC COLORIMETERS AND METHODS OF COUNTING BACTERIA, MEASURING BACTERIAL GROWTH AND PREPARING CELL-FREE EXTRACTS

CENTRIFUGES

THE best method for the separation of a microorganism from its suspending fluid is that of centrifugation. This is carried out in the centrifuge, an apparatus for the separation of two substances of different density by centrifugal force.

The rate of settling r (cm./sec.) of spherical particles of density dp and of radius a (cm.) in a medium of viscosity η (c.g.s. units) and of density dm is given by Stokes' law:

$$r=\frac{2a^2\text{G}(dp-dm)}{9\eta},$$

where G is the acceleration due to gravity (981 cm./sec.^{2}).

From this equation, it is evident that the rate of settling of a particle will be increased by the following factors:

(1) An increase in the size of the particle. Thus, larger microorganisms like yeast and fungi will sediment faster than bacteria which, in turn, will sediment faster than viruses. Note that the size of the particles is squared in the equation and thus an increase of the radius of the particles by a factor of 2 will increase the rate of settling by a factor of 4.

(2) An increase in the difference between the density of the particles dp and that of the medium dm. Thus a capsulate bacterium will have a lower average density and be more difficult to sediment than its non-capsulate variant.

(3) A decrease in the viscosity of the medium. For example, when defibrinated blood is being washed (*vide* p. 935), the first sedimentation of the corpuscles from the viscous serum takes much longer than when the corpuscles are suspended in saline.

(4) An increase in the force due to gravity. This force is increased artificially in the centrifuge. The degree by which this force is increased is measured by the relative centrifugal force (RCF) which can be obtained by the following formula:

$$\text{RCF (in G)}=1{\cdot}118\times 10^{-5}\times R\times N^2,$$

where R = the radius of the centrifuge in cm., being the distance from the centre of the centrifuge shaft to the tip of the centrifuge tube: N = revolutions per minute (r.p.m.).

From this equation, it is evident that the speed of the centrifuge, being squared, is very important in determining the rate of sedimentation. Although an increase in the radius of the machine will increase the rate of sedimentation, it is more efficient and simpler practically to increase the speed. However, it is most important to express the efficiency of a centrifuge according to the maximum RCF rather than the speed itself, which, without specification of the radius of the centrifuge, is meaningless. The calculation is simple. Thus, a centrifuge with a radius of 10 cm. and a speed of 4000 r.p.m. has an RCF of $1{\cdot}118 \times 10 \times (4000)^2 \times 10^{-5} = 1788$ G., say 1800 times the force of gravity. Consequently, particles will sediment in this centrifuge at a rate 1800 times faster than in a tube on the bench.

Types of Centrifuges

A variety of centrifuges is now available and the choice of a suitable model depends upon the following factors.

(1) The size of the particles to be sedimented. As shown previously, the smaller the particle, the greater will be the RCF and time required for centrifugation. Machines can be obtained commercially with speeds up to about 60,000 r.p.m. and RCFs of up to about 200,000 G. Generally speaking, yeasts and fungi require a centrifuge with a maximum RCF at least 1000–2000 G., bacteria about 2000–4000 G., and viruses about 50,000–150,000 G. At higher speeds (RCF above about 4000 G.), glass tubes are apt to break even if surrounded by a rubber sleeve or a layer of water. Stainless-steel tubes may be supplied for the most exacting strength requirements, that is for the very highest speeds and centrifugal forces and for maximum resistance to corrosion. However, for most purposes, plastic tubes of cellulose acetate, nylon or polythene can be used. In order to prevent deformation of these tubes under high centrifugal forces, caps should always be used and the tubes should be fully filled. The main disadvantage of plastic tubes in microbiological work is that they cannot be sterilised in a hot-air oven like glass tubes. Even boiling tends to cause deformation and it is recommended that the insides of the tubes and caps be exposed to ultra-violet light for sterilisation.

(2) The volume of material. Centrifuges can be obtained with capacities of up to at least 15 l. The fluid to be centrifuged is contained in tubes or buckets, the number and size of which is subject to a wide variation. For very large amounts of material, continuous-flow machines are available. The fluid to be centrifuged is normally continuously passed along the inside of a rotating tube. The particles sediment very quickly in the thin layer of liquid passing along the sides of the tube and the supernatant passes out of the machine to be collected. Continuous flow centrifuges (*e.g.* Sharples) of this type are common in industry, but are not often used in the laboratory.

(3) The ease with which the particles form a hard pellet at the bottom of the tube. Many centrifuges are of the angle type in which the tubes, instead of being allowed to swing out and rotate in a horizontal plane, are fixed at an angle (from 20°–45°) on the rotating head. The advantage of the angular position is that particulate matter is rapidly separated and concentrated, with consequent saving of time. This is because the particles have to traverse only a short distance before deposition on the sides of the tube, after which they slide to the bottom. The tubes are encased in a metal head, which in its rotation offers slight resistance to air and so obtains greater speed and is less liable to warm up due to friction. A disadvantage is that a "line" of deposited material may remain adherent on the peripheral wall of the tube, and when the suspending fluid is removed it is difficult to avoid contamination caused by turbulence.

(4) The temperature required for centrifugation. In most biological systems it is advantageous and often essential to centrifuge at low temperatures. This prevents metabolism, loss of viability or enzyme activity during

centrifugation. Consequently, refrigeration units are built into many of the larger centrifuges. This is particularly important in high-speed centrifuges where the temperature may rise due to friction unless refrigeration is used. In many machines it is possible to obtain temperatures down to about −15° C.

For a routine bacteriological laboratory, a small bench centrifuge taking 10–20 tubes of capacity 10–30 ml. at a maximum RCF of about 3000 G. is essential. It is, however, convenient to have a centrifuge that will hold the standard 5-in. test-tube and stopper used in routine bacteriological culture, thus avoiding the need for transference to a proper centrifuge tube. For more general and research purposes, larger machines are available, with or without refrigeration and with speeds up to about 6000 G. To centrifuge rickettsias and viruses and for special research purposes, speeds up to about 150,000 G. are required. For such high-speed ultracentrifuges (above about 20,000 r.p.m.), the centrifuging compartment must be held *in vacuo* in order to reduce friction, and vacuum pumps are included.

Method of using the Centrifuge

(1) Tubes must be put in the centrifuge in pairs that have been accurately balanced. The members of a pair of tubes must be placed diametrically opposite each other. If there is an odd number of tubes, a balance tube containing water must be prepared. If the buckets are removable from the centrifuge, they should be balanced with the tubes. With a pipette or plastic washing bottle add a little water to the lighter bucket, not the tube, until the two sides are balanced.

(2) Before putting tubes into the buckets, make sure that the rubber cushions or sleeves are in position at the bottom of the buckets. Otherwise breakages are liable to occur.

(3) Precautions must be taken to ensure that the cotton-wool plugs of culture tubes are not forced down into the tube during centrifugation. In a swing-out head, fold the upper portion of the plug over the mouth of the tube and secure it with a rubber band. With an angle centrifuge, it is sufficient to splay out the top of the plug. However, even when the cotton-wool plug is secured in this way, cotton fibres become detached and can be seen microscopically in the centrifugate. In order to avoid this, aluminium or stainless-steel caps can be used to keep the tubes sterile. Alternatively a screw cap without a washer can be placed over the mouth of the tube, the size being a loose fit. (For ordinary 15 ml. tubes, the M2 screw cap of a ¼-oz. "bijou" bottle is convenient.)

(4) After the tubes have been placed in position, make sure that the metal buckets in a swing-out head are properly seated on the rings and are free to swing.

(5) Close the lid and make sure it is secure. The lid must not be removed when the centrifuge is running. Apart from the danger of an open lid, a decrease in speed due to "winding" will ensue.

(6) Make sure that the rheostat is back to the zero position. (Some centrifuges have an automatic switch-off unless this is so. This prevents strain by inadvertently switching on with the resistance out of circuit.)

(7) Start the motor and *gradually* increase the speed by taking the resistance out by means of the rheostat. Pause at intervals to allow the machine to gather speed until the required r.p.m. are reached. Unless this process is carried out slowly, the life of the centrifuge will be considerably curtailed.

Some machines have a built-in revolution counter, while in others the rheostat must be calibrated by placing a tachometer on the rotating spindle.

(8) When the tubes have been centrifuged sufficiently, switch off the motor and *then* bring the rheostat back to the zero position. Some centrifuges have an automatic timer built in which will switch off after the required time-interval.

(9) Allow the centrifuge to come to a stop. Never slow the rotating head with your hand as brake. This will tend to redisperse the centrifugate due to turbulence and may cause serious injuries. Wait until the machine has stopped before attempting to remove the tubes.

(10) Periodically (*e.g.* once a week or once a fortnight) a centrifuge should be lubricated according to the maker's instructions.

The Washing of Bacteria and Other Cells: "Washed Suspensions"

The cell suspension is centrifuged at a suitable speed and preferably at a low temperature. Microorganisms grown on a solid medium are first suspended in liquid by scraping off the surface of the agar with a curved glass rod into a small volume of a suitable suspending fluid. (This suspension may be contaminated with lumps of agar which can be removed by filtration through cheesecloth.) The pellet of cells at the bottom of the centrifuge tube is resuspended and centrifuged. This washing process is repeated once or more to free the cells from the original suspending medium. The cells are finally made up to the required volume in the required solution.

For metabolic experiments, the cells are washed in a medium similar in composition to the culture medium but with one or more components omitted so that growth does not occur. The "washed suspension" so obtained is particularly suitable for experiments on catabolism; a substrate and buffer are added so that the breakdown of the substrate can be studied uncomplicated by growth processes or by the metabolism of other substrates. However, it must be realised that some activities "decay" rapidly after, or during, the preparation of the washed suspension.

PHOTOELECTRIC COLORIMETER AND SPECTROPHOTOMETER

One of the simplest and most accurate methods of measuring the quantity of a microorganism depends upon a turbidity measurement, just as many of the quantitative micro-methods used in biochemistry depend upon the measurement of the depth of colour in a solution. For such measurements, a photoelectric colorimeter or spectrophotometer is simpler and more accurate than visual comparison. It is also much quicker and free from many personal factors, such as eye fatigue, colour blindness, etc., which are inherent in visual methods.

The theory of the instrument as a colorimeter depends upon the application of Beer's Law, which states that the extent of diminution in light intensity on passing through an absorbing material depends upon the nature and concentration of the absorbing material and upon the length of the light path. This can be expressed as follows:

$$\log \frac{Io}{I} = acl$$

where I is the intensity of the beam after passing through the solution, Io is the incident intensity, a is the extinction coefficient depending upon the particular chromogen, c is the concentration of the chromogen and l is the length of the light path through the solution.

It is possible, therefore, to determine the concentration of a substance by measuring Io/I in a vessel of standard dimensions. In photoelectric colorimeters and spectrophotometers, light intensity is measured by photoelectric response which can be made directly proportional to the quantity of light falling on the photoelectric cell.

Two main types of instrument are available.

(1) Single-cell Apparatus

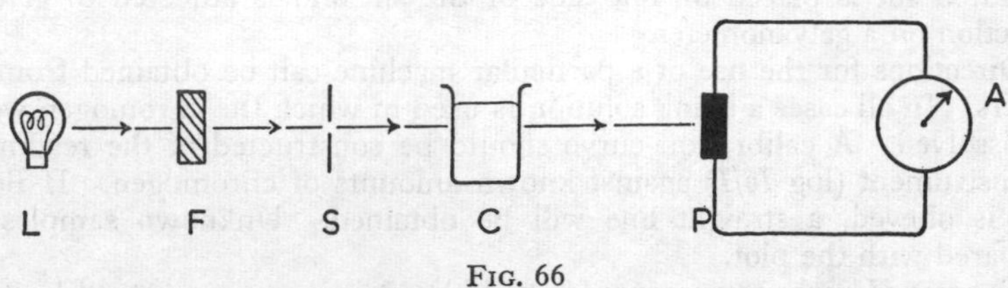

FIG. 66

(2) Twin-cell Apparatus

The following points should be noted:

(1) It is essential that the intensity of the source of light L should remain constant during a reading. A mains supply is subject to sudden changes of voltage and should be used only with a constant-voltage transformer.

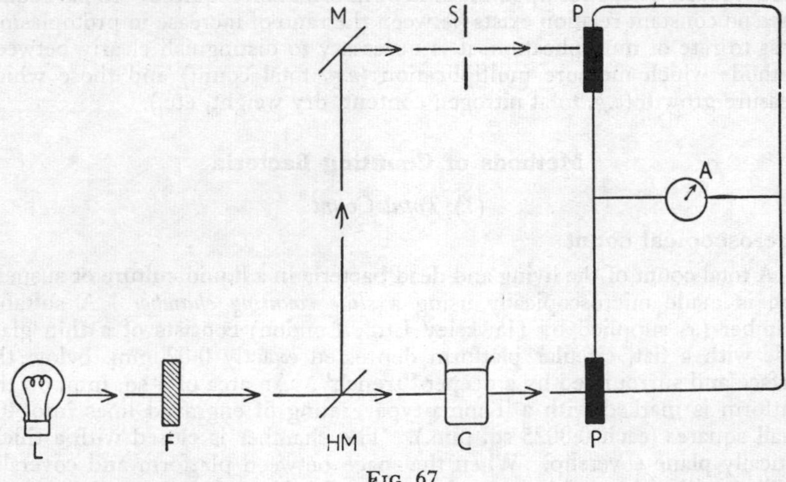

FIG. 67

Alternatively, an accumulator can be used. With a twin-celled instrument, changes in light intensity affect both cells equally and therefore no error is involved. In a single-celled instrument it is necessary to check the reading with the blank solution after each determination.

(2) The colour filter F isolates the part of the spectrum where absorption by the chromogen is greatest. A filter is selected that gives a colour of light complementary to the colour of the chromogen. Thus, if the solution

is blue, a red filter should be used. The narrower the range of wavelength transmitted, the more can interference by other compounds be eliminated. In a spectrophotometer, a prism is built into the machine and selects light of a small wavelength band.

(3) In the twin-celled instrument, a half-silvered mirror *HM* and a mirror *M* are used to split the light into two approximately equal beams.

(4) There is an adjustable slit *S* in the light path.

(5) The cuvette or tube *C* containing the solution should be of standard length of light path.

(6) Light falls on the photoelectric cell or cells *P* and the current generated is measured by a microammeter *A* which is usually calibrated in a log scale permitting direct reading of log Io/I. In some two-celled apparatus, a calibrated slit is placed on one side of the slit and is adjusted to give no deflection on a galvanometer.

Directions for the use of a particular machine can be obtained from the makers. In all cases a blank solution is used in which the chromogen would be dissolved. A calibration curve should be constructed of the reading of the instrument (log Io/I) against known amounts of chromogen. If Beer's Law is obeyed, a straight line will be obtained. Unknown samples are compared with the plot.

The use of such instruments for turbidimetric measurements of bacterial numbers is considered later (pp. 873-5).

COUNTING BACTERIA AND MEASURING BACTERIAL GROWTH

The method used for determining the amount of a micro-organism present in a suspension depends upon the kind of information required. In particular, since no constant relation exists between the ratio of increase in protoplasmic mass to rate of multiplication, it is necessary to distinguish clearly between methods which measure multiplication (*e.g.* total count) and those which measure growth (*e.g.* total nitrogen content, dry weight, etc.).

Methods of Counting Bacteria

(1) *Total Count*

Microscopical count

A total count of the living and dead bacteria in a liquid culture or suspension is made microscopically using a *slide counting chamber*. A suitable chamber (as supplied by Hawksley Ltd., London) consists of a thin glass slide with a flat, circular platform depressed exactly 0·02 mm. below the surface and surrounded by a deeper "trench". An area of 1 sq. mm. on the platform is marked with a Thoma-type grating of engraved lines into 400 small squares (each 0·0025 sq. mm.). The chamber is closed with a thick, optically-plane coverslip. When the space between platform and coverslip is filled with a bacterial suspension, the volume over each small square is $0{\cdot}02 \times 0{\cdot}0025$ c.mm., *i.e.* 0·000,000,05 ml. The average number of bacteria per square is calculated from counts made in sufficient squares (*e.g.* 100) to yield a significant total number of bacteria (*e.g.* 100–1000, preferably over 300). Counts are best made in preparations having between 2 and 10 bacteria per square (*i.e.* 40–200 million per ml.). For bacteria occurring in pairs, chains or clusters, an "individual cell count" may be made of all the cells, or a "group count" of the groups plus any isolated single cells.

Procedure.—(1) Fix the bacterial suspension by adding 2 or 3 drops of 40 per cent. formaldehyde per 10 ml. Mix thoroughly. If the suspension is too dense, prepare a measured dilution in the range 40–200 million bacteria per ml.

(2) Wash, rinse, drain and dry the counting chamber and coverslip. Keep them covered until use, free from grit and dust.

(3) Place a small drop or loopful of the suspension on the centre of the chamber platform and apply the coverslip. The size of the drop must be such that it will fill the whole space between platform and coverslip, yet not extend across the "trench" to float the coverslip from the slide. The coverslip must be applied closely and evenly; it is pressed down until coloured "Newton's rings" are seen uniformly distributed over the areas of contact.

(4) Examine the preparation with a phase-contrast microscope, using the dry, $\frac{1}{6}$ in. objective; this shows the unstained bacteria clearly and enables their distinction from detritus. Alternatively, a dark-ground microscope may be used, or an ordinary microscope with the iris diaphragm closed or the condenser slightly defocussed (it may then be helpful to stain the bacteria by prior addition of freshly filtered methylene blue to a concentration of 0·1 per cent.).

(5) Count the bacteria in a sufficient number of squares to obtain a total of several hundred bacteria, selecting the squares in a pre-arranged pattern (*e.g*. all in every fifth row). Focus at different levels for the bacteria that have not settled; most settle on the platform in 5 or 10 min., but some adhere to the coverslip and a few remain in suspension.

(6) Calculate the average number of bacteria per square. Multiply this by 20,000,000 and by the dilution factor, if any, to obtain the count per ml. in the original suspension. Count two further preparations of the same suspension, and unless discordant, take an average of the three results.

If the original suspension contains much less than 40,000,000 bacteria per ml., a haemocytometer with a 0·1 mm. chamber may be used so as to obtain a significant count in fewer squares. An ordinary microscope is used, the bacteria are stained and the preparation is left for twenty minutes before counting so that most bacteria may settle on the platform.

(2) *Viable Count*

(*a*) **Pour-plate method**

The number of living bacteria or groups of bacteria in a liquid culture or suspension is counted by a cultural method such as the *pour-plate method*. A measured amount of the suspension is mixed with molten agar medium in a Petri dish. After setting and incubation, the number of colonies is counted. As a compromise between sampling and overcrowding errors, counts of pure cultures should be made on plates inoculated to yield between 50 and 500 colonies (ideally 200–400).

Procedure.—(1) Prepare serial tenfold dilutions of the bacterial suspension over a range ensuring that one dilution will contain between 50 and 500 viable bacteria per ml. Use a diluent suitable for the organism concerned, *e.g*. buffered saline, Ringer or Locke's solutions. Pipette 9·0 ml. amounts of diluent into each of several (6–9) sterile test tubes. Mix uniformly the bacterial suspension (vigorous shaking may disrupt cell groups and increase the viable count). With a sterile 1-ml. delivering pipette, transfer 1·0 ml. suspension into the first tube of diluent (fill and empty the pipette with suspension several times before withdrawing from the original container, remove any excess drop from the outside of the pipette and then slowly deliver its contents into the tube of diluent, touching the wall of the tube but not dipping into the diluent). With a fresh sterile 1-ml. pipette, mix the first dilution by filling and emptying several times, and then transfer 1·0 ml. into the next tube of diluent. Make the remaining dilutions in the same way, using a fresh pipette for each.

(2) Starting with the greatest dilution, pipette 1·0 ml. amounts of each dilution into each of three 4-in. Petri dishes. Then pour into each dish about 10 ml. of clear nutrient agar, melted and cooled to 45–50° C. At once mix by rapidly moving the plate, while flat on the bench, in a combination of side-to-side and circular movements in different directions; continue for about ten seconds, taking care not to spill any of the contents. Allow the agar to set and incubate inverted for two days at 37° C., or as most suitable for the species examined.

(3) Count the colonies in the three plates that were inoculated with the dilution giving between 50 and 500 colonies per plate (see p. 970 for counting methods). Multiply the average number per plate by the dilution factor to obtain the viable count per ml. in the original suspension.

(*b*) Surface viable count by spreading method

A surface viable count is made when the bacterium is best grown in surface culture or on an opaque medium. Prior to inoculation, the plate of medium is dried for at least two hours at 37° C. with the lid ajar; it should then be able to absorb all the water of the inoculum within about fifteen minutes, *i.e.* before the bacteria can multiply. Tenfold dilutions of the bacterial suspension are made as for the pour-plate method. A suitable volume of each dilution, *e.g.* 0·1 ml., is pipetted on to the surface of each of three plates and at once spread widely with a fine wire loop. The viable count is calculated from the average colony count per plate.

(*c*) Surface viable count by Miles and Misra method

Alternatively, by the method of Miles and Misra (1938), the inoculum is deposited as drops from a calibrated dropping pipette. Each drop, 0·02 ml. in volume, is allowed to fall from a height of 2·5 cm. on to the medium, where it spreads over an area of 1·5–2·0 cm. diameter. Each of six plates receives one drop of each dilution in separate numbered sectors. Counts are made in the drop areas showing the largest number of colonies without confluence (up to 20 or more); the mean of the six counts gives the viable count per 0·02 ml. of the dilution.

Because of variations in average cell size, bacterial counts do not bear a constant relationship to the amount of protoplasmic growth. The amount of protoplasm is better gauged by an opacity measurement, weighing or a total nitrogen estimation.

Methods of Measuring Growth

(1) Centrifugation

A specified volume of the suspension is centrifuged in a special tube, usually a capillary tube. The height of the packed organisms provide a measure of the total protoplasmic mass. However, the method is only useful if very thick suspensions of cells are available.

(2) Wet Weight

Amounts of culture for inoculation of animals are sometimes measured by wet weight. The moist surface growth on a solid medium is scraped from the medium and weighed at once. However, such estimations are inaccurate because of the difficulty of evaluating the relative contributions of water wetting the bacterial surface and intracellular water. Further, in bacteria forming capsules and slime, the wet weight may greatly overestimate the amount of protoplasm, since it includes the weight of these highly hydrated extracellular substances.

(3) Dry Weight

The weight of the dried solid matter of bacteria affords a better measure of their protoplasm. The cells from a known volume of culture are washed free from soluble salts, nutrients and waste products by centrifugation in distilled water (p. 868). It is assumed that no lysis occurs during this process. The whole or a known proportion of the washed cells is placed in a weighed vessel and weighed again after drying to a constant weight by heating in an oven, *e.g.* at 120° C. for about three hours. Cool after each heating in a desiccator over P_2O_5 and weigh quickly to prevent absorption of water.

(4) Total Nitrogen

One of the most reliable and constant methods of measuring the amount of bacterial protoplasm for metabolic measurements is by an estimation of the nitrogen present in the nitrogenous components of the cells, *i.e* mainly proteins and nucleic acids (nitrogen content about 16 per cent.). The cells from a known volume of culture are washed by centrifugation to free them from nitrogenous constituents of the medium and from extracellular excretion products. The total nitrogen of the cells is then estimated by the micro-Kjeldahl method. The cells are digested with sulphuric acid using a $CuSO_4$-K_2SO_4-selenium catalyst. The ammonia produced is removed after making the solution alkaline by steam distillation in a suitable still (*e.g.* a Markham still), trapped in 2 per cent. boric acid and estimated either by titration or colorimetrically after the addition of a suitable reagent (*e.g.* Nessler reagent).

Instead of measuring the total nitrogen content of the cells, it may be preferable to measure the total non-dialysable nitrogen content. A measured volume of a washed bacterial suspension is placed in a length of dialysis cellophane tubing tied off at its lower end. The bacterial enzymes are inactivated and the cell membranes burst by immersing the sack in boiling water for a few minutes. The sack is then closed tightly on its contents by tying the upper end. It is placed for a period of 24 hours in a jar of running tap water, or in a large volume of distilled water. The fluid inside the dialysis sack is removed by cutting one end and the volume noted for any changes during dialysis. The nitrogen content is then determined as described.

(5) Turbidity

Brown's Opacity Tubes.—A simple method of determining the *approximate* number of bacteria in a suspension is by means of standard turbidity tubes such as the Brown series (Brown, 1919-20). This consists in comparing the opacity of the suspension with that of a series of ten standard tubes containing different dilutions of suspended barium sulphate. The suspension may be made up in liquid, in which case it must be well shaken before use. Alternatively a stable suspension in gelatin can be used provided a preservative is added. In making comparisons the bacterial suspension should, of course, be placed in a tube of similar dimensions to the standards. The matching is facilitated by reading printed letters through the suspensions.

The table gives the numerical equivalents of the opacity standards for certain organisms according to Cunningham and Timothy (1924).

It must be realised, however, that these figures may be inaccurate owing to the method of counting that was used. Further, the opacity of a bacterial suspension will depend not only on the number of bacteria and the species of bacterium but also on the strain and the conditions of growth, which both affect cell size and density. It is advised that if opacity tubes are used, they should be calibrated for the particular organism and growth conditions being studied.

Showing the Relation of the Opacity of Brown's Standards to the Numerical Equivalent of various Bacteria estimated by means of the Haemacytometer Method

Opacity Tube No.	*Staphylococcus aureus*	*Streptococcus pyogenes*	*Pneumococcus*	*Gonococcus*	*Esch. coli*	*S. typhi*	*S. paratyphi B*	*N. catarrhalis*	*H. influenzae*
10	3·8	3·0	7·1	3·6	3·8	4·6	4·2	3·6	11·4
9	3·4	2·7	6·3	3·2	3·4	4·1	3·8	3·3	10·3
8	3·0	2·4	5·6	2·9	3·0	3·7	3·3	2·9	9·1
7	2·7	2·1	4·9	2·5	2·7	3·2	2·9	2·5	8·0
6	2·3	1·8	4·2	2·1	2·3	2·7	2·5	2·2	6·8
5	1·9	1·5	3·5	1·8	1·9	2·3	2·1	1·8	5·7
4	1·5	1·2	2·8	1·4	1·5	1·8	1·7	1·4	4·6
3	1·1	0·9	2·1	1·1	1·1	1·4	1·3	1·1	3·4
2	0·8	0·6	1·4	0·7	0·8	0·9	0·8	0·7	2·3
1	0·4	0·3	0·7	0·4	0·4	0·5	0·4	0·4	1·1

The figures represent thousands of millions per ml.

Standard opacity tubes with the corresponding tables are supplied by Burroughs Wellcome & Co.

USE OF A PHOTOELECTRIC COLORIMETER OR SPECTROPHOTOMETER.—The turbidity of a suspension is caused by the light scattered by particulate matter during its passage through the suspension. Clearly, accurate measurements of turbidity and hence bacterial growth, can be obtained in two ways.

(1) By measuring the amount of light scattered directly, a procedure occasionally called nephelometry. This is rarely used in practice.

(2) By measuring the light lost from the beam by scattering. Light absorption is assumed to be absent. This loss can be measured accurately in a photoelectric colorimeter or spectrophotometer where a relation similar to Beer's Law applies. The expression is the same as that on p. 868 except that the term extinction coefficient is replaced by a constant called the turbidity coefficient. A standard plot can be made of log Io/I against either the total nitrogen content or the dry weight. The concentration factor applies mainly to protoplasmic mass as the size of the organisms as well as their number determines turbidity.

The following points should be noted:

(1) The calibration curve applies only to *a particular organism grown under a particular set of growth conditions.* A new curve must be prepared if a change is made in either of these. It should be noted that the shape of an organism as well as its size will alter turbidity. Further, cells grown in a medium to give a high carbohydrate or fat content generally have a high turbidity per cell.

(2) Use a neutral or a blue filter. In a spectrophotometer use a wavelength of 5400 Å. Light scattering increases very greatly as the wavelength decreases, although it is not advisable to use too low a wavelength since light absorption will become increasingly apparent.

(3) For the blank use the suspending fluid. The growth medium can be used provided the absorption is not altered by growth of the organisms. If it is altered, the cells must be washed and resuspended in fresh solutions.

(4) At low concentrations, a linear calibration plot should be obtained, but at higher concentrations a considerable departure from a straight line will normally occur. High cell populations cannot be determined unless they are first diluted to a suitable range.

(5) The suspending fluid must be the same as that used for the preparation of the calibration curve.

Turbidity estimations in this way are the easiest and the quickest way of calibrating a bacterial population and they are accurate for comparative studies provided the above points are borne in mind.

THE PREPARATION OF CELL-FREE EXTRACTS OF MICROORGANISMS

In order to study the chemical and antigenic components of microorganisms and particularly to study their enzymology, it is necessary to lyse the cell and to liberate their internal contents. This lysis will be accompanied by varying degrees of disintegration and solubilisation of cell components (*e.g.* the cell wall, cytoplasmic membrane, nucleus, etc.). It is preferable to use methods which avoid too much denaturation of the high molecular weight cell components. Thus, any raising of the temperature during lysis should be avoided. After lysis, intact cells and cell debris can be removed by centrifugation together with any abrasives added to aid disintegration. Before this process, it is often useful to add a small quantity of deoxyribonuclease to reduce the viscosity due to deoxyribonucleic acid.

Various methods have been devised and are discussed in more detail by Hugo (1954).

(1) **Autolysis**

Many cells undergo autolysis under suitable environmental conditions. The rate of this autolysis varies according to the nature of the organism and the surrounding medium. However, due to their mechanically strong cell wall, autolysis in bacteria is usually slow and is rarely an effective method for preparing a cell-free extract.

(2) **Induced Lysis**

Various agents have been used to induce lysis in cells. The best methods for studying components of the protoplast depend upon the use of agents specific for cell-wall destruction. The enzyme lysozyme obtainable from egg-white, tears, saliva and other body fluids breaks down links in the cell wall so that, in the absence of an osmotic stabiliser, the cell bursts. However, lysozyme acts only on a restricted range of bacteria. Other enzymes have also been used for this purpose as has bacteriophage "lysis from without" and complement in presence of the specific antibody.

(3) **Extraction of Dried Cells**

When a cell suspension is dried, the cytoplasmic membrane is usually damaged so that the permeability properties of the cells are changed and intracellular constituents can be extracted by suitable buffer solutions. Two methods of drying have been used commonly.

(*a*) Preparation of acetone powders. A thick bacterial suspension is added to at least ten volumes of acetone previously cooled to $-10°$ C. Stir the mixture vigorously. Allow to settle for ten minutes and decant the supernatant. Filter on a Buchner funnel and wash with cold acetone and ether. Dry in air on a filter paper.

(*b*) Lyophilisation (*i.e.* freeze-drying; see pp. 808-811).

(4) **Grinding with an Abrasive**

A very simple method of producing a microbial cell-free extract is by grinding in a pestle and mortar with a suitable abrasive. A thick paste of bacteria is mixed with two to ten parts by weight of abrasive, the proportions varying with the organism concerned. Suitable abrasives are powdered Pyrex glass, polishing alumina or carborundum and the particles should have an average diameter of about 1 μ. About 5 g. of the mixture is chilled in the mortar and is ground vigorously for about 5 min. in a cold room or ice-bath. A suitable buffer is added before centrifugation.

There are also a number of machines available that will carry out a mechanical grinding by movement of the mixture of abrasive and bacteria between opposing glass surfaces.

(5) **Shaking with Glass Beads**

The cells are shaken vigorously with smooth glass beads. A suitable machine is the Mickle disintegrator[1] and suitable beads are those incorporated into beaded projection screens.[2] A roughly equal weight of glass beads and a fairly thick bacterial suspension are placed in the disintegrator tube and are shaken for 15–60 min. depending on the organism. It is preferable to place the whole disintegrator in a cold room for this stage. The beads can then be separated on a sintered glass filter.

This method, although it causes inactivation of many enzymes, is particularly suitable for the preparation of cell walls.

(6) **Extrusion through a Small Orifice under Pressure**

If cells are driven through a narrow orifice under a very high pressure applied for a short interval of time, disruption and lysis often occurs. The Hughes' press[3] can be used for this purpose. A thick paste of cells prepared with or without a suitable abrasive, is placed in a stainless-steel block previously cooled to about $-20°$ in a deep-freeze unit. A close-fitting piston is forced on to the cells with a series of blows on a fly-press.[4] The high pressure liquefies the frozen suspension and forces it through a narrow orifice into a reservoir chamber in the block, where it freezes again. During this process, the cells are disrupted at a low temperature, therefore causing a minimum

[1] Manufactured by H. Mickle, 4 Ormond Drive, Hampton, Middlesex.
[2] *E.g.* Ballotini beads manufactured by the English Glass Co. Ltd., Leicester.
[3] Obtainable from Shandon Scientific Co. Ltd., 6 Cromwell Place, London, S.W.7.
[4] *E.g.* Denbigh No. 4 Fly-press, manufactured by Thomas Ward, Ltd., Sheffield.

of denaturation. The halves of the block are separated and the preparation is recovered.

(7) **Exposure to Sound Waves**

When a microbial suspension is subjected to sonic or ultra-sonic waves, breakage of cells occurs due to the creation of local areas of low and high pressure. Thick suspensions of bacteria can be disrupted within a short interval of time and at low temperatures. Ultrasonic disintegrators producing frequencies between 400 and 600 kilocycles/sec. have been largely replaced by magnetostricture sonic disintegrators giving about 8–20 kilocycles/sec. An example is the M.S.E.-Mullard Disintegrator[1] giving a frequency of about 20 kilocycles/sec. A relatively thick suspension of bacteria is placed in a suitable tube (up to about 20 ml. at a time) and the probe of the disintegrator is placed so that it just touches the surface of the bacterial suspension. After tuning the instrument (see instructions provided with the machine), the apparatus is left running for between five and thirty minutes, depending upon the organism being disrupted. Cooling may be necessary and the tube can be placed in an ice-bath.

This method is one of the simplest and most reproducible methods of preparing cell-free extracts of bacteria and it is coming into increasing use in the laboratory.

(8) **Freezing and Thawing**

A series of freezing and thawing operations may cause lysis of a sensitive organism. Although this method has not been much used in the preparation of cell-free extracts, it has been useful in the liberation of toxins *e.g.* of *Bord. pertussis*.

METHODS FOR THE FRACTIONATION OF BACTERIAL COMPONENTS

In order to fractionate the components of a bacterial cell, it is first necessary to grow the organism in large amounts. It is then separated from the surrounding medium and washed by centrifugation or filtration. This surrounding medium will contain unutilised metabolites, intermediate metabolites produced in excess, the end products of metabolism (*e.g.* fermentation products) and the results of any autolysis which has gone on during growth. In addition, there will usually be high molecular weight substances which often have important biological properties and are usually of protein, polypeptide or polysaccharide nature (*e.g.* extracellular enzymes, exotoxins, antibiotics, levans, dextrans, type-specific polysaccharides, etc.).

The washed cells so obtained can then be fractionated in two general ways.

(1) **Structural Fractionation**

The cell is fractionated into its various morphological components, whose chemical and functional properties can then be determined. For example, methods have been developed for the separation and purification of the cell wall, the cytoplasmic membrane, the nuclear body and some of the many types of inclusion bodies (lipid and glycogen granules, ribosomes, chromatophores, etc.). The medical bacteriologist has been particularly interested in those surface structures which are responsible for the antigenic character of the organism, some of its toxic properties and its resistance to the antibacterial

[1] Details obtainable from the manufacturers, Measuring and Scientific Equipment Ltd., Spenser Street, London, S.W.1.

mechanisms of the host organism and to bacteriophage. Thus, the capsule, microcapsule and cell wall have received particular attention (Salton, 1960). Components of the capsule can be removed from the cell wall by treatment with solvents or enzymes, whilst a concentrate of the walls can be prepared after rupture of the cells by shaking with glass beads.

(2) **Molecular Fractionation**

The various types of molecule that make up the bacterial cell can be fractionated and their structure and function determined in the pure isolated state. We may distinguish two types of compounds within the cell, those in solution separately within the cytoplasm and those integrated into more complex structures. The soluble substances can be separated by breaking down the cell wall and cytoplasmic membrane by one of the methods described in the previous section. If the resultant suspension is subjected to high-speed centrifugation, the complex structures will be found in the centrifugal deposit, *i.e.* complexes of high molecular weight proteins, polysaccharides, lipids and nucleic acids. The supernatant will contain many of the enzymes, together with inorganic ions and a pool of organic metabolites and metabolic intermediates. Further methods are available that separate high and low molecular weight compounds. The most commonly used are:

(a) *Acid extraction.*—The cells are extracted with 5 per cent. trichloracetic acid or 10 per cent. perchloric acid in the cold so as to minimise hydrolysis. The low molecular weight intermediates together with some polysaccharides and lipids are obtained in solution after centrifugation.

(b) *Production of acetone powders.*—A thick suspension of cells is squirted rapidly into about 10 volumes of pure acetone cooled to −20° C. The high molecular weight compounds in the precipitate are separated by centrifugation and washed with cold acetone and ether.

In order to purify the components of the complex structures within the cell, it is necessary to break down the loose bonds joining the various molecules together. As an example, polysaccharides, lipids and lipopolysaccharides can be obtained by comparatively drastic procedures which denature much of the protein. Alcohol and alcohol-ether at 40° C. to 50° C. will extract much of the lipid, although a preliminary hydrolysis by sulphuric acid may be necessary for some lipids. The lipopolysaccharide components at the surface of the cell wall in Gram-negative bacteria can be extracted using trichloracetic acid (Boivin, Mesrobeanu & Mesrobeanu, L., 1933) or 45 per cent. phenol solution (Westphal, Luderitz & Bister, 1952). These lipopolysaccharides have the toxic pyrogenic and immunologically specific properties of the O antigen of smooth-colonied cells, although the ability to produce antibody rests with the "complete" antigen which can only be extracted from the cell using mild procedures such as extraction with diethylene glycol in the cold. This O antigen consists of a high-molecular weight complex of protein, polysaccharide and two types of lipid.

REFERENCES

Boivin, A., Mesrobeanu, I. & Mesrobeanu, L. (1933). *C. R. Soc. Biol. (Paris)*, **114**, 307.

Brown, H. C. (1919-20). *Indian J. med. Res.*, **7**, 238.

Cunningham, J. & Timothy, B. (1924). *Indian J. med. Res.*, **11**, 1253.

Hugo, W. B. (1954). *Bact. Rev.*, **18**, 87.

Miles, A. A. & Misra, S. S. (1938). *J. Hyg. (Lond.)*, **38**, 732.

Salton, M. R. J. (1960). In *The Bacteria*, p. 97. Ed. Gunsalas, I. C. & Stanier, R. Y. New York: Academic Press.

Westphal, O., Lüderitz, O. & Bister, F. (1952). *Z. Naturforsch.*, **7b**, 148.

CHAPTER 52

BIOLOGICAL STANDARDISATION AND MEASUREMENT

BIOLOGICAL METHODS OF MEASURING VIRULENCE

Bio-assay

BIOLOGICAL assay is the estimation of the amount of some material in a preparation by observation of its activity on a living population, usually laboratory animals, but occasionally microorganisms, plants, men or tissue cells. The procedure involves (i) a test preparation of unknown potency, (ii) a standard preparation of known potency, (iii) a test population, and (iv) a detectable response that is specifically produced by the substance concerned in the assay. The potency of the test preparation is determined by ascertaining the mean response to a certain dose and comparing this dose with the amount of the standard preparation that produces the same mean response, or "*standard indicating effect*", under the same experimental conditions.

In assessing the potency of a biologically active substance, a *unit* of measurement must first be defined and the particular activity of the substance is then compared with that of a known standard preparation in terms of this unit. If no standard preparation exists, a stable form of the new preparation is submitted when possible and this may be regarded as a provisional standard, of which a fixed weight or volume is said to contain one unit of the particular activity. A unit is thus defined as the specific biological activity contained in a given weight or volume of the standard preparation. If it is attempted to define a unit otherwise, *e.g.* as the smallest amount of the substance producing a specified effect in an experimental animal, the wide variation in susceptibility between individual animals of the same species generally introduces many difficulties and sources of error. It will be evident that experiments involving such comparisons of test populations frequently demand a careful statistical approach and proper planning.

Many methods of measurement in microbiology have much in common with bio-assay methods and involve comparisons of the responses of sample groups of a test population to different stimuli or agents. If the responses are to be properly comparable, all of the samples or groups of the test population used in the experiment should be identical. It can be shown that haphazard selection of animals, for example, may result in the inclusion of a significantly higher proportion of more robust animals in the early groups. There are also well recognised sources of observer and selector bias in unconscious preferences for certain numbers and other factors so that it is essential to adopt a correct *random sampling procedure* in selecting comparable population samples or groups.

Randomisation affords some insurance against selecting unequivalent groups of individuals from a test population. Replication of observations increases the precision of the average values and gives some measure of the degree of random variation within the group. It may be that the effect of random variation can be reduced by making comparisons between subgroups that are more comparable. For example, animal experiments may be designed in which the responses of littermates to two different treatments are compared and, in this case, each of a pair of littermates of the same sex and similar weight may be randomly assigned to one treatment or the other.

Since variation between individual responses is inevitable there is bound to be unpredictable variation in the results of an assay. This variation is referred to as *sampling error* and the ways of measuring its effect are fully described elsewhere (see Hill, 1961). When average results are given it is useful to give the *mean* result, *i.e.* the arithmetic average of all the results. This value may, however, be affected considerably by the presence of a few extreme values, and where this is the case the *median* result may be given instead, *i.e.* the middle result of all the results when these are arranged linearly in ascending order. The median is not affected by a few extreme results.

In bio-assay work, a sample of a standard preparation is routinely included in each assay. Laboratories may hold their own local standard materials and these are checked periodically against recognised standards that are held in stable form by a central laboratory. The International Laboratories for Biological Standards at the Statens Seruminstitut, Copenhagen, Denmark, and at the National Institute for Medical Research, London, England, hold all International Biological Standards and International Biological Reference Preparations. These include (*a*) immunological substances such as tuberculin, tetanus toxoid, diphtheria toxoid, pertussis vaccine, tetanus antitoxin and diphtheria antitoxin; and (*b*) pharmacological substances such as antibiotics, hormones, vitamins and drugs.

Biologically active substances that can now be estimated quantitatively by physico-chemical methods may be assayed independently of biological methods. This is true of many substances that used to be assayed biologically, *e.g.* vitamin C.

Assay Methods

Direct Assay.—The amounts of the standard and test preparations required to produce a specified response are directly compared. For example, the dose of a substance that on average kills the test animal within a specified time (or that which, when infused at a constant rate, just kills the test animal) may be measured and compared with that of a standard preparation tested simultaneously. Since animals vary in susceptibility, the mean of several experiments is taken in each case and the potency of the test substance in relation to the standard is indicated by the ratio of the two means. Direct measurement of the critical dose required to elicit a particular response is frequently not possible and indirect assay methods are more usually employed.

Indirect Assay.—Responses produced by different doses are observed. This type of assay may involve observations of: (i) the presence or absence of a typical response, such as death of the test animal. This "all-or-nothing" result is referred to as a *quantal response*; or (ii) degrees of magnitude of the response, such as increase of weight or time of survival of the test animal. This is a *quantitative response.*

When the responses of similar groups of the test population to graded doses of the standard and test preparations are measured in parallel and the means of each series are plotted against the logarithm of each dose (log. dose), a *dose-response curve* is obtained for each preparation. This is frequently linear in its mid-portion (see Wilson and Miles, 1964: p. 1209).

Microbiological Assay.—Under appropriate conditions in a synthetic medium, the amount of bacterial growth (*e.g.* the number of cells when the growth is completed) is linearly proportional to the concentration of a growth factor or essential amino acid whose supply is deficient in relation to the other nutrients. Thus the amount of a growth factor or amino acid may be measured according to the amount of the growth that it supports, as in the assay of vitamin B_{12} using *Lactobacillus leichmannii.* The method has the advantage of specificity and high sensitivity. In the case of vitamins it is possible to determine as little as 0·001 μg. per ml., and in some cases (biotin and B_{12}) considerably less. It should be noted that the response in these assays, *e.g.* production of turbidity or acidity by a growing culture, is usually linearly related to the dose and not to the logarithm of the dose.

Microbiological assays are also of use in assaying antibiotics, and various methods have been devised. In these assays, the degrees of inhibition of growth of a culture of bacteria by different concentrations of the test preparation are compared with the degrees of inhibition produced by known concentrations of a standard preparation of the antibiotic.

Measurement of Virulence

The minimum lethal dose ("*MLD*").—This is the dose of a bacterial suspension or toxin that just kills the test animal (or all of several test animals) within a specified time after administration by a given route. The use of this measure assumes that all animals in the same species are equally susceptible, but since there may be differences in susceptibility between animals the accuracy of the determination is partly dependent upon the number of animals used. In a procedure recommended for the determination of diphtheria toxin in terms of MLD, final testing is considered probably correct within 10 per cent. if at least three doses not differing more than ±10 per cent. are used with two guinea-pigs per dose (see Boyd, 1956; p. 642); the smallest dose killing both guinea-pigs is the MLD.

*LD*50.—The LD50 (50 per cent. lethal dose) of a bacterial culture or toxin is the dose that kills 50 per cent. of the test animals within a specified time. In view of the variation in the susceptibility of different animals of the same species, the LD50 is usually a more practical and reliable measurement than the MLD. The LD50 of a particular preparation is usually estimated by reference to the linear mid-section of the dose-response curve in which percentage responses (deaths) between 25 and 75 are plotted against the logarithms of the doses administered. It should be stressed that this method of determining the LD50 involves assumptions regarding the linearity of the mid-section of the particular dose-response curve and ignores observations outwith the 25–75 per cent. response range. Furthermore, misleading conclusions may be drawn if such an experimental determination is not performed with adequate numbers of animals in each group. The problems involved are discussed extensively by Boyd (1956: p. 694).

The measurement of 50 *per cent. end-points*.—In testing the potency of a bacterial toxin, or the lethal dose or infective dose of a bacterial or viral suspension, varying amounts of the test preparation (differing by a constant dilution factor) may be inoculated into groups of susceptible animals. As described above, it is more accurate to take the end-point of the titration as that dilution at which 50 per cent. of the animals react, and to work in terms of the LD50, ID50 etc. When the standard indicating effect is not death but some other response, the dose that is *effective* in 50 per cent. of the test animals is referred to as the ED50. The dose *infecting* 50 per cent. of animals is the ID50. The dose *protecting* 50 per cent., as in testing immunising agents (*q.v.*), is the PD50. In many virus titrations it is possible to use chick embryos or tissue cultures instead of animals. The TCD50 is the dose causing a *cytopathic effect* in 50 per cent. of the inoculated tissue cultures.

The most reliable assay method involves testing large numbers of animals or tissue cultures with many closely spaced dilutions near the value for 50 per cent. reaction. Especially when animals are used, this is seldom economically possible and it is often necessary to use rather widely spaced dilutions (*e.g.* decimal or doubling dilutions) and groups of moderate numbers of animals.

The method of Reed and Muench (1938) allows a more precise determination of the 50 per cent. end-point than is possible by simple interpolation between two critical dilutions and gives an effect as if larger groups of animals had been used than were actually inoculated. There is, moreover, a tendency to equalise chance variations.

Reed and Muench's method for estimation of LD50

In Reed and Muench's method it is assumed that animals dying at a stated dose would also have been killed by greater amounts of the agent and conversely that those surviving would also have survived smaller doses. An accumulated value for the animals affected is obtained by adding the number dying at a certain dilution to the number killed by lesser doses; a similar addition, but in the reverse direction, is made for the survivors (see example).

The accumulated values of the two critical dilutions between which the 50 per cent. end-point lies are now substituted in the formula and the LD50 is obtained.

In making these calculations it is assumed that the doses used are equally placed on the logarithmic scale, that the 50 per cent. end-point falls somewhere in the middle of the range of dilutions used and that the same number of animals was used for each dilution.

Example:

Virus dilution	Mortality Ratio	Died	Survived	Accumulated Values: Died (D)	Accumulated Values: Survived (S)	Accumulated Values: Mortality Ratio	Accumulated Values: Per cent. $\frac{(D)}{(D+S)} \times 100$
10^{-1}	10/10	↑ 10	0	31	0	31/31	100
10^{-2}	10/10	10	0	21	0	21/21	100
10^{-3}	8/10	8	2	11	2	11/13	85
10^{-4}	3/10	3	7	3	9	3/12	25
10^{-5}	0/10	0	10 ↓	0	19	0/19	0

The arrows indicate the direction of addition for the accumulated values.

In this titration the 50 per cent. end-point is seen to lie between 10^{-3} and 10^{-4}. It will be located at the proportionate distance from 10^{-3}.

$$\text{Proportionate distance} = \frac{\text{mortality above 50 per cent.} - 50}{\text{mortality above 50 per cent.} - \text{mortality below 50 per cent.}}$$

$$= \frac{85-50}{85-25} = \frac{35}{60} = 0{\cdot}58$$

Negative logarithm of LD50 titre = Negative logarithm of dilution above 50 per cent. mortality + Proportionate distance

$$= 3{\cdot}0 + 0{\cdot}58$$

$$\text{LD50} = 10^{-3{\cdot}58}$$

Kärber's method for estimation of LD50

An alternative and slightly simpler method is that of Kärber (1931):

$$\text{log. LD50 titre} = 0{\cdot}5 + \text{log. of greatest virus concentration used} - \frac{\text{Sum of percentage of dead animals}}{100}$$

For the above example:

$$\text{log. LD50 titre} = 0{\cdot}5 + (-1{\cdot}0) - \frac{100+100+85+25}{100}$$

$$= 0{\cdot}5 - 1{\cdot}0 - 3{\cdot}1$$

$$= -3{\cdot}6$$

$$\text{LD50 titre} = 10^{-3{\cdot}6}$$

Litchfield and Wilcoxon's method for estimation of LD50

This method (1949) is a rapid graphic procedure for estimating the median effective dose (ED50, LD50, etc.) and the slope of the dose-per cent. effect curve. It gives confidence limits of both these parameters for 19/20 probability. It is highly recommended. The original paper should be consulted for detailed instructions.

For guidance in choosing methods of estimating the LD50 in quantal response data, the reader is referred to the paper by Armitage and Allen (1950).

Toxin-Antitoxin Assay

The unit of diphtheria antitoxin was originally defined as that amount of antitoxin (or antitoxic serum) that just neutralises 100 MLD of a certain diphtheria toxin. The MLD was defined as the minimum amount of toxin that kills a guinea-pig of 250 grams weight in 4 days. It is not feasible, however, to preserve a standard toxin for testing antitoxin, but by means of a preserved standard antitoxin any toxin preparation can be standardised by neutralisation tests in guinea-pigs, and the value of a new antitoxin can then be estimated. The usual method is to ascertain first the "*L+*" *dose* of the toxin; this is the quantity of diphtheria toxin that, when mixed with 1 unit of standard antitoxin, is just sufficient to kill a 250-gram guinea-pig within 4 days. Varying dilutions of the new antitoxin are then mixed with the L+ dose and injected into guinea-pigs. In this way the neutralising power of the new antitoxin can be compared quantitatively with the standard and the number of units in a given volume stated. Antitoxin may also be titrated by the neutralisation of the *reaction* following the intracutaneous injection of mixtures of toxin and antitoxin in the guinea-pig or rabbit, using an "*Lr*" *dose* of toxin. This is the amount of toxin that, when injected intradermally along with 1 unit of antitoxin, causes a localised erythema 5 mm. in diameter within 36 hours. The amount of the unknown antitoxin producing the equivalent result when injected with the same dose of toxin will contain 1 unit of antitoxin. In practice, several skin tests may be done simultaneously on one animal and, in order to avoid injecting a lethal dose of toxin, these neutralisation tests may be performed with dilutions equivalent to specified fractions of units (provided that the test dose of toxin injected is not diluted beyond its active titre).

It will be evident from the above example that in toxin-antitoxin testing, some effect such as death within a stated time, or production of a stated area of erythema or necrosis, is the specified response or *standard indicating effect*. Antiserum is routinely calibrated by determining the dilution that, when mixed with a fixed amount of the particular toxin (the *test dose*), just allows it to produce the standard indicating effect. In other words, the antitoxin in the serum is serially diluted in the presence of a test dose of toxin, the effect of which becomes demonstrable at the end-point of the titration. The amount of the test antiserum contained in the end-point dilution is then regarded as equivalent in the number of units to the amount of a standard antitoxin that allows the same standard indicating effect when mixed with a test dose of toxin in a parallel titration.

The test dose of toxin is determined by adding a constant volume of the standard antitoxin, containing x units, to graded doses of the toxin. The mixture that subsequently produces the standard indicating effect contains the test dose at the x-units level of testing. It is important that the proposed level of testing, *i.e.* the number of units contained in the fixed amount of standard antitoxin used, should be such that the appropriate test dose of toxin is indeed capable of producing the standard indicating effect. A simple control titration of toxin should always be included to demonstrate this.

The *Lo dose* of a toxin is the amount of toxin that is just neutralised by 1 unit of antitoxin. This is technically difficult to measure exactly and titrations are generally based instead on the *L+ dose*, *i.e.* the amount of toxin that, when mixed with 1 unit of antitoxin, produces the standard indicating effect.

Danysz phenomenon.—Antibody and antigen combine in different proportions according to the amount of each in a mixture. The addition of a relatively small amount of toxin to a large amount of antitoxin results in the combination of many more antitoxin molecules per molecule of toxin than would occur if more toxin had been available in the initial mixture. Thus, if an amount of toxin and a minimum amount of antitoxin are chosen, such that they would give a non-toxic mixture if they were mixed together all at once, and if the toxin is split into several portions and these are added to the anti-toxin one after the other, the final mixture will be found to be toxic. The initial combination of relatively large numbers of antitoxin molecules with relatively few toxin molecules leaves insufficient free antitoxin for the prompt neutralisation of the fractions of toxin subsequently added. The final mixture therefore remains toxic, at least until a spontaneous rearrangement takes place in the combining ratio of the antibody and antigen molecules. For this reason, when mixtures of antitoxin and toxin are made in neutralisation experiments, antitoxin is added to toxin and not *vice versa*.

In-vitro testing.—Toxin and antitoxin may be assayed by in-vitro methods if an indicating effect of the toxin, such as haemolysis, can be specifically neutralised by the homologous antitoxin. The conditions under which such tests are performed may be critical and it is important to define them when reporting results. For example, the lecithinase (alpha toxin) of *Clostridium welchii* may be assayed in terms of its haemolytic activity. In this case, the species of red cell and the composition of the diluent greatly influence the result of the test.

Optimal Proportions in precipitation or flocculation reactions.—When a series of mixtures of antigen and antibody is set up in tubes with a constant amount of antiserum and increasing amounts of antigen, precipitation and flocculation occur most rapidly and most markedly in the tube in which antibody and antigen occur in *optimal proportions* (Dean & Webb, 1926). The ratio is constant for all dilutions of a given antiserum and antigen, and usually all of the antigen is precipitated at this point. The antibody content of different sera may therefore be compared by ascertaining the amounts required to produce most rapid and complete flocculation with a given antigen.

Thus antitoxin may be assayed *in vitro* by the Ramon flocculation method based on the rapid precipitation obtained when optimal proportions of toxin and antitoxin are mixed. The *Lf dose* of toxin is first determined as the amount of toxin that flocculates most quickly with 1 unit of antitoxin. The unknown antitoxin is then tested to find the dilution that flocculates most rapidly with 1 Lf dose of toxin. This dilution will contain 1 Lf unit of antitoxin.

Avidity of antiserum.—In addition to the actual content of antitoxin in an antiserum, the combining power of the antitoxin in terms of rate and firmness of combination with toxin, *i.e.* its *avidity*, significantly influences its effective neutralising power. The antitoxin in an avid serum combines quickly and firmly with toxin. The protective effect of an antiserum, as judged by animal experiments, may not always exactly parallel estimates of its potency based upon in-vitro experiments. One explanation for this is that slight differences may exist in a group of components that normally act as a single antibody complex but may consequently participate to different degrees in various in-vitro reactions. It is also clear that in-vitro procedures may not give a true estimate of the relative therapeutic values of two antisera containing equal amounts of antitoxin if one serum is much more avid than the other.

The Evaluation of a Protective Antigen

Mouse protection test.—In the evaluation of immunising agents it is usual to give groups of animals graded doses of the test preparation and to give similar groups the same doses of a standard preparation. After a suitable period the animals in the two series are then challenged with, for example, a normally lethal dose (*e.g.* 100 LD50) of the bacteria or toxin against which they were presumably protected. The size of the challenge dose should be adjusted so that it is likely to produce a significant mortality but it must not be so great that there are no survivors in either of the series. The percentage of survivors in each group is subsequently recorded and the logarithms of the doses of the test and standard preparations associated with 50 per cent. survival are estimated. The difference between these is the log. potency ratio, and the antilogarithm of this figure gives the actual potency ratio of the two preparations in terms of the amounts that produced 50 per cent. protection (PD50) against the challenge dose.

In assessing the protective value of vaccines for human use, controlled field and laboratory studies should be done. The principles are discussed in Chapter 43 (p. 594).

REFERENCES

ARMITAGE, P. & ALLEN, I. (1950). Methods of estimating the LD50 in quantal response data. *J. Hyg. (Lond.)*, **48**, 298.

BOYD, W. C. (1956). *Fundamentals of Immunology*. 3rd ed., pp. 642, 694. London and New York: Interscience Publishers.

DEAN, H. R. & WEBB, R. A. (1926). The influence of optimal proportions of antigen and antibody in the serum precipitation reaction. *J. Path. Bact.*, **29**, 473.

HILL, A. B. (1961). *Principles of Medical Statistics*. p. 108. London: *Lancet*.

KÄRBER, G. (1931). Beitrag zur kollektiven Behandlung pharmakologischer Reihenversuche. *Arch. exp. Pathol. Pharm.*, **162**, 480.

LITCHFIELD, J. T. & WILCOXON, F. (1949). A simplified method of evaluating dose-effect experiments. *J. Pharm. exper. Therap.*, **96**, 99.

REED, L. V. & MUENCH, H. (1938). A simple method of estimating fifty per cent. endpoints. *Amer. J. Hyg.*, **27**, 493.

WILSON, G. S. & MILES, A. A. (1964). *Topley & Wilson's Principles of Bacteriology & Immunity*. 5th ed. p. 1209. London: Arnold.

CHAPTER 53

ANTIMICROBIAL AGENTS

SUBSTANCES that are used against microorganisms may be described as *cidal* if they kill cells quickly, or *static* if their effect is predominantly one of inhibiting growth. Most substances that are static, however, are cidal if their concentration is raised, or if the exposure is sufficiently prolonged. *Disinfectants* are substances that are strongly bactericidal in the concentrations usually used and sometimes they also destroy bacterial spores. They are generally used to eradicate microorganisms from inanimate material. *Antiseptics* are less irritant substances that destroy or inhibit the growth of microorganisms and that may be applied locally against pathogenic organisms growing in living tissues. They are in most cases, however, general protoplasmic poisons and therefore tend to be toxic to tissues as well as to bacterial cells. Clearly the difference between disinfectants and antiseptics is one of degree only, and some disinfectants may be used as antiseptics. The terms *germicide* and *bactericide* are used to describe both disinfectants and antiseptics.

Antimicrobial drugs are chemotherapeutic substances that destroy or inhibit the growth of microorganisms in living tissue. They usually differ from antiseptics and disinfectants in possessing a high *therapeutic index*, i.e. they are much more toxic to microbes than to tissues, and they have a more selective range of antimicrobial action. They may be given parenterally or orally against deep-seated or systemic infections. *Antibiotics* are substances produced by some living organisms that kill or inhibit the growth of other organisms and some are sufficiently non-toxic to be used as antimicrobial drugs.

DISINFECTANTS AND ANTISEPTICS

A great variety of compounds can act as disinfectants and antiseptics. Those most commonly used include the following: *acids and alkalis*; *metallic salts—e.g.* mercuric salts; *organic metallic compounds—e.g.* merthiolate; *halogens—e.g.* chlorine and iodine; *alcohols, ethers and aldehydes—e.g.* ethanol and formaldehyde; *phenols—e.g.* phenol and cresols; *oxidising and reducing agents—e.g.* hypochlorites, hydrogen peroxide and sulphurous acid; *organic dyes—e.g.* brilliant green, crystal violet and proflavine; *soaps and synthetic detergents—e.g.* quaternary ammonium salts. These substances are usually general protoplasmic poisons and act relatively non-specifically on bacteria (with the exception of the organic dyes, which are more selective and are used in connection with selective methods of cultivation). They will also kill mammalian cells such as phagocytes, often at concentrations lower than those required to kill bacteria. The non-specific action of these substances is due to their activity in destroying or denaturing compounds or structures common to all living organisms. Thus mercuric salts react with the $-SH$ groups in proteins, rendering them biologically inactive, while phenols, soaps and detergents probably act by destroying the semi-permeable plasma membrane at the surface of all cells.

A variety of factors will affect the activity of a disinfectant or antiseptic and these should be borne in mind during use. The most important are:

(1) *Concentration.*—The higher the concentration of the germicide the greater will be the rate of killing. This is particularly important with the phenolic group of compounds, whose activity falls off very rapidly with dilution.

(2) *Time and temperature.*—In general, germicidal activity is increased

with time and a sufficient exposure is imperative for efficient disinfection. An increase of temperature will also raise the rate of killing.

(3) *Organic matter.*—Most germicides are reduced in activity by the presence of organic matter and particularly by the presence of proteins such as those in body fluids.

(4) *Number of organisms.*—The larger the number of organisms, the greater will be the time required for disinfection.

(5) *The presence of spores.*—Spores are exceptionally resistant to the great majority of disinfectants.

Testing of Disinfectants

A simple way to test the effect of a particular antiseptic is to incorporate a series of different concentrations of the antiseptic in 10 ml. amounts of nutrient agar, pour the medium in plates and then make a stroke inoculation from a bacterial suspension. This should be prepared in sterile distilled water from a young culture on solid medium and should show just a faint turbidity to the naked eye. Different organisms can be tested at the same time by making stroke inoculations on each of the various plates. The plates are incubated for 48 hr., when observations can be made.

Instead of solid medium, tubes of broth or serum (sterile ox serum previously heated at 56° C.) may be substituted. To a series of such tubes varying concentrations of the antiseptic are added and then each is inoculated with a standard amount of bacterial suspension. The effect is observed after incubation at 37° C. for 48 hr., the presence or absence of living organisms being decided by subculturing; one stroke is made from a loopful of each mixture. In this way one agar plate will serve for subcultures from a series of tubes.

In the case of slowly acting bactericidal substances, such as the flavine and other antiseptic dyes, it is often found that concentrations that have entirely inhibited growth, as shown by the absence of turbidity in the relevant fluid cultures, still contain a few living organisms which may be revealed by subculture from the fluid cultures on to solid media. The lowest concentration of antiseptic that produces this result (inhibitory concentration) yields a satisfactory index of the bacteriostatic potency.

The efficiency of disinfectants is most frequently assessed by measuring the rate of kill against a selected range of organisms under specified circumstances. The majority of methods employ phenol as a standard reference so that a *phenol coefficient* is frequently quoted for disinfectants. It may be said to express the bactericidal power of a particular substance as compared with pure phenol. The principal techniques are the Rideal-Walker, Chick-Martin and United States (FDA) test.

Their chief application is in comparing disinfectants composed of coal-tar derivatives which are water-soluble or water-miscible. They are of no use in assessing the relative merits of different classes of compounds—*e.g.* coal-tar in comparison with quaternary ammonium compounds.

Rideal-Walker Test[1]

Materials required:

(1) Standard loop of 28 SWG wire, 4 mm. internal diameter, bent

[1] For full details of technique, see *Technique for Determining the Rideal-Walker Coefficient of Disinfectants*, British Standards Specification, No. 541, 1934, with amendments dated 1943 and 1951; obtainable from British Standards Institution, 28 Victoria Street, London, S.W.1

almost at a right angle to the wire, so that in the subsequent manipulations the plane of the loop is horizontal.

(2) Culture of *S. typhi*. It is of the utmost importance to use a standard culture.[1]

Subcultures should be made in the standard broth at 24 hr. intervals, three times before the test is carried out, and a 24 hr. broth culture used for the test proper.

Method of Testing:

(1) Determine beforehand the inhibition concentration of the particular germicide for the standard strain of *S. typhi* and make up a series of five graded concentrations in distilled water, the lowest being slightly greater than the inhibition concentration.

(2) Make up 100 ml. of a 5 per cent. stock solution of pure phenol in sterile distilled water, and from it prepare the following dilutions of phenol: 1 in 95, 1 in 100, 1 in 105, 1 in 110 and 1 in 115.

(3) To 5 ml. (in stoppered sterile test-tubes) of each of the solutions prepared from the germicide to be tested, add with a sterile pipette 0·2 ml. of the 24 hr. broth culture of *S. typhi* and shake the mixtures. The tubes containing the solutions should be kept during the test in a water-bath at 18° C.

(4) At intervals of 2½ min. up to 10 min. remove a large loopful from each mixture, using the standard wire loop and transfer to tubes of 5 ml. standard broth. The bacterial suspension in (3) should be added to the tubes of antiseptic in succession at definite intervals, *e.g.* 30 sec. The loop-transfers to broth from each tube, after 2½, 5, 7½ and 10 min. respectively, can then be accurately timed.

(5) and (6) Carry out with the phenol solutions the same procedure as in (3) and (4).

(7) Incubate the broth tubes for 48 hr. and note those in which growth has occurred.

(8) The coefficient is calculated by dividing the figures indicating the degree of dilution of the disinfectant that shows life in 2½ and 5 min., but no life thereafter, *by* that figure indicating the degree of dilution of phenol that shows life in 2½ and 5 min. but no life thereafter. *E.g.*, see table.

Dilution		Time in Minutes			
		2½	5	7½	10
Unknown Germicide	1 : 400	−	−	−	−
	1 : 500	−	−	−	−
	1 : 600	+	−	−	−
	1 : 700	+	+	−	−
	1 : 800	+	+	+	+
Phenol	1 : 95	+	−	−	−
	1 : 100	+	+	−	−
	1 : 105	+	+	+	−
	1 : 110	+	+	+	−
	1 : 115	+	+	+	+

(+ = growth, − = no growth) Phenol coefficient $= \frac{700}{100} = 7{\cdot}0$.

[1] Obtained from The National Collection of Type Cultures, Central Public Health Laboratory, Colindale Avenue, London, N.W.9; the purpose for which the culture is required should be stated.

The Rideal-Walker test compares the action of the antiseptic with that of phenol on *S. typhi* in distilled water only and does not necessarily give any indication of the disinfecting action under practical conditions where much organic matter is usually present.

The Chick-Martin Test has been advocated in which the disinfectant is tested in the presence of organic material, which is the quantity of solid matter present when heat-sterilised liquid faeces containing 10 per cent. of solids is mixed with twice its volume of disinfectant. The use of faeces in this test is open to several objections, and Garrod has devised a modification of the Chick Martin test with yeast instead of faeces.[1] The yeast is made up in suspension in distilled water equivalent to 5 per cent. of dry yeast, and for the test 48 ml. is added to 2 ml. of the *S. typhi* broth culture. 2·5 ml. of this mixture is added to 2·5 ml. of separate parallel dilutions, varying by 10 per cent., of the disinfectant and of phenol. After 30 min., samples are taken exactly as in the Rideal-Walker test. The phenol coefficient is calculated by dividing the mean of the highest concentration of phenol permitting growth and the lowest concentration producing sterility with the corresponding mean of the disinfectant. Thus, supposing there was no growth with 2·0 per cent. phenol, but growth with 1·8 per cent., the mean is 1·9. Similarly, suppose there was no growth with 0·457 per cent., but growth with 0·411 per cent. of the disinfectant, the mean is 0·434. The result is expressed in the following form:

$$\text{Phenol coefficient} = \frac{1{\cdot}9}{0{\cdot}434} = 4{\cdot}4.$$

The rapidly expanding use of disinfectants and antiseptics for removing microorganisms from surfaces has focussed attention on tests which allow the antimicrobial agent to act upon the microorganism on the surfaces of objects. Recent techniques utilise glass cylinders (Mallman and Hanes, 1945) and squares of test material such as steel, linoleum or tile (Stedman, Kravitz and Bell, 1954) and the original papers should be consulted for details.

ANTIMICROBIAL DRUGS

Antimicrobial drugs must have a selective action against microorganisms as compared with mammalian tissues, *i.e.* they must possess a high therapeutic index. This specificity may depend upon the target mechanism being peculiar to the microbe, or being more accessible, or more immediately vital to the microbe than to the mammalian tissue. The basis for such activity is probably often the specific inhibition of particular enzymes.

The mode of action of the sulphonamides—competitive inhibition

The sulphonamide series of drugs are all based upon the molecule of sulphanilamide, usually with various organic groupings substituted on the $-SONH_2$ grouping. The first clue to their mode of action came in the

[1] *Modified Technique of the Chick-Martin Test for Disinfectants*, British Standards Specification, No. 808, 1938; see footnotes, p. 396.

finding that natural extracts (*e.g.* yeast extract) would reverse the inhibitory effect of the sulphonamides on bacterial growth; the substance responsible for this action proved to be *p*-aminobenzoic acid (PABA).

$NH_2C_6H_4SO_2NH_2$ — Sulphanilamide

$NH_2C_6H_4COOH$ — *p*-aminobenzoic acid

PABA was found to be a growth factor for many microorganisms, whilst a conjugated form related to folic acid was of universal occurrence in living organisms, being concerned as a coenzyme in certain enzyme systems essential for growth. Sulphanilamide was shown to inhibit an enzyme concerned in the transformation of PABA to this coenzyme form. The inhibition was of the competitive type, PABA and the sulphonamide competing for the active site on the surface of the enzyme. This is because of their similar structure and therefore the ability of both to "fit" into the enzyme surface. It should be noted that the inhibitory effect on bacterial growth is observed only when the ratio sulphonamide/PABA in the environment exceeds a certain value, irrespective of the absolute concentration of the two substances. Thus the inhibitory effect of the sulphonamides carried over from body fluids to culture media may be reversed by the addition of PABA (see p. 749).

Competitive inhibition of this kind may be the mechanism of action of many other antimicrobial drugs.

Antibiotics[1]

Most antimicrobial drugs used today are antibiotics. These substances are produced mainly by microorganisms living in the soil where they may play a part in overcoming competing species in their natural habitat. The most important antibiotic-forming group of microorganisms are the Actinomycetes, although some fungi and aerobic spore-forming bacilli are also active. Although most antibiotics are too toxic to the host tissues to be used as antimicrobial drugs, or are rapidly inactivated in the animal body, a large number of therapeutically useful agents has been isolated and manufactured recently. Those most commonly used include the following (the name of the antibiotic-producing organism is given in brackets): penicillin (*Penicillium notatum* or *P. chrysogenum*); ampicillin, cloaxacillin, carbenicillin and oxacillin (prepared by modification of the side chain of the penicillin molecule); streptomycin (*Streptomyces griseus*); chlortetracycline (*Streptomyces aureofaciens*); oxytetracycline (*Streptomyces rimosus*); tetracycline (prepared from chlortetracycline); demethylchlortetracycline (mutant of *Streptomyces aureofaciens*); chloramphenicol (*Streptomyces venezuelae*); erythromycin (*Streptomyces erythreus*); neomycin (*Streptomyces fradiae*); polymyxin or aerosporin (*Bacillus polymyxa*); bacitracin (*Bacillus subtilis*); cycloserine (*Streptomyces orchidaceus*); kanamycin (*Streptomyces kanamyceticus*); colomycin (*Bacillus colistinus*); gentamycin (*Micromonospora purpurea*).

Many antibiotics will inhibit the growth of a wide range of bacteria and these are usually called *broad spectrum antibiotics*, e.g. the tetracyclines; others have a more restricted antibacterial spectrum, *e.g.* penicillin is active against Gram-positive bacteria, neisseriae and spirochaetes, whereas streptomycin is most active against Gram-negative and acid-fast bacteria. One of the most characteristic structures in bacteria is the cell wall, which is quite different

[1] For further general details on antibiotics, see *Brit. med. Bull.*, **16**, pt. 1

from those of higher organisms. It is probable that many antibiotics owe their specificity to an inhibition of bacterial cell-wall synthesis (*e.g.* penicillin and bacitracin). Although chloramphenicol is active by inhibiting protein synthesis, the initial site of its action has not yet been determined.

Drug Resistance in Bacteria

In species that are normally susceptible to a particular drug, some strains or variants may occur that are specifically resistant to it. The choice of a drug to be used for treatment may therefore have to be based not only on a species identification of the causal organism isolated from the patient but also on the results of in-vitro sensitivity tests made with this particular strain. The likelihood of encountering resistant strains, and thus the importance of sensitivity testing, varies in the different bacterial species. For example, it may be assumed for practical purposes that strains of *Strept. pyogenes*, pneumococcus or meningococcus will be sensitive to penicillin, but that strains of *Staph. aureus* will include many that are resistant to this antibiotic.

Drug resistant infections originate in two distinct ways of very different epidemiological significance. (1) *Drug resistant variants due to genetic mutation* (p. 96) *may occur in a sensitive strain in a patient undergoing treatment.* After a favourable initial response to the drug, associated with destruction of the sensitive parent-type organisms, the infection relapses as a result of proliferation of the drug-resistant mutants. Variation of this kind is particularly liable to occur during treatment with streptomycin, *e.g.* in the tubercle bacillus and many kinds of Gram-negative bacilli. Tubercle bacilli are also liable to mutations conferring resistance to isoniazid and *p*-aminosalicylic acid. However, it is found that *simultaneous* treatment with two of these drugs generally prevents the emergence of resistant variants. Apparently this is due to the almost negligible chance of a given cell undergoing simultaneously the two mutations required to confer the two kinds of resistance. This is "double-drug" therapy.

(2) *Infection may occur with an already resistant strain derived from an exogenous source.* Some bacterial species rarely or never undergo resistance mutation to a particular drug in patients receiving treatment, yet include many naturally resistant strains that are disseminated throughout the host community. Thus the *Staph. aureus* strains found in patients and healthy carriers include a proportion that are naturally resistant to penicillin by virtue of their capacity for producing penicillinase, an enzyme that destroys penicillin. Strains resistant to a given drug occur most frequently in communities where the drug is widely used, *e.g.* in hospitals, since their survival and spread is selectively favoured. Patients undergoing drug treatment in hospital are thus very liable to suffer cross-infection with a "hospital strain" which is resistant to a multiplicity of drugs and in some cases may be highly virulent from frequent passage in infected tissues. The skin and nostrils of hospital staff are subject to frequent contamination with traces of spilt antibiotics, and this may result in a high proportion of healthy carriers harbouring drug-resistant strains.

TESTING THE SENSITIVITY OF BACTERIA TO ANTIMICROBIAL AGENTS

These tests are carried out by the same methods as used in other forms of microbiological assay, the principles of which are shown in Fig. 68.

A concentration gradient of the antibiotic is prepared in a medium fully adequate to support the growth of the test organism, which is added uniformly to the mixture. Following incubation, growth occurs in the medium in concentrations of antibiotic below the inhibitory level and ceases where this level is reached, thus allowing assessment of the susceptibility of the microorganism.

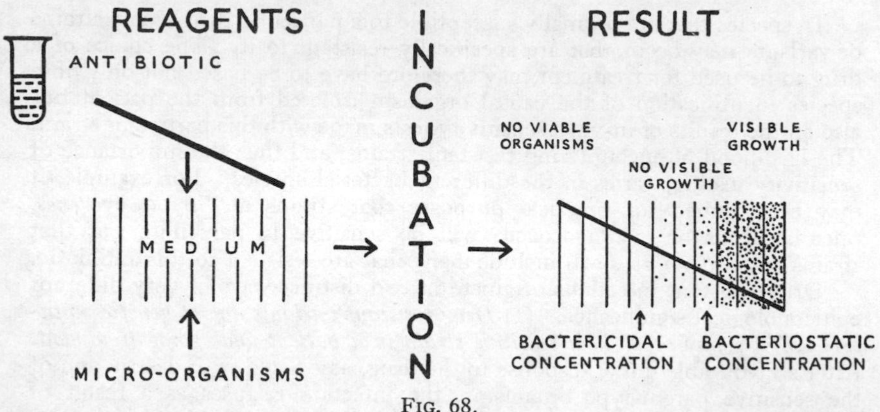

Fig. 68.

Principles of antibiotic sensitivity tests and microbiological assays. (Gould, J. C. (1960). *Brit. med. Bull.* **16**, 29).

Specific antimicrobial therapy may be instituted if the species of infecting microorganism is one whose drug-resistant variants are known not to assume clinical importance, and to this end a working knowledge of the antimicrobial spectra of each of the antimicrobial drugs in general use is of advantage. Thus a number of important pathogens have "fixed" antibiograms, *i.e.* are invariably sensitive or resistant to certain antibiotics, and treatment may proceed on the basis of bacteriological diagnosis and clinical judgment without recourse to *in vitro* sensitivity tests. Such organisms are:

Streptococcus pyogenes—sensitive to penicillin, erythromycin and chloramphenicol and resistant to streptomycin.

Pneumococcus—sensitive to penicillin, erythromycin and chloramphenicol, resistant to streptomycin.

Haemophilus influenzae—sensitive to streptomycin, chloramphenicol and tetracyclines.

Salmonella spp.—sensitive to ampicillin and chloramphenicol.

However, it must be emphasised that strains within many other species of bacteria are not alike in their antibiotic susceptibility so that the only reliable guide to the therapeutic use of antimicrobial agents is an *in vitro* sensitivity test coupled to clinical experience. In most infections the sensitivity of the causative organism should be determined before specific therapy has begun and if a specimen is available the most vital information concerning bacteriological diagnosis and antibiotic susceptibility can usually be available within 24 hr. This requires speed in the preliminary bacteriological investigations, and antibiotic sensitivity tests must be considered as part of these preliminary investigations. Diffusion tests on solid media have been adopted by most laboratories to cope with the demand for a simple, expeditious and reliable *in vitro* technique.

Diffusion Tests.—In these the antimicrobial agent is held in a reservoir from which it diffuses through agar medium to form a diffusion gradient to which the microorganisms, growing in or on the agar, are exposed. Diffusion of the antimicrobial agent takes place continuously from the reservoir outwards through the surrounding agar so that the concentration gradient is continuously changing. Zones of inhibition of growth are formed when the organism is susceptible, and these are frequently complex showing the effect of different concentrations on the microorganisms during growth (Fig. 69).

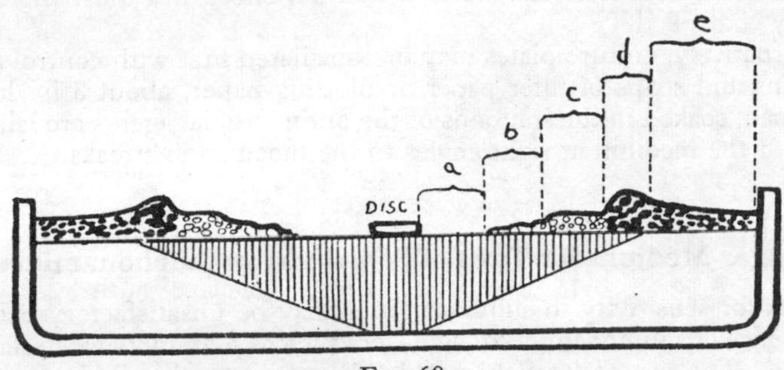

FIG. 69.

(*a*) Zone of complete inhibition. (*b*) Zone of delayed growth.
(*c*) Zone of lysis. (*d*) Zone of stimulated growth.
(*e*) Zone of normal growth.

Petri dish in section showing in diagrammatic form the theoretical concentration gradient of antibiotic after diffusion from the disk. Also diagrammatically represented are the various zones of inhibition and growth that may occur. (Gould and Bowie, 1952.)

The size of these zones depends upon factors that influence the diffusion of the antimicrobial agent, such as pH, depth, hydration and concentration of the agar, and nutrients and other substances in the gel, as well as the rate of growth of the organism. However, since the rate of growth of the majority of the pathogens encountered in the clinical laboratory is similar, and the experimental conditions can be standardised, diffusion tests can give results of a high standard of reproducibility as well as a reasonable degree of accuracy. Replicate tests are easily set up and a number of antimicrobial agents can be tested on a single plate.

The reservoir may be a hole or gutter cut out of the medium and filled with antimicrobial agent in solution or mixed with agar. Alternatively, the antimicrobial agent may be placed in a cylinder of glass, porcelain or steel resting on the surface of the medium, or in absorbent paper disks.

Agar Strip Diffusion Test for Sensitivity to Antibiotics

A simple technique originally used by Fleming is as follows. A strip of agar about ½ in. wide is cut from the centre of a plate of suitable culture medium (nutrient or blood agar) and discarded. An appropriate amount of antimicrobial agent (sulphonamide 200 μg. per ml.; penicillin 5–10 units per ml.; streptomycin 100 μg. per ml.; tetracycline 50 μg. per ml.; chloramphenicol 50 μg. per ml.) is added to 5 ml. of molten agar and pipetted into the gutter in the medium. The surface of the agar is inoculated by stroking loopfuls of cultures to be tested at right angles to the gutter and it is desirable to control the test by including known sensitive and resistant strains.

During incubation growth is inhibited for a distance varying with the sensitivity of the strain to the antimicrobial agent under examination. The size of the inoculum is relatively unimportant in testing the susceptibility of most species to the antibiotic agents though generally speaking the larger the inoculum the more resistant the organism appears. The apparent variation in the sensitivity of penicillinase-producing strains of staphylococci to penicillin is related to the size of the inoculum. With the sulphonamides the size of the inoculum may have a marked effect and must therefore be carefully controlled.

Alternatively, culture plates may be inoculated first with control and test organisms and strips of filter paper or blotting-paper, about 3 in. long and ½ in. broad, soaked in the solutions of the antimicrobial agents are laid on the surface of the medium at right angles to the inoculation streaks.

Agar Medium for Tests of Sensitivity to Sulphonamides

Tests for sensitivity to sulphonamides may be unsatisfactory because of the presence of sulphonamide antagonisers such as *p*-aminobenzoic acid in the medium. The use of lysed horse blood overcomes this difficulty (Harper and Cawston, 1945).

The following medium is useful in carrying out diffusion sensitivity tests with sulphonamides:

Peptone (Evans) . . .	20 g.
Sodium chloride . . .	2·5 g.
Sodium glycerophosphate .	2·0 g.
Agar powder (Davis) . .	10 g.
Water	1000 ml.

Dissolve the ingredients in water and add 11 ml. of sodium carbonate per litre. Adjust the pH to 7·2–7·4, bottle in 100 or 500 ml. amounts and steam for 40 min., or autoclave at 121° C. for 20 min. Before use, melt the medium and add 6 per cent. of oxalated horse blood which has been freshly lysed with saponin (2 ml. of a 10 per cent. saponin solution per 100 ml. of blood). Mix thoroughly, pour plates and store in the refrigerator for at least 12 hr. before use to allow complete neutralisation of the antagoniser.

DIFFUSION TESTS WITH FILTER-PAPER DISKS FOR DETERMINING SENSITIVITY TO ANTIBIOTICS

This constitutes a simple and reliable technique specially applicable in routine bacteriological work. It consists in impregnating small disks of a standard filter paper with given amounts of an antibiotic, placing them on plates of culture medium inoculated with the organism to be tested and, after incubation, determining the degree of sensitivity by measuring the easily visible areas of inhibition of growth produced by the diffusion of antibiotic from the disks into the surrounding medium (Gould and Bowie, 1952).

These disks are 6·25 mm. in diameter punched from No. 1 Whatman filter paper and sterilised by dry heat at 140° C. for one hr. in batches of 100 in screw-capped bottles. The required antibiotic solutions are prepared quantitatively in sterile distilled water from the preparations issued for therapeutic use; 1 ml. of the solution is added to each bottle of 100 disks, and as the whole of this volume is absorbed, it can be assumed that each disk contains approximately 0·01 ml. The solutions are therefore made up so that 1 ml. contains 100 times the required amount of antibiotic (*vide infra*). When large numbers of disks are being used it is convenient to bottle in batches of 200 or 500, the appropriate amount of antibiotic solution being added.

The disks are used in the wet condition. They can be stored at 4° C. and will retain their moisture and potency for at least three months in screw-capped bottles (the caps being carefully screwed down so that the bottles are air-tight). The disks are placed on culture medium with sterile fine-pointed forceps.

Standard graphs for each antibiotic are prepared by testing disks containing varying amounts with a standard organism of known sensitivity, e.g. *Staph. aureus*, Oxford "H" strain, NCTC 6571. The organism is grown for 18 hr. in broth and diluted to approximately 100 million bacterial cells per ml. by comparison with opacity standards (p. 873). Agar or blood-agar plates are inoculated uniformly from this broth culture (a sterile capillary pipette being used) by flooding the surfaces and then removing the excess. The open plates are then allowed to dry in the inverted position in an incubator for 30 min. or open on the bench for one hour. Finally, the disks are placed on the medium suitably spaced apart and the plates are incubated overnight at 37° C. For each antibiotic the diameters of the circular areas of inhibition are plotted against the logarithms of the antibiotic concentrations and the resultant graph is approximately a straight line. It should be noted that the areas of inhibition measured include that of the disk as well as the surrounding zone.

Quantitative Interpretation of the Disk Diffusion Test

The zones of inhibition of growth may be related to the amounts of antimicrobial agent required for inhibition of growth in the following manner.

The sensitivity (Minimum Inhibitory Concentration, MIC) of an organism may be calculated from the prepared graphs by reference to the amount of antibiotic required to inhibit the standard organism to the same degree (diameter). The sensitivity of the standard organism (*Staph. aureus*, NCTC 6571) is known (*e.g.*, MIC penicillin=0·03 units per ml.); therefore the calculation of the sensitivity of the test organism is as follows:

$$\text{Sensitivity} = \frac{\text{Amount per disk required to inhibit test organism}}{\text{Amount per disk required to inhibit standard organism to same degree}} \times \text{sensitivity of standard organism.}$$

For all routine tests, disks containing the same amount of antimicrobial agent are used, therefore the amount used to inhibit the test organism is constant. The amount required to inhibit the standard organism is constant. The amount required to inhibit the standard organism is obtained from the prepared graphs as in the following example for penicillin. Suppose the diameter of the zone of inhibition of a test organism using a 1 unit penicillin disk is 13 mm. The graph for penicillin (Fig. 70) indicates that a disk containing 0·05 units penicillin will inhibit the standard organism to 13 mm., therefore the sensitivity of the test organism is $\frac{1}{0{\cdot}05} \times 0{\cdot}03 = 0{\cdot}6$ units per ml.

In this way the sensitivity in units or μg. per ml. is denoted along the abscissae of the graphs (see graph for penicillin).

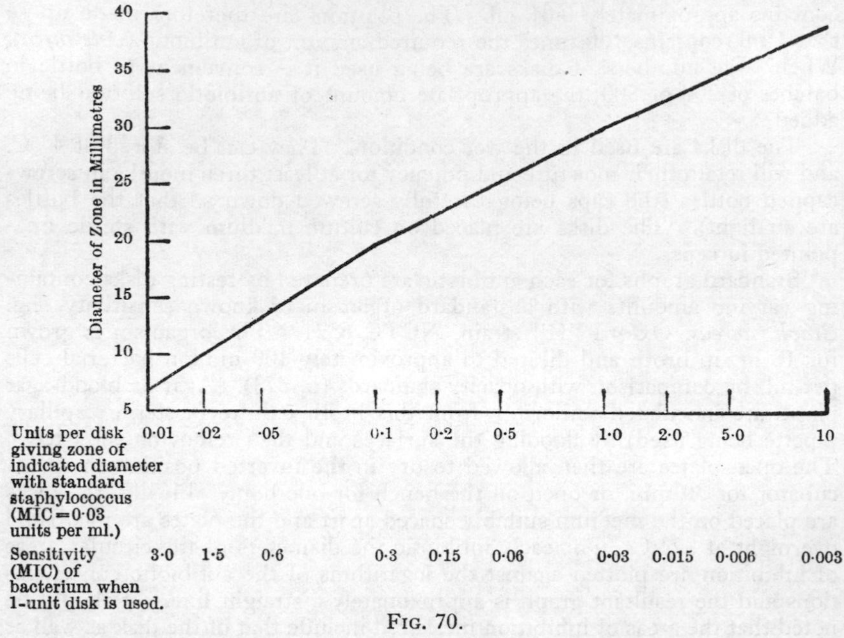

FIG. 70.

PREPARATION OF DISKS FOR ROUTINE USE

Disks containing the following amounts of antibiotics and other chemotherapeutic agents are used in routine tests;

benzyl-penicillin	1, 10 and 100 units each.
ampicillin	10 and 100 μg.
penicillinase-resistant penicillins (*e.g.* methicillin) 10 μg.	
streptomycin	10 and 100 μg.
kanamycin	10 and 100 μg.
neomycin	10 μg. (Diagnostic for *Clostridium* 100 μg.)
bacitracin	10 units (Diagnostic for Group A *Str. pyogenes* 2·5 units).
chloramphenicol	25 μg.
tetracycline	10 and 25 μg.
erythromycin	10 μg.
framycetin	100 μg.
cycloserine	100 μg.
colomycin and polymyxin	1000 units.
nystatin	100 μg.
nitrofurantoin	100 μg.
sulphonamide	250 and 500 μg.
novobiocin, ristocetin and vancomycin 10 μg.	
fucidic acid	10 μg.
gentamicin	10 μg.
carbenicillin	10 μg.

After overnight incubation the diameters of the zones of inhibition are measured and the sensitivity obtained from the corresponding graphs. The amounts of each antibiotic recommended above have been found to give with sensitive organisms, zones of inhibition which are easily measurable.

Identification of the Disks.—The large number of different antibiotics and chemotherapeutic agents makes identification of individual disks necessary. For this the disks may be coloured using "cotton" dyes which are "fast" to the paper and do not interfere with the activity of the antimicrobial agents nor exert any antibacterial activity themselves in the concentrations recommended (Bowie & Gould, 1952). As there is a limited range of easily distinguishable colours an extended range of disks can be made by using filter paper overprinted with dots or lines which is simply done by cutting a stencil with dots or lines and putting the filter paper sheets through a duplicator.

Colouring Agents.—Stock solutions of the following dyes containing 25 mg. per ml. are prepared in distilled water and autoclaved. These may be stored indefinitely and are used to identify the various antibacterial agents.

"Chlorazol" sky blue ICI FF 200 . .	BLUE
"Clayton" aniline tolamine pink . . .	RED
"Durazol" fast orange ICI R 150 . .	ORANGE
"Durazol" scarlet ICI 4B, 150 . . .	SCARLET
"Durazol" turquoise blue ICI FBF . .	TURQUOISE
"Durazol" yellow ICI GR 200 . . .	YELLOW

The stock solutions are diluted to 5 mg. per ml. before use.

Antimicrobial Agent	*Dye Solutions*	*Colour*
Ampicillin	red diluted 1 : 10	PINK
Bacitracin	2:2:1 mixture of scarlet: orange: blue	BROWN
Benzyl-penicillin	red	RED
Chloramphenicol	3:1 mixture of yellow: blue	GREEN
Colistin	blue diluted 1:10	PALE BLUE with SPOTS
Cycloserine	1 : 4 mixture of orange : yellow	ORANGE
Erythromycin	1:1:8 mixture of orange: blue:red	PUCE
Framycetin	1:10 dilution of blue	LIGHT BLUE
Fucidic acid	none	WHITE with SPOTS
Gentamicin	red diluted 1 : 10	PINK with SPOTS
Kanamycin	Scarlet	SCARLET with SPOTS
Methicillin	turquoise	TURQUOISE
Neomycin	1:9 mixture of blue: yellow	LIGHT GREEN
Nitrofurantoin	yellow	YELLOW with SPOTS
Polymyxin	1: 5 blue: red	PURPLE with SPOTS
Streptomycin	none	WHITE
Sulphonamide	blue	BLUE
Tetracycline	1:1 mixture of orange: scarlet	TERRA-COTTA

With the exception of the agents mentioned below solutions or suspensions of the antibacterial agents, twice the final potency per ml. required to prepare the disks are made by adding sterile water to commercial preparations; *i.e.* benzyl-penicillin, 200 units per ml. (for 1 unit disks); 2000 units per ml. (for 10 unit disks) etc.

Equal parts of the antibacterial solutions and dye solutions are mixed and 1 ml. of the colour mixture added to 100 disks (2 ml. to 200 disks and *pro rata*).

For Streptomycin, Polymyxin, Bacitracin and Sulphonamides.—These antibiotics precipitate the dyes in solution, and although this does not interfere with the activity of the antibiotic the colouring of the disks is not satisfactory. Uncoloured disks are used for streptomycin; the disks for polymyxin and bacitracin are first coloured with the dye, dried and then impregnated with antibiotic solution. Solutions of these antibiotics are made up therefore as follows: streptomycin 1000 μg. per ml.; polymyxin 10,000 units per ml.; and bacitracin 1000 units per ml. 1 ml. of these solutions are added to each bottle of 100 disks.

Disks for sulphonamides are dyed blue and then impregnated with solutions of the sodium salts of sulphonamides containing 12·5 mg. per ml.

Commercial disks are available, impregnated with antibiotic and marked to indicate the nature of the drug. Some of these are of absorbent paper, others consist of a vehicle with antibiotic and binding agent compressed into a tablet (Sleigh, 1958). The amount of antibiotic in these preparations has been found to vary. For ease of placing multiple disks simultaneously on a plate some are made available with a mechanical dispenser. Others are manufactured with the disks joined together and prolonged storage under variable conditions may result in a falling off in potency. The substances used as vehicles or binding agents in the tablets may be biologically active and under test conditions become antibacterial or interfere with the action of the antibiotic. For these reasons the standardisation of commercial disks for antibiotic sensitivity tests is desirable (see Greenberg *et al.*, 1957). If commercial disks are used it is recommended that they be compared with fresh disks of known potency prepared in the laboratory.

SENSITIVITY TESTS

Primary.—In testing organisms of unknown sensitivity a result adequate for clinical purposes can be obtained from a primary sensitivity test in the majority of cases.

Indeed the results may be more relevant to the case since the inoculum may represent more correctly conditions pertaining in the patient's tissues, and when multiple species are present any interaction between them and the antibiotics will be detected. Further it is often easier to appreciate which antibiotic is most effective against all the flora isolated.

An additional advantage of the use of the disks on the diagnostic plates is the creation of locally selective zones which often allow separation of mixed species and therefore facilitate identification.

When these tests are carried out under anaerobic conditions the apparent activity of some antibiotics is changed; *e.g.* streptomycin has usually reduced zones of inhibition.

The area of initial inoculation (reservoir) of the specimen on the diagnostic culture plate is made so that it covers a sufficient area of the medium and the material is spread as uniformly as possible. Disks containing antimicrobial agents are applied within this area, their centres separated by two or more centimetres. After incubation the zone of inhibition, if any, is measured. These may be compared with the results of subculture tests if desired. There will be a number of primary tests in which the inoculum is so sparse that the result cannot be assessed properly, and in such cases recourse to a subculture test is necessary.

Secondary.—Subcultures of the test organisms are made in broth and incubated for 6–18 hr. Any density of inoculum may be used, but in most cases the surfaces of culture plates may be sown as already described with broth containing approximately 100 million cells per ml. After drying, the surface disks are applied, the plates incubated and zones of inhibition measured.

Replica Plate Method to show Bacteriostatic and Bactericidal Action

A zone of inhibition of growth around a disk in the preceding test may indicate that the antimicrobial agent is either bactericidal or merely bacteriostatic. The presence or absence of living organisms within the zones of apparent complete inhibition of growth on antibiotic diffusion plates may be shown by the replica plate method (Elek & Hilson, 1954). Bacteria are transferred from the surface of the sensitivity test plate to a second (replica) plate containing no antibiotic, without disturbing their spatial relationships. This is done by means of a "stamp". Cylindrical wooden blocks, 3 cm. in height and of a diameter slightly less than the Petri dish used, are made from seasoned, close-grained wood. The surfaces should be as even and smooth as possible. An even layer of latex adhesive is brushed over one face and a piece of good-quality furnishing velour of about 2·5 mm. thickness, with a close pile, is smoothed over the surface with the pile facing away from the wood. Trim the edge of the velvet to the block. These "stamps" are autoclaved and stored in pairs with their faces in contact. They may be used repeatedly until the velvet becomes matted or uneven, when the fabric must be replaced.

The velvet surface of a sterilised "stamp" is pressed evenly and firmly on the surface of a sensitivity plate, avoiding lateral movement. The stamp is then lifted off and pressed firmly on the replica plate. This plate is incubated and examined for growth within the areas corresponding to the zones of inhibition on the sensitivity plates. Approximately 1 per cent. of the organisms are transferred from plate to plate by this technique.

Serial Dilution Tube Technique

Serial dilution tests in which the concentration gradient is discontinuous are frequently used to determine the antibiotic sensitivity of strains of bacteria and to assay the antibiotic activity of body fluids during treatment.

To each of a series of sterile stoppered test-tubes a standard volume of medium that will support the growth of the test organism is added. A solution of the antimicrobial agent is prepared in broth and a series of doubling dilutions prepared (Fig. 71) with sterile pipettes. The range of concentrations should extend from at least twice the highest concentration likely to be found in the tissues during treatment to half that which inhibits the growth of the most sensitive member of the species being tested. Control tubes contain (*a*) medium without antibiotic and (*b*) uninoculated medium. The inoculum, consisting of a suitable dilution of an overnight broth culture of the test or standard control organism, is added, one loopful to each tube.

The tubes are incubated at 37° C. for 18–24 hr. and examined for turbidity. The tube with the highest dilution showing no visible turbidity is the minimum inhibitory concentration (bacteriostatic concentration). To measure the bactericidal concentration it is necessary to subculture from the tubes showing no visible growth on to agar or into broth free of antimicrobial agent. The highest dilution yielding no growth is the bactericidal concentration. Where available, a specific neutraliser of the antimicrobial agent should be used in the subculture medium, *e.g.* penicillinase for penicillin. Wherever possible, replicate tests should be set up and control titrations with control organisms of known sensitivities carried out.

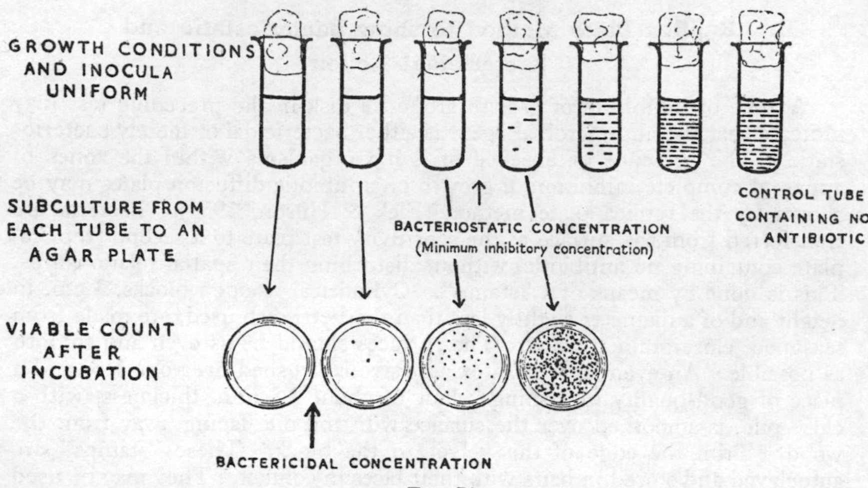

FIG. 71
Serial dilution tube test. (Gould, J. C. (1960). *Brit. med. Bull.* **16**, 29.)

TESTS FOR ANTIBIOTIC SYNERGISM AND ANTAGONISM

Mixtures of antibiotics may show greater or lesser bactericidal effects than equivalent concentrations of the individual components alone. Methods to determine these effects are used to help in the selection of antimicrobial drugs in the treatment of some infections such as cases of subacute bacterial endocarditis in which a single drug does not control the growth of the infecting microbe. The exact concentrations of component antimicrobial drugs in a mixture having the greatest bactericidal effect may be ascertained only by setting up large series of tubes containing combinations of different concentrations of each drug. However, for most clinical purposes either of the following tests gives an adequate result.

Tube Test to measure Combined Antibiotic Action

This comparatively simple test uses a limited number of tubes and a single concentration of each drug to be tested in combination, the concentration being that most likely to be attained in the tissues during therapy (Chabbert, 1953).

Antibiotics in their appropriate concentrations are added to tubes containing serum or digest broth. The combinations that appear on p. 903 have been found useful.

The inoculum is a drop of a 1 in 100 dilution of an overnight broth culture of the test organism added to each tube. Immediately after mixing, a loopful from each tube is spread over a segment of a culture plate. The tubes and plates are incubated for 18–24 hr. at 37° C. and another loopful is plated from each tube on to a second series of culture plates. After the second set of plates have been incubated, the two sets are compared and any increased or decreased killing effect of the combinations measured by counting the number of colonies.

Tube 1 Penicillin	*Tube* 2 Penicillin + Streptomycin	*Tube* 3 Penicillin + Chloramphenicol	*Tube* 4 Penicillin + Tetracycline
	Tube 5 Streptomycin	*Tube* 6 Streptomycin + Chloramphenicol	*Tube* 7 Streptomycin + Tetracycline
		Tube 8 Chloramphenicol	*Tube* 9 Chloramphenicol + Tetracyline
	Tube 11 Control No Antibiotic		*Tube* 10 Tetracycline

A duplicate set of tubes may be set up, but with a more dilute inoculum, *e.g.* a 1 in 10,000 dilution of an overnight broth culture, since increased bactericidal effects, if any, may be more easily observed under these conditions.

The Disk Test to measure Combined Antibiotic Action

Some information on the combined effect of two or more antibiotics *in vitro* can be obtained by using the disk technique after the manner of Lamanna and Shapiro (1943). The disks are placed with their centres at a suitable distance apart so that the respective antibiotics will diffuse into one another to produce a continuous range of concentrations in the early hours of incubation. This is best done after subculture tests have determined the sensitivity of the test microorganism to individual antibiotics, *e.g.* "A" and "B", and the position of the disks containing these antibiotics can be predetermined to effect the desired concentration mixtures; for example, disks A and B can be placed x mm. apart when $x=a+b$, a being the radius of the zone of inhibition with A and b the zone with B. After incubation, the two zones of inhibition will make contact and there will be a thin wedge of growth on either side of the point of contact of the zones. When there is appreciable additive or synergisitic effect by individually sub-inhibitory concentrations of A and B, the growth in the area of these wedges is inhibited. On other occasions resistant growth within the zone of inhibition produced by one drug may be inhibited by relatively small concentrations of the other which has diffused into the area. The concentration of the individual components producing these inhibitory effects can be inferred from the standard graphs in the usual way by measuring the distances from the individual disks to the area of inhibition.

Mutual interference (antagonism) between antibiotics is similarly shown by decrease in the size of the zones of inhibition.

METHODS FOR TESTING THE SENSITIVITY OF MYCOBACTERIUM TUBERCULOSIS TO ANTIMICROBIAL DRUGS

Several antimicrobial drugs such as streptomycin, para-amino-salicylic acid (PAS) and isonicotinic acid hydrazide (isoniazid) have a beneficial effect in cases of tuberculosis infection if the organism is sensitive to the drug. Unfortunately, tubercle bacilli may become resistant to these drugs in a few months, especially when they are given alone, so that it is customary to administer two or more drugs simultaneously. It is essential therefore to test strains before and at intervals during treatment, to determine that the organism is and remains sensitive to the drugs used.

The criteria for interpreting resistance from the tests to be described have been determined by closely correlating the results of sensitivity tests with clinical findings.

Sensitivity to Streptomycin.—The testing of strains of tubercle bacilli for sensitivity to streptomycin is carried out on Löwenstein-Jensen medium. Dihydrostreptomycin is used because of its greater heat stability. The antibiotic concentrations used are 1 μg. per ml. by twofold increments to 64 μg. per ml. These are the actual concentrations in the medium before inspissation. A control without the drug is included. Dispense the medium in 1·25 ml. amounts into $\frac{1}{4}$-oz. screw-capped bottles. Inspissate for one hr. at 85° C. to produce a firm medium and store in the refrigerator at 4° C. They may be kept for at least one month without loss of potency of the antibiotic.

To prepare the inoculum, sterilise $\frac{1}{4}$-oz. screw-capped bottles containing 0·1 ml. water and six $\frac{1}{4}$-in. glass beads. Make a suspension of the culture to be tested by shaking a loopful of the growth in the 0·1 ml. water on a mechanical shaker for a few min. and dilute to a standard suspension. Use an inoculating loop of 2·5 mm. internal diameter of 22 SWG wire diameter and streak a loopful of the suspension up the centre of the control and each antibiotic-containing L.J. slope. This will give an inoculum of 10^4–10^5 particles per slope. In each batch of tests include a control test using the standard drug-sensitive strain of *Myco. tuberculosis* H37 Rv. Read at the end of 28 days' incubation at 37° C.

The end-point is the lowest concentration of the antibiotic that inhibits growth. Growth is considered to be inhibited if fewer than 20 colonies appear on the slope. The result is expressed as a ***resistance ratio*** by comparison with the control as follows:

$$\text{Resistance ratio} = \frac{\text{Lowest concentration of the antibiotic that inhibits patient's strain of } \textit{Myco. tuberculosis}}{\text{Lowest concentration of the antibiotic that inhibits the standard drug-sensitive strain, H37 Rv}}$$

For example, if the patient's strain is inhibited by 16 μg. per ml., and the standard, drug-sensitive strain by 4 μg. per ml., then the resistance ratio is $\frac{16}{4} = 4$.

Strains are considered resistant to streptomycin if the resistance ratio is 8 or more. A ratio of 4 is suggestive of resistance, but not conclusive. In such a case, other cultures from the patient's strain should be tested and the previous chemotherapy considered.

Sensitivity to Para-aminosalicylic Acid (PAS).—Sensitivity tests to *PAS* are performed in the same way as for streptomycin using twofold differences of concentration of PAS ranging from 0·25–16 μg. per ml. The result is again expressed as a resistance ratio. Sodium PAS is used because it is more stable and more soluble.

Strains are considered resistant to PAS if the resistance ratio is 8 or more. A ratio of 4 is suggestive, but not conclusive. In such a case, other cultures from the patient's strain should be tested and the previous chemotherapy considered.

Sensitivity to Isoniazid.—The following method is that recommended by the Medical Research Council (1953). The medium, method of inoculation and period of incubation are the same as for testing streptomycin sensitivity and the concentrations of isoniazid 0·2; 1; 5 and 50 μg. per ml. The end-point is the lowest concentration inhibiting growth to 20 colonies or less. Strains are resistant to isoniazid if growth occurs on 1 μg. per ml. or more. Growth on 0·2 μg. per ml. is suggestive of resistance, but is not conclusive. In such a case other cultures from the patients strain should be tested and previous chemotherapy considered.

Alternatively, a closer range of isoniazid concentrations (from ·025 to 0·8 μg. per ml.) may be used and the results reported as the resistance ratio. A ratio of 4 indicates resistance.

For alternative methods for estimating the sensitivity of *Myco. tuberculosis* to these drugs see Canetti *et al.* (1963).

Sensitivity tests for other Antitubercular Drugs.—Tests for viomycin, cycloserine and oxytetracycline may be carried out in a manner similar to that for testing streptomycin.

TITRATION OF ANTIMICROBIAL AGENTS IN BLOOD AND OTHER BODY FLUIDS

It may be desirable to estimate the amount of antibiotic or other antimicrobial agent in body fluids during treatment to ensure that an adequate dosage is being administered. The methods employed are similar to those used to determine the sensitivity of bacteria to antibiotics. A simple method suitable for most clinical purposes is as follows.

The fluid to be examined is collected aseptically. If it is likely to be contaminated with microorganisms, these must be removed, *e.g.* by filtration. Blood is withdrawn by venepuncture and the serum separated, being centrifuged if necessary to free it completely from suspended red cells. The test should be carried out as soon as possible after collection of the fluid.

Suitable dilutions of the fluid under examination are prepared in broth and inoculated with a standard organism of known sensitivity such as the Oxford strain of *Staph. aureus* which is sensitive to concentrations of all the commonly used antimicrobial agents that can be easily attained in the tissues. A control tube containing the medium alone is included. The tubes are incubated for 18–24 hr. and examined to find the tube with the highest dilution that has no turbidity.

A control test is set up in parallel using a fresh sample of the same body fluid known to contain no antimicrobial agent and to which a known amount of the agent being assayed has been added. By comparing the dilutions that inhibit the growth of the standard organism an exact estimation of the amount of antimicrobial agent can be made, taking into account the bacteriostatic action of the fluid under test, *e.g.* if the unknown fluid inhibits growth at a dilution of 1 : 60 and the control fluid containing 5 μg./ml. at a dilution of 1 : 120, the unknown contains $\frac{60}{120} \times 5 = 2{\cdot}5$ μg./ml.

Estimation of streptomycin in serum and cerebrospinal fluid

The method recommended by the MRC Subcommittee (MRC Report, 1948) can be used when a rapid clinical assay is required. When a more precise determination is required, the method of Mitchison and Spicer (1949) may be used.

There are many detailed techniques, both chemical and biological, for assaying individual antibiotics, and for these appropriate textbooks should be consulted (*e.g.* Kavanagh, 1963).

PRODUCTION OF PENICILLINASE

Penicillin is rapidly destroyed by the products of growth of many organisms, and such material has been termed "penicillinase". Some strains of *B. subtilis* produce it in large quantities. Penicillinase is useful when it is desirable to destroy penicillin present in body fluids from which cultivation tests are carried out: for example, blood culture, when ascertaining the survival times of organisms subjected to the action of penicillin or when testing preparations of penicillin for sterility.

B. subtilis (strain NCTC 6346) is grown in broth, the culture is filtered and the resultant fluid constitutes "penicillinase". The filtrate is tested for potency, with penicillin and the standard Oxford strain of staphylococcus.

Preparation of Penicillinase

Distribute digest broth in shallow layers in 20- or 32-oz. flat bottles. Inoculate the broth with a culture of *B. subtilis* (strain 6346).

Incubate the bottles horizontally for 14 days at 26° C. A pellicle forms which is shaken down each day.

At the end of incubation, filter the culture through a Seitz disk. The filtrate contains 100,000 units or more of penicillinase per ml.

Tests for Potency

Make up a solution of penicillin, 1000 units per ml.

Prepare in tubes or bottles a series of 10 ml. amounts of broth containing 1000 units of penicillin, and add varying amounts of penicillinase.

Inoculate each tube or bottle with a loopful of an overnight culture of the standard strain of staphylococcus, and incubate for 48 hr.

The end-point is the least amount of penicillinase that allows growth. This amount neutralises 1000 units of penicillin and thus contains 1000 units of penicillinase. For example, if the least amount of filtrate permitting growth is 0·005 ml., then the penicillinase content is 200,000 units per ml.

REFERENCES

Bowie, J. H. & Gould, J. C. (1952). Colouring agents for use in disc-antibiotic sensitivity tests. *J. clin. Path.*, **5**, 356.

Canetti, G., Froman, S., Grosset, J., Haudoroy, P., Langerová, M., Mahler, H. T., Meissner, G., Mitchison, D. A. & Sula, L. (1963). Mycobacteria: Laboratory methods for testing drug sensitivity and resistance. *Bull. Wld. Hlth. Org.*, **29**, 565.

Chabbert, Y. (1953). Action des associations d'antibiotiques sur les germes aérobies. *Ann. Inst. Pasteur*, **84**, 545.

Elek, S. D. & Hilson, G. R. F. (1954). Combined agar diffusion and replica plating techniques in the study of antibacterial substances. *J. clin. Path.*, **7**, 37.

Gould, J. C. & Bowie, J. H. (1952). The determination of bacterial sensitivity to antibiotics. *Edinb. med. J.*, **59**, 178.

Greenberg, L., Fitzpatrick, K. M. & Branch, A. (1957). The status of the antibiotic disc in Canada. *Canad. med. J.*, **76**, 194.

Harper, G J. & Cawston, W. C. (1945). The in vitro determination of the sulphonamide sensitivity of bacteria. *J. Path. Bact.*, **57**, 59.

KAVANAGH, F. (1963). *Analytical Microbiology.* New York and London: Academic Press.

LAMANNA, C. & SHAPIRO, I. M. (1943). Sulfanilamide bacteriostasis in the presence of mercuric chloride and *p*-aminobenzoic acid. *J. Bact.*, **45**, 385.

MALLMAN, W. L. & HANES, M. (1945). The use-dilution method of testing disinfectants. *J. Bact.*, **49**, 526.

MITCHISON, D. A. & SPICER, C. C. (1949). A method of estimating streptomycin in serum and other body fluids by diffusion through agar enclosed in glass tubes. *J. gen. Microbiol.*, **3**, 184.

Medical Research Council Sub-committee Report (1948). Specific laboratory tests in streptomycin therapy of tuberculosis. *Lancet*, **2**, 862.

Medical Research Council Report (1953). Laboratory techniques for the determination of sensitivity of tubercle bacilli to isoniazid, streptomycin, and PAS (M.R.C. Isoniazid Trial: Report No. 3). *Lancet*, **2**, 213.

SLEIGH, J. D. (1958). Difficulties encountered in reporting the penicillin sensitivity of staphylococci. *Scot. med. J.*, **3**, 454.

STEDMAN, R. L., KRAVITZ, E. & BELL, H. (1954). Studies on the efficiencies of disinfectants for use on inanimate objects.

I. Relative activities on a stainless steel surface using a new performance test method.

II. Relative activities on porous surfaces.

Appl. Microbiol., **2**, 119 and 322.

CHAPTER 54

IMMUNOLOGICAL AND SEROLOGICAL METHODS

The classical techniques for detecting antibody-antigen reactions—precipitation, agglutination, and complement-fixation have been described in Chapter 7. These techniques are of considerable value in identifying unknown antigens and detecting the presence of antibody in the serum of an immunised subject. They have provided a basis for precise quantitation of antibody and antigen and for qualitative studies of high resolution and specificity. The last few years have seen the introduction of refined precipitin methods by the use of gels and other forms of support media, and the technique of immunodiffusion has become widely used in immunological work. The application of the agglutination phenomenon has been extended to include the use of non-particulate soluble antigens in the reaction. This has been achieved by the use of tannic acid treated red cells, or the inert particles polystyrene latex, bentonite and collodion. These particulate materials are coated with the soluble antigen and become susceptible to agglutination by the appropriate antibody. Complement fixation techniques are available with a high degree of sensitivity and micro methods can be used where only small quantities of reactants are available. Extensions of this procedure, making use of non-haemolytic complement and the conglutination phenomenon, have been devised with further increase in sensitivity. Other techniques are now available which are not derived from the classical test tube reactions of antigens and antibodies. Thus the introduction of the fluorescent antibody and isotope labelling techniques has enabled the study of the fate of injected antigens and antibody, the localisation of invading microorganisms and the distribution of tissue antigens. The passive cutaneous anaphylaxis tests will detect minute quantities of antibody injected into guinea-pig skin.

The next section of this chapter consists of a general discussion of the basis and use of some of these methods. Detailed consideration of a wide range of the newer immunological techniques are described by Weir (1967).

The sensitivity of each of the main types of reactions is indicated in the appropriate sections and is expressed in terms of the minimal quantity of antibody nitrogen that can be detected by the method. As nitrogen is an integral constituent of all proteins, quantitative analysis for protein is conveniently carried out by estimation of the nitrogen. The antibody nitrogen estimations are made from the analysis of the washed specific precipitates by the micro-Kjeldahl method after complete precipitation of the antibody by addition of antigen in slight excess (Kabat & Mayer, 1961). Thus in a particular serological test if an antiserum containing 1 mg. of antibody nitrogen per ml., as estimated by the micro-Kjeldahl method, gives an end point in the test at a dilution in 1 ml. of 1/1000 the test dilution can detect as little as 1 microgram (μg.) of antibody expressed as nitrogen.

AGGLUTINATION

The aggregation of cells or particles is brought about by antibody molecules linking across from one cell or particle to another and so forming visible aggregates. This is possible only when the antigen against which the antibody is directed is at or near the surface of the cell or particle (in certain cases special treatment of cells, *e.g.* by enzymes, is employed in order to expose antigens below the cell surface).

Agglutination tests are performed by mixing a dilution series of antiserum with a suspension of the cells or particles. The method is used to examine sera for antibodies (particularly IgM macroglobulin antibodies) against salmonella and brucella and, using standard antisera, to identify cell suspensions.

In general the underlying principle of the technique of agglutination tests in enteric infections is to examine serum *quantitatively* for agglutinins towards the particular organism. For this purpose the method usually adopted is to mix varying dilutions of serum (made up in saline solution) with a fixed quantity of a uniform and stable suspension of the organism, the mixtures being placed in narrow tubes, kept at 37° C. or 50°–55° C. in a water-bath for a certain length of time, and then examined for *visible* agglutination or flocculation of the suspension. The agglutinated organisms tend to sediment, and the reaction can also be gauged by the amount of deposit in the tubes and the clarity of the supernatant fluid. The strength of the reaction can be stated in terms of the highest dilution ("titre") that produces agglutination.

The Meaning of Titre.—The titre of an antiserum is a measure of the number of antibody units per unit volume of the original serum; thus if the last tube showing a reaction *e.g* agglutination or lysis, contains 1 ml. volume and is a dilution of 1 in 128 of the original serum, the titre of the serum is 128 units of antibody per ml. of serum. Titre is often mistakenly expressed as a function of dilution without reference to unit volume.

Blood specimens for agglutination tests are taken by vein puncture, so as to obtain a satisfactory amount of serum for the complete test. At least 5 ml. of blood should be obtained, and the blood immediately transferred from the syringe to a dry stoppered sterile tube or screw-capped bottle and allowed to clot. When the serum has separated, it is pipetted off into a sterile tube.

THE WIDAL TEST

The nature of the *Widal agglutination reaction* and its applications in the diagnosis of enteric fever are referred to on p. 227 *et seq.*

In the routine Widal reaction the patient's serum is tested simultaneously with each of the organisms likely to be responsible for enteric fever in the particular region, *e.g.* in Great Britain at the present time, *S. typhi* and *S. paratyphi B*. In other parts of the world *S. paratyphi A* or *C* may require to be included. As explained later, additional information can be obtained by testing separately for H and O agglutinins (p. 912). Thus, the Widal test generally involves parallel tests with different *Salmonella* group organisms, and also different forms of the same organism.

In addition to the tests with typhoid-paratyphoid organisms, it is the practice in many laboratories to test also for *Br. abortus* agglutinins, and, if considered necessary, with *Proteus* X19, X2 and XK for typhus infection (p. 490), thus increasing the number of parallel tests carried out.

To simplify description a single test will be referred to.

Requisites

1-ml. pipette graduated to the tip in 1/10ths and 1/100ths; 0·1 ml. pipette graduated to the tip in 1/100ths and 1/500ths; a rubber teat, or preferably a mouth-piece for pipetting by suction, *i.e.* 3 in. of 5–7 mm. bore glass tubing with 9–12 in. of rubber tubing attached which can be fitted to the top of the pipette (*vide infra*). The free end of the mouth-piece is "smoothed" in the Bunsen flame.

Sterile 0·85 per cent. saline; test-tubes $3 \times \frac{1}{2}$ in.; agglutination tubes

$3 \times \frac{1}{6}$ in., or Dreyer's agglutination tubes with rounded bottoms (not conical as originally made); test-tube racks suitable for the tubes used; small beaker or similar container for saline solution; grease pencil for marking tubes; capillary pipette. Automatic syringes (see p. 943) containing 1·0 ml. and adjusted to deliver 0·4 ml. are convenient and save much of the time required in the usual pipetting method.

Bacterial Suspension

The strain used must be carefully selected and known to be suitable for the diagnostic agglutination tests. It must be a motile "smooth" form of the particular type, and if the organism is "diphasic", e.g. *S. paratyphi B*, must represent the specific phase. Since the antigens of fimbriae (p. 247) are similar in different types of *Salmonella*, the use of suspensions prepared from fimbriate cultures may lead to confusing cross-reactions. Non-fimbriate cultures may be obtained by two or three successive subcultivations on well dried agar plates; liquid media should not be used.

It is now a general practice to use standard suspensions such as those described later; but if it is desired to prepare a small quantity of suspension for immediate use the following method can be adopted: add in fractions 5 ml. of physiological saline to a well-grown 24 hours' agar slope culture, and emulsify the growth with the aid of a wire loop. This suspension can be standardised to a suitable opacity, *e.g.* tube 1, Brown's opacity standards (p. 873). The suspension is decanted and allowed to stand for half an hour until bacterial clumps and fragments of agar have sedimented. Alternatively, it may be centrifuged for one minute.

Serum Dilutions

First make up a 1 in 15 dilution of the patient's serum, and from this prepare a series of doubling dilutions in small ($3 \times \frac{1}{2}$ in.) test-tubes:

1	2	3	4	5	6	7
1 in 15	1 in 30	1 in 60	1 in 120	1 in 240	1 in 480	CONTROL—NO SERUM

The actual procedure is as follows.

In the rack place seven tubes as above; add 0·4 ml. saline to each of the tubes 2 to 7; in a separate tube add 0·1 ml. patient's serum to 1·4 ml. saline, *i.e.* a 1 in 15 dilution; wash out the pipette thoroughly in saline solution; add to tubes **1** and **2** 0·4 ml. of the 1 in 15 dilution of patient's serum; the dilution of serum in tube **2** is now 1 in 30; after thorough mixing withdraw 0·4 ml. from tube **2** into tube **3**, making now in tube **3** a 1 in 60 dilution of serum; withdraw 0·4 ml. from tube **3** into tube **4**, *i.e.* 1 in 120, and so on till a dilution of 1 in 480 is obtained in tube **6**; withdraw and discard 0·4 ml. from tube **6**; tube **7** contains saline only.

0·4 ml. of the bacterial suspension is added to each tube and the pipette is then sterilised. The dilutions of serum are now:

1	2	3	4	5	6	7
1 in 30	1 in 60	1 in 120	1 in 240	1 in 480	1 in 960	CONTROL—SUSPENSION—NO SERUM.

If the amount of serum available is insufficient to allow of 0·4 ml. being used for the various serum dilutions, a small volume, *e.g.* 0·3 or even 0·2 ml., may be employed with, of course, the same volume of bacterial suspension.

The mixtures are transferred with a capillary pipette to agglutination tubes, starting with tube **7**.

An *alternative method of preparing doubling dilutions of serum* and making mixtures of serum and bacterial suspension is to use a "constant-volume" pipette made by slightly constricting a capillary pipette so that the volume of fluid contained in it from the tip to the constriction is about 0·25 ml., the capillary stem being 3½ to 4 in. long and not too fine in calibre. This pipette is actuated by a teat, and with it the serum dilutions can be made directly in the narrow agglutination tubes; thus, after preparation of the 1 in 15 dilutions, the constant volume measured with the capillary pipette is substituted in the directions above for the 0·4 ml. volume of serum dilution, saline or bacterial suspension measured with a graduated pipette. The contents of the tubes are mixed by gently bubbling air through the fluid by means of the pipette, starting with tube **7**. A convenient dilution procedure employs an automatic pipette (p. 943).

To observe agglutination of the H type (p. 912) it is usually sufficient to incubate at 37° C. for two hours and then leave for half an hour at room temperature. (Some workers prefer incubation at 50–55° C.). "Large-flake" clumping or agglutination can easily be detected with the naked eye in a satisfactory light. The flocculi also sediment rapidly and the deposit is quite perceptible in the narrow tubes.

When agglutination of the O type (p. 912) is tested for, readings should be made after 4 and 24 hr. as this form of reaction develops slowly. It was at one time considered advisable to incubate at 50°–55° C., but it has been shown that prolonged exposure of O agglutinins at this temperature level may weaken the agglutination reaction, and it is preferable therefore to incubate for 2–4 hours at 37° C. and then to keep the tubes at 4° C. in a refrigerator for 20–22 hr. The clumps are small and "granular" and observations are aided by the use of a hand-lens and a strong illuminant.

Pipetting with a Graduated Pipette and Mouth-Piece

The glass mouth-piece is held between the teeth at the right corner of the mouth, and the top of the pipette is supported between the second and third fingers of the right hand so that the rubber tube immediately above the end of the pipette can be compressed between the thumb and the first finger (see Fig. 72). The fluid is drawn up, *e.g.* from a test tube, into the pipette by suction until the column extends just above the required graduation mark. The end of the mouth-piece is then closed with the tongue, and the column of fluid is depressed to the particular level by gentle pressure on the rubber tubing between the thumb and fore-finger. *With the tongue still firmly applied to the mouth-piece* this exact volume of fluid can be transferred from the original tube and then expelled from the pipette into another tube.

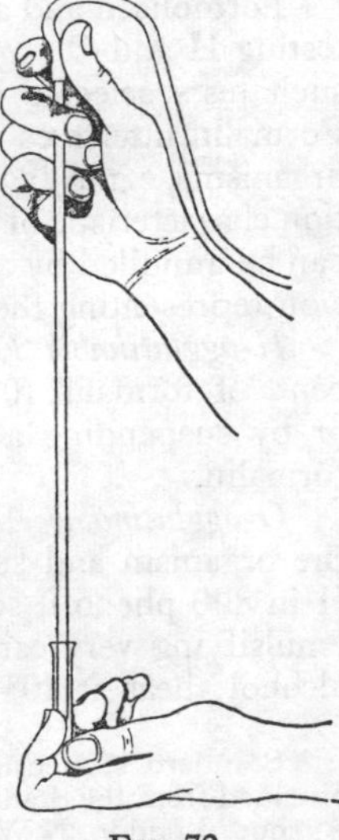

FIG. 72

This method, for which the necessary skill is soon acquired by practice, permits of *accurate* and *rapid* measurements of even small volumes.

The glass-tube of the mouth-piece can be sterilised by flaming.

Measurement of Serum and other Fluids by Drops

Some serological workers prefer to make measurements of serum, saline, etc., in terms of drops delivered from a suitable dropping pipette. This consists in its simplest form of a piece of glass tubing drawn out to capillary dimensions (as in the capillary pipette). Alternatively, special dropping pipettes can be purchased. The pipette is actuated by a teat. When used it is held vertically and the fluid in it is allowed to drop slowly from the capillary stem.

The following exemplifies the carrying out of an agglutination test by this method. In a suitable rack place a row of five Dreyer's agglutination tubes and a test-tube (about 3 × ⅜ in.) which may be called the "dilution tube". Into this tube measure with the dropping pipette 18 drops of normal saline. Similarly, add 2 drops of the serum and mix. This yields a 1 in 10 serum dilution. Saline, serum dilution and bacterial suspension are now added to the five agglutination tubes as follows:—

Tube	1	2	3	4	5
	Drops				
Saline	0	5	8	9	10
Serum, 1 in 10	10	5	2	1	0
Bacterial suspension . . .	15	15	15	15	15
Final dilution of serum . . .	1 in 25	1 in 50	1 in 125	1 in 250	Control

The tubes are incubated and the observations then made (*vide supra*).

Full details of the preparation and use of dropping pipettes is given by Fildes (1931).

Bacterial Suspensions for Testing H and O Agglutinins

Formolised and alcoholised suspensions supply the necessary reagents for testing H and O agglutinins respectively,[1] and it is also advisable to use for such tests selected strains which are sensitive to H and O agglutination. Formalin interferes with O agglutination, and in the case of motile flagellate organisms, e.g. *S typhi*, formolised suspensions show the large-flake agglutination characteristic of the H antigen (p. 115). The reactivity of the H antigen can be annulled by alcohol, and if cultures are treated with alcohol a suspension representing the O antigen alone can be obtained.

H-agglutinable Formolised Suspensions are prepared by adding 0·1 per cent. of formalin (0·04 per cent. formaldehyde) to a 24 hr. broth culture or by suspending a young agar culture in saline containing 0·1 per cent. formalin.

O-agglutinable Alcoholised Suspensions are prepared as follows: plate out the organism and select a smooth colony; subculture this on phenol agar (1 in 800 phenol); scrape off the growth in the minimum amount of saline, emulsifying very carefully, and add about 20 times the volume of absolute alcohol; heat at 40°–50° C. for half an hour; centrifuge (if necessary) and

[1] Standard suspensions for the Widal and other agglutination reactions may be obtained from the Standards Laboratory, Central Public Health Laboratory, Colindale Avenue, London, N.W.9.

suspend the deposit in saline to the proper density, with chloroform as a preservative. This emulsion keeps moderately well, but if an old suspension is used, it should be centrifuged and re-suspended in fresh saline. The original practice of keeping O suspensions in alcohol and diluting when ready for use is not recommended as the alcohol eventually annuls the agglutinability of the organisms.

The Typhoid Bacillus Vi Agglutination Test.—This test has a limited application in the diagnosis of suspected cases of enteric fever, but is of value in the recognition of carriers of the typhoid bacillus.

The bacterial suspension should be prepared from a selected strain that responds only to the Vi agglutinin and is not acted on by the H and O agglutinins. It loses sensitiveness on keeping, and should not be used after two months. The test mixtures are made up and incubated in $3 \times \frac{1}{2}$ in. test-tubes. A series of doubling dilutions of the serum is prepared, the initial dilution being 1 in 10 and the last tube in the series being 1 in 640. An additional tube is included, for control purposes, containing saline only. The amount of each dilution should be 1 ml. One drop (0·05 ml.) of the suspension is then added to each tube. Incubation is carried out at 37° C. for two hours and the tubes are then allowed to stand at room temperature overnight. To observe the result, the tubes are examined in ordinary daylight, being held somewhat tilted, and the type of sediment determined with the aid of a hand-lens. In the control the sedimented organisms should form a small, circular, well-defined, compact deposit. If marked agglutination has occurred, the deposit, consisting of clumped organisms, is scattered over the foot of the tube. Intermediate degrees are also observed. "Standard agglutination" is denoted by absence of the central deposit and bacterial clumps occupying about half the area of the foot of the tube. It has been pointed out that sera with haemolysed red cells may give false positive reactions in low dilutions.

In cases of suspected typhoid fever, standard agglutination in a titre of 10 (dilution 1 in 10) is considered significant, but repeated tests and demonstration of a rising titre would make the result more conclusive. In suspected typhoid carriers a titre of 10 would also be regarded as suggestive.

OTHER AGGLUTINATION TESTS

The agglutination techniques described above are also applicable to diagnostic tests with various *Salmonella* group organisms, *Br. melitensis* or *Br. abortus*, *Proteus* X19 (Weil-Felix reaction of typhus fever), etc. These may be carried out at the same time and in parallel with the Widal test. The series of dilutions tested can, of course, be varied according to the range within which agglutination is likely to occur. It is essential in all cases to make these tests quantitative so that the "titre" or highest dilution in which agglutination occurs, can be estimated.

STREPTOCOCCUS MG AGGLUTINATION TEST

Reagents

(1) *Patient's serum.* 1·0 ml. is required. Two samples of serum should be tested: the first taken during the acute phase of the illness and the second after an interval of 12–18 days.

Note. The sera must not be inactivated at 56° C. as this lowers the titre.

(2) *Streptococcus "MG" Suspension.* Remove the growth from a 48 hour digest broth culture of the organism by centrifugation and wash it three times with sterile saline. Kill the suspension by heating in a water bath at 100° C. for 30 min. After one further washing with saline make the suspension up to a standard density (Brown's opacity tube No. 5, see p. 873) and add merthiolate 1 in 10,000 as a preservative.

(3) *Standard positive rabbit antiserum.*

(4) *Physiological saline.*

The Test

Use 3×½ in. tubes: Set up a rack containing 7 tubes. In the first tube place 0·8 ml. saline and 0·5 ml. in the remaining tubes. Add 0·2 ml. serum to the first tube, mix thoroughly and transfer 0·5 ml. of the mixture to the second tube and continue preparing doubling dilutions to the end of the row. Include a control tube containing 0·5 ml. saline only. To each tube add 0·5 ml. Streptococcus MG suspension. Final serum dilutions are 1 in 10, 1 in 20, 1 in 40, 1 in 80, 1 in 160, 1 in 320, and 1 in 640.

With each batch of tests a titration of the positive rabbit serum should be included.

The tubes are incubated overnight in the water bath at 37° C.

A rising titre between acute and convalescent sera (at least four-fold) is regarded as significant. A titre of 20 or over is regarded by some workers as suggestive.

Sera should not be screened by using a single low dilution tube method as a *prozone* is frequently observed.

"COLD AGGLUTINATION" REACTION

It has been shown that in cases of primary atypical pneumonia the serum may agglutinate at low temperatures human erythrocytes of the blood group O. This reaction is absent in other types of pneumonia, other infections of the respiratory passages and normal individuals, and has been suggested as a means of confirming a diagnosis of atypical pneumonia. The reaction, however, tends to be late in its appearance during the illness. The test can be carried out quantitatively by preparing a series of nine doubling dilutions of serum from 1 in 8 to 1 in 2048 and adding to each an equal volume of a 0·2 per cent. suspension of washed group O human red cells. The mixtures are placed in a refrigerator at 0°–4° C. overnight after which readings of agglutination are made by shaking the tubes and observing clumped cells with the naked eye. As the agglutinin is readily absorbed by erythrocytes at low temperature, the serum should be separated from the blood specimen at a temperature above 20° C. A titre of 32 or 64 (in terms of the final dilution of serum after addition of red cells) may be considered significant, but much higher titres have been recorded.

A high proportion of the cases of primary atypical pneumonia (85–90 per cent.) that have positive cold agglutination reactions are associated with infection with Eaton's agent (*Mycoplasma pneumoniae*, see p. 496).

THE PAUL-BUNNELL REACTION

During and after an attack of infectious mononucleosis an agglutinin for sheep red blood cells is present in the serum and is of diagnostic significance.

The test is performed as follows. Heat the serum at 55° C. for 20 minutes. Make a series of doubling dilutions of the serum with saline in 0·5 ml. amounts in 3-in. × ½-in. tubes, ranging from 1 in 16 to 1 in 1024, as described on p. 910 for agglutination tests. A control tube containing only saline is included. Add to each tube 0·5 ml. of a 1 per cent. suspension of sheep red corpuscles in saline, washed as for the Wassermann test. Shake the tubes thoroughly and incubate at 37° C. for four hr. Note which tubes show agglutination of the red cells, and state the titre of the reaction in terms of the final dilution of the serum: 1st tube, 1 in 32; 2nd, 1 in 64; etc. Normal serum may agglutinate in low dilutions. A suggestive titre is 128. Repeated tests may reveal a rising titre. A significant tire is 256.

If a second reading of results is made after the tubes have stood overnight at room temperature or in the refrigerator, they should be replaced at 37° C. for one or two hr. This avoids fallacious results from "cold agglutination" (p. 914) which is reversible at 37° C. and, so far as is known, is not associated with infective mononucleosis.

It should be noted that the reaction is negative in tuberculosis, leukaemia and Hodgkin's disease.

In persons who have recently received an injection of a therapeutic serum (from the horse), an apparently similar heterophile antibody (Forssman's antibody) may be present in considerable amount in the blood, since horse serum contains the appropriate heterophile antigen and stimulates the production of an antibody for sheep red cells.

It has been pointed out by certain authors that the type of antibody present in infective mononucleosis differs in certain respects from the Forssman antibody, and also from that found in normal serum, and that this difference can be determined by agglutinin-absorption tests as follows:—

Antibody	Treated with emulsion of guinea-pig kidney	Treated with ox red cells
Normal serum	Absorbed	Not absorbed
After serum therapy	Absorbed	Absorbed
Infective mononucleosis	Not absorbed	Absorbed

It may be found, however, that the antibody present after serum therapy is not absorbed by ox red cells and only partially absorbed by guinea-pig kidney tissue, *i.e.* more closely resembles the antibody in normal serum.

The following method, a modification of Barrett's (1941) technique, may be adopted for determining these absorption effects.

Reagents

1. *Patient's serum.*—1·0 ml. is required. Heat the serum in a water-bath at 56° C. for 30 min.

2. *Physiological saline.*

3. 20 *per cent. guinea-pig kidney emulsion in saline.*—Take several fresh guinea-pig kidneys and, after removing any fat, cut into small pieces with scissors. Wash several times with saline to remove all the blood, and mash

the tissue into a fine pulp in a mortar. To the pulp add four times its volume of saline and boil in a water-bath for 1 hr. Allow to cool, and add sufficient 5 per cent. phenol to give a final concentration of 0·5 per cent. Make up to original volume with distilled water.

4. 20 *per cent. ox red cell suspension in saline.*—Make a 20 per cent. suspension of washed ox cells in saline and treat in exactly the same way as the 20 per cent. guinea-pig kidney emulsion described above.

(*Note*: Both these antigens keep well at 4° C.)

5. 2 *per cent. suspension of sheep red cells.*—Wash the sheep cells in saline and make a 2 per cent. suspension in saline. The cells should be more than one day and less than seven days old.

The Test

Use 3-in. × $\frac{3}{8}$-in. test-tubes.

In three separate test-tubes (*a*), (*b*) and (*c*) place:

(*a*) 1·0 ml. saline.
(*b*) 1·25 ml.[1] of guinea-pig kidney emulsion.
(*c*) 1·25 ml.[1] of ox cell suspension.

To each tube add 0·25 ml. of heated serum. Allow to stand for one hr. at room temperature, and then centrifuge tubes (*b*) and (*c*).

Set up a rack containing three rows of 10 tubes. Into the last 9 of each row put 0·25 ml. saline. Into the first 2 tubes of the front row place 0·25 ml. of the diluted serum (*a*). From the mixture in the second tube carry over 0·25 ml. to the third tube, and continue doubling dilutions to the end of the row. Repeat this process using the supernatant fluid from (*b*) and (*c*) in the middle and back rows respectively.

To every tube add 0·1 ml. of the 2 per cent. suspension of sheep cells and mix thoroughly by shaking.

The final serum dilutions are 1 in 7, 1 in 14, 1 in 28, 1 in 56, etc.

The test is read, after the tubes have stood for 24 hr. at room temperature, by removing the tubes from the rack and attempting to re-suspend the cells by flicking the tubes with the finger. The end-point is the highest dilution of serum in which the cells cannot be evenly suspended. The end-point can be made more clear-cut if the tubes are centrifuged for 2 min. before re-suspension of the cells is attempted.

A preliminary report can be made after the test has been set up for an hour, if the tubes are centrifuged before making the reading, but a final report should be postponed until the following day.

A typical report in a case of glandular fever would be:

Heterophile agglutinin for sheep cells present in dilutions up to 1 in 448. The agglutinin is completely absorbed by ox cell suspension, but unaffected by guinea-pig kidney emulsion. Using the absorption technique, as detailed above, even a titre of 28 in rows (*a*) and (*b*) is significant.

TESTS FOR RHEUMATOID ARTHRITIS SERUM FACTOR

Sheep red blood cells sensitised with a rabbit anti-sheep erythrocyte serum are agglutinated by the sera of 70–80 per cent. of patients with rheumatoid arthritis and positive reactions occur in some 2–5 per cent. of normal

[1] The extra quantity of material in these tubes is because 1·25 ml. of a 20 per cent. emulsion or suspension contains only 1·0 ml. of fluid.

subjects. It is known that the serum factor concerned is a macroglobulin which may represent an index of some inherited metabolic disturbance which predisposes the individual to rheumatoid arthritis (Kellgren & Ball, 1959).

The factor behaves in many respects as an antibody to denatured γ globulin (see Glynn, 1963) and this property is used to detect its presence in serum. Either sheep red cells coated with rabbit anti-sheep cell serum or latex particles coated with human γ globulin are agglutinated by serum containing the factor.

Rose-Waaler test or *Differential sheep cell agglutination test* (*DAT*).

Reagents.—The sensitising serum is prepared by the method on p. 936. The neat rabbit-serum is stable in the frozen state for several months. In the test the serum is used at a dilution that just fails to agglutinate erythrocytes but which contains as high a haemolytic titre (see p. 936) as possible. Its haemagglutinating activity is determined by adding a 2 per cent. suspension of sheep red blood cells to two series of four doubling serum dilutions, one beginning at 1 in 50, and the other at 1 in 70. After incubation for 1 hr. at 37° C. a reading is taken. The end point is the first tube in which cells show no agglutination and in which the cells have settled into a completely negative button.

Sensitised red cells are prepared by mixing equal volumes of the haemolytic antiserum at its determined requisite dilution and a 2 per cent. suspension of sheep cells. Sensitisation is rapid and the cells may be used within a few minutes.

The Test.—The patient's serum, previously inactivated for 30 min. at 56° C., is serially diluted in two-fold steps from 1 in 2 to 1 in 1024. Two sets of these dilutions are required; to one set is added an equal volume of sensitised cells while the second set serves as a serum control and receives an equal volume of 1·0 per cent. unsensitised sheep cells. The tubes are incubated for one hour at 37° C. and then placed in the refrigerator until the cells have completely settled. The reading is according to the pattern of sedimented cells and the end point is taken as the last tube to show definite haemagglutination.

Instead of the saline diluent some workers prefer to use 2·5 per cent. sheep serum in saline. This has the effect of increasing the sensitivity of the test without loss of specificity. The titre of positive sera is increased by this method from two- to eight-fold but the test is rather more difficult to read and end points are not so clear cut.

Serum titres of 16 or more are taken as positive and are found in rheumatoid arthritis in 70–80 per cent. of cases, and also in some cases of disseminated lupus erythromatosis, scleroderma, and erythema multiforme.

AGGLUTINATION TESTS USED FOR THE SEROLOGICAL IDENTIFICATION OF CERTAIN ORGANISMS BY MEANS OF SPECIFIC ANTISERA

In this case the series of dilutions depends on the titre of the serum for the homologous organism. Thus, if the titre were 16,000, the following range of dilutions might be tested: 1 in 1000 *to* 1 in 32,000 in a series of doubling dilutions. In general, for identification of an unknown organism it should agglutinate in approximately as high a serum-dilution as a known homologous organism.

If the organism is a motile species and it is desired to identify both H and

O antigens, formolised and alcoholised suspensions respectively are tested with H and O agglutinating antisera (*vide infra*). It should be noted that in the *Salmonella* group the H antigen may occur in two phases, one of which may have non-specific characters. The serological identification of these organisms is considered more fully on p. 233 *et seq.*

Special applications of the agglutination technique, *e.g.* in the identification of serological types, are referred to elsewhere.

SLIDE AGGLUTINATION

This method is useful where only small quantities of culture are available, as in the identification of the whooping-cough bacillus, or where agglutination is carried out with undiluted serum, *e.g.* in typing pneumococci or typing streptococci by Griffith's method, and it is necessary to use as small a quantity as possible. The method may be applied likewise for identifying organisms of the *Salmonella* and dysentery groups. Slide agglutination is only practicable when the clumping of organisms occurs within a minute or so; it is not suitable where the mixture of organisms and serum has to be incubated.

The procedure can be carried out quite readily on an ordinary slide, but where a number of agglutination tests have to be made it is more convenient to use a piece of ¼-in. polished plate glass about 6 in.×2 in. A long horizontal line is ruled with a grease pencil through the middle of the glass from end to end and then a number of lines are ruled at ½-in. intervals at right angles to this line, thereby dividing the glass into a series of divisions.

A drop of saline is placed in one of the divisions and a small amount of culture from a solid medium emulsified in it by means of an inoculating loop. It is then examined through a hand-lens (8 or 10×), or the low-power microscope, to ascertain that the suspension is even and that the bacteria are well separated and not in visible clumps. With a small loop, 1½ mm. diameter, made from thin platinum wire take up a drop of the serum and place it on the slide just beside the bacterial suspension. Mix the serum and bacterial suspension and examine with the hand lens, or place on the stage of the microscope. Agglutination when it occurs is rapid and the clumps can be seen with the naked eye, but the use of some form of magnification is an advantage. For control purposes, two drops of saline can be placed in adjacent divisions and bacterial culture emulsified in both, one only being mixed with the serum. With streptococci a broth culture is used, and methods for obtaining suitable suspensions for the agglutination test are described on p. 161. Two drops of suspension are placed on the slide and a small loopful of the serum mixed with one of them and examined as described above.

While the slide agglutination test is rapid and convenient, its limitations must be realised. In order to obtain rapid agglutination the serum is used undiluted or in low dilutions. In consequence, it may contain normal agglutinins which give non-specific agglutination with organisms other than that against which the serum was prepared. Thus, with regard to the *Salmonella* group particularly, slide agglutination with its high concentration of agglutinins may show low-titre reactions with organisms outside the group, *e.g.* '*paracolon bacilli*' which may also have somewhat similar biochemical reactions. It is important therefore to confirm the slide test by quantitative tests in tubes, particularly when any doubt arises or where precise results from agglutination tests are desired.

PREPARATION OF AGGLUTINATING ANTISERA

The instructions given here apply particularly to organisms of the *Salmonella* and dysentery groups.

Rabbits are used for immunisation, and large healthy animals should be selected, not under 2000 g. in weight.

The purity and identity of the culture used should be carefully ascertained beforehand, and in view of variability in antigenic composition the culture selected should be such that it represents the motile "smooth" form and the specific phase of the particular species (pp. 115, 235).

The rabbits are injected intravenously (p. 1010) at intervals of five to seven days with a suspension in saline of a 24 hr. slope culture killed by exposure for one hour at 60° C. The following series of doses may be given: 1/20, 1/10, 1/5, 1/3, and 1/2 culture. These doses are easily measured by emulsifying a slope culture in a given volume of saline and then injecting the appropriate fraction.

In the case of organisms of high toxicity, e.g. *Sh. shigae*, it is necessary to start with even lower doses, *e.g.* 1/100 of a culture.

Other methods for standardising dosage may be used, *e.g.* where the doses are stated in terms of the number of organisms, as in the administration of vaccines, but the system indicated above is simple and sufficiently accurate for ordinary purposes.

With certain organisms, e.g. *Salmonella* group, higher titres may be obtained if living organisms are injected. To commence with, very small amounts, *e.g.* 0·01 ml., of a young living broth culture should be injected intravenously. As the animal becomes immune larger doses may be given until several ml. of the living culture can be tolerated.

When separate H and O agglutinating antisera are required for motile bacteria, immunisation is best carried out with selected strains known to be suitable for the purpose. For the production of the O agglutinin a culture boiled for 2½ hr. is used as the antigen. A non-motile variant also serves well as a pure O antigen.

Seven to ten days after the last injection a specimen of blood is withdrawn from an ear vein (p. 1010) and the serum is tested for its agglutinating power towards the strain used for immunisation. In making tests with H and O antisera, formolised and alcoholised suspensions respectively are used. A series of dilutions is tested and if agglutination occurs in a 1 in 1600 or higher dilution,[1] the animal is bled from the neck vessels or by cardiac puncture (p. 1011), the blood is allowed to coagulate in a sterile stoppered or screw-capped bottle, placed overnight in the refrigerator, and the serum is then separated. 0·1 ml. of a 5 per cent. solution of phenol in physiological salt solution is added for each ml. of the serum—equivalent to 0·5 per cent. pure phenol. This prevents bacterial growth resulting from any accidental contamination. (Glycerol may also be used as a preservative, an equal volume being added to the serum, or 0·1 per cent. *p*-chloro-*n*-cresol.) The serum may be stored in 1-ml. or 5-ml. stoppered or screw-capped bottles, or ampoules may be used. Alternatively, it may be kept in sterile glass tubes (5–7 mm. bore), about 1 ml. in capacity, drawn out at both ends to capillary dimensions; the tubes are filled by suction, applying the mouth-piece used in pipetting (p. 911), and the ends are sealed in the Bunsen flame. The serum should be kept in the refrigerator (about

[1] More powerful agglutinating sera may, of course, be obtained; 1600 is merely the *minimum* titre that should be aimed at.

4° C.) and will retain its potency for long periods (three years). The temperature should not be allowed to fall below 0° C. if phenol is used as a preservative, as the solidification of the serum by freezing may be deleterious owing to the separation out of the phenol in the pure state. If a refrigerator at −30° C. is available, antisera frozen solid can be preserved over a long period. In this case no preservative is added to the serum.

Antisera can be preserved in the dry state by freeze drying (p. 808). The potency of antisera is retained over a considerably longer period when freeze-dried than when stored in fluid form.

AGGLUTININ-ABSORPTION TESTS

Agglutinins, like other antibodies, combine firmly with their homologous antigens, and by treating an agglutinating antiserum with the homologous bacteria and then separating the organisms by centrifuging, it is found that the agglutinin has been "absorbed" or removed by the organisms from the serum.

In certain cases, to prove the serological identity of an unknown strain with a particular species, it may be necessary to show not only that it is agglutinated by a specific antiserum to approximately its titre but also that it can absorb from the serum the agglutinins for the known organism. This becomes necessary owing to the fact that, on immunising an animal with a particular bacterium, "group antibodies" for allied organisms are developed, and in some cases these may act in relatively high titre. "Absorption" with a heterologous strain would remove only the group agglutinins without affecting the specific agglutinin. These effects are exemplified in the *Salmonella* and *Brucella* groups. The general method of carrying out such absorption tests is to mix a dense suspension of the organism—*e.g.* 24 hours' growth on a 4-in. plate of nutrient agar, suspended in 1 ml. saline and killed at 60° C. (30 min.)—with an equal volume of a suitable dilution of the serum, *e.g.* 64 times the concentration of the known titre. (The bacterial growth must have been thoroughly washed with normal salt solution, *i.e.* by mixing with several volumes of saline, centrifuging and repeating the process 2–3 times). Thus, if the titre is 1600, the dilution used would be 1 in 25. The mixture is incubated for three to four hr. at 37° C. and the serum is then separated from the bacteria in a high-speed centrifuge. (In some cases for complete absorption the process may require to be repeated with a similar fresh quantity of bacteria.) The dilution of the serum would now be approximately double the original dilution—in the example taken (*vide supra*) 1 in 50. From the treated serum a series of doubling dilutions is prepared as in direct agglutination tests, so that, when an equal volume of bacterial suspension is added, the series will reach to the known titre of the serum. In the example taken above, the following series of dilutions would be tested:

1 in 50   1 in 100   1 in 200   1 in 400   1 in 800,

and after the addition of bacterial suspension these would become

1 in 100   1 in 200   1 in 400   1 in 800   1 in 1600

A control tube is also included, containing suspension but no serum, and the general technique is that employed in direct agglutination tests.

Thus, the identity or non-identity of an unknown culture (*X*) with a known (*A*) may be investigated by agglutinin-absorption as follows:

1. Absorb, as above, antiserum to *A* with a dense suspension of organism *X*=*X*-absorbed serum.

2. Test the agglutinating power of *X*-absorbed serum for *A* and *X*.

(A control test would show that the antiserum to *A* after absorption with *A* agglutinates neither organism.)

Results

(*a*) The absorbed serum agglutinates neither *A* nor *X*. This indicates that the organisms are identical, because *X* has absorbed agglutinins for *A*; to establish this conclusion completely an antiserum to *X* after absorption with *A* should agglutinate neither organism.

(*b*) The absorbed serum fails to agglutinate *X*, but still agglutinates *A*. This shows that the organisms are not identical, because *X* has not absorbed the agglutinins for *A*, though it has removed the heterologous agglutinins.

COATED-PARTICLE AGGLUTINATION REACTIONS

The inert particles of polystyrene latex, collodion and bentonite, and red cells both treated with tannic acid and untreated, can be coated with a variety of protein antigens and also in the case of untreated red cells, with polysaccharide antigens. They can then be used for the detection of antibody as shown by the agglutination of the coated particles. The haemagglutination tests are the most sensitive and can detect as little as 0·003 μg. of antibody measured as antibody nitrogen, which is about 10 times more sensitive than the most sensitive gel diffusion techniques (see p. 948).

The value of these tests has increased considerably with the development of techniques for storing antigen-coated red cell preparations. A large batch of cells can be coated with antigen and a standardised preparation is then available for use for some months afterwards. Of the various methods available probably the most useful is that described by Csizmas (1960) in which the cells are formalinised by placing a dialysis bag of formalin into a beaker of carefully washed cells. After recovery from the formalin, the cells can be stored in the refrigerator and after tanning and coating with the antigen, they may be stored at −20° C. These techniques have the advantage that in common with other agglutination reactions they can be used as antibody titration methods. A large variety of antigens can be adsorbed on to cells or particles, and even two different antigens have been applied to the same red cells (Lecocq & Linz, 1962) or latex particles (Singer *et al.*, 1961). The methods are simple to use and once a particular test is standardised reproducible results can be obtained.

Tanned Red Cell Agglutination Tests

The surfaces of red blood cells are altered and the cells rendered much more agglutinable by treatment with tannic acid. This enables cells coated with various antigens—proteins and viruses—to be agglutinated by specific antibody. The method here described employs thyroglobulin but this could be replaced by any one of a large number of antigens. (For detailed consideration of the application of the test to the detection of thyroglobulin autoantibodies see Fulthorpe *et al.*, 1961.)

Reagents

(1) Phosphate buffered saline 0·15 *M* KH_2PO_4, 0·15 *M* Na_2HPO_4 mixed in suitable proportions (see Chapter 50) to give the pH required—

e.g. pH 7·2 for the thyroglobulin antibody test. One volume of this buffer is added to 9 volumes of 0·85 per cent NaCl.

(2) Tannic acid solution, 1 in 20,000 made up fresh before use (12·5 mg. of analytical grade tannic acid[1] dissolved in 250 ml. of the buffer).

(3) Defibrinated sheep blood not more than 1–2 days old.

(4) Antigen at a concentration of 2 mg./ml. in the buffered saline *e.g.* human thyroglobulin prepared by the method of Derrien, Michel and Roche (1948).

(5) 0·85 per cent. NaCl.

(6) Rabbit or horse serum which has been inactivated for 30 min. at 56° C. and absorbed for 10 min. at room temperature with washed sheep red blood cells (approx. 0·1 ml. of packed cells to 10 ml. of serum).

Method[2]

(1) Wash about 20 ml. of the sheep blood three times (twice with 0·85 per cent. NaCl and once with the phosphate buffered saline) in a one-ounce universal container. Centrifuge finally at 750 *G.*[3] for 15 min. to pack the cells.

(2) Pipette 0·6 ml. of the packed cells into each of two universal containers and add 10 ml. of buffered saline to each bottle to resuspend the cells.

(3) Add 10 ml. of the 1 in 20,000 tannic acid solution to each container, shake and incubate for 15 min. at 37° C.

(4) Centrifuge the bottles at 750 *G.* for 5 min. and discard the supernatant, resuspend cells in each container in 20 ml. of buffer, centrifuge for a similar period and discard the supernatant.

(5) Lay one container of cells aside; this will be used as the source of uncoated cells for absorbing the heterophile agglutinins in the sera to be tested, and for various controls.

(6) Resuspend the cells in the other container in 10 ml. of buffer and then add 10 ml. of buffer containing the antigen to be coated on to the cells. Incubate for 30 min. at 37° C. shaking occasionally.

(7) Centrifuge the coated cells for 5 min. at 750 *G.* and remove the supernatant.

(8) Wash these cells and the cells set aside (5) three times with the buffered saline made up to contain 1 per cent. normal rabbit or horse serum (previously inactivated and absorbed), centrifuge for 5 min. at 750 *G.* on each occasion and discard the supernatant. (Make sure each bottle is correctly labelled.)

(9) Finally make up both batches of cells, *i.e.* the coated and the uncoated, to 50 ml. with the buffer to which has been added the 1 per cent. serum as in (8).

The Test

(1) Inactivate the test sera for 30 min. at 56° C. (not necessary for formalinised cells *vide infra.*).

(2) Add 0·1 ml. of inactivated serum to 0·9 ml. of the uncoated cell preparation, leave on bench for 15 min. and centrifuge for 5 min. at 750 *G.* to recover the serum—which is now diluted 1 in 10.

[1] Obtainable from Merk Biochemical Corp., U.S.A. or Hopkin and Williams, Freshwater Road, Chadwell Heath, Essex.

[2] As modified by W. J. Herbert, 1967.

[3] About 2300 r.p.m. in an MSE Minor bench centrifuge—see conversion formula page 867.

(3) Make 8 or more doubling or trebling dilutions of the serum in the buffered saline in 0·1 ml. volumes using a WHO plate. Add 0·1 ml. of the 1 per cent. coated cells to each well and to a control well containing 0·1 ml. of buffer only. Set up controls using uncoated cells with and without serum.

Read first for agglutination after 2 hr. on the bench (20° C.) and after leaving overnight at 4° C. The end point is taken as the last cup showing a smooth mat of agglutinated cells with a crenated rim. Doubtful results appear as a smaller circle of cells having a dark outer rim and a negative result shows as a closely packed button of cells. The controls should always be negative.

Formalinisation of red cells (prior to tanning and coating)

Mammalian or avian red blood cells can conveniently be preserved by the method of Csizmas (1960). The treated cells are morphologically identical to normal red cells and withstand treatment with water or freezing and thawing. They may even be freeze dried without damage. They retain most of the surface properties of fresh red cells and can be tanned and coated with antigens or agglutinated by viruses.

Method

(1) Fresh (sheep) blood is washed five times with 0·85 per cent. saline and the cells packed after the final wash (for 15 min. at 750 *G*.). (It is important to avoid any lysis).

(2) 25 ml. of packed cells are resuspended to 200 ml. in phosphate buffered saline pH 7·2 and placed in a 500 ml. conical flask.

(3) 50 ml. of formalin (40 per cent. formaldehyde) is introduced into a length of dialysis tubing and tied off so that the tubing is only $\frac{2}{3}$ full, but air is excluded, *i.e.* the knot is tied in the tubing which has not been distended with air one third of the total length of the tubing above the top of the formalin.

(4) The two-thirds filled dialysis tube is submerged in the cell suspension in the conical flask, stoppered, and the whole *gently* agitated for 3–4 hr. at o om temperature (20° C.) . Gross foaming should be avoided (a Matburn blood cell suspension mixer with a wire mesh glassware crate attached is a suitable arrangement).

(5) After 3–4 hr. the swollen dialysis sac is punctured, the formalin allowed to mix directly with the cells and the empty sac removed. Gentle mixing is continued overnight.

(6) At the end of this period the dark brown cell suspension is carefully decanted from the flask into centrifuge bottles, leaving the surface scum of froth and damaged cells behind (the cells may be filtered through gauze to achieve this). The cells are then washed 5 times with 0·9 per cent. saline to remove the formalin (for 10 min. at 750 *G*.). Gentle stirring of the deposit with a glass rod helps to ensure adequate resuspension at each wash.

(7) The cells are finally made up to a 25 or a 50 per cent. suspension in 0·85 per cent. saline and stored at 4° C. or at −20° C. to be made up to a 1 per cent. suspension before use.

The supernatant from the first wash after formalinisation is normally very dark.

Latex Fixation Test for Rheumatoid Factor

The following is a simplification of the method of Singer and Plotz (1956).

Reagents

(1) Polystyrene latex uniform sized particles 0·81 μ in diameter (Difco Bacto-latex).[1] Add 20 ml. of distilled water to 2 ml. of the latex suspension and filter through Whatman 40 filter paper (the suspension will keep for months at 4° C.).

(2) Borate buffer pH 8·2 (see page 855).

(3) Stock gamma-globulin solution—0·5 per cent. in borate buffer. To 0·1 g. of lyophilised human fraction II gamma-globulin[2] add borate buffer in small increments, mixing well until 20 ml. have been added and the gamma globulin completely dissolved. This preparation will keep for several weeks at 4° C.

The Test. (Bywaters & Scott, 1960)

(1) Add 1 ml. of the borate buffer to a series of $3 \times \frac{1}{2}$ tubes, include one tube for each test serum and one for a positive control and another for a control with buffer only.

(2) Inactivate the sera for 30 min. at 56° C. and add 0·05 ml. of serum to each tube (*i.e.* a dilution of 1 in 21 of the serum).

(3) To each serum dilution and to the controls add 1 ml. of a mixture containing 1 per cent. stock latex and 5 per cent. stock gamma globulin in borate buffer (for 10 ml. add 0·1 ml. of stock latex and 0·5 ml. of stock gamma-globulin to 9·5 ml. of buffer).

(4) Shake the tubes carefully and incubate in a 56° C. water bath for 2 hr.

(5) Prior to reading the tests centrifuge for 3 min. at 1000 *G*.

Readings

Opaque suspension, no deposit, −ve.

Opaque suspension, minimal deposit, ± doubtful

Partially cleared suspension, granular deposit, +

Clear or almost clear supernatant, granular deposit, ++

A reading of + or ++ is regarded as positive, ± is of doubtful significance.

FLOCCULATION TESTS FOR SYPHILIS

The direct mixture of syphilitic sera with antigens of the type used in the Wassermann reaction results in the appearance of a flocculent deposit which is easily seen with the hand lens and which may also be visible to the naked eye. Such reactions, however, may occur in non-syphilitic infections (*e.g.* tuberculosis, leprosy, malaria, hepatitis, infectious mononucleosis, etc.) and the tests are therefore sensitive to many different types of infection. It is, however, possible to reduce the sensitivity of the reaction by adjusting the conditions under which the test is performed and to render the test almost specific for syphilis; many flocculation reactions give results that are closely parallel to those of the complement-fixation technique. The value of flocculation tests lies in the simplicity of the technique employed and the fact that they can be carried out in places where complement and the reagents of the haemolytic system of the Wassermann test are not available. Ideally the tests are used as a first screening investigation and any positive sera are then subjected to the full Wassermann test. Many varieties of the flocculation reaction are described and the Meinicke, Hinton, Mazzini and Kahn tests are all in common use together with the test employing the cardiolipid

[1] Baird & Tatlock Ltd., London.

[2] Nutritional Biochemical Corporation, U.S.A., obtainable through L. Light & Co., Colnbrook, Bucks. or Kodak Ltd., Kirkby, Liverpool.

antigen devised by the Venereal Disease Research Laboratory. This latter test has been in use in the Bacteriology Department of Edinburgh University and can be recommended as a simple and reliable technique.

THE VDRL FLOCCULATION TEST

A rapid screening test which is simple to perform is of great value in dealing with large numbers of sera. The following method is that described in the Bulletin of WHO (1951) and is very satisfactory. The following reagents are required.

(1) *Antigen.* This has the following composition:

Cardiolipin . . .	0·03 per cent.
Lecithin . . .	0·24 per cent.
Cholesterol . . .	0·9 per cent.

It may be purchased from Messrs. Burroughs Wellcome & Co., London.

(2) *Diluent.* Buffered saline prepared as follows:

Formaldehyde, neutral reagent grade . .	0·5 ml.
Na_2HPO_4, $12H_2O$	0·093 g.
KH_2PO_4	0·170 g.
NaCl	10·0 g.
Distilled water	1000 ml.

This solution has a pH of $6 \cdot 0 \pm 0 \cdot 1$.

(3) *Unbuffered Saline.* 1·0 per cent. sodium chloride.

(4) *Serum under test.* Prepared and inactivated as for the Wassermann test.

(5) *Antigen Emulsion.* In a stoppered bottle place 0·4 ml. of the buffered saline and add to it drop by drop from a pipette 0·5 ml. of antigen. Ensure that the antigen is added during a period of approximately 6 sec. and that the bottle is continuously rotated during this time. After the addition, the bottle is rotated vigorously for a further 10 sec. Now add 3·6 ml. of 1·0 per cent. unbuffered saline. Mix well and allow to stand for 5 min., but not longer than 2 hr., before use.

The Qualitative Serum Test

Use $3 \times \frac{1}{2}$ in. tubes. Transfer 0·5 ml. inactivated serum to a tube and add to it 0·5 ml. diluted antigen. Place in a rack in the Kahn shaker and shake for 5 min. The tubes are now spun at about 2000 r.p.m. for 10 min. in a straight-headed centrifuge. After this the tubes are shaken again for exactly one minute and the test is read at once. Visible aggregation in a clear or very faintly turbid medium are read as positive. A slightly turbid appearance with a "silken swirl" on gentle shaking is the typical negative appearance. All borderline reactions should be reported as negative. The test can be used quantitatively with serial doubling dilutions of the patient's serum, ranging from 1 in 2 to 1 in 64. The weakest dilution giving a positive reaction is reported as the titre of the serum.

THE KAHN FLOCCULATION TEST

Apparatus required

(1) Small test-tubes, $3 \times \frac{1}{2}$ in., as used in the Wassermann test; these tubes should be of perfectly clear glass and thoroughly clean.

(2) Flat-bottom glass cylinders, $1\frac{1}{2} \times \frac{1}{2}$ in., for the preparation of the diluted antigen.

(3) 1 ml. and 0·1 ml. graduated pipettes as used in the Wassermann test.

(4) Special pipettes: one graduated from the tip to deliver 0·0125, 0·025 and 0·05 ml. respectively; the other with one graduation to deliver 0·15 ml.

(5) Suitable racks for the tubes.

Reagents

(1) Patient's serum—at least 0·5 ml. required.

(2) Antigen[1]—"Bacto" Kahn standard antigen which can be obtained commercially[2] is also recommended as being satisfactory in stability and sensitivity. Alternatively, it can be made from "Bacto" Beef Heart.[2]

(3) 0·85 per cent. sodium chloride in distilled water.

(4) Control sera—at least four should be included in any set of tests; these should be selected according to previous results as follows: Negative, +, + +, + + + (*vide infra*). All sera tested are heated at 55° C. for 30 min. before testing. For full details of the test and the preparation of the antigen see Kahn (1928).

Dilution of antigen

The antigen is diluted with saline in the proportions prescribed for the preparation—usually 1 to 1·1.

(1) Ascertain the total volume of diluted antigen required for the set of tests by multiplying the number of sera by 0·0875 ml. (the volume of diluted antigen required for one serum) and adding to this figure 0·3 ml. for loss in pipetting, etc. No more than is sufficient for 40 tests should be made up at one time.

(2) Pipette *separately* into each of two small cylinders (referred to above) the volumes of normal saline and undiluted antigen required to yield in the prescribed proportions the total bulk of diluted antigen.

(3) Add the saline from one cylinder rapidly to the antigen in the other and mix by pouring from one cylinder to the other five or six times.

The diluted antigen should be used for the test not less than 10 min. and not more than 30 min. after mixture.

The *test* for each serum is set up as follows:

Tube	1	2	3
Add *diluted antigen* . .	0·05 ml.	0·025 ml.	0·0125 ml.
Add *serum*	0·15 ml.	0·15 ml	0·15 ml.

The tubes are shaken by hand or preferably in a special shaking machine at 270 oscillations a minute for 3 min. (After shaking, incubation in a water-bath at 37° C. for 15 min. or an incubator at 37° C. for 20 min. is advantageous.)

Then add *saline* . .	1·0 ml.	0·5 ml.	0·5 ml.

Readings are now made.

The following *antigen control* is included in each set of tests:

Tube	1	2	3
Add *diluted antigen* . .	0·05 ml.	0·025 ml.	0·0125 ml.
Add *saline* . . .	0·15 ml.	0·15 ml.	0·15 ml.

[1] Obtainable from Medical Research Council Venereal Diseases Reference Laboratory, Ashfield Street, Whitechapel, London, E.1.

[2] Obtainable from Baird & Tatlock Ltd., London.

Shake tubes as above.
Incubate as above.
Then add *saline* . . 1·0 ml. 0·5 ml. 0·5 ml.

Note.—Instead of using a calibrated volumetric pipette for the antigen dilution, a dropping pipette, external diameter at the tip equivalent to a No. 55 Morse gauge hole of a Starrett plate, may be substituted. One drop from this pipette equals 0·025 ml., two drops equal 0·05 ml., and four drops equal 0·1 ml. For patient's serum a pipette with external diameter of 2·8 mm. will deliver 0·15 ml. of serum in three drops at the rate of one drop per sec. (Khairat, 1952).

Reading of results.—The tubes should be held in a sloped position and the fluid viewed (if necessary with an 8× hand-lens) in a strong light against a dark background or the concave surface of a microscope mirror.

The following results may be observed in individual tubes:
− = the fluid remaining uniformly opalescent.
+ = minute floccules just visible to the naked eye throughout the fluid.
+ + + + = large floccules sedimenting completely in the tube.
+ + and + + + = intermediate degrees of flocculation.

The interpretation of results is illustrated as follows:

Tube	1	2	3	Average Result	Diagnostic interpretation
Serum A	++++	++++	++++ }	++++	Strongly positive
,, B	+++	++++	++++ }		
,, C	++++	+++	+++ }	+++	Strongly positive
,, D	+++	+++	++++ }		
,, E	+++	++	++ }	++	Positive
,, F	+	++	++ }		
,, G	+	+	++	+	Weakly positive
,, H	−	±	++	±	Doubtful
,, I	−	−	−	−	Negative

THE KAHN VERIFICATION TEST

This test was introduced by Kahn (1940, 1941) with the object of ascertaining whether weak or doubtful reactions obtained by his standard flocculation test are non-specific or definitely significant of syphilitic infection. From studies of "false positive" reactions he concluded that a positive result may in some cases be related to biological changes apart from syphilic infection but that this non-specific reaction can often be differentiated from the true syphilis reaction by the occurrence of a stronger effect at 2° C. than at 37° C. or the absence of flocculation at the higher temperature. He has called this the "general biologic type" of reaction and regards it as non-syphilitic, the reaction in the syphilitic case being usually stronger at 37° C. than at lower temperatures.

In carrying out such comparative tests at different temperatures the reagents before mixing must be adjusted to the particular temperature. Thus, for the test at 37° C., pipettes, tubes and racks are placed in a 37° C. water-bath for fifteen minutes before performance of the test, and likewise the diluted antigen, serum and saline are similarly kept at 37° C. before the mixtures are made; further, at all stages of the test the required temperature is maintained as far as possible. In carrying out the test at the low temperature, an ice-water bath can be used in the same way as the 37° C. water-bath, the working temperature being about 2° C. Otherwise the test is performed as in the standard procedure (p. 925).

The various types of comparative results are illustrated in the following Table:

At 37° C.	At room temperature.	At 2° C.	Classification of result
++++ or +++ ++	++ −	+ or − −	Syphilitic
+ or − −	++ −	++++ or +++ ++	General Biologic
++ − ++	++ + −	++ − ++	Inconclusive
−	−	−	Negative

It may be noted that the application of this "verification" test has shown that the sensitivity of the syphilitic reaction is increased at 37° C. as compared with room temperature, *i.e.* the temperature of the standard test.

The comparative test at 37° C. and 2° C. is of value when the usual Kahn reaction is weak or doubtful or when there is some discrepancy between the serological result and the clinical findings. It is of similar value when other syphilis serum tests also give a weak or doubtful result. Of course, it must be recognised that in a proportion of such cases even the "verification" test is inconclusive.

COMPLEMENT FIXATION METHODS

Complement fixation techniques are among the most frequently used serological methods and can be employed with either soluble or particulate antigens for the detection either of antigen or of antibody, Fig. 73 (see Chapter 8 for a description of the general mechanism). The great sensitivity of the complement fixation test is useful for the detection of antibodies to soluble antigens where visible precipitates usually only form with quantities of over 1 μg. of antibody nitrogen. As little as 0·08 μg. of antibody nitrogen has been detected by means of complement fixation. The quantitative complement fixation method of Mayer *et al.* (1948) has been widely used for the quantitative determination of antigens and to study their physical and chemical character. Studies of this type employed photometric methods for the measurement of haemolysis and have taken into account the role of calcium and magnesium ions in the reaction. It was pointed out by Wallace, Osler and Mayer (1950) that the complement fixing titre of antiserum is not strictly a reflection of the antibody content of the serum since different samples of rabbit antisera to bovine serum albumin containing the same amount of antibody nitrogen may vary in their capacity to fix complement. Correlation with the immunisation schedules showed that the animals which had received two courses of immunisation fixed more complement per unit of antibody than less highly immunised animals. Thus the complement fixing titre of an antiserum is a reflection of both the quantity and quality of an antibody.

One of the important problems associated with complement fixation tests is that of the anti-complementary activity of the serum. Anticomplementary effects may result from the aggregation of gamma-globulins such as takes place on heating or other forms of denaturation or when abnormal or raised gamma globulins are present as in myelomatosis and systemic lupus erythematosus. The anti-complementary activity that may develop in normal serum kept at room temperature for a few days, presents no problem as it can be eliminated easily by heating at 56° C. for 30 minutes. Unfortunately other anticomplementary activities of antisera and antigens are not sufficiently understood to enable the serologist to overcome them regularly. It is, however, very important to take into account these anticomplementary effects when carrying out the determination of the amount of complement for use in any particular test.

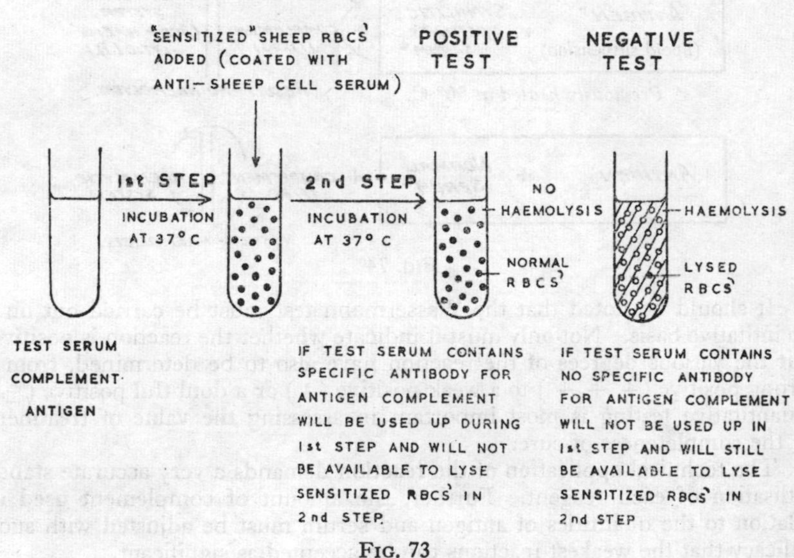

FIG. 73

The conglutinating complement adsorption test.—When sheep red cells coated with anti-sheep cell antibody are mixed with fresh horse serum, the horse complement is bound to the antibody coated cells but will not lyse the cells as horse complement is non-lytic. If these cells are exposed to bovine serum they will be agglutinated due to the presence of a globulin component known as *conglutinin.* Should the horse complement have been bound by another antigen antibody system it will not be available to react with the sensitised sheep cells and thus on the addition of bovine serum the cells will not be agglutinated. This is the basis of the conglutinating complement absorption test re-developed by Coombs and his associates (see Coombs, Coombs, and Ingram, 1960).

WASSERMANN SYPHILIS REACTION

This reaction depends on the "fixation" of complement by a suspension of a phosphatide lipoid (similar to lecithin and extracted from certain normal animal tissues) along with the *heated* serum of a person infected with syphilis, and constitutes an important diagnostic test.

For complement-fixation tests, an indicator of the presence of complement is required. The "haemolytic system" used in these tests serves this purpose (p. 935). It consists of the red corpuscles of a particular animal species "sensitised" with the corresponding haemolytic antibody, *e.g.* the red cells of the ox or sheep *plus* the serum of a rabbit that has been immunised with the red cells of the species used. The immune body in the serum is thermostable. The serum is heated at 56° C. to annul the natural complement, and stored in bottles or tubes or preserved in the dry state (*vide infra*). The heated serum is non-haemolytic by itself, but in the presence of a suitable complement brings about lysis of the homologous red corpuscles. Fixation of complement is denoted by the absence of lysis in the haemolytic system.

In its simplest form the Wassermann reaction can be represented as follows:

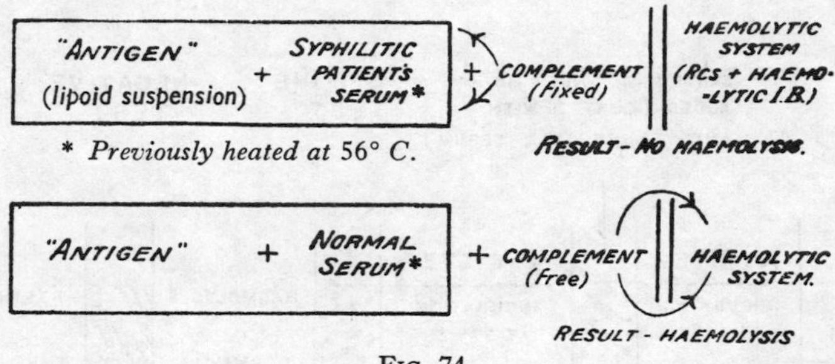

Fig. 74

It should be noted that the Wassermann test must be carried out on a quantitative basis. Not only must it indicate whether the reaction is positive, but the various degrees of the reaction have also to be determined, from a strong positive (+ + +) to a weak positive (+) or a doubtful positive (±). Quantitative testing is most important in assessing the value of treatment or the completeness of cure.

The technical application of the reaction demands a very accurate standardisation of each reagent. Further, the amount of complement used in relation to the quantities of antigen and serum must be adjusted with such delicacy that the weakest reactions can be accepted as significant.

Several modifications of the test are employed, although the essential principles are the same. Some workers use constant amounts of antigen and of the patient's serum with varying amounts of complement. An example of this method is Harrison's technique as modified by Wyler and described in previous editions. Other workers hold the amounts of antigen and complement constant and employ varying amounts of patient's serum. Two examples of the latter procedure are described. Method I (Price's (1950b) modification of the Wyler (1929 and 1934) technique) is a convenient and rapid one-tube screening procedure in which small volumes of the reagents are added by a dropping technique.

Method II (Kolmer) employs larger volumes measured by graduated pipettes. Overnight fixation in the cold at 4° C. is used. This method has the advantage that it can be adapted readily for use with other antigens such as those prepared from the Reiter spirochaete or from other bacteria and viruses.

Method I

Antigen[1]

Fresh ox hearts are obtained from the slaughter house and are freed of fat and connective tissue. They are cut into pieces no longer than 1 cm. and weighed. About 50 g. of the cut muscle is pounded with powdered glass in a mortar for a minute of two. This mixture is transferred to a 2 litre flask and 9 ml. absolute alcohol are added for every gram of muscle. Not more than 100 g. muscle should be treated in one flask. The flask is now tightly stoppered, shaken thoroughly, and left for five days at room temperature in a dark cupboard. The flask must be shaken well every day. The mixture is now filtered through No. 1 Whatman filter paper at room temperature and is stored in the refrigerator overnight. Filter once again through Whatman No. 1 filter paper while still cold in the refrigerator. Store the filtrate in amber glass bottles away from the light in a cool place.

For use, 6 parts of the alcoholic extract are added to 4 parts of a 1 per cent. solution of cholesterol and this mixture is then diluted with saline according to the optimal titre of the antigen. If, for example, the optimal titre is 320, 0·25 ml. of the cholesterol antigen mixture is accurately pipetted to the bottom of a 100 ml. measuring cylinder and 80 ml. saline is measured into a similar cylinder. The saline is now poured *rapidly* into the measure containing the antigen and the mixture is completed by pouring from one cylinder to the other six times. The resultant opalescent mixture is the antigen to be used in the test; it should stand for 20 min. before use and can be used throughout the working day. It should not be used after 8 hr.

Human heart muscle has always been reputed to make a very sensitive Wassermann antigen but recent work indicates that it may give non-specific results.

Before use the antigen must be tested in the following three ways: (1) it must be shown to have complement-fixing ability; (2) the anti-complementary action of the antigen must be determined by itself and also in the presence of normal serum; and (3) the antigen must be titrated by the method of optimal proportion to discover the appropriate dilution to be used in the test. With commercially prepared antigens these steps have usually been carried out by the makers who supply instructions for the use of their product in the test. Full details of the method of titration of antigens are given by Price (1950a) but the essential steps are as follows. First, the anticomplementary activity of the antigen in the presence of normal serum is determined. To accomplish this a chess-board titration is set up with a series of antigen dilutions and a series of complement dilutions. The antigen is prepared in seven doubling dilutions from 1 in 20 to 1 in 1280 and the complement in seven dilutions ranging from 1 in 10, 1 in 20 and so on to 1 in 70. Each tube also contains normal human serum and the haemolytic system (*vide infra*). When the titration is read the complement titre for each antigen dilution is recorded and from these figures the "diagnostic doses" of complement needed in the next step is calculated by the method on p. 934.

The Optimal Proportion Titration of the Antigen.—Employs the same series of antigen dilutions that were used in determining the anti-comple-

[1] A suitable antigen (Maltaner Cardiolipin Antigen) is available commercially from Messrs. Burroughs Wellcome, London.

mentary activity. They are set up in a fresh chessboard titration against a series of seven dilutions of a positive serum ranging from 1 in 10, 1 in 20 to 1 in 70. To each serum-antigen mixture the appropriate "diagnostic dose" of complement, and (after an interval for fixation) the haemolytic system is added. The known positive serum is preferably of moderate strength with a titre of about 1 in 40. The end point of the titration is that antigen dilution which reacts with the greatest dilution of the serum. It is often necessary to read the result by interpolation and since the reactivity may be spread over a zone of antigen dilutions it is permissible to take the mid-point of the zone as an end point. As a final step this antigen dilution is taken as a working suspension and retitrated to determine the amount of it to be used in the test proper. The antigen suspension is now diluted in saline in a series of seven doubling dilutions ranging from 1 in 2 to 1 in 64. It is next set up in a chessboard titration against the positive serum diluted 1 in 2, 1 in 4 and so on to 1 in 64. The volumes of reagents used and the technical procedures are those described on p. 937.

Cardiolipin (as Antigen in the Syphilis Serum Reactions)

This substance, isolated from the phosphatide fraction of lipoidal extracts of heart muscle, has been extensively used in recent years in the Wassermann and flocculation tests for syphilis. It has been claimed that cardiolipin yields more specific results than those obtained with the unpurified lipoid preparations usually employed as antigen in these reactions. It is also supposed that the specific activity of these lipoid preparations with syphilitic sera depends on "cardiolipin". This substance contains phosphorus but no nitrogen; on saponification it yields fatty acids, a non-reducing carbohydrate, and phosphoric acid.

In the syphilis reactions it is used along with lecithin and cholesterol, and preparations containing an appropriate admixture of these constituents are available for diagnostic tests, *e.g.* the cardiolipin (Whitechapel) antigen, obtainable from Burroughs Wellcome & Co., London, which has the following composition: cardiolipin 0·05 per cent., lecithin 0·05 per cent., and cholesterol 0·5 per cent. The titre in which the antigen should be used is specified by the makers. This antigen is suitable for the Wassermann test, in substitution for the original antigen employed in this method.

Patient's Serum

A specimen of blood is obtained by vein puncture as for blood culture. The blood is then placed in a sterile stoppered test-tube or screw-capped bottle and allowed to coagulate. It is advisable to obtain about 5 ml. of blood. The serum is pipetted off after separation and heated in a waterbath at 56° C. for 30 min. Heating *eliminates the fallacy of non-specific fixation effects which may occur with normal unheated sera* plus *the antigen*; it also deprives the serum of its complementing property.

It is thought that the albumin fraction in unheated syphilitic serum may act as a protective colloid and that it tends to reduce precipitation in flocculation reactions. Heating the fraction eliminates this effect.

Complement

Fresh or specially preserved guinea-pig serum is used. It contains an active haemolytic complement for the red corpuscles of the ox or sheep sensitised with the homologous haemolytic antibody. When fresh serum is used, the blood is obtained 12 to 18 hr. before the test by severing the large vessels of the neck over a 6-in. funnel, from which the blood is collected in a measuring cylinder; it is allowed to coagulate and stand overnight in the refrigerator. The complement in serum too recently withdrawn is apt to be excessively "fixable", and in consequence is unsuitable for the Wassermann test.

If possible the pooled serum of several guinea-pigs should be used.

It should be noted that complement is unstable and deteriorates on keeping at ordinary temperatures. It is advisable throughout the experiment to keep the guinea-pig serum on ice. If storage at −30° C. is available the fresh serum may be divided into small portions and kept frozen for a few weeks.

It is now a general practice to use specially preserved serum pooled from a number of animals and it is recommended that it should be absorbed with packed sheep erythrocytes (0·1 m. cells/ml. guinea-pig serum for 30 min. at 4° C.

Preservation of Complement

For the preservation of complement two principles have been applied: (1) rapid drying of the serum from the frozen state *in vacuo* ("freeze-drying") and the reconstitution of the serum when required by dissolving the dried material in the appropriate amount of distilled water; this is exemplified by *Rayner's method* for the preservation of bacterial cultures and serum as described on p. 810; and this technique is also recommended for complement-serum, particularly when the complement may not be used for some time; (2) addition to the liquid serum of sodium chloride or other salts in hypertonic concentration; this is exemplified by *Richardson's method* and the *sodium acetate boric acid method.* Preservation of the complement-serum in the liquid state constitutes a simple and convenient procedure.

Richardson's Method.—Preservation of liquid complement-serum in hypertonic salt solution is effective provided the pH is adjusted to 6–6·4. A convenient method, employing borate-buffer-sorbitol for control of pH, is described here (Richardson, 1941).

Two stock solutions, which keep indefinitely, are used:

(*A*) Boric acid (H_3BO_3) 0·93 g., borax ($Na_2B_4H_7$, $10H_2O$) 2·29 g., and sorbitol ($C_6H_{14}O_6$, $\frac{1}{2}H_2O$) 11·74 g. are dissolved in and made up to 100 ml. with saturated NaCl solution. The *resulting* molar concentrations are: 0·27 *M* boric acid, 0·12 *M* sodium borate, 0·6 *M* sorbitol in saturated sodium chloride.

(*B*) Borax 0·57 g. and sodium azide (NaN_3) 0·81 g. are dissolved and made up to 100 ml. with saturated NaCl solution. The *resulting* molar concentrations are: 0·03 *M* boric acid, 0·03 *M* sodium borate, 0·125 *M* sodium azide in saturated sodium chloride.

To preserve complement-serum, mix 8 parts of serum with 1 part of solution *B*, followed by 1 part of solution *A*. This treated serum keeps very well even at room temperature. At 0°–3° C., loss of titre is not noticeable until after six to nine months. The mixture contains 0·03 *M* boric acid, 0·015 *M* sodium borate, 0·06 *M* sorbitol, and 0·0125 *M* sodium azide.

For use as 1 in 10 complement, 1 part of preserved serum is diluted with 7 parts of distilled water. Any further dilution from this 1 in 10 mixture is made with saline. Diluted serum should not be kept more than an hour or two. According to Richardson, no case of faulty behaviour in the Wassermann reaction attributable to preserved serum has come to notice.

Preservation by Sodium Acetate.—A very simple and most convenient method of preserving complement is to add to the serum an equal volume of a solution of 12 per cent. sodium acetate and 4 per cent. boric acid in distilled water (Sonnenschein, 1930). The serum is kept in sterile screw-capped bottles at approximately 4° C. The full haemolytic activity of the serum and the fixability of the complement in the Wassermann reaction are maintained for about six months. It should be noted in using this preserved complement that it represents a 1 in 2 dilution of the original serum.

It should be noted that traces of zinc reduce the haemolytic activity of complement. Since Analar preparations of sodium chloride do not at present limit the presence of zinc, it is a wise precaution to check the diluents and solutions used in preparing complement. Traces of zinc are detected by turbidity on the addition of a freshly prepared solution of 0·1 per cent. sodium di-ethyl-dithiocarbamate (Wilkinson, 1950).

Titration of Complement

Price's method (1949) is recommended. A pool of six or more normal sera and another of strongly reacting positive sera are required. Prepare a series of ten dilutions of complement in saline ranging from 1 in 10, 1 in 20, and on to 1 in 100. Set out five rows of $3 \times \frac{1}{2}$ in. tubes as follows:

Row 1 has 10 tubes, to which are added:
1 volume complement at dilutions 1 in 10 to 1 in 100
2 volumes saline.

Row 2 has 5 tubes, to which are added:
1 volume complement dilutions at 1 in 10 to 1 in 50
1 volume saline
1 volume antigen diluted as in test

Row 3 has 5 tubes, to which are added:
1 volume complement dilutions at 1 in 10 to 1 in 50
1 volume saline
$\frac{1}{5}$ volume pooled normal serum
1 volume antigen.

Row 4 has 7 tubes, to which are added:
1 volume complement dilutions at 1 in 10 to 1 in 70
2 volumes saline
$\frac{1}{5}$ volume pooled positive serum.

Row 5 has 7 tubes, to which are added:
1 volume complement dilutions at 1 in 10 to 1 in 70
2 volumes saline
$\frac{1}{5}$ volume normal serum.

Plastic plates of the WHO type are a convenient alternative to the $3 \times \frac{1}{2}$ tubes. The usual volume employed in the test is 0·11 ml., as in the Wyler technique, and the reagents are conveniently added by standard dropping pipettes attached to suitable separating funnels. Droppers of three different sizes are required (Donald's Method) (1) for *saline*, *complement* and *sensitised cells* a piece of glass tubing is drawn out, inserted into a Rawco gauge and cut squarely at a point where its outside diameter is 0·75 cm. (2) For the *antigen* suspension a dropper is cut in the same manner with an outside diameter of 0·9 cm. (3) For *undiluted human sera* the pipette dropper is inserted into the No. 56 hole in the Starrett gauge and cut as near to the surface of the gauge as possible. Pipettes (1) and (2) deliver per drop 0·11 ml. of the reagents for which they are designed. Pipette (3) delivers in 1 drop 0·022 ml. of inactivated human sera, *i.e.* $\frac{1}{5}$ the volume of that discharged by (1) and (2). It is necessary to check the pipettes for accuracy before use.

When the reagents have been added, the rack is incubated for 1 hr.

in a 37° C. bath. At the end of this period, the rack is removed from the bath and to every tube is added 1 volume of sensitised red blood cells. The rack is returned to the bath for a further 30 min. and the results are then read. The last tube in the serial dilutions to show complete sparkling haemolysis is taken as the end-point.

Two amounts of complement will be needed in the test proper: (A) *For the Serum Controls.*—This dilution of complement is the highest to show complete haemolysis in Row 4 or 5. *This is the serum control dose.*

(B) *For the Diagnostic Test.*—This dose is calculated by taking the end-point in Row 3 and multiplying it by $\frac{5}{4}$. For example, if 1 in 40 were the end-point then the complement would be used at a dilution of $\frac{1}{40}\times\frac{5}{4}=\frac{5}{160}=\frac{1}{32}$. *This is the diagnostic dose.* The 25 per cent. margin of extra complement used is sufficient to cover the occasional anti-complementary activity of normal sera.

Haemolytic System

With guinea-pig complement, a haemolytic system consisting of sheep red corpuscles sensitised with the appropriate haemolytic antibody is used.

Defibrinated blood is obtained at the abattoir (p. 739). The required quantity is thoroughly mixed with several volumes of normal saline and then centrifuged to separate the corpuscles, the supernatant fluid being pipetted off. This process has generally been designated "washing" the blood corpuscles and is repeated three or four times. The centrifuged deposit of corpuscles after the final washing is suspended in normal saline to form a 6 per cent. suspension. Sheep cells should not be used until one week old when they are uniformly susceptible to lysis.

Standardisation of the Red Blood Cell Suspension

Transfer exactly 1·0 ml. of the suspension to a special haematocrit tube (Price & Wilkinson, 1947).[1] After centrifuging for ten minutes at 2500 r.p.m the height of the column of packed cells is read off. The standard packed cell volume required in the test is 0·05 ml. and the original 6 per cent. suspension is adjusted to this content by dilution by simple proportion. The following example shows the method of calculation:

6 per cent. suspension packed volume = 0·057
Desired packed cell volume . . = 0·050

Dilution factor $\frac{0{\cdot}057}{0{\cdot}050}$ . . . = 1·14

Thus, 0·14 ml. saline should be added to each 1·0 ml. of the original 6 per cent. cell suspension.

Equal volumes of this standard suspension and saline containing 12 MHD of the haemolytic serum per unit volume are mixed, shaken vigorously, and incubated in the water-bath for 30 minutes at 37° C. Some workers prefer to ensure complete mixing by passing a current of air through the suspension during the period of incubation.

Preservation of Sheep Red Blood Cells

Sheep blood for complement fixation tests may be preserved at 4° C. in an equal volume of sterile modified Alsever's solution (Muschel & Lowe, 1955) consisting of:

[1] Obtainable from Messrs. R. B. Turner & Co. Ltd., London.

Glucose	2·05 per cent.
Sodium chloride	0·42 per cent.
Trisodium citrate	0·8 per cent.
Citric Acid	0·055 per cent.
in Distilled Water	

Sheep cells have been satisfactory for use for a period of six weeks after collection in this solution.

Haemolytic Antiserum

The following method (Darter, 1953) is recommended. Rabbits receive on alternate days a series of five *intracutaneous* inoculations of whole sheep blood in the following doses: 0·5, 1·0, 1·5, 2·0, 2·5 ml. These are followed on the twelfth and fifteenth days by the intravenous inoculation of 1·0 ml. of a 20 per cent. suspension of sheep red blood cells in normal saline to which has been added 0·01 per cent. magnesium sulphate. A trial bleeding is taken from the rabbit's ear on the eighteenth day and if the haemolysin content of the serum is satisfactory (the titre should be over 10,000) the rabbit is exsanguinated and the serum is separated. If the titre is not high, further intravenous injections are given. High-titre serum is usually preserved by adding to it an equal volume of sterile glycerol.

The haemolysin titre of the serum (sometimes referred to as its minimum haemolytic dose) is estimated as follows: Set out ten tubes and add to them saline according to the following table.

	Tube No.									
	1	2	3	4	5	6	7	8	9	10
Saline solution	None	ml. 0·5	ml. 1·0	ml. 1·5	ml. 2·0	ml. 0·5	ml. 0·5	ml. 0·5	ml. 0·5	ml. 0·5

Prepare a 1 in 1000 dilution of the haemolytic serum and add 0·5 ml. of it to the first five tubes of the titration. Then proceed as follows:

Tube No.	Procedure	Final haemolysin dilution: 1 in
1	None	1000
2	Mix. Discard 0·5 ml.	2000
3	Mix. Transfer 0·5 ml. to tube 6. Discard 0·5 ml. .	3000
4	Mix. Transfer 0·5 ml. to tube 7. Discard 1·0 ml. .	4000
5	Mix. Transfer 0·5 ml. to tube 8. Discard 1·5 ml. .	5000
6	Mix. Transfer 0·5 ml. to tube 9	6000
7	Mix. Transfer 0·5 ml. to tube 10	8000
8	Mix. Discard 0·5 ml.	10,000
9	Mix. Discard 0·5 ml.	12,000
10	Mix. Discard 0·5 ml.	16,000

Now add to each tube 0·5 ml. of a 1 in 10 dilution of complement and 0·5 ml. of 3 per cent. suspension of red blood cells prepared as above. Incubate for one hour at 37° C. in a water-bath; the last serum dilution to show complete haemolysis is taken as the end-point. The lowest titre which is acceptable for the purpose of sensitising red blood cells for the Wassermann reading is 1000.

Burroughs Wellcome haemolytic serum for *sheep* red corpuscles may conveniently be used in preparing a haemolytic system for the test. This anti-sheep haemolytic serum is obtained from the horse. It tends to exert a pronounced agglutinating effect on the homologous corpuscles, with rapid sedimentation of the cells. It is advisable therefore to add the serum to the corpuscles just before the haemolytic system is required.

An alternative method for the preparation of a haemolytic antiserum for sheep's red blood cells is that of Sawyer and Bourke (1946) which employs the stroma of lysed erythrocytes as the antigen and a shorter inoculation schedule thereby minimising the shock reactions that are liable to occur with the usual immunisation procedures.

Sensitised cells for the test are made by mixing equal volumes of the standard 6 per cent. suspension (p. 935) and the haemolytic serum diluted to contain 12 MHD per unit volume. After vigorous shaking, the mixture is incubated for one hour in a 37° C. water-bath.

The Test (the method is that of Price, 1950b)

Small test-tubes $3 \times \frac{1}{2}$ in. or WHO plates are used and the reagents are added to them either with graduated pipettes or according to Donald's dropping method (see p. 934).

The first step, before commencing the test, is to titrate the complement using the sensitised red blood cell suspension to be used in the test (see p. 934). This is necessary because even pooled preserved complement-serum may vary in activity against different specimens of red blood cells.

The test proper is a screening procedure and each serum has two tubes allocated to it. The reagents are added as follows:

Tube 1. Serum Control Tube:

Patient's serum	$\frac{1}{5}$ volume
Saline	2 volumes
Complement serum control dose . .	1 volume

Tube 2. Diagnostic Tube:

Patient's serum	$\frac{1}{5}$ volume
Saline	1 volume
Complement diagnostic dose . .	1 volume
Antigen	1 volume.

After adding the reagents the racks are shaken thoroughly and placed in a water-bath for 1 hr. at 37° C. At the end of this time the racks are placed on the bench and to each tube is added one volume of sensitised red blood cells. After shaking again, the racks are replaced in the water-bath for a further 30 min., after which the test is read.

Complete haemolysis in both tubes is read as negative reaction. No haemolysis in the diagnostic tube with complete haemolysis in the control tube is read as a positive reaction. Partial haemolysis in the serum diagnostic tube and complete haemolysis in the control tube is read as a weakly positive reaction. No result can be given if the serum control tube of any particular specimen of serum fails to show complete haemolysis. Positive and weakly positive sera are set aside to be put up for a quantitative test.

Quantitative Tests.—In this method doubling dilutions of the serum in saline from 1 in 5 to 1 in 160 are used. Seven tubes are required for each serum and they are set up as follows:

Tube 1. Serum Control Tube:

Serum diluted 1 in 5	1 volume
Saline	1 volume
Serum control dose of complement .	1 volume.

Tubes 2–7. Diagnostic Quantitative Tubes:
Serum appropriate dilution (1 in 5 to 1 in 160) . . . . . 1 volume
Complement diagnostic dose . . 1 volume
Antigen . . . . . . 1 volume.

The sensitised red blood cells are added in the same manner as in the test proper and the incubation times are the same. The end-point is taken as that tube which just fails to show sparkling haemolysis.

The results are reported in terms of the serum dilutions, *e.g.* "Positive with serum diluted 1 in 30".

Cerebrospinal Fluid.—In this test the procedure is closely similar to that used for serum. Neat cerebrospinal fluid is used in the test proper and one volume is added to both the diagnostic and control tubes instead of the one-fifth volume used for sera. The test is made quantitative by making doubling dilutions from neat cerebrospinal fluid and results are recorded as "Positive, fluid diluted 1 in 2, 1 in 4" and so on.

Each batch of tests should include known positive sera of varying degrees of reactivity and a known negative serum. Controls should be set up for each of the reagents used.

Method II (Kolmer's Method)

It is not possible to include the minutiae of details described by Kolmer, and workers who use this method are referred to Kolmer's own papers (*e.g.* Kolmer, Spaulding & Robinson, 1952).

The main essentials of reagents and technique are, however, given below.

Antigen.—A cardiolipin antigen containing 0·03 per cent. cardiolipin, 0·05 per cent. lecithin and 0·3 per cent. cholesterol is used. The antigen dilution is indicated on the label of the bottle; usually it is 1 in 150.

Saline.—0·85 per cent. NaCl containing 0·01 per cent. magnesium sulphate.

Sheep red blood cell suspension.—A 2 per cent. washed suspension of red cells is used. It is standardised, using the haematocrit as in Method I to contain 0·02 ml. packed cells per ml.

Haemolytic serum.—Dilute with saline to contain 4 MHD per ml.

Patient's sera.—Treat as in Method I.

Complement.—Preserved complement is titrated in the presence of diluted antigen, and after 1 hr. in the water-bath at 37° C. the haemolysin and the sheep cell suspension are added separately.

Tube No.	Complement 1 in 30	Diluted antigen	Saline Solution		Haemolysin	Sheep cell suspension (2 per cent.)	
	(ml.)	(ml.)	(ml.)	37° C. water-bath for 1 hour	(ml.)	(ml.)	37° C. water-bath for ½ hour
1	0·20	0·5	1·3		0·5	0·5	
2	0·25	0·5	1·3		0·5	0·5	
3	0·30	0·5	1·2		0·5	0·5	
4	0·35	0·5	1·2		0·5	0·5	
5	0·40	0·5	1·1		0·5	0·5	
6	0·45	0·5	1·1		0·5	0·5	
7	0·50	0·5	1·0		0·5	0·5	
8	None	None	2·5		None	0·5	

Remove rack from waterbath and read complement titration. The smallest amount of complement giving complete haemolysis is the exact unit. The full unit is 0·05 ml. more than the exact unit.

For the complement-fixation tests, complement is diluted so that 2 full units are contained in 1·0 ml.

Example:

	ml.
Exact unit . . .	0·3
Full unit . . .	0·35
Dose (2 full units) .	0·7

Dilution of complement to be employed in the test proper may be calculated by dividing 30 by the dose, *i.e* $\frac{30}{0{\cdot}7}=43$ or 1 in 43 dilution of guinea-pig serum.

The Test

Two tubes are used for each serum to be treated and in each batch sera of graded reactivity from negative to strong positive are included. Additional controls are needed for the reagents used in the test, *i.e.* the antigen, the haemolytic system and the complement. The test is set up as follows:

	Diagnostic Tube	*Serum Control Tube*
Serum	0·2 ml.	0·2 ml.
Antigen	0·5 ml.	Nil
Saline	Nil	0·5 ml.
Stand at room temperature 10-30 min.		
Complement containing 2 full units per ml.	1·0 ml.	1·0 ml.

Mix by thorough shaking and place overnight in the refrigerator at 6°–10° C. for 15 to 18 hr. The following day remove the racks and place them for 10 min. in a 37° C. water-bath. Remove from the bath and add to all tubes except the red cell control tube, 0·5 ml. of the diluted haemolytic serum, and then add 0·5 ml. of the 2 per cent. sheep cell suspension. Mix thoroughly by shaking the tubes and return the racks to the 37° C. water-bath. Begin to read the tubes after 10 min. and watch the known sera controls and the antigen controls with care. When the known pattern of the reactions of these sera appears the final reading is made. Usually this occurs within 30 min. and should certainly be present in less than one hour. The results are interpreted in the same manner as in Method I.

An outline of the Kolmer Method for sera and cerebrospinal fluids including the amounts contained in the reagent control tubes is as shown in the table on p. 940.

This method is used quantitatively with serum serial doubling dilutions from 1 in 2 to 1 in 64 on all positively reacting sera.

The Kolmer Test is readily adaptable to virological work and the Reiter Protein Test (see p. 349). In these and other circumstances, when only small amounts of antigens are available, the test is carried out with volumes one-fifth the size of those above.

Tube No.	Saline solution	Antigen	Shake rack well. Allow to stand at room temperature for 10 to 30 minutes	Complement 2 full units	Shake rack well. Primary incubation 15 to 18 hours at 6°-10° C. followed by 10 minutes in 37° C. water-bath.	Haemolysin 2 units	Sheep cell suspension (2 per cent.)	Shake rack well. Secondary incubation in 37° C. water-bath.
Serum (ml.)	(ml.)	(ml.)		(ml.)		(ml.)	(ml.)	
1. 0·2	None	0·5		1·0		0·5	0·5	
2. 0·2	0·5	None		1·0		0·5	0·5	
Spinal fluid (ml.)								
1. 0·5	None	0·5		1·0		0·5	0·5	
2. 0·5	0·5	None		1·0		0·5	0·5	
Controls								
Antigen .	0·5	0·5		1·0		0·5	0·5	
Haemolytic system .	1·0	None		1·0		0·5	0·5	
Corpuscle .	2·5	None		None		None	0·5	

The Complement-Fixation Test in Gonorrhoea

The general technique of this test is very similar to that of the Wassermann test.

Antigen.—This is made from cultures of several freshly isolated strains of gonococci. It may be prepared and titrated by Cruickshank's (1947) modification of Price's method or may be purchased from Burroughs Wellcome & Co.

The Test employs the haemolytic system and complement in precisely the way described in Method I of the Wassermann tests. The test proper is also carried out in this way except that one volume of inactivated patient's serum is used instead of one-fifth volume employed in the Wassermann test.

The gonococcal complement-fixation test is of limited practical value in acute uncomplicated cases but it is a useful diagnostic aid in chronic infections especially those with closed lesions such as salpingitis, prostatitis and arthritis.

COMPLEMENT-FIXATION TESTS IN VIRUS DISEASES

The Preparation of Viral Antigens

Suspensions of the infected tissues of animals or eggs, or infected tissue cultures are used as the source of the virus antigen which is then extracted and purified by such methods as differential centrifugation, adsorption and elution from erythrocytes, or concentration in a density gradient. Because these processes inevitably involve the loss of a certain amount of the virus the starting material must always contain a large amount of actively growing virus, the minimal acceptable infectivity titre is usually $10^{-6.5}$ but much higher figures than this are desirable.

Negative Control Antigens.—Whenever a viral antigen is being prepared it is always necessary to process alongside it, using precisely similar steps, a small amount of normal uninfected tissue. In this way a control antigen is obtained for comparison with the viral antigen.

Yolk Sac Antigens are suitable for work with rickettsiae, and members of the psittacosis, lymphogranuloma, trachoma and inclusion conjunctivitis group. A psittacosis group antigen is prepared by inoculating the yolk sac of six eight-day chick embryos with 0·25 ml. of egg adapted virus diluted

10^{-4}. (Dilutions of the seed psittacosis virus of 10^{-8}–10^{-10} should kill the embryos in 4 days.) On the death of the embryos the yolk sacs are harvested and impression smears are stained by Castaneda's stain (only those which are rich in elementary bodies are used). The yolk sacs are rinsed in saline once to free them from adherent yolk, and a suspension is prepared by grinding them with 1·0 ml. Ca-Mg-buffered diluent (*vide infra*) for each yolk sac in a Ten Broeck grinder. The emulsion is clarified by centrifuging for 10 min. at 100 *G* and the supernatant fluid is taken off to be centrifuged again in an angle centrifuge for three hours at 1500 *G*. The deposit is resuspended in the diluent to one quarter of its original volume. Finally, the antigen is placed in boiling water for 20 min. and phenol is added to give a concentration of 0·5 per cent.

Allantoic fluid (*V*) *antigens* are principally used in work with the influenza and mumps viruses. They contain mature virions and are sometimes referred to as "V" antigens. Influenza A or B antigens are prepared by inoculating nine-day embryos by the allantoic route using 0·4 ml. seed virus (titre 10^{-6} or above). The eggs are incubated for 40–44 hours at 35° C. Next the eggs are chilled for an hour in the refrigerator at 4° C. and the allantoic fluids are harvested, pooled, and spun lightly to remove debris. If the haemagglutinating titre of the pooled fluids is 1280 or above it can be used without further processing. The antigen can be preserved by adding 0·08 per cent. sodium azide and storing at −30° C. or by freeze drying in ampoules. A mumps antigen can be prepared in a very similar way but six to eight days embryos are inoculated and must be incubated for five to seven days before harvesting the allantoic fluid. Influenza "V" antigens are sometimes associated with strain specific reactions and for diagnostic work some workers prefer to use "Soluble" or "S" antigens prepared from extracts of infected allantoic membranes.

Allantoic membrane (*S*) *antigens* are used in work with the influenza and mumps virus. Influenza viruses A2/Singapore/57 and B/England/939/59 are passed in small doses (*e.g.* 0·1 ml. of a 10^{-3} dilution of seed virus having a haemagglutination titre of 10^{-7}) by the allantoic route to batches of 11–13 day chick embryos. After 24 hr. incubation at 36° C. the allantoic fluids are harvested without pre-chilling, and used undiluted in a dose of 0·1 ml. to inoculate the allantoic cavities of batches of 13-day embryos. A number of eggs are left uninoculated to provide allantoic membranes for the preparation of the negative control antigen.

After 24 hours' incubation the eggs are killed by chilling, and the shell over the air sac is removed. Through a cross-shaped incision in the chorio-allantoic membrane the embryo and its yolk sac can be evacuated leaving the membrane behind and lightly adherent to the shell. The membranes are then removed from the shell, rinsed free of blood and split yolk in three changes of 0·08 per cent. sodium azide in physiological saline, dried between filter-papers, and finally weighed in bulk.

The membranes are now suspended in 5–10 ml. azide-saline and are frozen and thawed three times by alternate immersion in a mixture of alcohol and solid carbon dioxide at −70° C. and in a water-bath at 37° C. For this purpose it is advisable to place the membrane emulsion in a plastic container. Now add sufficient azide-saline to make a 40 per cent. w/v suspension of membrane and homogenise in a blender. The suspension is now lightly centrifuged to remove the coarse debris and a few drops of chloroform are added. After standing overnight at 4° C. a precipitate of egg proteins is formed and this is removed, without significant loss of the soluble antigen, by centrifuging for 1 hr. in an angle centrifuge at 1500 *G*.

The resultant, somewhat opalescent, fluid contains the soluble antigen and is best preserved by freeze-drying small volumes of it in ampoules. Alternatively, the fluid antigen may be kept without marked deterioration for about one month at –30° C.

Strain specific influenza antigens.—Hoyle (1952) showed that when influenza virions are exposed to ether they disintegrate and the inner S antigen which is common in all influenza A virus strains is freed. It is possible to extract the strain specific V antigen from such a preparation by adsorption to and elution from erythrocytes, and strain specific complement fixing antigens can thus be made for use in serodiagnostic procedures. Antisera prepared in the guinea-pig against these strain specific antigens are valuable in the antigenic analysis of freshly isolated viruses. (Lief & Henle, 1956; Henle, Lief & Fabiyi, 1958).

Tissue culture antigens are used principally in the serodiagnosis of infections with the *picorna* group of viruses (enteroviruses etc.) but they are also employed in measles, and in infections with the para-influenza and respiratory syncytial viruses. They are obtained from tissue cultures in which very rapid multiplication is proceeding. One method commonly used for preparing an antigen is to take large monolayers of primary or secondary monkey kidney cells, HEp2, or HeLa cells and to inoculate them with a virus dose calculated to supply 5–10 virions for each cell of the monolayer. When the maximal cytopathic effect of the virus is seen the cells are scraped off the glass with a rubber policeman and harvested together with the culture fluid. This suspension is now alternately frozen at $-70°$ C. in a mixture of acetone and solid carbon dioxide and thawed at 37° C. in the water-bath. After freezing and thawing three times, the preparation is spun lightly to throw down coarse cellular debris, and the infectivity of the supernatant is estimated by titration of its cytopathic effect in tissue cultures. Effective antigens require to have infectivity titres ranging from $10^{-6 \cdot 5}$ to 10^{-8} TCD50 per 0·1 ml.

Animal tissue antigens are sometimes used, especially in circumstances when the viruses do not multiply actively in eggs or tissue cultures. Thus a suspension of the carcases of suckling mice infected with strains of Group A Coxsackie viruses may be purified and concentrated by differential centrifugation and the use of one of the density gradient techniques. Similarly the brains of suckling mice infected with members of the group of arboviruses provide a rich source of virus for making serological antigens (Clarke & Casals, 1958).

Complement Fixation Test for Viral Antibodies

The method described is recommended as the standard technique for use by the WHO Expert Committee on Respiratory Virus Diseases (1959). The method is the small volume method originally described by Hoyle (1948) but is modified for use with antigen prepared from infected chick embryos and adapted for the WHO perspex plates.

Apparatus

(1) Plastic plates with 80 wells (WHO type) are used throughout. They can be obtained from Messrs. Prestware Ltd., Southdown Works, Kingston Road, London, S.W.1. The plates after use are cleansed by overnight immersion in 2 per cent. sodium hydroxide followed by rinsing under running tap water; next a rinse in 2 per cent. hydrochloric acid is followed by a further washing in tap water and a final rinse in ion-free distilled water. These steps can be carried out conveniently by transferring the plates through

a series of plastic buckets containing the fluids. Finally the plates are shaken, inverted and drained at room temperature until they are dry.

(2) Automatic syringes containing 1 ml. and delivering 0·1 ml. are used throughout. (Obtainable from Messrs. R. B. Turner Ltd., Inocula House, Church Lane and Hobbs Green, East Finchley, London, N.2.)

Reagents

(1) Sera are inactivated at 56° C. for 30 min. Positive control sera from naturally occurring infection and negative control sera are included.

(2) Diluent. The veronal-NaCl diluent described on page 861 is used throughout.

(3) Haemolytic system. Washed packed sheep red blood cells are prepared as for the Wassermann Test, and an accurate 2 per cent. suspension is made and checked in the haematocrit (see p. 935). The cells are sensitised by the addition of an equal volume of haemolytic antiserum (see p. 936) diluted to contain 10 MHD and the mixture should be incubated for 30 min. at 37° C. before use.

(4) Complement preserved by Richardson's method (see p. 933) is used throughout. It should be noted that the serum from some guinea-pigs is known to contain antibodies to the para-influenza viruses and only complement known to be free of such antibodies should be used in tests for these viruses. Complement of this preserved type is available commercially from Messrs. Burroughs Wellcome.

Titration of Complement

This is carried out in the presence of the antigen to be used. Prepare a 1 in 10 dilution of a complement by adding 0·5 ml. of preserved complement to 3·5 ml. of distilled water. Next prepare a series of 13 complement dilutions in $3 \times \frac{1}{2}$ in. tubes according to the following plan:—

Tube No.	1	2	3	4	5	6	7
Diluent in ml.	1·0	1·25	1·5	1·75	2·0	2·25	2·5
Complement 1 in 10 in ml. .	0·25	0·25	0·25	0·25	0·25	0·25	0·25
Reciprocal of complement dilution	50	60	70	80	90	100	110
Tube No.	8	9	10	11	12	13	14
Diluent in ml.	2·75	3·0	3·25	3·5	3·75	4·0	4·25
Complement 1 in 10 in ml. .	0·25	0·25	0·25	0·25	0·25	0·25	0·25
Reciprocal of complement dilution	120	130	140	150	160	170	180

Proceed as follows:—

(1) Transfer 0·1 ml. of each complement dilution to a series of cups in a WHO plate.

(2) Add to each cup 0·1 ml. of the antigen at the dilution to be used in the test.

(3) Add to each cup 0·1 ml. of diluent.

(4) Add to each cup 0·2 ml. of sensitised sheep cells.

(5) Incubate the plate for 30 min. at 37° C.

(6) Make a reading of the cup containing the highest complement dilution giving 100 per cent. haemolysis.

For use in the tests dilute the 1 in 10 complement to contain 2·5 MHD by the 100 per cent. haemolysis reading.

Titration of the Antigen

Each new antigen before use is titrated against an excess of a known positive serum. The unit volume used throughout is 0·1 ml. Two rows, each of eight cups, in a WHO plate are used together with three more for the controls.

Proceed as follows:—

(1) To all the eight cups in each of the two rows, but omitting the first cup, add with an automatic pipette one volume of the diluent.

(2) To control cup A (serum control) add one volume of diluent, to control cup B (complement control) add two volumes, and control cup C (haemolytic system) add three volumes.

(3) Add to the first two cups of both rows one volume of neat antigen.

(4) Make a series of doubling dilutions by mixing the contents of the second cup in the first row thoroughly with the pipette and transferring one volume to the third cup; proceed in this fashion to the end of the row and discard the volume remaining in the pipette. Repeat the same process with the second row. The antigen dilutions in the rows are 1 in 1, 1 in 2, 1 in 4, 1 in 8, 1 in 16, 1 in 32, 1 in 64 and 1 in 128.

(5) Rinse the pipette thoroughly and add 1 volume of diluent, in place of serum, to each of the cups in the first row which now constitutes the antigen control.

(6) Dilute the positive control serum to eight times its known titre (*e.g.* a serum with a titre of 1 in 128 would be diluted to 1 in 16).

(7) Add one volume of the diluted serum to the cups of the second row and to control cup A.

(8) Add one volume of complement diluted to contain 2·5 MHD to all cups *except* cup C.

(9) Incubate the plate for 60 min. at 37° C.

(10) Add *two* volumes of sensitised sheep red cells to all cups.

(11) Incubate again for 30 min. at 37° C.

(12) Read the results as soon as the cells have settled. Any cup showing less than 50 per cent. haemolysis is regarded as positive. More than 50 per cent. haemolysis is regarded as negative.

For use in the test the antigen is used at a concentration four times the figure obtained from the end point in this titration (*e.g.* if the maximal antigen titre were 16 the antigen would be used at 1 in 4).

The Test for the Titration of Serum Antibodies

This is carried out using the methods and reagents described above. The unit volume is 0·1 ml.

Preliminary screening is generally practised to save unnecessary labour and to conserve laboratory reagents. The convalescent serum *only* is tested at a single dilution usually 1 in 8. Only in cases where the finding is positive is the full test with both acute and convalescent sera set up.

The Full Test requires serum dilutions of 1 in 2, 1 in 4, 1 in 8 and 1 in 16 for the acute serum and 1 in 2, 1 in 4, 1 in 8, 1 in 16, 1 in 32, 1 in 64, 1 in 128, 1 in 256 for the convalescent serum. Controls for each serum diluted to 1 in 2 and 1 in 4 are included. Each cup in the test contains one volume of diluted serum, one volume of antigen at the required dilution, and one volume of complement containing 2·5 MHD complement. Antigen, complement and haemolytic system controls are required. The subsequent procedure and the reading of the results are as described in the method of antigen titration (step 9 onwards).

A method designed for use with the freeze-dried antigens supplied by the Public Health Laboratory Service is described by Bradstreet and Taylor (1962).

Reduced volumes of reagents may be employed in a technique in which drops of the fluids used are placed on ruled perspex plates that are incubated in a special humidified cabinet (Fulton & Dumbell, 1949).

A microtechnique which employs special loops to prepare the dilutions and which permits at least an eight-fold saving of reagents has been described by Takatsy (1955). A report on a trial of this apparatus is given by Sever (1962).

HAEMAGGLUTINATION-INHIBITION TESTS IN INFLUENZA

The value of these tests lies in their extreme specificity and the fact that they can be used to distinguish antibodies to the various substrains and variants of the influenza viruses. The reaction is of great importance also in the identification of freshly isolated strains of influenza viruses. Haemagglutination-inhibition tests thus differ from the complement-fixation reactions described on p. 942 for the latter are group specific and will do no more than distinguish the antibodies to influenza viruses A, B and C.

Saline Diluent.—Throughout the tests the buffered calcium saline is used at pH 7·2–7·4 (see p. 861). Alternatively, the veronal saline diluent with added calcium and magnesium may be used (see p. 861).

Standard Erythrocyte Suspension.—Blood is obtained from the wing vein or the heart of a fowl (see p. 1022) and added to a suitable anticoagulant. Human "Group O", or guinea-pig erythrocytes may also be used. The cells are washed thoroughly in the centrifuge and then the volume of the packed cells is determined in a graduated centrifuge tube by spinning in a straight-headed centrifuge for 10 min. at 1000 *G*.

The cells are then suspended to make a 0·5 per cent. suspension.

Standard antigens are prepared from high-titre pools of infected allantoic fluid. At present it is recommended that the following should be used: A2/Singapore/57 and B/England/939/59.

Titration of Virus.—Set up two rows of $3 \times \frac{1}{2}$ in. tubes, 10 tubes in each row. Place 1·0 ml. amounts of saline solution in each tube in the front row. With a 1·0 ml. pipette add 1·0 ml. of the viral antigen to the first tube of the front row. Discard the pipette. Mix well with a clean pipette and transfer 1·0 ml. to the second tube of the front row and 0·25 ml. to the first tube of the back row. Take a fresh pipette and mix the contents of the second tube of the front row and then transfer 1·0 ml. to the third tube of the front row and 0·25 ml. to the second tube of the back row. Continue through the series until all the tubes of the back row contain 0·25 ml. of doubling dilutions of the virus. *It is extremely important to take a fresh pipette to make each virus dilution.* Discard the front row of tubes. Add to each tube 0·25 ml. saline solution and 0·5 ml. of the 0·5 per cent. red cell suspension. Include an erythrocyte control tube containing 0·5 ml. saline and 0·5 ml. of the red cell suspension. Stand for 1 hr. at room temperature and read the results according to the haemagglutination pattern. The 0·25 ml. volume of the virus dilution which completely agglutinates the red cells contains one haemagglutination unit. For the test four haemagglutinating units are required and the viral antigen is diluted to one fourth of the titre obtained.

Test Sera.—Pairs of sera obtained during the acute and convalescent phases of the illness are absolutely essential. Both sera must be examined at the same time. It is important to remove the non-specific inhibitors of viral haemagglutination usually present in normal serum.

Preparatory Treatment of Sera for Haemagglutination-Inhibition Tests.—Since the presence of non-specific virus inhibitors in many human and animal sera renders difficult the interpretation of serological findings, it is a matter of importance to eliminate this source of error. Inhibitors may be removed from human sera without affecting the titre of specific antibody by the following methods:

Treatment with a crude filtrate of V. cholerae

The filtrate is prepared as follows: Semi-solid tryptic digest heart agar, spread in a thin layer in Petri dishes, is inoculated with 0·2 ml. of an 8 hr. broth culture of *V. cholerae* (4 Z strain). After 16 hours' incubation at 37° C. the soft agar cultures are filtered through cotton wool and paper, clarified by slow centrifugation, Seitz filtered, and adjusted to pH 7·2. Filtrates are titrated by estimating the minimal amount that will, in a given amount of normal rabbit serum, eliminate the inhibition of virus haemagglutination.

Sera, of which 0·1 ml. amounts are required for each virus antigen to be used, are treated as follows:

To 0·1 ml. serum add 0·5 ml. of an appropriate calcium saline dilution of cholera filtrate, incubate for 18 hr. in a water-bath at 37° C., and finally heat for 1 hr. at 56° C. to inactivate the receptor-destroying enzyme in the cholera filtrate. Add 0·2 ml. saline, and the serum now diluted 1 in 8 is ready for examination.

Treatment with Periodate

Make up a solution by dissolving 0·127 gram of potassium metaperiodate in 50 ml. distilled water. To 1 volume of serum add 2 volumes of periodate solution and store overnight at 4° C. The following morning add two volumes of 1·0 per cent. glycerol in saline and then adjust the serum dilution to 1 in 8 by adding 3 volumes of saline. The serum is now ready for use in the test.

Titration of Antibodies in Serum

For each serum to be tested set up four rows of ten $3 \times \frac{1}{2}$ in. tubes. Into all the tubes of the front row place 1·0 ml. saline solution. To the first tube of the front row add 1·0 ml. of a 1 in 8 dilution of the patient's serum. Mix well and transfer 1·0 ml. to the second tube of the front row and continue this procedure until the tenth tube. Discard the remaining serum dilution in the pipette. Now transfer 0·25 ml. of the contents of the tenth tube to the last tubes of the other three rows and using the same pipette carry out the same step with the ninth, eighth and the other tubes until all have received their appropriate serum dilutions. Discard the front row of the tubes which are not used in the test.

Now add the test viral antigens diluted to contain four haemagglutinating doses (*vide supra*) in 0·25 ml. amounts to their appropriate rows (*e.g.* influenza viruses A_1, A_2 and B). Finally to these virus serum mixtures add 0·5 ml. of the 0·5 per cent. red cell suspension and shake thoroughly to mix the reagents. Stand at room temperature for 60 min. and then read the tests on the basis of the haemagglutination pattern. The titre of the serum is expressed as the highest initial dilution that completely inhibits viral haemagglutination. Tubes showing partial haemagglutination are ignored. In any batch of haemagglutination-inhibition tests the viral antigens must always be re-titrated and known positive and negative sera must be included. Other controls include a serum control of 0·25 ml. 1 in 8 serum+0·25 ml. saline +0·5 ml. erythrocyte suspension and also a cell suspension control as used in the virus titration.

Haemagglutination-Inhibition Test in Influenza C Infections

Influenza C grows poorly in the allantoic cavity and this virus must be cultivated in the amniotic cavity of 10-day chick embryos for 26 to 30 hr. at 35° C. A suitable inoculum is 0·1 ml. of a 1 in 100 dilution of the seed virus.

Since influenza virus C elutes rapidly at room temperature, haemagglutination and haemagglutination-inhibition titrations must be carried out in the cold at 4° C.

Modification of the Haemagglutination-Inhibition Test for use with Plastic Plates

Plastic plates of the type recommended for the complement-fixation test are used. For virus titrations the volume of antigen used is 0·25 ml. to which is added directly 0·25 ml. of 0·5 per cent. red blood cells and 0·25 ml. diluent.

For the titration of antibodies serial dilutions of 0·25 ml. volumes of the serum are made; this is followed by the addition of an equal volume of red blood cell suspension and then 0·25 ml. of the virus antigen diluted to contain four haemagglutinating units. The reading of the test is similar to that described above.

THE MEASUREMENT OF ANTIVIRAL ACTIVITY IN SERA BY NEUTRALISATION TESTS

In only a limited number of virus diseases is there an *in vitro* test which can be relied on to give an estimate of the level of immunity in the individual and it is therefore necessary in some cases to use animal protection tests to gauge the level of antibody in the serum. The protective action of an antiserum may also be demonstrated in eggs or tissue cultures. Neutralisation tests are at present chiefly used in yellow fever, Coxsackie virus infections, poliomyelitis, other enterovirus infections and the arthropod-borne encephalitides.

In one method a fixed quantity of inactivated serum is added to falling dilutions of the virus and the mixtures are held at room temperature for 30 min. or longer before being inoculated into groups of animals, eggs, or tissue cultures. Acute and convalescent phase sera are included in the same batch of tests and a control virus titration is set up. The neutralisation index is then determined by comparing the 50 per cent. end-point of the control virus titration with that of the virus-serum mixture.

$$\text{Logarithm of neutralisation index} = \text{Negative logarithm of control titre} - \text{Negative logarithm of virus-serum mixture}$$

Neutralisation index = Antilogarithm of the figure thus obtained.

Neutralisation indices below 10 are regarded as negative, and between 10 and 49 as doubtful; over 50 they are usually indicative of an infection. In a second method a fixed amount of virus, sufficient to affect 100 per cent. of the controls, is added to progressive dilutions of serum. In this case the Reed and Muench or Kärber methods (see p. 882) are used to determine the 50 per cent. protective or neutralising end-point of both acute and convalescent phase sera. In calculating these end-points it is necessary to reverse the direction of addition of the appropriate columns dealing with the "deaths" and "survivals". By converting the logarithm of the 50 per cent. serum titre to its anti-logarithm the neutralisation index is obtained. For diagnostic purposes the increase in the neutralisation index during convalescence should be at least 100.

The Measurement of Virus Infectivity

The usual procedure for estimating the potency of a suspension of living virus particles is to inoculate groups of susceptible animals with varying amounts of the preparation differing by a constant dilution factor. The end-point of the titration is taken, for accuracy, as that dilution of the virus at which 50 per cent. of the animals react. In many such virus titrations it is possible to use chick embryos or tissue cultures instead of animals, but the principle remains the same.

End points are calculated by the method of Reed and Muench (1938), see page 882.

IMMUNODIFFUSION

The present status of immunodiffusion techniques as analytical procedures of high resolution and specificity followed the new interpretation of precipitate formation in gels by Oudin in 1946. He showed that concentrated antigen layered over an agar-antiserum mixture in a tube will form a precipitin band in a position directly related to the concentration of the antigen and its diffusion coefficient and inversely proportional to the concentration of the antibody. Following these observations methods were developed in which antigen and antibody were allowed to diffuse towards each other in agar and one or more precipitin bands were formed according to the number of specific reactants present. This method is known as double diffusion, and may be carried out in tubes or Petri dishes. The most suitable temperature at which to carry out immunodiffusion tests is 4° C. since at higher temperatures although more rapid precipitation occurs, there is decreased resolution of the precipitin bands and precipitation is less complete. In addition denaturation of labile reactants is less likely at the lower temperature. The time taken for visible precipitin bands to form depends upon the diffusion rates of the two reactants and their relative concentrations. Precipitin bands when they are first formed are at their sharpest and tend to broaden with time. A further development of the double diffusion procedure uses preliminary electrophoresis (the movement of charged particles in a conducting solvent subjected to a direct current p. 954) in agar of a mixture of antigens, the separation of the individual components which occurs allows the easy identification of precipitin bands which form after a specific antiserum has diffused towards the different components. For further information on the mechanics of immunodiffusion the reader is referred to Crowle (1961).

Double diffusion carried out in tubes 5 cm. × 2 cm. in which the antigen and antibody diffuse towards each other in a layer of agar is the basis of the Oakley and Fulthorpe (1953) and Preer (1956) techniques. The antigen and antibody solutions may be introduced in liquid form particularly when the concentration of either is low and dilution is not desirable. More conveniently the antigen and antibody can be mixed with agar. The three layers of the system then consist of antigen and antibody mixed with agar separated by a layer of agar. The concentration of the agar used is commonly 0·6 per cent. The precipitin bands form in the middle layer and with strong antisera may be seen within a few hours. Dilution of the antisera or antigen causes displacement of the band towards the antiserum-agar or antigen-agar interface respectively. This type of immunodiffusion technique in tubes has the distinction of being the most sensitive type of precipitin test available with respect to the quantities of reactants required for the formation of

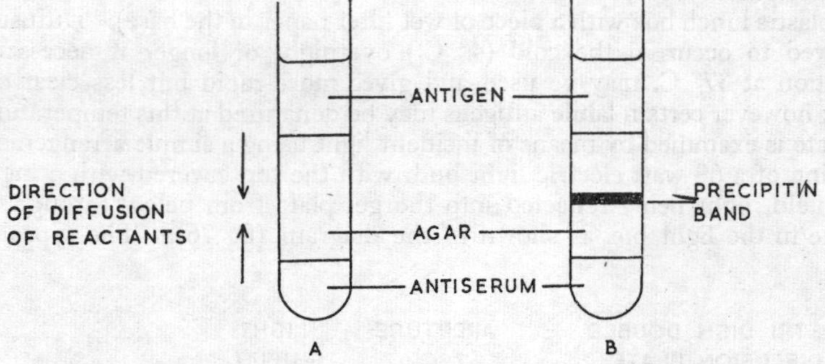

DOUBLE DIFFUSION IN TUBES. A BEFORE DIFFUSION HAS TAKEN PLACE.
B AFTER DIFFUSION HAS TAKEN PLACE.

FIG. 75

visible precipitates. Quantities of reactants too small to form visible precipitates if they were simply mixed together are concentrated in a very narrow zone and can thus form an observable precipitate (Crowle, 1961). The number of precipitin bands observed in the agar tubes does not necessarily indicate the total number of systems present as some of the bands in complex mixtures may be hidden by others and would only be identified by procedures of high resolving power such as immuno-electrophoresis (see page 954).

Immunodiffusion has been extensively used in microbiology for the identification of different types and strains of bacteria and viruses.

The smallpox virus can be detected in the exudate from the skin lesions (see page 372) and poliomyelitis virus can be typed (Grasset, Bonifas & Pongratz, 1958). Fungi can be identified by immunodiffusion and a diagnostic test has been developed for histoplasmosis (Heiner, 1958).

Immuno-electrophoresis can be used for the identification of myeloma proteins for increase in globulin, and the changes in such diseases as virus hepatitis, cirrhosis and the reticuloses are distinct enough to suggest the appropriate diagnosis. Techniques have been developed for the simple quantitation of γ globulin in patients being treated by passive transfer of this protein (Gell, 1957). The use of immuno-electrophoresis in analysis of human pathological sera has been reviewed by Scheiffarth and Goetz (1960) and Crowle (1961).

Double diffusion in plates

Sufficient 1 per cent. agar in 0·85 per cent. NaCl or 0·2 *M* phosphate buffer pH 7·2 containing 0·1 per cent. sodium azide is poured into a small flat bottomed Petri dish to give a perfectly level surface (about 10 ml.). When this has solidified, wells are cut in the agar with a cork borer in positions determined by a pattern drawn on a piece of paper which is placed under the Petri dish. More conveniently wells are cut with a gel cutter with for example a central well surrounded by six satellite wells (Shandon Scientific Company). A very large number of different sizes and shapes and arrangements of wells have been used in this technique, the circular central well with equidistant satellite wells is perhaps the most popular. After the wells have been filled, using separate clean Pasteur pipettes, with the antigen and antiserum solutions, *e.g.* the antiserum in the central well and the antigens in the peripheral wells, the plate is covered and placed in a damp chamber (*e.g.* a plastic lunch box with a piece of wet filter paper in the base). Diffusion is allowed to occur in the cold (4° C.) overnight or longer if necessary. Incubation at 37° C. may be used and gives more rapid but less clear cut results; however certain labile antigens may be denatured at this temperature. The plate is examined by means of incident light using a simple arrangement consisting of a 60 watt electric light bulb with the top covered with a metal light shield, light being reflected into the gel plate from below through an aperture in the light box as shown in the diagram (fig 76). The types of

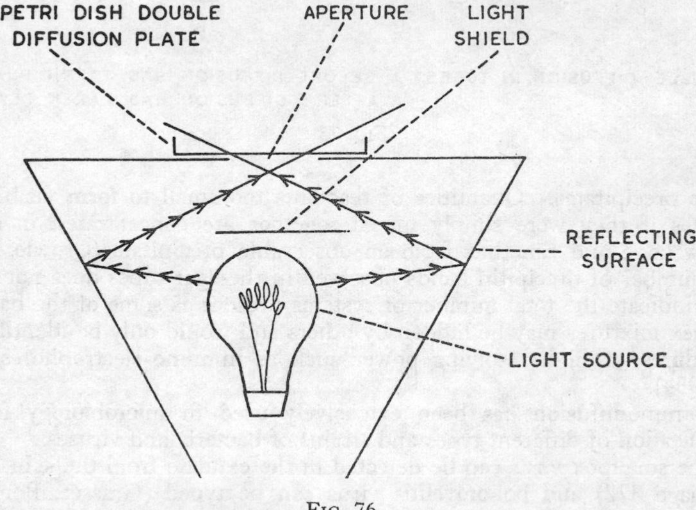

FIG. 76
Immunodiffusion viewing box.

precipitin bands commonly observed are shown in fig. 77. They take the form essentially of one of three different patterns; (1) the reaction of identity where the lines are continuous from one well to the next; (2) the reaction of non-identity where the lines cross each other and (3) the reaction of partial identity which is similar to (1) except for spur formation at the junction of the precipitin bands.

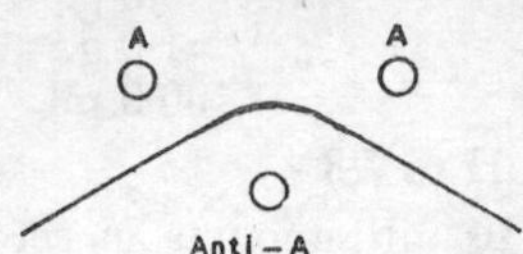

REACTION OF IDENTITY, MAY BE SLIGHTLY SKEWED IF DIFFERENT CONCENTRATIONS IN A WELLS.

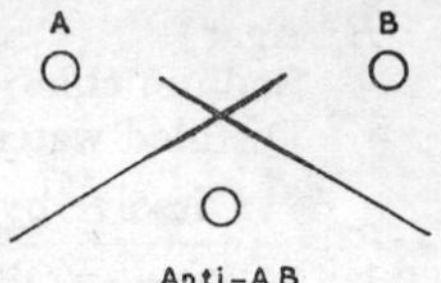

REACTION OF NON IDENTITY, PATTERN OBTAINED WHEN TWO SEROLOGICALLY DIFFERENT ANTIGENS ARE USED WITH AN ANTISERUM CONTAINING ANTIBODY TO BOTH.

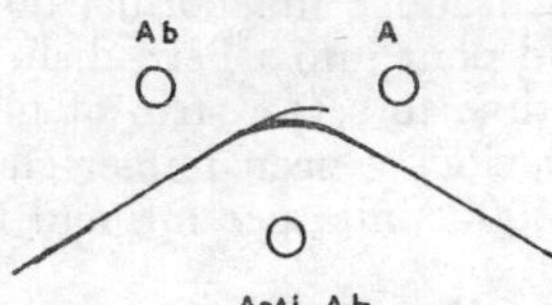

REACTION OF PARTIAL IDENTITY, 'SPUR' FORMATION AT JUNCTION OF PRECIPITIN BANDS.

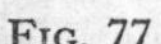

FIG. 77

Commonly observed patterns found in double diffusion plates where two antigen solutions are compared using antiserum as the analytic agent.

Demonstration of Precipitating Antibodies in Farmer's Lung

A double diffusion test is used to demonstrate precipitating antibodies in the serum of patients with Farmer's Lung disease, Pepys *et al.* (1963). About 85 per cent. of these patients can be shown to have antibodies against an antigenic extract of *Thermopolyspora polyspora.*

Requisites.—(1) Petri dishes prepared for double diffusion as described on page 950 with a well pattern consisting of a central well surrounded by 6 equidistant satellite wells (a suitable cutter is manufactured by the Shandon Scientific Company, London—type 1812).

(2) Extract of *Thermopolyspora polyspora,* is distributed by the Mycological Reference Laboratory, London School of Hygiene and Tropical Medicine, Keppel Street, London and is available commercially from Bencard Ltd. London.

(3) Patient's serum.

Method.—The test serum is placed in the central well with a clean Pasteur pipette and doubling dilutions of the antigen starting at 10 mg./ml. in 0·85 per cent. saline in the peripheral wells. A positive is indicated by the appearance after incubation at 37° C. of 1 to 7 lines of precipitation. Strong sera show reactions in 24 hr. but several days' incubation may be needed with other sera.

The Gel-Precipitation Test for Diphtheria Toxin

The following method shows the production of diphtheria toxin in an agar plate culture and can be used as a substitute for the animal virulence test.

Culture Medium.

A.	Peptone (Difco proteose)	4·0 g.
	Maltose	0·6 g.
	Lactic acid (B.P.)	0·14 ml.
	Distilled water	100·0 ml.

Adjust pH to 7·8

B.	Agar	3·0 g.
	Sodium chloride	1·0 g.
	Distilled water	100·0 ml.

Dissolve by heat, filter, adjust pH to 7·8

Mix equal parts of A and B, distribute in 10 ml. amounts in screw-capped bottles, sterilise by steaming for 30 min. on each of three successive days.

The Test.

(1) Melt 10 ml. agar medium, cool to 55° C., add 2 ml. normal horse serum, Burroughs Wellcome No. 2, and pour into a Petri dish.
(2) Introduce immediately (before agar has time to set) a strip of filter paper 60 mm.×15 mm. which has previously been immersed in diphtheria antitoxin of a strength of 1000 units per ml. and the surplus antitoxin allowed to drain off.
(3) Dry the surface of the medium for 45 min. in the incubator.
(4) Inoculate the plate by stroking a heavy inoculum of the diphtheria bacillus to be tested across the plate at right angles to the paper strip. Two or three strains can be thus stroked, and a known virulent (toxigenic) strain is also inoculated at the same time. The line of inoculum should be as narrow as possible.
(5) Incubate and examine after 24 and 48 hr.

Note.—Plates should be freshly prepared immediately before each test.

A positive reaction is denoted by fine white lines commencing from the stroke about ½ in. from the filter-paper (see illustration facing p. 182). It appears at about 24 hours' incubation and in its early stages must be looked for with a hand lens. The plate is best examined against a dark background. After 48 hours the white line of precipitation is easily seen. The toxin diffuses sideways from the stroke, and the antitoxin diffuses from the filter paper and where these meet at optimum neutralising concentration, a precipitate is formed. If the plate is then left at room temperature, secondary lines may be seen representing the interaction of other bacterial substances, diffusing out from the growth, with antibodies corresponding to them in the antitoxic serum. It should be realised that the diphtheria toxin used for the production of antitoxin is not a pure substance but may contain several antigens in addition to the actual toxin itself.

It should be noted also that not all makes of peptone are suitable and that some samples of horse serum prevent the development of the reaction.

ELECTROPHORESIS

When charged particles are introduced into a conducting solvent and subjected to a direct current, they can be separated electrophoretically by virtue of the fact that they move at rates dependent on their charge at the particular pH of the solvent used.

Electrophoresis is used in immunology: (1) For the identification of abnormal serum proteins. (2) For the determination of gamma globulin levels in sera or other fluids, and for the preparation of globulin from such fluids. (3) As a preliminary to immuno-electrophoresis.

Fig. 78 shows the main normal serum components that can be identified by electrophoresis and immuno-electrophoresis.

The apparatus in its simplest form consists of a power supply for direct

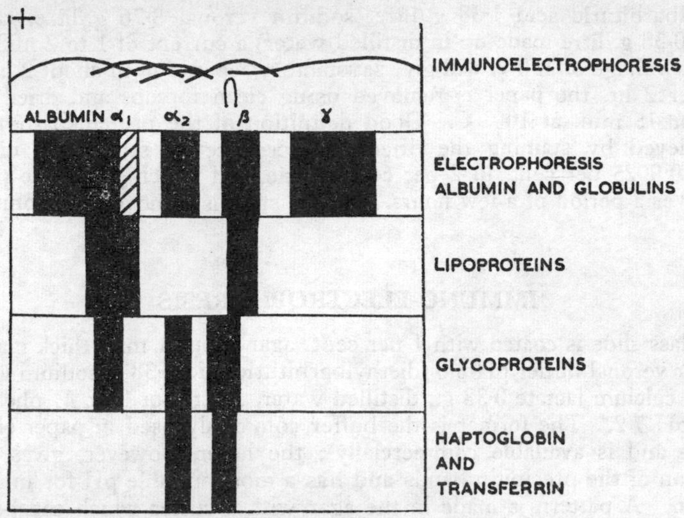

FIG. 78

Diagram showing major serum components.

current,[1] positive and negative non-polarising electrodes (platinum) and vessels for each electrode (plastic lunch boxes are suitable). The electrophoresis paper (either filter paper or cellulose acetate paper) forms a bridge between the two vessels and before use is soaked in the electrophoresis buffer and blotted before the serum or other material to be electrophoresed is applied. It is advisable to separate the electrodes from the part of the vessel into which the filter paper wicks (connecting the ends of the paper to the buffer) are dipping to prevent electrolysis products from the electrodes changing the pH of the buffer in contact with the wicks. This can be achieved as shown in the diagram by using two vessels connected by wicks on each side, with the electrode in one vessel and the electrophoresis paper

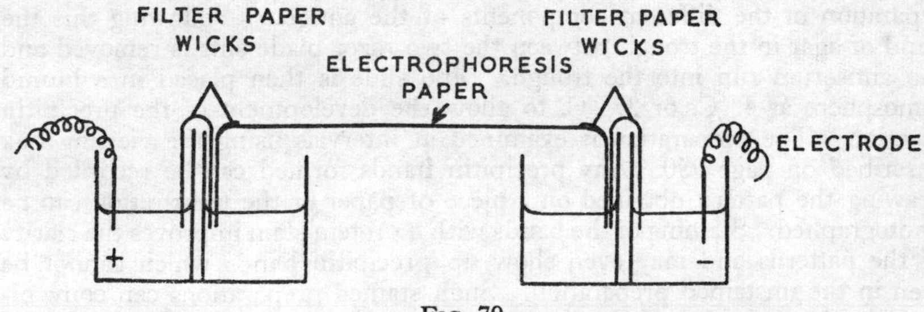

FIG. 79

Diagram of simple electrophoresis apparatus.

connected to the other. Alternatively a sponge can be placed across the width of each box just in front of the electrode. The current required will depend on the material to be electrophoresed and the type of buffer used. With serum on cellulose acetate paper (Oxoid) and veronal buffer pH 8·2

[1] A suitable power supply can be obtained from the Shandon Scientific Company, London or L.K.B. Produktur, London & Stockholm.

(diethylbarbituric acid 1·38 g./litre, sodium veronal 8·76 g./litre, calcium lactate 0·38 g./litre made up in distilled water) a current of 1 to 2 milliamps giving a voltage of 150 v. will give satisfactory separation in about 2 hr.

After 2 hr. the paper is removed using clean forceps and dried in an oven for 15 min. at 100° C. Good definition of the protein patterns can be achieved by staining the dried cellulose acetate strip with nigrosin (Gurr) 0·0025 per cent. in 2 per cent. acetic acid which stains the protein black over a period of a few hours. Excess stain is removed in running tap water.

IMMUNO-ELECTROPHORESIS

A glass slide is coated with 1 per cent. agar about 1 mm. thick made up in either veronal buffer pH 8·6 (diethylbarbituric acid 1·38 g. sodium veronal 8·76 g., calcium lactate 0·38 g., distilled water, 1 litre) or 0·02 *M* phosphate buffer pH 7·2. The former is the buffer commonly used in paper electrophoresis and is available commercially[1]; the latter, however, gives better resolution of the precipitin bands and has a more suitable pH for immunodiffusion. A pattern is made in the agar with a cutter which can be constructed by forcing two large gauge hypodermic needles (1–2 mm. internal diameter) with their points sawn off through the centre area of a large cork stopper 4 cm. in diameter about 7 mm. apart. Between the needles are placed the two halves of a razor blade inserted into the cork so that they are parallel and separated from each other by 1 mm. The cutter is lowered onto the agar on a slide to cut the required pattern and the agar plugs are removed from the wells cut with the needles (a fine Pasteur pipette on a water pump is suitable). The agar between the two parallel cuts made by the razor blades is left *in situ* until after electrophoresis. The prepared slide is used as a bridge between the two compartments of the electrophoresis apparatus, and is connected to the buffer at each end by means of filter paper wicks. It is important that the wicks are kept damp as they tend to heat up and dry due to the passage of the current. Electrophoresis of the antigen (placed in the peripheral wells) is carried out using about 50 volts requiring approximately 2·5 ma. per slide for a period (45 min.–4 hr.) sufficient to give adequate separation of the different components of the antigen. Following this the band of agar in the trough between the two razor blade slits is removed and the antiserum run into the trough. The slide is then placed in a humid atmosphere at 4° C. or 37° C. to allow the development of the precipitin reaction. The preparation is examined at intervals using the viewing box described on page 950. Any precipitin bands formed can be recorded by drawing the pattern obtained on a piece of paper or the preparation can be photographed. Staining of the bands with a protein stain improves the clarity of the patterns and may even show up precipitin bands which cannot be seen in the unstained preparation. Such stained preparations can conveniently be dried and kept for reference. A suitable procedure for staining and drying is as follows:—

(1) The unprecipitated protein is washed out of the agar by immersion of the slide for 24 hr. in the buffer used to make up the agar solution.

(2) The slide is then washed for 15 min. in 1 per cent. acetic acid to remove excess salts.

(3) Staining is carried out with a protein stain such as naphthalene black made up to a 1 per cent. solution in a solvent containing glacial acetic acid

[1] L.K.B. Produktur, London & Stockholm.

1 ml., distilled water 49 ml., and methylated spirit 50 ml. Staining should be carried out for about 30 min. with this stain.

(4) Excess stain is washed out with the solvent to give a preparation with dark blue precipitin bands on a clear background.

(5) The preparation is finally soaked in 1 per cent. acetic acid containing 1 per cent. glycerol for 15 min. and dried at 37° C. in an incubator.

ANTIGEN-ANTIBODY REACTIONS USING FLUORESCENT LABELS

The precise localisation of tissue antigens or of the antigens of infecting organisms in the body, of anti-tissue antibody and of antigen-antibody complexes was achieved by the introduction of the use of fluorochrome labelled proteins by Coons and Kaplan in 1950. This immunofluorescence technique combines the sensitivity and specificity of immunology with the precision of microscopy; it has yielded new information that could hardly have been discovered in any other way. The absorption of ultraviolet light between 290 and 495 mμ by fluorescein and its emission of longer-wavelength green light (525 mμ) is used to visualise protein labelled with this dye. The technique is more sensitive than precipitation or complement fixation techniques, and fluorescent protein tracers can be detected at a concentration of the order of 1 μg. protein per ml. of body fluid (Nairn, 1962). Of the variety of fluorescent dyes available fluorescein isothiocyanate which emits a green light and lissamine rhodamine B (RB200) emitting an orange yellow colour are most commonly used. In both cases the conjugation process is very simple. There are two main methods used in immunofluorescent work, the direct method and the indirect method (Fig. 80).

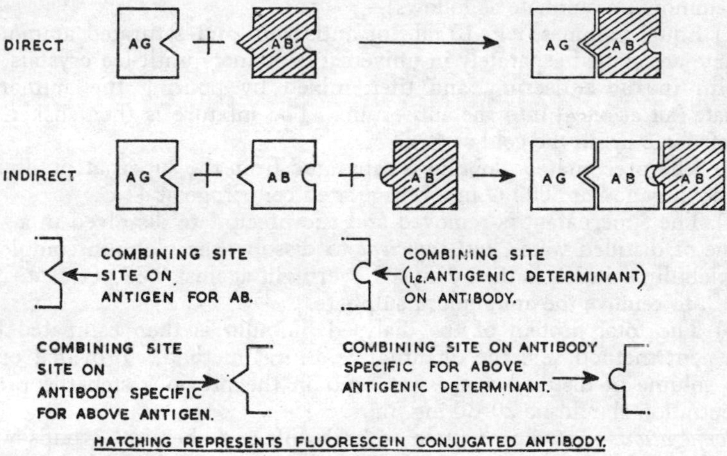

FIG. 80

Diagram illustrating the direct and indirect fluorescent antibody methods.
AG = Antigen. AB = Antibody.

The direct method consists of bringing fluorescein tagged antibodies into contact with antigens fixed on a slide, allowing them to react, washing off the excess antibody and examining the slide under the fluorescence microscope. The site of union of the labelled antibody with its antigen can be determined by the apple green or orange yellow fluorescent areas on the slide.

The indirect method is used both for detecting specific antibodies in sera or other body fluids and also as a direct method for identifying antigens. For the detection of antibodies (for example those in serum to a particular antigen), a slide to which a preparation of the antigen is fixed, is flooded with the specific serum, and after an interval the excess serum is washed off. The localisation of the antibody on the antigen preparation is then visualised microscopically by layering the slide with a fluorescein labelled antibody specific for the serum proteins of the serum under test. The most suitable type of labelled antibody is that directed primarily against the globulin (antibody containing) fraction of the test serum, *i.e.* a fluorescein labelled antiglobulin serum. Such an antiglobulin serum can be used to detect antibody globulin in sera to a variety of different antigens. Identification of an unknown antigen by the indirect immunofluorescence method is accomplished by layering a known antibody on to a slide on which there is a preparation of the unknown antigen. After washing off the excess antibody the preparation is layered as in the above example with a fluorescein conjugated antiglobulin serum specific for the globulin of the known antibody. Fluorescence indicates a reaction between the unknown antigen and the known antibody globulin.

The indirect technique is substantially more sensitive (4 to 12 fold) than the direct method due to the additional combining sites which are made available by the antibody molecules of the middle layer acting as antigen for the fluorescent antiglobulin.

Conjugation of Antiserum with Fluorescein Isothiocyanate

Prior to conjugation it is necessary to separate the globulin fraction from the antiserum and this is conveniently carried out by 50 per cent. saturation with ammonium sulphate as follows:—

(1) Equal volumes, *e.g.* 10 ml., of antiserum and saturated ammonium sulphate are chilled separately in universal containers until ice crystals start to form in the antiserum, and then mixed by pouring the ammonium sulphate (all at once) into the antiserum. The mixture is then shaken well and left for 2 hr. in the cold at 4° C.

(2) The precipitated globulin is separated from the supernatant albumin by centrifugation at 3000 *G* in a refrigerated centrifuge at 4° C.

(3) The supernatant is removed and the precipitate dissolved in a small volume of distilled water, *just sufficient* to dissolve the globulin completely. The globulin solution is then dialysed overnight against 0·85 per cent. NaCl at 4 °C. to remove the ammonium sulphate.

(4) The total protein of the dialysed globulin is then estimated by a convenient method, *e.g.* the quantitative Biuret method. Provided only a small volume of distilled water was used in the previous step the protein concentration should be 20–30 mg./ml.

Conjugation.—Proteins contain several different chemical groups which can be used for the attachment of fluorochromes. These include the free amino and carboxyl groups at the ends of each protein chain and free amino groups in the lysine side chains. The optimal quantity of fluorescein has been estimated by Coons and Kaplan (1950) as 0·05 mg./mg. of protein. Above this level no further conjugation takes place and progressively larger amounts of protein are denatured.

Conjugation with Fluorescein Isothiocyanate

(1) The globulin fraction prepared as indicated above is diluted to 10 mg.

of protein per ml. with 0·5 *M* carbonate-bicarbonate buffer pH 9·2 (p. 856) (made up fresh before use) so that the final mixture contains 10 per cent. buffer.

(2) The solution is chilled to 4° C. and 0·05 mg. of fluorescein isothiocyanate (British Drug Houses) per mg. of protein is added. During the addition of the fluorochrome and for the next 18 hr. the mixture should be stirred continuously, *e.g.* with a magnetic stirrer, and kept at 4° C.

(4) Following conjugation excess fluorescein is dialysed away against phosphate buffered saline (physiological 0·85 per cent. NaCl buffered with 0·01 *M* phosphate) in the cold, changing the buffer frequently until the dialysate contains no further dye.

(5) The conjugate is finally centrifuged for 45 min. at 3000 *G* at 4° C. to remove any precipitated denatured protein.

Conjugation with Lissamine Rhodamine B (*RB*200)

The fluorochrome is used as the sulphonyl chloride prepared by grinding 0·5 g. of RB200 with 1 g. of PCl_5 in a mortar (using a fume cupboard). After mixing, 5 ml. of acetone is added with stirring for a few minutes and the mixture filtered. This solution should be used within 48 hr. of preparation. The conjugation process is similar to that for fluorescein isothiocyanate except that 0·2 ml. of the solution is used for every 100 mg. of protein and after mixing with the globulin stirring need only be continued for 30 min.

Storage of Conjugates

Conjugates may be stored at 4° C. with the addition of preservative, *e.g.* merthiolate 1/10,000; alternatively they may be stored at −20° C. or freeze dried. Prior to use non-specific fluorescence will require to be absorbed out from the conjugate.

Anti-nuclear Factor Test

The application of the indirect fluorescent antibody technique to the study of sera that are able to induce the formation of LE cells showed that these sera contain an antibody—*the antinuclear factor* (ANF)—which reacts with the nuclei of tissue cells. The method is so valuable in the diagnosis of systemic lupus erythematosus (SLE) that it is generally agreed that a diagnosis of SLE would be difficult to sustain in the absence of a positive test. It is necessary to point out however that positive tests can be found in other disease states and in occasional normal sera—usually in low titre—and that a positive test does not necessarily imply that the patient is suffering from SLE.

Method (Weir, Holborow & Johnson, 1961):

Reagents:—

(1) A source of cell nuclei—sections of animal tissue are commonly used, *e.g.* mouse liver, calf thyroid. The freshly taken tissue is snap frozen in a sealed container and CO_2 snow at −70° C. and sections approximately 6 μ thick are cut in a cryostat.[1] The sections are air dried in front of a small electric fan.

[1] South London Electric Company, Hither Green, London, S.E. 13 and Prestcold Ltd., Swansea, manufacture suitable models.

(2) Anti-human globulin conjugated with fluorescein isothiocyanate. Unconjugated serum can be obtained from Burroughs Wellcome and conjugated by the method described on page 956 or a Difco conjugated serum can be obtained from Baird & Tatlock (London).

(3) Buffered saline pH 7·1 (physiological saline buffered by 0·01 *M* phosphate).

(4) Clean slides and coverslips.

(5) Buffered glycerol mounting medium (one part of the buffered saline to 9 parts of glycerol).

Absorption of conjugates.—To remove "non-specific" fluorescence of the conjugate it is absorbed with liver powder prepared from fresh rabbit or mouse liver homogenised in a Waring blender, repeatedly washed with acetone and finally dried and finely powdered in a mortar and pestle. Approximately 100 mg. of the resulting powder is used for absorbing 1 ml. of conjugate. The carefully shaken mixture is left for 1 hour, after which the conjugate is recovered by centrifugation (1500–2000 *G* for 10 min.). A further absorption may be required with some conjugates.

The Test

Each section is covered with a few drops of test serum (*see controls*) and incubated in a moist chamber for 30 min. at 37° C. After incubation, the serum is washed off carefully in two changes of the buffered saline for a total of 20 min., fixed in 90 per cent. alcohol for 5 min., washed again in buffer, and stained with the fluorescein conjugated anti-human globulin serum by covering the section with a few drops of the conjugate and incubating as before. After 30 min. the sections are again washed and mounted in buffered glycerol. Examination of these sections under the fluorescence microscope (see p. 633) will show apple green fluorescence of the cell nuclei in a positive preparation and unstained spaces in negative sera.

Controls.—Each series of tests should include a known positive serum and a negative serum control. It will be found necessary to dilute the test serum with buffer in this test as in the FTA 200 technique (*vide infra*) in order to dilute out the "non-specific" adherence of serum proteins to tissues. The actual dilution necessary may vary with different anti-human globulin conjugates and a trial will have to be carried out using a group of 10 normal sera diluted, *e.g.* 1 in 2 to 1 in 20, to establish the most suitable dilution required to give an unstained background. (See Holborow & Johnson, 1964.)

FTA 200 test

The indirect fluorescent antibody technique is used for the detection of specific antibodies to *Treponema pallidum* and is a simple alternative to the Treponema Pallidum Immobilisation Test. The test is based on that described by Deacon, Falcone and Harris (1957) and utilises a desiccated standardised killed suspension of *Trep. pallidum* and fluorescein conjugated goat anti-human globulin serum. The reagents (Difco) required can be obtained commercially from Baird & Tatlock (London). The conjugate may require to be absorbed with liver powder (*vide supra*).

The Test

(1) Draw a circle 1 cm. in diameter on a clean dry microscope slide.

(2) Place approximately 0·01 ml. of the reconstituted treponemal antigen solution on the slide covering the encircled area. Allow to dry.

(3) Fix the smear of organisms with anhydrous acetone for 10 min. and allow to dry.

(4) Layer the smear of organisms with about 0·03 ml. of the patient's serum diluted 1 in 200 in phosphate buffer pH 7·0 (page 854). Known positive and negative controls should be set up at the same time.

(5) Place the slide in a damp chamber for 1 hr. at 37° C.

(6) Wash off excess serum in the buffer for 10 min., change the buffer twice during this time. Blot the slide gently with absorbent paper.

(7) Add one drop of the fluorescein conjugated goat anti-human globulin to the serum treated smear of organisms, and leave in a damp chamber for 30 min. at 37° C.

(8) Wash off excess conjugate in the buffered saline for 10 min. changing the buffer once. Remove the slides, blot, place a drop of buffered glycerol (page 958) on the smear and cover with a glass coverslip.

(9) Examine under the fluorescence microscope (see p. 633) using dark ground illumination. Careful comparison of the negative control with the positive control will show green fluorescent treponemata distinctly visible in the positive control only. If tungsten lighting is available on the microscope a useful check of what appear under UV to be fluorescent organisms can be made by examination of the same field under the tungsten light. In routine use, and once the worker is familiar with the appearances with positive and negative sera, the test should be carried out so as to include, amongst the sera under test, positive and negative controls which should be examined without prior knowledge of their origin. When the tests have all been read the results can then be checked with the actual origin and labelling of the preparations.

LE Cell Test

A sample of clotted blood (2 ml. or more) is taken into a clean dry container and incubated at 37° C. as soon as possible after having been taken from the patient. After 2 hr. the container is shaken (in order to damage some of the leucocytes and make them more susceptible to LE cell formation) and re-incubated for a further 20 min. At the end of this period, using a Pasteur pipette, the mixture of serum and cells is separated from the clot, and centrifuged for 5 min. in a Wintrobe tube at approximately 1000 *G* The superficial layer—"the buffy coat" containing the leucocytes—is carefully removed using a *fine* Pasteur pipette and films prepared on clean glass slides. After staining with Leishman's stain the slides are examined under the low power objective for 10 min. and the oil immersion objective used to examine suspicious cells closely. Only polymorphs containing homogeneous inclusions which stain a pink purple colour and which show no residual chromatin pattern should be accepted as LE cells. The polymorph nucleus is displaced to one side of the cell by the large inclusion which is surrounded by a thin rim of polymorph cytoplasm. More darkly staining inclusions (ingested unaltered leucocyte nuclei) with well marked chromatin pattern and phagocytosed red cells must be differentiated from a true LE cell.

Antistreptolysin-O Test

Titration of antibody to the streptolysin-O of *Strept. pyogenes* is helpful in the diagnosis of acute rheumatic fever, and acute glomerular nephritis. A titre of 200 units per ml. or more indicates recent streptococcal infection. One of 50 units per ml. or below practically excludes rheumatic fever and is commonly found in normal individuals. A method has been described by Gooder & Williams (1959).

REFERENCES

BARRETT, A. M. (1941). Serological diagnosis of glandular fever (infectious mononucleosis); new technique. *J. Hyg. (Lond.)*, **41**, 330.

BRADSTREET, C. M. P. & TAYLOR, C. E. D. (1962). Technique of complement-fixation test applicable to the diagnosis of virus diseases. *Mth. Bull. Minist. Hlth. Lab. Serv.*, **21**, 96.

BYWATERS, E. G. L. & SCOTT, F. E. T. (1960). Rheumatism and connective tissue diseases. p. 279 in *Recent Advances in Clinical Pathology*. Ed. S. C. Dyke. London: Churchill.

CLARKE, D. H. & CASALS, J. (1958). Techniques for haemagglutination and haemagglutination-inhibition with arthropod-borne viruses. *Amer. J. trop. Med. Hyg.*, **7**, 561.

COOMBS, R. R. A., COOMBS, A. M. & INGRAM, D. G. (1960). *The Serology of Conglutination and its Relation to Disease*. Oxford: Blackwell.

COONS, A. H. & KAPLAN, M. W. (1950). Localization of antigens in tissue cells. *J. exp. Med.*, **91**, 1.

CROWLE, A. J. (1961). *Immunodiffusion*. New York: Academic Press.

CRUICKSHANK, R. (1947). In *Recent Advances in Clinical Pathology*. London: Churchill.

CSIZMAS, L. (1960). Preparation of formalised erythrocytes. *Proc. Soc. exp. Biol. (N.Y.).*, **103**, 157.

DARTER, L. A. (1953). Procedure for production of antisheep haemolysin. *J. Lab. clin. Med.*, **41**, 653.

DEACON, W. E., FALCONE, V. H. & HARRIS, A. (1957). A fluorescent test for treponemal antibodies. *Proc. Soc. exp. Biol. (N.Y.)*, **96**, 477.

DERRIEN, Y., MICHEL, R. & ROCHE, J. (1948). Recherches sur la préparation et les proprietés de la thyroglobuline pure. *Biochem. biophys. Acta. (Amst.)*, **2**, 454.

Diagnostic Procedures for Virus and Rickettsial Diseases (1964). 3rd Edition. Edited by E. H. Lennette & N. J. Schmidt. New York: American Public Health Association.

FILDES, P. (1931). The measurement of small quantities of fluid. *A System of Bacteriology*, **9**, 174. London: Medical Research Council.

FULTHORPE, A. J., ROITT, I. M., DONIACH, D. & COUCHMAN, K. (1961). A stable sheep cell preparation for detecting thyroglobulin auto-antibodies and its clinical application. *J. clin. Path.*, **14**, 654.

FULTON, F. & DUMBELL, K. R. (1949). The serological comparison of strains of the influenza virus. *J. gen. Microbiol.*, **3**, 97.

GELL, P. G. H. (1957). The estimation of individual human serum proteins by an immunological method. *J. clin. Path.*, **10**, 67.

GLYNN, L. E. (1963). Rheumatoid arthritis and the rheumatoid factor. P. 593 in *Clinical Aspects of Immunology*. Eds. Gell, P. G. H. & Coombs, R. R. A. Oxford: Blackwell.

GOODER, H. & WILLIAMS, R. E. O. (1959). Titration of Antistreptolysin-O. *Broadsheet No. 25. (New Series)*, Assoc. Clin. Pathologists.

GRASSET, E., BONIFAS, V. & PONGRATZ, E. (1958). Rapid slide precipitation microreaction of poliomyelitis antigens and antisera in agar. *Proc. Soc. exp. Biol. (N.Y.)*, **97**, 72.

HEINER, D. C. (1958). Diagnosis of histoplasmosis using precipitin reactions in agar gel. *Paediatrics*, **22**, 616.

HENLE, W., LIEF, F. S. & FABIYI, A. (1958). Strain-specific complement-fixation test in antigenic analysis and serodiagnosis of influenza. *Lancet*, **1**, 818.

HERBERT, W. J. (1967). In *Handbook of Experimental Immunology*. Ed. D. M. Weir. Oxford: Blackwell.

HOLBOROW J. & JOHNSON, G. D. (1964). Antinuclear factor in Systemic Lupus Erythematosus. A consideration of the immunofluorescent method of detecting antinuclear antibodies, with results obtained in a family study. *Arthritis and Rheumatism*, **7**, 119.

HOYLE, L. (1948). Technique of the complement fixation test in influenza. *Mth. Bull. Minist. Hlth. Lab. Serv.*, **7**, 114.

HOYLE, L. (1952). Structure of the influenza virus. *J. Hyg. (Lond.)*, **50**, 229.

KABAT, E. L. & MAYER, M. M. (1961). *Experimental Immunochemistry*. 2nd Ed. p. 476. Springfield, Illinois: Thomas.

KAHN, R. L. (1928). *The Kahn Test.* Baltimore: Williams & Wilkins.
KAHN, R. L. (1940). The serology of syphilis. *J. Lab. clin. Med.*, **26**, 139.
KAHN, R. L. (1941). Serologic verification tests in the diagnosis of latent syphilis. *Arch. Derm. Syph.* (*Chic.*), **41**, 817.
KELLGREN, J. H. & BALL, J. (1959). Clinical significance of the rheumatoid serum factor. *Brit. med. J.*, **1**, 582.
KHAIRAT, O. (1952). Kahn tube test with dropping pipettes. *Brit. med. J.*, **1**, 582.
KOLMER, J. A., SPAULDING, E. H. & ROBINSON, H. W. (1952). *Approved Laboratory Technique.* London: Lewis.
LECOCQ, E. & LINZ, R. (1962). Agglutination d'hématies tannées traitées par deux antigenes. *Ann. Inst. Pasteur, Lille*, **102**, 437.
LIEF, F. S. & HENLE, W. (1956). Studies on the soluble antigen of influenza virus. *Virology*, **2**, 753, 773, 782.
MAYER, M. M., OSLER, A. G., BIER, O. G. & HEIDELBERGER, M. (1948). Quantitative studies in complement fixation. *J. Immunol.*, **59**, 195.
MUSCHEL, L. H. & LOWE, K. M. (1955). New complement-fixation test for syphilis. *J. Lab. clin. Med.*, **46**, 147.
NAIRN, R. C. (1962). *Fluorescent Protein Tracing.* 2nd Ed. Edinburgh: Livingstone.
OAKLEY, C. L. & FULTHORPE, A. J. (1953). Antigenic analysis by diffusion. *J. Path. Bact.*, **65**, 49.
OUDIN, J. (1946). Methode d'analyse immunochemique par précipitation specifique en milieu gelifie. *C.R. Acad. Sci.* (*Paris*), **222**, 115.
PEPYS, J., JENKINS, P. A., FESTENSTEIN, G. N., GREGORY, P. H., LACEY, M. E. & SKINNER, F. A. (1963). Farmer's lung. *Lancet*, **2**, 607.
PREER, J. R. (1956). A quantitative study of a technique of double diffusion in agar. *J. Immunol.*, **77**, 52.
PRICE, I. N. O. (1949). Complement-fixation technique; estimation of complement doses. *Brit. J. vener. Dis.*, **25**, 157.
PRICE, I. N. O. (1950a). Complement-fixation technique; titration of Wassermann antigen. *Brit. J. vener. Dis.*, **26**, 33.
PRICE, I. N. O. (1950b). Complement-fixation technique; Wassermann reaction. *Brit. J. vener. Dis.*, **26**, 172.
PRICE, I. N. O. & WILKINSON, A. E. (1947). A rapid method of standardisation of the sheep-cell suspension used in the Harrison-Wyler Wassermann technique. *Brit. J. vener. Dis.*, **23**, 124.
REED, L. J. & MUENCH, H. (1938). A simple method of estimating fifty per cent. end points. *Amer. J. Hyg.*, **27**, 493.
RICHARDSON, G. M. (1941). The preservation of liquid complement serum. *Lancet*, **2**, 696.
SAWYER, H. P. & BOURKE, A. R. (1946). Anti-sheep amboceptor production with elimination of rabbit shock. *J. Lab. clin. Med.*, **31**, 714.
SCHEIFFARTH, F. & GOETZ, H. (1960). Significance of immuno-electrophoresis in differentiation of pathological sera. *Arch. Allergy.* (*N.Y.*), **16**, 61.
SEVER, J. L. (1962). Application of a microtechnique to viral serological investigations. *J. Immunol.*, **88**, 320.
SINGER, J. M., ALTMANN, G., ORESKES, I. & PLOTZ, C. M. (1961). The mechanism of particle carrier reactions. *Amer. J. Med.*, **30**, 772.
SINGER, J. M. & PLOTZ, C. M. (1956). The latex fixation test. *Amer. J. Med.*, **21**, 88.
SONNENSCHEIN, C. (1930). Komplementkonservierung durch Natriumazetat und Borsaure. M. *Immun.-Forsch.*, **67**, 512.
TAKÁTSY, G. (1955). The use of spiral loops in serological and virological micromethods. *Acta microbiol. Acad. Sci.* (*hung.*), **3**, 191.
WALLACE, A. C., OSLER, A. G. & MAYER, M. M. (1950). Quantitative studies of the complement-fixation. V. Estimation of complement-fixing potency of immune sera and its relation to antibody nitrogen content. *J. Immunol.*, **65**, 661.
WEIR, D. M. (1967). *Handbook of Experimental Immunology.* Oxford: Blackwell.
WEIR, D. M., HOLBOROW, E. J. & JOHNSON, G. D. (1961). A clinical study of serum antinuclear factor *Brit. med. J.*, **1**, 933.
WILKINSON, A. E. (1950). Destructive effect of traces of zinc salts on complement. *J. clin. Path.*, **3**, 363.
WORLD HEALTH ORGANIZATION (1951). Cardiolipin antigens. *Bull. Wld. Hlth Org.*, **4**, 151.
WORLD HEALTH ORGANIZATION (1959). Expert Committee on respiratory virus diseases. *Wld. Hlth. Org. techn. Rep. Ser.*, No. 170, p. 41.

Wyler, E. J. (1929). The Wassermann Test. *Spec. Rep. Ser. med. Res. Coun. (Lond.)*, No. **129**.

Wyler, E. J. (1934). Certain practical considerations concerning haemolytic system in complement fixation tests; with a note on the standardisation of droppers for Wassermann test. *J. Path. Bact.*, **39**, 521.

CHAPTER 55

BACTERIOLOGY OF WATER, MILK, ICE-CREAM, SHELL-FISH, OTHER FOODS, AIR

BACTERIOLOGICAL EXAMINATION OF WATER

DRINKING-WATER supplies liable to contamination with sewage or other excreted matter may cause outbreaks of intestinal infections such as typhoid fever. In safeguarding public water supplies, health authorities and water engineers rely on information obtained from the results of frequent bacteriological tests. The demonstration of pathogenic bacteria, *e.g.* the typhoid bacillus, would obviously constitute the most direct proof of a dangerous impurity, but these pathogens, if present, are usually so scanty that the technical difficulty of their isolation makes the test impracticable for ordinary purposes (but see p. 977). Instead we rely on tests that will reveal the presence of commensal bacteria of intestinal origin such as those of the coliform group, *Streptococcus faecalis* and *Clostridium welchii.* These do not themselves constitute a hazard, but they indicate that faecal matter has entered the supply and that the water is therefore liable to contamination with more dangerous organisms. The coliform bacilli are the most reliable indicators of faecal pollution. Although the presence of streptococci is strong evidence of faecal pollution, their absence does not exclude such impurity. The sporing anaerobes, on the other hand, being highly resistant, would in the absence of the other intestinal organisms indicate pollution of some remote period rather than one of recent occurrence.

Since the coliform group of bacteria may be derived from the intestines of various animals and birds they are likely to occur in small numbers even in water supplies far removed from the possibility of human contamination. Water grossly polluted with human excretal matter, *e.g.* sewage, contains them in larger numbers. The test for their presence as an index of the degree of pollution must therefore be carried out on a quantitative basis. The coliform group of lactose-fermenting Gram-negative bacilli includes a number of different organisms (Enterobacteriaceae). Those referred to as "typical" or "faecal" (e.g. *Esch. coli*) are essentially commensals of the intestine and are derived almost exclusively from this source. Others, known as "atypical" (e.g. *Kl. aerogenes*), may grow also in the soil and on vegetation, and by derivation from these sources often come to be present in waters that are not subject to excretal pollution. The typical faecal bacilli (*Esch. coli*) die in water during the course of several days or weeks after leaving the animal intestine; thus, their presence in water is an indication of recent faecal contamination, whereas the presence of the hardier atypical coliforms is not necessarily so. In carrying out the test for coliform bacilli in water it is therefore advisable to determine whether the strains present are typical or atypical.

A determination of the total number of viable bacteria in a water sample is a useful supplementary test, although of limited value by itself. It gives an indication of the amount and type of organic matter present in the supply. The test is carried out in duplicate at 37° C. and 20°–22° C. The bacteria that grow at 37° C. are those most likely to be associated with organic material of human or animal origin, whereas those growing at the lower temperature are mainly saprophytes that normally inhabit the water or are derived from soil and vegetation.

The routine tests generally used in bacteriological examination of water are:

1. A quantitative test for all coliform bacilli known as the *presumptive coliform count.*

2. A differential test for typical coliform bacilli (*Esch. coli*) known as the *differential coliform test.*

3. An enumeration of viable bacteria known as the *plate count*; this is done in duplicate, cultivating at 37° C. and 22° C.

Chemical analyses are sometimes used for judging the quality of water supplies. They are not, however, as sensitive as bacterial tests for detecting dangerous pollution.

Collection of Specimens

Specimens are taken in bottles, of *c.* 230 ml. capacity, with ground-glass stoppers having an overhanging rim; they are sterilised by autoclaving, the stopper and neck of the bottle being covered over by two layers of kraft paper. Alternatively, 6-oz. screw-capped bottles may be used. These are wrapped in kraft paper and sterilised in the autoclave. The opening and closing of the bottle in the process of collecting a sample must be carried out with meticulous care to avoid any bacterial contamination from an outside source. When water is drawn from a tap, the mouth of the tap should be flamed, *e.g.* with a blow-lamp or spirit lamp, and the water allowed to run for 5 min. before filling the bottle. In the case of streams, rivers and lakes, the stopper should be removed carefully with one hand, and with the other the bottle held at its base should be inserted, mouth downward, a foot below the surface of the water; the bottle is then turned so that the mouth is directed to the current and water flows into the bottle without coming into contact with the hand. If there is no current the bottle should be moved horizontally, the mouth foremost, so that water flows into it. The bottle is then brought to the surface and the stopper is replaced. Care must be taken that the stopper is not contaminated during the sampling process. This method of sampling avoids the collection of surface water, which may contain a good deal of decomposing vegetable matter.

When a sample is to be obtained from a depth, a bottle weighted with lead is used, having two cords attached—one to the neck, the other to the stopper; the bottle is lowered to the required depth, and is filled by jerking out the stopper by means of the attached cord; the bottle is then quickly raised to the surface and re-stoppered.

When 3 hr. or more must elapse before the laboratory examination can be carried out, the bottles should be kept on ice. Special insulated boxes for the purpose can be obtained and are essential where specimens have to be transported some distance.

Neutralisation of Chlorine.—If a sample is taken from a chlorinated water supply it is important that any traces of free chlorine should be neutralised immediately as otherwise killing of bacteria may proceed in the time elapsing before the specimen is examined in the laboratory. A crystal of sodium thiosulphate introduced into the sampling bottle prior to sterilisation serves to effect neutralisation.

Immediately before testing, the water sample should be mixed by inverting the bottle 25 times. Thereafter some of the contents are poured off, the stopper is replaced and the bottle is shaken vigorously 25 times with an up-and-down movement.

Presumptive Coliform Count (Multiple Tube Technique)

An estimation of the number of coliform bacilli in a water supply is usually made by adding varying quantities of the water (from 0·1 ml. to 50 ml.) to bile salt lactose peptone water (with an indicator of acidity) contained in bottles with Durham tubes to show the formation of gas; acid and gas formation (a "positive" result) indicates the growth of coliform bacilli. In this way it is possible to state the smallest quantity of water containing a coliform bacillus and thus to express the degree of contamination with this group of organisms.

This method requires examination by culture of several samples of several different quantities of the water so that an average result can be stated. It has been shown that if one 50 ml., five 10 ml. and five 1 ml. volumes, or five 10 ml., five 1 ml. and five 0·1 ml. volumes are tested, the probable number of coliform bacilli in 100 ml. can be computed according to the various combinations of positive and negative results, tables compiled by McCrady being used for the purpose (p. 966). This is the method recommended for routine use.

Method.—Measured amounts (*vide infra*) of single and double strength modified MacConkey's fluid medium (see p. 783) are sterilised in bottles containing a Durham tube for indicating gas production. The size of the bottle varies with the quantity of medium and water to be added to it.

With sterile graduated pipettes the following amounts of water are added:

One 50 ml. quantity of water to 50 ml. double strength medium
Five 10 ml. quantities each to 10 ml. double strength medium
Five 1 ml. ,, ,, 5 ml. single ,, ,,
Five 0·1 ml. ,, ,, 5 ml. ,, ,, ,,

This range of quantities may be altered according to the likely condition of the water examined; thus, the 50 ml. quantity is included when testing filtered or chlorinated water, and in this case it is unnecessary to examine 0·1 ml. volumes. This amount, *i.e.* 1 ml. of the sample diluted 1 in 10 (for dilution technique, see p. 970), is tested only when the water supply is suspected of being highly contaminated.

The bottles are incubated at 37° C. and examined after 18-24 hr. Those that show acid and sufficient gas to fill the concavity at the top of the Durham tube are considered to be "presumptive positive" as a result of the growth of coliform bacilli. Any remaining negative bottles are reincubated for another 24 hr., and if acid and gas develop they too are regarded as being positive. In reporting the results of the presumptive test reference is now made to McCrady's probability tables (pp. 966-68). According to the various combinations of positive and negative results obtained the probable number of coliform bacilli in 100 ml. of the water can be read.

According to the older system of notation, these results can be stated alternatively as "coliform bacillus present in . . . ml.", the number of ml. being 100 divided by the figure in the last column; thus, if the number of coliform bacilli in 100 ml. is 5, the result can be stated as "coliform bacillus present in 20 ml.", 20 ml. being the smallest amount of water in which a coliform bacillus is likely to be present.

Probability Tables (according to McCrady)

Quantity of Water	50 ml.	10 ml.	1 ml.	Probable number of coliform bacilli in 100 ml. of water.
No. of samples of each quantity tested	1	5	5	
Number giving positive reaction (acid and gas).	0	0	0	0
	0	0	1	1
	0	0	2	2
	0	1	0	1
	0	1	1	2
	0	1	2	3
	0	2	0	2
	0	2	1	3
	0	2	2	4
	0	3	0	3
	0	3	1	5
	0	4	0	5
	1	0	0	1
	1	0	1	3
	1	0	2	4
	1	0	3	6
	1	1	0	3
	1	1	1	5
	1	1	2	7
	1	1	3	9
	1	2	0	5
	1	2	1	7
	1	2	2	10
	1	2	3	12
	1	3	0	8
	1	3	1	11
	1	3	2	14
	1	3	3	18
	1	3	4	20
	1	4	0	13
	1	4	1	17
	1	4	2	20
	1	4	3	30
	1	4	4	35
	1	4	5	40
	1	5	0	25
	1	5	1	35
	1	5	2	50
	1	5	3	90
	1	5	4	160
	1	5	5	180+

Quantity of Water	10 ml.	1 ml.	0·1 ml.	
No. of samples of each quantity tested	5	5	5	
Number giving positive reaction (acid and gas).				Probable number of coliform bacilli in 100 ml. of water.
	0	0	0	0
	0	0	1	2
	0	0	2	4
	0	1	0	2
	0	1	1	4
	0	1	2	6
	0	2	0	4
	0	2	1	6
	0	3	0	6
	1	0	0	2
	1	0	1	4
	1	0	2	6
	1	0	3	8
	1	1	0	4
	1	1	1	6
	1	1	2	8
	1	2	0	6
	1	2	1	8
	1	2	2	10
	1	3	0	8
	1	3	1	10
	1	4	0	11
	2	0	0	5
	2	0	1	7
	2	0	2	9
	2	0	3	12
	2	1	0	7
	2	1	1	9
	2	1	2	12
	2	2	0	9
	2	2	1	12
	2	2	2	14
	2	3	0	12
	2	3	1	14
	2	4	0	15
	3	0	0	8
	3	0	1	11
	3	0	2	13
	3	1	0	11
	3	1	1	14
	3	1	2	17
	3	1	3	20
	3	2	0	14
	3	2	1	17
	3	2	2	20
	3	3	0	17
	3	3	1	20
	3	4	0	20
	3	4	1	25
	3	5	0	25

Quantity of Water	10 ml.	1 ml.	0·1 ml.	Probable number of coliform bacilli in 100 ml. of water.
No. of samples of each quantity tested	5	5	5	
Number giving positive reaction (acid and gas).	4	0	0	13
	4	0	1	17
	4	0	2	20
	4	0	3	25
	4	1	0	17
	4	1	1	20
	4	1	2	25
	4	2	0	20
	4	2	1	25
	4	2	2	30
	4	3	0	25
	4	3	1	35
	4	3	2	40
	4	4	0	35
	4	4	1	40
	4	4	2	45
	4	5	0	40
	4	5	1	50
	4	5	2	55
	5	0	0	25
	5	0	1	30
	5	0	2	45
	5	0	3	60
	5	0	4	75
	5	1	0	35
	5	1	1	45
	5	1	2	65
	5	1	3	85
	5	1	4	115
	5	2	0	50
	5	2	1	70
	5	2	2	95
	5	2	3	120
	5	2	4	150
	5	2	5	175
	5	3	0	80
	5	3	1	110
	5	3	2	140
	5	3	3	175
	5	3	4	200
	5	3	5	250
	5	4	0	130
	5	4	1	170
	5	4	2	225
	5	4	3	275
	5	4	4	350
	5	4	5	425
	5	5	0	250
	5	5	1	350
	5	5	2	550
	5	5	3	900
	5	5	4	1600
	5	5	5	1800+

Differential Coliform Test

To ascertain whether the coliform bacilli detected in the presumptive test are *Esch. coli*, the Eijkman test is usually employed. This depends on the ability of *Esch. coli* to produce gas when growing in bile-salt lactose peptone water at 44° C., and the inability of atypical coliform bacilli to do this. After the usual presumptive test, subcultures are made from all the bottles showing acid and gas into fresh tubes of single strength MacConkey's medium. It is advisable to heat the tubes to 37° C. in a water-bath before inoculating them. They are then incubated at 44° C. and examined after 24 hr. Those yielding gas may be regarded as containing *Esch. coli* and a computation of the number in 100 ml. of water can be made as before. This is the "confirmed *Esch. coli* count".

An alternative medium for use in the Eijkman test is ***brilliant green bile broth*** (p. 784). This was found by Mackenzie *et al.* (1948) to be superior to MacConkey's fluid medium for detecting typical coliform bacilli, since the brilliant green tends to suppress the growth of anaerobic lactose-fermenting organisms such as *Cl. welchii*, which otherwise might give false positive reactions at 44° C. Positive results in this medium are indicated by gas production and turbidity. There is no colour change.

Two types of atypical coliform bacilli are known to give rise to gas production at 44° C. They are Irregular Type II and Irregular Type VI as classified by Wilson *et al.* (1935). Unlike typical coliform bacilli these types are unable to produce indole at 44° C. Although they rarely occur in water supplies in this country, it is advisable when carrying out Eijkman tests to inoculate at the same time tubes of peptone water from the positive "presumptive" tubes. All tubes are incubated at 44° C.

The following interpretation of results is given by Mackenzie *et al.*

Gas in brilliant green bile broth at 44° C.	Indole production at 44° C.	
+	+	Typical coliform bacilli
+	−	Irregular Type II / Irregular Type VI
−	+	Other coliform organisms
−	−	Other coliform organisms

It is very important that incubation at 44° C. should be carried out in a thermostatically controlled water-bath that does not deviate more than 0·5° C. from 44° C. An incubator is not satisfactory.

For fuller differentiation of the coliform group by means of the methyl-red, Voges-Proskauer, citrate-utilisation and sugar fermentation reactions, reference should be made to Chapter 18.

The Plate Count

With a sterile graduated pipette place 1 ml. water in a sterile Petri dish (4 in. diameter) and add 10 ml. yeast extract agar (see p. 783), melted and cooled to 50° C.; mix thoroughly and allow to solidify. The agar should be as transparent as possible.

If the water is suspected of contamination, plate out a smaller quantity, *e.g.* 0·1 ml., and in dealing with specimens which may be highly polluted it is advisable to make a series of plate cultures with further decreasing quantities of the water. Serial dilutions may be made from the sample, *e.g.* 1 in 10, 1 in 100, etc., using sterile quarter-strength Ringer's solution as a diluent. In preparing the 1 in 10 dilution, 10 ml. of the well-mixed sample is added to 90 ml. of Ringer's solution contained in a screw-capped bottle of 120 ml. capacity. After thorough mixing, further tenfold dilutions can be prepared by transferring 10 ml. of the 1 in 10 dilution to a second bottle of 90 ml. Ringer's solution and so on. One ml. quantities of each dilution are then plated.

Prepare duplicate plates from each volume or dilution, and incubate one at 37° C. for one day and the other at 20°–22° C. for three days. Those organisms that grow rapidly at 37° C. are mainly parasitic and are derived from excremental contamination, while those growing best at 20°–22° C. are the natural saprophytes of water and soil. It is customary in some laboratories to extend the incubation period at 37° C. to 48 hr. This is not recommended since after two days certain saprophytic bacteria capable of growing more slowly at 37° C. may have developed into visible colonies.

After incubation, the colonies that have developed in the medium are counted using a hand lens, if necessary, to detect small colonies. Each colony may be taken to represent one viable bacterium in the original specimen.

To facilitate the counting of colonies, to prevent eye-strain and to minimise inaccuracies, it is desirable that a special illuminated counting box fitted with a magnifying glass should be used and a mechanical hand tally counter. As each colony is recorded it should be "spotted" by pen and ink on the under surface of the plate. If there are large numbers of colonies present divide the plate into sections by ruling lightly on the under surface with a grease pencil and count the colonies in each section. If the plates prepared from the undiluted water show between 30 and 300 colonies, these should be counted. If there are more than 300 colonies and the sample has been diluted, then the plates giving counts between 30 and 300 should be selected and the other discarded. If all plates show more than 300 colonies, then the result should be reported as more than 300 multiplied by the reciprocal of the highest dilution used; *e.g.* if the sample was diluted 1 in 100, the result would be given as "more than 30,000". Alternatively, provided no more than 500 colonies are present, a count of more than 300 colonies may be made as accurately as possible and the result given as an approximate one. Since only a proportion of the bacteria originally present in the water are capable of developing under the conditions of the test, the total colony count represents the number of organisms per ml. of the sample, which have grown at the specified temperature (*i.e.* 37° C. or 22° C.) in the specified time (*i.e.* one day or three days). The result is expressed briefly as the plate count per ml. at 37° C. and 22° C.

Interpretation of Results

It must be realised that it is not possible to lay down rigid bacteriological standards to which all drinking-water supplies should conform. The bacteriological flora of water varies widely according to the nature of the supply, *i.e.* whether it is derived from a well, river, lake or reservoir, and to the climatic conditions prevailing in the gathering grounds. The aim of the authorities should be to obtain a thorough knowledge of the topography of the catchment area and in the light of this to establish a standard for that particular supply, based on regular and frequent bacteriological examinations. Any later deviation from that standard should be viewed with suspicion.

Generally speaking, the results of plate counts are by themselves of little value in estimating the hygienic quality of a water supply, though where regular observations are made on the same supply, a high count on a particular occasion may draw attention to a fault requiring investigation. A slight rise in the count of water from a deep well which is normally very pure may be the earliest indication that a defect has occurred in the structure of the well and is allowing its pollution from outside. The plate count is also of value in judging the efficacy of water treatment processes and in indicating whether a particular supply is suitable for use in the preparation of food and drink, where a high bacterial content may lead to food spoilage.

The test for coliform bacilli is of much greater value in assessing the quality of a water supply. In interpreting the results, however, the nature of the supply must still be taken into account. Heavy rain after a dry spell may cause flooding of the countryside carrying soil and vegetation into a water supply or give rise to flooding of drains and cesspools with the risk of more serious contamination. Bacteriological examinations therefore should always be carried out after a sudden climatic change of this kind.

Chlorinated Supplies.—The water supplied to most large cities is treated by chlorination. In Report No. 71 Ministry of Health (1956) it is recommended that if tests reveal the presence of coliform bacilli (of any kind) in 100 ml. of chlorinated water as it enters the distribution system, the treatment should be considered inefficient. Since, however, spore-bearing bacilli such as *Cl. welchii* may survive chlorination and give a positive reaction in the presumptive test, it is advisable, before condemning the supply, to confirm the result by plating out all the positive bottles on MacConkey's agar and discarding those that fail to produce colonies of coliform bacilli.

Non-chlorinated Piped Supplies.—In the same report it is recommended that non-chlorinated piped water supplies, sampled on entering the distribution system of any community of more than minimal population, should be classified as follows:

		Presumptive coliform count per 100 ml.	*Esch. coli* count per 100 ml.
Class 1	Excellent	0	0
Class 2	Satisfactory	1-3	0
Class 3	Suspicious	4-10	0
Class 4	Unsatisfactory	greater than 10	0, 1 or more

The presence of *Esch. coli* immediately places the sample in Class 4.

Thus it is considered that the presence of *Esch. coli* in 100 ml. of water in a supply of this nature renders it unfit for drinking purposes. On the other hand, a certain degree of latitude with regard to the coliform count is permitted, since it is difficult to prevent the occasional presence of atypical coliform organisms in untreated water. The following standards, based on the results of frequent tests, are suggested. Throughout the year 50 per cent. of samples should fall into Class 1, 80 per cent. should not fall below Class 2, and the remainder should not fall below Class 3. With deep well or other pure waters that normally fall into Class 1, a sudden deterioration in quality even to Class 2 would have to be considered significant.

It has been emphasised that the above standards only apply to the water as it enters the distribution system. Between that point and the consumers' premises there may be many sources of contamination (*e.g.* defective washers on taps, packing in joints of water pipes, service reservoirs or cisterns may all harbour coliform organisms). If a comparison of the water before and after distribution reveals wide differences in the quality, then steps should be taken without delay to detect and remove the cause. The W.H.O. (1961) have recommended certain minimum requirements regarding the frequency of testing of water within the distribution system depending on the size of population.

Unpiped Rural Supplies.—In small rural communities where no piped water supply is available, a private supply *e.g.* a shallow well adequately protected from obvious sources of pollution, should be considered adequate if the coliform count lies between 10 and 25 per 100 ml. If it fails repeatedly to keep within that limit, if it reaches 50 or more per 100 ml. or if *Esch. coli* appears in more than minimal numbers, the supply should be condemned for drinking purposes.

Pollution resulting from Heavy Rain.—It is particularly advisable to test all water supplies at short intervals after heavy rain follows a dry spell. A sudden increase in the number of coliform bacilli after rain might indicate flooding of the surrounding countryside and the potential danger of water-borne disease often associated with flood water.

Examination for Streptococci.—The type of streptococcus indicative of faecal pollution is *Streptococcus faecalis.* This organism grows in the medium used for the test for coliform bacilli and by itself ferments the lactose but without gas production. Its presence in water can therefore be determined by further examination of the contents of the bottles showing acid or acid and gas fermentation in the above mentioned test.

In order to isolate *Strept. faecalis* from other organisms which may be present, several methods have been advocated. The Metropolitan Water Board have obtained the most satisfactory results from the use of a medium containing sodium azide (Hannay & Norton, 1947). Subcultures from all positive bottles in the presumptive coliform test are made into tubes containing 5 ml. of sterile sodium azide medium (see p. 784).

The presence of *Strept. faecalis* is indicated by the production of acid in the medium within 18 hr. at an incubation temperature of 45° C. Their presence in any tubes which become acid should be confirmed by plating out a heavy inoculum on MacConkey's agar. *Strept. faecalis* produces characteristic minute red colonies.

The demonstration of *Strept. faecalis* is of value in confirming the faecal origin of coliform bacilli in cases where there may be difficulty in interpreting the results of the coliform test.

Examination for Clostridium welchii.—50 ml. of water are added to 100 ml. of sterile milk (or litmus milk medium) in a stoppered bottle of suitable size. The bottle is then heated at 80° C. for 15 min. to destroy non-sporing organisms. Sterile liquid paraffin is run on to the surface of the medium to maintain anaerobiosis.

The tubes should be incubated for at least five days at 37° C., although the "stormy clot" reaction which is indicative of the presence of *Cl. welchii* may develop within 24 to 72 hr. If varying quantities of water are examined as in the presumptive coliform test, an estimate of the probable number of *Cl. welchii* in 100 ml. of water can be made.

Although in recently contaminated water *Cl. welchii* occurs in much smaller numbers than *Esch. coli*, it is able to survive for much longer periods than the non-sporing bacteria of faecal origin. The chief value of the test therefore is in detecting pollution of some previous time or to confirm the faecal origin of atypical coliform bacilli in the absence of *Esch. coli.*

Bacteriological Examination of Sewage and Sewage Effluents

The bacteriological examination of sewage may be carried out to determine the purity of an effluent from a sewage purification process. The procedure is the same as in water examination; an estimation of the viable bacteria present is made by plating and counting colonies, and the test for coliform bacilli is carried out as with a specimen of water; much smaller amounts, however, are tested than in the case of water, depending on the likely extent of pollution of the effluent. The numbers of bacteria per ml. in crude sewage vary greatly, *e.g.* from 1 million to 100 million. Sewage may also be examined by the membrane filter technique (p. 974).

For isolation of typhoid-paratyphoid bacilli from communal sewage either the sewer swab (Moore, 1948) or the membrane filter method (p. 977) is used.

Bacteriological Control of Swimming Baths

Public swimming pools and indoor swimming baths may become infected with pathogenic organisms derived either from contaminated water entering the pool or from the bathers. Unless adequate means of purifying the water are provided, this contamination may lead to outbreaks of diseases, such as gastro-enteritis, infections of the respiratory tract, otitis media, infections of the conjunctiva and the skin.

Most modern swimming pools are operated on a system which provides a continuous circulation of the water from the bath at the deep end through a purification plant where it undergoes filtration, clarification and chlorination before entering the pool again at the shallow end. The amount of chlorine introduced into the water is accurately measured and controlled so that the free residual amount present in the bath is maintained between 0·2 and 0·5 p.p.m. (Ministry of Health, 1951).

The results of bacteriological examinations of samples of water taken from the inlet and outlet of the bath give an indication of the effectiveness of the treatment in maintaining the water free from undesirable contaminants. The methods usually employed are those used for testing samples of drinking-water, viz. an estimation of the number of viable bacteria by the plate counts at 37° C. and 22° C. and the presumptive test for coliform bacilli followed by the differential tests for *Esch. coli* (p. 969). The bacteriological quality of the water should approximate to that of high purity drinking-water.

The following standards for water purity were recommended by the Water Subcommittee of the Public Health Laboratory Service (Gray *et al.*, 1953):

"No samples examined from a bath should contain any coliform organisms in 100 ml. of water; and in 75 per cent. of the samples examined from the bath the plate count at 37° C. from 1 ml. of water should not exceed 10 colonies and in the remainder should not exceed 100 colonies."

Amies (1956) maintains that "before a swimming pool can be pronounced as satisfactory, the surface water should be examined bacteriologically as well as the main body of the water", and describes a method for doing this. He presents evidence to show that oral or nasal bacteria collect in the surface film of fatty substances derived from the skin and hair of the bathers, and are protected by it from the action of the chlorine. He considers that this surface film may be a contributory factor in the spread of bacterial and viral diseases by swimming pools.

Swimming pools should be provided with overflow gutters into which the polluted film can drain. The method by which the surface film may be removed for bacteriological examination involves the use of calcium alginate gauze which is commercially available as sterilised surgical dressings measuring 4 × 7 in. and weighing 1·2 g.[1] The gauze is laid on the surface of the pool so that the layer of water beneath it is absorbed. It has been calculated that 8·8 g. of water is absorbed in this way. The wetted gauze is then placed in a jar containing 50 ml. 10 per cent. aqueous solution of sodium hexametaphosphate in which it readily dissolves, thus liberating the bacteria. (In order to neutralise the effect of any residual chlorine, 0·1 ml. of 10 per cent. solution of sodium thiosulphate is added to the jar shortly before the sample is taken.)

The number of bacteria which were present in the surface film can be estimated by a viable count on the solution in the jar. The Miles and Misra technique (p. 872) is suitable for this purpose, blood agar and MacConkey's agar plates being inoculated with standard drops. If necessary the colonies which develop can be readily identified. For further details, reference should be made to the original paper.

THE MEMBRANE FILTER TECHNIQUE FOR THE BACTERIOLOGICAL EXAMINATION OF WATER AND SEWAGE

This method is based on the use of a highly porous cellulose membrane, the pore structure of which enables fairly large volumes of water or aqueous solutions to pass through rapidly under pressure, but prevents the passage of any bacteria present in the sample. These are retained on the surface of the membrane which is then brought into contact with suitable liquid nutrients. These diffuse upwards through the pores thereby inducing the organisms to grow as surface colonies which can be counted.

The technique was first described in this country by Windle Taylor *et al.* (1953). Since then much investigational work had been done in the laboratories of the Metropolitan Water Board in order to devise modifications suitable as standard techniques for the examination of water samples of all types, both treated and untreated. (Windle Taylor *et al.*, 1955; Windle Taylor, 1955-56; 1957-58; 1959-60; 1961-62.) A review of the progress that has been made in membrane filtration technique has been published (Windle Taylor & Burman, 1964) and further progress described by Windle Taylor (1963-64).

Membrane filters may also be used for the isolation of pathogens from water and sewage and for the demonstration of tubercle bacilli in cerebrospinal fluid and other fluid specimens including sputa from cases of tuberculosis. (Haley & Rosty, 1957.)

Apparatus

Various types of filtering apparatus suitable for water and sewage examination are now available. A German-made funnel has been used extensively by the Metropolitan Water Board. It may be obtained in Britain from Hudes Merchandising Corporation.[2] It is known as the "Coli 5" model and consists of a funnel of nickel-plated brass of 500 ml. capacity attached by means of a bayonet-locking device to the base of the apparatus which contains a disk of sintered glass on which the membrane is supported. The outlet is provided with a tap and fits into the rubber stopper of a suction jar.

[1] Calcium alginate gauze of the required dimensions is obtainable from Medical Alginates Ltd., Wadsworth Road, Perivale, Middlesex, England.

[2] Hudes Merchandising Corporation Ltd., 52 Gloucester Place, London, W.1.

Some of the other types of funnel do not have this outlet tap and are therefore not so convenient to handle. It is also an added advantage to have the inside of the funnel provided with graduation marks for easy measurement of the water sample.

The special "Coli 5" German-manufactured membranes for use with the apparatus described above are paper-thin, porous disks, 5 cm. in diameter, composed of a cellulose derivative which forms the framework for a thin gelatinous layer of suitable porosity. They are quite tough and elastic even when dry, white in colour and opaque with a glazed surface. They may be obtained marked with a grid to simplify the counting of the colonies. British-made membranes manufactured by Courtaulds Ltd., and marketed by Oxoid Ltd., have been found in some ways more satisfactory for the culture of the bacteria, though they tend to be brittle and more readily damaged than the German ones. Membranes that have been used for the coliform count may be washed in running water, dried between blotting-paper and sterilised for further use. This may be done up to twelve times, but damaged membranes should always be discarded.

Sterilisation

The filtering apparatus is assembled without the membrane, wrapped in kraft paper and sterilised by autoclaving at 121° C. for 15 min. Thereafter, between each test, it is sufficient to apply a jet of live steam, or alternatively a pad of cotton-wool attached to a metal rod, dipped in alcohol and ignited. Both the inner and outer surfaces of the funnel as well as its base and the sintered glass disk require to be sterilised in this way. The routine examination of large numbers of water samples is facilitated by the use of several funnels for each piece of apparatus. While one sample is being filtered, the spare funnels for subsequent samples can be sterilised and cooled.

The membranes may be sterilised by either of two methods.

(1) Gentle boiling in prefiltered distilled water on two occasions each of 20 min. duration. Vigorous boiling tends to make the membranes buckle. This method not only sterilises but washes out residual solvents and air present in the pores.

(2) Autoclaving at 115° C. for 10 min. For this purpose bundles of 10 membrane filters are interleaved with disks of good quality absorbent paper (subsequently to be used for holding the liquid medium). The bundles are secured between two pieces of thin card held in position by adhesive tape and the whole is wrapped in kraft paper and sterilised.

Media for culture on membrane filters

1. *M-Yeast extract broth (for the enumeration of viable bacteria).*

In order to obtain results comparable with those of the agar plate count for all types of water, it is necessary to use nutrient broth of the following composition:

Yeast extract (see p. 783)	6 g.
Peptone	40 g.
Distilled water	to 1000 ml.
pH	7·4

2. *M-MacConkey broth (for estimations of Esch. coli).*

MacConkey's bile-salt lactose broth is the medium of choice in this country but it has been necessary to modify the original composition for use with membranes. The following formula is found to give the most satisfactory results, but it is recommended that the optimum proportion of bile salts (commercial sodium taurocholate or other satisfactory bile salt) should be determined for each new batch obtained (Burman, 1955).

Peptone	10 g.
Lactose	30 g.
Bile salts	4–10 g. (according to quality)
Sodium chloride (NaCl.)	5 g.
Bromocresol purple (1 per cent. alcoholic solution)	12 ml.
Water (distilled)	to 1000 ml.
pH	7·4

Bile salts No. 3 (Oxoid or Bacto) should be used at the lower concentration.

3. *Teepol* 610 *phenol red broth* (*for estimations of coliform bacilli other than Esch. coli*). Higher numbers of coliform bacilli can be recovered from membranes by using phenol red instead of bromocresol purple (which tends to be somewhat inhibitory to certain types of coliform bacilli) and by using 3 per cent. Teepol 610 instead of bile salts.

Peptone (Evans)	10 g.
Lactose	30 g.
Teepol 610	30 ml.
Sodium chloride (NaCl)	5 g.
Phenol red 0·4 per cent. alkaline solution	50 ml.
Water (distilled)	to 1000 ml.
pH	7·4

4. *M-resuscitation broth* (*vide infra*)

Peptone	40 g.
Yeast extract	6 g.
Lactose	30 g.
Water (distilled)	to 1000 ml.
pH	7·2

Oxoid Ltd. supply media suitable for use with membrane filters.

Method of Filtration

After sterilisation, the filtering apparatus is inserted into the suction jar attached to the vacuum pump, the outlet tap being closed. The funnel is removed, and with sterile forceps one of the membranes is laid, grid-side up, on the top of the sintered glass disk. By turning on the pressure and opening the tap carefully, the membrane is sucked down and comes to lie quite flat against the disk. (In order to protect the membrane and hasten filtration, a disk of filter paper should be inserted between the supporting glass disk and the membrane.) After closing the tap and releasing the pressure, the funnel is screwed into place and a suitable amount of the water to be examined is poured into it. The actual amount depends on the likely degree of pollution. If there is doubt about this, two or more different volumes of the sample should be filtered. The following amounts are recommended:

Purified tap water	250–500 ml.
Well water	10 and 100 ml.
River water	1 and 10 ml.

Water which is highly contaminated should be diluted to 1 in 10, 1 in 100 and 1 in 1000 and each dilution filtered. Quantities smaller than 20 ml.

should be made up to that amount with sterile distilled water before being passed through the filter.

When the water has been filtered and a small amount of sterile distilled water allowed to pass through as a final rinse the funnel is removed and the vacuum released. The membrane is then transferred with sterile flat-bladed forceps to a 2-in. Petri dish containing a sterile absorbent pad (Whatman's No. 17 pads, 5 or 6 cm. in diameter, are suitable), saturated with about 2 ml. of the appropriate liquid medium. The membrane should be placed on the moist pad in such a way as to exclude any air bubbles. The Petri dish is then inverted with the pad and membrane adhering to the base and incubated in a moist atmosphere.

Incubation. For total colony counts at 37° C. incubation for 18 hr. on yeast extract broth gives results that are comparable with the agar plate counts at that temperature. For colony counts at 22° C. incubation for 3 days is necessary. All the colonies that develop on the membranes are counted and the number of bacteria per ml. of undiluted water may then be calculated. For membrane coliform counts, the cultures on 3 per cent. Teepol phenol red broth are incubated for 4 hr. at 30° C. followed by 14 hr. at 35° C. The number of yellow colonies is then counted. These merely represent lactose fermenting organisms that may or may not be gas producers. Their identity is presumed to be that of coliform bacilli for the purpose of routine water examination, but this can be confirmed by the usual tests (see p. 249) if required.

Windle Taylor states that it is possible to obtain directly an accurate count of *Esch. coli* by first incubating the membrane at 37° C. in contact with a pad soaked in M-resuscitation broth (*vide supra*). After 2 hr. at that temperature the membrane is transferred to a pad soaked in M-MacConkey broth and incubated for 16 hr. at 44° C. The preliminary incubation is thought to encourage the growth of organisms that may have become attenuated as a result of the inhibitory action of inorganic salts present in the water supply. (Allen, Pasley & Pierce, 1952).

For further studies on the Membrane Filter Technique reference should be made to the reports of the Metropolitan Water Board quoted above.

Isolation of Pathogenic Organisms from Water and Sewage

(*a*) **By Membrane Filter Technique.**—Relatively large amounts of the fluid to be tested, *i.e.* 500 ml. or more, depending on the amount of suspended matter present, can be passed through the membrane filter fairly rapidly. If pathogenic organisms are present, even in small numbers, they will be retained on the surface of the membrane, and by transferring it to a suitable differential medium there is a reasonable chance of isolating them.

For isolating typhoid and paratyphoid bacilli Wilson and Blair's bismuth sulphite medium has been reported as giving satisfactory results by this method. The membrane may be placed directly on the agar medium in a small Petri dish, the proportion of agar having been reduced to 1·5 per cent., but Kabler and Clark (1952) recommend the use of absorbent pads impregnated with double-strength liquid medium (agar omitted). Characteristic convex black colonies with a paler periphery appear within 30 hr. at 37° C. If discrete, each one is surrounded by a halo, showing a metallic sheen. Blackening of the medium underneath the membrane is suggestive of typhoid colonies. In such a case, it is necessary to transfer the membrane to a tube or bottle of liquid medium such as tetrathionate broth or selenite enrichment medium (p. 765) subculturing from this after 18 to 24 hr. incubation at 37° C. on desoxycholate citrate agar.

In order to isolate intestinal pathogens, other than typhoid and paratyphoid bacilli, Kabler and Clark recommend a preliminary incubation of the membrane for 3 hr. in contact with single-strength tetrathionate broth without chalk before transferring it to a differential medium. Incubation of the membrane for 3 hr. on this medium tends to inhibit coliform bacilli and enhances the growth of salmonellae other than *Salmonella typhi.* Characteristic colonies may then be recognised and subcultured for the usual confirmatory tests.

(*b*) **By a Concentration Technique, using a membrane filter apparatus with pulverised diatomaceous earth.**—The Metropolitan Water Board have reported satisfactory results from the use of a modification of the method of Hammerström and Ljutov (1954) and Ljutov (1954) for isolating pathogenic intestinal organisms from water and sewage. The technique is so simple and quickly carried out that its use is to be recommended rather than that mentioned above: Windle Taylor (1955-56).

A layer of diatomaceous earth (Hyflo Super-Cel) is substituted for the membrane at the bottom of the filter funnel, supported on a disk of stainless steel wire micro-mesh. After setting up the filtering apparatus with the micro-mesh in place, a small amount of sterile distilled water is poured into the funnel and to this is added a quantity of 1 per cent. sterile Hyflo Super-Cel suspension to give the required thickness. The pressure is turned on and the measured sample poured in before all the sterile water has gone through. (Up to 100 litres of water can be filtered in thirty minutes, sewage from 3 to 10 ml. suitably diluted, and effluent 50–500 ml.). After all the fluid has been sucked through, the wire-mesh support is lifted off with sterile forceps and the paste tipped into 100 ml. selenite F medium in a screw-capped bottle (4 in. in depth by 2 in. in diameter). This is incubated at 42° C. After 18 hr. subcultures are made on selective media.

(Hyflo Super-Cel is a diatomaceous silica filter-aid preparation obtainable from the Johns-Manville Company Ltd., 20 Albert Embankment, London, S.W.1.)

BACTERIOLOGICAL EXAMINATION OF MILK

In hygienc work the bacteriological examination of milk generally consists of:

(1) An enumeration of viable bacteria present in a given quantity.

(2) A quantitative estimation of contamination by coliform bacilli.

(3) The determination of the presence of specific pathogenic organisms, e.g. *Myco. tuberculosis.*

Since 1936 the *methylene blue reduction test* has been used as a standard official method in England for gauging milk purity, *i.e.* as a substitute for the bacterial count. It depends on the reduction and decolourisation of the dye by the bacteria in the milk, and the rate of reduction affords a measure of the degree of bacterial contamination.

As a check on the pasteurisation of milk, the *phosphatase test* is now a standard procedure; it determines the inactivation by heat of the enzyme phosphatase, which is normally present in cow's milk. Activity of this enzyme implies that the milk has not been adequately heated for the destruction of pathogenic organisms present.

The *turbidity test* is the official test for "sterilised" milk, *i.e.* milk that has been heated to 212° F. (100° C.) or over for such a period as to ensure that it will satisfy the turbidity test. The test depends on the fact that by heating to the degree necessary for sterilisation the heat-coagulable proteins are precipitated, so that if ammonium sulphate is then added and the mixture filtered and boiled for 5 min. no turbidity results. The test also distinguishes between pasteurised and "sterilised" milk.

Under the Milk (Special Designation) Regulations, 1963 and 1965 of England, and the Milk (Special Designations) (Scotland) Order, 1965 and 1966, standard methods for testing milk have been prescribed in official memoranda. These should be consulted for full details of the methods recommended. Recently, a new special designation, "*Ultra Heat Treated*," has been prescribed in relation to milk that has been retained at a temperature of 270° F. (132·2° C.) for not less than one second.

Bacteriological Standards

England and Wales

The following standards have been laid down under the Milk (Special Designation) Regulations, 1963:

"*Untreated*" *milk* and "*Pasteurised*" *milk* when tested by the prescribed method at 9.30 a.m. on the day following that on which the sample was taken, must fail to decolourise methylene blue in 30 min. Before testing the samples must be maintained at atmospheric shade temperature when tested during the period 1st May to 31st October and at atmospheric shade temperature until 5 p.m. on the day of sampling and thereafter at a constant temperature of 17° C. to 20° C. when tested during 1st November to 30th April. The test is not carried out if the atmospheric temperature exceeds 21° C.

"*Pasteurised*" *milk* must also satisfy the phosphatase test (*vide infra*), *i.e.* when tested under the prescribed conditions the milk must give a reading of 10 μg. or less of *p*-nitrophenol per ml. of milk.

"Sterilised" milk must satisfy the turbidity test described on p. 984.

"*Ultra Heat Treated*" *milk* must satisfy a colony count test by yielding less than 10 colonies per standard loop (approx. 0·01 ml. capacity) when grown in yeastrel milk agar at a preselected temperature of between 30° C. and 37° C. for 48 hr.

Scotland

The special designations that may be used in Scotland are "*Premium*", "*Standard*", "*Pasteurised*", "*Sterilised*" and "*Ultra Heat Treated*". The standards required by the milk (Special Designations) (Scotland) Order when tested according to the provisions laid down in the Order are as follows:

"*Premium*" *milk* must contain not more than 15,000 bacteria per ml. and no coliform bacteria in 0·01 ml.

"*Standard*" *milk* must not contain more than 50,000 bacteria per ml. and no coliform bacteria in 0·001 ml.

"*Pasteurised*" *milk* must contain no coliform bacteria in 0·01 ml. and on submission to the phosphatase test must give a reading not exceeding 10 μg. of *p*-nitrophenol per ml. of milk.

"*Sterilised*" *milk* must satisfy the turbidity test.

"*Ultra Heat Treated*" milk must contain not more than 1000 bacteria per ml.

Sampling.—If the milk is contained in retail bottles, one unopened bottle delivered to the laboratory constitutes the sample. When the milk is in a bulk container it must be carefully mixed before a sample is taken. This can be done by means of a sterile plunger which is moved up and down several times in the milk. The specimen is then obtained with a sterile dipper from well below the surface of the milk and placed in a sterile 4 oz. stoppered or screw-capped bottle. Bottles containing the milk samples should be dispatched to the testing laboratory without delay in an insulated box and should be examined as soon as possible after arrival except in the cases of "Untreated" milk tested by the methylene blue test which requires special storage temperatures depending on the time of the year and "Ultra Heat Treated" milk samples which are retained at 30° C. for 24 hr. before being tested for the bacterial count.

Technique of Estimating the Number of Viable Bacteria.—The medium recommended in the regulations is yeast extract milk agar (see p. 783).

A series of dilutions of the milk sample is made up in sterile stoppered bottles with sterile tap water as follows:

1 in 10 .	90 ml. water *plus* 10 ml. milk
1 in 100 .	90 ml. „ „ 10 ml. of the 1 in 10 dilution
1 in 1000 .	90 ml. „ „ 10 ml. of the 1 in 100 dilution

Before these dilutions are made, the specimen should be carefully mixed by inverting the sample bottle about 25 times. The dilutions must also be mixed, but without vigorous shaking. The pipettes used should be straight-sided and appropriately graduated. For each dilution a separate sterile pipette should be used.

For testing *premium* milk under the Scottish regulations 1 ml. of the 1 in 100 dilution is plated, duplicate or preferably triplicate plates being made; in examining *standard* milk 1 ml. of the 1 in 1000 dilution is plated as above. The diluted milk is placed with a sterile pipette in a sterile Petri dish (4 in. diameter) and 10 ml. of melted agar cooled to 45° C. is added and mixed with the milk by rotating the plate carefully first to the right, then to the left, so that the organisms are uniformly distributed throughout the agar.

The time between the preparation of the dilutions and the mixing with the medium should not exceed 15 min.

After the medium has solidified, the plates are incubated in the inverted position for 72 hr. at 30° C. ± 0·5° C.

The number of colonies including "pin-point" colonies, is counted in each plate and the mean calculated; this multiplied by the dilution is reported as the "number of viable bacteria per ml.". The count is made as described on p. 970. If the number of colonies in a plate is over 300, a count may be made of those in a given part of the plate and the total is then calculated; but it is advisable in examining a milk of unknown quality to plate 1 ml. of each dilution (*vide supra*) and use for the count those showing 30 to 300 colonies.

Ultra heat-treated milk samples are maintained in the unopened sample bottle in an incubator at a temperature of between 30° C. and 37° C. (in Scotland at 30° C. ± 0·5° C.) for 24 hr. Under the Scottish milk regulations at the end of the 24 hr. incubation period, 1 ml. of 1 in 10 dilution of the milk is plated as above and the Petri dish cultures are then incubated at 30° C. ± 0·5° C. for 48 hr. and the colonies counted. In England the milk is withdrawn from about 1 ml. below the surface by means of a standard iridium platinum loop. (The loop has an internal diameter of 4 mm. and is made of wire conforming to British Standard 19 containing 10 per cent. iridium. It will withdraw about 0·01 ml. milk.) The loopful of milk is transferred to 5 ml. melted yeastrel milk agar cooled to between 45° C. and 50° C. contained in a test tube or screw-capped bottle of 1 oz. capacity. The contents are carefully mixed and allowed to solidify in a sloping position. The bottle or tube is then incubated at a temperature of between 30° C. and 37° C. for 48 hr. after which time the colonies are counted.

Under the most favourable conditions a specimen of raw milk may contain at least 500 bacteria per ml.; but under bad conditions the numbers may reach even several million per ml. The standards given on p. 979 indicate the degree of bacterial contamination allowable in the case of designated milks.

Test for Coliform Bacilli.—Varying amounts of milk are added to tubes or bottles of bile-salt lactose medium (p. 783). The range of amounts that require to be tested depends on the likely degree of contamination. In the case of milk of unknown quality the following series is suggested:

1·0 ml. of a 1 in 10 dilution of the milk
" " 1 in 100 " "
" " 1 in 1000 " "
" " 1 in 10,000 " "

The decimal dilutions are prepared in series (*vide supra*).

The smallest amount that yields acid *and gas* is ascertained.

Under the Scottish regulations, for *premium* and *pasteurised* milk three tubes or bottles containing 10 ml. of the above medium are inoculated (by means of a sterile pipette) each with 1 ml. of the 1 in 100 dilution of the sample and incubated at 37° C. for 48 hr. For *standard*, three tubes are inoculated each with 1 ml. of the 1 in 1000 dilution. The tubes are examined for acid and gas production; the milk is taken to have passed the test if acid and gas are absent from two of the three tubes.

Methylene Blue Reduction Test.—Standard methylene blue tablets must be used. (The names of manufacturers who supply such tablets are furnished by the Ministry of Health.) A standard solution is prepared as follows: one tablet is dissolved in 200 ml. cold sterile glass-distilled water in a sterile flask with a rubber stopper. The solution is then made up to 800 ml. with distilled water and stored in a cool, dark place. This solution gives a final concentration of methylene blue of approximately 1/300,000, and should not be used after two months.

Test-tubes conforming to the British Standards Specification 625:1959, nominal size 150 × 16mm. and a mark indicating 10 ml. are used. They are stoppered with cotton-wool or aluminium caps and sterilised in a hot air oven (160° C. for 1 hr). Rubber stoppers to fit the tubes are also required. These are sterilised in boiling water before use.

A thermostatically controlled, covered water-bath, with a rack to hold the tubes immersed in the water, is required; the water should be at 37°–38° C.

1-ml. straight-sided pipettes are used for measuring the methylene blue solution (these should conform to a prescribed specification). They are sterilised in the hot air oven.

The sample is mixed thoroughly, as prior to making the bacterial count (*vide supra*).

The milk is poured, with the usual aseptic precautions, into a test-tube up to the 10 ml. mark, and 1 ml. of methylene blue solution is carefully added. The tube is closed with a sterile rubber stopper which should be inserted with sterile forceps. It is then inverted slowly once or twice and placed in the water-bath.

The following controls should be put up: (1) 10 ml. mixed milk *plus* 1 ml. methylene blue solution, (2) 10 ml. mixed milk *plus* 1 ml. tap water.

These control tubes are placed for 3 min. in boiling water to destroy the natural reducing system of the milk. Comparison with (1) indicates when decolourisation is beginning and with (2) when it is complete.

Decolourisation is considered complete when the whole column of milk is decolourised or decolourised up to within 5 mm. of the surface. The time of complete decolourisation is recorded. For the purposes of the Milk (Special Designation) Regulations *untreated* milk is considered satisfactory if it fails to decolourise methylene blue in 30 minutes (standards given on p. 979).

Rationale of the Various Bacteriological Tests used for the Examination of Milk

Whichever test is adopted for the routine examination of milk it should be capable of indicating the degree of bacterial contamination and thereby of showing whether the conditions under which the milk is produced and handled are hygienically satisfactory.

The advantage of the plate count for this purpose is that it gives a direct assessment of the number of viable bacteria in the supply. The results are readily understood by the dairyman, and since it is as suitable for milk of low bacterial content as for grossly contaminated supplies, it will indicate any changes in conditions of production leading to either an improvement or deterioration in quality. On the other hand, the plate count test is costly in time and material, the results are not available for 72 hr. and owing to the fact that a very small amount of milk is tested and that some of the bacteria are distributed in small clumps and chains, the error of sampling is high.

The coliform test is usually carried out in conjunction with the plate count. It indicates mainly the degree of contamination by coliform organisms arising from dust or unsterile utensils. Since adequate pasteurisation destroys the majority of coliform bacilli, the presence of these in milk that passes the phosphatase test is an indication of contamination after pasteurisation.

The methylene blue test is simple to carry out and requires a minimum of equipment. In general, the greater the number of bacteria in the milk, the greater their metabolic activity and consequently the shorter the reduction time.

However, milk heavily contaminated with inert bacteria may give a long reduction time, while short reduction times may be the result of non-bacterial reducing systems which are sometimes present in freshly produced milk, milk obtained late in the lactation period and milk containing leucocytes or other cells.

The time required to reduce the dye is also dependent on the temperature at which the milk is held prior to testing; thus, in the winter, milk gives a longer reduction time than it would in the summer, with the same bacterial content. Allowance is made for this in the higher standard required in the winter time by the English regulations.

It is difficult to compare high-quality milks by means of the standard methylene blue test, since the reduction time is very long for all of them, but the test will readily detect milk of poor hygienic quality. With *pasteurised* milk, provided the milk is kept for at least 24 hr. at a temperature not exceeding 18° C. (65° F.) before being tested, the correlation between the reduction time at 37° C. and the degree of bacterial contamination is fairly good. The test is of no value for freshly pasteurised milk.

The Resazurin Test. This test which is also a dye reduction test is sometimes used to determine the hygienic quality of a milk supply. One ml. of a standard solution of resazurin is added to 10 ml. of the well-mixed sample in a sterile test-tube which is then fitted with a sterile rubber stopper and placed in a water bath at 37·5° C. Unlike methylene blue, the dye resazurin passes through a series of colour changes: blue, lilac, mauve, pink mauve, mauve pink, pink before it is finally reduced to the colourless state by bacterial action; thus a reading may be made at any specified time after the test has been set up and the milk graded according to the amount of reduction that has taken place. A set of colour standards are used in a Lovibond comparator against which the colour of the dye and milk mixture may be matched and the amount of reduction measured. Alternatively, the result may be expressed as the time required for complete reduction of the dye.

The Ten Minute Resazurin Test is used as a "platform" test in creameries to detect unsatisfactory milk supplies as they arrive. Other modifications of the test are used for special purposes, *e.g.* the Temperature-Compensated Resazurin Test is used to off-set the effect of variations in atmospheric temperature on the metabolic activity of the bacteria prior to testing the milk. The time of incubation varies, according to the mean atmospheric shade temperature, from 120 min. to 15 min. for a temperature range of 40° and under to 4°–15·5° C. (60° F.) (For further details see Chalmers, 1962.)

Phosphatase Test for Pasteurised Milk

The statutory test for pasteurised milk is the Aschaffenburg and Mullen phosphatase test. This test determines inactivation of the enzyme phosphatase, normally present in cow's milk, by such degree and time of heating as to destroy non-sporing pathogenic organisms, *e.g.* 62·8° C. (145° F.) for 30 min. or 71·6° C. (161° F.) for 15 sec., as in the recognised methods of pasteurisation. The standard method for detecting the presence of the enzyme is based on its ability to liberate *p*-nitrophenol from disodium *p*-nitrophenyl phosphate. This yields a yellow coloration and the result is expressed in arbitrary units that can be read by viewing the degree of colour in a Lovibond comparator.

Apparatus required:

A Lovibond "all purpose" comparator complete with stand for work in reflected light and a comparator disc APTW or APTW 7.
Two fused glass cells 25 mm. deep.
A waterbath or incubator at 37·5° C. ± 0·5° C.
A pipette to deliver 5 ml.
A supply of 1·0 ml. straight-scaled pipettes of an accuracy equal to NPL grade B.
A 1000 ml. graduated flask.
A 100 ml. measuring cylinder.
A supply of test tubes of British Standard 625:1959, nominal size 150 × 16 mm. with rubber stoppers.

New glass-ware should be carefully washed in chromic acid solution and after use test tubes and pipettes should be thoroughly washed in hot soda water, rinsed in warm water, and then distilled water, and dried. Glassware used for the test should not be used for any other purpose and should be stored separately from other laboratory apparatus.

Buffer-substrate solution:

(*a*) Buffer solution: 3·5 g. anhydrous sodium carbonate and 1·5 g. sodium bicarbonate are dissolved in distilled water and made up to one litre. (*b*) Substrate: 0·15 g. disodium *p*-nitrophenyl phosphate is placed in a 100 ml. measuring cylinder and made up to 100 ml. with buffer solution.

Method:

5 ml. of the buffer-substrate solution is transferred to a test tube which is then stoppered and brought to a temperature of 37° C. by placing in a water-bath. 1 ml. of the milk to be tested is added, the test tube stopper is replaced and the contents shaken to mix. The test tube is then replaced in the waterbath for exactly 2 hr. at 37° C. A blank prepared from boiled milk is incubated with each series of samples. Highly coloured milk such as that of Channel Island cows requires a separate blank of the same type of milk. After incubation the tubes are removed from the waterbath and their contents well mixed. The blank is placed on the left hand of the stand and the test sample on the right. Readings are taken in reflected light by looking down on the two apertures with the comparator facing a good source of daylight or a daylight type of artificial illumination. The disc is revolved until the test sample is matched. Readings falling between two standards are reported as plus or minus the figure of the nearest standard.

Interpretation:

Milk that gives a reading of 10 μg. or less of *p*-nitrophenol per ml. of milk is considered to be properly pasteurised.

The Turbidity Test for Sterilised Milk.—Add 20 ml. of the well-mixed milk to a 50-ml. conical flask containing 4 gm. ammonium sulphate (AR). Shake thoroughly for 1 min. to dissolve all the ammonium sulphate. Allow to stand for 5 min. and then filter into a test-tube through a Whatman No. 12 folded filter paper (12·5 cm. in diameter). Collect at least 5 ml. of clear filtrate and place the tube in a beaker of boiling water for 5 min. Cool in cold water and examine the tube for turbidity, holding it in front of an electric light suitably shaded from the eyes. It is advisable to compare it with a tube of milk heated in a boiling water bath for 20 min. and then treated with ammonium sulphate in the same way.

An absence of turbidity indicates that the milk has been heated to at least (100° C.) 212° F. for a period of at least 5 min., which denatures the soluble proteins in the milk so that they can no longer be precipitated by ammonium sulphate. The test will detect the presence of 0·6 to 0·8 per cent. raw milk, but owing to the heat resistance of some sporing organisms it gives no indication of the probable keeping quality of the "Sterilised" milk.

Examination for Tubercle Bacillus.—The sample is thoroughly mixed and a quantity of 100 ml. is divided into 50 ml. amounts and centrifuged for 30 min. at a minimum speed of 3000 r.p.m. The sediment in each tube is suspended in 2·5 ml. of sterile saline solution. It is advisable to add some of the cream to this inoculum. Two guinea-pigs are injected subcutaneously on the inner side of one thigh with the suspended sediment and kept under observation to ascertain whether tuberculous lesions result (p. 195). One guinea-pig is killed at the end of four weeks and an autopsy carried out; if it shows no tuberculous lesions, the other animal is kept for eight weeks, when it is killed and examined.

Lesions should be examined microscopically for the tubercle bacillus to confirm their tuberculous nature. (It has been shown that *Br. abortus* which may occur in cow's milk, produces (tubercle-like lesions in guinea-pigs. It is advisable to inoculate at least two animals from one specimen, as inoculated guinea-pigs may die sometimes from infection with other organisms present in the milk, *e.g.* sporing anaerobic bacilli, or some intercurrent disease —*e.g.* pneumonia, enteritis, etc.—may also cause death before tuberculous lesions have developed and so nullify the test if only one animal is injected.

A direct microscopic examination of the deposit of centrifuged milk for tubercle bacilli may be made.

The absence of tubercle bacilli in films, however, does not exclude their presence in the specimen. On the other hand acid-fast bacilli other than the tubercle bacilli may be revealed. The microscopic test, therefore, is not a valid method of demonstrating tubercle bacilli.

The method of *direct cultivation* described on p. 202 can very suitably be applied to unmixed milk taken directly from the cow, but the animal inoculation test is the standard procedure for demonstrating tubercle bacilli in milk samples generally.

Examination for Brucella Infection in Milk.—In infected cows the brucella organisms tend to localise in the udder and to be excreted in the milk. They may be isolated by plating out thickly several loopfuls of cream taken directly from the top of the milk on to the surface of plates of serum dextrose agar containing various antibiotics to inhibit contaminants (see p. 767). Alternatively, the milk may be centrifuged for 15 min. at 1000 r.p.m. The milk from below the cream is removed for the Whey Agglutination Test (*vide infra*) and the sediment mixed with some of the cream is plated out on the selective medium. One ml. of the cream and sediment mixture may also be inoculated intramuscularly into 2 guinea-pigs. After 6 weeks both animals are killed. Blood is removed to provide serum for agglutination tests with *Br. abortus* suspension. This may give evidence of infection without the need to isolate the organism. The spleen is cut in two aseptically and the cut surface rubbed over a plate of serum dextrose agar. In infected animals the spleen is often considerably enlarged. Care should be exercised in handling the guinea-pigs at post-mortem since faulty technique may readily lead to accidental infection. Inoculated plates are incubated at 37° C. in an atmosphere of 10 per cent. CO_2 for at least 5 days. Colonies with the characteristics of brucella organisms should be subcultured on serum dextrose agar slopes and identified by the appropriate means (see p. 283). A slide agglutination test with standard brucella antiserum may be carried out in the first instance to identify the colonies as those of brucella organisms.

Milk Ring Test (*MRT*) *for Brucella.*—The milk of cows suffering from brucella infection of the mammary gland may contain brucella agglutinins. On the addition of a concentrated suspension of *Br. abortus* stained with haematoxylin the bacteria are agglutinated by the antibodies and rise up with the fat globules to form a deep blue ring in the cream layer. The test is very sensitive and may be applied to bulk milk of individual herds since a positive milk continues to give a blue ring reaction even when highly diluted with negative milk from non-infected cows. Care must be taken in interpreting a positive result, however, since the milk of animals immunised against brucellosis when adult may give a positive ring reaction for 2 years or more. On the other hand vaccination of calves during the 6th to 8th month does not interfere with this test although conferring a high degree of immunity to infection for several years.

The technique is as follows:

(1) Mix the milk thoroughly and pour into a $3 \times \frac{3}{8}$ in. test-tube sufficient

to give a column of milk about 1 in. high. (2) Add 1 drop of stained antigen (*vide infra*) and mix thoroughly by shaking. Avoid frothing which interferes with the reading of the test. (3) Incubate in a 37° C. water-bath for about 40–50 min., *i.e.* sufficient time for the cream to rise.

The stained antigen[1] is prepared as follows:—Make a concentrated suspension of *Br. abortus* by washing off mass cultures of a smooth aerobic strain with 0·5 per cent. phenol in saline; heat at 60° C. for 30 min. in a water-bath; wash the cells and pack by centrifuging; stain with haematoxylin diluted 1 in 5 (Ehrlich's or Delafield's) for 5 min.; 10 ml. of packed cells require 1200 ml. of diluted stain; finally suspend the washed stained cells as a 4 per cent. suspension in equal parts of glycerol and phenol-saline.

In milk containing brucella agglutinins the bacteria are agglutinated and rise with the cream, forming a blue cream line leaving the skim-milk white. In samples in which there are no agglutinins there is a white cream line and the rest of the milk remains blue.

The results may be interpreted thus:

Positive (+ + +). Cream layer forms a deep blue ring on top of a completely white column of milk. This indicates a high concentration of agglutinins.

Positive (+ +). Cream layer deeply coloured and milk column slightly blue.

Doubtful or weak positive (+). The cream layer has a definite blue ring but the column of milk is distinctly blue.

Negative (±). The cream layer is the same colour or slightly more coloured than the milk column.

Negative (−). The cream layer is white and the milk column blue.

Whey Agglutination Test.—This is usually applied to the milk of individual cows. Since it is not considered to be influenced greatly by previous vaccination of the animals it is often used to confirm a positive Milk Ring Test.

A few drops of cheese-making rennet are added to 10 ml. skim milk. The tube is incubated for 30 min. at 37° C. to hasten the coagulation of the casein and the liberation of the water-clear whey. Agglutination tests are carried out on the whey in the usual manner using a standard brucella suspension. A titre of 10 or more is considered diagnostic of udder infection.

Other Pathogens in Milk.—The methods for demonstrating typhoid-paratyphoid bacilli and other pathogens correspond to those used for isolating those organisms from other infected material. The sediment after centrifugation is plated out on the appropriate media and some of the milk added to tubes of selective or enrichment broth. For the methods of identifying the organisms isolated by these means reference should be made to the relevant chapters dealing with the organisms being looked for.

BACTERIOLOGICAL EXAMINATION OF ICE-CREAM

The general principles and methods applicable to milk can be adopted for the bacteriological examination of ice-cream. This subject has been reported on by the Public Health Laboratory Service Staff of the Medical Research Council (Gillespie *et al.*, 1947, 1948, 1949, 1950).

[1] Obtainable from the Ministry of Agriculture, Fisheries & Food, Central Veterinary Laboratory, New Haw, Weybridge, Surrey.

In a circular (No. 69/47) issued by the Ministry of Health with reference to the Ice-Cream (Heat Treatment, etc.) Regulations of 1947, attention is drawn to a form of the methylene blue reduction test for grading ice-cream from the hygienic standpoint. This is described in the first of the above reports.

The test should be commenced at 5 p.m. on the day on which the sample is taken. With a graduated pipette, 7 ml. of one-quarter strength Ringer's solution are added to the reduction tube, as used for milk (p. 981), and 1 ml. of standard methylene blue solution; the sample is then added up to the 10 ml. mark (*i.e.* 2 ml. and constituting a 1 in 5 dilution). With precautions to avoid bacterial contamination the tube is closed with a sterile rubber stopper and inverted once. The tube is placed in a water-bath at 20° C. until 10 a.m. on the following day. It is then placed in a water-bath at 37° C. and inverted once every half-hour until decolourisation is complete, as compared with the control, the time for decolourisation being recorded. This control consists of a tube to which are added 8 ml. one-quarter strength Ringer's solution, and ice-cream to the 10 ml. mark, and incubated at 20° C. and 37° C. as in the actual test. A methylene blue control should also be included as in milk testing (*q.v.*).

According to the time taken at 37° C. for complete decolourisation the sample is graded provisionally as follows:

Grade 1. over 4 hours
Grade 2. 2½ to 4 hours
Grade 3. ½ to 2 hours.
Grade 4. Decolourised at time of removal from the 20° C. bath.

In the Ministry of Health Circular it is suggested that if ice-cream consistently fails to reach grades 1 and 2, it would be reasonable to regard this as indicating defects of manufacture or handling which call for investigation.

The Department of Health for Scotland in a Circular No. 43/1948 advises the use of the plate count and the test for coliform bacilli in the bacteriological examination of ice-cream. Although no test is considered to be sufficiently valid as a statutory test, it is suggested that a bacterial count of more than 100,000 per g. and the presence of coliform bacilli in 0·01 g. would indicate faults in the manufacture and handling of ice-cream.

BACTERIOLOGICAL EXAMINATION OF SHELL-FISH

The method used by Bigger (1934) for examining mussels is recommended with a few slight modifications. It may also be adapted to the examination of all types of shellfish including other bivalves such as oysters and univalves such as winkles and cockles.

Bigger's procedure for preparing the mussel emulsion is as follows:

(1) Ten mussels of average size are selected.
(2) These are washed with running tap water, using a boiled nail brush.
(3) One is grasped with sterile ovum forceps, rinsed under the tap and then with sterile water.
(4) It is placed on a piece of sterile parchment paper in which it is grasped with the left hand. The shell is held with the flat edge towards the body, the anterior (pointed) end to the left and the left valve of the shell upwards.

(5) A small portion of the shell at the broad (posterior) end is nibbled away with sterile nibbling forceps, and through the opening the blade of a sterile scalpel is inserted. With this the posterior adductor muscle and the other attachments of the mussel to the left valve are cut, and, holding them with the paper interposed between them and the hands, the two valves of the shell are separated and the left one removed.

(6) All the fluid in the shell is poured off and, with the help of the scalpel, the body is transferred to a small beaker provided with a graduation at the 25 ml. level.

(7) The body of the mussel in the beaker is thoroughly minced with a sterile pair of scissors. Sterile saline is added up to the 25 ml. mark and mixed thoroughly with the minced body, the scissors being used for this purpose.

It has been found advisable to include the shell fluid in the test and to make up the volume to 25 ml. with sterile water instead of saline in order to counteract the high salt content already present.

Varying amounts, viz. 0·5, 0·1 and 0·02 ml. of the minced mussel emulsion are then added to tubes of bile-salt lactose medium (p. 783). The following technique is suggested:

Add 25 ml. sterile water to the beaker containing the 25 ml. minced mussel emulsion, thus making a dilution of 1 in 2. With a sterile pipette, 1 ml. of this dilution is added to 10 ml. of bile-salt lactose medium; 2 ml. of the dilution are next transferred with the same pipette to 8 ml. sterile water in a test-tube giving a second dilution of 1 in 10. Using a fresh sterile pipette, 1 ml. of the 1 in 10 dilution is added to a second tube of bile salt lactose medium and 0·2 ml. of the same dilution to a third tube of the medium. For greater accuracy duplicate tubes of bile-salt lactose medium are recommended for each dilution. This procedure is repeated with each mussel and the cultures are incubated at 37° C. for 24 hr. when they are examined for acid and gas production. An additional reading is made after a further 24 hr. When two tubes of medium are employed for each dilution, results are reported as positive only when acid and gas are produced in both tubes.

It has been found advantageous to use Eijkman's test (p. 969) to confirm the presence of typical or "faecal" coliform bacilli. Subcultures are made from each "positive" tube into fresh tubes of bile-salt lactose medium and are incubated at 44° C. The development of gas at this temperature within 24 hr. is considered to be evidence of the presence of *Esch. coli.*

Interpretation of Results.—According to Bigger's suggested standard, a batch of mussels should be considered undesirably contaminated if more than seven out of the ten tested have coliform bacilli in 0·5 ml. of minced mussel emulsion or more than three in 0·1 ml., or more than one in 0·02 ml.

Consignments of shellfish should not be condemned on the result of one examination alone, but only on a series of results combined with what is known of the condition of the source of the supply and the methods of treatment and handling after harvesting.

BACTERIOLOGY OF CANNED FOOD

Deleterious changes in canned food known as "spoilage" may be brought about through the development of microorganisms. These may be present in the food either as a result of their resistance to the heating process or through being introduced after processing through defects in the structure of the can.

Heat-resistant organisms and the types of spoilage caused by them vary according to the nature of the food they infect. Foods preserved by canning can be divided broadly into two groups: (*a*) medium, low and non-acid foods with pH above 4·5, including meat, fish, vegetables, soup, milk and starch foods; (*b*) high acid foods with pH of less than 4·5. The border-line of pH 4·5 has been chosen because spores of the most heat-resistant of the food poisoning organisms, viz. *Clostridium botulinum*, will not germinate in conditions of acidity higher than this. For this reason it is not usual to heat the foods in group (*b*) above 100° C., which is sufficient to destroy all vegetative forms. Pressure heating on the other hand is necessary to render safe all foods with pH above 4·5. The actual amount of heating employed varies with the food to be processed and is determined by careful laboratory tests carried out by specialists in the canning industry, the main considerations being that although it should be sufficient to destroy spores of pathogenic organisms in the centre of the contents it should not be so great as to alter the appearance and palatability of the food in question.

The minimum degree of heat necessary to destroy the spores of *Clostridium botulinum* may not be adequate to sterilise completely the food and where extremely heat-resistant spores remain, and the temperature of storage is such that germination and growth of the organisms can take place, spoilage will occur.

Organisms that bring about spoilage of food as a result of their heat-resistance are aerobic and anaerobic spore formers of the genera *Bacillus* and *Clostridium*. Many are thermophilic, having an optimum temperature for growth of 55° C. but have the ability to grow slowly at temperatures considerably below this. The type of spoilage gives an indication of the organisms responsible. The following are the main types of spoilage that may occur in group (*a*) foods.

A. *Saccharolytic Spoilage*

1. Acid without gas, known as "flat sour" spoilage, produced by certain species of the genus *Bacillus*, e.g. *B. megaterium*.

2. Acid with gas production sufficient to cause "swelling" of the can, "Hard Swell", due to saccharolytic species of the genus *Clostridium*, e.g. *Cl. multifermentans*.

3. Slight acid production with hydrogen sulphide. No "swelling" occurs since the gas is soluble, but the contents become dark in colour. The organism usually responsible is *Clostridium nigrificans*.

B. *Putrefactive Spoilage*

Digestion of the food with gas production results from the growth of putrefactive species of the genus *Clostridium*, e.g. *Clostridium botulinum* and *Clostridium sporogenes*.

Spoilage of acid foods of group (*b*) is brought about by acid tolerant bacteria and occasionally by yeasts and moulds, which survive the short periods of heating at temperatures below 100° C. The bacteria responsible include sporing aerobes and anaerobes as well as non-sporing species, all capable of developing in high concentrations of acid. Gas may or may not be produced. Examples are *Bacillus thermoacidurans*, *Clostridium pasteurianum*, *Lactobacillus lycopersici* and *Leuconostoc*.

Contamination after Processing

Microorganisms may enter leaking cans and infect the food after processing. They may include a variety of sporing and non-sporing bacteria, often derived from the water used for cooling the cans. If pathogenic organisms gain entrance in this way, cases of food poisoning will result. Staphylococci and organisms of the genus *Salmonella* have occasionally been incriminated in food poisoning outbreaks due to canned food, probably contaminated in this way.

Technique for examining Canned Food

To test the sterility of canned food, and where spoilage has occurred or the food is suspected of causing food poisoning, the following procedure, based on that of Tanner (1944), is recommended for the isolation of the organisms responsible.

Unless the can shows visible signs of spoilage through "swelling" it is advisable to stimulate the multiplication of heat-resistant organisms which may be present in only small numbers, and probably in a "dormant" condition, by incubating it, before opening, at 37° C. for at least one week for mesophilic and 55° C. for thermophilic organisms. Acid foods should be incubated at 25° C. for ten days.

Before being opened the can is carefully examined for physical defects, particularly round the seams. Any signs of "swelling" are noted, and where rustiness or dents have occurred these are scrutinised for pin holes. After examination the can is scrubbed with soap and water and rinsed with alcohol or ether to remove the grease. The area where an opening is to be made is then sterilised by flaming or by treatment with 70 per cent. alcohol. If heat is applied it should be carefully distributed in such a way as to avoid overheating the contents, which may then spurt out when the can is opened. If the can is swollen, it is advisable not to sterilise by heating but rather by the use of alcohol. The point of a sterile opener is then inserted into the sterilised area and an opening is cut sufficiently large to enable a portion of the food to be withdrawn in the following aseptic manner:

Liquid food is withdrawn with a sterile pipette or an untapered glass tube and inoculated directly into the culture medium. 15–20 ml. should be tested in this way. Solid food is sampled with a modified cork borer, 10 in. long and $\frac{3}{4}$ in. in diameter, having a rod inserted to expel the contents. The sample should include food from the centre of the contents, where heat-resistant organisms are likely to occur, and from the surface, where contamination through leakage may have taken place. The solid food should then be thoroughly emulsified in sterile water by grinding with a sterile pestle and mortar or by shaking in a screw-capped bottle with pieces of broken glass (Baumgartner, 1945).

Technique for Culture

Tubes containing 10 ml. amounts of suitable fluid media are inoculated with 1 ml. of the liquid food and incubated at 37° C. and 55° C., both aerobically and anaerobically. Cooked meat medium is recommended for culturing anaerobic bacilli, and glucose broth is suitable for aerobic mesophilic and thermophilic organisms. In order to culture spoilage organisms from acid foods, tomato glucose broth is recommended by Tanner. This consists of tomato juice and nutrient broth in equal parts with the addition of 1 per cent. glucose. The tubes are examined after 24 and 48 hr., and where growth has occurred the organisms may be identified by microscopic examination of stained films and by further culture tests. If the food is suspected of causing food poisoning through infection with organisms of the Salmonella and Staphylococcus groups, media selective for these organisms should also be inoculated with portions of the food. For salmonellae, tetrathionate broth and selenite medium are suitable; for staphylococci, cooked meat medium to which 10 per cent. sodium chloride has been added is recommended.

Organisms developing in these selective media should be further examined by the methods described in the appropriate sections dealing with them.

It is advisable to make direct films of the food for microscopic examination although no significance should be attached to organisms seen unless the cultures confirm that they are viable.

After removing samples for culture, the food is turned out of the can and examined carefully for any abnormalities in appearance and smell. The inside of the can too should be inspected for defects in its manufacture.

The Bacteriological Examination of Milk Bottles

To test the adequacy of the cleansing and sterilisation of milk bottles at farms and creameries, the following technique, based on the recommendations of the Ministry of Agriculture and Fisheries (1947) is advocated.

At least four bottles should be picked at random immediately after washing. They should be capped or fitted with a sterile rubber bung and sent immediately to the laboratory so that testing may be begun within 4 hr. of sampling.

To each bottle, irrespective of its size, 20 ml. of sterile quarter-strength Ringer solution are added and the cap or bung replaced. The bottle is then laid horizontally on the bench and rotated by rolling so that the whole of the internal surface is rinsed with the solution. This process is repeated at intervals over a period of half an hour, the bottle being kept on its side during that time.

Five ml. of the solution are then plated in duplicate using 20 ml. yeast extract milk agar (p. 783), this large amount being necessary to produce solidification. One plate is incubated at 37° C. for 48 hr. and the other at 22° C. for 3 days. (For greater accuracy duplicate plates may be prepared for both temperatures.) The results are reported as the colony count per bottle, *i.e.* the individual plate count multiplied by 4.

Based on the 37° C. count, the following scheme of classification was suggested:

Average Colony Count per bottle	*Classification*
Not more than 200	Satisfactory
Over 200 to 600	Fairly satisfactory
Over 600	Unsatisfactory

In addition, a test for the presence of coliform bacilli should be carried out by inoculating each of two bottles containing 10 ml. double-strength MacConkey's broth with 5 ml. rinse solution. These are examined for acid and gas production after 48 hr. incubation at 37° C. If adequate methods are employed in cleansing and sterilising the bottles, no coliform bacilli should be present.

The Bacteriological Examination of Washed Crockery and Cutlery

The adequacy of washing-up methods employed in the kitchens of catering establishments, schools and other institutions may be tested by bacterial examinations of swabs taken from freshly washed crockery and cutlery.

Preparation of Swabs.—Absorbent cotton-wool swabs ¾ in. long, as used for clinical purposes may be employed. It is more generally convenient to have them on wooden applicator sticks 6½ in. long than on wires, so that after the specimen has been collected the swab may be broken off above the cotton-wool and allowed to drop down into a container of quarter-strength Ringer's solution. The swabs are inserted into test-tubes 5 in. by ½ in. plugged with cotton-wool and are sterilised by autoclaving at 115° C. for 15 min.

Higgins (1950) obtained a greater recovery of organisms by using swabs made of calcium alginate wool instead of cotton-wool, the advantage being that the alginate swabs may be completely dissolved in Ringer's solution containing sodium hexametaphosphate. In this way all the bacteria contained in the swab are liberated into the solution. Not more than 50 mg. of wool should be used for each swab to ensure complete solution even in cold weather, when larger amounts tend to form crystals. It is important that the calcium alginate wool should be declared by the manufacturer to be free from bactericidal substances such as "Fixanol C", a quaternary ammonium compound which was originally impregnated into the wool for use in the manufacture of certain textiles.

Method of Swabbing.—One swab is used for five similar articles. It is first moistened by dipping in sterile quarter-strength Ringer's solution, the surplus liquid being squeezed out against the inside of the screw-capped container. The swab is then rubbed thoroughly over the whole of the appropriate areas, which are as follows:

the inner surfaces of plates and bowls that come in contact with food;
the inner and outer surfaces of cups, mugs and glasses to a depth of 3 cm. below the rim ;
bowls and the backs of spoons and the back and front surfaces of forks and between the prongs.

After swabbing five similar articles in this way, the swab is returned to the test-tube and sent to the laboratory without delay.

Method of Testing

(*a*) If cotton-wool swabs have been used, the swab is broken off the wooden stick with sterile forceps and allowed to drop into a screw-capped bottle of 1 oz. capacity containing 10 ml. of sterile quarter-strength Ringer's solution. If delay in transporting the sample to the laboratory is unavoidable, this should be done by the person taking the sample. In the laboratory the bottle is shaken vigorously to disintegrate the swab and liberate as many as possible of the bacteria contained in it. 1 ml. quantities of the test solution are plated out in duplicate on yeast extract agar (p. 783), one plate of each being incubated at 37° C. for 48 hr. and the other at 22° C. for 3 days. The results are reported as the bacterial counts per utensil for each temperature (*i.e.* count per ml. × 2). (*b*) If calcium alginate swabs are used, it is recommended by Higgins and Hobbs (1950) that two swabs should be employed for each test, one being moistened in Ringer's solution before use and the other used dry. The surfaces of five articles are rubbed over, first with the moistened swab and then with the dry one. Both swabs are then broken off the sticks with sterile forceps and allowed to drop into 9 ml. quarter-strength Ringer's solution. 1 ml. of 10 per cent. sodium hexametaphosphate solution (sterilised by autoclaving) is then added and the bottle shaken until both swabs have dissolved. The solution is plated out either by the method described under (*a*) or by the Miles and Misra technique, using blood agar plates on which the test solution is inoculated in the form of drops of 0·02 ml. volume delivered from a calibrated Pasteur pipette.

Standards

There is no standard officially recognised in Great Britain, but attention is drawn to the United States Public Health Standard (Tiedman *et al.*,1944) for washed crockery. Based on the swabbing technique followed by the standard plate count test it allows a maximum of 100 colonies per utensil examined. If the Miles and Misra method is used, specimens giving 2 colonies orless per 6 drops of undiluted test suspension on blood agar plates may be considered to conform to the American standard.

EXAMINATION OF FOODSTUFFS IN OUTBREAKS OF FOOD POISONING

Bacterial Food Poisoning (acute gastro-enteritis) results from the consumption of food infected with certain pathogenic organisms which are capable of proliferating in food if conditions are favourable. They fall into two categories depending on the manner in which they produce their harmful effects, viz: (*a*) those which infect the body (notably the salmonella group), and (*b*) those which produce a toxin during their growth in the food, the main cause of this type being certain coagulase-positive staphylococci. Certain types of *Clostridium welchii*, characterised by the heat resistance of their spores, are also responsible for a type of food poisoning but their mode of action has not yet been clarified.

Specimens of food for Bacteriological Examination

Meat preparations (ham, brawn, sausages, etc.), and made-up dishes such as sandwiches prepared by hand, have been responsible for outbreaks of salmonella and staphylococcal food poisoning, and pre-cooked meat, stews, beefsteak pies, etc., prepared the day before serving, frequently cause outbreaks of *Cl. welchii* food poisoning. Eggs used in the preparation of uncooked or only partially cooked foods, have caused salmonella infections, and unpasteurised milk and milk products have in the past been responsible for both staphylococcal and salmonella food poisoning. Any of the above foodstuffs should be viewed with suspicion if they have been eaten by the patients shortly before the commencement of symptoms, and samples should be examined bacteriologically for the three main food poisoning organisms.

For the methods of isolation and identification of the various specific bacteria, reference should be made to the appropriate sections in Part II. The following points should be observed.

Non-specific Contamination.—The examination of food samples should commence with a careful inspection to determine if there are any abnormalities in appearance or smell. This is followed by a microscopic examination of stained preparations which will indicate any gross contamination. It is also useful to determine the total count of viable bacteria per gram of food at 37° C. and 22° C., by means of the *plate count method* (see p. 969) applied to a suspension of 1 g. of the food in 10 ml. of sterile Ringer's solution. This test should be combined with an examination for coliform bacilli as in the examination of milk samples (see p. 980). These preliminary tests will indicate whether or not the food has been subjected to contamination of a non-specific nature arising from poor standards of kitchen hygiene.

Salmonella Infection.—In testing foodstuffs for organisms of the salmonella group, both direct culture and enrichment techniques should be carried out (see p. 226). In order to isolate salmonellae from frozen liquid whole egg the Food Hygiene Laboratory of the Central Public Health Laboratory recommend the following technique. Two 25 g. amounts of the egg (liquid or frozen) are weighed in sterile jars with screw caps, and after the addition of 25 ml. of quarter-strength Ringer's solution the mixtures are incubated for 1–2 hr. at 37° C. before the addition of 50 ml. double strength selenite enrichment broth to one lot and 50 ml. double-strength tetrathionate broth to the other. These enrichment cultures are incubated at 37° C. and subcultured on to both desoxycholate citrate agar and Wilson & Blair's agar after 24 hr. and again after 3 days' incubation. Suspicious colonies are picked for identification.

This method may be applied to the examination of any liquid foods.

Staphylococcal Intoxication.—There is no reliable laboratory method for identifying the enterotoxin of *Staphylococcus aureus*, and diagnosis of this type of food poisoning can only be made if coagulase-positive staphylococci are isolated from the food. By the Miles and Misra counting technique (see p. 872), using 10 per cent. salt milk agar (p. 750) as a selective medium, it is possible to determine the approximate number of staphylococci per gm. of suspected food. Although it is not known how many staphylococci are necessary to cause food poisoning, large numbers growing in direct culture from suspected food would be highly suggestive of it being the cause. In order to isolate *Staphylococcus aureus* from foodstuffs heavily contaminated with other organisms, the use of cooked-meat medium containing 10 per cent. salt (see p. 750) may be advantageous. Any coagulase-positive staphylococci isolated by the above methods should be typed by bacteriophage or serological methods. In order to determine the source of the infection, all persons engaged in the preparation and handling of the food should be examined to determine whether they are harbouring the same organism in their noses or in skin lesions.

Cl. welchii Food Poisoning.—This form of food poisoning, which has been increasingly recognised in recent years, is caused by a variant of Type A *Cl. welchii* characterised by being non-haemolytic, feebly toxigenic and having spores that can survive boiling for several hours.

Anaerobic culture on blood agar plates inoculated by the Miles and Misra technique will indicate the degree of contamination by anaerobic or facultative anaerobic organisms. Unless they grow in relatively pure culture it may not be easy to distinguish the colonies of non-haemolytic *Cl. welchii* from those of non-sporing organisms. They may be more readily isolated by inoculating small portions of the food into an enrichment medium such as cooked-meat medium and incubating for 18 hr. before culturing on blood agar, but it should be borne in mind that such indirect culture does not have the same significance as direct culture. Use may be made of the selective medium of Willis & Hobbs (p. 759). The identity of any possible *Cl. welchii* colonies isolated by the above methods should be further confirmed (see p. 318 for further details).

Cl. botulinum Intoxication.—Botulism, a rare type of food poisoning has an incubation period which varies from less than 24 hr. to 72 hr. The highly potent exotoxin formed during the proliferation of *Cl. botulinum* in the food is absorbed through the gastric mucosa and affects the nervous system rather than the gastro-intestinal tract. This subject is dealt with more fully on p. 337-41.

Foods which have been incriminated include improperly processed canned and preserved meat, meat and game pastes, and vegetables that are eaten uncooked or only partially cooked (the toxin is destroyed by heating to 90° C.). The spores of *Cl. botulinum* may survive boiling for several hours but are destroyed within 15 minutes by a temperature of 120° C. They fail to germinate if the pH of the food is less than 4·5.

BACTERIOLOGICAL EXAMINATION OF AIR

Settle plates.—In the past the procedure frequently adopted for determining the relative numbers and species of microorganisms present in air has been to expose open plates of culture medium for given periods of time, *e.g.* ½ or 1 hr. A count of the colonies after incubation of the plates for 24 hr. at 37° C. yields a relative estimate of the number of organisms present, and if blood agar is used, the occurrence in the air of pathogenic staphylococci and streptococci can be determined. This method has proved valuable in demonstrating the presence of such organisms in the air and dust of hospital wards in which they are being spread. Such findings have also thrown light on cross-infection in hospitals.

Slit Sampler.—It is recognised, however, that this simple method of exposing plates has certain limitations as a means of studying the bacteriology of air; for example, it is not a satisfactory method of detecting bacteria in very small suspended particles such as droplet-nuclei. More elaborate procedures have therefore been adopted. A technique introduced by Bourdillon, Lidwell and Thomas (1941) involves the use of a special instrument, the "slit sampler", by which a known volume of air is directed on to a plate through a slit 0·25 mm. wide, the plate being mechanically rotated so that the organisms are evenly distributed over it. One cubic foot of air per minute is allowed to pass through the slit, and samples of 1 to 10 cubic feet, or more, may be tested. More advanced models of the slit sampler have a timing arrangement that allows the number of colonies on each sector of the plate to be related to the number of bacteria-carrying particles sampled in a particular part of the sampling period. These instruments can be obtained commercially.[1]

The slit sampler and other air samplers have been used in examining the amount of bacterial contamination in the air of hospitals, schools, factories and other places, with a view to determining the danger of air-borne infection and the factors that increase and decrease numbers of air-borne bacteria (Bourdillon *et al.*, 1948). Observations have been made in surgical operation rooms in relation to the efficacy of different ventilation systems in minimising aerial contamination, and in schools, hospitals and other places in tests of the efficacy of ultraviolet irradiation and chemical vapours for air disinfection.

[1] C. F. Casella & Co. Ltd., Fitzroy Square, London, W.1.

Cascade Impaction Sampler.—Lidwell (1959) has described an impaction sampler that operates on the cascade principle and collects air-borne infected particles in four ranges of size on four separate culture plates. The size ranges (diameters) of the particles are: less than 4 μ, between 4 and 10 μ, between 10 and 18 μ, and greater than 18 μ. In hospitals and other occupied places, the air-borne particles carrying pathogenic organisms such as *Staph. aureus*, *Strept. pyogenes*, *Candida albicans* and ringworm fungi, are mostly in the range of 10–18 microns in diameter (Noble, Lidwell and Kingston, 1963). Especial interest attaches, however, to the smaller proportion of infected particles (e.g. *c.* 5 per cent.) that are under 5 μ in diameter and are thus able to remain airborne for long periods (e.g. for more than 30 min.) and, if inhaled, to penetrate deeply into the respiratory tract and reach the lung alveoli.

Levels of air infection.—These are generally expressed in terms of the counts of bacterial colonies of all kinds made on blood agar plates incubated for 24 hours at 37° C. When plates are incubated for a much longer period at room temperature the counts are often very much higher as a result of the slow growth of saprophytic organisms that do not grow well at 37° C. The counts are expressed as the number of bacteria-carrying particles per cubic foot (28·3 litres) of air when the examination is made with a slit sampler, and as the number of bacteria-carrying particles settling on a 3½ in. (88 mm.) Petri dish per minute, or per hour, when it is made with settle plates.

Since we still lack knowledge of the relative dangers of infection that are presented by different levels of bacterial contamination of air, and since the levels of contamination vary very greatly from time to time and from place to place within occupied premises, it is not possible as yet to define the limits of the levels of contamination that may be regarded as acceptable.

Under conditions of normal occupation, the air in hospital wards, offices, schools, and private houses commonly shows levels of contamination in the range of 5 to 100 bacteria-carrying particles per cu. ft., and in the range of 0·05 to 5 bacteria-carrying particles per 3½ in. (88 mm.) settle plate per min.; the higher levels are found when there is much bodily movement or other disturbance, such as bed-making, that is liable to raise dust into the air. Bourdillon *et al.* (1948) have suggested, as provisional standards of air hygiene, that the following may be regarded as the limits to the levels of infection that are acceptable: in factories, offices, homes, etc., 50 per cu. ft.; in surgical operating theatres providing for most forms of surgery, 10 per cu. ft.; in surgical theatres where operations on the central nervous system or dressings of burns are done, *c.* 1 per cu. ft. Peak levels of contamination limited to short periods of exceptional disturbance and movement are disregarded in applying these standards.

The great majority of the bacteria found in the air are harmless saprophytes or commensals, and even in hospital wards and other rooms occupied by patients and carriers, usually not more than 1 per cent., and commonly only 0·01–0·1 per cent., of the air-borne bacteria are pathogens. *Staph. aureus* is the pathogen most commonly found in the air. It is present in most occupied premises. Occasionally up to 10, or more, *Staph. aureus*-carrying particles are found per cu. ft. of air, but much more commonly between 0·01 and 1·0 per cu. ft. *Strept. pyogenes* is sometimes found in large numbers (e.g. *c.* 10 per cu. ft.) in the air of rooms occupied by patients with tonsillitis, scarlet fever or infected wounds and burns, but usually the level of contamination is between 0·01 and 1 per cu. ft. in such places.

Whilst the higher levels of air contamination with pathogenic organisms are obviously the most dangerous, it should be noted that there is no level of contamination, however low, that can be regarded as certainly safe. Little is known about the minimum size of dose of organisms required to initiate infection on inhalation. It is quite possible that a man may be infected if he inhales only a single infected particle in the 500 or so cubic feet of air that he respires in the course of a day. In an investigation described by Riley (1957) the number of tubercle bacillus-carrying particles present in the air in a tuberculosis hospital ward was calculated, from infection rates in guinea-pigs exposed to the ward air, to be on average only about 0·00008 per cu. ft. Such a level of contamination was considered to be sufficient to account for the infection of a considerable proportion of originally tuberculin-negative nurses during 6 months of duty in a tuberculosis hospital, since each nurse would in this time inhale a volume of air sufficient to contain one infective particle.

Bacteriological Examination of Environmental Dust

Sweep plates.—The sweep plate method is used to examine personal clothing, bed-clothes, carpets, curtains, soft furniture and other domestic fabrics for the presence of pathogenic bacteria liable to be liberated in dust. An ordinary Petri dish containing nutrient agar, blood agar or a selective culture medium is removed from its lid and rubbed to and fro on the surface of the fabric. The medium faces the fabric and the edges of the plate are made to scrape the fabric so that dust is thrown up on to the medium. About 10 sweeps may be made with a plate of non-selective medium, and more with one of selective medium.

Dust on floors and hard surfaces.—This may be collected on a cotton-wool swab moistened with broth and the swab is plated out in the usual way on a suitable medium. For large areas, a more representative sample may be obtained by sweeping the dust together and suspending a portion in broth and plating out different dilutions of the broth.

REFERENCES

ALLEN, L. A., PASLEY, S. M. & PIERCE, M. S. F. (1952). Conditions affecting the growth of Bacterium coli on bile salts media. Enumeration of this organism in polluted water. *J. gen. Microbiol.*, **7**, 257.

AMIES, C. R. (1956). Surface Film on Swimming Pools. *Canad. J. Pub. Hlth.*, **47**, 93.

BAUMGARTNER, J. G. (1945). *Canned Foods.* London: Churchill.

BIGGER, J. W. (1934). The bacteriological examination of mussels. *J. Hyg. (Camb.)*, **34**, 172.

BOURDILLON, R. B., LIDWELL, O. M. & THOMAS, J. C. (1941). A slit sampler for collecting and counting air-borne bacteria. *J. Hyg., Camb.*, **41**, 197.

BOURDILLON, R. B., LIDWELL, O. M., LOVELOCK, J. E., CAWSTON, W. C., COLEBROOK, L., ELLIS, F. P., VAN DEN ENDE, M., GLOVER, R. E., MACFARLAN, A. M., MILES, A. A., RAYMOND, W. F., SCHUSTER, E. & THOMAS, J. C. (1948). Studies in air Hygiene. *Spec. Rep. Ser. med. Res. Coun. (Lond.)*, No. 262, H.M.S.O.

BURMAN, N. P. (1955). The standardisation and selection of bile salt and peptone for culture media used in the bacteriological examination of water. *Proc. Soc. Water Treat. Exam.*, **4**, 10.

CHALMERS, C. H. (1962). *Bacteria in Relation to the Milk Supply.* London: Arnold.

DEPARTMENT OF HEALTH FOR SCOTLAND (1948). Ice-cream (Scotland) Regulations D.H.S. Circular No. 43/1948.

GILLESPIE, E. H., KING, G. J. G., MOORE, B. & TOMLINSON, A. J. H. (1947); (1948); (1949); (1950). Bacteriological examination and grading of ice-cream. *Mth. Bull. Minist. Hlth. Lab. Serv.*, **6**, 60; **7**, 84; **8**, 155; **9**, 231.

GRAY, R. D., JEBB, W. H. H., MCCOY, J. H., MORRISON RICHIE, J., KINGSLEY SMITH, A. J., WATKINSON, JOAN M., WINDLE TAYLOR, E. & SUTHERLAND, J. (1953). The choice of an indicator organism for the bacteriological control of swimming-bath purification. *Mth. Bull. Minist. Hlth. Lab. Serv.*, **12**, 254.

HALEY, L. D. & ROSTY, A. (1957). Use of millipore membrane filters in the diagnostic tuberculosis laboratory. *Amer. J. clin. Path.*, **27**, No. 1, 117.

HAMMERSTRÖM, E., & LJUTOV, V. (1954). Concentration technique for demonstrating small amounts of bacteria in tap water. *Acta path. microbiol. scand.*, **35**, 365.

HANNAY, C. L. & NORTON, I. L. (1947). Enumeration, isolation and study of faecal streptococci from river water. *Proc. Soc. appl. Bact.*, No. 1, p. 39.

HIGGINS, M. (1950). A comparison of the pour plate and surface plate methods in estimating bacterial infection of table crockery and kitchen utensils. *Mth. Bull. Minist. Hlth. Lab. Serv.*, **9**, 52.

HIGGINS, M. & HOBBS, B. C. (1950). Kitchen hygiene: the effectiveness of current procedure in cleansing tableware. *Mth. Bull. Minist. Hlth Lab. Serv.*, **9**, 38.

KABLER, P. W. & CLARK, H. F. (1952). The use of differential media with the membrane filter. *Amer. J. publ. Hlth.*, **42**, (1), 390.

LIDWELL, O. M. (1959). Impaction sampler for size grading air-borne bacteria-carrying particles. *J. Scientif. Instrum.*, **36**, 3.

LJUTOV, V. (1954). Filtering methods for demonstration of Salmonella bacteria in water. *Acta path. microbiol. scand.*, **35**, 370.

MACKENZIE, E. F. W., TAYLOR, E. W. & GILBERT, W. E. (1948). Recent experiences in the rapid identification of bacterium coli Type I. *J. gen. Microbiol.*, **2**, 197.

MINISTRY OF AGRICULTURE & FISHERIES (1947). (National Milk Testing & Advisory Scheme). The bacteriological examination of milk bottles. Technique No. B743/TPB.

MINISTRY OF HEALTH (1947). Ice-cream (Heat Treatment, etc.) Regulations Circular 69/47.

MINISTRY OF HEALTH (1951). *The Purification of the Water of Swimming Baths.* London: H.M.S.O.

MINISTRY OF HEALTH (1956). *The Bacteriological Examination of Water Supplies.* Report No. 71. London: H.M.S.O.

MOORE, B. (1948). The detection of paratyphoid carriers in towns by means of sewage examinations. *Mth. Bull. Minist. Hlth. Lab. Serv.*, **7**, 241.

NOBLE, W. C., LIDWELL, O. M. & KINGSTON, D. (1963). The size distribution of air-borne particles carrying micro-organisms. *J. Hyg., Camb.*, **61**, 385.

RILEY, R. L. (1957). Aerial dissemination of pulmonary tuberculosis. *Amer. Rev. Tuberculosis*, **76**, 931.

TANNER, F. W. (1944). *Microbiology of Foods*, 2nd ed. Champaign, Ill.: Garrard Press.

TIEDMAN, W. D., FUCKS, A. W., GUNDERSON, N. O., HUCKER, G. J. & MALLMANN, W. J. (1944). A proposed method for control of food utensil sanitation. *Amer. J. publ. Hlth.* **34**, 255.

WILSON, G. S., TWIGG, R. S., WRIGHT, R. C., HENDRY, C. B., COWELL, M. P. & MAIER, I. (1935). The Bacteriological Grading of Milk. *Spec. Rep. Ser. med. Res. Coun. (Lond.)*, No. 206.

WINDLE TAYLOR, E. (1955-56). Membrane filtration. *37th Ann. Rep. Dir. Water Exam. Met. Water Bd. London*, pp. 13-20.

WINDLE TAYLOR, E. (1957-58). Progress in Membrane Filtration. *38th Ann. Rep. Dir. Water Exam. Met. Water Bd. London*, p. 26.

WINDLE TAYLOR, E. (1959-60). Further Progress with Membrane Filtration. *39th Ann. Rep. Dir. Water Exam. Met. Water Bd. London*, pp. 20-27.

WINDLE TAYLOR, E. (1961-62). Further Progress with Membrane Filtration. *40th Ann. Rep. Dir. Water Exam. Met. Water Bd. London*, pp. 15–17.

WINDLE TAYLOR, E. (1963-64). Progress with Membrane Filtration. *41st. Ann. Rep. Dir. Water Exam. Met. Water Bd. London*, pp. 17-21.

WINDLE TAYLOR, E. & BURMAN, N. P. (1964). The application of membrane filtration techniques to the bacteriological examination of water. *J. appl. Bact.*, **27**, 294.

WINDLE TAYLOR, E., BURMAN, N. P. & OLIVER, C.W. (1953). Use of the membrane filter in the bacteriological examination of water. *J. appl. Chem.*, **3**, 233.

WINDLE TAYLOR, E., BURMAN, N. P. & OLIVER, C. W. (1955). Membrane filtration applied to the routine bacteriological examination of water. *J. Inst. Water Engineers*, **9**, No. 3, 248.

WORLD HEALTH ORGANIZATION (1961). *European Standards for Drinking-Water.* Geneva: Palais des Nations.

CHAPTER 56

THE CARE AND MANAGEMENT OF EXPERIMENTAL ANIMALS

LABORATORY animals in Great Britain are protected by the Cruelty to Animals Act (1876), under which only workers who hold a licence granted by the Home Secretary are permitted to experiment on them. Advice on the procedure to obtain a licence may be got from the Research Defence Society, 11 Chandos Street, London, W.1. The licence authorises the licensee to carry out experiments in the stated registered place only. All registered places are approved by the Home Office before registration is granted, and are thereafter visited from time to time without notice by the Home Office Inspector for the area. Depending on the scope of his experiments, the licensee may require a certificate (or certificates) in addition, for in any experiment authorised by licence alone, the animal must be anaesthetised before the experiment begins and must be killed before recovery from the anaesthetic. Certificate A must be obtained if no anaesthetic is to be used; this covers most of the bacteriologist's usual laboratory work with animals: namely, procedures that do not exceed the equivalent of injection or superficial venesection. It can authorise, for example, inoculation of the animal subcutaneously, intravenously, intraperitoneally, or by scarification. For experiments requiring procedures which exceed the equivalent of the above in severity, an anaesthetic must be used. Certificate B must be obtained to authorise any experiment whose object would be frustrated unless the animal is allowed to recover from the anaesthetic. Further certificates must be obtained to authorise experiments in which cats, dogs or the equidae are used. In all cases of doubt about animal experiments, and the law relating to them, the worker is strongly advised, in his own interest, to seek the advice of the Home Office Inspector for his area, whose name and address can be got by application to the Under Secretary of State, Home Office, London, S.W.1.

GENERAL DIRECTIONS FOR THE CARE OF ANIMALS

The health and well-being of laboratory animals depend almost entirely on the care, humanity and watchfulness of the staff of the animal house. To keep laboratory animals healthy and contented requires a high degree of technical skill, a genuine liking for animals, and a full understanding of their ways of life. Animals in cages are deprived of their own ways of fending for themselves and they are completely dependent on their attendants for all their necessities and comforts; it is impossible for them to find their own food or water, to move to a cooler or a warmer place, to seek fresh air or to obtain exercise or companionship. To make good these deficiencies in their life a number of general principles must be observed in the day to day running of an animal house.

Fluid

No animal should ever be deprived of a plentiful supply of fresh clean drinking water. It is wrong to assume that wet mashes and moistened diets supply enough fluid although it is true that in the case of guinea-pigs and rabbits, a plentiful supply of fresh cabbage or lettuce may obviate the need for drinking bottles. Animals kept short of water lose condition, eat less, waste, and are prone to cannibalise their young.

Drinking water can be conveniently supplied to the animals from a bottle attached to the outside of the cage. Suitable and inexpensive bottles are medical flats, blood transfusion bottles, ginger-beer bottles; wide mouthed pathological specimen jars are particularly recommended as being easily cleaned. The bottles should hold 250–500 ml. of water, smaller bottles are more liable to leakage through agitation. The water is led in 6–9 mm. glass tubing through a rubber bung to an accessible position inside the cage; the outlet of the tubing should be narrowed to about 3 mm.

Diet

A balanced diet which contains carbohydrate, fat, proteins, vitamins, mineral salts, and trace elements in appropriate proportions must be given regularly. Usually such a diet can be obtained commercially in the form of cubes or pellets and can be placed in hoppers attached to the sides of the cages so that food is available at all times to the animals. When cage hoppers are not available the pellets may be placed in dishes inside the cages or a dry or wet mash may be given in the same manner. The latter method, however, is time consuming and much food-stuff is wasted by spilling and contamination. The condition of many animals is improved by supplementing pellet diets with small quantities of greenstuffs.

Cleanliness

Animals will not thrive under dirty conditions and unless they are kept clean there is a considerable risk of epidemic disease. Once each week the animals should be transferred to clean cages and the dirty cages should be removed to a special room set aside for them where they should be scraped free from all litter and droppings, scrubbed thoroughly in soap and water and sterilised in the autoclave or hot air oven. The animals, especially when breeding, should not however have their cages changed too frequently because they are disturbed by the process and as a result often lose weight. With adequately absorbent litter such as peat moss the cages remain hygienic for a week. Where heat sterilisers are not available the cages can be boiled in soapy water or, failing that, immersed overnight in a solution of disinfectant such as 3 per cent. lysol. Lysol, however, should not be used for rabbit cages because its smell distresses the animals. The cages should be perfectly dry before being used again. Clean cages should then be stacked on a trolley to be transferred for storage in a special clean room where clean litter can be placed in them and clean sterile hoppers or dishes of food and drinking bottles added to them before they are taken into use again. A special trolley should be reserved for the clean cages and another for dirty cages.

Litter

A layer of absorbent material should be spread to a depth of ½ to 1 inch on the bottom of the cages. For this purpose fine soft wood sawdust, wood shavings, peat moss or sugar-cane pith are all satisfactory. Pregnant animals must also be supplied with nesting material; shredded paper is recommended for mice and clean hay for rabbits and guinea-pigs.

Cages

Each species of animal requires its own type of cage and the design must ensure that there is enough room to give free movement and space for resting when the animal lies down fully stretched out. The cage should be large enough for the animal to take some exercise; this is especially important for monkeys. To facilitate cleaning many cages are provided with coarse wire-mesh floors through which the excreta fall on to a tray which can easily be removed for cleaning without disturbing the occupants. Such cages do however inflict some discomfort on the animals and it is usually necessary to place some litter (*e.g.* paper shavings) within the cage in order to prevent the animals developing sores on the pads of the feet.

Labelling of Cages

Every cage should have attached permanently to it a socket or holder for a small card about $2\frac{1}{2} \times 3\frac{1}{2}$ inches, on which is recorded the name of the experimenter, the identifying marks of the animals, the date, the nature of the experiment and any other relevant matter. The card must not be removed before the conclusion of the experiment and must be placed in such a position that it cannot be chewed or defaced by the animal. Breeding cages should also be labelled so that each animal can be identified especially if a breeding programme (*e.g.* inbreeding) is being carried out.

Ventilation

Ideally the animal house should be air-conditioned; at least ten changes of air in each hour are needed. When there is no air conditioning adequate ventilation from windows must be ensured but great care must be taken not to expose the cages to draughts. Animals kept in badly ventilated rooms are more liable to respiratory diseases.

Temperature and Humidity

Each animal has its own optimum temperature and animal rooms must be kept close to this level if the stock is to remain healthy and able to breed. Sudden fluctuations of temperature must be avoided since they may result in the death of whole colonies of animals. If animals such as guinea-pigs or rabbits are kept in open runs, sufficient litter or hay must be provided for them to make nests in which to keep warm. The humidity of the animal house should range between 45 per cent. for rabbits to 65 per cent. for mice.

Handling

If animals are handled frequently and sympathetically they soon become tame and easily managed; it is only when they are frightened that they bite and then only in self-defence. Loud noises such as the clattering of metal cages and the slamming of doors must be avoided in the animal house which should be as quiet a place as possible. When it is necessary to handle an animal, place the cage on the bench and allow the creature to know what is happening; open the cage door gently, introduce the hands slowly and deliberately, and pick up the animal with firm unhurried movements. Give the animal a sense of complete security by fully supporting its weight and eliminating the risk of dropping it. Avoid all sudden grabbing movements and approach the animals with a steady confidence. It is seldom necessary to wear leather gloves when handling animals except when new stock is introduced into the colony and their confidence has not yet been won. An exception is made, however, with rats and monkeys, where a bite is accompanied by the risk of a severe infection to the handler.

Breeding

Porter and Lane-Petter (1962) give detailed instructions for the breeding of common laboratory animals.

Marking Animals

White or lightly coloured animals can be temporarily marked by staining the fur with a strong dye. Marking ink of the type contained in commercial glass ink-pens is very convenient and the dye persists on the fur for two months or more. Alternatively strong carbol fuchsin can be used. Rabbits can be marked by tattooing the ears either with a special instrument designed for the purpose or with a needle dipped in India ink. For rats and mice ear punching is a simple method; a special ear punch can be obtained from veterinary instrument makers and this cuts holes about $\frac{1}{8}$ in. in diameter in patterns arranged according to an identification code. For fowls, numbered metal tags are clipped through the loose skin of the wing.

The Detection of the Signs of Disease in Animals

It is easy to miss the early signs of illness in caged animals and in order to make sure that the stock is healthy a routine tour of inspection of the occupants of every cage should be made at least once a day but preferably twice, early in the morning and again in the evening. Attention must be paid to the general condition of the animals, the amounts of food and water consumed and the nature of the faeces. The position and movements of the animals should be noted and any animal that remains quiet and still or seems listless should be removed from its cage and exercised. A quiet animal left undisturbed may appear to be normal and yet may be found to be paralysed or ataxic when made to move. The appearance of the fur is of particular importance; when the animal is generally in poor condition or is suffering from a chronic illness it lacks its normal lustre and when acutely ill the fur may be staring or ruffled. Acute illnesses are often accompanied by inflammation of the conjunctiva and nasal mucosa which often are also the sites of a muco-purulent discharge. Ulceration of the skin, the tail, and the pads may indicate ectromelia in mice, and localised lesions of this type may indicate parasite infestations. Full details of the commoner diseases of laboratory animals are given by Harris (1962), Worden & Lane-Petter (1957) and Parish (1950). Sometimes there may be no obvious clinical signs of illness and the only sign manifest in the animal is fever (*e.g.* rickettsial infections). Thus it may be necessary to record an animal's temperature daily or at more frequent intervals.

Taking an Animal's Temperature

An ordinary clinical thermometer smeared liberally with sterile petroleum jelly may be used though the blunt ended rectal thermometer is to be preferred as being less easily broken. It is introduced into the rectum or vagina to a depth of about three-quarters of an inch; the depth must be the same on every occasion and the mercury bulb must always be completely inserted. Whenever possible the animal's temperature should be taken before feeding and it must be remembered that the temperature of a frightened or struggling animal may be raised without any pathological cause being present.

Prevention of Disease

When new animals are purchased and introduced into the animal house they should be placed in a special quarantine room and kept there under observation for 10–14 days. If, during this period, any animals sicken or die the stock should be held in quarantine and necropsies must be made to investigate the cause of the trouble.

Animals infected experimentally with bacteria or viruses should be held in separate isolation rooms and full precautions taken to prevent the spread of infection to other animals. Bedding and unused foodstuffs from these animals should be removed and burned. The cages should be removed on a special trolley reserved for the purpose, handled separately, and autoclaved before being placed in contact with clean cages. People who have handled infected animals, cages, or any contaminated material should immediately wash their hands thoroughly with soap and water, and change to a clean coat before proceeding to handle clean animals.

Some potentially pathogenic organisms may be harboured by apparently healthy animals and can readily be transmitted to other animals whose resistance is lowered by overcrowding in cages, lack of ventilation, temperature fluctuation, or by inadequate diets. It is only by constant attention to all the rules of animal hygiene that infection can be prevented.

Insect Pests

Care must be taken in the animal house to control insect pests. General cleanliness, sterilisation, and the proper design of cages and racks so that small crannies and crevices are eliminated are often sufficient, but special methods are occasionally needed. Bed bugs, fleas, lice, mites, ticks and flies, mosquitoes and cockroaches may all infest the animal house and can be controlled by the use of insecticidal sprays such as 0·5 per cent. DDT or 10 per cent. Lethane applied to focal points. To destroy fleas in the fur or feathers of animals an effective dusting powder containing 0·5 per cent. of pyrethrin may be used. Insecticides such as dieldrin, aldrin, DDT or benzene hexachloride incorporated in a urea formaldehyde resin can be obtained in the form of a quick drying transparent lacquer. They can be sprayed or painted on to cages and racks and are very effective. Because the spray is inflammable great care is required in its use (Worden & Lane-Petter 1957).

General Anaesthesia

Ether is one of the most satisfactory drugs for short periods of anaesthesia because its action is rapid and the depth of narcosis can be controlled from minute to minute. Chloroform has marked toxic properties for many species of animals, especially mice, and is best avoided. It is wise to fast animals for twelve hours before anaesthetising them. For small animals a simple method is to place them on the wire tray of a glass desiccator which contains an ether-soaked pad in its lower compartment. Larger animals, such as rabbits may be placed in a box which has a hinged door and a glass inspection window; an ether-air mixture is pumped slowly into the box through a rubber tube leading from a wash bottle containing ether with rubber bellows attached to its inlet. Whatever method is used for anaesthesia great care must be taken that liquid ether does not touch the animal because mucous membranes can easily be burned in this way.

When the animal has lost consciousness and is lying quietly with deep, even, respiratory movements it should be removed from the container without delay and placed on the bench. During the next 3–4 min. simple inoculations or small operations can be carried out, but for more lengthy procedures the anaesthesia must be continued. For this purpose a suitable mask can be made by replacing the base of a conveniently sized tin with wire gauze and by shaping it to fit comfortably over the animal's nose. A pad soaked with ether is placed deep in the tin touching the wire gauze and the depth of anaesthesia is controlled by varying the distance between the mouth of the tin and the animal's nose.

For longer periods of anaesthesia barbiturate anaesthetics may be injected intraperitoneally or intravenously. The drug of choice is pentobarbitone sodium (Nembutal) and is usually used in a dose of 28 mg./kg. body weight. A stock solution containing Nembutal 60 mg./ml. is convenient and may be diluted to required strengths with 10 per cent. ethyl alcohol. Thiopentone sodium (Pentothal sodium) may also be used but its action is less certain. Anaesthesia with these drugs may take 15–30 min. to develop and lasts 1–2 hr.; complete recovery may take up to 12 hr. during which time the animal may pass through a phase of incoordination during which it may injure itself or tear out stitches if it is left unsupervised. It is important to keep the animal warm during the recovery phase (particularly mice) and the cage may be placed close to a radiator for this.

A useful introduction to anaesthetic methods for laboratory animals is given by Croft (1962).

Humane Ways of Killing Animals

Physical Methods

Most methods involve breaking the spinal cord in the cervical region or damaging the brain itself. They are used only for small animals which are easily handled and which have relatively thin skulls. Mice and guinea-pigs may be quickly and painlessly killed by bringing the head suddenly against a hard object such as the edge of a sink, but it is emphasised that this method requires some manual dexterity and must be learned from an experienced person. Birds can be killed by breaking the cervical cord; the legs are held in the left hand and the head in the right and the neck is then quickly extended and bent back with a sharp jerk.

Chemical Methods

(a) *Volatile Agents.*—An overdose of some volatile agent such as ether, chloroform, nitrogen, or coal gas is commonly employed for euthanasia. Ether alone, however, is not reliable; it is too irritant and excitant for large animals and very young mice and rats may recover many hours after appearing to die from its effects. Chloroform is suitable for most animals other than the dog in which it causes over-excitement. For small animals a pad of cotton wool soaked in chloroform is placed in the lower compartment of a desiccator and the animal is placed on a wire mesh tray above the pad. For larger animals the chloroform may be applied on an anaesthetic mask but care must be taken that it does not actually touch the face of a conscious animal because the liquid is irritant. If coal gas is used an easy death is achieved but only if it is introduced slowly into the chamber.

(b) *Non-volatile Agents.*—Where the intravenous route of injection is practicable animals can be quickly and painlessly killed by the injection of a saturated solution of magnesium sulphate but it must be remembered that this substance is lethal only if injected into a vein. Pentobarbitone sodium (*e.g.* Nembutal) or thiopentone (*e.g.* Pentothal sodium) can also be used to kill animals but is rather expensive; the dose is three to four times that required for anaesthesia and the drugs may be injected by the intravenous, intraperitoneal or intramuscular routes. Rabbits may be killed by the rapid intravenous injection of 40–50 cc. of air.

Disposal of Dead Animals

The best way to dispose of animal carcases is to burn them in the incinerator, but before this can be carried out it is absolutely essential to be sure that the animal is dead. *In order to ensure against the possibility of accidentally burning a live animal no carcases should be put in the incinerator unless one of the following conditions applies*: (1) The body is cold, still and rigor mortis has set in. (2) The animal has been decapitated. (3) A complete necropsy has been performed. (4) The heart has been removed.

Fuller details of the care and manipulation of laboratory animals are given by Smith (1931).

Material Inoculated

Urine, *cerebrospinal fluid*, *blood* and *serous fluids* are easily inoculated with a medium-bore needle. Tenacious material such as *pus* and *sputum* is injected through a wide-bore needle.

Cultures.—Fluid cultures are easily drawn through a medium-bore needle. It may be found advantageous first to pour the culture into a small (2-in.) Petri dish, or a wide-mouthed 1-oz. screw-capped bottle. Growths on solid media may be scraped off and suspended in broth or saline, or the diluting fluid may be poured on the culture which is then emulsified with a wire loop.

Tissues.—Small fragments of soft tissues such as brain, liver, spleen and kidney are readily homogenised by crushing them with a suitable diluent in a Ten Broeck grinder. If larger volumes of tissue suspensions are needed or if firmer tissues such as muscle or lung have to be used, an electrically powered blender of the Waring type is recommended. Tough and fibrous tissues such as skin or chronically inflamed lymph glands should be cut into small pieces in a sterile porcelain mortar by means of scissors sterilised by boiling. Some clean coarse sand, previously washed with acid to remove carbonates, or fine powdered sintered glass, contained in a stoppered bottle and sterilised by hot air, is then added to the mortar and the whole thoroughly ground with the pestle. When the tissue has been well ground up, saline is added and the mixture further triturated. On standing for a short time, the sand and tissue rapidly settle to the bottom of the mortar and the supernatant fluid can be drawn into the syringe. When intravenous inoculation of a tissue suspension has to be employed, care must be taken that no large particles are injected. To avoid this, the suspension must be centrifuged at low speed and only the supernatant fluid used.

Necropsy

All experimental animals, whatever the cause of death, should be examined *post mortem* as a routine. When a virulent organism such as the bacillus of plague or of anthrax has been used, special care must be taken, otherwise the infection may be disseminated, with danger to the operator and other workers.

Details will be given of the procedure in conducting a necropsy in the usual manner, and also the method used when dealing with highly infectious organisms.

As a primary reason for the necropsy is to recover organisms previously injected into the animal, the examination must be conducted with strict aseptic precautions.

Materials required:

A suitable animal board or *table*, on which the carcase can be fixed in the supine position.

Instruments.—Three scalpels; scissors, ordinary size, four pairs; mouse-toothed forceps, four pairs; small bone forceps, if the skull is to be opened; a searing iron—a 4-oz. soldering bolt is suitable for the purpose; sterile capillary pipettes; sterile Petri dishes; sterile test-tubes, and tubes, bottles or plates of media.

The knives are sterilised in strong lysol (about 20 per cent.) and then placed in a weaker solution (2 per cent.), and the metal instruments by boiling in a sterilising bath, *e.g.* an enamelled "fish-kettle". When ready for use, the tray of instruments is lifted out of the steriliser and laid on a spread towel which has previously been soaked in 1 : 1000 solution of mercuric chloride.

It is a useful practice, where cultures have to be made, first to immerse the animal completely in weak lysol solution (3 per cent.) for a few moments. This not only destroys most of the surface organisms, but prevents the dust in the fur from getting into the air and contaminating other materials. The animal is now fixed to the board and towels moistened with antiseptic are placed over the head and lower extremities.

The instruments are removed from the steriliser. A long median incision through the skin of the abdomen and chest is now made and the skin widely dissected, exposing the abdominal and chest muscles. With another set of instruments the peritoneal cavity is opened and the abdominal wall is reflected to each side. With fresh instruments the spleen is removed and placed in a sterile Petri dish. Other organs such as the liver and kidneys may be similarly removed. The ensiform cartilage is now tightly gripped with a pair of strong forceps, and by means of a sterile pair of strong scissors a cut is made on either side of the chest through the costal cartilages. The sternum is raised and pulled towards the head. The heart is now exposed. A sterile capillary pipette, furnished with a teat, is passed through the heart wall. Blood can thus be withdrawn and inoculated into various media. If the necropsy has been properly performed, it is not necessary to sear the surface of the heart. The lungs are then removed with fresh instruments by cutting each organ free at the hilum. Care must be taken not to open into the oesophagus if the lungs are to be used for cultivation.

After the organs to be used for culture have been removed and placed in separate Petri dishes, the necropsy can be completed.

While the instruments are again being boiled the naked-eye appearances of the organs should be studied. For culture the spleen gives the best results, but the other solid viscera may similarly be used. The organ is cut with sterile instruments and a small portion is taken up with a stiff wire and smeared on the surface of solid media. Liquid media are inoculated with a small fragment of the tissue.

In conducting post-mortem examinations, various animal diseases, such as worm infestation, coccidiosis, pseudotuberculosis, etc., may be noticed, and the worker should be familiar with their appearances.

When the animal is infected with highly pathogenic organisms the worker *must* wear rubber gloves. The carcase is soaked in antiseptic solution as before and nailed to a rough piece of board of the appropriate size. This board is then placed in a large enamelled iron tray. The necropsy is carefully performed in the usual way. The carcase is finally covered with 10 per cent. lysol, which flows over the board and into the tray. The whole contents of the tray—board and carcase—are then destroyed in a furnace or incinerator. The rubber gloves, instruments and tray are thoroughly sterilised. When performing animal necropsies we strongly advise the wearing of a large overall made of waterproof material, and in addition, the use of some form of glasses or goggles to protect the eyes.

RABBITS

Data

Rectal temperature . . .	38·7–39·1° C.; 101·6–102·4° F.
(No temperature below 40° C. or 104° F. is regarded as pathological)	
Normal respiration rate . .	55 per min.
Pulse rate	135 per min.
Gestation period . . .	28–31 days.
Weaning age	6–8 weeks.
Mating age	6–9 months.
Litters	4 yearly; average litter, 4.
Room temperature . . .	15·5–18·5° C.; 60–65° F.
Humidity	40–45 per cent.
Weight—adult . . .	0·9–6·75 kg.

Cages

Individual cages are best made of galvanised iron. The minimum size for a medium sized rabbit is $2 \times 2 \times 1\frac{1}{2}$ ft., but larger cages may be needed for the bigger breeds. Young rabbits up to 3 months of age may be housed together but after that time the sexes should be separated. From 8 to 10 young rabbits may be kept together in a pen similar to that used for guinea-pigs.

Feeding

The pelleted Diet 18 of Bruce and Parkes (1947) or commercial breeders pellets are suitable for rabbits. Alternatively a daily supply of 2·5 oz. (72 g.) of a mixture of one part oats and three parts bran may be fed as a slightly moist mash. Either diet may be supplemented with green stuffs or root vegetables and hay. A liberal supply of clean drinking water is essential at all times.

Handling

Smooth the ears of the rabbit back and then pick up the ears and the loose skin at the back of the neck with one hand in a firm grip, place the other hand under the hind quarters to support the weight and lift gently. A rabbit must never be lifted by the ears alone. When a rabbit is removed from its cage it should always be placed on a non-slippery surface because otherwise it feels insecure and becomes frightened; for this purpose the bench may be covered with a piece of sacking. Most rabbits remain quiet and still if they are handled by people they know; if restraint is required during anaesthesia or inoculation, they can be wrapped in a roller towel or placed in a special box so constructed that the head only protrudes at one end.

Breeding

When the doe is on heat the vulva becomes moist, red and swollen. At this time she is taken to the buck for mating; do not introduce the buck into the doe's cage as she may attack and injure him. Small-size strains of rabbits may be mated for the first time at the age of 6 months, larger strains at about 9 months. The gestation period is 28 days and at about the 24th day the doe is transferred to a clean breeding cage, preferably with a screened breeding compartment where the animal can produce its young in seclusion. Liberal bedding and hay must be provided for nesting. In order to avoid the risk of cannibalism the doe and her new litter should be disturbed as little as possible during the first 10 days. The young are weaned at 6–8 weeks, sexed, and then separated into male and female pens.

Common Diseases

Coccidiosis is a common disease of rabbits taking two forms, hepatic and intestinal. The symptoms are a ravenous appetite with diarrhoea, progressive emaciation, and gradually increasing weakness of the hind limbs. The diagnosis is easily confirmed by the finding of the oocysts of *Eimeria stediae* in wet films of the faeces. In fatal cases yellowish white nodules and haemorrhages are seen at necropsy in the liver and intestine. Treatment with sulphadimidine included in a mash in a concentration of 1 per cent. is effective if given within 10 days of infestation.

Pseudotuberculosis is a chronic infection with *Pasteurella pseudotuberculosis* and is characterised by loss of weight, emaciation and eventually by death. At necropsy primary caseous nodules are present in the intestine and are most marked in the caecum; metastatic lesions are seen as well defined yellow areas, like those of miliary tuberculosis, in the liver, spleen, and lymph glands.

Respiratory tract infections.—The most common is "Snuffles", which is so-called from the characteristic nasal discharge. The disease is due to *Pasteurella septica* and is highly infectious; animals suffering from this infection should be removed from the animal house and destroyed at once. Rabbits are also liable to infection with pneumococci and streptococci which may cause a rapidly fatal pneumonia with pericarditis.

Intestinal infections.—Mucoid enteritis, a disease of obscure origin may be responsible for epizootics in the animal house. Severe diarrhoea and marked emaciation are the principal symptoms and the condition may be mistaken for coccidiosis. The mortality of very young rabbits is 100 per cent., that of adults about 30 per cent. Diarrhoea may also be caused by organisms of the *Salmonella* group, e.g. *S. typhimurium.*

Rabbit syphilis.—A relatively common condition characterised by papules or discharging ulcers on denuded areas of the genitalia. It is caused by *Treponema cuniculi*, a spirochaete very similar to *Treponema pallidum* (q.v.). The condition responds well to treatment with penicillin.

Ear canker is the commonest form of mange in the domestic rabbit. It is caused by two species of mites *Psoroptes communis* and *Chorioptes communis.* The condition can be easily cleared up by softening the scabs with vegetable oil, removing them and then applying a 20 per cent. emulsion of benzyl benzoate (National Formulary).

Worms.—The cysticercus stage of the dog tapeworm, *Taenia pisiformis*, is the commonest type of infestation and is characterised by numerous cysts in the omentum and liver.

Experimental Procedures

The chief use of the rabbit lies not so much in diagnostic work as in its value for experimental purposes. It is, also, extensively used for the production of immune sera, such as agglutinating and neutralising sera, which are used in diagnostic work.

Antisera.—There is no agreement on the best inoculation schedule for the production of antisera in rabbits. One method employs four to six intravenous injections of gradually increasing amounts of the antigen spaced at two to three day intervals. (Many workers complete the course within ten days to minimise the risk of anaphylactic shock.) A sample of blood should be taken before beginning the course and a second six to eight days after finishing it. The antibody titres of both samples are estimated and if that of the second sample has not risen to a high level further injections may be given. Although this method gives good results (*e.g.* in the preparation of antisera to salmonellae) many other schedules using other routes of inoculation in various combinations, different doses of antigen, longer or shorter time intervals, may all give equally satisfactory results. It is, however, wise to reduce the number of inoculations to the minimum needed to produce the required antibody titres because a prolonged series of injections may harm the animal and may also result in the appearance of unwanted or non-specific antibodies. In general, the worker will be guided in the choice of a schedule by such factors as the toxicity and purity of the antigen, whether living or dead microorganisms are to be injected, and by the condition of the animal being immunised.

It is possible to produce high levels of antibodies with a single subcutaneous inoculation if the antigen is mixed with Freund's complete adjuvant. Freund's adjuvant (Difco) can be obtained commercially with or without (incomplete) added mycobacteria; it comprises 9 parts of an oil, Bayol F, and one volume of an emulsifying agent, Arlacel A, with the addition, if required, of 2 mg. per ml. of heat-killed *Mycobacterium butyricum.* Equal volumes of a saline suspension of the antigen and Freund's adjuvant are mixed to make a water in oil emulsion. In making the emulsion successive small amounts of the antigen are squirted below the surface of the adjuvant with a syringe and the mixing is continued by filling and emptying the syringe through the needle until the emulsion has assumed an opaque appearance and a syrupy consistency. Considerable care must be taken to obtain the correct consistency to give a ***water in oil emulsion***, which is achieved when a drop let fall on the surface of a beaker of water remains as a discrete drop. Oil in water suspensions, which are not so effective antigenically, are detected when a drop allowed to fall on the surface of water spreads out to form a diffuse film.

Anaesthesia	Short-acting.	Ether.
	Long-acting.	Pentobarbitone sodium 28 mg/kg. body-weight intravenously.

With pentobarbitone, anaesthesia develops rapidly and there are 45–60 minutes of unconsciousness followed by some abnormality of the central nervous system lasting up to 24 hours.

Scarification.—The hair is removed from the flank of the animal by first clipping and then shaving, or by means of the depilating mixture described on p. 1013. The skin is cleansed with alcohol, which is allowed to evaporate. A number of parallel scratches are made with a sharp sterile scalpel, just sufficiently deep to draw blood. The infective material is rubbed into the scarified area with the side of the scalpel. This method is mainly used for the propagation of vaccinia virus.

Subcutaneous inoculation may be made either into the abdominal wall or into the loose tissue about the flank or at the back of the neck. The hair is clipped, the skin is sterilised with iodine and then pinched up, and the needle is inserted. The technique is the same as that for the guinea-pig.

Intravenous inoculation is employed when material has to be introduced directly into the circulation. The marginal vein of the ear is the most convenient site. The rabbit may be held by an assistant or placed in a special box so that only its head protrudes. The hair over the vein should be dry-shaved with a sharp razor. The vein may be distended for ease of inoculation either by vigorous rubbing with a piece of cotton-wool or by holding the ear over an electric-light bulb, when the heat causes a dilatation of the blood vessels. According to the amount of material to be injected, a suitable sterile syringe is selected. The operator faces the animal and the ear is held horizontally by means of the left hand. The needle is kept as nearly parallel as possible to the vein and the point inserted towards the head of the animal. When the injection is completed, the needle is withdrawn and a small piece of cotton-wool placed on the vein, which is then compressed between the thumb and finger.

Intraperitoneal inoculation is carried out as in the guinea-pig.

Intracerebral inoculation.—The animal is anaesthetised with ether, the hair over the head shaved, and the skin disinfected with alcohol and tincture of iodine. A short incision is made through the scalp at a point situated 2 mm. lateral to the sagittal suture and 1·5 mm. anterior to the lambdoidal suture. The skull is then perforated with a trephine or a mechanical drill, and the needle, which is cut down to $\frac{5}{16}$ in. long, introduced through the opening. About 0·45 ml. of material can be inoculated into the occipital lobe of a large rabbit. After injection the needle is rapidly withdrawn, the skin sutured and the area covered with collodion solution.

Rabbits may also be inoculated in the frontal lobe, at a point situated 2 mm. lateral to the median plane on a line joining the two external canthi of the eyes.

Intra-testicular.—If the testes are not palpable in the scrotum they are made to descend from the abdominal cavity by steady pressure on the belly while the animal lies on its back. They are then fixed by an assistant who places a finger over each abdominal ring. The scrotal skin is cleansed with methylated spirit and is stretched tightly over one of the testicles. A hypodermic needle is now plunged directly into the centre of the organ and 0·2–0·4 ml. of inoculum can be injected.

Ophthalmic.—Material may be dropped into one eye from a Pasteur pipette leaving the other untreated as a control. Under anaesthesia the cornea of one eye may be scarified before the instillation of infected material. Only one eye is inoculated as the procedure should never give any risk of blinding the animal.

Collection of Blood.—From the ear vein of a large rabbit 20–30 ml. of blood may be obtained easily and without causing any distress to the animal. The ear is shaved and sterilised with sterile gauze soaked in 70 per cent. alcohol. Meanwhile a small vessel containing petroleum jelly has been heated over the Bunsen to render it sterile, and when cool, but still fluid, the petroleum jelly is painted over the vein, and on the margin and under-side of the ear. The ear is held forward and the vein is made prominent by means of a small spring clip at the base of the ear, and then incised with a small sharp sterile scalpel.

The blood flows over the petroleum jelly, and is allowed to drop into a sterile flask containing glass beads or a suitable anticoagulant according to requirements. The vessels of the ear can be dilated by holding an electric bulb below it or by rubbing the part not covered by petroleum jelly with a pledget of wool moistened with xylol. When sufficient blood has been obtained the clip is removed and a piece of cotton-wool pressed firmly over the cut in the vein. The xylol is removed from the ear with alcohol, and some petroleum jelly then lightly smeared on. *Water should always be provided in the cage of the animal after bleeding.*

Larger amounts of blood can be obtained by *cardiac puncture.* The anaesthetised animal is fastened to a board with the body axis quite straight and the fur clipped over the left side of the chest; the area is shaved and then sterilised with alcohol and ether. A 100 ml. bulb pipette (*vide* diagram) is cut down at both ends to 9 in. in length, one end being slightly tapered and the other end stoppered with cotton-wool. It is wrapped in kraft paper and sterilised in the hot-air oven. A wide-bore transfusion needle is fitted into

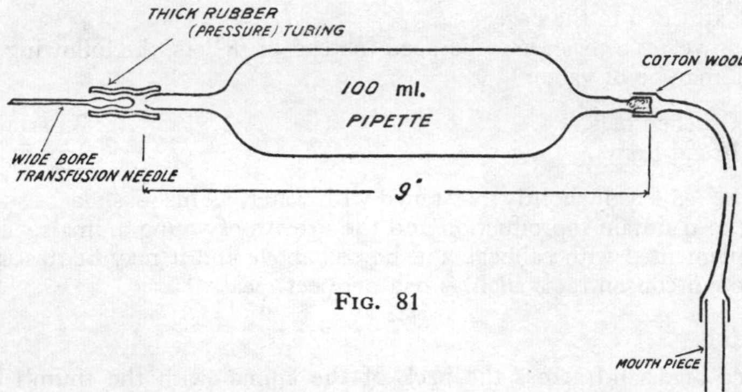

Fig. 81

a short length ($1\frac{1}{2}$ in.) of thick rubber tubing and sterilised by boiling. When the animal is anaesthetised, the rubber tubing is attached to the tapered end of the pipette and to the other end is fitted a mouth-piece such as that used in pipetting (p. 911). The needle is inserted into the left side of the chest and suction applied. The needle should lie in the right ventricle of the heart, and blood rapidly flows into the pipette. About 50 ml. of blood per kg. of body-weight can be obtained. The blood is then transferred to a sterile 500-ml. flask or bottle containing glass beads for defibrination.

GUINEA-PIGS

Data

Rectal temperature . .	37·6–38·9° C.; 99·6–102° F.
Normal respiration rate . .	80 per min.
Pulse rate	150 per min.
Gestation period . . .	59–72 days; average 63 days.
Weaning age	14–21 days.
Mating age	12–20 weeks.
Litters	3 yearly; average litter, 3.
Room temperature . .	18·5–21° C.; 65–70° F.
Humidity	45 per cent.
Weight—weaning . .	120 g.
adult . . .	200–1000 g.

Cages

Stock runs should be about 4×6 ft. and 1 ft. 8 in. high. One square foot of space should be allowed for each animal and not more than 25 animals should be kept in any one pen.

For experimental animals galvanised-iron cages are recommended as they can be readily cleaned and sterilised. A convenient size is 14×9×8 in. fitting in a tray 1½ in. deep.

Feeding

A diet in pelleted form is recommended in preference to mashes. Pellets are placed in a hopper in the animal cage and provide a continuous source of food. Diet 18 of Bruce and Parkes (1947) contains balanced proportions of protein, fat and carbohydrate with added vitamins, salt and trace elements. This diet is recommended and to it must be added 2 oz. of cabbage or kale and 2 oz. hay daily for each animal. In winter, carrots, swedes or mangold may be substituted for the green food. Fresh water must be provided from a bottle attached to the cage.

If, however, a mash is to be used instead of pellets, the following simple formula may be of value:

Crushed oats	2 parts
Broad bran	1 part

It may be fed dry or slightly moistened with water. This mash lacks sufficient protein to maintain reproduction and the growth of young animals. It must be supplemented with cabbage and hay as above and it may be necessary to add protein concentrates such as fish or meat meal.

Handling

Place one hand across the back of the animal with the thumb behind the shoulders and the other fingers well forward on the opposite side; lift the animal gently and support its weight with the other hand placed palm uppermost under the hind quarters.

Breeding

The boar is fertile at the age of 8–10 weeks when it weighs about 500 g.; the sow can be mated for the first time at the age of 12 weeks when it weighs about 450 g. One boar is placed in a breeding pen with 5–10 sows and one square foot of space allowed for each animal. As the sows approach parturition they are isolated in individual cages. After weaning at 14–21 days the young are weighed, sexed and the sows and boars are placed in different pens. The mother is then returned to the breeding pen.

Common Diseases

Pseudotuberculosis (p. 277).—May be either acute or, more commonly, chronic. In the acute type the animal dies in a few days. In the chronic type the liver, spleen and mesenteric glands show very numerous yellowish-white areas scattered through them, somewhat suggestive of tuberculosis. Often a whole stock becomes infected, and experimental animals frequently die before the experiment is completed.

Abscesses in lymphatic glands, due to haemolytic streptococci of group C, are not uncommon. (These organisms may also produce septicaemia.)

Respiratory tract infections.—Guinea-pigs are liable to pneumonia and pleurisy, often haemorrhagic, and septicaemia due to such organisms as the pneumococcus, pneumobacillus, haemolytic streptococcus, *Pasteurella* group.

Intestinal infections.—Organisms of the *Salmonella* group, e.g. *S. typhimurium*, are the cause of the most lethal of all guinea-pig diseases. Explosive epizootics may occur in which practically the whole of a colony is destroyed.

Protozoan diseases.—Coccidiosis is of common occurrence. Toxoplasmosis is found infrequently.

Virus diseases, such as guinea-pig paralysis and pneumonia, may be met with.

Experimental Procedures

For general purposes an adult guinea-pig weighing about 400 g. is satisfactory.

Anaesthesia

Short acting. Ether. Excessive post-operative mucous secretions are common but can largely be prevented by the use of 0·5 ml. of a 0·5 per cent. solution of atropine sulphate (2·5 mg. or 1/25 grain) given at least half an hour preoperatively by the subcutaneous route.

Long acting. Pentobarbitone sodium 28 mg./kg. body-weight intraperitoneally. 56 mg./kg. body-weight is the fatal dose.

With pentobarbitone sodium anaesthesia may take about 15 minutes to develop, lasts 1–2 hours, and complete recovery may take up to 12 hours during which time the animal must be kept warm.

Subcutaneous inoculation.—An assistant holds the animal during the operation, and the injection is made under the skin of the flank. The animal is grasped across the shoulders in one hand, with the thumb curved round the animal's neck so that it rests on the lower jaw. The hind legs are secured between the first and second, and second and third fingers of the other hand, the knuckles being uppermost, and the animal is held so that the flank is presented for inoculation. The skin may be disinfected with tincture of iodine. The operator picks up a fold of skin and introduces the point of the needle into the base of the fold so that it lies in the subcutaneous tissue. Amounts up to 5 ml. can be introduced. A 2-ml. or a 5-ml. syringe is convenient for the purpose.

Some workers inoculate by picking up a fold of skin about the mid-abdomen. The needle is introduced into the base of the fold and passed down in the subcutaneous tissue until it reaches the groin, where the injection is made. This method obviates superficial ulceration when tuberculous material is injected.

Intracutaneous inoculation.—This method is used chiefly in testing cultures of the diphtheria bacillus for virulence. The hair is removed from the flanks of the animal by plucking or alternatively by means of a fresh 5 per cent. solution of sodium sulphide or a depilating powder. White guinea-pigs (300–400 grams weight) are used, as the skin is unpigmented and the results of the test can easily be read.

The depilating powder is made as follows:

Barium sulphide, commercial powder	7 parts
White household flour	7 parts
Talcum powder	7 parts
Castile soap powder	1 part

Remove the hair from the flanks as closely as possible with hair clippers. Make up the depilating powder into a smooth paste with water, and rub into the animal's hair with a wooden spatula or toothbrush. Allow the paste to act for one minute and renew the application. After two minutes remove the paste with the spatula or handle of the toothbrush. Now wash the animals' skin and surrounding hair with warm water and dry with a cloth. The depilated surface should be quite smooth and white. It is advisable not to leave the paste on too long as the skin becomes red and excoriated in patches, making the subsequent observation of reactions very difficult. The depilating powder should be used at least one hour before the intracutaneous injection is carried out.

For the test a 1-ml. all-glass tuberculin syringe, fitted with a short needle of No. 25 or 26 gauge (exactly as used for Schick and Dick tests), is employed. The skin of the animal is pinched up between the thumb and forefinger, and the point of the needle is inserted at the top of the fold so that the bevel of the needle is towards the surface of the skin. The needle passes only into the dermis, as near the surface as possible, *and not into the subcutaneous tissue*; when the injection has been correctly made a definite and palpable bleb appears in the skin. The usual amount injected is 0·2 ml. and when several tests are to be made the injections should be about one inch apart and not too near the middle line of the abdomen. No more than ten injections should be made on one animal. The results are read 24–48 hr. later.

Intraperitoneal inoculation.—The animal is held in a similar manner. The inoculation is made in the mid-line in the lower half of the abdomen. The assistant holds the animal with its head downwards, so that the intestines fall towards the diaphragm. The skin is pinched up, the point of the needle is first passed into the subcutaneous tissue and then downwards through the abdominal wall into the peritoneal cavity. There is no risk of damage to the intestines. Not more than 5 ml. can safely be inoculated intraperitoneally.

Collection of Blood.—Small amounts, up to 0·5 ml., may be taken by simple incision of the marginal ear vein. Cardiac puncture is, however, the only satisfactory way of obtaining larger volumes. The animal is lightly anaesthetised with ether and then laid on its back with its front limbs drawn forwards. An area over the fourth and fifth left intercostal spaces is plucked and the skin painted with tincture of iodine. The position of the apex beat of the heart is defined by digital palpation and at this point a needle (No. 20 gauge mounted on a syringe) is inserted between the ribs. A sharp downward movement inclined towards the mid-line then takes the needle point through the ventricular wall. As much as 15 ml. of blood may be obtained from a 350–400 g. animal, though smaller amounts are advisable if the guinea-pig is to survive. Very sharp needles are essential for the success of this operation.

MICE

Data

Normal temperature	37·4° C.; 99·3° F.
Pulse rate	120
Oestrous cycle	4–5 days.
Gestation period	19–21 days.
Weaning age	19–21 days.
Mating age	6–8 weeks.
Litters	8–12 yearly ; average litter, 7–8.

Room temperature	20–21° C.; 68–70° F.
Humidity	50–60 per cent.
Weight—weaning	7 g.
adult	25–28 g.

Cages

There are many different designs of mouse cages and no one pattern is the standard. A common form is an aluminium box approximately 6 × 12 × 6 in. deep, with tapering sides to facilitate stacking. The lids are made of sheet metal or of strong wire mesh and are designed so that a food hopper is built into them and accommodation provided to hold the drinking bottle. The cages are light, durable and easily sterilised by dry or moist heat. Similar cages made of polypropylene are now available and are quieter to handle and, since the plastic material is not a good conductor of heat, are warmer for the animals. Plastic cages are less expensive than metal and appear to be equally satisfactory; they can be sterilised in the autoclave but not in the hot air oven. Up to six mice can be housed in cages of this type which are suitable for breeding purposes. Larger cages to hold up to 100 mice approximately 30 × 18 × 6 in. can be used for stock rearing or holding purposes but overcrowding in such cages carries a great risk of epidemic disease.

Feeding

Pelleted diets such as diet 86 of Howie (1952) or diet 41 of Bruce (1950) are satisfactory. Fresh water in drinking bottles must be provided *ad lib.*

Handling

An assistant takes a grip on the middle of the tail of the animal with the left hand and gently raises the hind limbs from the floor of the cage. A mouse held in this position cannot turn round and bite. Then with the right finger and thumb a fold of skin is taken up as close as possible to the head. The animal can now be lifted into a convenient position for the operator to carry out simple inoculation procedures. When an assistant is not available a mouse can be manipulated single handed: place the animal on a rough surface and hold it by its tail with the right hand, then pick up the loose skin at the base of the neck with the left forefinger and thumb, lift and turn the left hand palm uppermost at the same time catching the tail and pressing it against the palm with the left little finger. The right hand is now free to pick up a syringe.

Breeding

Two methods may be used (1) *Monogamous mating* when one male and one female aged 8–12 weeks are placed permanently in a cage together. Three to four weeks later the first litter is produced and mating occurs again in the immediate post-partum period. The young mice must be weaned just before the next litter is expected. Thus litters may be expected every 3–4 weeks. (2) *Polygamous mating* when one male is placed in a cage with up to four females. When it is established that a female is pregnant she is transferred to a separate cage and allowed to nest and nurse her young until they are weaned at the age of three weeks, after which she is mated again. Both systems have advantages and disadvantages; the first produces double the number of mice but the young mice produced by the second method are heavier and reach maturity and suitability for experimental use in a shorter time.

Common Diseases

Salmonellosis.—Intestinal infections termed "Mouse typhoid" are common and are usually caused by the Salmonella group (e.g. *S. typhimurium* and *S. enteritidis*).

Severe epizootics may follow the introduction of new stock into a colony especially when the animals are overcrowded or where animal hygiene is inadequate. It seems impossible to control an epizootic with chemotherapy and the only satisfactory procedure is to destroy existing animals, sterilise their cages, and then to obtain a fresh clean stock.

Ectromelia (Mouse pox) is the most troublesome of mouse diseases; it takes two forms: (*a*) the acute form characterised by necrosis of the liver and spleen with a rapidly fatal result, (*b*) a chronic form with generalised skin eruption and characterised by ulcers which are covered by crusts of dried serous discharges. These lesions may occur anywhere on the body but are most obvious on the tail. In the most chronic form there is enlargement of one of the foot pads due to oedema and scab formation followed by gangrene either of a digit or the whole foot. The disease is caused by a pox virus related to the vaccinia virus. When this infection is established it is extremely difficult to control and may necessitate the destruction of the whole colony. If valuable stocks are threatened by ectromelia it is, however, possible to protect them by vaccination on the tail with the calf lymph used against human smallpox.

Streptobacillus moniliformis infection may be epizootic or sporadic. The acute form of the disease has no characteristic lesions but the organism can readily be recovered from the blood and organs. The chronic form is commoner and is characterised by swelling of the ankles and tail with ulceration of the foot. The condition may closely resemble ectromelia.

Miscellaneous Virus Infections.—Among the many virus infections affecting mouse colonies are the pneumonia virus of mice (PVM of Curnan & Horsfall, 1946), Nigg's pneumonitis virus (Nigg & Eaton, 1944), and the lymphocytic choriomeningitis virus (Traub, 1939 ; Haas, 1954).

Worms.—Occasional infestation with the tape-worm *Taenia taeniae-formis* may occur with large cysts formed in the liver. The primary host of this helminth is the cat which should be excluded from mouse rooms. Cats may infect oats, maize and pellets with tape worm ova in the mill and these feeding stuffs should not be purchased unless they have been sterilised and packed in paper bags by the makers.

Experimental Procedures

Anaesthesia

Short acting.	Ether.
Long acting.	Pentobarbitone sodium stock solution 60 mg./ml. diluted 1 in 25 with 10 per cent. ethyl alcohol 0·8 ml. per 100 g. body-weight intraperitoneally.

Mice are particularly sensitive to cold while they are unconscious, and it is important that the animals be kept warm until they have returned to consciousness.

Subcutaneous inoculation.—An assistant grasps the loose skin at the nape of the neck in one hand and the tail in the other. In this manner the animal is held in a fixed position while the needle is introduced under the skin near the root of the tail. Amounts up to 1 ml. may be injected.

Intraperitoneal inoculation may be carried out if the animal is similarly held and then turned over. For steadiness, the assistant's arms should rest on the table. The injection is made to one side of the middle line in the lower half of the abdomen and amounts up to 2 ml. can be introduced.

Intravenous inoculation may be made into a vein at the root of the tail if a fine needle be used and the vein dilated by placing the tail of the animal in water at about 45° C. The maximum amount that can be injected is 0·5 ml. for a mouse of 20 grams. A small cylindrical cage made of perforated zinc, and just large enough to hold the mouse with its tail protruding, is useful for this procedure.

Intracerebral inoculation.—The skin over the head is cleansed with 70 per cent. alcohol and the animal is lightly anaesthetised with ether for the inoculation. A fine-bore needle attached to a 1-ml. syringe (as used for intracutaneous inoculation) is employed and easily penetrates the skull. The site of injection is midway between the outer canthus of the eye and the point of attachment of the pinna of the ear at about 3 mm. from the mid-line. The point of the needle is carried through the skull for $\frac{1}{8}$ in. to $\frac{1}{4}$ in. Up to 0·03 ml. of fluid can be injected with safety.

Intranasal inoculation.—This should if possible be carried out in an inoculating chamber designed for the purpose for there is a risk that the operator may himself inhale infective material. Failing this, a mask should be worn. The mouse is lightly anaesthetised with ether and as soon as its breathing has become deep and automatic 0·1 ml. of the inoculum is introduced into the anterior nares on one side only.

Collection of Blood.—Under deep anaesthesia the animal is pinned out and the skin over the thorax and abdomen is reflected as for necropsy (*vide infra*). The great vessels in the axilla are incised and the blood which wells out is taken up in a sterile Pasteur pipette. An alternative and less time-consuming method is to displace the globe of the eye forwards and to puncture the retro-orbital plexus of veins with the tip of a fine Pasteur pipette which is then used to take up the free-flowing blood. About 1·0 ml. may be obtained and the mouse may be permitted to recover from the anaesthetic and to survive. Small samples of blood can be obtained by clipping thc tail as in the rat.

Inoculation of Infant Mice.—Suckling mice no older than 48 hr. are used for the isolation of the herpes simplex, enteric, and arboviruses. Great care and cleanliness is required in handling the litters if cannibalism by the mothers is to be avoided. The following injections can be used: 0·03 ml. subcutaneously, 0·05 ml. intraperitoneally, 0·03 intracerebrally. Sometimes the intraperitoneal and the intracerebral routes are used together in the same animals.

Snell (1941) gives full details of the biology of the laboratory mouse.

RATS

Data

Normal temperature	37·5° C.; 99·5° F.
Normal respiration rate	210 per min.
Oestrous cycle	4–5 days.
Gestation period	21–23 days.
Weaning age	23–28 days.
Mating age	70–84 days.
Litters	7–9 yearly; average litter, 7.

Room temperature . . . 18·5–21° C.; 65–70° F.
Humidity . . . . 45–55 per cent.

Cages

Rats can be housed in cages similar to those used for guinea-pigs. For details of stock and breeding cages see the UFAW Handbook (1967).

Feeding

The dry pellet diet No. 86 (Howie, 1952) used for mice can be used without supplementation. A plentiful supply of drinking water is essential.

Handling

Docile rats can be handled by an experienced operator in exactly the same way as guinea-pigs. Wild or vicious rats, however, should be handled with the hand covered by a leather glove because the sharp incisor teeth can inflict a deep wound. Alternatively the animal may be picked up by gripping the loose skin at the base of the neck with tongs or broad bladed forceps.

Breeding

As in mice monogamous mating may be practised or alternatively polygamous mating used when two males which have been living together for some weeks are placed in a breeding cage with six females; the animals should be 10–12 weeks old. Each female, when pregnant, is removed to a separate cage where she nests and nurses her young until they are weaned at the age of 3–4 weeks. After resting for two weeks the female may be mated again.

Common Diseases

Bronchopneumonia and more rarely suppurative otitis may occur due to *Bord. bronchiseptica*, *Streptobacillus moniliformis*, *streptococci*, *diphtheroids*, etc. Salmonellosis (often due to *S. typhimurium* or *S. enteritidis*) causes a severe form of enteritis which may spread rapidly in a colony. Mange is a common parasitic infestation and is characterised by brownish scales on the skin of the ears and tail which are often encrusted with dried blood.

Anaesthesia

Short acting:	Ether.
Long acting:	Ether or
(*a*) Adult rats.	Pentobarbitone sodium stock solution (60 mg./ml.) diluted 1 in 10 with 10 per cent. ethyl alcohol. 0·75 ml. per 100 g. body-weight intraperitoneally.
(*b*) Young rats. (under 50 g. body-weight).	Pentothal sodium stock solution (60 mg./ml.) diluted 1 in 25. 1 ml. per 100 g. body-weight intraperitoneally.

Experimental Procedures

Inoculation by the subcutaneous and intraperitoneal routes is made in a manner similar to those described for the guinea-pig. Intravenous inoculation may be made into the vein at the root of the tail. The vein should be dilated by immersing the tail in warm water. Blood may be collected by cardiac puncture as in the guinea-pig. Small samples of blood can be obtained on repeated occasions, by snipping off with very sharp scissors or a razor blade a very small portion of the tip of the tail.

HAMSTERS

Data

Rectal temperature . . .	36·7–38·3° C.; 98–101° F.
Oestrous cycle . . .	4–5 days.
Gestation period . . .	16–17 days.
Weaning age . . .	3–4 weeks.
Mating age	7–9 weeks.
Litters	3–4 yearly; average litter, 6.
Room temperature . .	20–22° C.; 68–72° F.
Humidity	40–50 per cent.

Cages

Galvanised-iron cages in sheet metal or mesh are satisfactory. A convenient size is 17×7×9 in. Cages of aluminium, zinc or wood are not suitable as hamsters may gnaw through them.

Feeding

Commercially available cubed diets for mice, rats or guinea-pigs are satisfactory for the basic diet but better health results when daily supplements of fresh green foods are given. Milk added to a bran and oats mash is valuable as an additional supplement for pregnant or lactating females. Fresh drinking-water must always be available.

Breeding

The mating of animals is best carried out under observation for the female after coitus may often attack the male and injure him severely.

Diseases

Golden hamsters are remarkably free from spontaneous disease. They may, however, acquire salmonella infections and mange in the animal-house.

The golden hamster (*Mecocricetus auratus*) is susceptible to many bacterial and viral infections. The animals should be handled gently and carefully, for they can inflict a deep biting wound if they are suddenly disturbed. *Intraperitoneal* and *subcutaneous inoculation* may be carried out in the manner used for rats or guinea-pigs. The susceptibility of the hamster to bacterial and viral infection is often markedly increased by the injection of cortisone acetate in a dose of 2 mg. per kilo body-weight prior to inoculation.

Anaesthesia

Short acting.	Ether.
Long acting.	Pentobarbitone sodium stock solution (60 mg./ml.) diluted 1 in 10 with 10 per cent. ethyl alcohol. 1 ml. per 100 g. body-weight intraperitoneally.

Experimental Procedures

Inoculation and bleeding is carried out in the manner used for guinea-pigs.

FERRETS

Data

Normal temperature . .	37·8–39·2° C.; 100–102·5° F.
Gestation period	41–42 days.
Weaning age	6–8 weeks.
Mating age	6–9 months.
Litters	2 yearly; average litter, 7–8.
Room temperature . .	15·5–18·5° C.; 60–65° F.
Humidity	50–60 per cent.
Weight at birth . . .	10 g.

Cages

A common form is a wooden hutch 3 ft. by 1 ft. 6 in. by 1 ft. 6 in. high ; it is divided into two compartments by a partition through which a circular hole 4 in. in diameter is cut. The inner compartment, which is for sleeping and breeding, is kept dark. The outer compartment serves as an exercise run and is provided with a hinged door with vertical metal bars. The hutch will house three adult ferrets. Individual animals under experiment may be housed in metal cages constructed of sheet zinc forming an 18 in. cube with a perforated lid for ventilation.

Feeding

Each ferret requires 4 oz. of raw meat (horse flesh, lights, etc., are satisfactory) and 4 oz. fresh milk daily.

Breeding

The oestrous condition is easily recognised by the redness, moisture and tense swelling of the vulva. At this time the bitch is brought to the dog for mating; if fertilisation occurs the vulvar swelling subsides in about a week, if not the mating should be repeated. As soon as it is certain that the bitch is pregnant she is isolated in a separate hutch. After the birth of the litter the animals should on no account be disturbed for the fear that the mother will eat her progeny. After five to six weeks when the young are able to move out into the exercise compartment it is safe to handle the animals.

Precautions against Infection

Because ferrets are highly susceptible to the influenza and canine distemper viruses, great care is needed to prevent their accidental infection. Those who work with ferrets must be constantly aware of the possibility of the risk of transferring on their persons the distemper virus from infected canine pets and of themselves infecting the ferrets with influenza during the early stages of an illness. The risk of the worker himself being infected from the ferrets must also be borne in mind.

There is a very great risk of cross infection in experimental animals inoculated with these two viruses and special measures required to prevent this occurring include the use of special isolation cages with solid walls and the use by the worker of rubber boots, waterproof overalls and rubber gloves all of which are washed down with lysol after use.

Handling

It is advisable for beginners to wear leather gloves, but once the confidence of the animals has been won they can be picked up with the bare hands. A ferret should be lifted with a steady and firm grip with the fingers encircling the neck, shoulders and fore limbs while the other hand supports the rump.

Common Diseases

Distemper.—Ferrets are highly susceptible to distemper and the mortality is almost 100 per cent. The manifestations of the disease are similar to those in the dog (p. 413). If distemper is accidentally introduced into the animal house all infected ferrets should be destroyed and the premises should be vigorously disinfected.

Foot rot is caused by mites and occurs only if the ferrets are kept in dirty conditions. It can be treated by cutting back the claws, bathing off the crusts on the swollen feet with warm soap and water, and by applying a 20 per cent. emulsion of benzyl benzoate (National Formulary) or a 10 per cent. sulphur ointment.

Staphylococcal and streptococcal infections and toxoplasmosis also occur.

Experimental Procedures

Anaesthesia

Short acting.	Ether.
Long acting.	Pentobarbitone sodium stock solution (60 mg./ml.) diluted 1 in 10 with 10 per cent. ethyl alcohol. 1 ml. per kg. body-weight intraperitoneally.

Intranasal inoculation.—Under light ether anaesthesia, as soon as regular respiration is established, 1–2 ml. of material can be introduced into the nares from a Pasteur pipette. Other methods of inoculation are those described for the guinea-pig.

FOWLS

Data

Rectal temperature	41·6° C.; 106·9° F.
Normal respiration rate	12 per min.
Normal pulse	140 per min.

Cages

Galvanised-iron wire cages about 24 in. tall and 20 × 20 in. are suitable for individual birds. For further information on the breeding and care of poultry the reader is referred to Ministry of Agriculture Bulletins No. 54 and 56.

Feeding

One of the pellet diets ("breeding" or "laying" diets) available commercially can be used; it should be properly balanced and contain vitamins and trace elements. Green foods may be fed two or three times a week and grit and fresh water must be provided *ad lib.*

Common Diseases

Intestinal infections due to salmonellae of various types (e.g. *S. typhimurium*) are not uncommon. *S. pullorum* is the cause of bacillary white diarrhoea of young pullets and *S. gallinarum* causes outbreaks of "Fowl typhoid". Coccidiosis is another cause of acute enteritis in young chicks. *Tuberculosis* due to the avian type of *M. tuberculosis* is now relatively uncommon.

Parasitic infections due to lice and red mites may be controlled by the use of an aerosol spray of 2·0 per cent. piperonyl hydroxide +0·4 per cent. pyrethrum. Two applications spaced seven to ten days apart should be used.

Avian leucosis of three different types, lymphoid leucosis, myeloid leucosis and erythroleucosis, is a very common cause of loss in poultry.

Virus diseases include infectious laryngotracheitis, fowl pest due in Great Britain to the Newcastle virus and also, elsewhere, to the fowl plague virus (see p. 407) and fowl pox.

Experimental Procedures

The red blood cells, serum and plasma of the domestic fowl are frequently required in virological work and it is often necessary to keep a number of cockerels in the animal house. For certain types of work hens' blood is unsuitable. Turkeys, ducks, geese and pigeons are occasionally used and the day-old domestic chicken is a valuable experimental animal in some types of infectivity studies. The use of the chicken embryo is described on p. 1025 *et seq.*

Anaesthesia.—It should be noted that *ether anaesthesia is seldom satisfactory* in birds and that the injection of pentobarbitone sodium in a dose of 25 mg. per kilo body-weight intramuscularly in the thigh region gives better results. The anaesthetic should be given about half an hour in advance.

Subcutaneous inoculation is carried out in the pectoral or thigh regions.

Intraperitoneal inoculation is carried out in the mid-line between the vent and the posterior end of the sternum.

Insufflation.—Infective material is dropped from a Pasteur pipette into the nostril.

Collection of Blood.—If clear plasma is required, the bird should be deprived of food for about eight hours before bleeding.

(a) *From the Wing Vein.*—A 10- or 20-ml. syringe with a No. 21 or 22 gauge needle is required and it is usually necessary to treat it and the tubes into which the blood is to be placed with a solution of heparin (see p. 1039). The bird is placed on its side and the upper wing is fanned out to expose its under-surface. Feathers are then plucked from an area over the "elbow" and the large brachial vein can be seen running over the bone and just beneath the skin. The area is cleaned with 70 per cent. alcohol, and when dry the vein is gently pierced with the needle. Great care must be taken to avoid passing the needle too deep and on through the far side of the vein for if this happens a large haematoma results and it becomes impossible to obtain any blood.

(b) *Cardiac Puncture: Method* (1).—The bird is anaesthetised and placed on its right side. The needle is inserted over the heart between the second and third ribs at a point close to where the edge of the breast muscle can be felt. At a depth of 1½ in. the needle enters the ventricle. This method carries a risk of lung pucture and requires experience before it can be used with confidence. *Method* (2) is perhaps easier. Place the bird on its back, ventral side uppermost, and stretch its neck over the edge of the table. Pluck the base of the neck and clean the skin with alcohol as before. A 20-ml. syringe with a No. 17 or 18 gauge needle 2 in. long is inserted horizontally just deep to the sternum; it should be tilted very slightly downwards and will enter the heart at a depth of 1½ in.

MONKEYS

Data

Normal temperature	38·3° C.; 101·0° F.
Normal pulse rate	100 per min.
Normal respiration rate . . .	20 per min.
Gestation period	$5\frac{1}{2}$–6 months.
Room temperature	20–22° C.; 68–72° F.

Cages

A galvanised iron cage having a floor space of approximately 3 × 4 feet and a height of 4 feet is required to give the animal sufficient space for exercise. A pair—male and female—can be kept together in such a cage. The floor may be of wire mesh with a tray fitted beneath it to catch the excreta. A wooden board may be fitted halfway up the cage for the monkey to perch and sleep on. The door fitted to the cage should be of the sliding type and it should contain at its base a small hinged door through which food trays can be put into the cage. Both the doors should be fitted with padlocks. A convenient addition to this cage is the fitting of a movable screen or false back to the cage which can be adjusted in position so that the monkey can be brought very close to the bars of the cage to receive a sedative injection before handling.

Feeding

A basic diet of boiled potatoes and slice of bread covered with Bemax (vitamin B) is fed once a day and vegetables such as carrots, lettuce, turnips or parsnips are added *ad lib.* Alternatively a pellet diet may be used (Short & Parkes, 1949). A lump of sugar soaked in a solution of vitamins A, C and D is given daily. Monkeys love oranges, bananas, grapes and tomatoes, and these may be fed several times a week. Fresh water is placed in a hopper high up on the side of the cage so that it escapes fouling.

Handling

Monkeys can be caught directly with the gloved hands, and are held with their arms clasped firmly behind their backs just above the elbows. Often, however, it is necessary to catch them with a net. The use of barbiturate drugs concealed in foodstuffs or given by injection to the animal pressed against the side of the cage has much to recommend it.

Common Diseases

The commonest diseases that monkeys contract in captivity are tuberculosis, bacillary dysentery and pneumonia. Newly arrived animals should be kept apart for several weeks and observed carefully for signs of disease; they should be tuberculin tested and their faeces should be examined for the presence of pathogenic bacteria. Tuberculous monkeys constitute a considerable risk to their attendants and if the disease is suspected on clinical grounds or because the tuberculin reaction is positive the diagnosis should be checked by X-rays and if confirmed the animal should be destroyed painlessly without delay. Bacillary dysentery may be treated by incorporating sulphaguanidine in the diet or by injecting streptomycin. Pneumonia, which is the least common of the diseases, can be treated with sulphadiazine.

Anaesthesia

Short acting. Ether or chloroform.
Long acting. Pentobarbitone sodium stock solution (60 mg./ml.) 25 mg. per kg. body-weight intraperitoneally.

For further information on the use of monkeys see the UFAW Handbook.

REFERENCES

Bruce, H. M. (1950). Feeding and breeding of laboratory animals. *J. Hyg.* (*Lond.*), **45**, 70.

Bruce, H. M. & Parkes, A. S. (1947). Observations on the feeding of guinea pigs. *J. Hyg.* (*Lond.*), **47**, 70.

Croft, P. G. (1962). *An introduction to the anaesthesia of laboratory animals*. London: The Universities Federation of Animal Welfare.

Curnen, E. C. & Horsfall, F. L. (1946). Studies on pneumonia virus of mice (P.V.M.). *J. exp. Med.*, **83**, 105.

Haas, V. H. (1954). Some relationships between lymphocytic choriomeningitis virus (L.C.M.) and mice. *J. inf. Dis.*, **94**, 187.

Harris, R. J. C. (1962). *The Problems of Laboratory Animal Disease.* London: Academic Press.

Howie, J. W. (1952). Nutrition experiments in laboratory animals. *J. anim. Tech. Ass.*, **2**, 7.

Lane-Petter, W., Worden, A. N., Hill, B. F., Paterson, J. S. & Vevers, H. G. (1967). *UFAW Handbook on the Care and Management of Laboratory Animals*, 3rd ed. Edinburgh: Livingstone.

Ministry of Agriculture, Fisheries and Food. *Bull. Nos.* 54 *and* 56. London. H.M.S.O.

Nigg, C. & Eaton, M. D. (1944). Isolation from normal mice of pneumotropic virus which forms elementary bodies. *J. exp. Med.*, **79**, 497.

Parish, H. J. (1950). *Notes on Communicable Diseases of Laboratory Animals.* Edinburgh: Livingstone.

Porter, G. & Lane-Petter, W. (1962). *Notes for Breeders of Common Laboratory Animals.* London: Academic Press.

Short, D. J. & Parkes, A. S. (1949). Feeding and breeding of laboratory animals. X. A compound diet for monkeys. *J. Hyg.* (*Camb.*), **47**, 209.

Smith, W. (1931). The breeding, maintenance and manipulation of laboratory animals. *A System of Bacteriology*, vol. 9, 236. London: H.M.S.O.

Snell, G. D. (Ed.) (1941). *The Biology of the Laboratory Mouse.* Philadelphia: Blakiston.

Traub, E. (1939). Epidemiology of lymphocytic choriomeningitis in mouse stock observed for four years. *J. exp. Med.*, **69**, 801.

Worden, A. N. & Lane-Petter, W. (Eds.) (1967). *The UFAW Handbook on the Care and Management of Laboratory Animals*, 3rd. ed. Edinburgh: Livingstone.

CHAPTER 57

THE CULTIVATION OF VIRUSES

Viruses multiply only within living cells and therefore cannot be grown on inanimate artificial culture media. Setting aside bacteriophages, which grow inside bacterial cells (p. 64), the viruses with which we are concerned may be propagated in three ways. They will grow in the body of a living animal, in the membranes and tissues of the chick embryo and in the cells of tissue cultures. Each of these host systems has its own special value, but no single one can be used successfully for all viruses. Since they are both more convenient and less expensive, chick embryo and tissue cultures have in recent years largely replaced the methods of animal inoculation. Animals still, however, provide the only susceptible hosts for a number of viruses; for example, the detection of the rabies virus in routine diagnostic work depends on the results of mouse inoculation experiments, and most Coxsackie group A viruses can be demonstrated only by the lesions they produce in suckling mice. The methods recommended for the infection of animals or their tissues with particular viruses are given under their appropriate headings. The techniques for the various routes of inoculation and instructions on the care of experimental animals are described in Chapter 56.

CULTIVATION OF VIRUSES IN THE EMBRYONATED EGG

Fertile hen eggs are used, preferably with light-coloured shells, *e.g.* from white Leghorn birds. The shells should be perfectly clean. Incubation of the eggs must begin not later than ten days, and if possible within five days after being laid, and in the interval they should have been kept at a temperature between 4·5° and 20° C. Incubation is carried out in a commercial incubator at 39° C. and the eggs are turned twice daily. Before inoculation, *e.g.* after seven to twelve days' incubation, the eggs are examined by trans-illumination ("candled"); for this purpose a 100-watt lamp enclosed in a box with an oval opening is used, and the candling is best done in a dark room. The embryo which is seen as a dark shadow must be alive, as demonstrated by its spontaneous movements and by the well-defined shadows of the blood vessels in the chorio-allantois. The air sac can be seen at the rounded pole of the egg and can be outlined, for later guidance, by pencil marking on the shell. For various methods of inoculation, the shell is cut through with a rotating disk operated by a dental drill. A vulcanite carborundum disk can be recommended. Special care must be taken to avoid damage to the underlying membranes and consequent bleeding. Mounted dissecting needles, forceps, scissors, syringes and capillary pipettes are required for the manipulations involved in inoculating the egg. Inoculation must be carried out by an aseptic technique and with sterilised instruments. In carrying out various manipulations it is found convenient to lay the egg on a triangular wooden stand (4×4×2 in.) which supports it at three points, with the area to be opened uppermost. After inoculation the eggs are incubated in a bacteriological incubator at 35°-36° C. They must be kept stationary, resting on special stands or trays.

Inoculation of the Chorio-allantoic Membrane.—The eggs are incubated, usually for twelve days. In candling, a circle about 12 mm. in diameter is pencilled over the area of densest opacity, *i.e.* where the chorio-allantois is best developed and opposite the area in which the chorio-allantois fails to line the inside of the egg. The circular area should not overlie any large blood vessel. The shell is drilled with the rotating disk along the sides of the circle so marked out, and is also drilled over the centre of the air sac so as to make a small perforation through the shell membrane into the sac. The drilled disk of shell is then carefully removed by inserting a dissecting needle at one angle and gently raising the cut piece of shell without damaging the shell membrane. A drop of normal saline is now deposited on the exposed shell membrane, and the membrane under the drop is split along the line of the fibres by means of a dissecting needle. Suction with a rubber teat is next applied to the opening in the air sac, and as a result the chorio-allantois recedes from the shell membrane, the saline being aspirated into the underlying space between chorio-allantois and shell membrane. The opening in the shell membrane is then

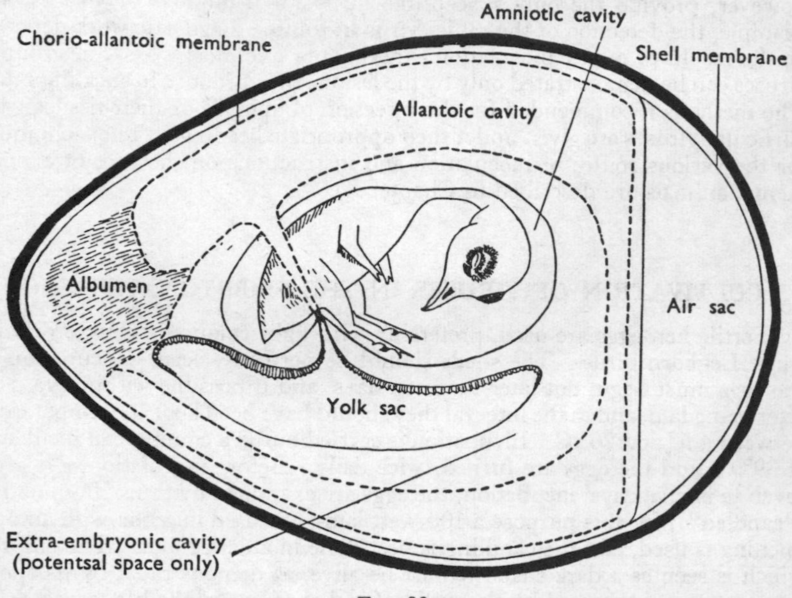

Fig. 82

Diagram of embryonated hen's egg after eleven days' incubation, to illustrate the various sites of inoculation with viruscs (*R.H.A.S.*).

enlarged and with a capillary pipette held vertically the inoculum (in an amount of 0·05 ml.) is dropped into the space, *i.e.* on to the chorio-allantoic membrane. The opening is finally sealed with commercial transparent adhesive tape ("Scotch tape") 1 in. wide. The inoculated egg is incubated for as long as necessary at the optimum temperature for the particular virus being cultivated. After this the egg is placed on a cotton-wool pad (moistened with antiseptic solution) in an open Petri dish; the seal is removed and the edge of the opening flamed with a Bunsen burner. The shell is broken off down to the level of the displaced chorio-allantois, which is then separated by cutting with scissors and carefully removed, spread out in buffered saline in a Petri dish and examined for pocks against a black background.

Allantoic inoculation.—For this purpose eggs are incubated for ten to eleven days. The outline of the air sac is pencilled in the process of candling and a point is marked on the shell where the chorio-allantois is well developed but without large vessels. A small perforation is cut through the shell *and* shell membrane over the centre of the air sac and a small groove (about 3 × 1 mm.) is drilled at the marked point on the shell. The egg is placed on the triangular stand with the groove uppermost and the inoculation is made by injecting, to a depth of 2 mm., 0·1–0·2 ml. through the groove with a tuberculin syringe. The opening is sealed with melted paraffin or nail varnish. Incubation is carried out for two days and the egg is then refrigerated for two to four hours to kill the embryo and obviate bleeding in later manipulations. For withdrawal of the allantoic fluid, the shell over the air sac is drilled and removed; the egg being supported in the upright position, *e.g.* in an egg-cup, the shell membrane and chorio-allantois in the floor of the air sac are cut away with scissors and forceps. The fluid of the underlying allantoic sac can then be aspirated with a capillary pipette.

Amniotic inoculation.—Eggs are used after thirteen to fourteen days' incubation. On candling, the densest part of the embryo is marked and a rectangular area (2 × 1·5 cm.) in the long axis of the egg is drilled at this point. Two further cuts of 1 cm. are made within the rectangle to form a triangle with the side of the rectangle towards the rounded pole of the egg, as the base. The triangular piece of shell is then removed, an opening is also made in the air sac and the same procedure as in chorio-allantoic inoculation is adopted to produce recession of that membrane. The remainder of the drilled rectangular area is finally removed and the underlying shell membrane is cut away. A part of the chorio-allantois which is free from large vessels is picked up with forceps and opened with scissors, avoiding any damage to the amnion. This membrane is now picked up with forceps through the opening in the chorio-allantois and pierced with a tuberculin syringe containing 0·05–0·25 ml. of inoculum and about 0·1 ml. of air; a little air is first introduced to ascertain if a bubble forms under the amnion, and if so the inoculation is completed. The amnion is allowed to fall back into position, and the shell opening is sealed with transparent adhesive tape.

In an alternative method a circle of shell 3 cm. in diameter is removed with its adherent shell membrane from over the air sac. Sterile liquid paraffin is applied to the inner layer of the shell membrane and through the resulting clear area a pair of forceps is inserted through the chorio-allantoic membrane and the amniotic sac is pulled upwards. The inoculation is then made in the manner described above and the egg is sealed with transparent adhesive tape. For this method the eggs must be incubated with the rounded end uppermost both before and after inoculation.

The egg is incubated for three to five days at 36° C. The shell is then removed down to the level of the receded chorio-allantois and the latter is cut away with scissors. The allantoic fluid is drained off and the amnion is picked up with forceps, and amniotic fluid for investigation aspirated with a capillary pipette.

Yolk-Sac inoculation.—Eggs are incubated for five to nine days. At the rounded pole of the egg over the air sac a small groove is drilled, and the yolk sac is inoculated with a syringe and 12 to 14 gauge needle, 3 to 3·5 cm. long. The needle is passed into the egg through the shell opening and in the long axis of the egg to a depth of about 3 cm., i.e. to just beyond the centre of the egg. 0·1 to 0·5 ml. of inoculum is introduced and the opening is sealed. Incubation is then carried out and the egg is candled daily. The yolk sac is removed when the embryo dies. The shell is drilled and separated over the air sac, and the shell membrane and chorio-allantois in the floor of the sac are cut away. The contents of the egg can then be turned out into a Petri dish;

and since the yolk sac membrane itself contains a large amount of virus, this is retained for further investigation.

For further details of the techniques of egg inoculation the reader is referred to a report by Beveridge & Burnet (1946).

TISSUE CULTURE

The simplification and refinement of tissue culture techniques in recent years has enabled many laboratories to adopt these methods and to apply them in a great variety of fields in microbiology. Among the advances are the isolation of pure lines of cells that can be propagated at will in defined culture media and the use of enzymes to disperse the cells of tissues and whole organs such as the monkey kidney.

Cultures of living cells provide an experimental host that possesses many advantages over the intact animal. It is possible to use pure clones derived from a single cell, to count the cells in a culture and to study the metabolic and morphological changes that result from infection. The cell surfaces are directly accessible to invasion and they are free from the immune defence mechanisms and the hormonal influences of the whole animal.

For full details of tissue culture techniques see Parker (1961) and Paul (1960).

Apparatus

Glassware of borosilicate glass made by Pyrex is generally preferred for all tissue culture work but soda glass as used in medical prescription bottles is also satisfactory. It may be mentioned that new glassware, even after very careful cleaning, may at first give a poor growth of cells. After it has been used once or twice, however, the difficulty disappears and satisfactory results are obtained. No explanation of this has yet been found. Tissue culture glassware requires to be cleaned by special methods (see p. 863) and to be rinsed very thoroughly with ion-free distilled water (see p. 859).

Stoppers for Tissue Culture Vessels.—Red or black rubber bungs and the rubber liners of screw-capped bottles contain substances that are toxic to cells in tissue culture. The surface impurities on these stoppers can to some extent be removed by boiling in weak alkali (*e.g.* 5 per cent. sodium carbonate), but even with this precaution it is always necessary to ensure that the rubber never touches any culture medium. This hazard can be overcome by using stoppers made of silicone rubber or grey virgin rubber, which are practically non-toxic for cells; they are greatly to be preferred.

Rubber tubing suffers from the same disadvantages and in general is best avoided. Silicone rubber tubing is recommended and is easily sterilised by heat.

Instruments must be kept scrupulously clean. They may be sterilised by dry heat or by boiling. New scalpel blades or razor blades are often covered by a protective layer of grease which is toxic to cells. They should be cleaned by wiping them with a cloth soaked in carbon tetrachloride before they are washed and sterilised.

Filters.—Before use, Seitz filter pads should be washed free of alkali and detachable asbestos fibres by the passage of considerable amounts of sterile demineralised water. Sintered glass filters should be cleaned after use by treatment with strong acid. Concentrated sulphuric acid to which a few crystals of sodium nitrate and sodium chlorate have been added is allowed to seep through the filter. Afterwards the filter must be rinsed thoroughly with a very large volume of de-ionised water.

Media for the Growth and Maintenance of Cells.—Most media employ for their base a balanced salt solution containing a number of essential inorganic chemicals. Since cells form acid as they grow, buffers are added to stabilise the pH and sodium bicarbonate is also included for this purpose. Glucose is added as a source of carbon and energy, and phenol red is used as a pH indicator.

Balanced Salt Solutions.—Double glass distilled water or demineralised water (see p. 859) should always be used in making up balanced salt solutions. The salts used should be of the highest analytical purity and the solutions should be kept in polythene bottles set aside specially for the purpose. Phenol red is added to the solutions as a pH indicator and is non-toxic to cells in concentrations up to 0·005 per cent. In preparing balanced salt solutions, care is required to avoid the formation of calcium and magnesium carbonate and phosphate. In order to achieve this, the calcium salt is dissolved separately and added slowly to the main solution in its final dilute stage. Hanks' solution is one of the most useful in tissue culture work and details are given of its preparation as an example of the procedure needed. The same procedure is adopted for Earle's and Gey's solutions.

Hanks' Solution

Stock solutions of the salt mixtures are convenient and are made up with ten times the concentration of all the components except for the bicarbonate solution, which is made up separately.

Phenol Red Indicator (0·4 per cent.).—Dissolve 1·0 g. phenol red in the minimum volume of 0·05 *N* NaOH and then bring the volume to 250 ml. by the addition of distilled water.

Stock Solution A:

(1)	NaCl	160·0 g.
	KCl	8·0 g.
	$MgSO_4 . 7H_2O$	2·0 g.
	$MgCl_2 . 6H_2O$	2·0 g.
	H_2O	800·0 ml.
(2)	$CaCl_2$	2·8 g.
	H_2O	100·0 ml.

Mix these two solutions slowly and adjust the volume to 1000 ml. with water. Add 2·0 ml. chloroform and store in a polythene bottle at 4° C.

Stock Solution B:

$Na_2HPO_4 . 12H_2O$	3·04 g.
KH_2PO_4	1·2 g.
Glucose	20·0 g.
Water	800·0 ml.

When dissolved add

Phenol red solution	100 ml.
Water to 1000 ml.	

Add 2 ml. chloroform and store as with Solution A.

Sodium Bicarbonate Solution:

$NaHCO_3$	1·4 g.
Water	100 ml.

Sterilise by autoclaving in a container with a tightly closed screw cap for 10 min. at 115° C. (9 lb. pressure).

Hanks' solution is made by adding 1 volume of stock solution A and 1 volume of stock solution B to 18 volumes of distilled water. It is sterilised by steaming for 1½ hr. Immediately before use add 0·5 ml. of sterile 1·4 per cent. $NaHCO_3$ solution to each 20 ml. of Hanks' solution. Hanks' solution is used when considerable fluctuations in pH are not anticipated and where a large buffering capacity is not required.

GEY'S SOLUTION (1936):

NaCl	7·00 g.
KCl	0·37 g.
$CaCl_2$	0·17 g.
$MgSO_4 . 7H_2O$	0·07 g.
$MgCl_2 . 6H_2O$	0·21 g.
$Na_2HPO_4 . 2H_2O$	0·15 g.
KHP_2O_4	0·03 g.
Glucose	1·00 g.
$NaHCO_3$	2·27 g.
Water	1000 ml.

EARLE'S SOLUTION

As in Hanks' solution the calcium salt should be dissolved separately and added slowly.

NaCl	6·80 g.
KCl	0·40 g.
$CaCl_2$	0·20 g.
$MgSO_4 . 7H_2O$	0·10 g.
$NaH_2PO_4 . H_2O$	0·125 g.
Glucose	1·00 g.
Phenol red solution	12·5 ml.
$NaHCO_3$	2·20 g.
Water to make	1000 ml.

Gey's and Earle's solutions contain greater amounts of sodium bicarbonate; they are useful when cultures produce much acid or have a large cell population. When used for cultures with small numbers of cells they may lose their CO_2 and become alkaline; such cultures need to be "gassed" with 5–10 per cent. CO_2 in air after the medium is changed and before stoppering.

Nutrient Media.—Many defined nutrient media have been devised incorporating amino acids, vitamins, enzymes, accessory growth factors, glucose and inorganic salts in varying proportions. They are used without supplementation to maintain established cultures for periods of three or four days when cell multiplication is not required. With serum or tissue extracts added they are used to promote the active growth of cells.

The most widely used defined medium is Morgan, Morton and Parker's Medium 199 (1950) or a modification of it; it is particularly useful in the maintenance of cells for virus production in vaccine manufacture and in diagnostic work with the enteroviruses.

Medium 199 (*Morgan, Campbell and Morton* (1955) *Modification M*150)

Solution		Mg. per 1000 ml.
	Amino Acids	
1	L-Arginine	70·0
	L-Histidine	20·0
	L-Lysine	70·0
	DL-Tryptophane	20·0
	DL-Phenylalanine	50·0
	DL-Serine	50·0
	DL-Valine	50·0
	DL-Alanine	50·0
	Glycine	50·0
	DL-Methionine	60·0
	DL-Threonine	60·0
	DL-Aspartic acid	60·0
	DL-Leucine	120·0
	DL-Isoleucine	40·0
	L-Proline	40·0
	DL-Glutamic acid	150·0
	L-Hydroxyproline	10·0
	Sodium acetate (anhydrous)	50·0
2	L-Tyrosine	40·0
	L-Cystine	20·0
3	*Vitamin B Group*:	
	Niacin	0·025
	Niacinamide	0·025
	Pyridoxine	0·025
	Pyridoxal	0·025
	Thiamine	0·010
	Riboflavin	0·010
	Ca-Pantothenate	0·01
	i-Inositol	0·05
	p-Aminobenzoic acid	0·05
	Choline chloride	0·50

Solution		Mg. per 1000 ml.
4	*Fat Soluble Group*:	
	Cholesterol	0·20
	Menadione (Vit. K)	0·10
	Calciferol	0·10
	Vitamin A	0·10
	Tween 80	20·0
5	*Vitamin C Mixture*:	
	L-Cysteine HCl	0·1
	Glutathione	0·05
	Ascorbic acid	0·05
6	Disodium tocopherol Phosphoric acid (Vit. E)	0·01
7	Folic acid	0·01
8	Biotin	0·01
9	Adenine sulphate	10·0
10	*Purine and Pyramidine mixture*:	0·30
	Guanine HCl	0·30
	Xanthine (monosodium)	0·30
	Hypoxanthine	0·30
	Thymine	0·30
	Uracil	0·30
11	Adenosine triphosphate (disodium)	10·8
12	$Fe(NO_3)_3 \cdot 9H_2O$	0·10
13	Adenylic acid	0·20
14	D-Ribose	0·50
	Deoxyribose	0·50
	Glutamine	100·0

Medium 199 is made up in Earle's balanced salt solution from the fourteen stock solutions given in the table. The glucose and the sodium bicarbonate of the Hanks' solution together with a solution of L-glutamine to give a final concentration of 100 mg. per l. are added immediately before sterilisation by passage through sintered glass filters. For the details of preparation of the stock solutions reference should be made to Morgan, Campbell and Morton's paper. (1955).

Many attempts have been made to simplify defined media of the 199 type and the best of these is that devised by Eagle. This medium contains only those ingredients that are essential for cell growth rather than those needed for optimal growth. It is unable to support growth in the total absence of added biological fluid. Although favoured by some workers, it has not found general acceptance, for, although simpler than 199, it is still complex enough to require much time in its preparation.

For details of Eagle's medium and other defined media the reader is referred to Paul (1960).

Antibiotics.—Nearly all the culture media in general use contain antibiotics to control chance contamination during the handling of cell cultures. For this purpose, stock solutions of penicillin and streptomycin are held available in the refrigerator and are added to the media immediately before use. Final concentrations of 50 units of sodium penicillin G and 50 μg. of streptomycin per ml. of the medium are sufficient for the purpose and are not toxic to the cells. Fungal contamination may be held in check by mycostatin (nystatin Squibb) added to give a concentration of 20–50 μg. per ml. but it must be remembered that this antibiotic is unstable at 37° C. and that after twenty-four hours its influence is lost. Neomycin or Kanamycin at concentrations of 20 μg. per ml. is also useful to control bacterial contamination and is particularly valuable against pleuropneumonia organisms which are often chronic contaminants of cell lines.

Antibiotics in high concentrations are valuable in elimination of bacteria from heavily contaminated tissues or from faecal material to be examined for the presence of viruses. Treatment of these materials for a short period with a solution containing 1000 units penicillin, 1000 μg. streptomycin is highly effective and neomycin 500 μg. per ml. is also valuable. The presence of antibiotic-resistant organisms contaminating material of this type can best be overcome by determination of sensitivity of the organisms to a range of antibiotics and subsequent choice of the most suitable agent. Occasionally in faecal emulsions, antibiotic-resistant bacteria can be removed by prolonged centrifugation at speeds of over 10,000 r.p.m. When attempting to isolate members of the psittacosis lymphogranuloma group sulphonamides, penicillin and tetracyclines must be avoided, but streptomycin in concentrations up to 2000 μg. per ml. will control most bacterial contaminants without harming the chick embryo.

The Preparation of Cultures of Cells from Fresh Tissues

Human Amnion Cell Culture—A placenta with its attached membranes is obtained following a normal delivery or preferably at a Caesarean section. It is important that the amnion should not be badly lacerated, that it should have been delivered with a minimum of handling, and that it should not have been in contact with any disinfectant. If possible the placenta should be received directly into a wide-mouthed, screw-capped sterile jar containing 200 ml. Hanks' solution with added antibiotics. It is convenient to use placentae delivered in the early hours of the morning; they should not be used after eight hours and on no account should they be placed in a refrigerator.

On receipt at the laboratory the placenta is suspended by the cord held by Spencer Wells forceps in a retort clamp over a large sterile bowl. If the placenta has many infarcts or if the amnion is badly lacerated, soft or oedematous, it should be rejected. Otherwise, dissection is begun at the point of entry of the cord and the amnion is stripped gently downwards from the underlying chorion. The whole amnion is separated and transferred to a sterile flask containing about 250 ml. Hanks' solution with added antibiotics. After agitation the membrane is rinsed in two changes of the solution and is then transferred to a sterile 6 in. Petri dish in which it is cut into inch wide strips with sterile scissors. Adherent blood and mucus are scraped off the surface of the strips using the edges of sterile microscope slides and the pieces of membrane are then placed in fresh Hanks' solution.

When this stage is completed the strips are transferred to a sterile flask containing 150 ml. of 0·25 per cent. trypsin (Difco "Trypsin 1:250") in Hanks' solution warmed to 37° C. After 30 min. the trypsin solution is removed and discarded and replaced with an equal volume of fresh solution. A sterile glass-covered magnet is now introduced into the flask which is placed on a magnetic stirrer in the 37° C. incubator. Stirring proceeds at the slowest possible rate and the tryptic digestion is continued for two and a half hours. At half-hourly intervals, on three or four occasions, the cloudy supernatant fluid which contains the detached cells is removed and replaced with fresh trypsin solution. The portions removed are bulked together in a flask and kept at 4° C. in the refrigerator. It is very important that the cells should not be damaged by exposure to trypsin at 37° C. for longer than is absolutely necessary.

When the last portion of cell suspension has been added the pool is filtered through a double layer of sterile gauze and the whole is spun for five minutes in a straight-headed centrifuge at 600 r.p.m. (80 G). The supernatant trypsin solution is now discarded and the cells are resuspended in 10 ml. of fresh Hanks' solution. Next, a count of the number of cells in the suspension is made in a haemocytometer chamber. For this purpose, 0·5 ml. of the suspension is added to 1·0 ml. of a 0·1 per cent. solution of crystal violet in 0·1 *M* citric acid. In making the count clumps of several cells adherent to each other are to be recorded as single cells. Cell counts may range from 50 to 80 million per ml. The suspension is now diluted with the culture medium to be used so that it contains 400,000 cells per ml.

The final step is to dispense the solution in 1·0 ml. amounts into $5 \times \frac{5}{8}$ in. tissue culture tubes. This is carried out while the cells are kept in continuous agitation by the magnetic stirrer and a syringe of the Cornwall[1] type for automatically pipetting fixed volumes is recommended for the purpose. Amounts of 50 ml. may also be placed in suitable bottles. Tubes and bottles are placed horizontally in the 37° C. incubator and are held stationary without further disturbance for three days.

The culture medium is changed twice weekly and it is recommended, though not essential, that, after the first change of medium on the third day, the tubes are transferred to a roller drum. By seven to ten days a sheet of cells has usually grown out and the cultures are ready for use. Some workers recommend the washing of the cell sheets twice with fresh medium before inoculation, but this step is not essential.

The medium recommended to promote amnion cell growth is Hanks' solution with 0·5 per cent. lactalbumin hydrolysate and 20 per cent. horse serum added. After the cells have been infected with virus they are maintained in a medium comprising Earle's solution which contains 0·5 per cent. lactalbumin hydrolysate, and 0·5 per cent. yeast extract (Yeastolate Difco). If the cells are to be maintained for longer than seven days, the medium should also contain 5 per cent. horse serum.

Secondary Cultures.—Bottle cultures of amnion cells are treated in the same way as tube cultures. It is sometimes convenient to use a confluent sheet of cells in a bottle to set up secondary tube cultures. For this purpose the cells are detached from the glass of the bottle by exposure for 30 min. to trypsin at 37° C. The suspension is then counted and transferred to tubes in the way described above for the primary cultures.

Monkey Kidney Cell Culture.—A kidney is removed from a rhesus or cynomolgus monkey under Nembutal anaesthesia, using full aseptic technique. One kidney is sufficient to provide over 1000 tissue culture tubes and

[1] Made by Becton, Dickinson & Co. Obtainable from R. B. Turner & Co., London.

it is a common practice to allow the animal to survive for about three weeks before killing it to obtain the other kidney. After this interval, the second kidney is often hypertrophied and provides an increased cell yield.

Once removed, the kidneys are immediately decapsulated with sterile instruments and the pelvis and calices are dissected away. With sterile long-handled scissors the kidney tissue is cut into 2–3 mm. fragments which are rinsed twice in Hanks' solution with added antibiotics. Next the fragments are transferred to 100 ml. of 0·25 per cent. trypsin solution in Hanks' solution warmed to 37° C. After gentle agitation for twenty minutes on a magnetic stirrer, the trypsin is discarded and replaced with fresh solution. At twenty-minute intervals on three or four occasions, the turbid solution with its suspended cells is removed, stored at 4° C. and replaced with fresh solution. The pooled cell suspensions are now gently centrifuged at 80 G and the cells are washed twice with Hanks' solution. The cell deposit is next resuspended in 10 ml. of the culture medium to be used and the cells are counted in a haemocytometer. The cell suspension is now diluted with culture medium so that it contains 300,000 cells per ml. The final step is to dispense the cell suspension in 1·0 ml. volumes into tissue culture tubes, in 15 ml. amounts in 16-oz. medicine bottles, or in 80 ml. amounts in Roux bottles according to requirements.

During active growth the cells are cultured in Hanks' solution containing 0·5 per cent. lactalbumin hydrolysate and 20 per cent. horse or human serum. (Human serum may, of course, contain antibodies that are able to inhibit virus growth.) During the first forty-eight hours the culture tubes are held stationary in a horizontal but slightly tilted position in racks or drums. Care must be taken that the culture medium does not come into contact with the corks of the tubes. Once the cells are adherent to the glass it is recommended, but not essential, that they are rotated in roller drums. When the cell growth has formed a confluent sheet, usually some four to six days later, the medium is changed to one of the maintenance type such as medium 199 and the tubes can then be inoculated with virus. If the cells are to be observed for more than three days, 2 per cent. calf serum should be added to medium 199.

Cell Strains.—The cells that are obtained from disaggregated tissues or from fragments growing in plasma clots can usually be carried in subculture for only a few transfers. After this the rate of multiplication declines and the cells die out. In some cases, however, after a variable static period there is a sudden outgrowth of new cells and thereafter proliferation is rapid. It is then possible to carry the strain in repeated serial transfers. After such a transformation occurs and when some dozen or more successful subcultures have been made it becomes apparent that the cells can be propagated indefinitely. In these circumstances the cells can be considered to constitute a strain or line.

Many cell strains have been derived from such normal human tissues as liver, kidney, intestines, embryonic skin and muscle (fibroblasts), and amnion. Other cell lines have been obtained from monkey kidney and sarcomatous tissue in the mouse. Three cell strains of great value in medical virology have originated in human malignant tissue. The HeLa strain of epithelial cells was obtained by Gey from a squamous cell carcinoma of the cervix uteri, the KB strain by Eagle from a carcinoma of the nasopharynx, and the HEp2 strain from an epithelioma. Every cell strain has its own characteristic pattern of susceptibility to infection by viruses. HeLa cells can be infected with an obvious cytopathic effect by the three types of poliovirus, the whole group of adenoviruses, the pox viruses, and by the herpes simplex virus; in general they are not susceptible to infection by the Coxsackie viruses of groups A or B or by the ECHO viruses.

The Cultivation of Cell Strains.—Cell strains grow uniformly as suspensions or as sheets on the surface of glass. Often it is important to be able to examine the cells during their growth and for this purpose they are manipulated so that a layer one cell thick (a "monolayer" is formed on the side of test-tubes ($\frac{1}{2}$ or $\frac{5}{8}$ in. diameter) which can be viewed with $\frac{2}{3}$ in. objective of the microscope. For other purposes they can be cultivated on the flat surfaces of Carrel flasks or Petri dishes and when required in greater numbers they are propagated on the sides of ordinary prescription bottles, Pyrex baby's bottles (4–8 oz.), or Roux bottles.

The Detachment of Cells from a Culture on Glass.—Cells can sometimes be brought into suspension simply by gentle scraping with a glass rod covered with silicone rubber tubing. This method cannot, however, be relied upon and it is usually necessary to detach the cells by one of the following two methods.

In the first method a chelating agent, "Versene", is used to bind divalent ions such as calcium and magnesium with the effect that the cells round up and leave the glass. "Versene" is diamino-ethane-tetra-acetic acid and its disodium salt is employed in the following solution:

Disodium versenate	0·2 g.
NaCl	8·0 g.
KCl	0·2 g.
Na_2HPO_4	1·15 g.
KH_2PO_4	0·2 g.
Glucose	0·2 g.
Water	1000 ml.

To suspend the cells remove the growth medium and wash the surface of the cell sheet with balanced salt solution (Ca and Mg free) warmed to 37° C. Replace the salt solution with the versene solution and incubate the culture for 10–15 min. at 37° C. As soon as the cells have left the glass add growth medium and disperse them by gentle pipetting. The cells in this suspension are then counted in a haemocytometer and diluted to give a concentration of the order of 100,000 per ml. With delicate or slow-growing cells, concentrations as high as 500,000 ml. may be required. This method is valuable for HeLa cells.

Proteolytic enzymes may be used to release the cells from the surface of the glass. A stock solution of 5 per cent. trypsin (Difco "Trypsin 1:250") in Hanks' solution is used for this purpose. Before use, the stock solution is diluted 1 in 10 (0·5 per cent.) with Hanks' solution and warmed to 37° C. The culture medium is removed from the monolayer culture and replaced by an equal volume of trypsin. After about ten minutes' incubation at 37° C., and as soon as the cells leave the vessel wall, they are spun down in a sterile tube for a few minutes at 80 G and the supernatant is replaced by culture medium. After the cells have been counted the suspension is diluted to give the required concentration in culture medium.

The second method is most commonly used. Some workers consider a lower concentration of trypsin (*e.g.* 0·025 per cent.) is desirable. During trypsinisation a careful watch must be kept on the pH. Below pH 7·0 trypsin is practically inactive and above pH 8·0 the cells are badly damaged. In centrifuging the cells, high speeds may cause damage and death of the cells, so that the slowest effective speed of the centrifuge should be used.

Maintenance and Feeding of Cells.—When the cell suspensions have been placed in the culture tubes, and vessels, they are incubated for forty-eight hours at 37° C. in the horizontal position until the cells are adherent to the glass. Thereafter tube cultures may be incubated in a rotating drum. The drum consists of sheet metal, or a plastic such as Perspex, pierced with holes of the appropriate size to hold the culture tubes and mounted on a horizontal shaft. The drum is tilted at an angle of 5 degrees in order to prevent the nutrient medium touching the stoppers of the tubes; it is rotated at a speed of 12–20 revolutions per hour by an electric motor fitted with a reduction gear.

The feeding of cell strains consists simply of pipetting off the old culture medium and replacing it with new. Medium may conveniently be removed by means of a pipette attached to a suction pump. A flask acting as a trap should be inserted between the pipette and the pump. A mechanical dispenser (*e.g.* an automatic syringe, see p. 943) greatly reduces the labour of adding medium to the tubes.

The medium used for growth of the cells varies with the cell strains but the following is in common use:

> Hanks' solution to which have been added 0·5 per cent. lactalbumin hydrolysate and 0·1 per cent. yeast extract (Difco). For HeLa cells an increased yield is obtained by supplementing with 5 per cent. tryptic digest broth (Tomlinson, 1962). To this mixture 20 per cent. serum is usually added. Horse serum is perhaps the best for most purposes, but human, calf, and rabbit serum may also be used either separately or in combination (*e.g.* 10 per cent. horse serum + 10 per cent. rabbit serum).

For maintenance of the cells medium 199 alone will suffice to keep the cells in good condition for periods of three to six days, but if maintenance for longer periods is needed, 2–5 per cent. horse serum should be added. If it is desired to slow the rate of cell multiplication, Earle's solution is used in making the medium and the concentration of serum is reduced by 50–75 per cent. Some workers also increase the sodium bicarbonate content of the medium. In the routine maintenance of cell strains it is convenient to handle them twice a week. On the first occasion they are fed and on the second they are detached from the glass and transferred to new vessels.

Plaque Techniques employ the method whereby a dilute suspension of virus is allowed to absorb, for a suitable time, to the cells of a growing monolayer which is then overlaid with molten nutrient agar or methyl cellulose. The overlay prevents the diffusion of the virus and its products in the way that occurs in fluid media; each infective particle, as it multiplies, is able to initiate a focus of necrosis spreading only to contiguous cells and ultimately gives rise to a clear, visible plaque. The value of the method is that it offers a precise means of titrating the infectivity of viruses which is then expressed in terms of plaque forming units (PFU). Thus, the virus neutralising activities of sera and also of anti-viral agents can be assessed by their abilities to inhibit plaque formation. The plaque is derived from a single infectious virus particle and is analogous to the bacterial colony. By the excision of a single plaque from a plate it is therefore possible to obtain a pure clone of the virus and also to separate it from a second virus in a mixed infection. Many viruses form plaques of different shapes and sizes and so the method is valuable in distinguishing and characterising them (Hsuing & Melnick, 1957).

In preparing cell cultures for virus infectivity titrations great care is required to ensure even monolayers of healthy cells growing on the glass of the bases of Petri dishes or Carrel flasks, or on the sides of bottles. If human serum has been used in the culture medium the cell sheet must be washed with a balanced salt solution to remove it. The virus for inoculation should be suspended in a fluid, selected according to the stability of the virus and buffered to near neutrality using, preferably, some system other than carbonate-bicarbonate.

Infection of the monolayers is carried out by allowing a predetermined virus dose in a suitable dilution of the infective suspension to disperse over the surface of the monolayer. Different viruses require varying times to absorb to their host cells; the time varies with the volume of the inoculum but should not exceed the length of the eclipse phase of the virus concerned. With increasing absorption periods the volume of the inoculum increases; thus, for a two-hour absorption period and a monolayer in a 2½-in. Petri dish, 0·5 ml. might be required for the vaccinia virus, whereas for overnight absorption 3·0 ml. would be needed. When the inoculum is large (*e.g.* more than 2·0 ml.) it should be removed with a pipette at the end of the period, but this is unnecessary with small inocula. After initial experiments the volumes and absorption times should be standardised to ensure that a constant proportion of the virus is absorbed by the cells.

To prevent subsequent absorption of the virus and also to inhibit secondary plaque formation, the infected monolayers are now covered with a semi-solid or viscous overlay. Two methods are used:

(*a*) Melt a 3 per cent. mixture of agar (Difco Noble agar) in balanced salt solution, cool to 43° C. and add it to an equal volume of culture medium at the same temperature (Hanks' solution containing 20 per cent. horse serum or a maintenance medium). Some workers add neutral red to give a final concentration of 0·002 per cent.; this vital dye stains the living but not the dead cells and thus renders the plaques more easily visible. Quickly cover the cell layer with the molten agar and set aside to solidify. Invert the bottles and incubate at 37° C. Examine the bottles daily in an oblique light for plaque formation.

This method suffers, however, from the disadvantage that the acid mucopolysaccharide present in agar tends to reduce plaque formation by a number of viruses (e.g. herpes simplex) (see Nahmias & Kilbrick, 1964).

(*b*) Make up Eagle's medium from the × 10 stock solution to 1·3 times its normal strength. To 7·5 ml. of this add 10 ml. calf serum and 15 ml. of a 5 per cent. w/v solution of carboxy-methyl cellulose in distilled water (Russell, 1962). Cover the monolayer with this solution to a depth of ¼ in. and incubate the plates in a moist atmosphere containing 5 per cent. CO_2, exercising great care not to disturb the cell layers. Plaques are produced in some three to six days and whenever they are apparent the fluid overlay is discarded and the monolayers are fixed with formaldehyde-saline and stained with Leishman's stain. A count can now be made of the plaques and from the figures obtained the content of infective virus particles can be calculated.

Cooper (1955) has described another method for plaque production, in which a cell-virus suspension is incorporated into molten agar. A suspension comprising about 15 million cells per ml. in a culture medium made up in Earle's solution is mixed with a dilute virus preparation and added to an equal volume of molten 1·8 per cent. agar at 44° C. The mixture is poured into 10 cm. Petri dishes and incubated, as soon as it has set, in an atmosphere containing 10 per cent. CO_2. Replacement of the bicarbonate buffer in the medium with 0·3 per cent. "tris buffer" (2-amino-2(hydroxy-methyl) 1 : 3-propanediol) enables the use of the CO_2 containing atmosphere during the incubation period to be dispensed with.

Plaque inhibition is frequently used to demonstrate the neutralising properties of antisera and other agents. Several methods can be employed:

(*a*) Immune serum and virus are mixed together and after a suitable interval residual virus activity is determined by plaque titration.

(*b*) Monolayers of cells infected with a standard dose of virus are overlaid with molten agar containing serial dilutions of the antiserum.

(*c*) Serum dilutions in molten agar are made as in (*b*) but used to overlay uninfected monolayers. Virus is applied in cups or beads, as in antibiotic assay work, and to produce plaques it must diffuse through the antisera contained in the agar.

(*d*) Monolayers of cells infected with a standard dose of virus are covered with an overlay of ordinary agar. Beads containing dilutions of antisera are now set on the surface of the agar and wherever antibodies are present they diffuse to the cells beneath to inhibit plaque formation (Busby, House & MacDonald, 1964).

Explantation in Plasma Clots.—A wide variety of human or animal tissues may be used to provide host cells for virus growth in tissue cultures. It is important that tissues removed at operation or at autopsy should be placed in a refrigerator at 4° C. without delay. As soon as possible the material should be sliced with very sharp instruments into small pieces about 5 mm. thick and then immersed in Hanks' solution containing penicillin and streptomycin. The cells in such slices remain viable at 4° C. for between eighteen and thirty-six hours. Mincing of the tissues into fragments of 1 mm. diameter is required for some types of cultures and may be undertaken with pieces of new razor blades held in a handle or by a fine pair of Spencer-Wells forceps. The fragments so made are rinsed several times in Hanks' solution to free them from amorphous debris and are then set up in cultures as follows.

A drop of chicken plasma is placed on the side of a test-tube and is spread out to cover the lower half of its length. Three or four tissue fragments are next placed at intervals on the plasma-coated tube. A drop of chick embryo extract is then flooded over the fragments and the plasma is allowed to clot during the next five to ten minutes. Next 0·5–1·0 ml. culture medium, which is similar in composition to that used for HeLa cells, is added to the tubes, which are then tightly stoppered and incubated at 37° C. in a rotating drum. The cultures are fed when the medium begins to become acid—usually every third day. After a few days, the growing cells, which may be epithelial or fibroblastic, migrate into the plasma and begin to grow. In three days the cells have often produced enough trypsin to digest the plasma clot and to form a large hole in it. This may be overcome by patching the hole with a drop of fresh plasma which is again made to clot by chick embryo extract. Alternatively the action of the trypsin can be entirely checked if the culture medium contains 0·05 mg. per ml. of a pure crystalline soya bean trypsin inhibitor.

BIOLOGICAL FLUIDS AND EXTRACTS

Serum is a valuable ingredient of the great majority of tissue culture media. Human, horse, calf and chicken sera are those most often used; they are obtained from whole blood after it has clotted. Serum must be tested for bacterial sterility before use and is best stored in a deep freeze cabinet at −30° C. Some sera are markedly toxic for growing cells and it is a wise precaution to test serial dilutions of each fresh batch of serum in a number of replicate cultures of cells. Human placental cord serum is regarded as being particularly good for promoting the growth of cells and is relatively free from toxic properties.

[1] Available commercially from V. & A. Howe, Pembridge Road, London, W.11

Ascitic and pleural fluids are useful culture media and are prepared and tested in the same way as sera.

Chicken Plasma.—Blood is taken from the wing vein into a sterile syringe containing sufficient heparin solution to give a strength of 5 units of heparin per ml. of blood. Greater strengths of heparin should be avoided as the plasma thus obtained may not clot. The blood is discharged into a clean dry test-tube and the plasma is separated by centrifuging at 80 G for 5 min. Store in small quantities at 4° C.

A convenient heparin solution is made by adding 1 ml. of heparin (Roche Liquemin, 1 ml. = 1000 international units) to 9 ml. Hanks' solution; it can be sterilised by autoclaving at 115° C. (10 lb.) for 10 min. and penicillin and streptomycin sulphate should be added to concentrations of 500 units/ml. and 500 μg./ml. 0·5 ml. of this solution is sufficient for 10 ml. of blood.

Bovine Amniotic Fluid.—This provides a valuable means of promoting the growth of tissue cultures without the interfering action of specific antibodies present in human serum.

An intact cow's uterus, some three months gravid is obtained from the slaughter house. The contained embryo should be between 8 and 12 inches long. The uterine surface is flamed and carefully incised at some dependent point away from the embryo. The amniotic fluid is allowed to escape into a sterile one litre measuring cylinder. Penicillin, 100 per ml., streptomycin 100 μg. per ml. and mycostatin 20 units per ml. are added together with sufficient stock phenol red solution (0·4 per cent.) to give a final concentration of 0·002 per cent. Using aseptic methods the fluid is filtered through gauze and then spun at 2000 r.p.m. in a straight headed centrifuge for 30 min. The resulting supernatant fluid is filtered through a Seitz E.K. filter, dispensed in small volumes in hard glass containers, stoppered, and stored at −30° C.

Chick Embryo Extract.—After chilling for two hours at 4° C. nine-day-old embryos are removed from the eggs and washed once in Hanks' solution. For some purposes it is necessary to remove the eyes of the embryos. Place the washed embryos in a homogenising flask and add 1·5 ml. per embryo of Hanks' solution. Add sufficient penicillin and streptomycin sulphate to give a final concentration of 100 units and 100 μg. per ml. Homogenise at medium speed for 10 min. Centrifuge the suspension at 1000 *G* for 10 min., transfer the supernatant to suitable tubes, stopper, and store at —25° C. Chick embryo extract is best used fresh but may be used for a week or more after its preparation.

Bovine Embryo Extract.—An embryo 4–6 in. long is obtained, cut into small pieces and placed in a Waring blender with an equal volume of Hanks' solution. It is homogenised at high speed for 2–5 min. and the resulting pulp is transferred to centrifuge bottles and spun down. The resultant somewhat turbid supernatant is used as the extract in culture media. Some workers prefer to purify it further by ultra-centrifugation and as a final step to pass it through a fine sintered glass filter.

Test for the Activity of Trypsin.—It is necessary to check from time to time the activity of the trypsin used in solutions to disaggregate the cells of tissues such as monkey kidney. This can be carried out by preparing a series of about 10 doubling dilutions from 1 in 10 onwards of the trypsin solution in Hanks' balanced salt solution. One drop of each dilution is placed on a strip of X-ray film together with one drop of Hanks' solution as a control. The strip is then placed on moist blotting-paper in a Petri dish, covered, and incubated for thirty minutes at 37° C. Remove the strip and allow to cool to room temperature or run cold water over the reverse side (no film) until the gelatin sets firmly. Now flood the whole film gently with cold water. Wherever trypsin was present the gelatin will have been digested to water-soluble products and a punched-out hole will appear in the film. The control area (Hanks' solution) is not dissolved at all.

REFERENCES

BEVERIDGE, W. I. B. & BURNET, F. M. (1946). The cultivation of viruses and rickettsiae in the chick embryo. *Spec. Rep. Ser. Med. Res. Coun. (Lond.)*, No. 256.

BUSBY, D. W. G., HOUSE, W. & MACDONALD, J. R. (1964). *Virological Technique.* London: Churchill.

COOPER, P. D. (1955). A method for the production of plaques in agar suspensions of animal cells. *Virology*, **1**, 397.

HSIUNG, G. D. & MELNICK, J. L. (1957). Morphologic characteristics of plaques produced on monkey kidney monolayer cultures by enteric viruses (poliomyelitis, Coxsackie and ECHO groups). *J. Immunol.*, **78**, 128.

MORGAN, J. F., CAMPBELL, M. E. & MORTON, H. J. (1955). Nutrition of animal tissues cultivated *in vitro*. Survey of natural materials as supplements to synthetic medium. *J. nat. Cancer Inst.*, **16**, 557.

MORGAN, J. F., MORTON, H. J. & PARKER, R. C. (1950). Nutrition of animal cells in tissue culture; initial studies on a synthetic medium. *Proc. Soc. exp. Biol. (N.Y.)*, **73**, 1.

NAHMIAS, A. J., & KILBRICK, S. (1964). Inhibitory effect of heparin on herpes simplex virus. *J. Bact.*, **87**, 1060.

PARKER, R. C. (1961). *Methods of Tissue Culture.* 3rd ed. London: Pitman.

PAUL, J. (1960). *Cell and Tissue Culture.* 2nd ed. Edinburgh: Livingstone.

RUSSELL, W. C. (1962). A sensitive and precise plaque assay for herpes virus. *Nature, (Lond.)*, **195**, 1028.

TOMLINSON, A. H. (1962). The culture of HeLa cells. *Mth. Bull. Minist. Hlth. Lab. Serv.*, **21**, 9.

APPENDIX 6

DIFFERENTIAL CHARACTERS OF THE THREE SPECIES OF THE GENUS BRUCELLA AND THEIR BIOTYPES

Species	Type	CO_2 requirement	H_2S production	Growth on dyes					Urease	Agglutination in monospecific sera		Phage Tb at RTD	Metabolic tests			
				Thiomin			Basic Fuchsin						Glutamic acid	Orni-thine	Ribose	Lysine
				a	b	c	d	e		A	M					
Br. melitensis	1	−	−	−	+	+	+	+	+ or ±	−	+	−	+	−	−	−
	2	−	−	−	+	+	+	+	+ or ±	+	−	−	+	−	−	−
	3	−	−	−	+	+	+	+	+ or ±	+	+	−	+	−	−	−
Br. abortus	1	+(−)	+	−	−	−	+	+	±	+	−	+	+	−	+	−
	2	+	+	−	−	−	−	−	±	+	−	+	+	−	+	−
	3	−(+)	+	−	−	+	+	+	±	+	−	+	+	−	+	−
	4	+(−)	+	−	−	−	+	+	±	−	+	+	+	−	+	−
	5	−	−	−	+	+	+	+	±	−	+	+	+	−	+	−
	6	−	−	−	+	+	+	+	±	+	−	+	+	−	+	−
	7	−	− or +	−	+	+	+	+	±	+	+	+	+	−	+	−
	8	+	−	−	+	+	+	+	±	−	+	+	+	−	+	−
	9	− or +	+	−	+	+	+	+	±	−	+	+	+	−	+	−
Br. suis	1	−	++	+	+	+	−	−	++	+	−	−	−	+	+	+
	2	−	−	−	+	+	−	−	++	+	−	−	+	+	+	−
	3	−	−	+	+	+	+	+	++	+	−	−	+	+	+	+

a = 1 in 25,000
b = 1 in 50,000
c = 1 in 100,000
d = 1 in 50,000
e = 1 in 100,000

Br. abortus, type 5 = British melitensis
Br. suis, type 2 = Danish suis

± = weak reaction

APPENDIX 7

ABBREVIATIONS AND CONVERSION FACTORS

Mass

g. = gram
kg. = kilogram (1 kg. = 1000 g.)
mg. = milligram (1 mg = 0·001 g.)
μg. = microgram (1 μg. = 0·001 mg.)
lb. = pound weight avoirdupois (1 lb. = 453·6 g.)

Length

m. = metre
cm. = centimetre (1 cm = 0·01 m.)
mm. = millimetre (1 mm. = 0·001 m.)
μ = micron (1 μ = 0·001 mm.).
mμ = millimicron (1 mμ = 0·001 μ = 10 Ångström unit, A.)
in. = inch (1 inch = 2·54 cm.)
ft. = foot (1 ft. = 12 in.)

Area

sq. in. = square inch (1 sq. in. = 6·45 sq. cm.)

Volume

l. = litre (1 l. = 1·76 pints)
ml. = millilitre (1 ml. = 0·001 l.)
μl. = microlitre (1 μl. = 0·001 ml.)
oz. = fluid ounce (1 oz. = 28.41 ml.)
cu. ft. = cubic foot (1 cu. ft. = 28·3 l.)

Temperature

X° C. = X degrees Centigrade
Conversion of X° Centigrade to X° Fahrenheit:

X° F. = 1·8X° C. + 32

Time

hr. = hour   min. = minute   sec. = second

Other Abbreviations

N = normal (*e.g.* 2 *N* HCl)
M = molar (*e.g.* 0·1 *M* Na_2CO_3)
r.p.m. = revolutions per minute
mv. = millivolt
p.p.m. = parts per million
LD50 = average lethal dose
MLD = minimum lethal dose
MHD = minimum haemolytic dose

per cent. The percentage concentration of solution is stated as g. of solute per 100 ml. of solution, *i.e.* as per cent. (w/v). Unless otherwise indicated the solvent is *water*. Per cent. (v/v) = ml. of substance per 100 ml. of mixture, as in gas mixtures.

G = force of gravity

INDEX